Everyone Has a Story.

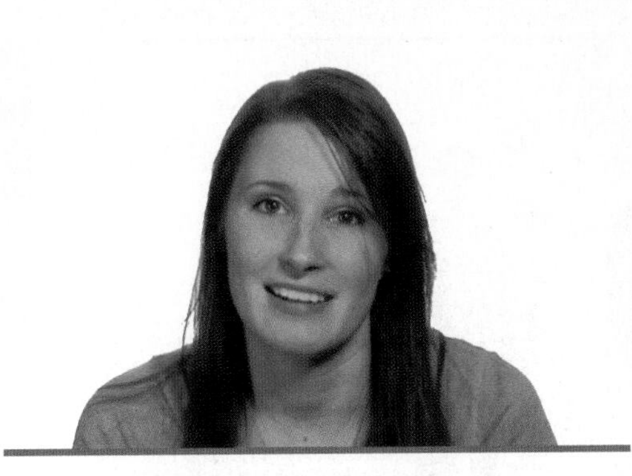

"Hi, I'm Rachel. When I was a freshman, I had major sleep issues. I would stay up all night long watching TV and I wouldn't think twice about going to sleep at four o'clock, waking up for class at ten, take a two hour nap in the afternoon, and then do it all over again."

(For more on Rachel's story, turn to page 99.)

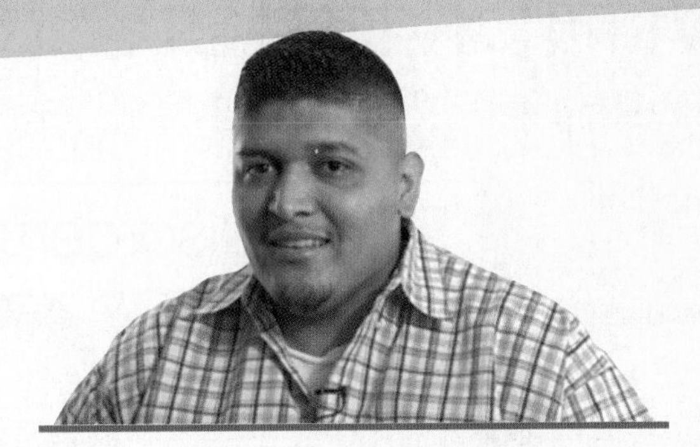

"Hi, I'm David. As a non-traditional student, some of the things that stress me out are maybe a little bit different than what other students go through…I have to pay a mortgage… put food on my kids' table… these things stress me out!"

(For more on David's story, turn to page 63.)

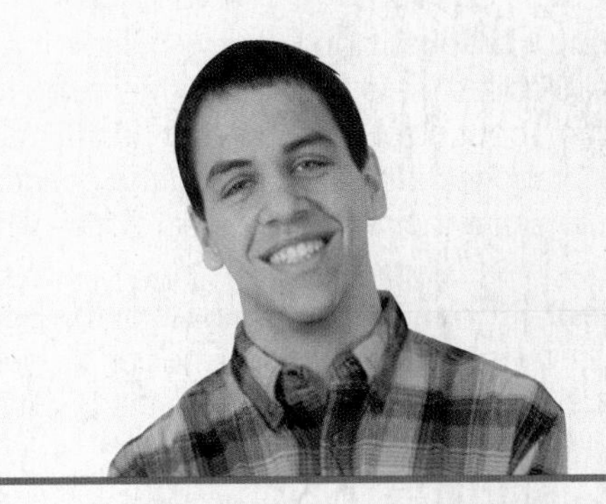

"Hi, I'm Addison. When I first started smoking I was 16 years old. I've tried to quit numerous times—always cold turkey. I'd last maybe a week if I was lucky."

(For more on Addison's story, turn to page 283.)

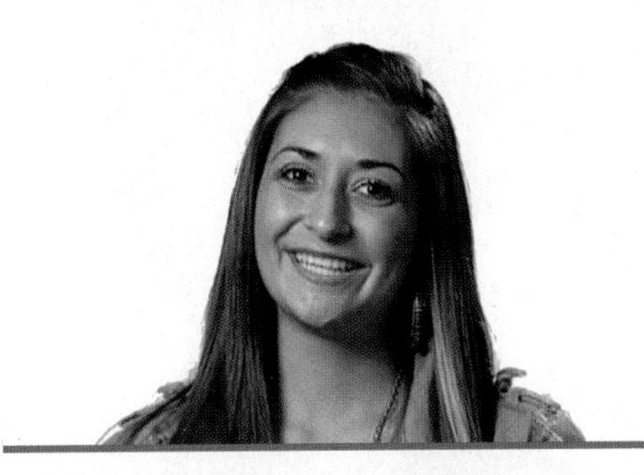

"Hi, I'm Nidya. I am a vegetarian and I decided to become one basically because of my cousin. She's also a vegetarian and she showed me a PETA video about how they treated animals when they kill them for food."

(For more on Nidya's story, turn to page 126.)

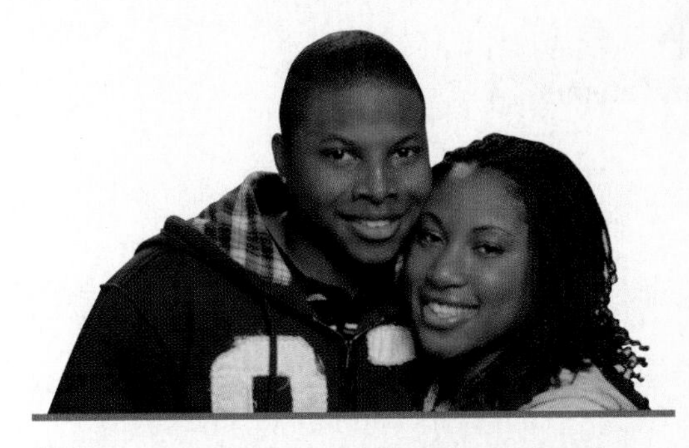

"We're Jonathan and Yeani, and we've been a couple for six months. There are a lot of obstacles that we face in our relationship, especially when it comes to juggling our schoolwork in addition to all the other aspects of our lives."

(For more on Jonathan and Yeani's story, turn to page 392.)

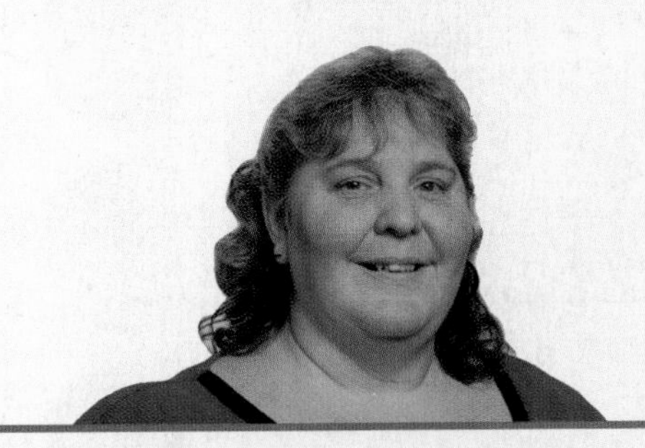

"My name is Holly. I am 45 years old. I was a single parent for about 12 years. I could not afford insurance for myself—it just wasn't in my budget. My kids always came first. If I got sick, I stayed at home and took care of myself."

(For more on Holly's story, turn to page 524.)

Student Stories and Student Stats

Highlight what Matters to Students

College students don't always believe that living a healthful lifestyle is something they need to start thinking about now. To show that health matters now, we approached students around the country and asked them to share their health-related stories with us.

Student Stories in every chapter of the book demonstrate that the lifestyle choices students make today can have lasting effects on the quality of their health in the future.

STUDENT STORY

Eating Disorders

"Hi, my name is Viege. My freshman year in college I had a friend named Lisa, who suffered from an eating disorder. She would always starve herself to try to look like other people or starve herself to get a guy. To be honest with you, I really didn't take it seriously. I just told her that it's just a phase she was going through. Everything will be all right. And then, as I saw her getting skinnier and skinnier, I was like, hey, maybe you do need to get some help. And all she would say is, I'm not crazy. I just want to be beautiful. So I just let it go. And that was the biggest mistake I've ever made because a couple months later, Lisa was rushed to the hospital because she had something wrong with her heart.

So, if you do have a friend that's struggling with eating disorders, you should probably talk to them. You may not think of it as serious but it can be, even if they're young."

1: What do you think was wrong with Viege's friend's heart? What could have caused her to be hospitalized?

2: Do you think it's common for people to take eating disorders seriously? What would prompt you to talk to a friend about a possible eating disorder? Do you think it's your place to convince a friend to get help?

Do you have a story similar to Viege's? Share your story at www.pearsonhighered.com/lynchelmore.

STUDENT STORY

Talking to a Friend about Alcohol

"Hi, I'm Charles. I have a friend that I've actually been really concerned with lately. He's been drinking probably every day, except for like Sunday, a significant amount, and he's kinda been worrying me about his habits. I haven't confronted him about it yet but I do plan on at least saying something in the next week or two if he keeps it up. I'm just going to word it as nicely as I can to not make him feel like he's already an addict, but I'm just going to give him a warning to let him know that he's getting himself into something that he really could regret."

1: How should Charles bring up his friend's drinking? Where and when do you think he should do it? What types of things should he say?

2: What organizations or resources could Charles look to for help with talking to a friend about drinking?

Do you have a story similar to Charles's? Share your story at www.pearsonhighered.com/lynchelmore.

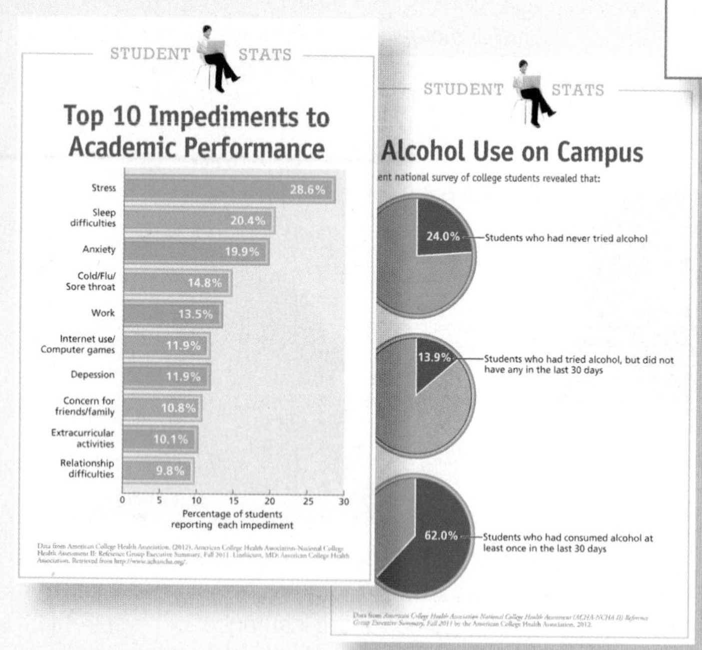

Student Stats throughout the book present up-to-date national statistics and research on key health topics as they apply to today's college population.

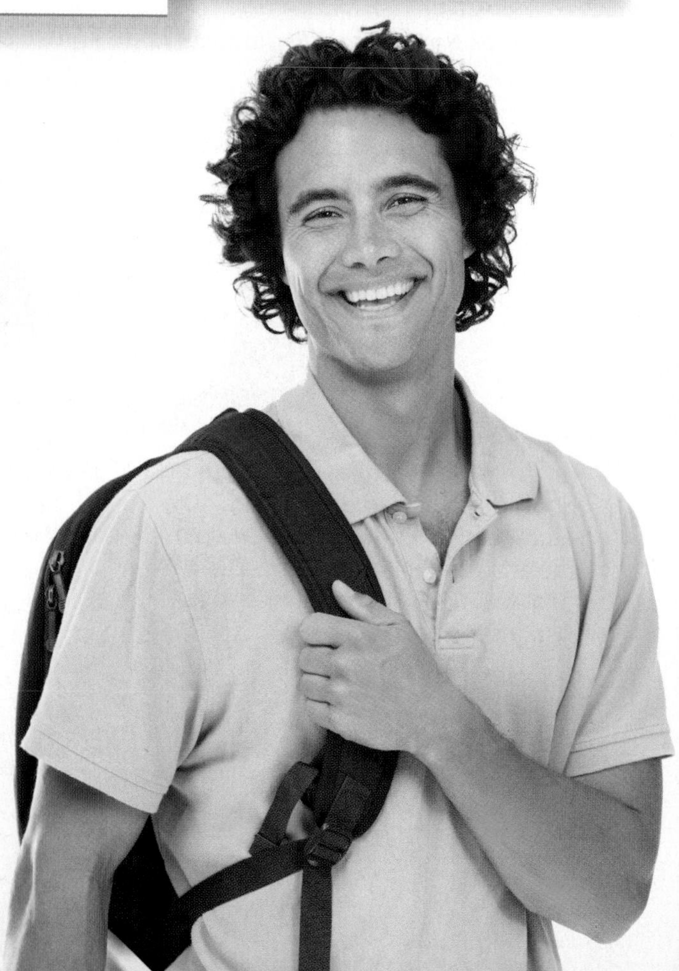

Student Stories Online

Students can view over 120 videos of real college students talking about health issues on the *Health: Making Choices for Life* Companion Website at **www.pearsonhighered.com/lynchelmore** or on our YouTube channel at **www.youtube.com/ch00singhealth.**

Students can submit their own stories, questions, or feedback for use in the book or online at **www.pearsonhighered.com/lynchelmore.**

Empowering Students

to Improve their Behaviors and their Environments

Each chapter of the text is full of information about health, but how can students implement it? **Consistent Change Yourself, Change Your World** sections at the end of each chapter give students solid, specific advice about how they can improve their own behaviors, help friends or family members, and advocate for changes in their environments to promote health for everyone.

Each Change Yourself, Change Your World section has a clear organization with subsections for **Personal Choices, Helping a Friend,** and **Campus Advocacy.**

This section empowers students to make changes in their own lives given the information in the chapter. → Personal Choices

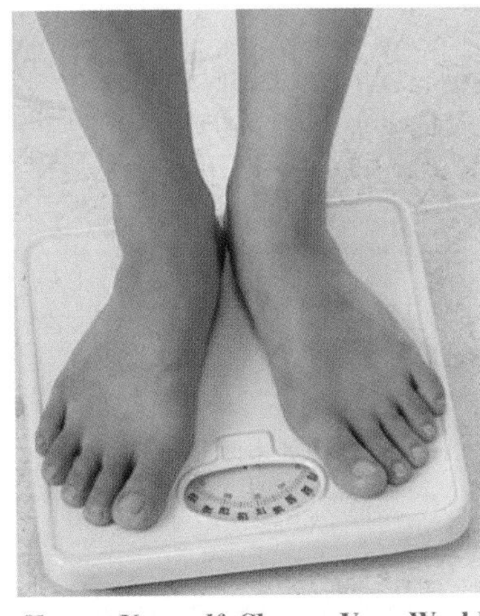

Change Yourself, Change Your World

For most people, the key to healthful weight loss lies in the ability to better control "energy in" and "energy out." If you want your body to use and reduce its fat stores, you need to make sure less energy is coming in and more energy is going out. This requires consistent work. Losing weight doesn't have to mean depriving yourself. But it does mean eating wisely and changing your lifestyle to be as physically active as possible.

Personal Choices

Did you grab a snack before sitting down to study this chapter? If so, what did you choose? Seemingly small decisions about what and how much you eat can support or undermine successful weight management. The nearby Practical Strategies box lists several helpful behaviors to practice.

Low-Fat Diets

Long-term weight loss is a challenge with low-fat diets, because dieters find them difficult to follow and to maintain. That said, we can all benefit from following these general fat intake guidelines:

- Cut trans fats from your diet. Trans fats are created when manufacturers add hydrogen to vegetable oil—a process called hydrogenation. Consumption of trans fats reduces your "good cholesterol" (HDL) and raises your "bad cholesterol" (LDL), thereby increasing your risk of cardiovascular disease.
- Consume more "good" fats. Fats found in plant oils, nuts, seeds, and fish should make up the majority of fats in your diet.

Low-Carbohydrate Diets

Most nutrition experts agree that Americans eat too many refined carbohydrates, especially from added sugars. But fiber-rich carbohydrates—including fruits, legumes and other vegetables, and whole grains—are nutritious foods that your body needs. Follow these guidelines:

- Choose fiber-rich carbohydrates. Carbohydrates found in whole grains, fruits, and vegetables are better options than refined carbohydrates found in white breads, cakes and other commercial baked goods, soft drinks, and candy.
- Watch your total Calories. Consuming lots of protein and fat won't help you lose weight. Total Calorie consumption is what matters. To lose weight, you need to consume fewer Calories than you expend, regardless of the type of diet you are following.
- When choosing protein-rich foods, look for leaner options. Fish, skinless chicken breasts, or rump, round, flank, and loin cuts of meat are choices lower in saturated fats. Better yet, choose plant proteins, which provide healthful unsaturated fats, and are high in fiber and micronutrients.

Take a small step toward achieving your target weight. Visit http://people.bu.edu/salge/52_small_steps/weight_loss/index.html for 52 tips on eating better, getting more active, and tracking your progress toward your goals.

Helping a Friend

An analysis of 500,000 users of the Calorie-tracking app MyFitnessPal revealed that the more friends users had, the more weight they lost. Moreover, people who gave friends access to their Calorie counts lost 50% more weight than the average user. If you want to help a friend shed pounds for good, try the following:

- Find non-food ways to celebrate successes together. Go to the movies, or catch a game. Find fun in something other than food.
- Don't coach—join in! Instead of suggesting your friend walk more often, arrange to walk to class together in the morning rather than drive.
- Cook a low-Calorie meal together. Cooking for one isn't always practical. Prepping meals for and with friends is more cost-effective and fun.
- Seek out a sport or activity you both enjoy. Hoops? Hiking? Zumba? Find something fun and share it regularly.

Campus Advocacy

College doesn't have to mean scary food in the dining hall and worrying about the "freshman 15." Get involved to help bring healthier options to your school that promote weight management and make it easier for you and your fellow students to avoid weight gain.

For inspiration, check out the Real Food Challenge (http://realfoodchallenge.org), a network of students working to improve the options students have at mealtime and bring better nutrition to campuses. This group, which has chapters at more than 360 colleges and universities so far, aims to "shift $1 billion of existing university food budgets away

66 Body Image, Body Weight: Achieving a Healthy Balance

Helping a Friend ← **Social support is key for many health issues. This section helps students learn how they can effectively support friends or family experiencing health problems or who are making positive changes.**

Campus Advocacy ← **Now more than ever we know that environments shape health. This section gives students ideas about how they can proactively improve their environments, to improve health for themselves and others.**

> **"I really like the part about helping a friend. I think the advocacy stuff is great too."**
>
> **—Karen N. Hunter, Eastern Kentucky University**

> **"I like that the students are challenged to critically think through the information especially to help someone else out."**
>
> **—Susan Stevenson, Northern Illinois University**

> **"I love the ending section on advocacy and how to get involved."**
>
> **—Melinda J. Ickes, University of Kentucky**

Behavior Change Tools

Help Students Put Plans into Practice

Choosing to Change Worksheets

Changing long-ingrained behaviors is tough. These worksheets help students implement behavior change for topics in every chapter of the book. The first step asks them to determine their stage of change based on the transtheoretical model of behavior change. The worksheets then walk students through articulating realistic goals and improving their behaviors based on their stage of change.

Interactive versions of the worksheets are available on the Companion Website and MyHealthLab.

Each student's first step is to determine his or her stage of behavior change based on the transtheoretical model of change: Precontemplation, Contemplation, Preparation, Action, or Maintenance.

Students might be asked to evaluate their current behaviors, through activities like keeping a sleep diary.

Choosing to Change Worksheet

To complete this worksheet online, visit www.pearsonhighered.com/lynchelmore.

In this chapter you learned about the importance of healthy sleep. To improve your sleep, follow the steps below.

Directions: Fill in your stage of change in Step 1 and complete Step 2 with your stage of change in mind. Then complete Steps 3, 4, or 5, depending on which ones apply to your stage of change.

Step 1: Your Stage of Behavior Change. Please check one of the following statements that best describes your readiness to obtain a good quality and quantity of sleep.

______ I do not intend to increase the quality or quantity of my sleep in the next 6 months. (Precontemplation)

______ I might increase the quality or quantity of my sleep in the next 6 months. (Contemplation)

______ I am prepared to increase the quality or quantity of my sleep in the next month. (Preparation)

______ I have been increasing my quality or quantity of sleep for less than 6 months. (Action)

______ I have been increasing my quality or quantity of sleep for more than 6 months. (Maintenance)

Step 2: Keep a Sleep Diary. A sleep diary is a useful tool for identifying sleep disorders and sleeping problems and pinpointing daytime and nighttime habits that may be contributing to your sleep struggles. Fill in the following chart for up to 7 days.

	Answer these Questions	Example	Monday	Tuesday	Wednesday	Thursday	Frida
Complete in the morning	Time I went to bed last night: Time I woke up this morning: Number of hours I slept last night:	11 p.m. 7 a.m. 8					
	Number of awakenings and total time awake last night:	5 times 2 hours					
	How long I took to fall asleep last night:	30 mins.					
	Medications taken last night:	None					
	How awake I felt when I got up this morning: 1 – Wide awake 2 – Awake but a little tired 3 – Sleepy	2					
Complete in the evening	Number of caffeinated drinks and time I had them today:	1 drink at 8 a.m.					
	Number of alcoholic drinks and time I had them today:	1 drink at 9 p.m.					
	Naptimes and lengths of naps today:	3:30 p.m. 45 mins.					
	Exercise times and lengths today:	None					
	How sleepy I felt during the day today: 1 – So sleepy I had to struggle to stay awake during much of the day 2 – Somewhat tired 3 – Fairly alert 4 – Wide awake	1					

After filling in the sleep diary, do you notice any habits, such as drinking alcohol or caffeine, taking medications, exercise, or napping, that could be negatively impacting your sleep?

______

Step 3: Precontemplation or Contemplation Stages. Answer the questions below to move toward improving your sleep patterns.

What are some reasons to improve your sleeping habits?______

What is holding you back from improving your sleeping habits?______

How can you overcome these obstacles to improving your sleep?______

Fill out the table in Step 4, below. Your confidence may be low for all strategies, but pick the one you feel may be the most helpful. How might you begin to implement that strategy?

______

Step 4: Preparation and Action Stages. The tips for getting to sleep more quickly provided on page 97 are listed below. On a scale of 1–5 (1 being the lowest and 5 the highest), rate your confidence in your ability to implement each strategy.

Practical Strategy	How confident are you in your ability to employ this technique? Low confidence				High confidence
1. Think of your bedroom as your "sleep cave."	1	2	3	4	5
2. Aim for a warm bed in a cool room.	1	2	3	4	5
3. Keep it quiet.	1	2	3	4	5
4. Cut caffeine.	1	2	3	4	5
5. Watch your food intake.	1	2	3	4	5
6. Hit the gym earlier in the day.	1	2	3	4	5
7. Get adequate exposure to natural light throughout the day.	1	2	3	4	5
8. Set stressors aside until morning.	1	2	3	4	5
9. Don't work in bed.	1	2	3	4	5
10. Give yourself time to wind down.	1	2	3	4	5
11. Don't stare at the ceiling.	1	2	3	4	5
12. Other	1	2	3	4	5

Select one strategy that you feel highly confident in implementing and set a start date. Start date:

______

Tell someone what you plan to do. Being accountable to others motivates you and also offers you the support and encouragement of others. Who did you tell?______

Based on their stage of change, students are walked through the process of improving their behaviors and moving toward the next stage of change.

Worksheets ask students to set specific goals, with timelines, and to tell others about their goals.

Mobile Tips

What's the one thing students never leave home without? Their smartphones. Now they can carry health tips covering everything from fitness to stress management with them wherever they go. Find them by going to **http://mobiletips.pearsoncmg.com** on any mobile device.

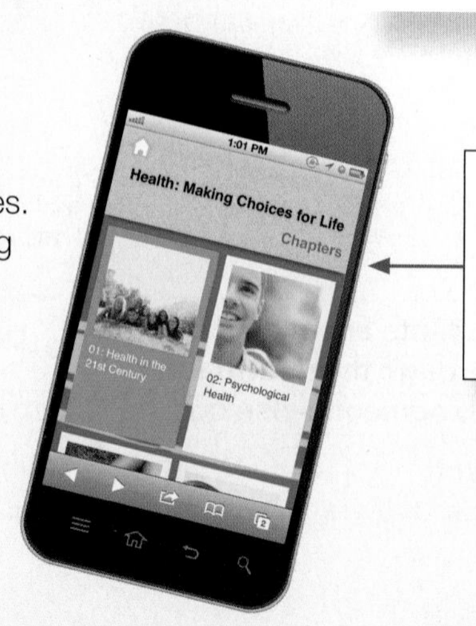

Or, for each chapter's tips, just scan the QR code at the end of the chapter using a QR reader app on your mobile device. There are many free QR readers available for all types of smartphones. Just search for "QR code reader" wherever you download apps.

Health Online

The One-Stop Shop for Each Chapter's Interactive Media

The **Health Online** section of the Companion Website for *Health: Making Choices for Life* is the one-stop shop for a wealth of videos, interactive versions of the Self-Assessments and worksheets from the text, weblinks, and social media tools for each chapter of the book. Access the Companion Website at **www.pearsonhighered.com/lynchelmore.**

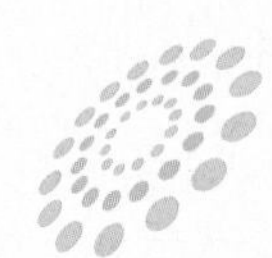

Any time you see the Health Online icon (at left) in the text, you can find the online version in the Companion Website's Health Online section for that chapter.

Over 120 videos of real college students talking about their health lets students see that health issues affect people just like them.

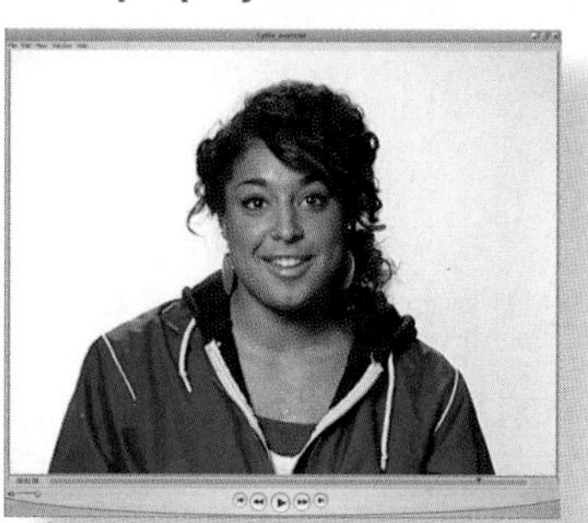

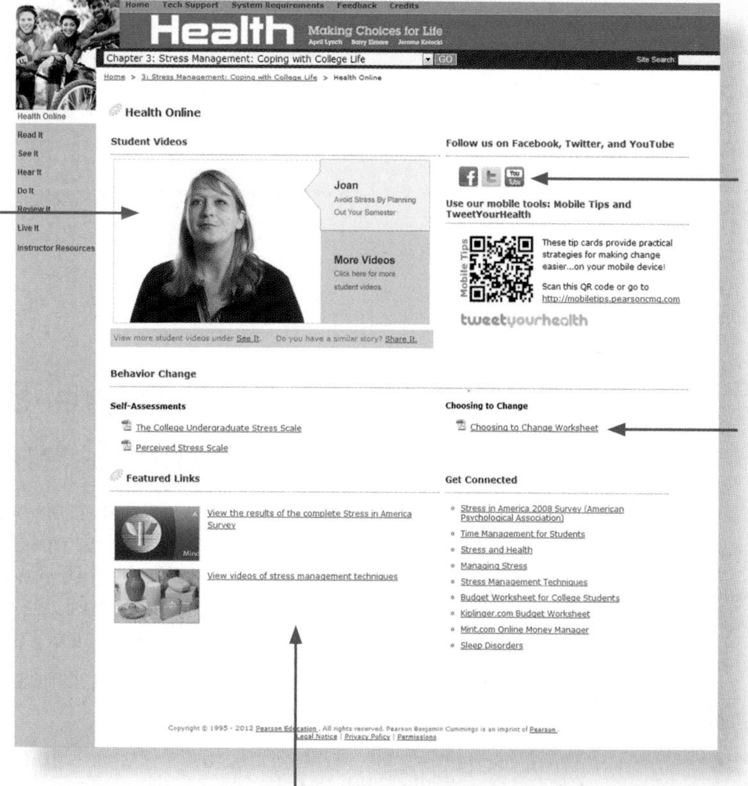

Links to powerful social media tools created for the text—such as our TweetYourHealth behavior tracking tool, Mobile Tips, Facebook page, YouTube channel, or Twitter feed—take health information to where students already are: online.

Interactive versions of the Choosing to Change Worksheets and Self-Assessments found in the chapters allow students to fill in these tools online and email or send to a professor's dropbox.

Choosing to Change Worksheet

Updated links to all the web pages listed within the text appear in the Health Online section for easy access to these internet resources.

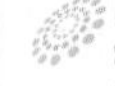

How many calories do *you* need each day? Find out in seconds using this simple tool: www.cancer.org/healthy/toolsandcalculators/calculators/app/calorie-counter-calculator.

Make Your Course Interactive

www.pearsonhighered.com/myhealthlab

The new MyHealthLab® from Pearson has been designed and refined with a single purpose in mind: To help educators create that moment of understanding with their students. The MyHealthLab system helps instructors maximize class time with customizable, easy-to-assign, and automatically graded assignments that motivate students to learn outside of class and arrive prepared for lecture. By complementing your teaching with our engaging technology and content, you can be confident your students will arrive at that moment—the moment of true understanding.

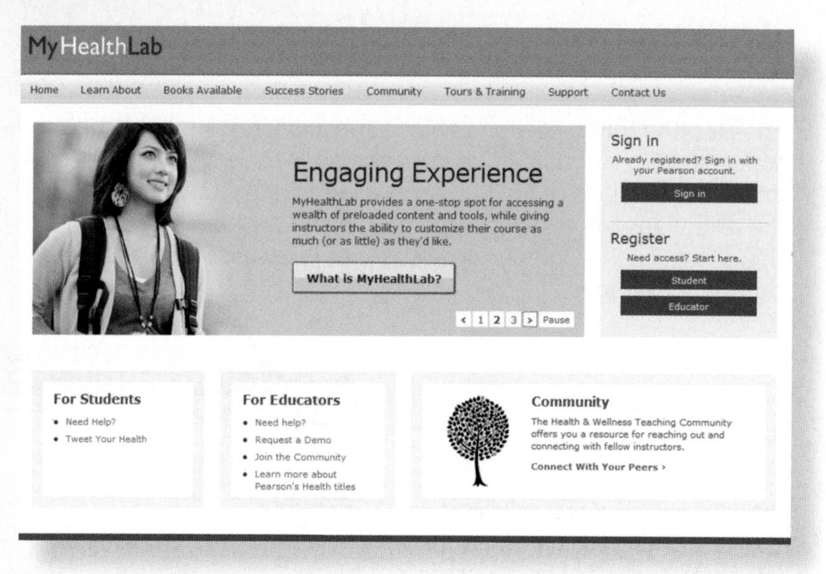

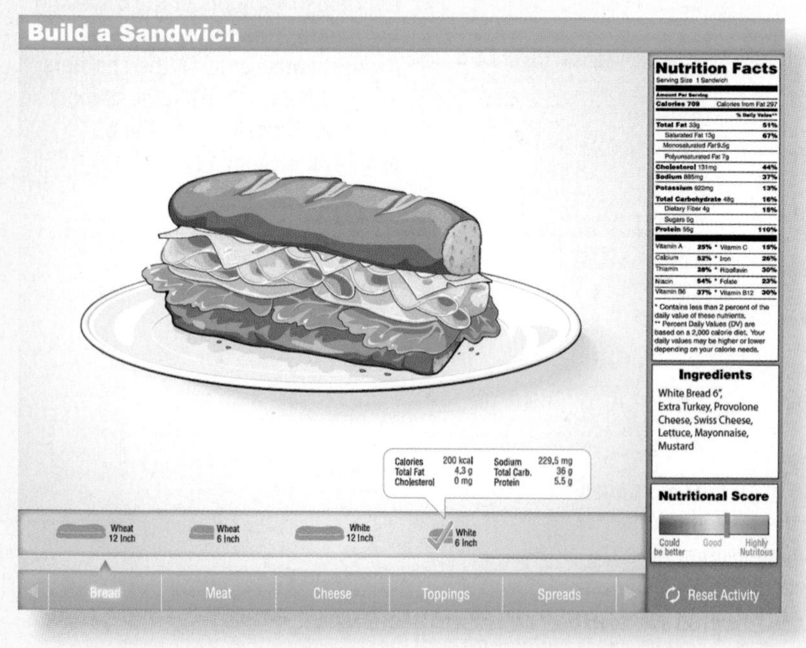

Over 150 Pre-Built, Publisher Created Assignments

Instructors can lessen their prep time and simplify their lives with preloaded quiz and test questions specific to the textbook that they can assign and/or edit, a gradebook that automatically records student results from assigned tests, and the ability to customize the course as much (or as little) as desired. Assignments include:

- student learning outcomes pre- and post-course exam.
- chapter tests.
- ABC News videos multiple choice quiz questions.
- NutriTools interactive nutrition activities with quiz questions (shown at left).
- MP3 case studies' assignable quizzes.
- entire content from the Test Library categorized by Bloom's Taxonomy.
- Self-Assessments that speak directly to the gradebook.
- gradable discussion board questions.

with MyHealthLab®

Assignable Choosing to Change Worksheets and Self-Assessments

All worksheets and Self-Assessments from the text are available online in interactive PDF format and are assignable through MyHealthLab. Additionally, Self-Assessments are available through the Assessment Manager so they can speak directly to the gradebook.

Pearson eText

Students can access the text whenever and wherever they have access to the Internet. The powerful functionality of the eText includes the ability to create notes, highlight text in different colors, create bookmarks, zoom, click on hyperlinked words to view definitions, and view in single-page or two-page view.

Pre- and Post-Course Evaluations

You can now easily measure how much each student learned in your course with pre- and post-course evaluations. A 50-question exam can be assigned at the start of the course, and again at the end, to effectively measure Student Learning Outcomes.

ABC News Videos

Over 60 videos from the ABC News team bring health topics to life. These 5-10 minute videos are available on MyHealthLab, the Instructor Resource DVD, and the Companion Website. Optional assignable video quiz questions are also available on MyHealthLab.

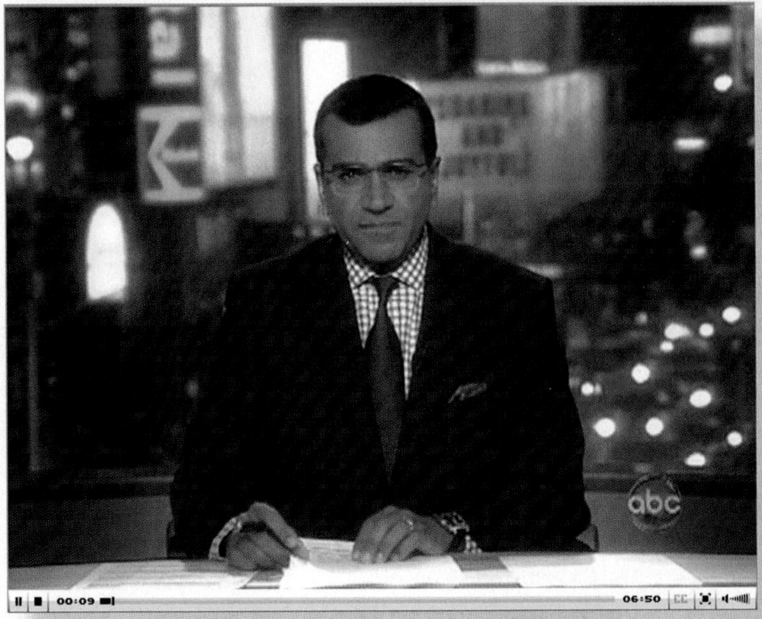

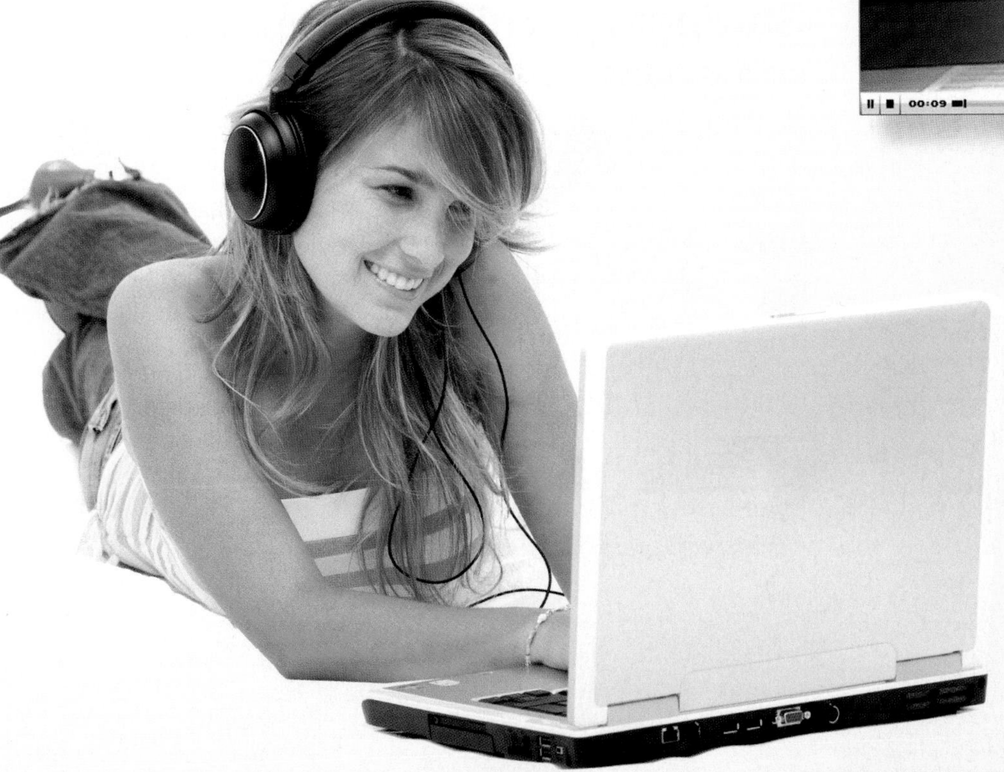

Dedicated instructor and student support via Internet chat at ***http://247pearsoned.custhelp.com*** *or the dedicated customer service line,* ***800-677-6337.***

Tools to Make Teaching Health Easier

Teaching Tool Box

978-0-321-85943-3 / 0-321-85943-X

Save hours of valuable planning time. In one handy box, instructors will find a wealth of resources that reinforce key learning from the text and suit virtually any teaching style. The Teaching Tool Box provides all the prepping and lecture tools an instructor needs:

- Instructor Resource DVD
- Printed Test Bank
- Instructor Resource and Support Manual
- User's Quick Guide
- MyLab Instructor Access Card
- Take Charge Self Assessment Worksheets
- *Teaching with Web 2.0*
- *Teaching with Student Learning Outcomes*
- *Great Ideas: Active Ways to Teach Health and Wellness*
- *Behavior Change Log Book and Wellness Journal* student supplement
- *Eat Right! Healthy Eating in College and Beyond* student supplement
- *Live Right! Beating Stress in College and Beyond* student supplement

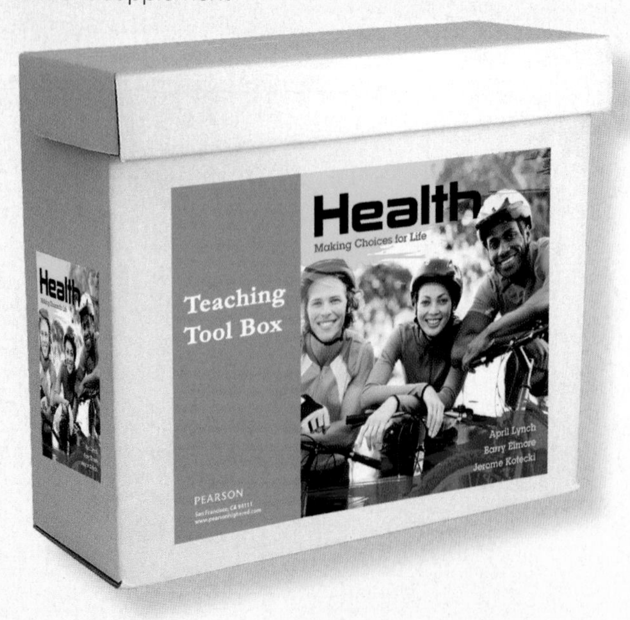

Instructor Resource DVD

Available in the Teaching Tool Box, the Instructor Resource DVD contains the Computerized Test Bank; over 60 ABC News videos; PowerPoint Lecture Outlines; PowerPoint step-edit image presentations; clicker questions; quiz-show questions; files for all art, tables, and selected photos from the book; transparency masters; and Word® files for the Test Bank and Instructor Resource and Support Manual.

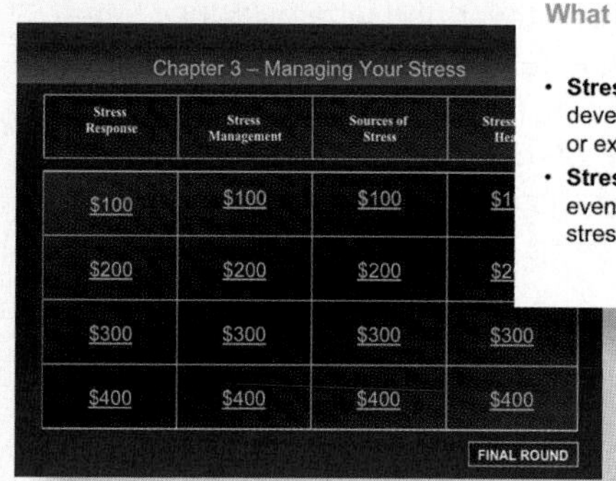

Teaching with Student Learning Outcomes

978-0-321-80265-1 / 0-321-80265-9

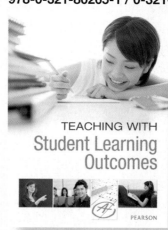

This new publication contains essays from 11 instructors who are using Student Learning Outcomes in their courses. They share their goals in using outcomes, the processes that they follow to develop and refine the outcomes, and many useful suggestions and examples for successfully incorporating outcomes into a personal health course.

Health

Making Choices for Life

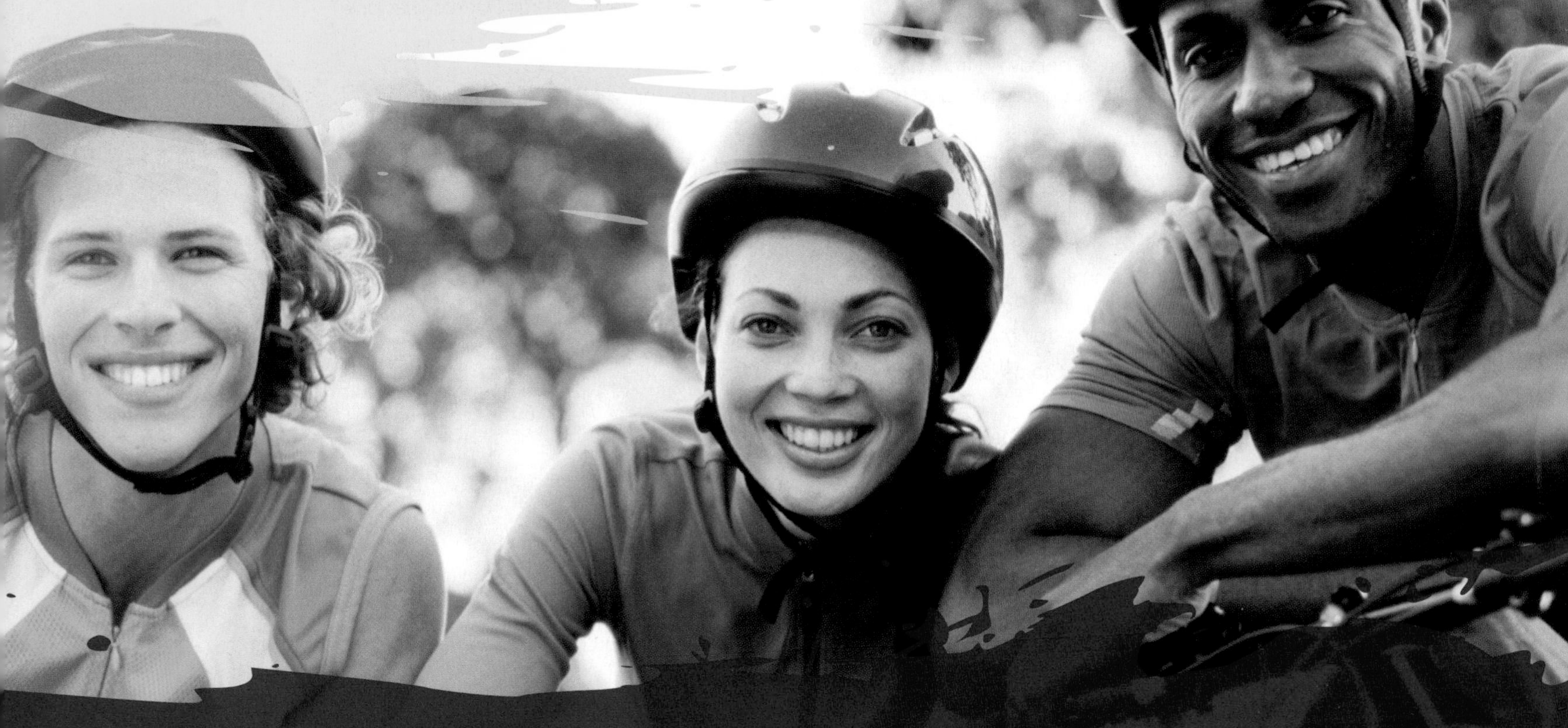

April Lynch

Barry Elmore, M.A.
EAST CAROLINA UNIVERSITY

Jerome Kotecki, HSD
BALL STATE UNIVERSITY

WITH CONTRIBUTIONS BY

Laura Bonazzoli

Tanya Morgan Gatenby, Ph.D., CPH
West Chester University

Sandra M. Walz, Ph.D., R.D.
West Chester University

Teresa Snow, Ph.D.
Georgia Institute of Technology

Karen Vail-Smith, M.S., M.P.A.
East Carolina University

Julie Sevrens Lyons

PEARSON

Boston Columbus Indianapolis New York San Francisco Upper Saddle River
Amsterdam Cape Town Dubai London Madrid Milan Munich Paris Montréal Toronto
Delhi Mexico City São Paulo Sydney Hong Kong Seoul Singapore Taipei Tokyo

Executive Editor: *Sandra Lindelof*
Director of Development: *Barbara Yien*
Senior Project Development Editor: *Marie Beaugureau*
Assistant Editor: *Meghan Zolnay*
Editorial Assistant: *Briana Verdugo*
Assistant Media Producer: *Sade McDougal*
Text Permissions Project Manager: *Alison Bruckner*
Text Permissions Specialist: *GEX, Inc.*
Senior Managing Editor: *Deborah Cogan*
Production Project Managers: *Lori Newman and Beth Collins*
Production Management: *S4Carlisle Publishing Services*
Copyeditor: *Anna Reynolds Trabucco*
Compositor: *S4Carlisle Publishing Services*
Design Manager: *Marilyn Perry*
Interior and Cover Designer: *Riezebos Holzbaur Design Group*
Illustrators: *Precision Graphics*
Photo Permissions Management: *Bill Smith Group*
Photo Researcher: *Bill Smith Group, Riezebos Holzbaur Design Group*
Senior Photo Editor: *Donna Kalal*
Senior Manufacturing Buyer: *Stacey Weinberger*
Executive Marketing Manager: *Neena Bali*
Senior Market Development Manager: *Brooke Suchomel*
Market Relations Manager: *Leslie Allen*
Cover Photo Credit: *George Doyle/Thinkstock*

Credits and acknowledgments for materials borrowed from other sources and reproduced, with permission, in this textbook appear on the appropriate page within the text or on page 637.

Library of Congress Cataloging-in-Publication Data is available upon request.

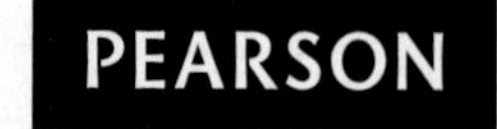

www.pearsonhighered.com

ISBN 10: 0-321-51641-9; ISBN 13: 978-0-321-51641-1 (Student Edition)
ISBN 10: 0-321-85942-1; ISBN 13: 978-0-321-85942-6 (Instructor's Review Copy)
ISBN 10: 0-321-89768-4; ISBN 13: 978-0-321-89768-8 (Books a la Carte Edition)
1 2 3 4 5 6 7 8 9 10—CRK—16 15 14 13 12

"This book is dedicated to my husband, Colin, daughter, Ava, and son, Van. In the ever-changing love and laughter project that is our family, I'm inspired to reach for better choices, every single day."

—April Lynch

"To Rick, Billie, and Sudie, my colleagues at ECU, and my students. Without you this book would not have been possible."

—Barry Elmore

"This book is dedicated to my friends and family for their continued support and love. They allowed me the time and energy to focus my passion and write this book."

—Jerome Kotecki

About the Authors

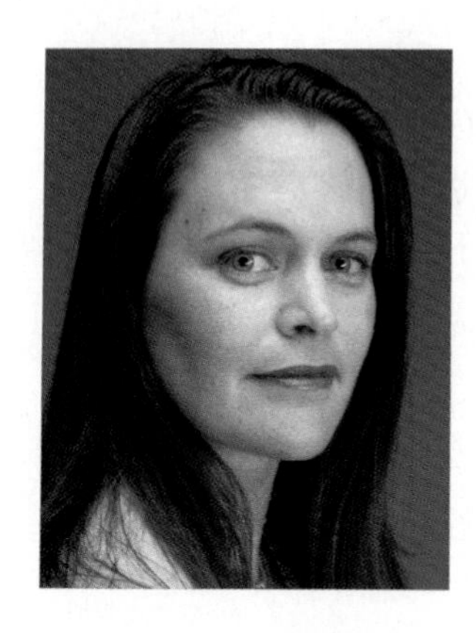

April Lynch

April Lynch is an award-winning author and journalist who specializes in health, science, and genetics. During her tenure with the *San Jose Mercury News,* the leading newspaper of Silicon Valley, she served as the Science and Health editor, focusing the paper's coverage on personal health and disease prevention. She has also worked as a writer and editor for the *San Francisco Chronicle.* April has written numerous articles on personal health, medical and scientific advances, consumer issues, and the ways that scientific breakthroughs are redefining our understanding of health. She has been a frequent contributor to leading university textbooks covering applied biology, nutrition, and environmental health and science. April co-authored *Choosing Health*, an innovative personal health textbook for users who desire a brief book for their course. Together with a leading genetic counselor, April is the co-author of *The Genome Book,* a hands-on guide to using genetic information in personal health decisions. Her work has won numerous awards from organizations such as the Society of Professional Journalists, the California Newspaper Publishers Association, and the Associated Press. Her current interests include a focus on how people receive and interact with health information online, as well as how complex scientific and medical information is best shared compellingly and effectively in digital media. She lives in the San Francisco Bay Area with her husband and children.

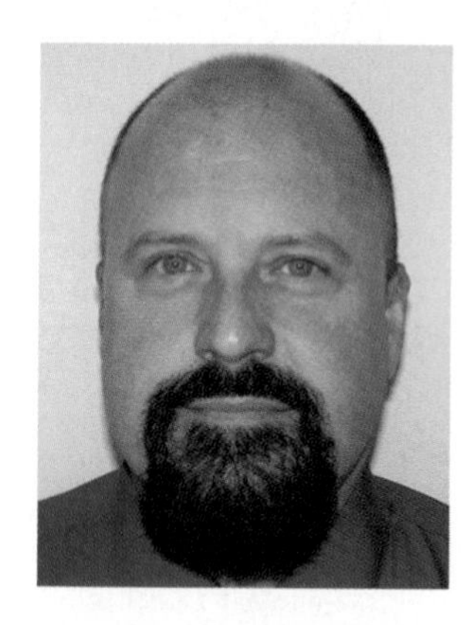

Barry Elmore, M.A.

East Carolina University

Barry Elmore is a faculty member at East Carolina University in the College of Health and Human Performance. He obtained a B.S. from Mount Olive College and an M.A. in Health Education at East Carolina University, where he was a merit scholar. Barry is co-author of *Choosing Health,* a brief textbook for the personal health course. Barry has extensive experience in the field of community health with particular focus on sexually transmitted diseases. He served as the executive director of an AIDS service organization before beginning his teaching career, and worked as a health educator in the nonprofit sector for nearly 20 years. Barry has been recognized for his commitment to advocating for and working with diverse populations and was awarded the first-ever Creed Award for Diversity at East Carolina University. He has been a leader in developing a service learning program at ECU. He continues to focus on health disparities and has worked with educators and health professionals on improving services to minority populations. Barry is a member of the American Public Health Association (APHA), the Society for Public Health Education (SOPHE), and the North Carolina Association for Research in Education (NCARE). Barry has been recognized for outstanding teaching by his department, college, and university.

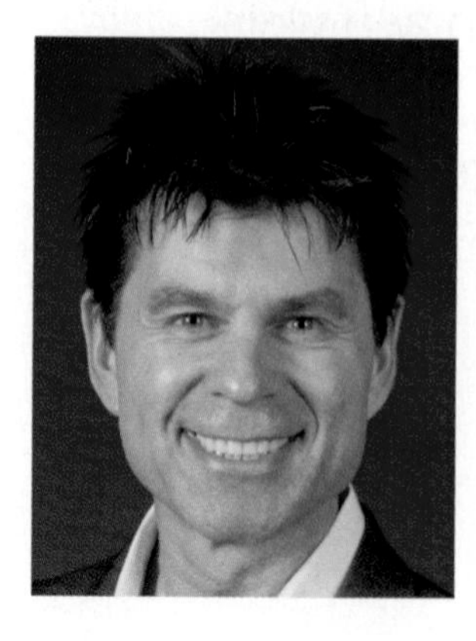

Jerome Kotecki, HSD

Ball State University

Jerome E. Kotecki is a professor of Health Science in the Department of Physiology and Health Science at Ball State University. Dr. Kotecki earned his doctorate in health education and his master's degree in exercise science from Indiana University. He has published more than 40 scientific research papers on the prevention, arrest, and reversal of the most common chronic diseases facing Americans today. Jerome has authored or co-authored multiple textbooks on the importance of healthy lifestyle habits to enhance the multidimensional components of human health and prevent cardiovascular disease, diabetes, cancer, and other chronic conditions. Jerome has extensive experience in health promotion, with particular focus on physical activity and health. An experienced teacher and researcher, he is devoted to helping students adopt and maintain healthy lifestyles. Jerome has been recognized for his contributions to the scholarship of teaching and learning by his department, college, and university. He is an avid fitness participant and enjoys cycling, resistance training, running, mountain biking, hiking, swimming, and yoga.

About the Contributors

Laura Bonazzoli

Laura Bonazzoli has been writing and editing in the health sciences for over 20 years. Her early work in human anatomy and physiology, chemistry, and other core sciences laid the foundation for writing projects in nursing, pathology, nutrition, complementary and alternative medicine, and personal health. Her commitment as a writer is to help her readers appreciate the power of small choices to improve their health and the health of their communities. In her free time, Laura and her daughter enjoy exploring the gardens, byways, and beaches of mid-coast Maine.

Teresa Snow, Ph.D.

Georgia Institute of Technology

Teresa Snow received an M.S. in Kinesiology and Health and a Ph.D. in Measurement and Statistics from Georgia State University. She coordinates the undergraduate wellness requirement at the Georgia Institute of Technology. Dr. Snow's research interests involve behavioral factors influencing disease and teaching strategies to improve learning. Teresa was selected as a 2009 Teaching Fellow by the Center for Enhancement of Teaching and Learning at Georgia Tech. She enjoys cycling and spending time with her dogs Rocky and Sam.

Tanya Morgan Gatenby, Ph.D., CPH

West Chester University

Tanya Morgan Gatenby is an Associate Professor and Masters of Public Health Program Director for Health Care Management at West Chester University. She received her Ph.D. in Health Policy and Administration from the University of North Carolina at Chapel Hill. Tanya has traveled around the world to teach and consult in the development of health curricula, in locations as diverse as Oxford University, England; Guizhou University, China; and La Paz, Bolivia. In addition to her global interests, Tanya's research focuses on health assessment of college students and the use of distance education in the classroom. Tanya is a member of West Chester University's Faculty Senate and serves as Vice President.

Karen Vail-Smith, M.S., M.P.A.

East Carolina University

Karen Vail-Smith received a B.S. from the University of North Carolina at Chapel Hill and an M.S. and M.P.A. from East Carolina University. She has been a faculty member in East Carolina University's Department of Health Education and Promotion for 22 years. She specializes in personal health and human sexuality. She has received numerous teaching awards, including the prestigious UNC Board of Governor's Distinguished Professor for Teaching award. She has published more than 25 articles in health professional journals.

Sandra M. Walz, Ph.D., R.D.

West Chester University

Sandra M. Walz, a Registered Dietitian, is an Associate Professor in Nutrition and Dietetics at West Chester University. She teaches foods, nutrition, and dietetics management courses. Sandra earned a B.S. in both Nutrition and Corporate and Community Fitness from North Dakota State University, an M.S. in Food and Nutrition from North Dakota State University, and a Ph.D. in Hospitality Management from Kansas State University. Her research interests include pedagogy (problem-based, experiential, and accelerated learning), adolescent obesity, and hospitality management. Sandra is devoted to engaging students in lifelong learning.

Julie Sevrens Lyons

Julie Sevrens Lyons is a communications expert based in the San Francisco Bay Area. She has worked as a personal health and science reporter at a number of publications, including the *San Jose Mercury News* and the *Contra Costa Times*. Her articles have been recognized by the Society of Professional Journalists and the California Newspaper Publishers Association, as well as by many leading health organizations. Julie received her M.S. in Mass Communications from San Jose State University—graduating with honors—and lives with her husband and young son.

Brief Contents

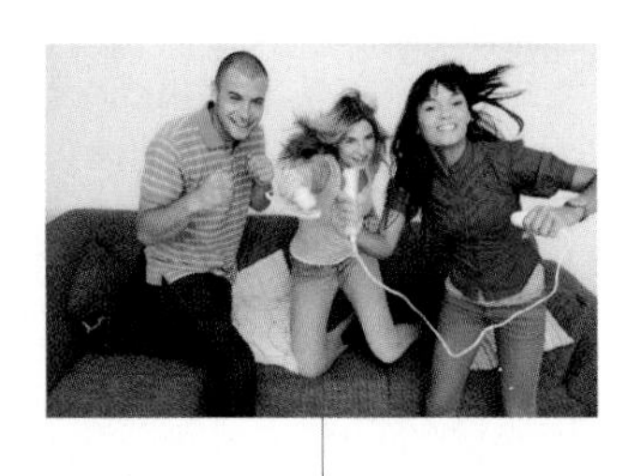

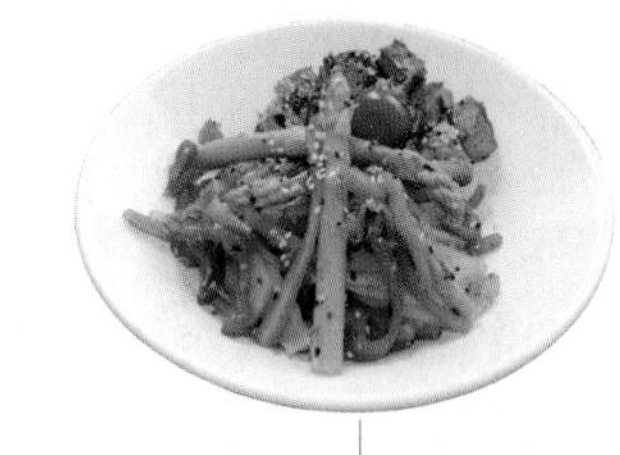

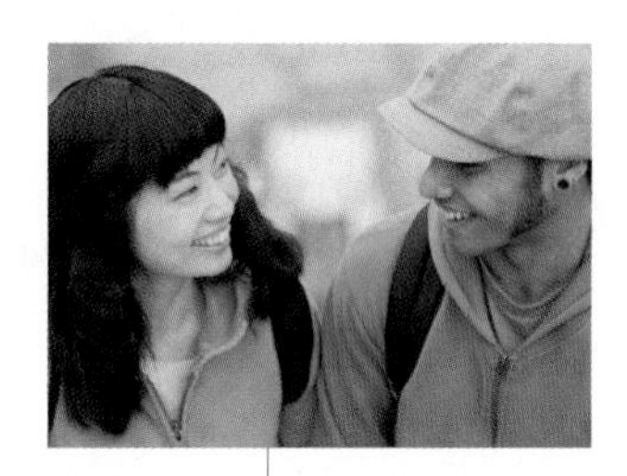

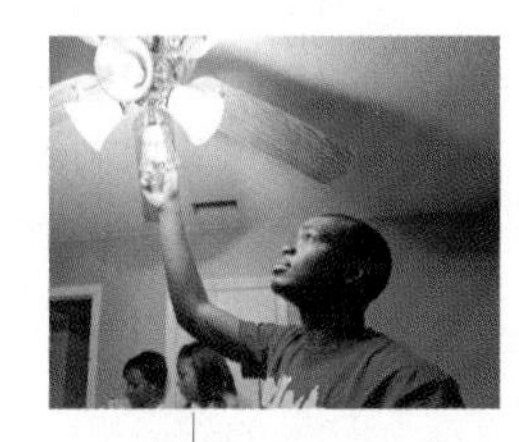

Contents

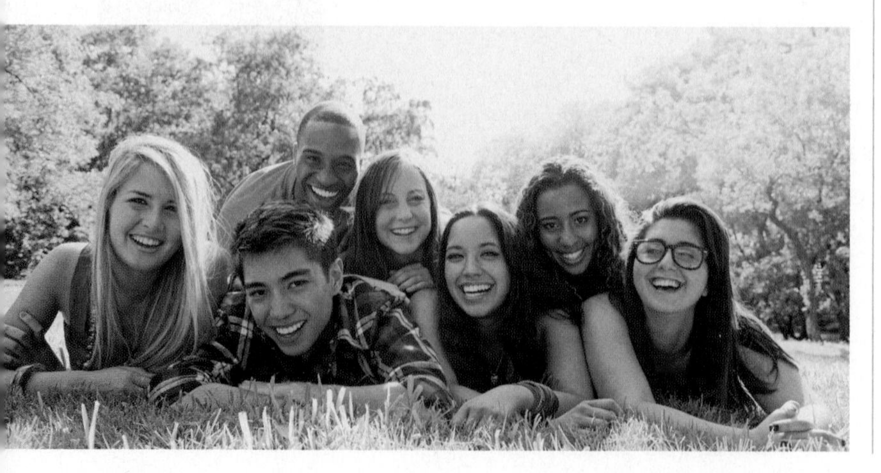

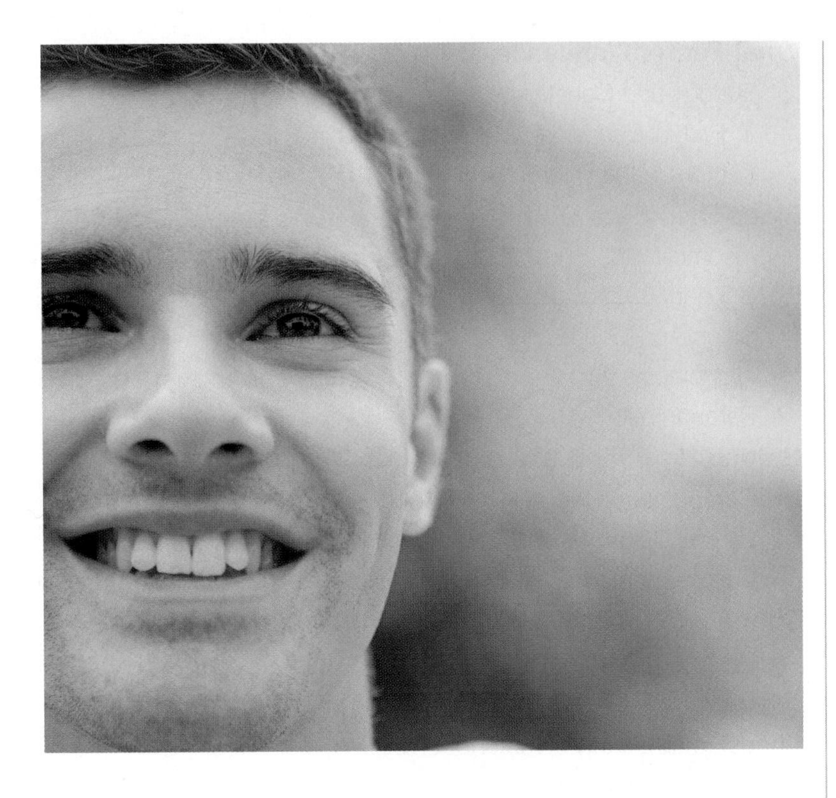

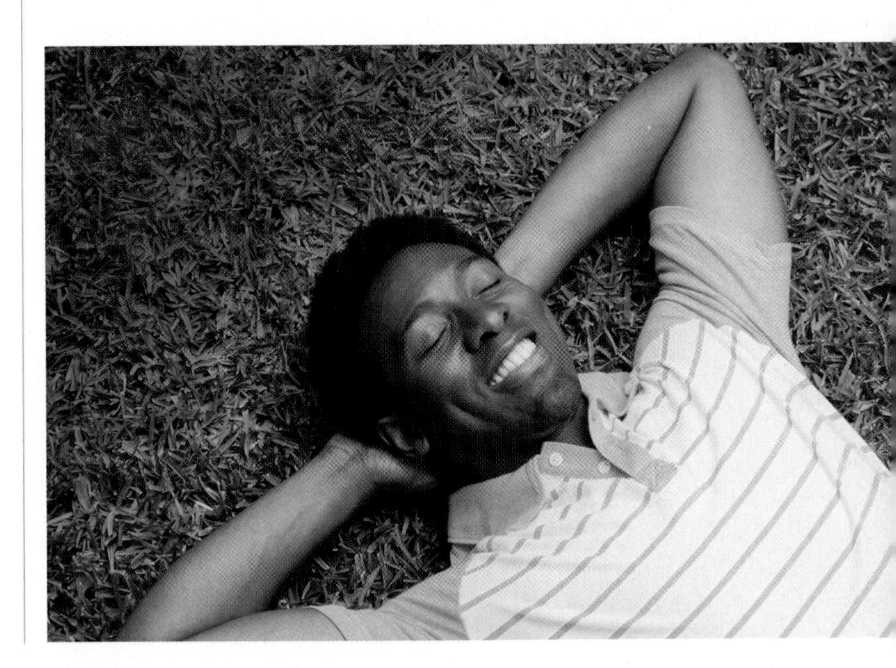

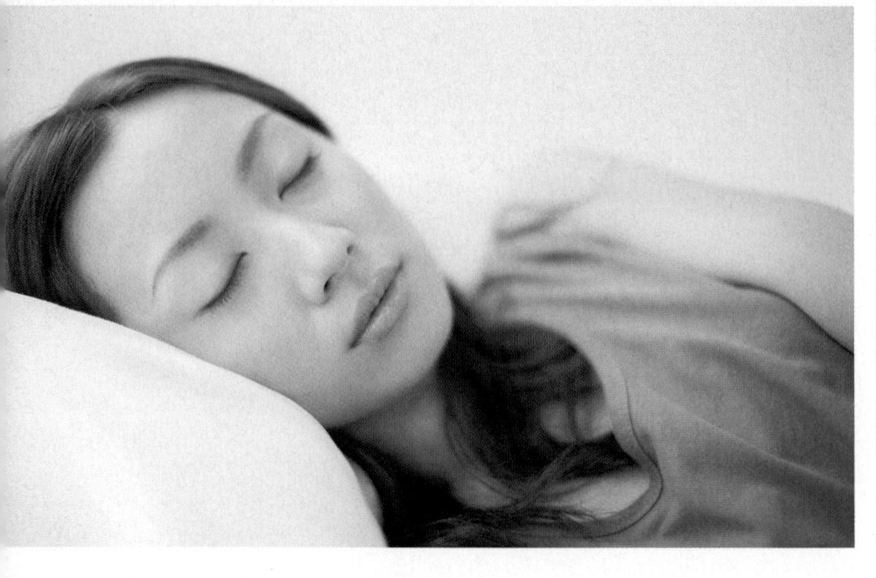

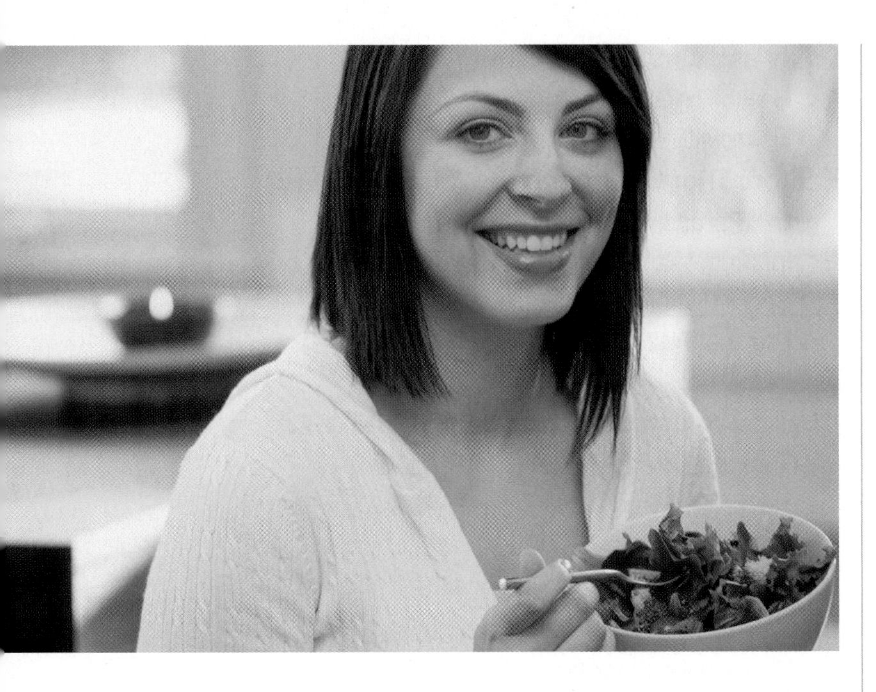

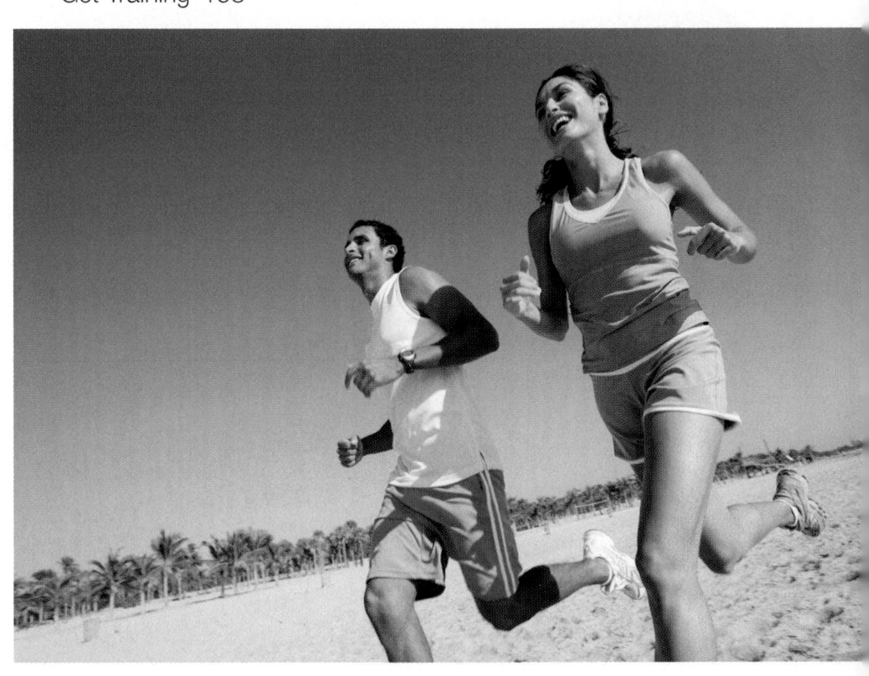

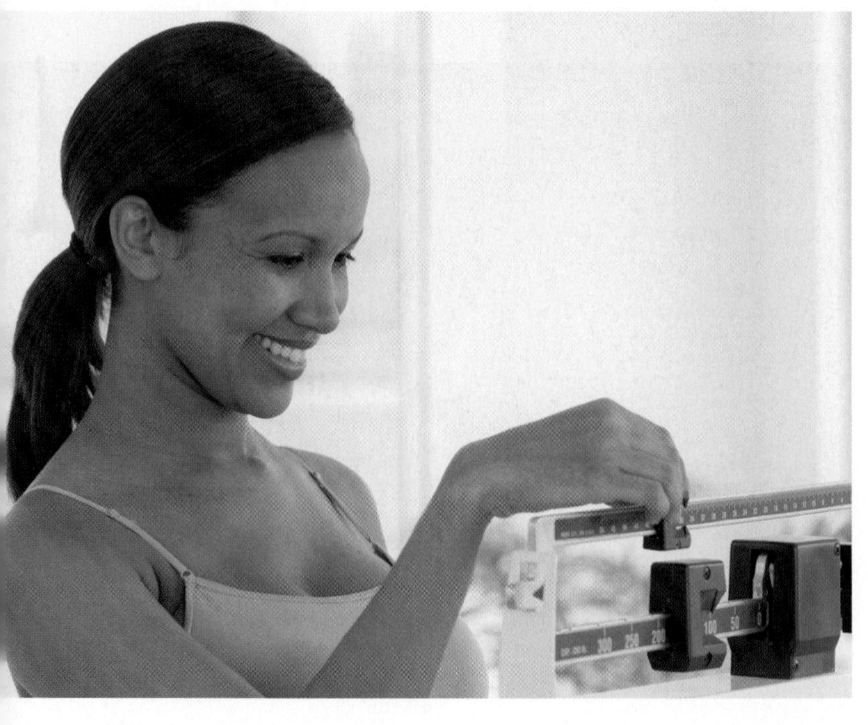

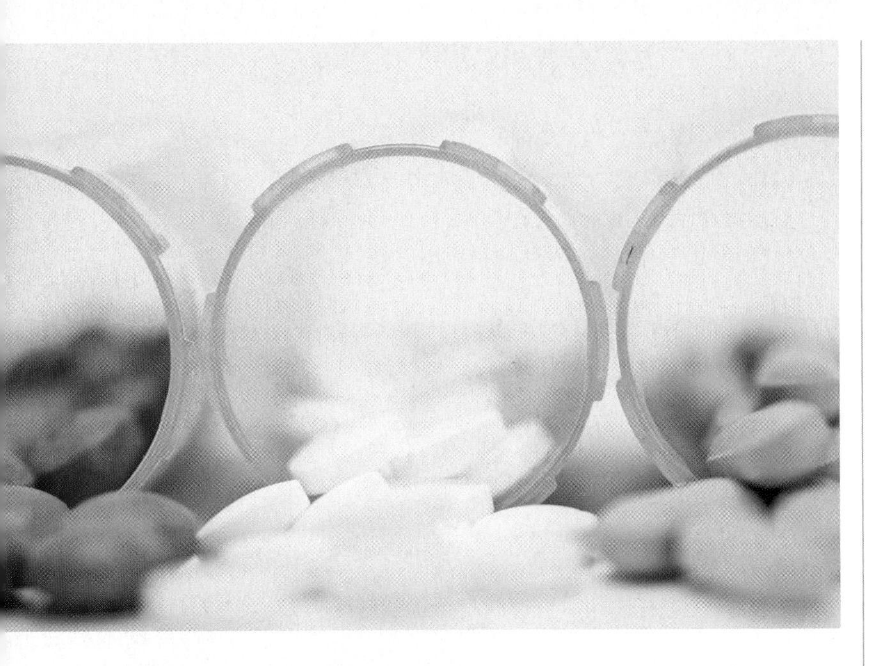

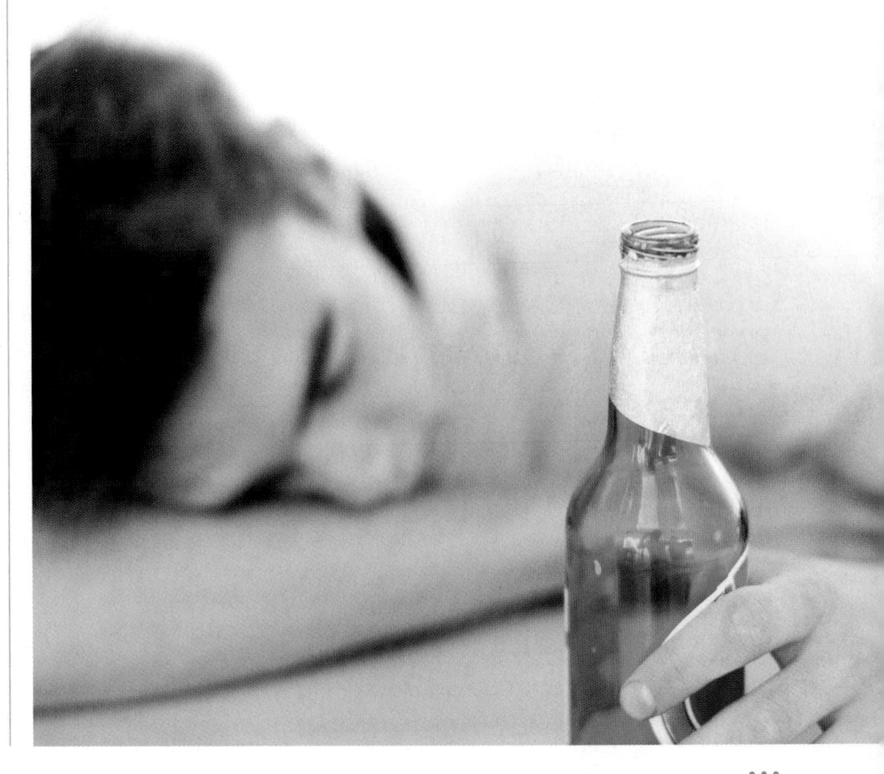

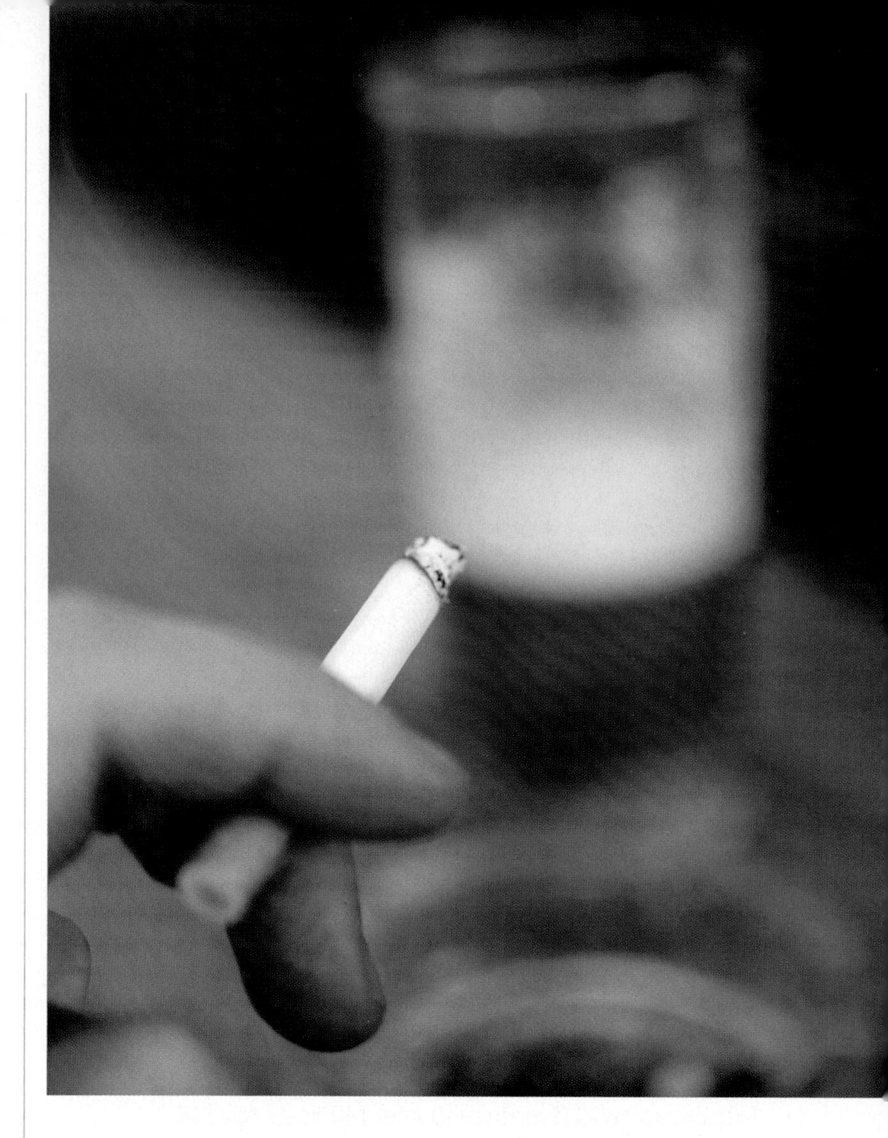

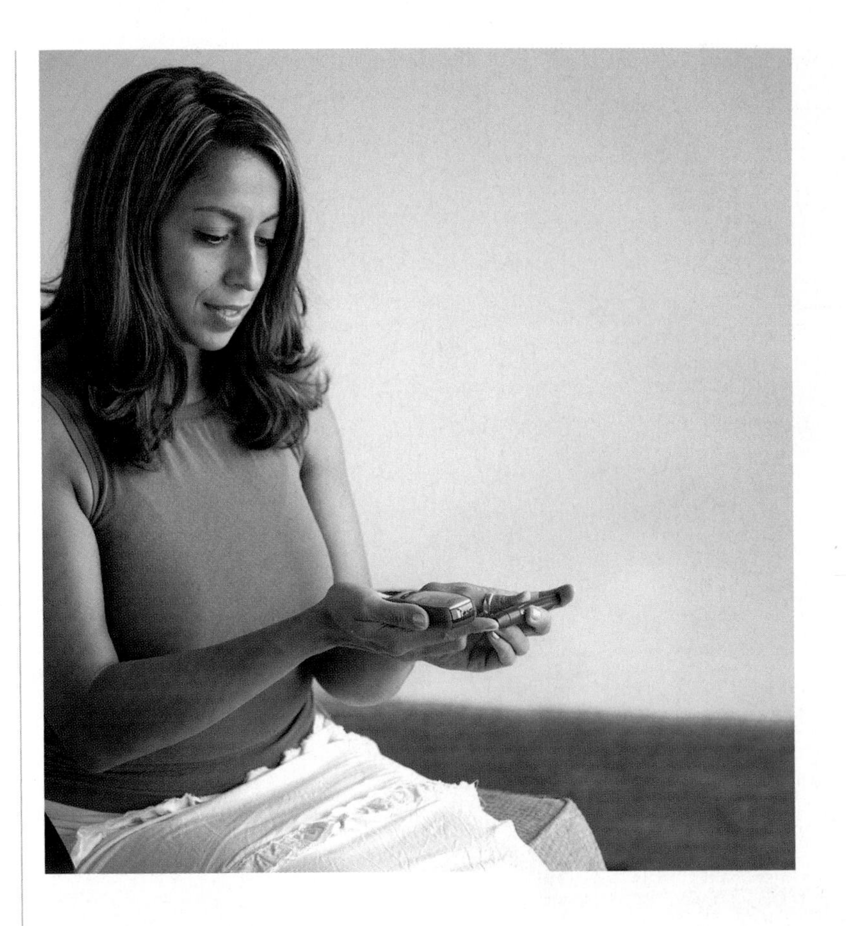

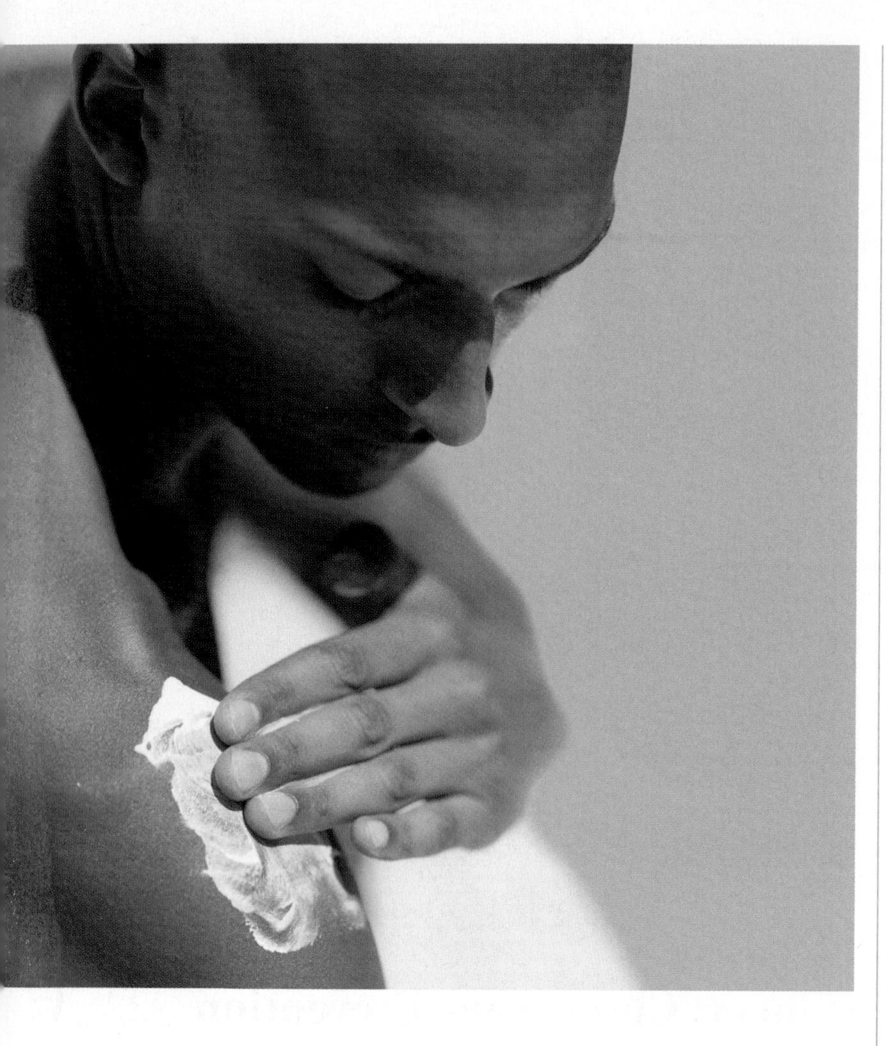

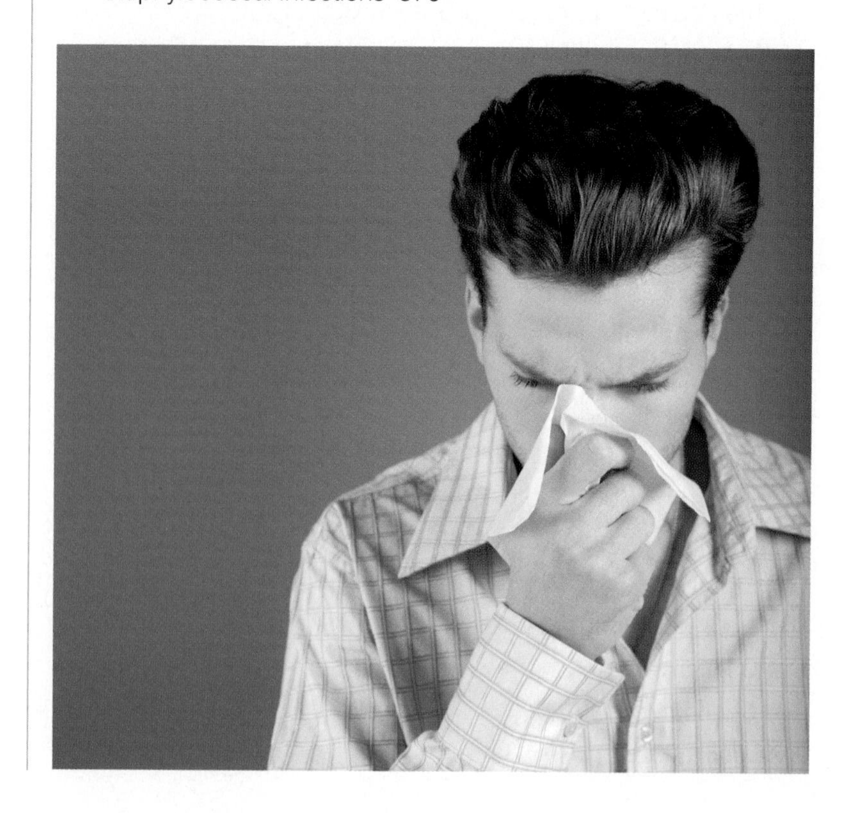

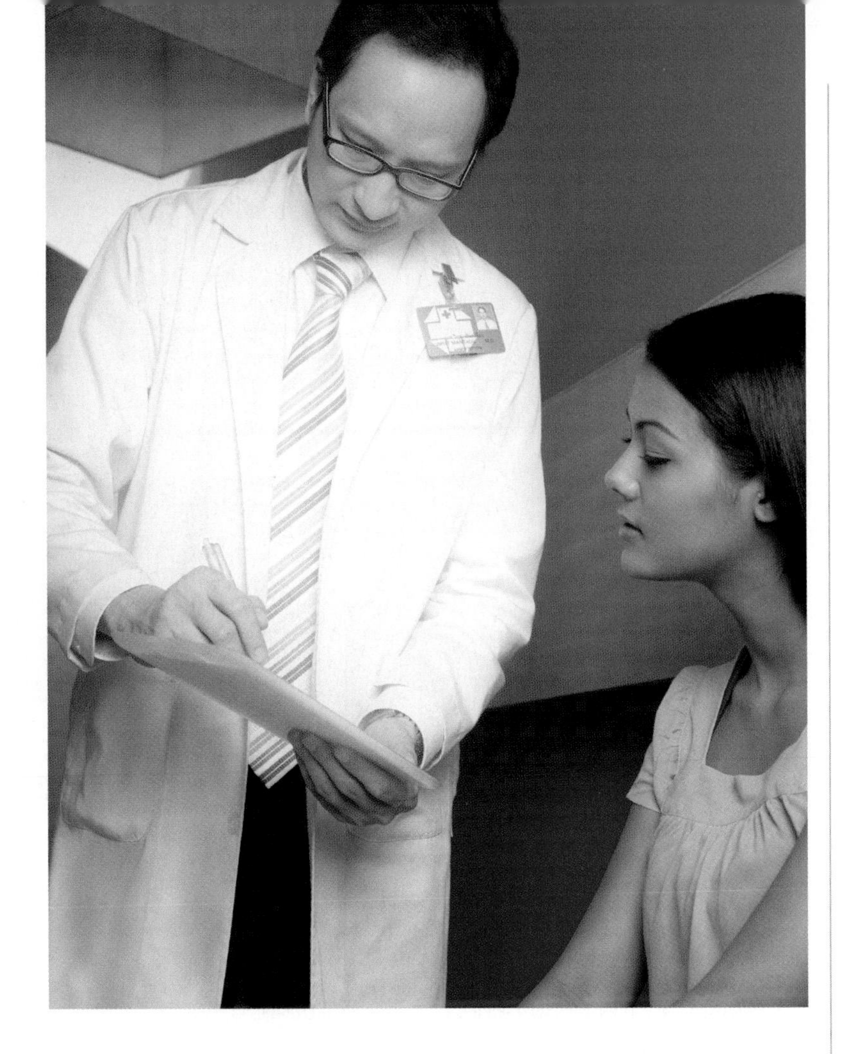

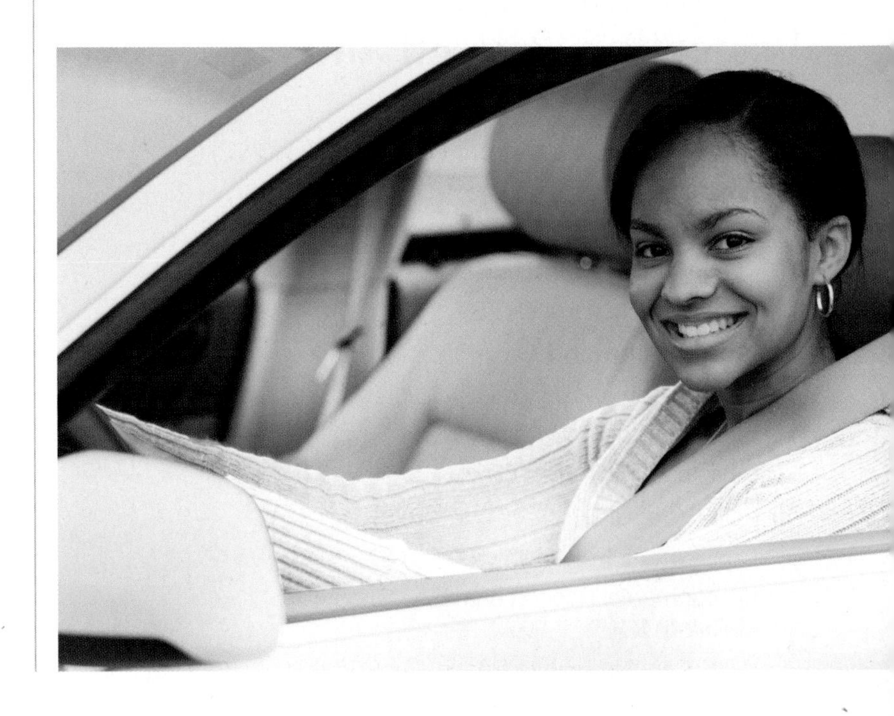

Chapter 21
Environmental Health: Protecting Yourself and Your World 575

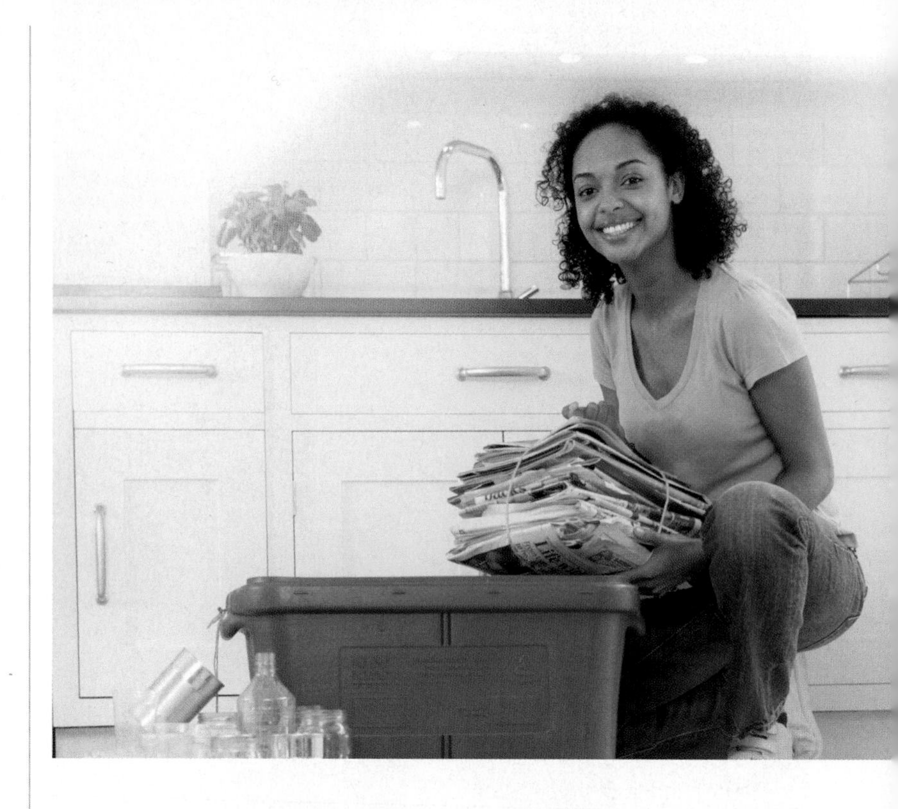

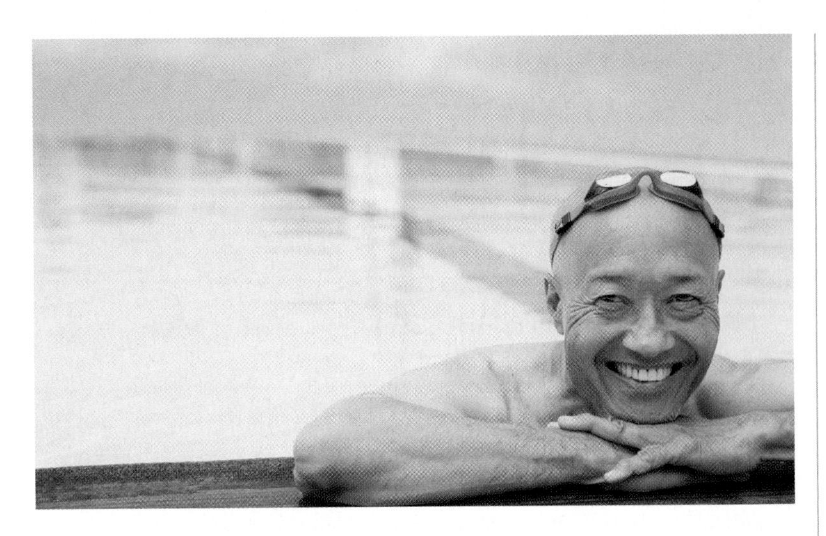

Chapter 22
Embracing Change: The Gifts and Challenges of Aging 604

Feature Boxes

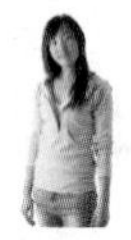

STUDENT STORIES

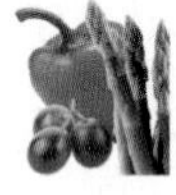

SPECIAL FEATURES

SELF-ASSESSMENT

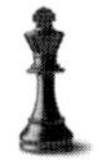

Practical Strategies for Change

Practical Strategies for Health

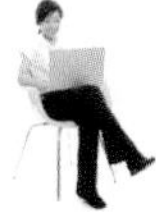

STUDENT STATS

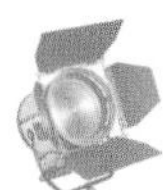

SPOTLIGHT

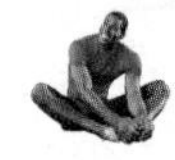

MYTH OR FACT?

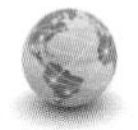

DIVERSITY & HEALTH

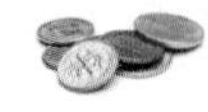

CONSUMER CORNER

Preface

Do the choices you make today affect your health?

If you're young and healthy you might not think so. Good health can feel like a given, something you don't need to worry about right now. But the truth is, in ways both large and small, what you choose today affects your health now, next year, and for the rest of your life. For example, if you choose to eat healthfully and keep your weight in check during college, you are instilling in yourself healthy habits that will make it easier to avoid becoming overweight as you age, and because of that you will reduce your risk for chronic disease later in life. Similarly, if you learn how to effectively manage the stress of your classes this semester, that will serve you not just during finals week, but as you build your career. And, if you make a habit of buckling your seat belt today, it could save your life tonight, tomorrow, or sometime in the future. So what do you think? Do these choices affect your health?

In an era when numerous factors compete for our time—school, work, family, friends, entertainment, social networking, and more—it can be hard to prioritize healthy habits. We all have to live with some factors we can't immediately control, such as our genetics, or contend with elements in our environment that may not promote healthy actions. But your decisions and lifestyle habits make a difference. You can make decisions now that greatly reduce your chances of developing health problems later. You can work to make your immediate environment more conducive to healthy lifestyles, improving health not just for you, but also for your peers. This book is called *Health: Making Choices for Life* to underscore that what you choose today *matters*. Good health is built through a series of choices, and making choices that encourage health is an essential part of creating the life you want, both on campus now and in the years to come.

Key Features of this Text

We wrote this book to help you make the best possible health choices, using the most recent and scientifically accurate information available. Other textbooks provide plenty of health information, but offer little guidance for actively improving your health. *Health: Making Choices for Life* makes health information more relevant for students, with unique features such as these:

- **Choosing to Change Worksheets** (also available online) in every chapter help you target a behavior you want to change, determine your stage of behavior change based on the transtheoretical model of behavior change, think through the steps necessary to make a positive change, and put yourself on a path to success.
- **Student Stories** appear throughout the text, and videos of real college students telling health-related stories stream on our Companion Website (www.pearsonhighered.com/lynchelmore). These stories reveal how students have dealt with health challenges, and may inspire you to make changes in your own life.
- **Health Online** links throughout the book guide you to relevant health-related quizzes, tools, websites, videos, and podcasts. These links can also be found on the Companion Website, where they will be updated as needed.
- **Change Yourself, Change Your World** sections at the end of each chapter show you how to implement the health information you've just learned. Each section offers advice on personal choices, helping a friend, and campus advocacy.
- **Self-Assessments** (also available online) enable you to evaluate your current health behaviors and identify areas you may wish to work on.
- **A magazine-style design** makes it fun to read!
- **The lively, engaging writing** is informative, scientifically reliable, and authoritative.

You will also find the following features:

- **Student Stats** throughout the book show you how health issues affect the college student population. Colorful graphs display statistics compiled by national surveys of college students.
- **Practical Strategies for Health** and **Practical Strategies for Change** boxes provide concrete tips you can use to develop and maintain healthful behaviors.
- **Consumer Corner** boxes examine consumer-related issues such as evaluating online health information, using over-the-counter medications safely, choosing athletic shoes, and deciding on whether to purchase organic produce.
- **Diversity & Health** boxes highlight how health issues can affect certain populations disproportionately, depending on sex, racial/ethnic background, socioeconomic class, and other factors.
- **Myth or Fact?** boxes provide scientific evidence supporting or refuting common health-related claims.

- **Special Feature** boxes highlight hot topics in health, including getting enough sleep, the effect of Facebook on social relationships and communication, emerging infectious diseases, and what health-care reform means for you.

Student Supplements

The student supplements for this textbook include:

- **The *Health: Making Choices for Life* Companion Website** (www.pearsonhighered.com/lynchelmore) is where you can view a complete set of student videos; view health-related *ABC News* videos; access online behavior change tools; access practice tests and self-assessments; view videos of author Barry Elmore responding to questions about health-related issues; find links to updated websites, videos, and podcasts; and access a rich suite of additional study tools, including NutriTools interactive activities, MP3 audio files, mobile tips you can access on your smartphone, audio case studies, an online glossary, and flashcards. You can also **send us your own videos, stories, or questions** via this website. If we decide to use your video or story for a future edition of *Health: Making Choices for Life,* you will receive both payment and publication credit!
- **Mobile Tips!** Now you can access health tips covering everything from stress management to fitness wherever you go, via your smartphone. A set of four different tip "cards" per chapter are available. Access them by navigating to http://mobiletips.pearsoncmg.com on any mobile device. Or go straight to each chapter's cards by scanning the QR code provided at the end of the chapter.
- **Facebook** (www.facebook.com/ChoosingHealth) **and Twitter** (http://twitter.com/choosing_health) **pages** provide up-to-the-minute health news as well as keep you informed of opportunities to submit your own videos and student stories.
- **A YouTube channel** (www.youtube.com/ch00singhealth) features selected student videos. If you send us a student video of your own that we like, you just might find it on this channel!
- **Access to TweetYourHealth** (www.tweetyourhealth.com), a powerful, easy-to-use, Twitter-based application, allows you to track and keep an online journal of everyday health behaviors (such as what you eat, how often you exercise, and how much sleep you get) via any mobile device with text messaging or Internet capabilities.
- **The Behavior Change Log Book and Wellness Journal** is a booklet you can use to track your daily exercise and nutritional intake and create a long-term nutrition and fitness prescription plan.
- **A Digital 5-Step Pedometer** measures steps, distance (miles), activity time, and calories.
- **MyDietAnalysis** (www.pearsonhighered.com/mydietanalysis) is an online tool powered by ESHA Research, Inc., that features a database of nearly 20,000 foods and multiple reports. It allows you to track your diet and physical activity, receive analyses of what nutrients you may be lacking, and generate and submit reports electronically.
- **Eat Right! Healthy Eating in College and Beyond** is a guidebook that provides practical tips, shopper's guides, and recipes so that you can start putting healthy principles into action. Topics include healthy eating in the cafeteria, dorm room, and fast food restaurants; eating on a budget; weight-management tips; vegetarian alternatives; and guidelines on alcohol and health.
- **Live Right! Beating Stress in College and Beyond** is a guidebook that provides useful strategies for coping with a variety of life's challenges, during college and beyond. Topics include sleep, managing finances, time management, coping with academic pressure, relationships, and being a smart consumer.
- **Take Charge! Self-Assessment Worksheets** is a collection of 50 self-assessment exercises that students can fill out to assess their health and wellness. Worksheets are available as a gummed pad and can be packaged at no additional charge with the main text.

Instructor Supplements

This textbook comes with a comprehensive set of supplemental resources to assist instructors with classroom preparation and presentation.

- **The Teaching Tool Box** contains everything you need to teach your course, all in one place. It includes *Teaching with Student Learning Outcomes,* a booklet of articles about how to use Student Learning Outcomes in your course; *Teaching with Web 2.0,* a booklet of ideas for incorporating Web 2.0 technologies into your classroom; an *Instructor Resource and Support Manual;* a printed *Test Bank;* an *Instructor Resource DVD* containing PowerPoint lecture outlines, "clicker" questions, quiz show questions, a computerized Test Bank, transparency acetate masters, NutriTools interactive activities, jpeg files of all the art, tables, and selected photos from the book, *ABC News* video clips, and student story videos; *Great Ideas! Active Ways to Teach Health and Wellness*; a *MyHealthLab* Instructor Access Kit (see the following page for details on *MyHealthLab*); *Take Charge! Self-Assessment Worksheets; Behavior Change Log Book and Wellness Journal;*

Eat Right! Healthy Eating in College and Beyond; and *Live Right! Beating Stress in College and Beyond.*

- **MyHealthLab** (www.pearsonhighered.com/myhealthlab) provides a one-stop shop for accessing a wealth of preloaded content and makes paper-free assigning and grading easier than ever. MyHealthLab contains all of the resources found on the *Health: Making Choices for Life* Companion Website, along with the Pearson eText version of *Health: Making Choices for Life* (which allows for instructor annotations to be shared with the class).

Electronic Editions

Health: Making Choices for Life is available in two electronic versions:

- **The Pearson eText** gives students access to the text whenever and wherever they can access the Internet. The eText pages look exactly like the printed text, and include powerful interactive and customization functions. Students can create notes, highlight text, create bookmarks, zoom in and out, click hyperlinked words and phrases to view definitions, and search quickly and easily for specific content. Instructors can add notes to guide students, upload documents, and customize presentations using Whiteboard mode. Contact your local Pearson sales representative for more information.
- **CourseSmart eTextbooks** are an exciting new choice for students looking to save money. As an alternative to purchasing the print textbook, students can subscribe to the same content online and save 40% off the suggested list price of the print text. Access the CourseSmart eText at www.coursesmart.com.

We are a team of health educators and communicators whose work reflects our deeply held belief that discussions of health are always a dialogue in progress. We hope this book will help you make changes toward better health. We also hope you'll let us know how those changes are going, and how we can make *Health: Making Choices for Life* even more useful. Find us on Facebook, Twitter, or our Companion Website, and share your stories with us!

April Lynch

Barry Elmore

Jerome Kotecki

Acknowledgments

Authoring a new textbook can feel like a solitary job during countless hours alone researching topics or drafting chapters. But in reality, we as authors were supported not only by each other, but by an amazing team of editors, publishing professionals, content contributors, supplement authors, and reviewers.

Collectively, the authors would like to thank everyone at Pearson Education for their support and belief in our vision and our book, and call out a few of the key players for special thanks. First off, this book would not be possible without the support of Vice President and Editorial Director Frank Ruggirello, who was always there to provide backing and funds for the project and to be our advocate to the highest reaches of the organization. Another lifeline for the book was Executive Editor Sandra Lindelof, who believed in our team from the start, provided creative and enthusiastic guidance for the book as a whole, and really fostered our student-centric approach to teaching health. This book would not be what it is today without the top-notch management and razor-sharp editorial skills of Director of Development Barbara Yien. Senior Project Development Editor Marie Beaugureau supplied even more editorial guidance, feedback, coordination, and management—her continuous contact with the team and excellent guidance in the face of tight schedules kept us all at the top of our game and on track, and this book wouldn't be here without her. We'd also like to thank Assistant Editor Meghan Zolnay, who commissioned and managed the impressive print supplement package for the book, and Sade McDougal, Assistant Media Producer, for her creativity and know-how in creating the robust and innovative interactive media and applications for the book. Editorial Assistant Briana Verdugo commissioned hundreds of reviews and provided administrative assistance that none of us could have done without. Beth Collins and Lori Newman, Production Project Managers, expertly coordinated the production aspects of the book, from coordinating the design to making sure manuscript was being sent to the correct places to double-checking all aspects of page proofs. We must also thank everyone at S4Carlisle Publishing Services, especially Senior Project Editor Norine Strang, for their wonderful work on the production and composition of the book—no matter how tight the schedule, they were always able to turn out the next round of page proofs. Manufacturing Buyer Stacey Weinberger researched all types of paper and printing methods for us, to help us produce the most beautiful printing of the book possible. And speaking of beautiful, a million thanks to the team at Riezebos Holzbaur Design Group, who designed the modern, engaging, and lively cover and interior for the book. Sarah Bonner and Donna Kalal provided invaluable expertise in the researching and coordinating of hundreds of photos for the book. A huge thanks goes out to Neena Bali, Executive Marketing Manager, who has worked tirelessly to get the message of *Health: Making Choices for Life* out to instructors across the country. In addition, Senior Market Development Manager Brooke Suchomel and Market Relations Manager Leslie Allen would not rest until they had spoken to as many instructors as possible about their teaching needs and determined what would make up a "perfect" textbook and supplement package. Many thanks for their awesome work. And last but not least, Laura Southworth developed a beautiful and engaging art program.

We would also like to thank our contributors, all of whom truly left their stamps on the book and whom we can't thank enough for their time and expertise. Without Laura Bonazzoli, this book would not have been made. Her creativity, attention to detail, and passion for explaining complex health issues show throughout the entire text. Her writing and editing have helped make this the book you see before you. Teresa Snow at Georgia Institute of Technology carefully examined every chapter of the book and provided extremely valuable feedback on accuracy, usefulness, and writing level. Karen Vail-Smith at East Carolina University was invaluable in helping create and vet the content this text is based on. Tanya Morgan Gatenby at West Chester University provided feedback and insight on much of the content that appears throughout the text. Sandra Walz at West Chester University shared nutrition and weight-management expertise that we could not have done without. Julie Sevrens Lyons played an important early role in the creation of the drugs, alcohol, tobacco, relationships, sexuality, and infectious diseases content.

The creation of the instructor and student supplements for *Health: Making Choices for Life* could not have been completed without the excellent work of our supplement team. Assistant Editor Meghan Zolnay worked with Denise Wright at Southern Editorial to create the excellent Test Bank, Instructor Resource and Support Manual, PowerPoint lecture outlines, "clicker" questions, and quiz show questions. Dr. John Kowalczyk at University of Minnesota, Duluth provided a taxonomy check of the Test Bank. Assistant Media Producer Sade McDougal worked with Dustin Childress of Ozarks Technical Community College to create the Test Your Knowledge and Chapter Reading online quizzes and with Susanne Wood of Tallahassee Community College to review the accuracy of the online quizzes. Sade also worked with Reizebos Holzbaur Design Group in the development of the dynamic and fun Mobile Tips website.

And finally, we'd like to thank all the reviewers who spent their time reading and commenting on our chapters—we listened to each and every one of your comments and are extremely grateful for your feedback. A full list of reviewers is included in the Acknowledgments.

From April Lynch

I have countless people to thank, beginning with those who helped with the heavy lifting of putting words to page. I'll always be grateful to long-time colleague and fellow writer Julie Sevrens Lyons. Julie's prose has a deft, highly approachable touch, and this book is far the stronger for her contribution.

This project would have never gotten off the ground without the deep knowledge, health expertise, teaching wisdom, and killer sense of humor held by co-author Barry Elmore. It wouldn't have stayed off the ground without the invaluable contributions of co-author Jerome Kotecki and contributor Laura Bonazzoli, who brought a new level of expertise and polish to our team. For particular guidance on the topic of human and clinical genetics, I'm indebted to Vickie Venne, M.S., C.G.C., an excellent genetic counselor, advisor, and friend. And for some occasional real-world perspective, student-style, there's no one I'd turn to before my niece Emma Lynch Marini, whose insights and help on this book have always been smart, funny, and spot-on. Maybe, Emma, you just might use this book when you reach college!

From Barry Elmore

I have so many people to thank for their hard work and contributions to this book. Thank you to all of the people at Pearson Education who worked so diligently on this book. I'd like to offer my sincere appreciation to April Lynch, Jerome Kotecki, Karen Vail-Smith, Dr. Sloane Burke, Sandra Walz, Julie Sevrens Lyons, Teresa Snow, Tanya Morgan Gatenby, and Laura Bonazzoli for their varied and invaluable contributions. It took a talented team of many players to bring this book to press, and I'd like to thank everyone who was a part of the effort.

From Jerome Kotecki

First, I am privileged to have had the opportunity to work with the extremely gifted team of April Lynch, Barry Elmore, and Pearson Education. Second, I am deeply grateful to those who continue to teach me on a daily basis: my students. The way in which they embrace learning—by being intellectually curious and inquisitive—provides a feedback loop that helps keep me focused on my own research and on investigating the latest findings in health research to expand my perspicacity as a professor. Third, I am fortunate to work with administrators who maintain that a well-written textbook based on expert knowledge reflects an important faculty contribution when it comes to the scholarship of teaching and learning. I appreciate the support of Dr. Michael Maggiotto, dean of the College of Sciences and Humanities, Dr. Terry King, provost and Vice President for Academic Affairs, and Dr. Jo Ann Gora, president, of Ball State University. Finally, I wish to extend my gratitude to my mentors. Thank you to Dr. James Stewart, my undergraduate advisor, for having faith in my abilities and encouraging me to stretch myself intellectually; and to Dr. Budd Stalnaker, Dr. John Seffrin, Dr. Mohammad Torabi, and Dr. Morgan Pigg, my graduate advisors, for your expertise and high standards and for guiding me on a path of enlightenment during my years at Indiana University and beyond.

REVIEWERS

Carol Cotton
University of Georgia

Deborah S. Dailey
Louisiana State University

Jennifer Susan Dearden
Morehead State University

Nicholas DiCicco
Camden County College

William Dunscombe
Union County College

LeAnne Farmer
Palomar College

Ari Fisher
Louisiana State University

Siah Fried
Las Positas College

Cari Goebel-Frahm
Montana State University

Anna Hanlon
Orange Coast College

Harvey Hellerstein
Bucks County Community College

Karen M. Hunter
Eastern Kentucky University

Melinda J. Ickes
University of Kentucky

Robert M. Isosaari
University of West Florida

Michelle Korb
California State University, East Bay

Robin Kurotori
Ohlone College

Erin Largo-Wight
University of North Florida

Krynn Larsen
Central Community College

Grace Lartey
Western Kentucky University

Jeri M. Lloyd
Piedmont Virginia Community College

Ayanna Lyles
California University of Pennsylvania

Kathleen Malachowski
Ocean County College

Tim Mead
University of St. Thomas

Susan Milstein
Montgomery College

J. Mike Misita
Holmes Community College

Scott Modell
California State University, Sacramento

Tracy Morris
Middle Tennessee State University

David Opon
Joliet Junior College

Heidi Paquette
Marquette University College of Nursing

Nicole Peritore
University of Kentucky

Patricia Popeck
The University of Scranton

Rodney J. Ragsdale
West Hills College Lemoore

Jill Riera
William Paterson University

Dan Ripley
Long Beach City College

Linda J. Romaine
Raritan Valley Community College

Khlood F. Salman
Duquesne University

Stephanie Sanders-Badt
Berkeley City College

Elissa Sauer
Reading Area Community College

John Seabolt
University of Kentucky

Diadrey-Anne Sealy
University of Georgia

Teresa Snow
Georgia Institute of Technology

Susan Stevenson
Northern Illinois University

Shirley Stewart
Southwest Tennessee Community College

David Stronck
California State University, East Bay

Eric Wickel
University of Tulsa

Trevor Winton
Chapman University

Barbara Wright
Virginia Western

Patricia Wright
The University of Scranton

PERSONAL HEALTH FORUM PARTICIPANTS

Vicki Armstrong
Fayetteville State University

Matt Barbier
Southwestern Community College

Brian Barthel
Utah Valley University

Jodi Brookins-Fisher
Central Michigan University

Sloane Burke
East Carolina University

Fay Cook
Lock Haven University

Shauna Dixon
East Carolina University

Kelly Falcone
Palomar College

Max Faquir
Palm Beach Community College

Joyce Fetro
Southern Illinois University

Brian Findley
Palm Beach Community College

Heidi Fowler
Georgia College

Gilbert Gibson
Virginia State University

Autumn Hamilton
Minnesota State University

David Harackiewicz
Central Connecticut State University

Melanie Healy
University of Wisconsin, La Crosse

Karen Hunter
Eastern Kentucky University

Tim Jones
Tennessee State University

Walt Justice
Southwestern College

Greg Kane
Eastern Connecticut State University

Cheryl Kerns-Campbell
Grossmont College

Ellen Larson
Northern Arizona University

Ayanna Lyles
California University of Pennsylvania

Mitch Mathis
Arkansas State University

Connie Mettille
Winona State University

Jennifer Musick
Long Beach City College

Jose Nanin
Kingsborough Community College

Kim Queri
Rose State College

Todd Sabato
James Madison University

Cindy Shelton
University of Central Arkansas

Mona Smith
Georgia Gwinnett College

Bernard Smolen
Prince George Community College

Debra Sutton
James Madison University

Amanda Tapler
Elon University

Ladona Tornabene
University of Minnesota, Duluth

Lisa Vogelsang
University of Minnesota, Duluth

Virginia White
Riverside Community College

Scott Wolf
Southwestern Illinois College

MARKET DEVELOPMENT PARTICIPANTS

Pamela Anderson
Georgia Gwinnett College

Elizabeth Ash
Morehead State University

Dipavali Bhaya
Bucks County Community College

K. C. Bloom
Salem State University

Becci Brey
Ball State University

Rick Cain
Southern Connecticut State University

Carol Cotton
University of Georgia

Jennifer Dearden
Morehead State University

Steven Dion
Salem State University

William Dunscombe
Union County College

Lorece Edwards
Morgan State University

Gerald Freedman
Essex County College

Siah Fried
Las Positas College

Marilyn Gardner
Western Kentucky University

Julie Gast
Utah State University

Carrie Gregory
William Paterson University

Charlene Gungil
William Paterson University

David Harackiewicz
Central Connecticut State University

Kyle Harris
Bucks County Community College

Joanna Hayden
William Paterson University

Janet Heller
Bronx Community College

Patrick Herbert
Towson University

Karen Hunter
Eastern Kentucky University

Doryce Judd
University of North Texas

Wade Kerr
Morehead State University

Joe Kersting
Glendale Community College

Jae Kim
Western Kentucky University

Grace Lartey
Western Kentucky University

Mary Lou McNichol
Bronx Community College

Courtney Miller
Seminole State College

Juli Miller
Ohio University

Scott Moe
Middle Georgia College

Marisa Moore
University of North Texas

Steven Owens
Tallahassee Community College

Scott Parker
Mayville State University

Sue Paul
Ball State University

Hector Quinones
Tallahassee Community College

Linda Rosskopf
Georgia Institute of Technology

Reineer Schelert
Central Texas College

Diadrey-Anne Sealy
University of Georgia

Sam Severo
Merced College

Adele Smith
University of Louisiana at Lafayette

Paul Villas
University of Texas—Pan American

Maryanne Walsh
William Paterson University

Kathy Werheim
William Paterson University

Twana Wilson
Lamar University

Ken Wolf
Anne Arundel Community College

Bonnie Young
Georgia Perimeter College

Thank You to Our Student Advisory Board

The *Health: Making Choices for Life* Student Advisory Board consists of students who submit stories, videos, questions, or feedback to us about *Health: Making Choices for Life.* Many of them are thanked on the Student Advisory Board page at the beginning of the book. The *Health: Making Choices for Life* team is constantly speaking to more health students and receiving more contributions from them. A continuously updated list of student advisors appears at www.pearsonhighered.com/lynchelmore.

Health matters.

LEARNING OBJECTIVES

IDENTIFY and describe the multiple dimensions of health.

COMPARE health challenges across America and around the world.

IDENTIFY four lifestyle choices that profoundly influence health.

PROVIDE examples of the six categories of determinants of health.

DESCRIBE three models of behavior change.

LIST seven steps for creating an effective behavior-change contract.

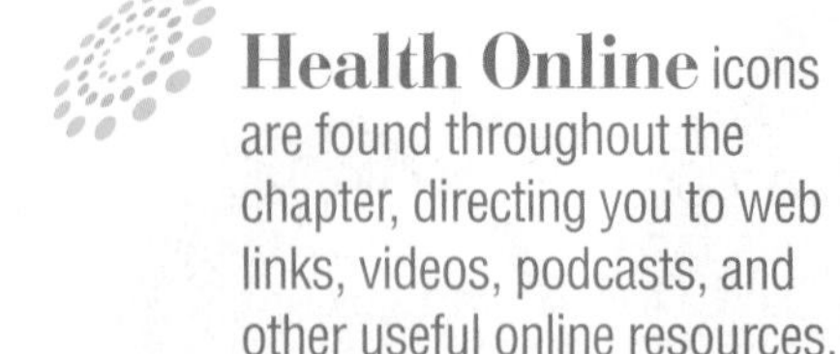

Health Online icons are found throughout the chapter, directing you to web links, videos, podcasts, and other useful online resources.

Have you ever noticed that, when you're ill, stressed, or sleep deprived, you're more likely to doubt yourself, argue with your roommate, and feel overwhelmed by even simple tasks? But when you're bursting with strength and stamina, you feel calm and confident. Even daunting challenges—like hiking a grueling trail or solving a complex calculus proof—can seem like fun.

Intuitively, you know health matters. But do your choices each day—what to eat, how much to sleep, whether to exercise, smoke, or abuse alcohol—really make health a priority? A theme of this textbook is that these so-called *lifestyle choices* can have a profound influence on your health. That's because, over many years, the cumulative effects of lifestyle choices can greatly increase or decrease your risk for disease, injury, disability, and early death. If health matters, then your choices matter, too.

This textbook provides the facts you need to begin evaluating your current lifestyle choices. But information is just a first step. Each chapter concludes by identifying a variety of practical strategies to improve your own health, as well as ways to get involved in promoting a more healthful environment on campus. With this support, you can start making healthy changes for yourself and your world.

Let's begin by exploring the concept of health: its definitions, dimensions, and unique terminology.

What Is Health?

A century ago, the term **health** was used to mean merely the absence of illness or injury. Then in 1948, the newly formed World Health Organization (WHO)—the global health unit of the United Nations—published a radical new definition of health as "a state of complete physical, mental, and social well-being, and not merely the absence of disease or infirmity."[1]

This holistic view of health acknowledges that, in a healthy person, many different dimensions of life are working harmoniously.

Although the WHO's definition of health has been broadly accepted for decades, some researchers have objected to the concept of "complete" well-being, or asserted that the definition lacks practical value. In 1986, in the Ottawa Charter for Health Promotion, the WHO offered the following context for its definition of health:[2]

> To reach a state of complete physical, mental, and social well-being, an individual or group must be able to identify and to realize aspirations, to satisfy needs, and to change or cope with the environment. Health is, therefore, seen as a resource for everyday life . . .

This emphasis on health as a resource we use to reach our goals and satisfy our needs helps us view health less as a stable state and more as an active process. This is true as well for the closely related concept of **wellness.** Some public health authorities view wellness as a state in which we realize our fullest potential as individuals and as members of our community. But others see wellness as a process in which we actively make choices to achieve optimal health.[3] People who have a high level of wellness continually make decisions that promote health in multiple areas of their lives. On the other hand, a low level of wellness is characterized by poor decisions that increase the risk of illness, injury, disability, and premature death.

health More than merely the absence of illness or injury, a state of well-being that encompasses physical, social, psychological, and other dimensions and is a resource for everyday life.

wellness The process of actively making choices to achieve optimal health.

The Illness-Wellness Continuum

In 1975, wellness pioneer John W. Travis, M.D., published a book on the *illness-wellness continuum*. He envisioned a continuum with two extremes: premature

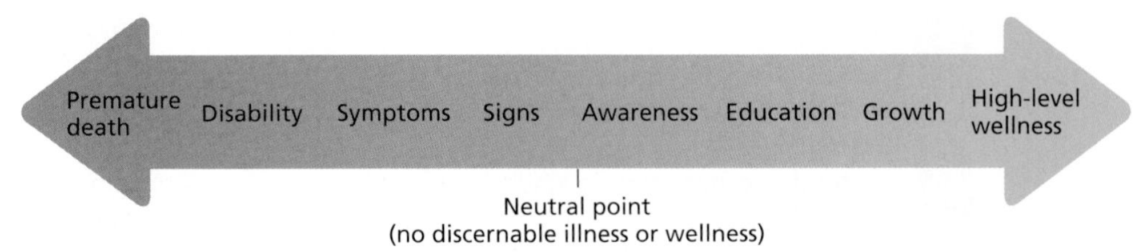

Figure 1.1 The illness-wellness continuum. Your general direction on the continuum matters more than your specific point on it at any given time.

Source: Adapted with permission, from *Wellness Workbook*, 3rd edition, © 2004 by John W. Travis, MD, and Regina Sara Ryan, Celestial Arts. www.thewellspring.com.

death at one end and high-level wellness on the other **(Figure 1.1).** Most of us fall somewhere in between, shifting between states of feeling sick, "neutral," and vibrantly healthy. Your general direction on the continuum (either toward optimal wellness or toward premature death) matters more than your place on it at any given time. You may have a cold, for instance, and not feel particularly well—but if you are taking care of yourself and have a positive attitude, your general direction will be toward greater wellness. Likewise, you may consider yourself healthy—but if you are under a great deal of stress, eating poorly, and drinking excessively, your general direction on the continuum will be toward reduced wellness.

Dimensions of Health and Wellness

Recall that the WHO definition of health identifies three dimensions—physical, mental, and social—all of which are working harmoniously. Though some researchers accept these three dimensions as adequate, others have identified more or different dimensions appropriate for the populations they serve. In this textbook, we acknowledge the following seven dimensions of health: physical, intellectual, psychological, spiritual, social, environmental, and occupational **(Figure 1.2).** (Note that because wellness is the process of achieving optimal health, wellness, too, is multidimensional.) Let's take a closer look at each of these dimensions.

Physical Health

Physical health focuses on the body: how well it functions, and how well you care for it. Optimal physical health includes being physically active, eating nutritiously, getting enough sleep, making responsible decisions about sex, drinking, and drugs, and taking steps to avoid injuries and infectious diseases.

Intellectual Health

Intellectual health is marked by a willingness to take on new intellectual challenges, an openness to new ideas and skills, a capacity to think critically, and a sense of humor and curiosity. People who have a high level of intellectual health not only recognize problems quickly, but also seek and create solutions. These characteristics are important not only during your years of formal education, but throughout your lifetime.

Psychological Health

Psychological health is a broad category encompassing autonomy, self-acceptance, and the ability to respond appropriately to our environment. It also includes the ability to maintain nurturing relationships with others and to pursue meaningful goals. Finally, people who are psychologically healthy sense that they are continually growing and developing as individuals.

Spiritual Health

Closely related to psychological health is spiritual health, which is influenced by the beliefs and values we hold and the ways in which we express them—for instance, in humanitarian activities, religious practices, or efforts to preserve nature and the environment. Spiritual health contributes to a sense of place and purpose in life, and can be a source of support when we face challenges.

Social Health

Social health describes the quality of our interactions and relationships with others. How satisfying are your relationships with your family, your friends, your professors, and others in your life? How do you feel about your ability to fulfill social roles, whether as a friend, roommate, or community volunteer? Good social health is also characterized by an ability to provide support to others and receive it in return.

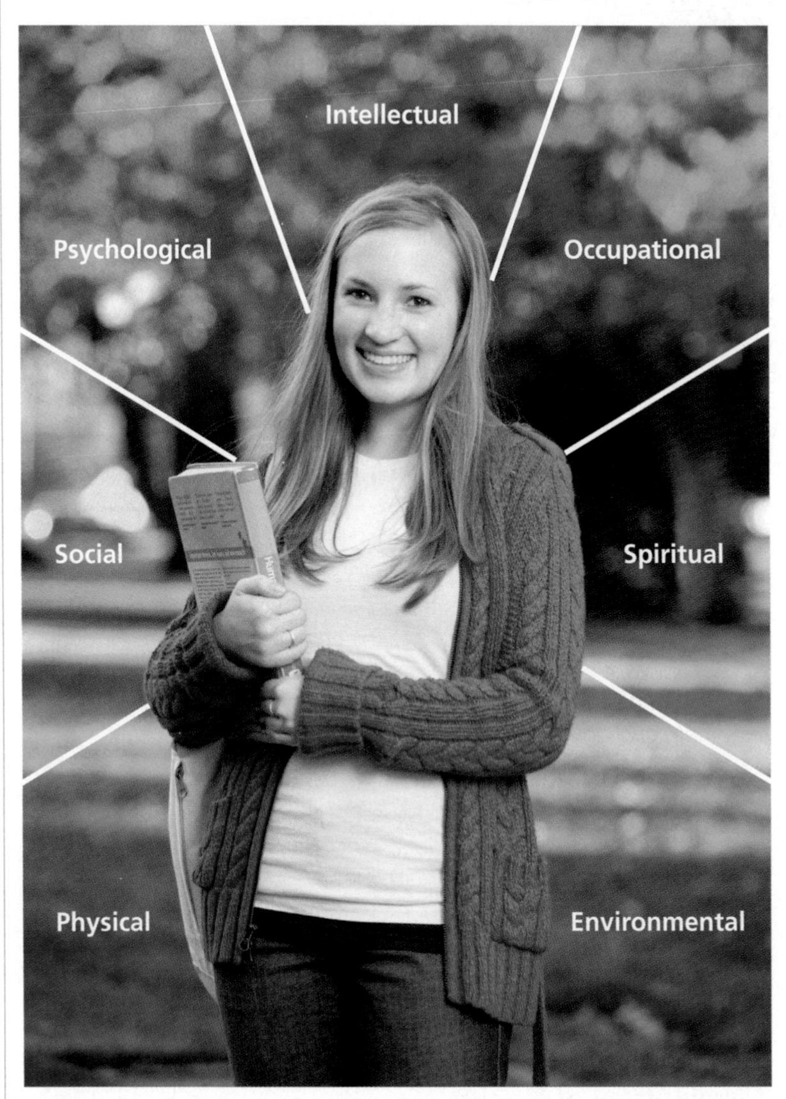

Figure 1.2 Dimensions of health. Health is more than just the absence of injury or illness; it encompasses multiple dimensions.

Proud of My Scars

STUDENT STORY

"Hi, I'm Corey. I'm 19 and I'm a sophomore park and rec management major. I was born with a skeletal condition where the left side of my body is bigger than the right side. The doctors had to even out my legs so that I could walk flat-footed and wouldn't have back problems later in life. I've had a total of three surgeries, which left me with some scars. I also have a scar from my belly button all the way to the side of my rib cage. Growing up, I was always self-conscious, especially during the summer when everybody was out at the beach in swimsuits, and all these guys had six-pack abs. I knew I'd never be able to have abs like that because I have this scar running straight through my abdominal muscle.

Now, though, I've realized that my scars are a great conversation starter. People will see me and ask 'Oh, cool scar, how'd you get it?' I've learned over the years that everybody has a fail point and mine just happens to be physical. I've just learned to live with it. Those scars are what make me 'me.' I also have friends who don't really care what I look like or whether I'm the strongest or best-looking guy in the world. My friends are there whether I'm having surgeries or I'm on top of the world."

1: Where do you think Corey falls on the wellness continuum?

2: Assess how Corey is doing in at least three different dimensions of wellness.

Do you have a story similar to Corey's? Share your story at www.pearsonhighered.com/lynchelmore.

Environmental Health

Environmental health describes the quality of our home, work, school, and social environments—as well as the health of our planet. Air quality, availability of clean water and nutritious food, crime rates, weather, pollution, and exposure to chemicals are just a few of the variables that factor into environmental health.

Occupational Health

Occupational health describes the quality of your relationship to your work. Rather than a paying job, your "work" may consist of your studies, an athletic endeavor, or an artistic pursuit—whatever it is that you consider your primary occupation. Does this work feel fulfilling? Do you have opportunities to advance and learn? Do you feel respected by your colleagues or peers? Challenges to occupational health include stress, lack of fulfillment in the work, poor relationships with colleagues, poor performance, inadequate compensation, and sudden unemployment.

Terminology of Health

As you can see, health and wellness are as broad as life itself. So it's not surprising that health-care providers and researchers in public health have developed an extensive vocabulary with which to communicate health-related concepts and statistics. The following are some of the most important of these terms, which you'll encounter not only throughout this textbook, but also in media reports on health-related topics:

- **Acute versus chronic illness.** An acute illness is one that comes on suddenly and intensely, like a headache or a bout of food poisoning. It typically resolves quickly, too, sometimes in a matter of hours, sometimes in a week or two. Medical treatment may or may not be required. Significant acute illnesses—like heat stroke or an infection involving the brain—can be fatal. In contrast, chronic illnesses become noticeable only gradually, often over months or years. They are initially very mild, and may continue that way, or may progress in severity. Examples are arthritis, heart disease, and age-related dementia.
- **Morbidity and mortality.** Morbidity is a clinical term meaning illness, especially the prevalence of a disease within a population. Mortality, of course, means death, but public health researchers use the term when referring to the number of deaths in a certain population or from a certain cause. For instance, a country's infant mortality rate—the percentage of babies who die before their first birthday—is often used as a general indicator of a nation's overall health status.

The U.S. Centers for Disease Control and Prevention publishes the *Morbidity and Mortality Weekly Report (MMWR)*. Listen to short podcasts from the MMWR on a variety of health topics, from salt intake to sleep, at www.cdc.gov/mmwr/mmwrpodcasts.html.

- **Signs and symptoms.** In the language of health care, a sign is an objective indication of a person's health status. For example, body weight, pulse, blood pressure, lab test results, and X-rays and scans are measures that can suggest the presence or absence of disease. Signs also include things we can't measure, but simply hear or see, such as wheezing, slurred speech, or a rash. In contrast, a symptom is a subjective experience reported by a patient—such as pain, shortness of breath, dizziness, or fatigue.
- **Health promotion and disease prevention.** At its simplest, health promotion is the process of helping people improve their health.[4] For instance, a campus campaign to get students to increase their hours of sleep each night qualifies as health promotion. So does reading this textbook. In contrast, disease prevention refers more specifically to actions taken to reduce the incidence of diseases. For instance, your campus health center might offer free latex condoms to reduce the incidence of sexually transmitted infections.
- **Causes and risk factors.** A cause is a factor that is directly responsible for a certain result. For example, a particular genetic defect is known to result in a disease called cystic fibrosis. And consuming food contaminated with a type of bacteria called *Salmonella* causes the infection salmonellosis. In contrast, a risk factor is a characteristic that increases the likelihood that an individual will develop a particular disease or experience an injury. For example, obesity is a risk factor for heart disease, and alcohol abuse is a risk factor for involvement in a motor vehicle accident. Notice that risk factors don't directly *cause* disease or injury; that is, not everyone who is obese develops heart disease, and many people who have heart disease are not obese. Instead, risk factors tell us about relationships; for example, 40% of deaths in motor vehicle accidents involve alcohol.[5]

Notice that, although you can reduce your risk for many health problems, few are entirely preventable. For example, for decades, a series of reports from the U.S. Surgeon General have stated unequivocally that smoking and exposure to secondhand smoke cause cancer; in fact, more than 440,000 Americans die each year as a direct result of their own or others' smoking.[6] But every day, people who have never smoked and have never lived with smokers learn that they have lung cancer. That's because many diseases, including cancer, are *multifactorial;* that is, they develop as a result of multiple factors, including some—such as your genetic inheritance and your age—that are not within your control. Still, the lifestyle choices you make—such as to avoid smoking and to eat a nutritious diet—can dramatically reduce your risk, or reduce the severity of your signs and symptoms should the disease develop.

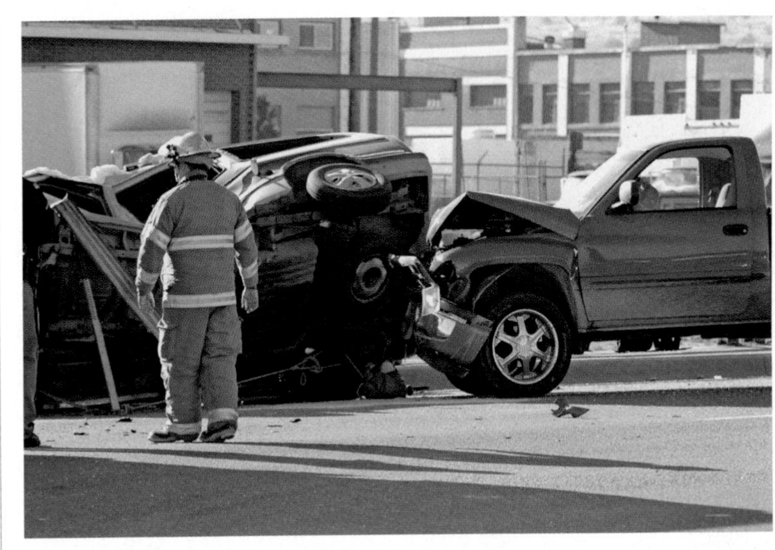

Motor vehicle accidents are the leading cause of death among people aged 15 to 24 in the United States.

Current Health Challenges

In the past century, dramatic technological advances have enabled people worldwide to enjoy longer, healthier lives. Advances in public health, such as municipal water purification, sanitation, and food service inspection, have decreased the prevalence of disease. At the same time, new diagnostic techniques such as MRI scans and DNA testing, as well as advances in vaccines, medications, radiation, and surgery, have helped us to treat disease earlier and more successfully when it does occur. Despite such progress, many health challenges remain.

Health Across America

By one very basic measure of health—how long the average person born in the United States can expect to live—we are in far better shape than our predecessors. The current **life expectancy** at birth in the United States is a record 78.7 years—more than 15 years longer than it was in 1940.[7] The causes of death have also changed dramatically over the years. In 1900, the leading causes of death were infectious diseases such as pneumonia, influenza, and tuberculosis.[8] Today, the leading causes of death in the United States are chronic diseases (see **Table 1.1**).[9]

life expectancy The average number of years a person may expect to live.

Want to know your life expectancy? Try an online longevity calculator like the ones at www.northwesternmutual.com/learning-center/the-longevity-game.aspx and www.livingto100.com.

Table 1.1: Top Five Causes of Death in the United States

	Cause of Death
All ages	1. Heart disease 2. Cancer 3. Chronic lower respiratory disease 4. Stroke 5. Accidents/unintentional injuries
15–24 years old	1. Accidents/unintentional injuries 2. Assault/homicide 3. Suicide 4. Cancer 5. Heart disease

Data from Deaths: *Preliminary Data for 2010* by S. L. Murphy, J. Xu, and K. D. Kochanek, 2012, *National Vital Statistics Reports,* 60 (4), pp. 1–69.

America's Health Challenges

In 2010, just two chronic diseases—heart disease and cancer—were responsible for almost half of all deaths (47.4%) in the United States.[9] Almost 1 out of every 2 adults has at least one chronic disease.[10] These statistics are all the more shocking when you realize that chronic diseases are among the most preventable of all health problems in the United States.[10] That's why one of the world's oldest and largest public health agencies—the U.S. Centers for Disease Control and Prevention (CDC)—is sponsoring a national initiative to reduce our rate of chronic disease. As part of this initiative, the CDC has identified four common behaviors that are responsible for most of the illness, suffering, and early death related to chronic diseases **(Figure 1.3).** They are:[10]

- Lack of physical activity
- Poor nutrition
- Tobacco use
- Excessive alcohol consumption

Are Americans paying attention, and if so, are we changing our behaviors? Recent national health surveys reveal the following trends among U.S. adults:

- More than 65% do not engage in regular leisure-time physical activity.[11]
- More than 34% are overweight and another 33.9% are obese.[12]
- Almost 20% smoke.[11]
- Almost 23% admitted to binge drinking within the last year.[11]

As these statistics suggest, it's time for Americans to make healthful lifestyle choices a priority.

Organizations That Promote America's Health

The U.S. Department of Health and Human Services (HHS) is the U.S. government's principal agency for protecting the health of all Americans and providing essential human services, especially for those who are least able to help themselves.[13] Its primary division is the U.S. Public Health Service (PHS), which is directed by the Office of the Surgeon General. The PHS includes a dozen operating divisions that

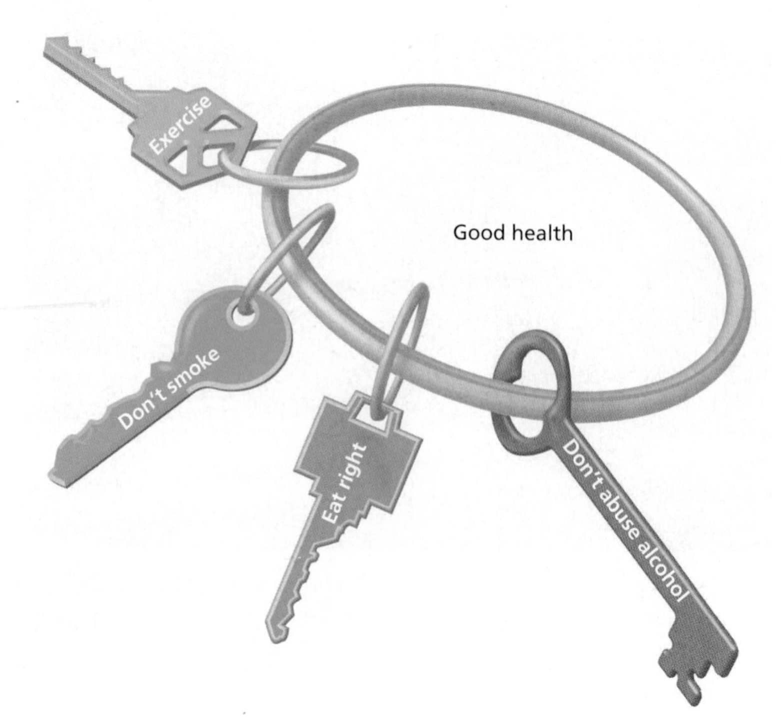

Figure 1.3 Four keys to good health. These four behaviors can significantly reduce your risk of chronic disease and early death.

work together to promote and protect the health of Americans. Among these is the CDC, as well as the following:[13]

- The *Food and Drug Administration (FDA)* is responsible for protecting the public health by assuring the safety, efficacy, and security of medications, medical devices, the food supply, cosmetics, and products that emit radiation.
- The *National Institutes of Health (NIH)* is the primary center for medical research in the United States. It comprises many institutes, such as the National Cancer Institute and the National Center for Complementary and Alternative Medicine.
- The *Substance Abuse and Mental Health Services Administration* is an agency whose mission is to reduce the impact of substance abuse and mental illness on America's communities.

Healthy People initiative A federal initiative to facilitate broad, positive health changes in large segments of the U.S. population every 10 years.

health disparities Gaps in the rate and burden of disease and the access to and quality of health care among various population groups.

The Healthy People Initiative

In 1979, HHS launched the **Healthy People initiative** with a report of the Surgeon General on health promotion and disease prevention efforts in the United States. This laid the groundwork for the publication in 1980 of *Healthy People 1990,* a set of 10-year objectives for improving the health of all Americans. Every decade since, HHS has updated *Healthy People* to include both new objectives and a report of the progress made over the previous decade. Called both a "road map and a compass for better health," the most recent effort, *Healthy People 2020*, was released in December 2010.[14]

Healthy People 2020 poses two main questions:[14]

- What makes some people healthy and others unhealthy?
- How can we create a society in which everyone has a chance to live long, healthy lives?

In exploring these questions, *Healthy People 2020* emphasizes an *ecological approach* to health, one that considers the relationship between an individual's health and the many factors that influence it—from biology and lifestyle choices to level of education, access to health-care services, and even the foods available in the individual's neighborhood. Later in this chapter, we'll discuss these influences in more detail.

One of the primary goals of the Healthy People initiative is to achieve *health equity*—the attainment of the highest level of health for all people.[14] This requires the elimination of **health disparities**—differences in the rate and burden of disease and the access to and quality of health care among various population groups. Health disparities adversely affect groups of people who have systematically experienced greater obstacles to health based on their racial or ethnic group; religion; socioeconomic status; sex; age; mental health; cognitive, sensory, or physical disability; sexual orientation or gender identity; geographic location; or other characteristics historically linked to discrimination or exclusion.[14] For example, gays and lesbians experience certain health disparities—including a lower quality of health care—associated with the discrimination they experience. The nearby **Diversity & Health** box examines health disparities specific to race and ethnicity, and we'll examine the role of poverty and other disparities as we continue in this chapter.

For more information on *Healthy People 2020,* visit www.healthypeople.gov.

Health on America's Campuses

Centers of higher learning, as microcosms of our larger society, have come to recognize that promoting students' health helps the institution meet its goal of providing the best education possible. Stress, sleep deprivation, poor nutrition, depression, anxiety, alcohol and tobacco use, and sexually transmitted infections are just a few of the health issues that can affect academic performance and achievement.

> *"The behaviors that increase the risk of developing chronic diseases—including unhealthy eating habits and a lack of physical activity—are common among college students."*

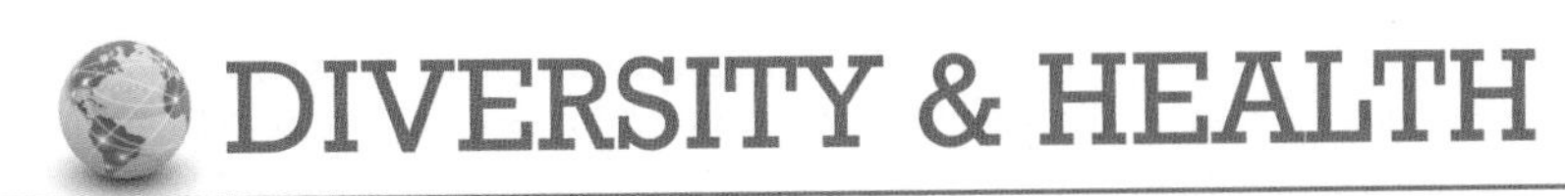

DIVERSITY & HEALTH

Health Disparities Among Different Racial and Ethnic Groups

Whether the causes are socioeconomic, biological, cultural, or still not well understood, health disparities exist among different racial and ethnic populations. For example:

- As a group, Hispanics are more likely to be overweight or obese than are Caucasians, more likely to die from complications of stroke or diabetes, less likely to receive all recommended childhood vaccinations, and less likely to receive prenatal care early in pregnancy.[1]
- African Americans experience the same leading causes of death as the general population, but tend to experience these illnesses and injuries more often and die of them at younger ages and higher rates than other groups. These differences start in infancy, when African American babies experience a higher infant mortality rate. Later in life, issues such as injury, violence, being overweight and obese, and chronic illnesses become especially pressing concerns. When it comes to cancer care, for example, African Americans are less likely to be diagnosed with many types of cancer early, when the disease is easier to treat, and less likely to survive 5 years after diagnosis.[2]
- Asians and Asian Americans, overall, tend to have a life expectancy longer than that of the general population. But as a highly diverse group with ancestries encompassing dozens of countries and regions throughout Asia and the Indian subcontinent, there are also significant differences in health concerns among subgroups of Asians. For example, people from parts of northeast Asia with high levels of hepatitis B tend to experience higher rates of this infectious illness (and the liver damage and liver cancer that can follow it) than other Asian subgroups.[3]
- Native Americans experience lower than average rates of some of the more common health concerns in the United States, such as heart disease or cancer.[4] But they also tend to have a shorter life expectancy than the general population, due to factors including unintentional injuries, substance abuse, and suicide.[4] Diabetes and its complications are an especially important concern—Native Americans as a group have the highest rate of diabetes in the world.[4]
- Caucasians are more susceptible to cystic fibrosis (a genetic disease) than are other populations.[5] In addition, Caucasian women have a higher incidence of breast cancer than other racial or ethnic populations.[6] One recent study found that middle-aged white men and women had the fastest growing rates of suicide compared with other ethnic groups, whose rates were holding steady or declining.[7]

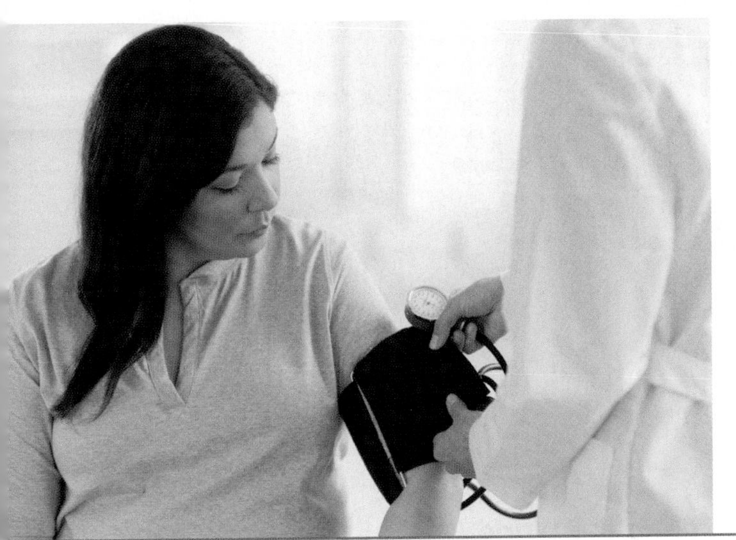

References: **1.** "Health Disparities Experienced by Hispanics—United States," by Centers for Disease Control and Prevention, 2005, *Morbidity and Mortality Weekly Report, 53* (4), pp. 935–937. **2.** "Health Disparities Experienced by Black or African Americans—United States," by Centers for Disease Control, 2005, *Morbidity and Mortality Weekly Report, 54* (1), pp. 1–3. **3.** "Hepatitis B" by S. Chavez, 2009, *Travelers' Health – Yellow Book,* retrieved from the Centers for Disease Control, http://www.nc.cdc.gov/travel/yellowbook/2010/chapter-2/hepatitis-b.aspx. **4.** "Health Disparities Experienced by American Indians and Alaska Natives," by Centers for Disease Control and Prevention, 2003, *Morbidity and Mortality Weekly Report, 52* (30), p. 697. **5.** "Cystic Fibrosis," by the U.S. National Library of Medicine, 2008, retrieved from http://ghr.nlm.nih.gov/condition/cystic-fibrosis. **6.** "Breast Cancer Rates by Race and Ethnicity," by the Centers for Disease Control and Prevention, 2009, retrieved from http://www.cdc.gov/cancer/breast/statistics/race.htm. **7.** "Mid-life Suicide: An Increasing Problem in U.S. Whites, 1999–2005" by G. Hu, H. Wilcox, L. Wisslow, and S. Baker, 2008, *American Journal of Preventive Medicine, 35* (6), pp. 589–593.

Campus Health Challenges

The **Student Stats** box lists common health issues reported by college students in a recent nationwide study.[15] The same study reported that nearly 60% of students describe their health as either "very good" or "excellent."

Among Americans aged 15 to 24, the leading causes of death are unintentional injuries, homicide, and suicide.[9] These sudden, traumatic deaths lead mortality in this age group because younger people do not experience the same high rates of chronic illnesses (such as heart disease and cancer) that increase mortality among the adult population as a whole. However, the behaviors that increase the risk of developing chronic diseases—including unhealthy eating habits and a lack of physical activity—are common among college students. Although 62.7% of students report being at a healthy weight, 21.4% are overweight and 11% are obese.[15] Furthermore, although 48.3% of college students meet national recommendations for physical activity (moderate exercise for at least 30 minutes at least 5 days per week or vigorous exercise for at least 20 minutes at least 3 days per week), more than half do not.[15]

Interestingly, research has shown that students tend to vastly overestimate how many of their peers are regularly using alcohol, tobacco, or other drugs.[15] For example:

- Students believe that 93.8% of their peers consumed alcohol during a given 30-day period. The actual percentage was 65.9%.
- Students believe that 81.8% of their peers had smoked cigarettes during a given 30-day period. The actual percentage was 15.2%.
- Students believe that 80.3% of their peers had smoked marijuana during a given 30-day period. The actual percentage was 15.9%.
- Students believe that 75.5% of their peers used illicit drugs (excluding marijuana) during a given 30-day period. The actual percentage was 12.9%.

The lesson here: When it comes to drugs and alcohol, it's simply not true that "everyone is doing it."

STUDENT 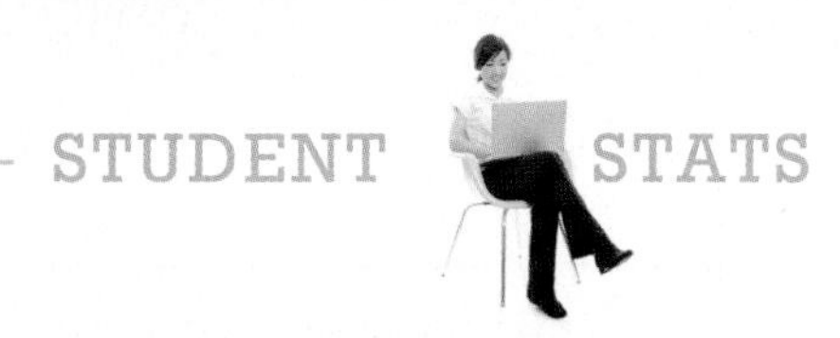 STATS

Common Health Problems Reported by College Students

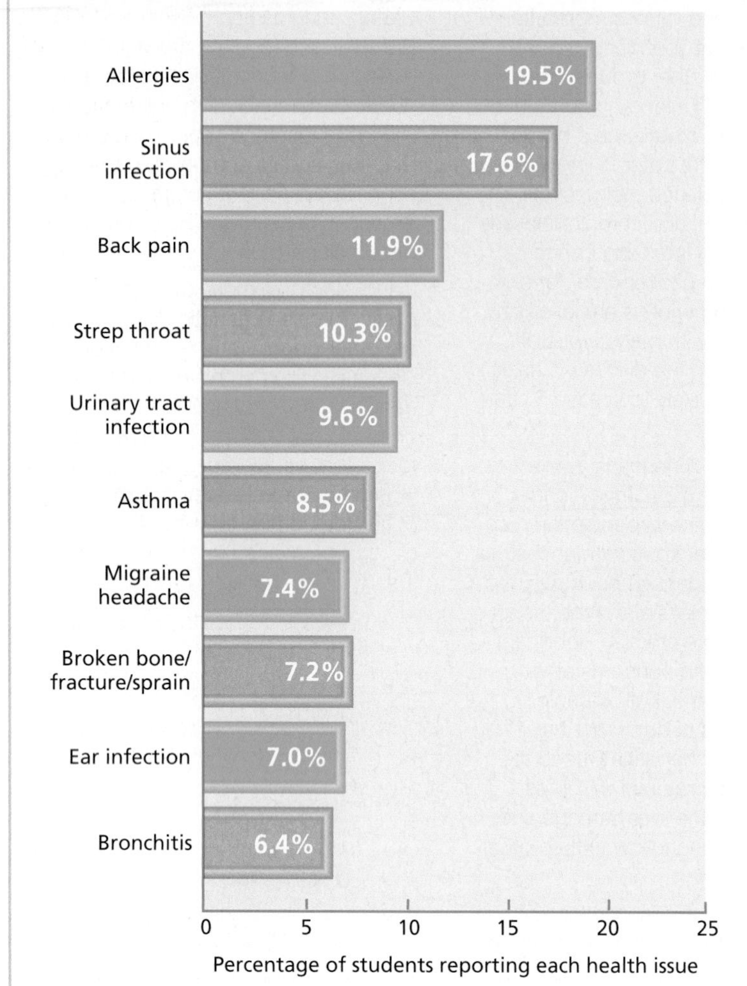

Data from *American College Health Association National College Health Assessment (ACHA-NCHA II) Reference Group Executive Summary, Spring 2011,* by the American College Health Association, 2011, retrieved from http://www.acha-ncha.org/docs/ACHA-NCHA_Reference_Group_ExecutiveSummary_Spring2011.pdf.

The Healthy Campus Initiative

In conjunction with the Healthy People initiative, the American College Health Association publishes an initiative called **Healthy Campus** for use in student settings. Colleges and universities participating in this program can choose to focus on improving health topics most relevant to them, such as:

- Reducing stress and depression
- Decreasing student abuse of alcohol and drugs
- Improving opportunities for daily physical activity on campus
- Improving sexual health among students

Specific objectives for *Healthy Campus 2020* are currently under development.

Healthy Campus An offshoot of the Healthy People initiative, specifically geared toward college students.

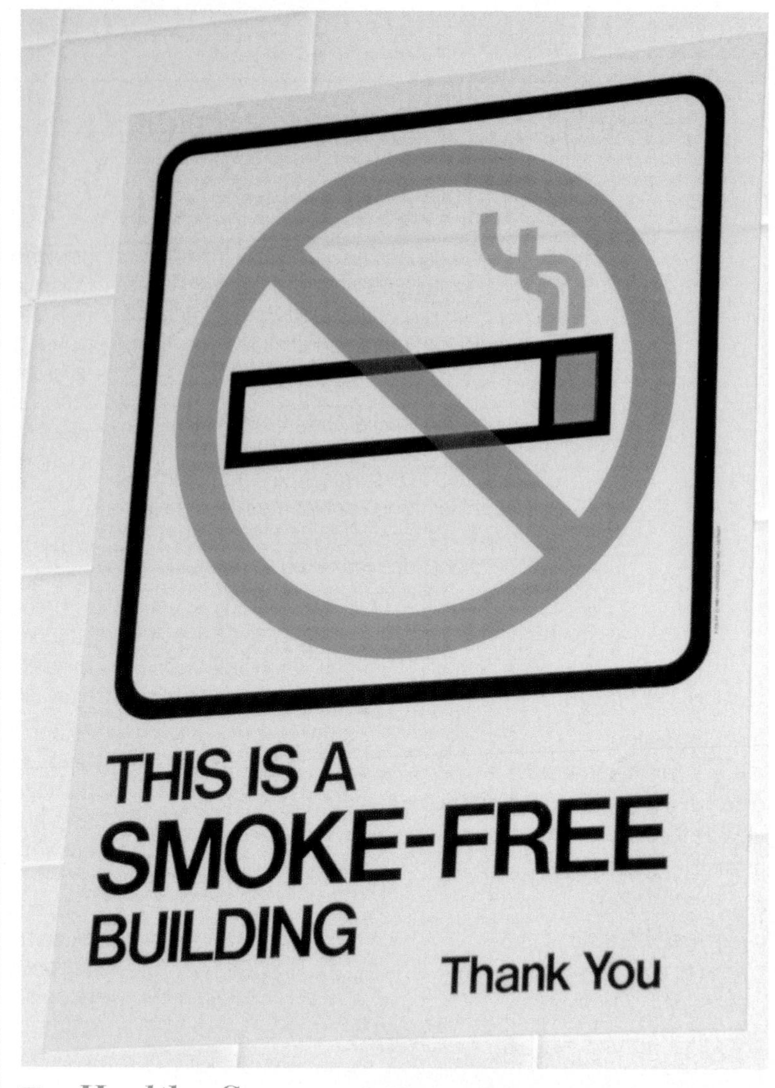

The **Healthy Campus** initiative aims to improve the health of college students nationwide.

Health Around the World

In our increasingly mobile and connected world, where a country experiencing a dangerous infectious disease is just a plane ride away, global health has become a top concern.

Some countries with lower levels of economic development and less stable political systems continue to experience high rates of infectious diseases that have largely been eradicated in other parts of the world. For example, parts of Africa, Asia, and South America continue to grapple with cholera, an infectious disease transmitted via unclean water supplies, and malaria, which is transmitted by mosquitoes. Although infections from the human immunodeficiency virus (HIV) have dropped in number in more-developed countries, HIV/AIDS continues to be a serious concern worldwide. More than 33 million people around the world are living with HIV infection; more than 67% of them live in sub-Saharan Africa. China, India, and Russia have seen a substantial increase in HIV infections in recent years.[16]

Some infections are now resisting conventional treatment with antimicrobial drugs. A wide range of disease-causing microorganisms—including the bacteria that cause tuberculosis and staph infections, the viruses that cause influenza, the parasites that cause malaria, and the fungi that cause yeast infections—are becoming resistant to the antimicrobial agents used for treatment.[17] People infected with resistant strains of microorganisms are more likely to have longer hospital stays and to die as a result of the infection.[17] This is a concern around the globe.

For more information on infectious diseases around the world, visit the World Health Organization website at www.who.int/topics/infectious_diseases/en.

Nutritional diseases are also still a concern in developing nations: More than 1 billion people in the world go hungry, and nearly 99% of these live in the developing world.[18] Deficiency of certain vitamins and minerals causes a variety of diseases rarely seen in the United States and Europe, such as night blindness, which develops when vitamin A is deficient, and a form of mental retardation called cretinism, which is due to iodine deficiency. Malnutrition also increases an individual's susceptibility to infection, as well as the risk that infection will result in death.

To address these global disparities, a number of privately funded international health organizations have joined with public efforts in recent years. Groups founded by prominent business leaders such as Microsoft founder Bill Gates and former U.S. presidents Jimmy Carter and Bill Clinton now provide funds for public health initiatives such as immunizations, mosquito nets, water filters, vitamin drops, and the addition of iodine to salt. In the next decade, it will become clear how well these initiatives are improving global health, and how well they complement the public health efforts carried out by international agencies such as the WHO.

Whereas global rates of HIV and certain other infectious diseases have begun to stabilize or decline, rates of chronic diseases such as heart disease and type 2 diabetes are rising worldwide, including in developing nations. That's because obesity—a risk factor for chronic diseases—is increasing. Two trends contribute to the rising prevalence of "globesity": A greater percentage of the world's population now has access to high-fat, high-sugar processed foods. At the same time, more people have access to motorized transportation, labor-saving devices, and sedentary forms of entertainment. These trends have contributed to an alarming statistic: The WHO estimates that in developing nations 115 million people now suffer from obesity-related disease.[19]

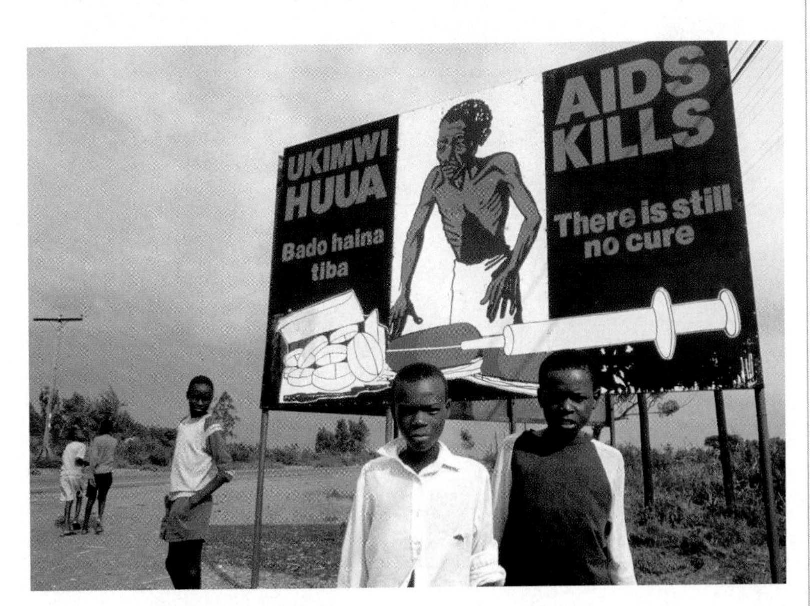
UKIMWI
HUUA
Bado haina
tiba
AIDS
KILLS
There is still
no cure

HIV/AIDS continues to be a serious concern worldwide, especially in sub-Saharan Africa.

Determinants of Health

Earlier we noted that *Healthy People 2020* takes an ecological approach to health—one that considers the relationship of individual human beings to their environment. In this view, individuals bear some, but not all, responsibility for the state of their health. A wide range of social, economic, and environmental factors are also recognized to influence heath. The WHO, as well as the CDC and other agencies of the HHS, refer to these factors as **determinants of health.** Any steps taken to improve health—both for individuals and for populations—are likely to be more successful when they target multiple determinants of health.[20]

determinants of health The range of personal, social, economic, and environmental factors that influence health status.

To watch a video explaining and providing examples of how determinants influence an individual's health, go to **www.healthypeople.gov/2020/about/DOHAbout.aspx.**

Determinants of health fall into six broad categories, all of which overlap to a greater or lesser extent **(Figure 1.4).** Let's take a closer look.

Biology and Genetics

Biologic and genetic determinants influence your health but are beyond your control. The following are the most significant determinants in this category:

- **Age.** Think back to childhood and your visits to the pediatrician. The kinds of health issues your doctor likely focused on then—ear infections, tooth eruption, and tracking your growth and development—

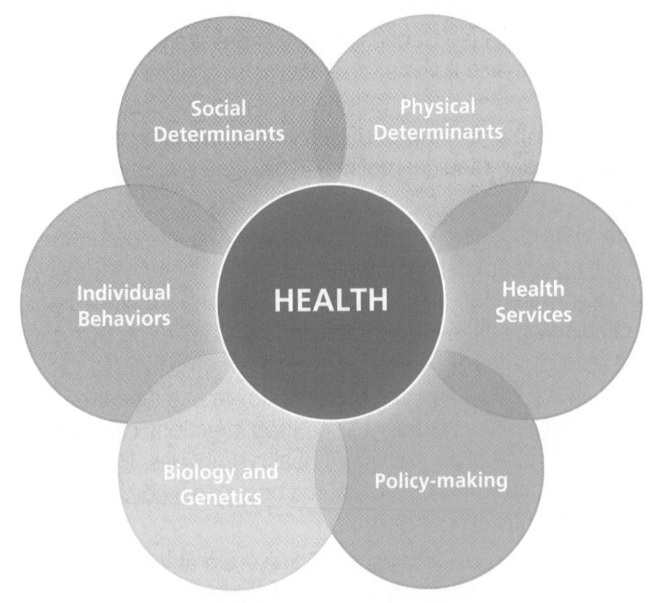

Figure 1.4 Determinants of health. An ecological approach to health acknowledges the influence of six categories of determinants on an individual's or population's health status. Notice that the categories overlap.

are not relevant for young and middle adults. At the other end of the age spectrum, the physical and cognitive effects of aging increase an older adult's vulnerability to poor health.[20] Chronic illnesses like heart disease, for example, are much more common among older adults, and infectious diseases like influenza can have far more serious consequences.

Create and print out your own family health history tree using the interactive tool *My Family Health Portrait* from the U.S. Surgeon General at https://familyhistory.hhs.gov/fhh-web/home.action.

- **Sex.** The genes you inherited at conception determined your sex—that is, the anatomical and physiological features that differentiate males from females. Sex has a powerful role on health, with biological differences between men and women resulting in many different health outcomes. Women tend to live about 4 years longer than men, for example, but have higher rates of some disabling health problems, such as arthritis and osteoporosis. Men are more likely to experience other serious chronic conditions, such as high blood pressure and cancer.[21]
- **Genetics.** Not only your sex, but many other aspects of your genetic inheritance influence your health. Most obviously, these include the presence or absence of any of a variety of genetic conditions such as color-blindness or hemophilia (a failure of blood clotting). You may also have inherited from one or both parents a particular gene or genes that increases your susceptibility to a disease. For instance, women who carry the BRCA1 or BRCA2 gene have an increased risk for breast and ovarian cancer.
- **Race/Ethnicity.** Although some researchers argue that race and ethnicity are social rather than biological concepts, certain population groups do have an increased or decreased risk for certain diseases when compared with the general population. (See the **Diversity & Health** box on page 7.) Awareness of these differences can prompt you to make better lifestyle choices, and can prompt your physician to provide more targeted care. For example, because African American men tend to develop aggressive prostate cancer at a higher rate than the general population, informed doctors may start screening these men for the condition earlier than others. Because Caucasians are more likely to carry genetic mutations for cystic fibrosis, doctors may consider making genetic screening before or during pregnancy a priority. Groups such as the National Coalition for Health Professional Education in Genetics are working to make medical professionals more aware of these diverse needs.
- **Health history.** Some conditions that you experienced in the past may still be influencing your health today. For instance, have you ever had chickenpox? If so, you're at increased risk for a disorder called shingles, which is characterized by a painful, itchy rash that forms blisters. After a person recovers from chickenpox, the virus remains in the body, and can become active at a later time as shingles. Similarly, many sexually transmitted infections can reduce your fertility and cause other persistent health problems. Past injuries—from a minor fracture to head trauma or a spinal cord injury—can also permanently affect health.
- **Family history.** You—and your children—are at increased risk for developing some of the same diseases that members of your family have experienced. This is true not only for recognized genetic diseases such as sickle-cell anemia and cystic fibrosis, but also for many chronic diseases such as high blood pressure, type 2 diabetes, and osteoporosis (low bone density), and even for some psychological disorders such as depression. It's important to know your family health history so that you and your health-care provider can monitor your risk. Moreover, if you know you're at risk for a particular condition, you may be able to change your lifestyle behaviors to reduce that risk.

Individual Behaviors

Although you can't turn back the clock on aging or select different genes, other health determinants—such as your individual lifestyle choices—are very much within your ability to control.

We noted earlier that the CDC has identified four behavioral decisions with a profound ability to influence your health. These are: (1) the level of physical activity you engage in, (2) the type of diet you eat, (3) your choice about whether or not to smoke, and (4) how much alcohol you consume. Making healthful choices in these four key areas can

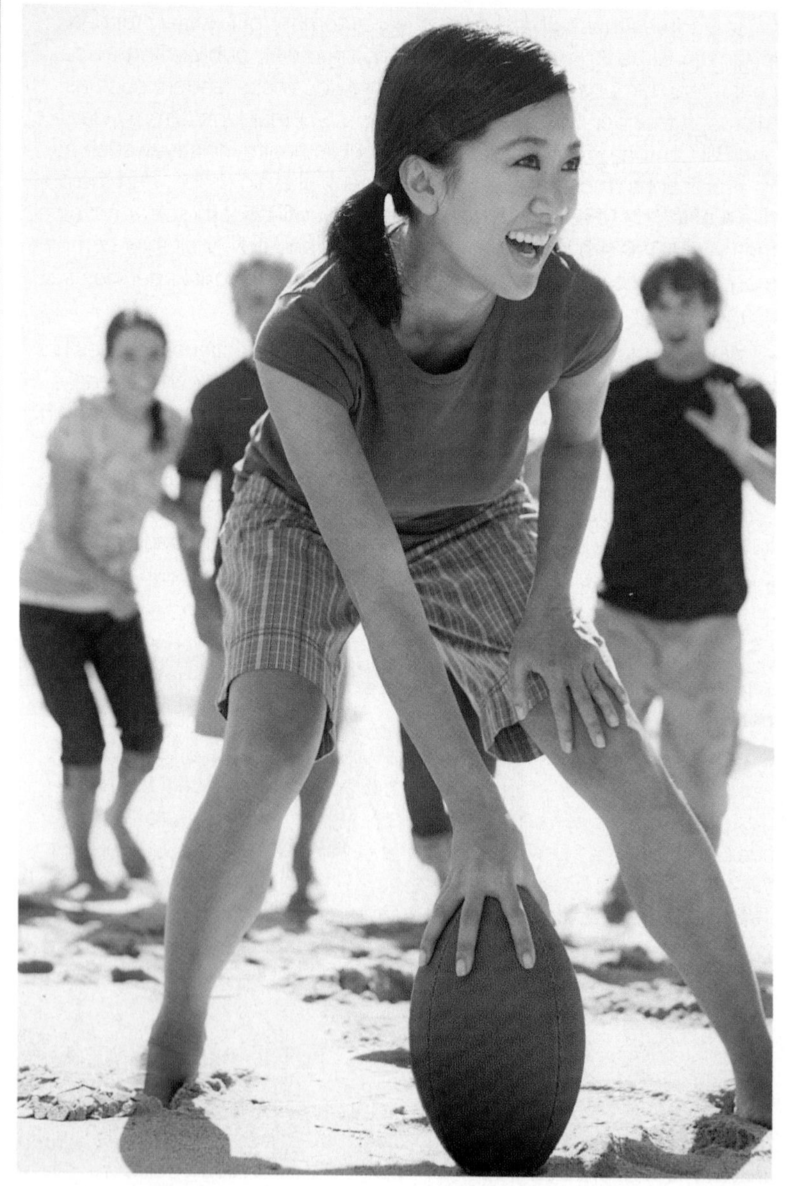

Regular **physical activity** is a key component of staying healthy.

greatly decrease your risk of developing serious illnesses later in life. On the other hand, poor choices in these areas can prematurely age you by up to 12 years![22]

Other lifestyle choices that play a significant role in promoting health include: managing your stress level, getting enough sleep, refraining from illicit drug use, developing supportive relationships with others, making responsible sexual health decisions, and taking basic steps to ensure your personal safety, such as wearing a seat belt. These behaviors are discussed later in this text.

Social Determinants

Individual behaviors are undeniably important in determining health, and are the emphasis of most personal health courses. But the ecological approach also recognizes the influence of a variety of social conditions that you can work to improve, but can't fully control. Social determinants are the economic and societal conditions in which people live—and which can impair their health or help them to thrive. They include, for example:[20]

- Availability of resources to meet daily needs, such as educational and job opportunities, living wages, or healthful foods
- Social attitudes, such as discrimination
- Public safety versus exposure to crime
- Social support and social interactions
- Exposure to mass media and emerging technologies, such as the Internet or cell phones
- Socioeconomic conditions, such as concentrated poverty
- Availability of quality schools
- Transportation options

Research over the past two decades has increasingly acknowledged the significant role that social determinants play in influencing health. For example, a family may understand the value of regular physical activity, but live in a high-crime area where they're afraid to go out walking or running, and can't afford the cost of membership in a fitness club. These social determinants limit their options for physical activity. In 2012, the American Academy of Pediatrics released a policy statement associating poverty, domestic violence, and other forms of "childhood adversity" with a wide range of physical and mental health problems across the lifespan.[23]

If you're getting the sense that poverty is a fundamental social determinant of health, you're right: Rates of both disease and premature death are dramatically higher among the poor than among the rich.[24] Called the **status syndrome,** this disparity in health and mortality has been observed not only in developing nations, but also in Europe and the United States. The status syndrome has traditionally been attributed to a poor person's reduced access to quality health care, health information, nutritious foods, safe, adequate shelter, and opportunities for physical activity. However, some researchers believe that it occurs because, in people who are poor, two fundamental human needs go unmet: These are the needs for autonomy and for full social participation. Deprived of a clean, safe neighborhood, meaningful work, opportunities for quality children's education, and freedom from violence and aggression, it is harder to have control over one's life or be a full social participant.[24] These factors—lack of control and low social participation—are known to dramatically increase stress, causing physiologic changes that can lead to a variety of diseases.[24]

status syndrome The disparity in health status and rates of premature mortality between the impoverished and the affluent within any given society.

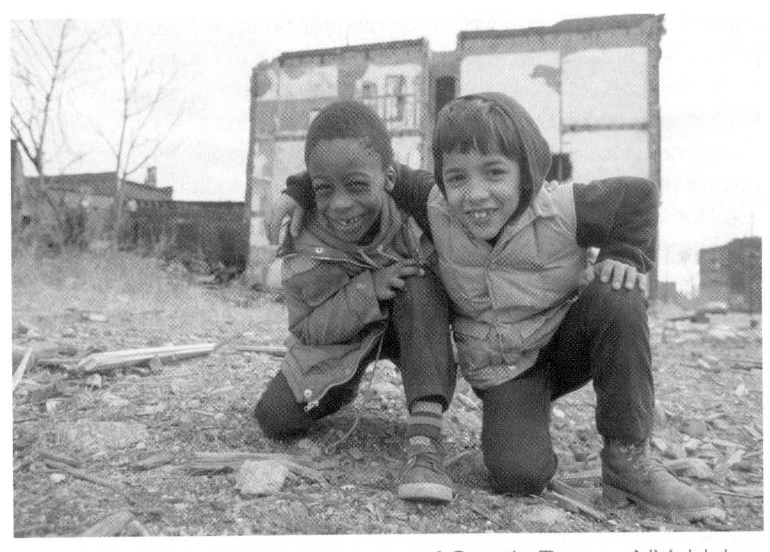

These boys live in a poor area of South Bronx, NY. Living in a neighborhood that **lacks access to resources** increases their risk for a variety of health problems.

Physical Determinants

Physical determinants are physical conditions in the environment. Examples include:[20]

- Aspects of the natural environment, such as plants, weather, or climate change
- Aspects of the so-called *built environment,* which includes all buildings, spaces, and products that are made or modified by people, such as homes, schools, factories, roads, subway systems, parks, and the tools, equipment, and objects within them
- Presence or absence of toxic substances and other physical hazards

For example, heat waves, floods, earthquakes, blizzards, and other natural hazards are aspects of the physical environment that influence health. Pollutants in the air, soil, and water are largely invisible, but can significantly increase disease rates. For instance, people living in regions with high levels of air pollution, such as Detroit, Michigan, or California's Central Valley, experience higher rates of asthma and other respiratory ailments.[25]

Health Services

Health services include availability of quality preventive and medical care as well as access to that care. Health literacy is also included in health services.

Access to Health Services

In countries with a national health service, health insurance status does not usually affect access to quality care. In the United States, health insurance status directly affects access to health services. People who lack adequate health insurance are less likely to have a regular doctor or place of care. They are also less likely to receive a wide range of health services, including preventive care, and more likely to delay medical treatment. Many uninsured wait until a condition has advanced to a crisis stage before visiting a local hospital emergency room—a habit that greatly increases the level of care required as well as the cost and outcome of that care. In one national survey, about 15% of respondents said they had no regular place where they sought or received health care.[11] And in 2011, the CDC reported that over 48 million Americans had no health insurance.[26] Not only people from lower socioeconomic brackets, but also members of ethnic minorities are generally less likely to have health coverage than the population overall.

Supporting the understanding that access to quality care is a key determinant of health, studies have found that while higher-income Caucasians have enjoyed a wide range of health gains, these improvements have not been shared by lower-income Caucasians and ethnic minorities.[27] In part to address this disparity, in 2010 the U.S. Congress passed into law a set of comprehensive new health-care reforms. Called the Affordable Care Act, the legislation aims to substantially reduce the number of Americans who do not have health insurance.[28]

 **For updates on the Affordable Care Act, visit www.healthcare.gov.**

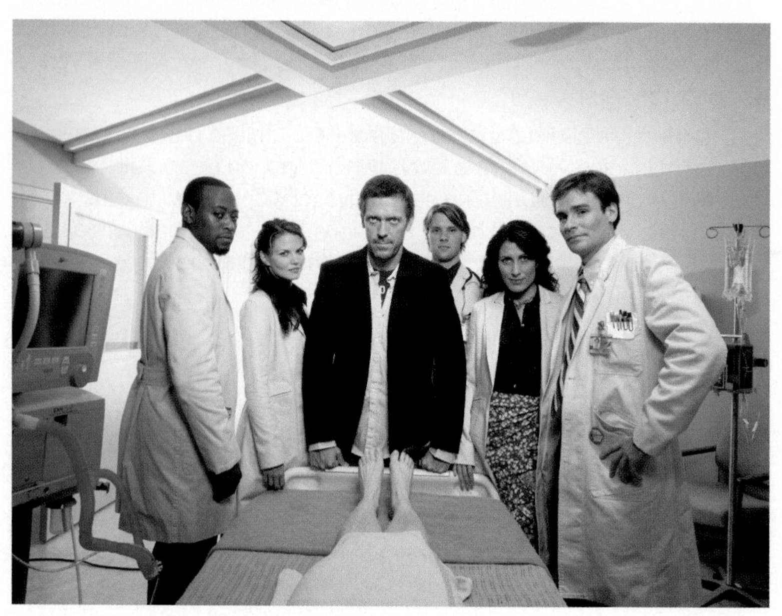

Can you trust **medical information** from doctors (real or fictional) on TV?

Regardless of your income, the region you call home also influences your access to quality care. For example, Americans living in rural areas (that is, places with fewer than 2,500 residents) have less access to specialized medical care or emergency services, and are more likely to die from heart attacks, serious injuries, and other medical emergencies.

Moreover, cultural and language barriers can limit access to quality care. All people deserve care provided by staff who understand relevant cultural concerns and can communicate with them effectively if they speak limited English. Medical translation services, available with a quick phone call, now help many care providers care for patients who otherwise might not be able to communicate with doctors or staff effectively.

Health Literacy

In the 21st century, quality health care increasingly depends upon **health literacy,** the ability to evaluate and understand health information and to make informed choices for your own care. It includes the ability to read, understand, and follow instructions in medical brochures and prescription drug labels; the ability to listen to health-care providers, ask good questions, and analyze the information you receive; and the ability to navigate an often-confusing and complex health-care system.[29] Increasingly, health literacy also requires a degree of computer literacy and media awareness. New health programs aimed at specific communities help build health literacy. In communities with sizeable Asian American populations, for example, targeted public awareness campaigns are emphasizing the need for screening and treatment for hepatitis B, which is more prevalent in several Southeast Asian countries and is often acquired in infancy or early childhood.[30]

health literacy The ability to evaluate and understand health information and to make informed choices for your health care.

Another goal of this text is to increase your health literacy by providing you with strategies to critically evaluate all the health information that you are exposed to—whether from books, magazines, newspapers, television, advertisements, or the Internet. Online search engines like Google are increasingly the first place many people turn when seeking health information, but search results don't distinguish between sites that provide unbiased, up-to-date, scientifically sound information and sites that contain inaccurate or misleading content. The accompanying **Spotlight** will help you evaluate health information in the media.

Policy-Making

Policies at the local, state, and federal levels also affect health. Increasing taxes on cigarettes, for example, improves health by reducing the number of people who smoke. Similarly, regulations to increase motor vehicle safety—for example, establishing speed limits, mandating seat belt use, and outlawing texting while driving—reduce traumatic injuries and deaths in motor vehicle accidents. Other examples of public policy-making include changes in city zoning ordinances to promote small gardens, state programs to provide free health screenings such as mammograms to low-income families, HHS provision of health insurance for older Americans (Medicare) and Americans in need (Medicaid), efforts by the FDA to improve food safety, and the establishment of standards for air, water, and soil quality set by the U.S. Environmental Protection Agency (EPA).

Policy-making also includes corporate initiatives. For example, in 2011, Walmart—the nation's largest grocer and the world's largest retailer—collaborated with First Lady Michelle Obama's efforts to reduce childhood obesity by announcing new policies to make fresh, local foods more affordable, and to increase support for nutrition programs.

Achieving Successful Behavior Change

We can't change our biology or genetics, but we can modify and change individual behaviors. Every day, we encounter opportunities to make choices that will benefit our health. Making the right choices, however, can be a challenge. We often have a good idea of what choices we *ought* to be making—for instance, eating more fruits and vegetables, setting aside time each day to exercise, or getting more sleep—but

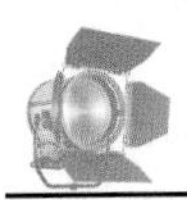

SPOTLIGHT

Evaluating Health Information in the Media

Is the health information you just researched on the Internet accurate? Can you trust your favorite actor's television advertisement for a weight-loss product? Was last week's episode of *The Dr. Oz Show* based on any kind of medical reality? How can you make sense of the endless stream of media headlines trumpeting health studies that sometimes contradict one another?

The term *media* can mean a variety of things. We use it here to include books, newspapers, magazines, television, and Internet/web programming, as well as advertisements. To get a sense of how frequently you're inundated with health information from the media, consider the following:

- How often do you encounter an advertisement for prepackaged snack foods or meals? In contrast, how often have you encountered an advertisement for fresh fruits and vegetables?
- How often have you seen an advertisement promoting prescription drugs—for everything from weight loss to social anxiety?
- How regularly are you exposed to images of seemingly perfect celebrities? How does this affect your feelings about your own body and your self-esteem?

Whenever you encounter information from the media, critically assess it. Is someone trying to sell you something? Are there other ways to solve problems like being overweight without resorting to pills? Do you realize that many of the images of celebrities you see in magazines have been digitally altered to make them look more attractive than they really are?

When you come across an article about the results of the latest health-related study, consider: Was the study conducted by an unbiased source, or was it carried out by an individual or organization with a vested interest in the outcome? Have the results been replicated by other researchers? Was the sample size of the study large or small? Was the study conducted over a short or long period of time? Is the study only showing what may be a coincidental *correlation* between two things, or is it truly showing that one variable is the direct result of another variable?

The Internet deserves special attention in discussions of health in the media, as it is increasingly where people turn for information. In one survey of more than 70,000 college students, students listed the Internet as their second most often used source of health information.[1] The only source they turned to more often was their parents. When you're evaluating health information online, ask yourself the following questions to determine whether or not the information is credible:

- Is the sponsor of the site identified? Is it a commercial, nonprofit, academic, or government site? In general, sites with URLs ending in ".gov" (signifying a U.S. government site) or ".edu" (signifying an educational institution) are more likely to provide credible information than those that end in ".com." Note that the domain ".org" is used by many credible, nonprofit, noncommercial sites, but it is sometimes used by commercial entities as well.
- What is the purpose of the site? Is it to inform and educate, or is it to sell you something? If it is to sell you something, be aware that the information presented is more likely to be biased.
- Does the site tell you where the information it presents is coming from? If so, is the content based on scientific evidence, or was it written by someone hired by the site to produce marketing information? Sites that are able to provide citations and links to scientific studies and journals are more likely to be credible than sites lacking these references.
- Does the site specify when its content was last updated? Health information can sometimes change quickly, so you want to seek out information that is as current as possible.
- Does the site list a reputable professional accreditation? Many reputable health sites, for example, are accredited by the Health on the Net Foundation, and bear an insignia reading "HON."

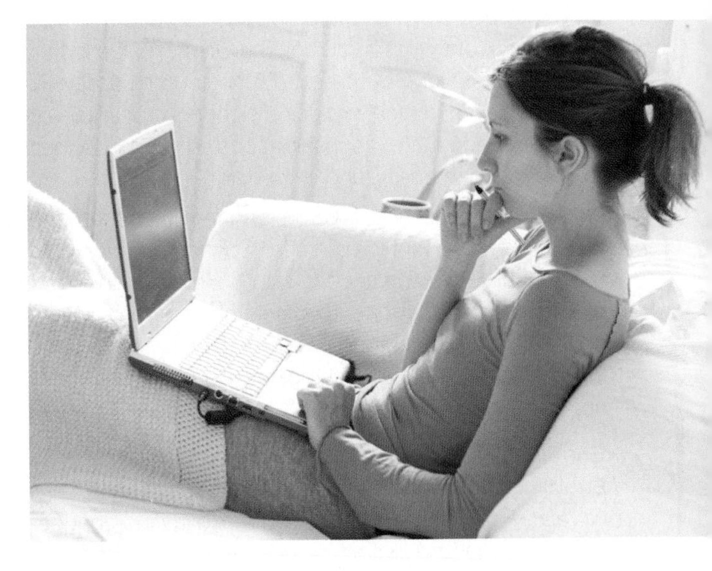

Throughout this text, the **Get Connected** feature lists health-related websites where you can obtain reliable health information. Still, keep in mind that information on the Internet is never a substitute for consulting a health-care professional. Do not rely solely on online information to make important decisions about your health! Make an appointment with your doctor and don't be afraid to ask questions to be certain that you are receiving the most accurate information about any health issue you may be facing

Reference: 1. *American College Health Association—National College Health Assessment Spring 2007 Reference Group Data Report (abridged)*, by the American College Health Association, 2008, *Journal of American College Health, 56* (5), pp. 469–479.

actually doing these things and achieving true **behavior change** is the hard part.

Factors That Influence Behavior Change

Let's begin our discussion of behavior change by taking a look at some factors that influence our success in making and maintaining change: *predisposing factors, enabling factors,* and *reinforcing factors*. Notice that these factors can help you make positive change, or can hinder your attempts to change.

behavior change A sustained change in a habit or pattern of behavior that affects health.

predisposing factor A physical, mental, emotional, or surrounding influence that shapes current behavior.

Predisposing Factors

Predisposing factors are the physical, mental, emotional, and environmental factors that shape current behavior. They include your knowledge of health issues, your beliefs about how susceptible you are to illness or injury, and your attitude toward how behavior change can benefit your health. For instance, someone whose best friend died in a car crash while driving intoxicated might be predisposed to avoid drunk driving.

The values you hold are predisposing factors that can and do shape behaviors—but what if you hold conflicting values? For instance, most people value a long life free of disease and disability. But what if you're a woman who so highly values a slender appearance that you deprive yourself of adequate, nourishing food—putting yourself at risk for anemia, low bone density, and even death?

Your age, sex, race, income, and family background can also be predisposing factors in your health behavior. If you have a family history of cancer, for instance, and you believe in the wisdom of regular screenings to allow for early detection, you may be predisposed to schedule and obtain these screenings yourself. On the other hand, if you grew up in a family of smokers, you may be more likely to take up smoking yourself.

Enabling Factors

Enabling factors are the skills, assets, capacities, and resources you have at your disposal to help you make lasting changes. Examples of individual enabling factors include strong motivation and willpower, as well as the understanding and physical health necessary to embark on a program of change, such as regular exercise.

Social factors can also enable change: The education you'll get in your personal health course is likely to help you make and maintain positive health behaviors. Your peers are key enablers: If you smoke, but start hanging out with nonsmokers, you're likely to quit. Of course, peer pressure often works the other way, prompting college students to adopt behaviors—like drinking too much or experimenting with drugs—that can initiate a pattern of increasingly negative behavior change.

Aspects of your physical environment can also enable change. If you wanted to eat more nutritiously, access to a neighborhood grocery store stocked with fresh, affordable produce would be an enabling factor.

Of course, access to health information and preventive care is a critical enabling factor. Access to a registered dietitian can enable you to design a healthful diet and stick to it, and access to a smoking cessation program can enable you to quit. Policy-making that supports such resources can be a powerful enabler within a population. If you smoked marijuana throughout high school, but now want to quit, enrolling in a college with a chemical-free campus would strongly enable that change.

Reinforcing Factors

Reinforcing factors include encouragements and rewards that promote positive behavior change. They include support and praise from others around you. A support group for anger management, encouragement from family members if you are trying to lose weight, or the companionship (and positive peer pressure) of a workout partner are all examples of reinforcing factors. Reinforcing factors also include barriers that can oppose, impede, or entirely derail your efforts to change. Perhaps you've begun a strength-training program to increase your level of fitness. All goes well for the first 3 weeks—but then you prematurely increase the weights and throw out your lower back. You'll need persistence and determination to overcome this negative reinforcer.

Think about a health behavior you'd like to change in your own life, and then consider the predisposing, enabling, and reinforcing factors that may affect your attitude and/or ability to implement that change.

enabling factor A skill, asset, or capacity that influences an individual's ability to make and sustain behavior change.

reinforcing factor An encouragement or a reward that promotes positive behavior change, or a barrier that opposes change.

transtheoretical model of behavior change A model of behavior change that focuses on decision-making steps and abilities. Also called the *stages of change* model.

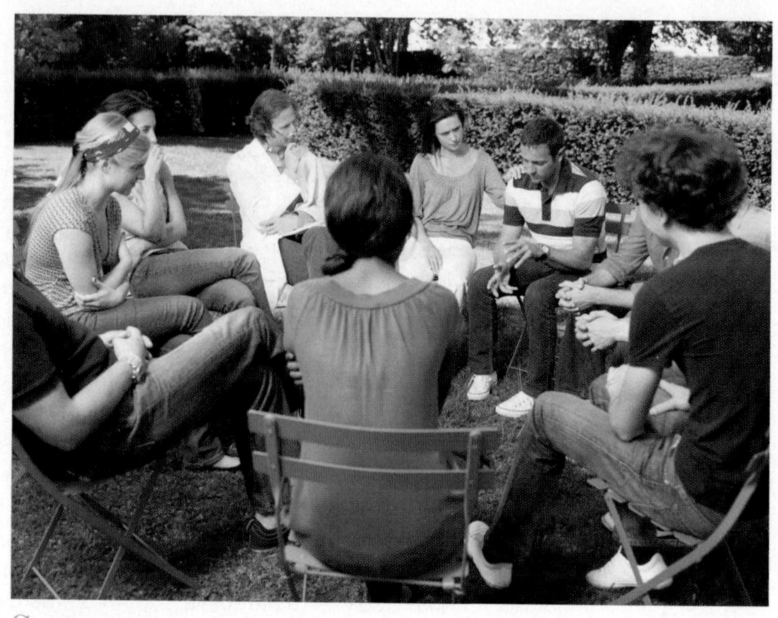

Support groups for quitting smoking or drinking can play a key role in lasting behavior change.

Models of Behavior Change

A *model* is a description that helps you understand something you can't directly observe. If you've ever attended a 5-year sobriety celebration or discovered that a formerly obese friend from high school has lost a lot of weight, you might have wondered how—exactly—they did it. And would the method they used work for you?

Over many decades, public health researchers have proposed at least a dozen different models identifying a method by which they believe lasting behavior change happens. They've based their models on their work with different populations facing different health challenges at different times. So as you might expect, no single model dominates.[31] Two of the oldest and most established models are the transtheoretical model and the health belief model. More recently, researchers have developed a variety of ecological models of behavior change. Let's take a look.

The Transtheoretical Model

The **transtheoretical model of behavior change,** also called the *stages of change* model, was developed by psychologist James Prochaska and his colleagues. Its basic premise is that behavior change is a process and not an event, and that individuals are at varying levels of motivation, or readiness, to change.[31] The model identifies six stages of change that a person progresses through before achieving sustained behavior change (see **Figure 1.5**).[32]

Precontemplation → Contemplation → Preparation → Action → Maintenance → Termination

Figure 1.5 The transtheoretical model of behavior change. Developed by James Prochaska, this model outlines six stages of behavior change.

- **Precontemplation,** during which a person may or may not recognize a health challenge, and in either case has no intention of making changes to address it in the near future (that is, within the next 6 months).
- **Contemplation,** during which a person acknowledges the health challenge and thinks about making a change within the next 6 months. At this stage, the person is still not ready to take action but is thinking about it.
- **Preparation,** during which a person intends to change the behavior within the next month and has a plan of action in mind (such as enrolling in a class or joining a support group).
- **Action,** during which a person modifies the behavior in an observable way—for example, quits smoking, begins jogging each week, etc. In this stage, the change is initiated, but is not yet consistent over time.
- **Maintenance,** in which a person has maintained the new behavior for 6 months or more, and continues to actively work to prevent relapse (reverting to old habits). Maintenance can last months or even years, and relapse is not unusual.
- **Termination,** during which a person has successfully achieved behavior change to the point where he or she is completely confident that relapse will not occur.

The transtheoretical model has its share of critics. The research is inconclusive, for instance, on whether application of the model truly results in lasting changes in behavior. However, the model is widely used as a framework for research studies in public health, and can be useful to consider when you think about embarking on a behavior-change plan in your own life.

The Health Belief Model

In the 1950s, researchers at the U.S. Public Health Service developed a model of behavior change called the **health belief model.**[31] This model identifies four factors as instrumental in predicting behavior change:[31]

- **Perceived threat.** The person perceives that he or she is at risk of a threat (such as illness or injury) and perceives that this threat is real.
- **Perceived severity.** The person understands that the threat could have serious consequences in terms of pain, lost work time, financial loss, or other consequences.
- **Perceived benefit.** The person believes that the benefits of making the behavior change will outweigh the costs, inconveniences, and other challenges, and that the change is possible for him or her to make and maintain.
- **Cues to action.** The person witnesses or experiences a precipitating force that causes him or her to commit to making the change. For example, a young person at risk for diabetes witnesses a parent attempting to cope following a foot amputation as a result of the disease.

Like the transtheoretical model, the health belief model has been widely studied and used in different research designs. One survey looked at how useful this model is in weight management, and found that the greatest motivation came from the perceived threat of obesity, while the greatest resource for change came from a person's belief in his or her ability to lose weight or to maintain a healthy weight.[33] Critics, meanwhile, say the model does not adequately gauge the effect that a person's family or friends, or other aspects of the environment, have on his or her ability to make successful changes. In any case, it may help to consider the health belief model when you are assessing your own readiness for changing a health behavior: Do you perceive a serious threat to your health? If so, can you identify real benefits to making changes—benefits that outweigh the time and other costs involved in change?

health belief model A model of behavior change emphasizing the influence of personal beliefs on the process of creating effective change.

STUDENT STORY

Sleep Deprived

"Hi, I'm Jasmine. I'm a freshman and I'm a child development major. Each night, I'm very lucky if I get 4 hours of sleep. I'm just a night owl. I like staying up at night. My father's the exact same way. It's like 3 o'clock in the morning and we'll still be up watching the food channel. Around exam time, I find myself awake at 7:30 in the morning, still up—knowing that I have a test at 9:30. Why, I don't know.

I don't think I'm doing my best right now because when I drag myself to class, I'm half asleep. I do need to change and get better rest so that I can do better in school. I don't think I've gotten 8 hours of sleep since I was 13. I'm 19, so that's 6 years of not getting a full night's sleep. That takes a toll on your body and your mind."

1: What stage of the transtheoretical model of behavior change would you guess that Jasmine is in?

2: Apply the health belief model to Jasmine's situation. What is the perceived threat? What is the perceived benefit to changing her behavior? What are the perceived barriers she may face?

3: Look at Jasmine's situation through an ecological model approach. What factors in her environment are reinforcing her late-night behavior? What factors are going against it?

Do you have a story similar to Jasmine's? Share your story at www.pearsonhighered.com/lynchelmore.

Ecological Models

A criticism of most models of behavior change is that they emphasize individual actions and disregard the influence of social and physical determinants, health services, and policy-making on the initiation and maintenance of behavior change. This has led to the development of a variety of **ecological models** of behavior change, in which the creation of a supportive environment is acknowledged to be as important to achieving change as an individual's acquisition of health information and development of personal skills.[34]

ecological model Any of a variety of behavior-change models that acknowledge the creation of a supportive environment as equally important to achieving change as an individual's acquisition of health information and development of personal skills.

Ecological models emphasize the following principles:[34]

- Multiple levels of factors—from individual behavior to family values, community support, and public policy—influence health behaviors **(Figure 1.6).**
- Influences at different levels interact in a positive way.
- For successful behavior change, interventions at multiple levels are most effective.

For example, an individual's motivation to lose weight might interact positively with a physician's advice to exercise, an employer's financial incentive for logging time at the company gym, and a city's construction of a new bike path. On the other hand, personal motivation is less effective when environments and policies make it difficult to choose healthful behaviors.

This means that, if you want to make lasting change, you shouldn't try to go it alone. You're more likely to succeed if you reach out for support from your health-care provider, your campus health services, and other resources in your community. In the next section, we talk more about recruiting support for your change. And if the resources you need don't currently exist—advocate for them! Every chapter of this text concludes with ideas on campus advocacy for health-related change.

Even with support, making healthful behavior change is still tough, so it helps to follow a systematic plan. The plan provided ahead uses an ecological framework to help you make effective and lasting behavior change.

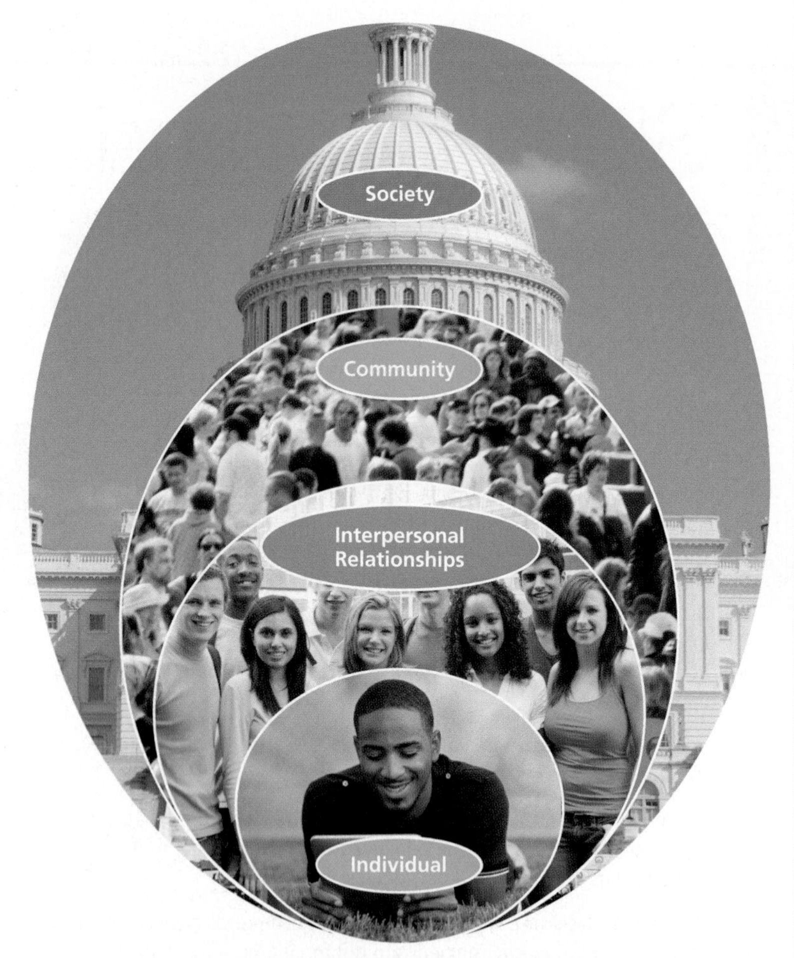

Figure 1.6 An ecological model of behavior change. Like ecological approaches to health itself, ecological models of behavior change acknowledge the influence of many factors at different levels, from individual to societal. They also emphasize the effectiveness of interventions at multiple levels.

Change Yourself, Change Your World

By enrolling in a personal health course and reading this textbook, you've already taken the initial step toward achieving better health and wellness. Throughout this book you'll find **Self-Assessments** that will help you assess your current health status, as well as **Choosing to Change Worksheets** that guide you on how to set appropriate goals and implement plans for behavior change. Each Choosing to Change Worksheet will prompt you to list your level of readiness for change—also known as your stage of behavior change—based on the transtheoretical model you read about earlier in this chapter. The Worksheets will then walk you through behavior-change techniques appropriate for your stage of change, promoting a greater chance of success. You can also find online versions of all of these worksheets at **www.pearsonhighered.com/lynchelmore.**

This chapter's **Self-Assessment: How Healthy Is Your Current Lifestyle?** is a general self-survey evaluating your current health behaviors. Complete the survey, then read the instructions for interpreting your score. Now, is there a particular area of health you'd like to turn around? Once you've identified the health behavior you most want to change . . . how do you begin? Let's look at the personal choices that help people succeed in making behavior change.

Personal Choices

Changing your targeted behavior will require more than a quick decision to "just do it." Effective change is a process and starts with information, a SMART goal, and a practical plan. You also need to identify and tackle your barriers, work your environment, promise yourself some rewards—and commit. Let's consider these seven steps one at a time.

Step 1. Get Informed

You've identified a goal—"Quit smoking" or "Get fit"—but how much do you really know about the behavior you want to change? For instance, what are the components of fitness, what are the benefits, how is it achieved, and how is it measured? If you're going to set a fitness goal and create a plan for reaching it, you need to be able to answer these questions. So your first step is to do some homework. The information in this text, together with the **Get Connected** links at the end of each chapter, are good resources for researching your health concerns. You can also find information at your campus health services center, from your health-care provider, and from reputable professional journals. Jot down the facts that seem most important for changing your targeted behavior. What rate of weight loss is reasonable per week, for instance? Or what's your target heart rate during aerobic exercise? Is it more effective to quit smoking "cold turkey" or gradually? Answering these questions will, among other things, help you identify a more effective behavior-change goal; that is, a SMART goal.

Step 2. Set a SMART Goal

If you don't know precisely where you're going, how will you know when you've arrived? Experts in business, education, health care, and personal development agree that goals are more likely to be achieved when they're SMART. The acronym SMART, which was first used in project management in the early 1980s, stands for the five qualities of an effective goal:[35]

- **Specific.** Your goal for change should be well-defined and entirely clear to you. For example, "I'm going to try to lose weight" is not a SMART goal. How much weight do you want to lose? Or if precise numbers don't motivate you, decide specifically how you want to look or feel: "When I'm wearing my new jeans, I want to be able to slide my finger comfortably between me and the waistband."
- **Measurable.** Include in your goal statement objective criteria for evaluating your success. What data would make it clear to anyone that you have succeeded? For instance, "By the end of this semester . . . I'll have lost 10 pounds . . . I'll be meditating for at least 20 minutes a day . . . I'll have paid off my credit card debt . . ."
- **Attainable.** Does the research you did earlier convince you that you can achieve your goal? If not, you probably won't. So make sure your goal isn't unreasonable. For instance, for most people who are overweight, it's sensible to aim to lose about ½–1 pound of body weight per week; however, 3 pounds a week is not attainable without putting your health at risk.
- **Relevant.** Don't borrow somebody else's health goal! Make sure that the goal you're working toward feels right for you. For instance, let's say you're overweight, and can't even climb a flight of stairs without feeling winded. You've been looking for some inspiration to get moving when a friend invites you to join him in training for a local marathon. Your friend has been involved in track since middle school. The goal is relevant for him, but it's not SMART for you.
- **Time based.** A SMART goal has a time frame. For instance: "For the next 6 months, each time I weigh myself—on the 15th and the 30th of each month—I'll have lost at least 1 pound. In 5 months' time, by December 30th, I'll have lost 10 pounds."

The National Institutes of Health also advises that your goal be *forgiving*.[36] That is, it should allow for the occasional intervention of unforeseen events. A goal of walking for 30 minutes a day, 5 days a week, is forgiving. A goal of walking for 30 minutes a day, every day, is not.

Step 3. Make a Plan

A SMART goal is like a guiding vision: "In 6 months, I'm going to get on that scale and see that I've lost 20 pounds!" But to make it happen, you need an action plan, and that means you need to break down your goal into specific, achievable, day-to-day actions that will enable you to accomplish it. In doing this, it helps to use a technique called **shaping;** that is, breaking a big goal into a series of smaller, measurable steps. If you'd like to eventually run a 10K, for instance, set yourself a goal of a shorter distance at first, and then gradually increase your distance a little each week.

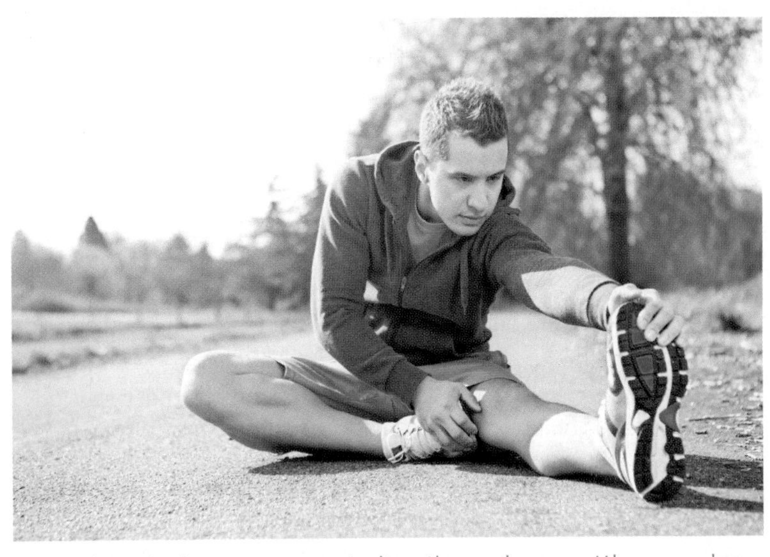

Keep in mind your current situation when setting goals. Set a goal that is **relevant** and **attainable** and you're more likely to reach it.

Many people who want to lose weight think that a good action plan would be: "I'll eat right and exercise every day." But what does it mean to "eat right"? And what kind of exercise? For how long? Where and when? When shaping, it can be helpful to ask yourself questions like: who, what, when, where, why, how, and how long? Here is an example:

- On Sunday morning, I'll weigh myself and write down my weight.
- Monday to Friday, on my morning break between classes, I'll skip the mocha and have a plain coffee with skim milk. At lunch, instead of a regular soda, I'll get a diet soda or water. And I'll skip the fries with my sandwich.
- Also, after my last class on M/W/F, I'll walk to the fitness center. I'll do at least 10 minutes on the treadmill, 10 minutes on the stationary bike, and 10 minutes on the stair-climber. On Saturday morning, I'll take the drop-in yoga class.
- On Sunday morning, I'll weigh myself again. If I've lost 1 pound or more, I'll continue with my plan for another week. And I'll call my best friend to celebrate! If I haven't, I'll increase my exercise next week to 15 minutes per machine.

Step 4. Identify Barriers and How You'll Overcome Them

Barriers are factors that stand in the way of successful change. You can think of them as the "disabling" factors and "negative reinforcers" we discussed earlier. In an ecological model of behavior change, barriers can emerge from any of the multiple levels of influence on human behavior. For instance, emotional factors like fear and anxiety are common barriers, as is a factor called low self-efficacy.[37] One of the most important psychological factors influencing our ability to change, **self-efficacy** is both the conviction that you can make successful changes and the ability to

shaping A behavior-change technique based on breaking broad goals into more manageable steps.

self-efficacy The conviction that you can make successful changes and the ability to take appropriate action to do so.

take appropriate action to do so. If you believe in your own ability to get in better shape, for example, you'll keep exercising, even if a few workouts leave you tired or frustrated. If you have low self-efficacy, you may give up, or never attempt an exercise program in the first place.

Your sense of self-efficacy, and the actions that stem from it, are closely tied to your **locus of control.** If you have an *internal* locus of control, you are more likely to believe that you are the master of your own destiny. When a barrier presents itself, you'll look for ways to overcome it. If you have an *external* locus of control, you are more likely to believe that events are out of your hands—that there's little you can do to overcome barriers.

What barriers might exist in your social environment? Let's say you want to lose weight, but your roommate is a culinary arts major who's constantly cooking and baking the most delectable treats—and asking you to try them. You might overcome this barrier by telling your roommate about your weight-loss plan, and asking him or her to create some low-calorie meals and snacks. Self-advocacy is an essential—though sometimes uncomfortable—skill to practice in demonstrating self-efficacy.

Aspects of your physical environment can act as barriers, too. But with some ingenuity, you can often find ways to overcome them. If you're trying to stop smoking, but there's an enticing smoke shop in your neighborhood with a variety of tobacco products from around the world, that's a barrier—especially if you tend to walk past it several times a day. A simple way to overcome this barrier would be to choose a different route. If you're trying to lose weight and struggle with binge eating, make sure you go through your apartment or dorm room and get rid of any junk foods.

We discussed earlier the significant disparity in access to health services in the United States. Lack of access to consistent, high-quality care is a barrier to change for millions of Americans. As a college student, you may have access to low-cost health services, from preventive and clinical care to counseling and support groups, as well as classes and programs in stress management, smoking cessation, and other health topics.

People with a high level of self-efficacy and an internal locus of control may be able to overcome most barriers to behavior change. You can increase your self-efficacy and shift your locus of control by turning to clearly defined techniques that help change behavior in positive ways specific to your health concerns. Throughout this book, we offer **Practical Strategies** boxes to help you do just that.

locus of control A person's belief about where the center of power lies in his or her life; it can be external or internal.

modeling A behavior-change technique based on watching and learning from others.

Step 5. Recruit Some Support

According to the ecological models of behavior change, your plan for change will be more likely to succeed if you have different levels of support. Start with your family members and friends. With whom do you feel comfortable sharing your plans for change? Give your support group specific instructions about how they can help; for instance, if you want to lose weight, you might ask your mom to stop sending you care packages loaded with cookies and other sweets. When your motivation wanes, call on your support group to cheer you on. If family members and friends can't provide the consistent support you need, consider joining a campus or community self-help group. Many such programs pair you up with a coach, mentor, or buddy you can call on for advice and caring.

A subtle form of social support comes through **modeling,** learning behaviors by watching others. This strategy enables you to learn from the experiences of others who have already made successful change. If you'd like to eat less junk food, for example, observe the habits of a health-conscious friend who has already scoped out the options for healthy eating on campus. A rarely acknowledged benefit of modeling is that it lets you imagine yourself engaging in the same healthful behavior—in a sense, it allows you to *rehearse* it. Frequent rehearsal through modeling helps you become more and more familiar and comfortable with the actions required for the behavior change. You don't have to be personally acquainted with your model, either: Reading a biography of someone who has successfully overcome alcohol addiction, for example, can help you understand how to change aspects of your personal life and your environment to achieve a similar change.

Don't ignore campus resources as a source of support for your plan for change. Remember all that campus-services information you got at the start of your freshman year? Take a look back through it, and you may be surprised to find a department or organization ideally suited to support your targeted change.

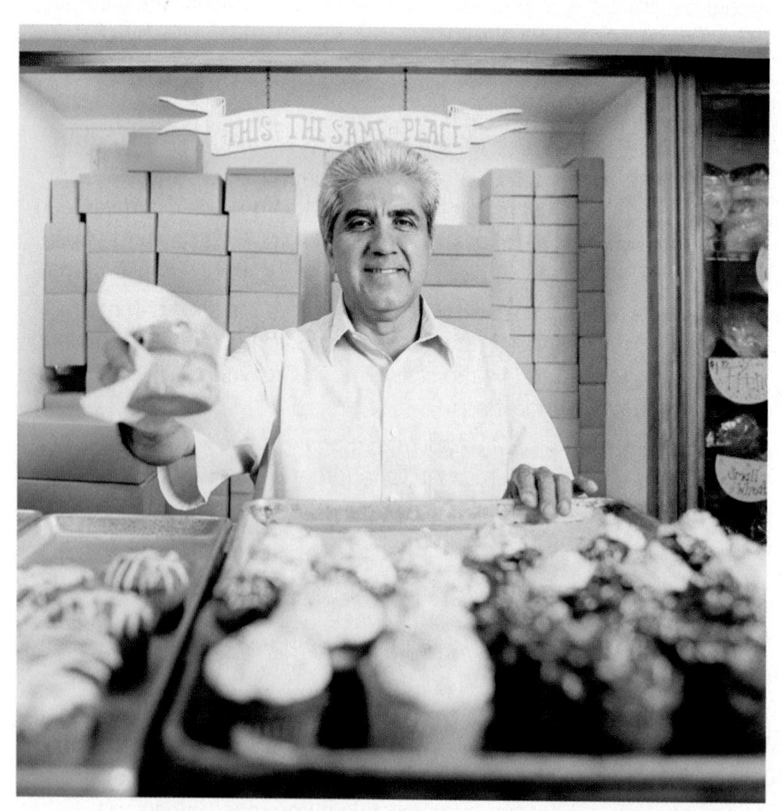

Factors in your **environment** can be barriers to behavior change. If you'd like to adopt a more healthy diet, you may want to limit your trips to the bakery!

Step 6. Promise Yourself Rewards

Rewards keep you motivated to sustain change. For example, you might promise yourself new clothing after you've reached a target weight goal.

However, **reinforcement** doesn't have to be a material object. For instance, the natural "high" people often feel after physical exercise can be its own positive reinforcement. Many people who are trying to quit smoking set aside the money they would have spent on cigarettes daily, with the promise of travel or another significant reward when they've reached a time goal—say, 6 months or a year—smoke free.

End-goal rewards are important, but it's also important to reward yourself for small steps along the way. For instance, if you enroll in an aerobics class held on T/TH throughout the current semester, you might promise yourself that, when you attend both sessions, you'll reward yourself with an act of "self-kindness," such as a long-distance call to a loved one that weekend.[36]

Step 7. Commit in Writing

Many people find it helps to write out and sign their name at the bottom of a behavior-change contract—indicating that they've made a pact with themselves that they intend to keep. So if you're ready to take the plunge, turn to the **Choosing to Change Worksheet** on page 22 for a form you can use. Notice that the steps in this contract follow those just discussed.

Make copies of your behavior-change contract, and place them anywhere you want support: on the refrigerator, your full-length mirror . . . or scan your contract and use it as your screensaver image on your laptop so you see it several times throughout the day!

Believe It!

Once you have your contract, it's time to make it happen. When barriers arise—and they will—don't give in to discouragement. Try to fill your mind with positive **self-talk**—thoughts that affirm your ability to change and acknowledge the help available to you from your environment. At all costs, avoid negative self-talk—the inner chatter that says you can't do this, or you don't have the time or money, or it's not important anyway. The nearby **Practical Strategies for Change** can help you turn negative chatter into positive self-talk.

Another tip for maintaining your belief in yourself is to engage in **self-monitoring;** that is, to observe and record aspects

reinforcement A motivational behavior-change technique that rewards steps toward positive change.

self-talk A person's internal dialogue.

self-monitoring A behavior-change technique in which the individual observes and records aspects of his or her behavior-change process.

> *"End-goal rewards are important, but it's also important to reward yourself for small steps along the way."*

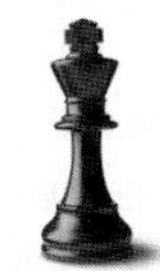

Practical Strategies for Change

Changing Your Self-Talk

Psychotherapists and personal development coaches know that a first step for changing your behavior is to change your thoughts about that behavior. Here are some proven strategies for becoming your own best behavior-change coach:

- **Bust the myth of "I can't."** You wrote a SMART—and forgiving—goal, right? That means it's *Attainable*, which in turn means, "You can." To bust the myth of "I can't," try expanding the statement with an action within your control. For instance, "I can, because I'm going to walk on the indoor track at the fitness center today, and whenever it snows." Or, "I can, because not even this friendship is worth more than my staying sober."
- **Affirm yourself, and then affirm yourself again.** Positive affirmations are often the subject of spoofs, but they can be highly effective in supporting change, because they force you to envision yourself as you plan to be. For instance: "I am fully able to handle anything that comes along today," or "My body is fit and strong," or, "Alcohol has no power over me." Experts suggest that you repeat your affirmation three or four times as soon as you wake up, and then several more times throughout the day. Tape your affirmation to your bathroom mirror, the glove compartment of your car, the back of your cell phone . . . anywhere you'll see it and say it.
- **Dump the disaster script.** Let's say you want to cut down on your drinking, but at a party after your last final exam, you blow it. Sick and discouraged the next day, you might be tempted to think of yourself as "a loser." Instead, recognize that what happened is not a disaster. You didn't drive while drunk and get in a car crash. Okay, you're sick, but not dangerously so. Switch your disaster script for a learning script: "I guess last night shows me that, when I'm letting down from stress, I'm more vulnerable than usual to binge drinking. I'm not a loser. I can control my drinking. From now on, I'm going to make sure I drink something non-alcoholic before going to a party, so I'm not thirsty when I get there, and I'll bring along a couple of bottles of non-alcoholic beer to have in between alcoholic drinks while I'm there."

In short, rather than dwelling on roadblocks, look for solutions. The result will help you feel better about yourself and solve your problems more effectively.

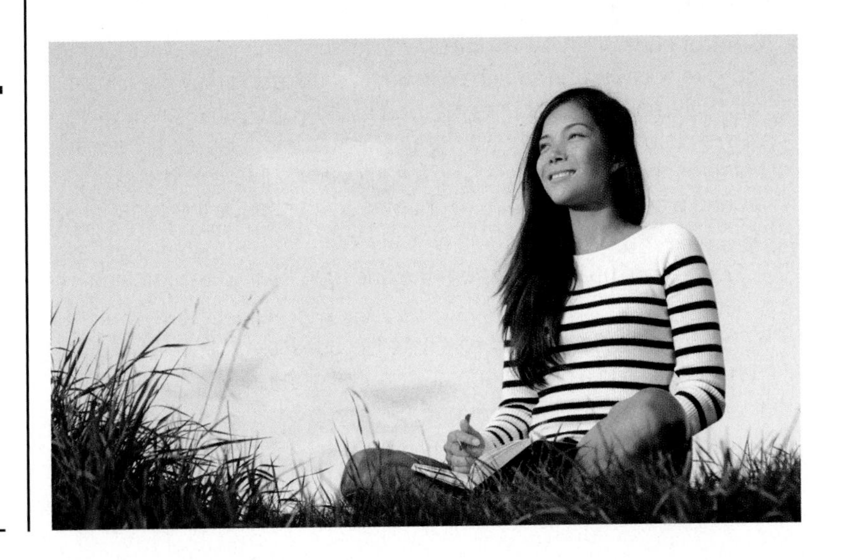

of your behavior-change process, such as how many servings of fruits and vegetables you eat each day, or how many hours of sleep you get each night. Such self-monitoring can provide solid evidence of improvement at times when you're not sure how you're doing, and can boost your confidence when it starts to slip. Your record can also show you when it's time to shift your change plan into higher gear. In all these ways, self-monitoring of a behavior can move you closer to your goal; for example, when the record shows that your level of physical activity is increasing, you'll be encouraged to keep it up.[36]

Cope With Relapse

When people attempt to change a long-term behavior, a lapse—a temporary "slip" back to the previous behavior—is highly likely.[38] For instance, a person trying to quit smoking who takes a drag on a friend's cigarette is experiencing a lapse. In contrast, a **relapse** is a return to the previous state or pattern of behavior: The person completely gives up the attempt to quit. Relapse is common; for example, according to the American Cancer Society, a majority of the people who successfully quit smoking have tried to quit—and relapsed—several times before.[39]

Certain conditions influence the likelihood that a lapse will devolve into a full-blown relapse. For instance, if the person views the lapse as due to external circumstances within the individual's control—"My roommate left an open pack of cigarettes out in full view, but from now on, has agreed to keep them out of sight."—then relapse is unlikely. By viewing a lapse as a learning experience, the person can then experiment with different strategies for changing or coping with the stimulus that provoked the lapse. In contrast, if a person views a lapse as due to factors that are internal, global, and/or uncontrollable—"My parents are alcoholics, so it's in my genes. I can't change."—then true relapse is more likely to occur.[38] See the **Practical Strategies for Change** for information on changing your self-talk to "dump the disaster script" and learn from your lapses.

Preventing a relapse is easy if you can prevent a lapse in the first place! To do it, take an inventory of the full ecological spectrum of factors that might trigger a lapse, and then identify strategies for coping. Two strategies for preventing lapses include the following:

- **Control cues.** With **cue control,** you learn to change the stimuli that provoke your unwanted behavior. For example, you may learn from your self-monitoring records that you're more likely to overeat while you're watching television, or whenever your mom leaves her latest batch of homemade cookies on the kitchen counter, or when you're around a certain friend. You might then try to change the behavior by:[36]
  - Separating the behavior from the cue (don't eat while watching television)
  - Taking action to avoid or eliminate the cue (ask your mom to put her cookies in a closed container out of sight)
  - Changing the environment or other circumstances surrounding the cue (plan to meet your friend in a nonfood setting)
- **Find a substitute.** For cue control to work, you have to have the capacity to change the stimulus. But in our complex lives, this isn't always possible. Fortunately, there's a technique called **counter-conditioning,** in which you learn to substitute a healthful or neutral behavior for the unwanted behavior when it's triggered by a cue beyond your control. One of the simplest examples is the urge to have something in their mouths that strikes most smokers repeatedly in the first few weeks after they quit. With counter-conditioning, the person replaces cigarette smoking with chewing on something, whether gum, licorice, or even a toothpick. Peer pressure commonly triggers lapses, but countering can be surprisingly effective in overcoming it. Write out and memorize one or more short, assertive statements such as, "No thanks, I've had enough." Then, in situations in which you'd usually give in, substitute your assertion.

relapse A return to the previous state or pattern of behavior.

cue control A behavior-change technique in which the individual learns to change the stimuli that provoked the lapse.

counter-conditioning A behavior-change technique in which the individual learns to substitute a healthful or neutral behavior for an unwanted behavior triggered by a cue beyond his or her control.

advocacy Working independently or with others to directly improve services in or other aspects of the environment, or to change related policies or legislation.

Campus Advocacy

When a barrier to change exists in your social or physical environment, or results from poor health services or policy-making, your best chance for change might just be in **advocacy;** that is, working independently or with others to directly improve services in or other aspects of your environment, or to change related policies or legislation. You may think of advocacy as lobbying to legislators, and while that's one form, there are many others available to you in your role as a college student. These include the following:

- Get better informed about the issue, especially what's happening on campus and within your community.
- Use your social networking pages to heighten awareness of the issue among your contacts.
- Meet directly with campus faculty or staff members to share your experiences, feelings, and suggestions on the issue.
- Write about the issue for campus news services.
- Speak about the issue at campus gatherings.
- Organize a letter-writing campaign to your dean of students or other decision-makers.
- Organize a petition drive or student demonstration related to the issue.
- Join a campus organization already working on the issue.
- Found an organization of your own.

Concluding every chapter of this book, you'll find suggestions for campus advocacy specific to the topics addressed in that chapter, from fitness to discrimination to climate change. These suggestions may or may not be appropriate for your campus. Still, we hope they'll provide you with practical examples of strategies that have worked for others, and some inspiration for advocacy of your own. The bottom line is, even in the face of health disparities that may seem beyond your personal control—poverty, pollution, lack of access to health services, restrictive policies—one voice can start a chain reaction that leads to change. Make it yours.

Watch videos of real students discussing their health at: www.pearsonhighered.com/lynchelmore.

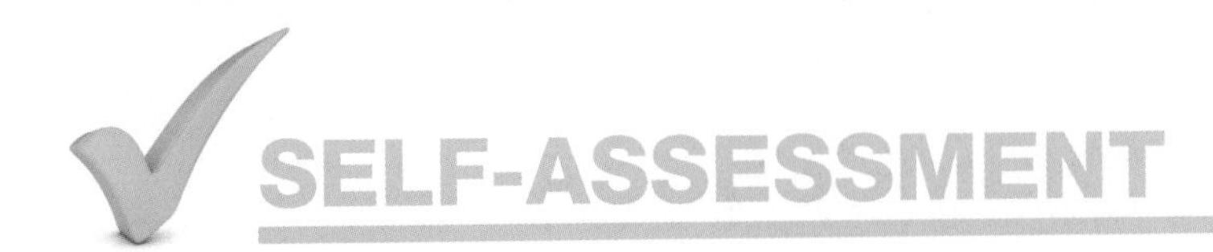

Take this self-assessment online at www.pearsonhighered.com/lynchelmore.

How Healthy Is Your Current Lifestyle?

Complete one section at a time by circling the number under the answer that best describes your behavior. Then add the numbers you circled to get your score for that section. Write the score on the line provided at the end of each section.

Cigarette Smoking	Almost Always	Sometimes	Almost Never
If you are currently a nonsmoker, enter a score of 10 for this section and go to the next section on Alcohol and Drugs.			
1. I avoid smoking cigarettes.	2	1	0
2. I smoke only low-tar and -nicotine cigarettes or I smoke a pipe.	2	1	0

Smoking Score 10

Alcohol and Drugs	Almost Always	Sometimes	Almost Never
1. I avoid drinking alcoholic beverages or I drink no more than 1 (for women) or 2 (for men) drinks a day.	4	1	0
2. I avoid using alcohol or other drugs (especially illegal drugs) as a way of handling situations or problems.	2	1	0
3. I am careful not to drink alcohol when taking certain medicines (for example, medicine for sleeping, pain, colds, and allergies) or when pregnant.	2	1	0
4. I read and follow the label directions when using prescribed and over-the-counter drugs.	2	1	0

Alcohol and Drugs Score 10

Eating Habits	Almost Always	Sometimes	Almost Never
1. I eat a variety of foods each day, such as fruits and vegetables; whole-grain breads and cereals; lean meats; low-fat dairy products; beans and legumes; nuts and seeds.	4	1	0
2. I limit the amount of fat, saturated fat, *trans* fat, and cholesterol I eat (including fat on meats, eggs, butter, cream, shortenings, and organ meats such as liver).	2	1	0
3. I limit the amount of salt I eat by cooking with only small amounts, not adding salt at the table, and avoiding salty snacks.	2	1	0
4. I avoid eating too much sugar (especially frequent snacks of sticky candy or soft drinks).	2	1	0

Eating Habits Score 5

Exercise/Fitness	Almost Always	Sometimes	Almost Never
1. I do vigorous exercises for 30 minutes a day at least 5 times a week (examples include jogging, swimming, brisk walking, or bicycling).	4	2	0
2. I do exercises that enhance my muscle tone for 15–30 minutes at least 3 times a week (examples include using weight machines or free weights, yoga, calisthenics).	3	1	0
3. I use part of my leisure time participating in individual, family, or team activities that increase my level of fitness (such as gardening, dancing, bowling, golf, baseball).	3	1	0

Exercise/Fitness Score 5

Stress Control	Almost Always	Sometimes	Almost Never
1. I have a job, go to school, or do other work that I enjoy.	2	1	0
2. I find it easy to relax and express my feelings freely.	2	1	0
3. I recognize early, and prepare for, events or situations likely to be stressful for me.	2	1	0
4. I have close friends, relatives, or others with whom I can talk about personal matters and call on for help when needed.	2	1	0
5. I participate in group activities (such as religious worship and community organizations) and/or have hobbies that I enjoy.	2	1	0

Stress Control Score 9

Safety/Health	Almost Always	Sometimes	Almost Never
1. I wear a seat belt while riding in a car.	2	1	0
2. I avoid driving while under the influence of alcohol and other drugs, or riding with someone else who is under the influence.	2	1	0
3. I obey traffic rules and avoid distractions like texting and talking on the phone when driving.	2	1	0
4. I am careful when using potentially harmful products or substances (such as household cleaners, poisons, and electrical devices).	2	1	0
5. I get at least 7 hours of sleep a night.	2	1	0

Safety/Health Score 9

HOW TO INTERPRET YOUR SCORE

Examine your score for each section and refer to the key below for a general assessment of how you are doing in that particular area of health.

Scores of 9 and 10

Excellent. Your answers show that you are aware of the importance of this area to your health. More important, you are putting your knowledge to work for you by practicing good health habits. As long as you continue to do so, this area should not pose a serious health risk. It's likely that you are setting an example for the rest of your family and friends to follow. Because you got a very high test score on this part of the test, you may want to consider other areas where your scores indicate room for improvement.

Scores of 6 to 8

Good. Your health practices in this area are good, but there is room for improvement. Look again at the items you answered with a "Sometimes" or "Almost Never." What changes can you make to improve your score? Even a small change can help you achieve better health.

Scores of 3 to 5

At Risk. Your health risks are showing. Would you like more information about the risks you are facing? Do you want to know why it is important for you to change these behaviors? Perhaps you need help in deciding how to make the changes you desire. In either case, help is available. You can start by contacting your health-care provider or a registered dietitian.

Scores of 0 to 2

Seriously at Risk. Obviously, you were concerned enough about your health to take this test. But your answers show that you may be taking serious risks with your health. Perhaps you were not aware of the risks and what to do about them. You can easily get the information and help you need to reduce your health risks and have a healthier lifestyle if you wish. Are you ready to take the next step?

Source: Bobroff, L.B. *"Healthstyle: A self-test."* Fact Sheet (FCS8553/he778). Gainesville, FL: University of Florida Institute of Food and Agricultural Sciences, 1999, 2011. From UF/IFAS Extension Data Information Source. http://edis.ifas.ufl.edu/he778.

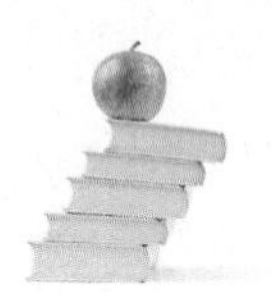

Choosing to Change Worksheet

To complete this worksheet online, visit **www.pearsonhighered.com/lynchelmore.**

The Choosing to Change Worksheets guide you on how to implement your behavior-change plans based on the stages of change identified by the transtheoretical model.

Stages of Behavior Change:

Precontemplation: I do not intend to make a change in the next 6 months.

Contemplation: I might make a change in the next 6 months.

Preparation: I am prepared to make a change in the next month.

Action: I have been making a change for less than 6 months.

Maintenance: I have been maintaining a change for more than 6 months.

After you have completed the Self-Assessment on the previous page, consider what stage of change you are in for each of the behaviors listed. Then, select one behavior—in which you are at either the contemplation or preparation stage—that you would like to target for change over the next few months. Next, fill out the Behavior Change Contract below. Make sure you sign it, and either display it where you'll see it often, or consider discussing it with your health instructor as part of your work toward your long-term goal.

Behavior Change Contract

My behavior change: ______________________________

1. Three important benefits of changing my behavior are:

   1. ______________________________

   2. ______________________________

   3. ______________________________

2. My SMART goal for this behavior change is:

   ____

   ____

   ____

3. Keeping my current stage of behavior change in mind, these short-term goals and rewards will make my SMART goal more attainable:

______________	______________	______________
Short-term goal	Target date	Reward
Short-term goal	Target date	Reward
Short-term goal	Target date	Reward

4. Barriers I anticipate to making this behavior change are:

   1. ______
   2. ______
   3. ______

   The strategies I will use to overcome these barriers are:

   1. ______
   2. ______
   3. ______

5. Resources I will use to help me change this behavior include:

   - a friend, partner, or relative: ______
   - a school-based resource: ______
   - a health-care resource: ______
   - a community-based resource: ______
   - a book or reputable website: ______

6. When I achieve the long-term behavior change described above, my reward will be:

______ ______
Target date

7. I intend to make the behavior change described above. I will use the strategies and rewards above to achieve the goals that will contribute to a healthy behavior change.

Signed: ______

Chapter Summary

- *Health* is more than merely the absence of disease or injury. In a healthy person, many different dimensions of life are working harmoniously.
- *Wellness* is the process of actively making choices to achieve optimal health.
- Although you can reduce your risk for many health problems, many are multifactorial, and some of the contributing factors are not within individual control.
- Although life expectancy in the United States is a record 78.7 years, many health challenges remain. For example, just two chronic diseases—heart disease and cancer—are responsible for almost half of all deaths in the United States.
- The four common behaviors responsible for most of the illness, suffering, and early death related to chronic disease in the United States are lack of physical activity, poor nutrition, tobacco use, and excessive alcohol consumption.
- The U.S. Department of Health and Human Services (HHS) is the U.S. government's principal agency for protecting the health of all Americans. Its primary division is the U.S. Public Health Service, and one of its leading agencies is the Centers for Disease Control and Prevention (CDC).
- The HHS initiative known as Healthy People takes an ecological approach to health that seeks to achieve health equity and the elimination of health disparities.

- Among Americans aged 15 to 24, the leading causes of death are unintentional injuries, homicide, and suicide. Stress, depression, anxiety, alcohol and tobacco use, and sexual health compromises are all common health concerns faced by college students.
- Global health problems include infection, malnutrition, and obesity-related diseases.
- The six broad categories of determinants of health include: biology and genetics, individual behaviors, social determinants, physical determinants, health services—including access to quality health care and health literacy—and policy-making.
- *Predisposing, enabling,* and *reinforcing factors* can all influence our success in making and maintaining health-related behavior change.
- The *transtheoretical model of behavior change* proposes six stages that a person progresses through before achieving sustained behavior change.
- The *health belief model* identifies four factors as instrumental in predicting health-related behavior change, including perceptions of threat, severity, benefit, and cues to action.
- Ecological models of behavior change acknowledge that the creation of a supportive environment is as important to achieving change as an individual's acquisition of health information and development of personal skills.
- After identifying a health-related behavior you want to change, seven steps for implementing that change include: becoming informed; setting a SMART goal; breaking down your goal into a sequential action plan; identifying barriers to change and how you'll overcome them; recruiting support; promising yourself rewards; and committing in writing.
- As you put your plan into action, identify thoughts constituting negative self-talk and replace them with affirmations and other examples of positive self-talk. Use self-monitoring to see your real progress and move closer to your goal.
- Prevent relapse by taking inventory of the full ecological spectrum of factors that might trigger a lapse, and then identifying strategies for coping, including cue control and counter-conditioning.
- Advocacy can be effective when a barrier to change exists in your social or physical environment, or results from poor health services or policy-making.

Test Your Knowledge

1. Which dimension of health is characterized by the quality of your interactions and relationships with other people?
   a. physical health
   b. intellectual health
   c. social health
   d. occupational health

2. The process of actively making choices to achieve optimal health is called
   a. psychological health.
   b. wellness.
   c. self-efficacy.
   d. precontemplation.

3. Which of the following behaviors can have profound health benefits?
   a. eating nutritiously
   b. being physically active
   c. not smoking and not drinking excessively
   d. all of the above

4. The ability to read, understand, and follow instructions in medical brochures and prescription drug labels is an example of
   a. health literacy.
   b. wellness.
   c. behavior change.
   d. occupational health.

5. You've decided to get fit. The fact that you live in a warm, sunny climate is an example of
   a. a predisposing factor for behavior change.
   b. an enabling factor for behavior change.
   c. a reinforcing factor for behavior change.
   d. none of the above.

Get Critical

What happened:

In the fall of 2009, British celebrity chef Jamie Oliver arrived in Huntington, West Virginia, and declared a "food revolution." With its soaring obesity rates, Huntington had recently been named the unhealthiest city in the United States by the Centers for Disease Control. Oliver's goal was to educate the residents of Huntington on the basics of good nutrition and to encourage behavior change at both the individual level and the community level (for example, making school lunches more nutritious), and to film his efforts for a nationally broadcast reality television show. Although the project had many supporters, critics charged that Oliver was a celebrity opportunist with a condescending attitude toward the citizens of Huntington.

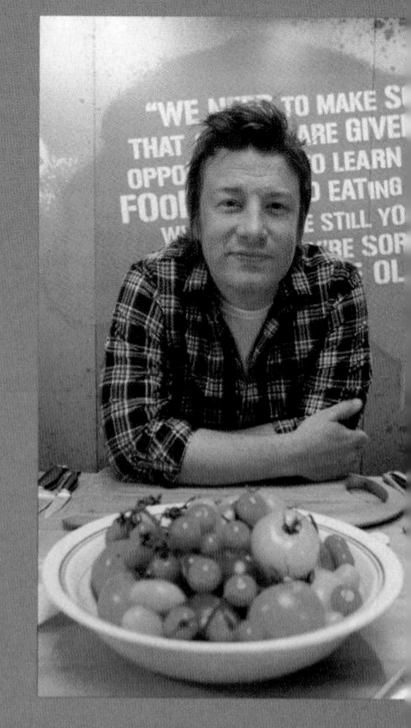

What do you think?

- **What's your opinion of Jamie Oliver's "food revolution"? Are you in favor of his efforts or do you find them offensive?**
- **Recall the ecological models of behavior change. With what principle(s) are Oliver's efforts aligned?**
- **Does a celebrity-driven health campaign make you more motivated to change a health behavior? Why or why not?**

6. In the transtheoretical model of behavior change, which stage indicates the period during which a person has modified the behavior in an observable way?
   a. precontemplation
   b. contemplation
   c. preparation
   d. action

7. Which of the following is a principle of the ecological models of behavior change?
   a. The individual's belief that making a change will reduce a threat to his or her health is the primary factor in behavior change.
   b. Interventions at multiple levels—from individual to society—are most effective in making health-related behavior change.
   c. Influences at multiple levels interact in a negative way.
   d. The individual must be able to admit the potential environmental consequences of changing a behavior.

8. The belief that events are out of your control is characteristic of
   a. self-efficacy.
   b. a strong internal locus of control.
   c. a strong external locus of control.
   d. the termination stage of behavior change.

9. Adopting a behavior by watching and learning from others is characteristic of
   a. modeling.
   b. shaping.
   c. reinforcement.
   d. changing self-talk.

10. Relapse is
   a. a temporary "slip" back to the previous behavior.
   b. uncommon.
   c. almost always due to circumstances beyond the person's individual control.
   d. less likely when the person views the lapse as due to external circumstances.

Get Connected

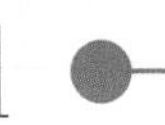

Mobile Tips!

Scan this QR code with your mobile device to access additional health tips. Or, via your mobile device, go to **http://mobiletips.pearsoncmg.com** and navigate to Chapter 1.

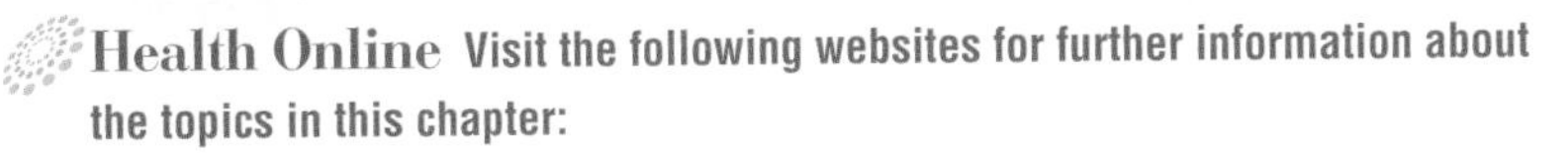

Health Online Visit the following websites for further information about the topics in this chapter:

- Centers for Disease Control and Prevention
  www.cdc.gov
- Go Ask Alice (answers to health questions, sponsored by Columbia University)
  www.goaskalice.columbia.edu
- U.S. Department of Health and Human Services' healthfinder.gov
  http://healthfinder.gov
- U.S. Department of Health and Human Services' *Healthy People 2020*
  www.healthypeople.gov
- Medline Plus
  www.nlm.nih.gov/medlineplus
- Mayo Clinic
  www.mayoclinic.com
- World Health Organization
  www.who.int/en
- New Mexico Media Literacy Project
  http://medialiteracyproject.org

Website links are subject to change. To access updated web links, please visit ***www.pearsonhighered.com/lynchelmore.***

References

i. Murphy, S. L., Xu, J., & Kochanek, K. D. (2012, January 11). Deaths: preliminary data for 2010. *National Vital Statistics Reports,* 60 (04). Available at www.cdc.gov/nchs/data/nvsr/nvsr60/nvsr60_4.pdf.

ii. Kvaavik, E., Batty, G., Ursin, G., Huxley, R., & Gale, C. (2010). Influence of individual and combined health behaviors on total and cause-specific mortality in men and women. *Archives of Internal Medicine, 170* (8), 711–718.

1. World Health Organization. (1948). Preamble to the Constitution of the World Health Organization as adopted by the International Health Conference, New York, 19–22 June, 1946; signed on 22 July 1946 by the representatives of 61 States (Official Records of the World Health Organization, no. 2, p. 100) and entered into force on 7 April 1948. Available at http://www.who.int/about/definition/en/print.html.

2. World Health Organization. (1986). Ottawa Charter for Health Promotion. First International Conference on Health Promotion. (21 November, 1986). WHO/HPR/HEP/95.1. Available at http://www.who.int/hpr/NPH/docs/ottawa_charter_hp.pdf.

3. National Wellness Institute. (2010). *Defining wellness.* Retrieved from http://www.nationalwellness.org/index.php?id_tier=2&id_c=26.

4. O'Donnell, M. P. (2009). Definition of health promotion. *American Journal of Health Promotion, 24* (1), iv. Available at http://www.healthpromotionjournal.com/index.html.

5. National Institute on Alcohol Abuse and Alcoholism. (2010). *Rethinking drinking: Alcohol and your health.* Retrieved from http://rethinkingdrinking.niaaa.nih.gov/WhatsTheHarm/WhatAreTheRisks.asp.

6. U.S. Department of Health and Human Services. (2010). *How tobacco smoke causes disease: The biology and behavioral basis for smoking-attributable disease. A report of the Surgeon General.* Retrieved from http://www.surgeongeneral.gov/library/tobaccosmoke/report/index.html.

7. World Bank. (2011, April 1). Life expectancy at birth: Total years. *World Development Indicators*. Retrieved from http://data.worldbank.org/indicator/SP.DYN.LE00.IN?cid=GPD_10.

8. Centers for Disease Control. (2000). *Leading causes of death, 1900–1998*. Retrieved from http://www.cdc.gov/nchs/data/dvs/lead1900_98.pdf.

9. Murphy, S. L., Xu, J., & Kochanek, K. D. (2012, January 11). Deaths: preliminary data for 2010. *National Vital Statistics Reports,* 60 (04). Available at www.cdc.gov/nchs/data/nvsr/nvsr60/nvsr60_4.pdf.

10. U.S. Centers for Disease Control. (2010, July 7). Chronic diseases and health promotion. Available at http://www.cdc.gov/chronicdisease/overview/index.htm.

11. U.S. Department of Health and Human Services. (2011). *Vital and health statistics: Early release of selected estimates based on data from the January–September 2010 National Health Interview Survey.* Available at http://www.cdc.gov/nchs/nhis/released201103.htm#9.

12. Ogden, C. L., & Carroll, M. D. (2010, June). Prevalence of overweight, obesity, and extreme obesity among adults: United States, trends 1976–1980 through 2007–2008. National Center for Health Statistics. Available at http://www.cdc.gov/NCHS/data/hestat/obesity_adult_07_08/obesity_adult_07_08.pdf.

13. U.S. Department of Health and Human Services. (2011). About HHS. Available at http://www.hhs.gov/about.

14. U.S. Department of Health and Human Services. (2010, December 2). What's new for 2020. Available at http://www.healthypeople.gov/2020/about/new2020.aspx.

15. American College Health Association. (2011). *ACHA-NCHA II: Reference group executive summary, Spring 2011*. Retrieved from http://www.achancha.org/docs/ACHA-NCHA-II_ReferenceGroup_ExecutiveSummary_Spring2011.pdf.

16. Joint United Nations Program on HIV/AIDS. (2009). *09 AIDS epidemic update.* Retrieved from http://data.unaids.org/pub/Report/2009/JC1700_Epi_Update_2009_en.pdf.

17. U.S. Centers for Disease Control. (2010, July 19). Antibiotic/Antimicrobial resistance. Available at http://www.cdc.gov/drugresistance/DiseasesConnectedAR.html.

18. Food and Agriculture Organization (FAO). (2009, October 14). The state of food insecurity in the world, 2009. FAO Media Centre. Available at http://www.fao.org/news/story/en/item/36207/icode/.

19. World Health Organization. (2011). Nutrition: Controlling the global obesity epidemic. Available at http://www.who.int/nutrition/topics/obesity/en/index.html.

20. U.S. Department of Health and Human Services. (2010, December 2). Determinants of health. Available at http://www.healthypeople.gov/2020/about/DOHAbout.aspx.

21. Williams, D. R. (2008). The health of men: Structured inequalities and opportunities. *American Journal of Public Health, 93,* 150–157.

22. Kvaavik, E., Batty, G., Ursin, G., Huxley, R., & Gale, C. (2010). Influence of individual and combined health behaviors on total and cause-specific mortality in men and women. *Archives of Internal Medicine, 170* (8), 711–718.

23. American Academy of Pediatrics. (2012, January). Early childhood adversity, toxic stress, and the role of the pediatrician: Translating developmental science into lifelong health. *PEDIATRICS, 129* (1), e224–e231. Retrieved from http://aappolicy.aappublications.org/cgi/reprint/pediatrics;129/1/e224.pdf.

24. Marmot, M. G. (2006, March 15). Status syndrome: A challenge to medicine. *JAMA, 295* (11). Available at http://www.psr.org/assets/pdfs/status-syndrome.pdf.

25. American Lung Association. (2010). *State of the air 2010.* Retrieved from http://www.stateoftheair.org/2010/assets/SOTA2010.pdf.

26. U.S. Centers for Disease Control and Prevention/National Center for Health Statistics. (2011). Health Insurance Coverage: Early Release of Estimates from the 2010 National Health Interview Survey, 2011. Available at http://www.cdc.gov/nchs/nhis/released201106.htm.

27. Krieger, N., Rehkopf, D., Chen, J., Waterman, P., Marcelli, E., & Kennedy, M. (2008). The fall and rise of U.S. inequities in premature mortality: 1960–2002. *Public Library of Science Medicine, 5* (2), e46.

28. The Henry J. Kaiser Family Foundation. (2010). *Focus on health reform: Summary of patient coverage provisions in the Patient Protection and Affordable Care Act.* Retrieved from http://www.kff.org/healthreform/upload/8023-R.pdf.

29. National Network of Libraries of Medicine. (2010). *Health literacy*. Retrieved from http://nnlm.gov/outreach/consumer/hlthlit.html.

30. American Liver Foundation. (n.d.). *Hepatitis B and Asian Americans.* Retrieved from http://www.thinkb.org/professionals/asianamericans.

31. Breslow, L., ed. (2002). Health-related behavior. In *Encyclopedia of public health*. Farmington Hills, MI: Gale Cengage Learning.

32. Prochaska, J., & Velicer, W. (1997). The transtheoretical model of health behavior change. *American Journal of Health Promotion, 12* (1), 38–48.

33. Daddario, D. (2007). A review of the use of the health belief model for weight management. *Medsurg Nursing, 16* (6), 363–366.

34. Sallis, J. F., Owen, N., & Fisher, E. B. (2008). Ecological models of health behavior. In Glanz, K., Rimer, B. K., & Viswanath, K. *Health behavior and health education*. San Francisco: John Wiley & Sons.

35. Doran, G. T. (1981). There's a S.M.A.R.T. way to write management's goals and objectives. *Management Review*, *70* (11) (AMA FORUM), 35–36.

36. National Institutes of Health. (2011, April 15). Guide to behavior change. Available at http://www.nhlbi.nih.gov/health/public/heart/obesity/lose_wt/behavior.htm.

37. Olson, J. M. (1992, February). Psychological barriers to behavior change. *Can Fam Physician, 38*, 309–319.

38. Marlatt, A., & Witkiewitz, K. (2005). Relapse prevention for alcohol and drug problems. In Marlatt, A., & Donovan, D. M., eds. *Relapse prevention: Maintenance strategies in the treatment of addictive behaviors*, 2nd ed. NY: The Guilford Press.

39. American Cancer Society. (2010, November 3). Helping a smoker quit: Do's and don'ts. Available at http://www.cancer.org/healthy/stayawayfromtobacco/helping-a-smoker-quit.

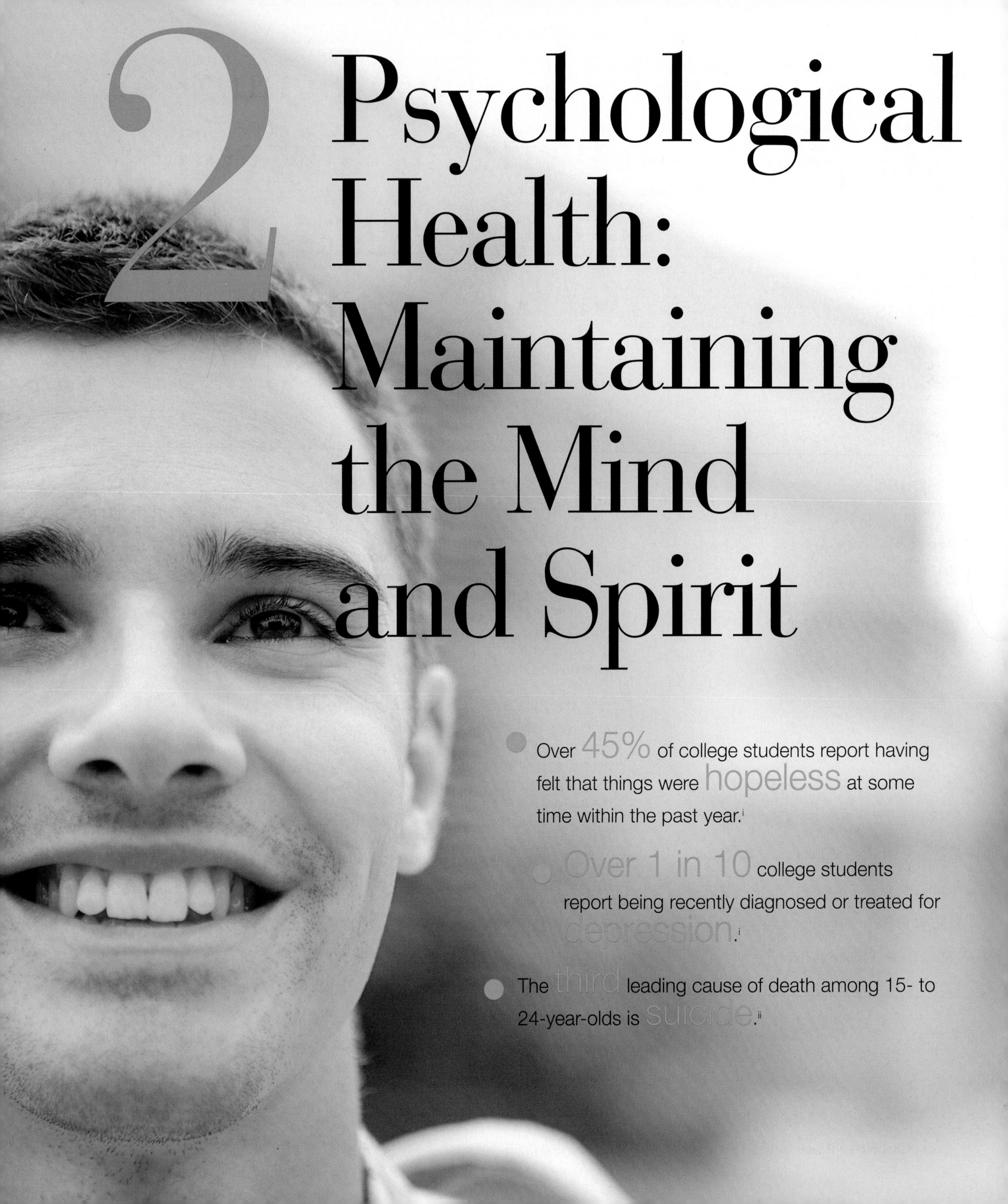

2 Psychological Health: Maintaining the Mind and Spirit

- Over 45% of college students report having felt that things were hopeless at some time within the past year.[i]
- Over 1 in 10 college students report being recently diagnosed or treated for depression.[i]
- The third leading cause of death among 15- to 24-year-olds is suicide.[ii]

LEARNING OBJECTIVES

IDENTIFY two components and six facets of psychological health.

DISCUSS a variety of factors that influence psychological health.

DESCRIBE common psychological challenges and ways to address them.

DISCUSS the controversies surrounding the issues of prevalence, origin, and treatment of mental disorders.

COMPARE AND CONTRAST mood disorders, anxiety disorders, attention disorders, and schizophrenia.

LIST the warning signs of suicide and describe suicide prevention methods.

DESCRIBE the different options for treatment of mental disorders.

IDENTIFY personal strategies for improving your psychological health.

Health Online icons are found throughout the chapter, directing you to web links, videos, podcasts, and other useful online resources.

Look at a brochure advertising any college in the country, and you'll find photos

of happy students enjoying their studies and having fun. But as you know, real life for college students is more complicated than such images suggest. When feelings of anxiety, shyness, frustration, anger, or loneliness arise, good psychological health can help you maintain your balance and resolve the challenge effectively.

So what does it mean to have "good" psychological health? How do you get it? If you're struggling to effectively nurture your mind or spirit, what strategies can help? We discuss these questions ahead.

What Is Psychological Health?

The field of psychology emerged as a separate discipline from philosophy in the late 19th century, when German and American scientists began conducting experiments to try to discover an anatomical or physiological basis for mental disorders. At the same time, the Austrian neurologist Sigmund Freud began exploring the role of past experiences of trauma in prompting unconscious conflicts that lead to mental disorders. But decades passed before researchers began to study the question of what constitutes psychological health. Here, we explore a few of the key concepts such work has revealed.

Components of Psychological Health

At its most basic, **psychological health** can be defined as the dimension of health and wellness that encompasses both mental and emotional components. **Mental health** can be described as the "thinking" component of psychological health. The term describes your ability to perceive reality accurately and respond to its challenges rationally and effectively. Good mental health is characterized by the intellectual capacity to process information, analyze choices, and respond appropriately. **Emotional health** refers to the "feeling" component of psychological health. It describes how you react emotionally to the ups and downs of life. Whereas we all experience difficult feelings and bad moods, people with good emotional health are better able to modulate their highs and lows and keep less happy times in perspective.

Mental and emotional health affect all other dimensions of health. Your physical health, for example—from the functioning of your gastrointestinal tract to the effectiveness of your immune response—is influenced by your thoughts and emotions. So is your social health: Rational thinking and an upbeat mood can draw others to you, whereas unrealistic expectations and stormy emotions can cause others to disengage.

psychological health A broad dimension of health and wellness that encompasses both mental and emotional health.

mental health The "thinking" component of psychological health that allows you to perceive reality accurately and respond rationally and effectively.

emotional health The "feeling" component of psychological health that influences your interpretation of and response to events.

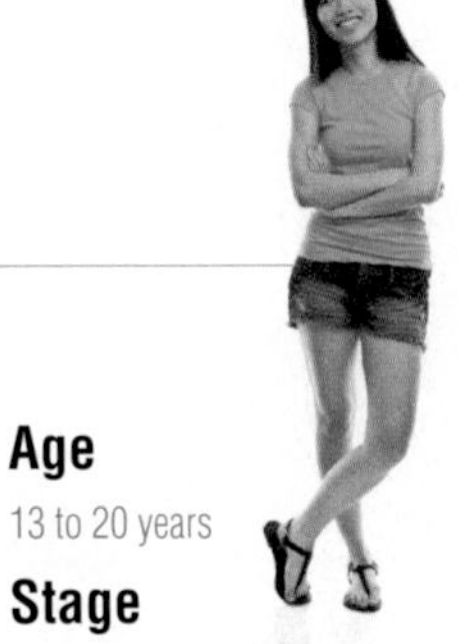

Age
13 to 20 years
Stage
Identity vs. Role Confusion
Developmental Tasks
The adolescent either carves out an authentic identity or develops role confusion and a weak sense of self.

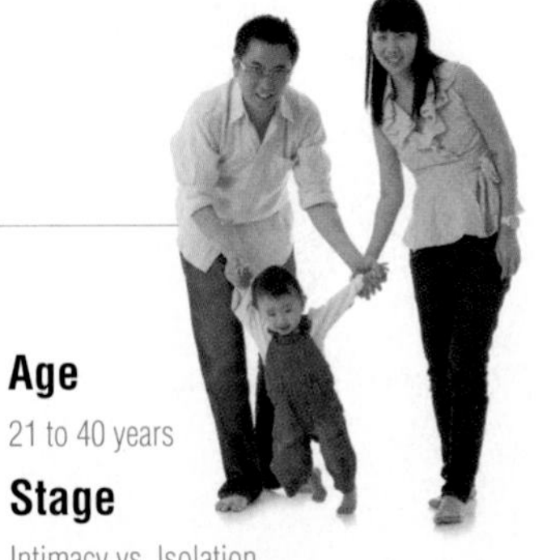

Age
21 to 40 years
Stage
Intimacy vs. Isolation
Developmental Tasks
The young adult either initiates and maintains intimate relationships or develops a sense of isolation.

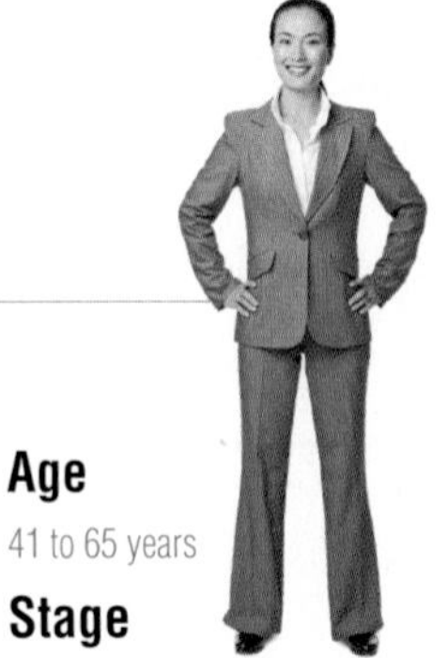

Age
41 to 65 years
Stage
Generativity vs. Stagnation
Developmental Tasks
The middle adult either creates or promotes positive change in the world, or develops a sense of futility and stagnation.

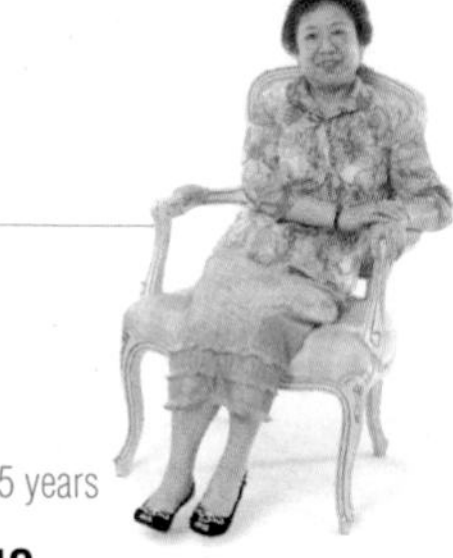

Age
Over 65 years
Stage
Ego Integrity vs. Despair
Developmental Tasks
The older adult either develops a sense of success, fulfillment, and wisdom, or dwells in regrets, experiencing bitterness and despair.

Defining Religion

A **religion** is a system of beliefs and practices related to the existence of a transcendent power. Religious beliefs are typically expressed in acts of service and devotion, either through an organized group or independently.

The 2007 U.S. Religious Landscape Survey found that over 83% of American adults say they are affiliated with a particular religion. Here's the breakdown:[19]

- Nearly 79% of respondents identify themselves as Christians.
- Nearly 5% of respondents practice Judaism, Buddhism, Islam, Hinduism, or another religion.
- Nearly 6% of respondents describe themselves as religious, but unaffiliated.
- The remaining 11% of respondents identify themselves as atheist, agnostic (that is, they claim neither belief nor disbelief in a divine being), secular, or uncertain.

The statistics for religious affiliation for young adults are somewhat lower: 75% of Americans aged 18 to 29 say they are affiliated with a particular religion.[19]

An ongoing analysis of more than 40 studies from countries across the globe suggests that religious belief and expression are common worldwide. The Cognition, Religion, and Theology Project at Oxford University, while taking no stance on the existence of God, finds that religion is universal, and deep-rooted in human nature.[20]

Benefits of Religion

A 2011 study found that more Americans are praying about their health: 49% in 2007, up from 43% in 2002.[21] Apparently, their prayers are effective: Studies have shown that "positive religious coping techniques" such as prayer improve both our subjective perception of our physical and mental health and objective clinical measurements of health. Moreover, in a 2009 study of university students, participants who scored high on "religiousness"—adherence to religious values and beliefs, and use of prayer and other religious practices in daily living—demonstrated levels of psychological well-being that were modestly higher than average and levels of psychological distress that were dramatically lower.[9]

Defining Spirituality

Although affiliation with an organized religion is common in the United States, it's just one expression of a broader approach to life commonly referred to as **spirituality.** The term is tough to define, in part because any definition—by its very nature—excludes, whereas spirituality is inclusive of just about everything. As Brian Luke Seaward, a pioneer in the field of health psychology, explains, spirituality is ageless, timeless, knowing no bounds and holding no allegiances.[22] The definition adopted by the World Health Organization identifies spirituality as "that which is in total harmony with the perceptual and non-perceptual environment."[23] For many, spirituality is a lifelong quest for the answers to life's biggest questions, such as "What is the nature of the cosmos?"; "What is my purpose in this life?"; and "What happens when we die?"

Although deeply individual and highly complex, spiritual well-being is generally said to rest upon three main "pillars" (**Figure 2.3** on page 34):[22]

- A strong personal value system
- Relationships: connectedness and community
- A meaningful purpose in life

Let's take a closer look at each.

Personal Values. Your term paper is due tomorrow and you haven't even started it. Should you buy one from an online site, stay up all night writing, or go to your instructor's office empty-handed, apologize, and ask for an extension? Questions like this force us to reflect on our **values,** the internal guidelines we use to make decisions and evaluate the world around us. Building your spirituality starts with

religion A system of beliefs and practices related to the existence of a transcendent power.

spirituality That which is in total harmony with the perceptual and nonperceptual environment.

values Internal guidelines used to make decisions and evaluate the world around you.

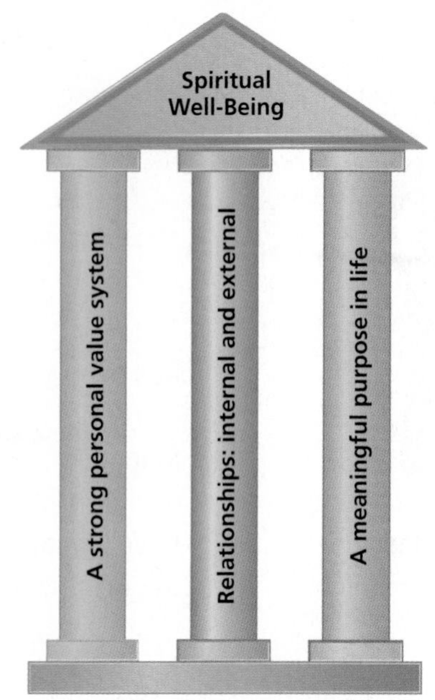

Figure 2.3 Seaward's pillars of spiritual well-being. A strong sense of values, meaningful relationships, and a sense of purpose together support spiritual well-being.

Source: Adapted from *Health of the Human Spirit: Spiritual Dimensions for Personal Health*, by B. L. Seaward, 2001, Boston: Pearson Education, p. 86.

knowing your values and putting them into practice. Your answers to the following questions will help reveal your values.

- What is important to me?
- What principles do I want to live by?
- What do I stand for?

Values evolve over the course of a lifetime. Many college students arrive on campus with values very similar to those of their parents. However, because of new relationships and experiences during the college years, many students find their values changing. Throughout adult life, a wide array of influences and circumstances requires you to refine your values repeatedly.

Living your values means reflecting them in the choices you make. For example, if you value the dignity of all human beings, you may be compelled to take action to reduce homelessness in your community. This might lead you to join a homeless outreach program or volunteer at a soup kitchen.

Relationships. Your first relationship is with yourself. How comfortable are you with your own company? Through reflection, prayer, or meditation, you can begin to develop a relationship with your "higher self," whatever you conceive this to be.[22] Developing an internal relationship leads you to see how you relate to everyone and everything in your environment: people, nature, institutions, and even nonphysical entities such as principles and laws.

Spiritual well-being also rests upon your connectedness with others. In your life as a college student, peer relationships may be critical, but you may also find spiritual support in your relationships with parents and siblings, old friends, romantic partnerships, or a spouse and children. Although these loved ones can't answer life's big questions for you, they can help you explore the answers for yourself.

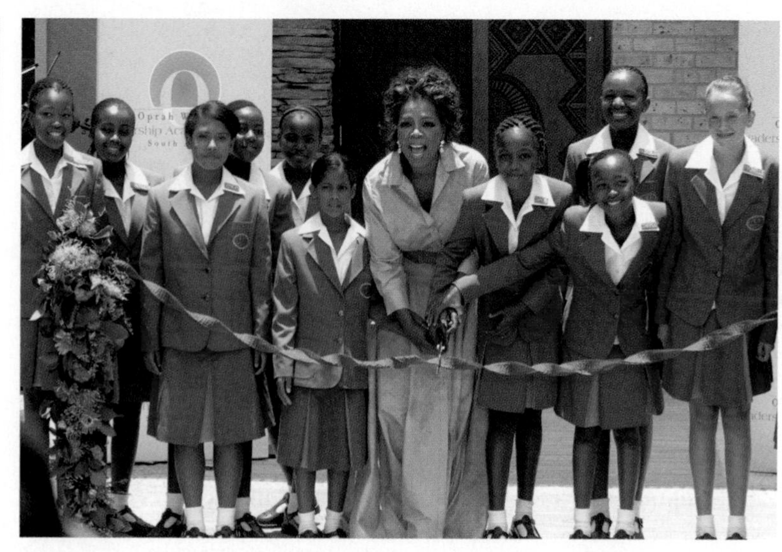

Oprah Winfrey acted altruistically when she started the Leadership Academy for Girls in South Africa.

As you work to clarify your internal and external relationships, avoid focusing on flaws. Instead, try starting from a place of gratitude. College may be tough, but at least you have the chance to attend. You may have caught a bad flu a couple of weeks back, but you've recovered. Even when a cherished relationship falls apart, you can still be grateful for the many other manifestations of enduring love in your life, and the opportunities for new commitments.

altruism The practice of helping and giving to others out of genuine concern for their well-being.

Adopting an "attitude of gratitude" can brighten your outlook on life. This, in turn, can lead to **altruism,** the practice of giving to others out of selfless concern for their well-being. Acts of altruism bring gifts to you: Helping others can put your own life in perspective, build self-esteem, and even help you manage stress.[24]

Purpose. Why do you exist? Thinkers throughout the ages have provided various answers for us, most of which focus on service to humanity. But how would you answer this question? Is it important to you to conduct your life in such a way that you know your living has made some difference? If so, given your unique values and gifts, how will you express your purpose?

Benefits of Spirituality

Studies of the benefits of spirituality on psychological health yield conflicting results. These differences may be due primarily to the way the studies are designed.

Studies that differentiate between religion and spirituality have found that respondents who score high on "religiousness" experience significantly lower rates of psychological distress than average, whereas respondents who score high on "spirituality" tend to have higher rates of psychological distress.[9] This might reflect the potential for people to turn to spirituality as a form of self-treatment for psychological challenges. It's also possible that some people scoring high on spirituality have turned away from organized religion and are thus experiencing psychological distress caused by a "crisis of faith."[9]

Studies that consider "religion and spirituality" as a single variable consistently find it strongly associated with improved psychological health.[25] Specific benefits include decreased anger, anxiety, and depression; a reduction in feelings of isolation; decreased substance abuse; and increased hope, optimism, a sense of satisfaction with life, and inner peace.[26]

Common Psychological Challenges

There may come times when you face challenges to your psychological well-being, just as you do to your physical health. This vulnerability does not mean there is something "wrong" with you. These challenges are common, and in almost every instance, there are steps you can take to feel more positive and in control.

Shyness

Shyness is characterized by a feeling of apprehension or intimidation in social situations, especially in reaction to unfamiliar people or new environments. Many people experience some degree of shyness, and an estimated 40–50% of college students consider themselves shy.[27] Shyness is common in creative people, from Albert Einstein to J. K. Rowling, and can prompt empathy, patience, a willingness to listen, and even success in leadership.

But shyness does have its challenges. Unlike introverts, who prefer to keep to themselves, shy people want to participate in social interactions, but find it difficult to do so because of self-consciousness, fear of embarrassment, or a negative self-image. Shyness can be confined to one type of situation, such as being in large groups or interacting with an authority figure, or it can be more general, materializing during many types of social events. Moreover, shyness can vary in severity from a slight feeling of discomfort to a pattern of avoidance that can limit personal and professional advancement—for example, if shy people hesitate to speak up for themselves or avoid situations where they need to be leaders or speak publicly.[28] Shyness can also lead to *social isolation,* a general withdrawal or avoidance of social contact or communication.

A common misperception is that you are "born" shy, but that's not necessarily true. There is some evidence that genes can contribute to shyness. In particular, one variation of a gene that helps regulate brain chemistry has been linked to some cases of being shy.[29] But this "shy" gene appears to be more significant when someone has been exposed to uncomfortable social pressures that also encourage shyness.[30] In other words, the gene doesn't work alone. Recall our previous discussion of early maladaptive coping patterns: For some people, life experiences alone are enough to make them shy.

Shyness can be a lifelong personality trait, or it may diminish with age. However, adults can develop shyness, especially during difficult transitions such as a divorce or getting laid off.[31]

Mild forms of shyness can usually be overcome with practice. Try making small talk with someone you'll probably never see again, like a person in line at the airport. If that feels reasonably comfortable, then try it again with a person you barely know, like the clerk at the bagel shop. In short, ease out of your comfort zone slowly. In addition, cognitive-behavioral therapy, discussed later in this chapter, can help.

shyness The feeling of apprehension or intimidation in social situations, especially in reaction to unfamiliar people or new environments.

loneliness A feeling of isolation from others, often prompted by a real or perceived loss.

> *Shyness is common in creative people, from Albert Einstein to J. K. Rowling, and can prompt empathy, patience, a willingness to listen, and even success in leadership."*

Loneliness

Loneliness is not a synonym for being alone. Many people are content to spend much of their time alone. Some even closely guard their solitude, honoring the creativity and insight it can bring. In contrast, **loneliness** is a feeling of isolation from others, a sense that you don't have—and don't know how to make—meaningful connections. It is often prompted by a real or perceived loss; for instance, when your best friend moves out of state, or you come to believe that your romantic partner would rather be spending time with someone else. Another common aspect is that lonely people often experience greater distress when they're with others than when they're actually alone.

Loneliness can do more than make you feel blue. It has been linked to higher levels of depression as well as physical disorders.[32] In fact, studies of older people have found that those who are unmarried and lonely may have shorter life expectancy than those in meaningful relationships.[33]

If you feel as though you need more meaningful connections in your life, you have many options:

- **Take advantage of the social and volunteer opportunities offered on campus or in your community.** Seek out groups that share your interests, such as sports organizations, civic organizations, or church groups. By focusing on activities of genuine interest to you, you are more likely to meet others who share your passions and values—and you're more likely to form meaningful relationships.
- **Express yourself openly and honestly.** Sharing your true feelings with someone can foster a feeling of connection that mere socializing cannot.
- **Look into college counseling center resources.** Campus counseling centers usually offer a variety of resources that can help you build your social skills and develop more meaningful relationships.

Anger

Anger is a completely normal and even healthy human emotion. Recognizing factors that make you angry can help you understand your values and assert yourself. Expressing anger is an important facet of the communication process.

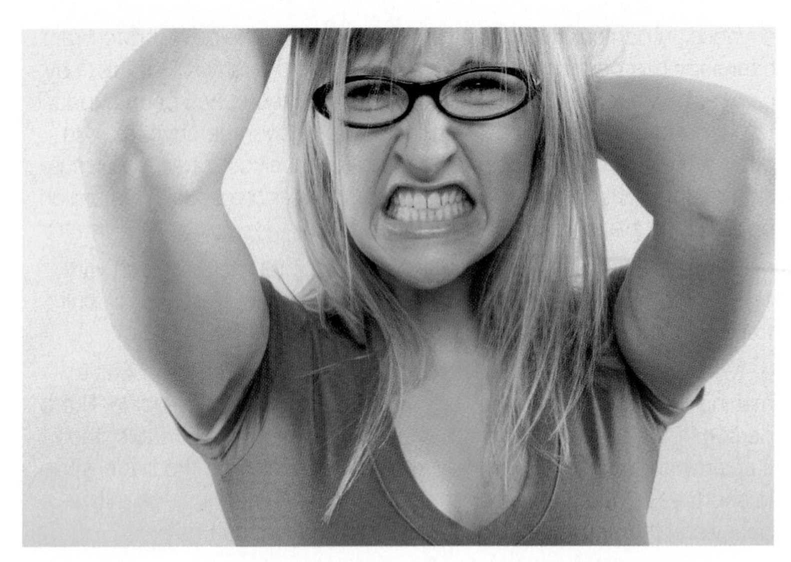

Although it may not feel like it, you can modify **anger** and **bad moods**.

However, anger that is out of control can be destructive. It can damage your relationships and may make it difficult for you to hold a job or participate in group activities. One study of anger found that people prone to irritability and aggressiveness were more likely to display hostility even when they weren't provoked.[34] Anger can even damage your health. The exploding rage you feel when you get really angry raises your blood pressure and appears to be associated with risk factors for heart disease.[35] In fact, studies suggest that the cardiovascular effects of anger can still be detected even a week after the angry outburst, if the person continues to dwell on the event.[36]

Anger that remains bottled up can also be harmful; it raises your levels of tension and stress and darkens your view of the world.[37] Harboring anger may also leave you feeling defensive, assuming you are being attacked more often than may actually be the case.

The key is to express your anger in a way that releases your emotions but doesn't damage your relationships. When you find yourself getting angry or defensive, take a step back and assess the situation objectively. Try to relax—a few deep breaths can often do the trick. Then explain, as calmly as you can, what's upsetting you. Speak honestly, but avoid criticism, blame, and threats. If necessary, step away from the person or situation to give yourself time to think. Once you're calmer, you may see solutions to the problem that you didn't notice before.

Bad Mood

Prolonged emotional states, or **moods,** can shape your view of the world for hours or days at a time. Although moods may often feel like they are caused by outside factors—a good or a bad grade on a paper, a fight with a friend—you have the ability to influence your moods. If you are in a bad mood, here are some strategies for breaking out of it:

- **Act, don't stew.** Dwelling on a problem or bad mood without taking action is unproductive and increases the chance that you will misdirect your frustrations at an innocent person later on.[38]
- **Change what has upset you.** If you have to miss a night out with friends in order to study, plan another one for a time you know you will be free. Taking action can reshape your mood.
- **If you can't change one thing, change another.** If a fight with a friend has put you in a bad mood, and there is no way to resolve the dispute right now, focus on calming yourself down. Go for a run, finish a project, or Skype your sister. You can work on resolving the fight when the time is right.
- **Don't drink or use drugs to cope.** Don't try to drown out your feelings with alcohol or drugs. You may feel better temporarily, but the circumstances that dragged down your mood will still be there after you have a couple of beers.

moods Prolonged emotional states.

mental disorders Significant behavioral and psychological disorders that disrupt thoughts and feelings, impair ability to function, and increase risk of pain, disability, or even death.

This National Public Radio program discusses mental health on campus: www.npr.org/templates/story/story.php?storyId=113835383.

Mental Disorders in the United States: An Overview

Everyone occasionally feels sad, worried, or "spaced out." The feelings may last a few hours or a few weeks, but eventually we get over it and move on with our lives. In contrast, **mental disorders** cause long-term disruptions in thoughts and feelings that reduce an individual's ability to function in daily life. These disruptions can impair functioning so much that the person becomes disabled. They also increase an individual's risk of pain, traumatic injury, and death. The American Psychiatric Association (APA) classifies and defines all the mental disorders it currently recognizes in its *Diagnostic and Statistical Manual of Mental Disorders* (DSM).

Like other aspects of your psychological health, your risk for developing a mental disorder is influenced by complex interactions among a vast number of genetic, biological, and environmental factors. And as we'll discuss shortly, aspects of our health care also play roles.

Mental Disorders in the United States and Around the World

Mental disorders are common. The National Institute of Mental Health (NIMH) estimates that more than 1 in 4 Americans over the age of 18 have experienced a diagnosable mental disorder at some time in the past year—a figure that translates to over 57 million people.[39] However, more than one-third of these cases are mild; that is, the disorder caused the person to feel unable to function in his or her normal role on fewer than four days during the year.[40]

College students face distinct academic and social pressures that can challenge their psychological health. In 2011, 21% of college students in the United States reported being treated for or diagnosed with some type of mental disorder in the past year.[41]

The NIMH reports that about 5% of all American adults have a *serious mental illness* (*SMI*), which is a mental disorder resulting in serious functional impairment that substantially interferes with or limits one or more major life activities.[39] Among Americans between the ages of 18 and 25, about 8% have an SMI.[39] Americans recognized as having an SMI are considered disabled, and typically receive some type of social security disability insurance

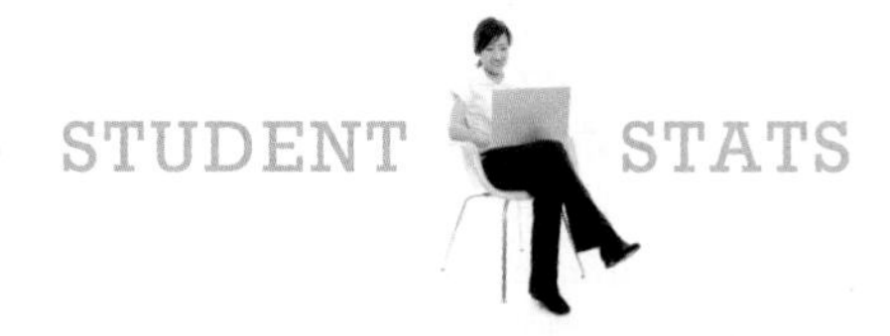

Psychological Health on Campus

Students reported feeling the following within the last 12 months:

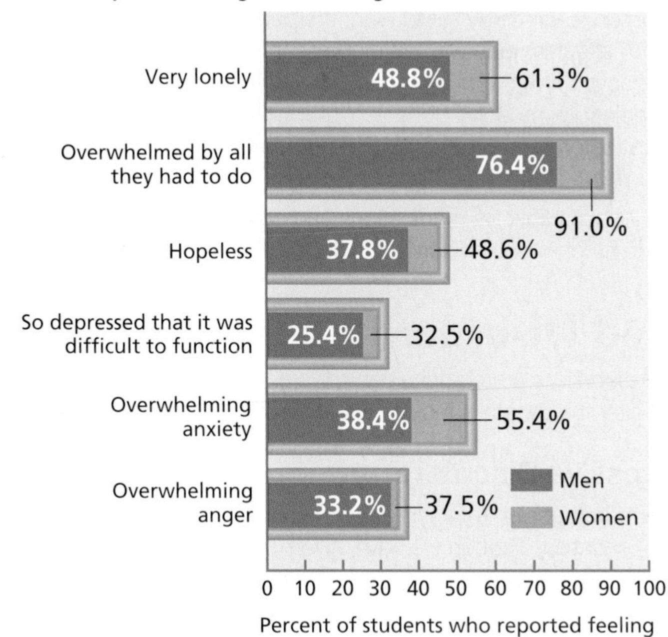

Data from *American College Health Association National College Health Assessment (ACHA- NCHA II) Reference Group Executive Summary, Fall 2011* by the American College Health Association, 2012, retrieved from http://www.acha-ncha.org/reports_ACHA-NCHAII.html.

(SSDI) payment. In 2002, the most recent year for which data is available, disability payments, health care, and lost income due to SMIs together cost the United States more than $300 billion.[42]

Intriguingly, a comparison of historical records suggests a startling increase in SMIs in the United States over the past 50 years. The available evidence suggests that in 1955, only 1 in 468 Americans (including adults and children) had a mental disorder that was serious enough to be disabling. By 2007, Social Security Administration reports showed that 1 in 76 American adults and children were disabled by mental disorders.[43]

A comparison of our rate of mental disorders with that of other countries is equally troubling. In 2004, the World Health Organization conducted a survey of mental disorders in 14 countries. Researchers used the same diagnostic interview tool in the same manner (face-to-face household surveys) in all 14 countries. The findings? The United States had the highest prevalence of mental disorders of all countries surveyed. Our rate of 26.4% was dramatically higher than the average range of 9–17%. From another perspective, the U.S. rate was more than double the rate in Mexico or Belgium, and triple the rate in Japan, Spain, Italy, or Germany.[40]

Do these variations reflect cross-cultural differences, either in people's willingness to admit to psychological distress or in psychiatrists' readiness to diagnose distress as a "mental disorder"? Are stronger family and community ties in countries like Italy and Japan protective? Could the variance reflect an over-reliance of American patients and physicians on a quick pharmaceutical "fix" for psychological distress that in some way is actually contributing to the higher rates of mental disorders in America? Health researchers have posed such questions for decades, but as more and more Americans, including children, are disabled by mental disorders, it's becoming increasingly urgent to find some answers.

The Theory of Chemical Imbalance

The increasing dominance of **psychoactive drugs** (drugs that affect the patient's mental state) as the primary form of treatment for mental disorders coincides with the increasing dominance of the *chemical imbalance theory* of psychiatric disorders.[44] The theory arose in the 1950s as drugs initially used to treat other disorders, such as tuberculosis or high blood pressure, were found to have psychological side effects.[45] Some produced sedation or even delusional depression. Others energized patients. Initially, researchers could not explain these effects, but over time, it became clear that the drugs were triggering mechanisms that caused the brain to be flooded with chemicals called **neurotransmitters.** These chemicals—including serotonin, epinephrine, dopamine, and others—are classified as neurotransmitters because they enable the transmission of messages from one nerve cell (called a *neuron*) to another.

> psychoactive drugs Drugs that affect the user's mood, perceptions, or other aspects of the mental state.
>
> neurotransmitters Chemicals including serotonin, epinephrine, dopamine, and others that enable the transmission of messages from one neuron to another.

To appreciate how neurotransmitters work, you need to understand some fundamentals of how your brain works. The human brain is a mass of tissue made up of about 100 billion neurons and perhaps 30 trillion supporting cells of other types.[46] Each neuron has many small extensions by which it communicates with other neurons. But these extensions don't actually touch: Instead, neurons send and receive messages across microscopic gaps called *synapses* (see **Figure 2.4** on page 38). Because each neuron has many extensions, your brain is thought to have more than 100 *trillion* synapses. When you hear your phone go off, or reach in your pocket to answer it, a vast network of neurons releases neurotransmitters into these synapses. The neurotransmitters cross the synapses and attach to *receptors* (think of them as loading docks) on adjacent neurons. When they do, they either activate the neuron or inhibit it. Once the neurotransmitter has exerted its effect, it is either quickly broken down by enzymes, or it is taken back up by the neuron that initially released it. In either case, the brain region returns to its initial state within a fraction of a second, ready to respond to new signals.

When it was discovered that psychoactive drugs cause an increase or decrease in the levels of neurotransmitters in the brain (sometimes by interfering with the enzymes that break them down, and other times by inhibiting their "reuptake"—their return to the sending neurons), psychiatrists theorized that mental disorders might be caused by having abnormally high or abnormally low levels of neurotransmitters in the brain. However, despite decades of research, scientists have failed to

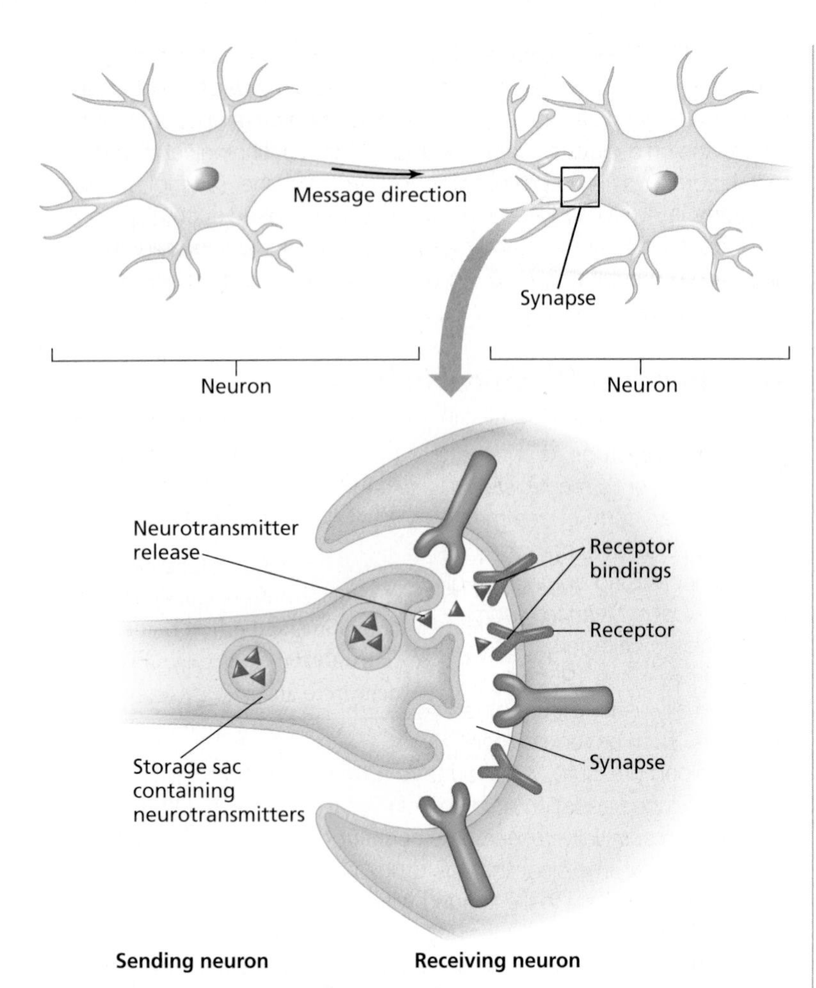

Figure 2.4 Transmission of messages in the brain. Neurotransmitters facilitate the transmission of messages across the gaps (called *synapses*) between adjacent neurons. After activating or inhibiting the receiving neurons, they are either broken down by enzymes or taken back up by the sending neurons. Psychoactive drugs alter the brain's mechanisms for maintaining its normal balance of neurotransmitters. This can produce a variety of effects, from euphoria to sedation.

find sufficient evidence to support this theory. Neurotransmitter levels and functioning appear to be normal in people with mental disorders before drug treatment; thus, a direct correlation between mood and neurotransmitters is now considered "too simplistic."[44, 45]

The current edition of the DSM states that the cause of most mental disorders is unknown, and makes no claims for any particular theory of underlying physiology. However, researchers have recently begun to investigate gene–environment interactions as the source. This line of study is focusing, for example, on the combined effects of genetic vulnerability and stressful or traumatic life experiences on a regulatory system involving the hypothalamus (a region of the brain) and two glands, the pituitary and the adrenal glands. Referred to as the *HPA axis*, this is proposed as a main site where genetic and environmental influences may converge to cause many mental disorders.[45]

What is not in doubt is that psychoactive drugs act by changing the levels of neurotransmitters in the patient's brain. After several weeks, this appears to prompt an effect that many physicians and patients interpret as beneficial: for example, anxious patients may feel calmer, and depressed patients more energized. However, in an attempt to compensate for the drug-induced imbalance, the brain begins altering its functions; for example, a brain flooded with serotonin may compensate by reducing the number of receptors for serotonin.

This means that getting off psychoactive medications can be challenging. For example, the brain of a person on anti-anxiety medications compensates by decreasing its own ability to manage anxiety, so if the medication is suddenly withdrawn, the person's anxiety can skyrocket. A similar effect is seen with antidepressants, antipsychotics, and other psychoactive drugs. For this reason, withdrawal from any psychoactive medication must be done very gradually, allowing time for the brain to restore receptor numbers and other aspects of its normal functioning.[47]

We discuss specific medications and other treatment options for the most common mental disorders in the next section.

Mood Disorders

Mood disorders are chronic, pervasive emotional states that significantly alter the person's thoughts, behavior, and normal functioning.

Depressive Disorders

The term *depression* refers to a mood state most commonly characterized by sadness. Though we have all felt depressed or lost interest in things that normally engage us, these feelings are usually temporary and in reaction to a sad event or loss. However, when a person is diagnosed with a **depressive disorder,** these feelings are more profound and long term, and interfere with daily life and normal functioning. Approximately 18 million, or about 8%, of adult Americans suffer from a depressive disorder every year.[39] The World Health Organization estimates that by the year 2020, depressive disorders will be the second most common health problem in the world.[48]

The most basic symptom of depressive disorders is persistent sadness. Other symptoms are:

- A feeling of being slowed down or lacking energy
- Feelings of helplessness, hopelessness, meaninglessness, or "emptiness"
- Feelings of worthlessness or guilt
- Loss of interest in school, work, or activities you once enjoyed
- Social withdrawal
- Difficulty thinking clearly or making decisions
- Sleep disturbances
- Changes in eating habits, eating more or less than you used to
- Restlessness, irritability
- In the most severe cases, recurring thoughts of death or suicide

Depressive disorders also often occur in conjunction with anxiety disorders and substance abuse.[39]

mood disorder Any chronic, pervasive emotional state that significantly alters the person's thoughts, behaviors, and normal functioning.

depressive disorder A mental disorder usually characterized by profound, persistent sadness or loss of interest that interferes with daily life and normal functioning.

Types of Depressive Disorders

Two of the most common forms of depressive disorder are major depressive disorder and dysthymic disorder.

Major Depressive Disorder. Also called *unipolar depression*, **major depressive disorder** affects more than 6% of American adults in a given year.[39] It is diagnosed when someone consistently experiences five or more depressive symptoms, including either depressed mood or loss of interest or pleasure, for at least 2 weeks straight.[49] In those cases, the person is said to be experiencing a "major depressive episode." These prolonged and severe symptoms prevent normal functioning. They can interfere with or completely impair a person's ability to study, work, eat, sleep, maintain relationships, and feel pleasure or joy. A major depressive episode may happen only once in a person's life, and may be prompted by the death of a loved one, job loss, divorce, or another stressful experience. In some people, the disorder occurs several times.

major depressive disorder (major depression) A type of depressive disorder characterized by experiencing five or more symptoms of depression, including either depressed mood or loss of interest or pleasure, for at least 2 weeks straight.

dysthymic disorder (dysthymia) A milder, chronic type of depressive disorder that lasts 2 years or more.

seasonal affective disorder (SAD) A type of depressive disorder caused by fewer hours of daylight during the winter months.

Students and teachers talk about how the pressures of college can lead to depression: www.depressioncenter.org/video/TheViewFromHere/default.asp.

Dysthymic Disorder. Also called *dysthymia,* **dysthymic disorder** is characterized by the same depressive symptoms listed earlier; however, the symptoms tend to be milder, and are chronic, occurring on a majority of days for at least 2 years in adults (1 year in children). The person may experience several days or weeks without symptoms, but not longer than 2 months. Those with dysthymia are more likely to suffer a major depressive episode in their lifetime. This type of depression is less common, affecting about 1.5% of American adults in a given year.[39]

Causes of Depressive Disorders

Depressive disorders can strike for a variety of reasons that are complex and interrelated; it is rarely possible to attribute a particular instance to a single source. When depressive disorders run in families, the pattern is likely influenced by both genetics and certain learned behaviors family members pass from one generation to the next. Earlier we mentioned the theory that genetic inheritance and stressful or traumatic life experiences affect a regulatory system called the HPA axis. Although researchers don't yet understand how, or to what extent, it seems clear that depressive disorders do arise from the interaction of several genes along with external influences.[50] Genetics alone will not cause depression. Indeed, the tendency toward depression and other mental disorders in minority groups is thought to be due to social determinants such as discrimination. (See the **Diversity & Health** box on page 40 for more information.)

There are several ways in which physical or biochemical problems can lead to depressive disorders as well. People with chronic pain or prolonged illness, for example, can experience a depressive disorder. Irregular hormone levels can also be a factor, which is why doctors will often test a patient's thyroid, a gland that regulates and secretes hormones, before diagnosing a depressive disorder. Paradoxically, both antidepressants and anti-anxiety medications can produce major depressive episodes. Even certain medications for physical illnesses can prompt them, and substance abuse is a common trigger.

External events linked specifically to depressive disoders include traumatic events, financial problems, and academic and career pressures. People with low self-esteem or a pessimistic view of the world also are at increased risk. If a person's network of emotional support is limited, or if it changes following the loss of a loved one, the person may be especially vulnerable.

Experiencing fewer hours of daylight during the winter months can lead to a form of depression known as **seasonal affective disorder (SAD).** SAD is normally worse in winter months and improves in the summer, and it is more common for people living in higher latitudes, where winter days are shorter and darker. Treatment for SAD usually involves *light therapy*—sitting near a special lamp that mimics sunlight (not a sun-tanning lamp)—for a certain length of time each day.

Depressive Disorders in Men and Women

Approximately 6 million men and 12 million women suffer from depressive disorders in any given year.[51] The causes and symptoms may vary between sexes.

Women and Depression. Until adolescence, girls and boys experience depressive disorders at about the same rate.[51] But after puberty, women's rates of both major depressive disorder and dysthymia rise relative to men's. Women are also more likely to have feelings of guilt when they are depressed, and depressive disorders in women are more likely to be associated with anxiety disorders and eating disorders than in men.[52]

Scientists continue to examine why there is an increased rate of depressive disorders in women. Physical factors may be partially to blame. Women experience hormonal changes in connection with the menstrual cycle, pregnancy, childbirth, the postpartum period, the years just before menopause, and menopause. These hormonal shifts appear to increase the risk of depressive disorders, but again, no precise cause for this increased risk is known.

In addition, a number of social and interpersonal factors increase women's stress, which contributes to depression. Women still tend to play a larger role than men in child care, while also pursuing professional careers. Women also experience higher rates of poverty and sexual abuse, and lower socioeconomic status, than men do. A few studies have also noted a tendency among women to pay more attention to difficulties and negative feelings, which can increase the risk for depressive disorders.[53] However, research in this area is not conclusive.

For women who have just had a baby, the combination of wildly shifting hormonal and physical changes, a radical change in lifestyle, the potentially overwhelming responsibility of a new baby, and a lack of sleep may contribute to *postpartum depression*. This is a depressive disorder that can make it difficult for a mother to bond with her new baby, or in the most serious cases, can promote thoughts of harming herself or her newborn. Women who have previously experienced depression or postpartum depression are more likely to suffer from it. When left untreated, postpartum depression can last up to a year. A recent report by the Centers for Disease Control estimates that about 12–20% of new mothers experience postpartum depression.[54]

Men and Depression. Depressive disorders in men are often underdiagnosed and under-treated. Because of that, the disparity in rates of depressive disorders between men and women may not actually be as

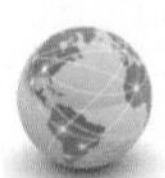

DIVERSITY & HEALTH

Mental Health Through the Lenses of Ethnicity and Sexuality

A deeply personal issue, mental health is shaped by our individual life experiences. As a result, race, ethnicity, and sexual orientation often have an effect on whether someone develops depression or other mental disorders and on the treatment that person receives.

Although there are not many large-scale studies on mental health in minority populations, it is known that in the United States many people of minority racial, ethnic, or sexuality status appear to be at greater risk for mental health problems than their Caucasian, heterosexual counterparts.[1, 2] A recent national survey shows that 8% of African Americans and 6.3% of Mexican Americans suffer from depression, compared with 4.8% of Caucasians.[3]

The tendency toward depression and other mental illness is no more inborn in minorities than in heterosexual Caucasians, but appears to be related to the obstacles and challenges that African Americans, Hispanics, Asian Americans, Pacific Islanders, Native Americans, and homosexuals face in society. Many minority groups experience higher rates of certain social factors that can contribute to mental illness, such as poverty, homelessness, incarceration, exposure to violence or trauma, refugee status, and childhood placement in foster care.[1] In addition, feelings of discrimination can exacerbate mental health issues. A recent study found that the increased likelihood of mental disorders in Latinos adapting to U.S. society is at least partially due to feelings that they are members of a group that is devalued and discriminated against.[4]

To make matters worse, minorities often lack access to culturally or linguistically appropriate mental health services. Only 2% of psychologists and psychiatrists in the United States are African American; most mental health providers in the United States speak only English; and the majority of mental health practitioners are not trained in the particular needs of homosexual clients.[1, 2] Minority groups are also less likely to have health insurance that would cover the cost of such services—for example, only 41% of Hispanics have private health insurance, compared with 75% of Caucasions.[5] Even when care is available, misdiagnosis of mental health disorders is more common in minorities than in Caucasians, and cultural stigmas against mental illnesses or distrust of mental health care can lead to underreporting of mental health problems or reliance on less-effective traditional remedies rather than medical treatment.

If you are interested in learning more about culturally compatible mental health services on your campus, contact your student health center or ask your health instructor.

References: **1.** "Mental Health: Culture, Race, and Ethnicity"; a supplement to "Mental Health: A Report of the Surgeon General," by the U.S. Department of Health and Human Services, 2001, retrieved from http://www.surgeongeneral.gov/library/mentalhealth/cre/sma-01-3613.pdf. **2.** "Mental Health Fact Sheets," by the National Alliance on Mental Illness, NAMI Multicultural Action Center, 2007. **3.** "Depression in the United States Household Population 2005–2006," by the U.S. Department of Health and Human Services, 2008, NCHS Data Brief No. 7. **4.** "Attributions to Discrimination Among Latino/as: The Mediating Role of Competence," by L. Torres, 2009, *American Journal of Orthopsychiatry, 79* (1), 118–124. **5.** "The Uninsured: A Primer. Key Facts about Americans without Health Insurance," by The Henry J. Kaiser Family Foundation, 2007, retrieved from http://www.kff.org/uninsured/upload/7451-03.pdf.

Listen to a radio story on mental health in the African American community: www.npr.org/templates/story/story.php?storyId=87952114&ft=1&f=88201937.

large as reported. Some of the lack of recognition may arise from the different ways men express their illness. Rather than appearing sad, they may be irritable, fatigued, or extremely cynical. Men with a depressive disorder may also be especially prone to physical effects like digestive problems, sleep disturbances, sexual problems, and headaches. Men may also have a hard time accepting their depression out of fear of social stigmatization, feeling that "real men" should be tough and not subject to feeling sad.

But though men's depression may be harder to recognize than women's depression, treating it is equally important. One study found that men with a depressive disorder are not only more likely to develop heart disease than other men, but also to die from it.[53] Depressed men are also more likely than women to self-medicate through destructive behaviors such as drug and alcohol abuse, or to engage in reckless, risky behavior.[51] Depression is also a risk factor for suicide, and suicide is the seventh leading cause of death for males in the United States.[55]

Prognosis for Depressive Disorders

For decades, researchers have acknowledged that many people recover spontaneously from depressive episodes—if given adequate time. A 2001 study of patients wait-listed for treatment showed that nearly 20% had recovered on their own, within a few months.[56]

With treatment, more than 80% of people recover from a depressive disorder.[52] One of the first steps in getting treatment should be an evaluation by a medical doctor to check for any physical causes. If physical sources have been ruled out, several types of treatments can help depressed people get their lives back on track.

Psychotherapy

Talking with a trained counselor or psychologist can make all the difference for many people with a depressive disorder. Talk therapies such as cognitive-behavioral therapy or psychodynamic therapy (discussed shortly) encourage depressed people to open up about their thoughts, feelings, relationships, and experiences in order to recognize problems that underlie their depression and work to improve them. Talk therapy may be the best treatment option for mild to moderate depressive disorders.[51]

Antidepressants

For those who are severely depressed or suicidal, the health-care provider may suggest medication as an adjunct to talk therapies. Like most psychoactive drugs, antidepressants prompt a change in the levels of neurotransmitters—typically serotonin—in the brain. The most prescribed types of antidepressants are called *selective serotonin reuptake inhibitors (SSRIs)* because they inhibit neurons releasing serotonin from taking it back up again. This leaves more serotonin at the synapse. The SSRIs include drugs like fluoxetine (Prozac), citalopram (Celexa), and sertraline (Zoloft). Antidepressants do not relieve symptoms immediately, and patients must take regular doses for at least 2 to 4 weeks before experiencing an effect.

These medications are not addictive, but as explained earlier, abruptly stopping them can cause withdrawal symptoms or lead to a relapse of depression. It's very important that, if you decide to stop taking antidepressants, you taper them off gradually and under a physician's supervision.

Although many depressed people report that they have been helped by antidepressants, these medications do come with risks and uncertainties. The most common side effects are headache, dry mouth, insomnia, tremors, anxiety, sexual dysfunction, nausea, and diarrhea. Severe side effects are less common, but include panic attacks, hostility, mania, delusions, seizures, and suicidal thoughts. In the 1990s, studies began warning physicians and patients of the increased risk of teenage suicides after starting SSRIs. In 2005, the U.S. Food and Drug Administration (FDA) required all antidepressant labels to carry a warning that alerts consumers about the suicide risk among this population. In 2007, this warning was extended to include young adults up to the age of 24.

In addition to such concerns, researchers have begun to question the rigor of the study data underlying the claims of antidepressants' effectiveness. In 2008, John Ioannidis, an internationally recognized authority on medical research, published an analysis questioning the effectiveness of antidepressants, in which he concluded: "Short-term benefits are small and long-term balance of benefits and harms is understudied."[57] Among the flaws Ioannidis identified in current studies of antidepressants were manipulated study design, biased selection of study participants, and selective and distorted reporting of results.

In 2011, Irving Kirsch, a researcher at Harvard Medical School, published similar findings. Kirsch and his colleagues spent 15 years analyzing 38 published clinical trials of antidepressants. To understand Kirsch's research, you need to understand the **placebo effect.** In drug studies, some participants receive the drug being studied, whereas other participants receive a placebo—typically a sugar pill with no active ingredients. Kirsch discovered that, overall, placebos were 75% as effective as antidepressants in relieving depression. He also found that when patients were given "active placebos," such as sugar pills that caused a side effect like dry mouth commonly associated with the drug being studied, there was *no* difference in response between the drug and the placebo.[58]

placebo effect Improvement in illness symptoms induced by the study participant's belief that he or she is receiving treatment when no treatment is actually given.

Watch a 60 Minutes report on the role of the placebo effect in treating depressive disorders at www.cbsnews.com/8301-18560_162-57380893/treating-depression-is-there-a-placebo-effect/?tag=currentVideoInfo;videoMetaInfo.

Certainly many studies have concluded that, for people suffering from severe depression, a course of supervised drug therapy can be helpful.[59] Such studies suggest that the best path forward is for psychiatrists and patients to weigh carefully the risk/benefit equation.

Currently, 25–50% of college students seen in counseling and student health centers are taking an antidepressant.[60] If your doctor suggests that an antidepressant may help you, check out the **Practical Strategies for Health** for some important questions to discuss

STUDENT STORY

Dealing with Depression

"Hi, I'm Javier. I first realized that I had depression when I started taking pills. I suffer from migraines and the pills make me go to sleep so I was kind of addicted to them. I took them all the time and I was practically asleep 24-7. I stopped going to school and I failed a lot of classes because of that. And so I went to a doctor and he told me that I suffer from mild depression and that I needed to do something about it. I needed to stop the medication I was on and take the medication that he prescribed. It was pretty hard for me to accept it. I mean, most guys don't think that there's something wrong with them until, you know, life hits them."

1: Javier self-medicated with his migraine pills when he was depressed. What are some other signs that can indicate depression in men?

2: What options does Javier have to deal with his depression?

3: If you had a friend who was experiencing symptoms like Javier's, would you say something to him? What would you say?

Do you have a story similar to Javier's? Share your story at www.pearsonhighered.com/lynchelmore.

Practical Strategies for Health

Questions to Ask Before Starting an Antidepressant

If your doctor thinks you might benefit from taking an antidepressant, discussing the following questions might help you to decide whether or not it's the right option for you:

- Why do you believe that an antidepressant is the right choice for me?
- Why do you suggest this particular antidepressant for me?
- How would I know if the antidepressant is really working, and I'm not just experiencing the placebo effect?
- When would I feel its effects? What should I do while I wait for it to work?
- What are the side effects? Am I at risk for them?
- What should I do if I decide to take this drug, and start experiencing side effects?
- What is your practice for following up with your patients on the effects of the antidepressants you prescribe?
- When do you anticipate that I could stop taking it? What would the withdrawal process entail?

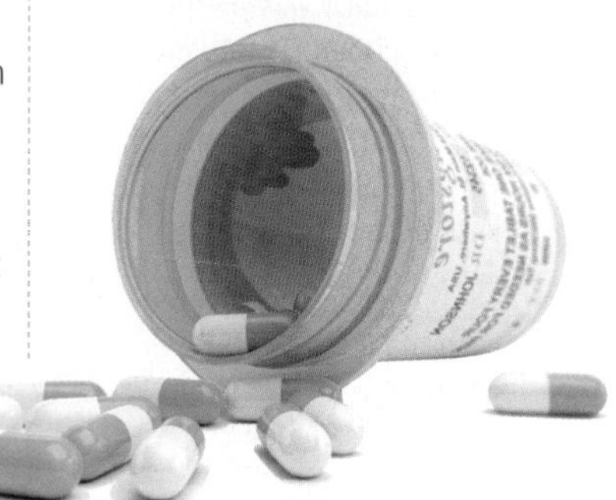

together. If you should decide against medication, talk to your doctor about other treatment options. These are discussed in detail later in this chapter.

Exercise

Can a daily aerobics class relieve your depression? It just might. Studies over two decades have concluded that regular exercise can relieve mild to moderate depression, and may play a supporting role in treating severe depression.[61] In one of many such studies, participants either engaged in a program of aerobic exercise, took an SSRI, or did both. After 16 weeks, depression had eased by essentially the same amount in 60–70% of the participants in all three groups. Moreover, a follow-up to that study found that exercise's effects lasted longer than those of antidepressants. Researchers checked in with 133 of the original patients 6 months after the first study ended. They found that the people who exercised regularly after completing the study, regardless of which treatment they were on originally, were less likely to have relapsed back into depression.

Why might exercise help? Researchers have long recognized that vigorous exercise prompts the body to produce certain hormones and neurotransmitters associated with increased feelings of well-being. Along with this "high," exercise increases strength and endurance, and builds self-esteem.[61] At the same time, it typically requires the person to enter into a different environment—the outdoors, or a fitness center—and often to interact with others. All of these factors can relieve isolation and help the person feel less stuck.

Bipolar Disorder

Bipolar disorder, also known as *manic-depressive disorder,* is characterized by occurrences of abnormally elevated mood (or *mania*) alternating with depressive episodes, with periods of normal mood in between. Mania can cause increased energy and decreased need for sleep, an expansive or irritable mood, impulsive behavior, and unrealistic beliefs or expectations. Manic people's thoughts race, their speech is rapid, their attention span is low, and their judgment is poor. Extreme manic episodes can sometimes lead to aggression or psychotic symptoms such as delusions and hallucinations. The alternating depressive episodes can be terrible, leading to thoughts of suicide.

Many people experience their first bipolar episode after abusing marijuana, stimulants, or other illicit drugs.[62] Others attempt to self-medicate with alcohol or other drugs, a habit that can make their symptoms worse and also make it harder for health-care providers to identify that they are bipolar. A psychotic break can be the first sign of bipolar disorder in some people.

Bipolar disorder usually develops in the late teens or early adult years and at least half of all cases start before the age of 25. It occurs equally among both sexes and in all races and ethnic groups.[63] The disorder has a tendency to run in families, and scientists are looking for genes that may increase a person's likelihood of developing the illness. However, most agree that many different genes are likely to act along with external factors to produce the illness.

Although bipolar disorder was once considered exceedingly rare, affecting no more than 1 in 5,000 Americans, it is now estimated to affect approximately 2.6% of the U.S. population.[39, 43] Why the rate spike? No one knows for sure, but one suspect is the increased use of prescription stimulants such as Ritalin among children diagnosed with attention deficit hyperactivity disorder (ADHD, discussed shortly). In 2006, the FDA issued a memorandum on the risk of "psychiatric adverse events," which include psychosis (loss of contact with reality) and mania, associated with drug treatment of ADHD.[64] The report stated that, although the numbers of episodes of such events with drug treatment were small, they occurred with all but one of the several ADHD drugs tested. In contrast, the FDA concluded, "the complete absence of such events with placebo treatment was notable."

bipolar disorder (manic-depressive disorder) A mental disorder characterized by occurrences of abnormally elevated mood (or mania), often alternating with depressive episodes, with periods of normal mood in between.

The most common treatment for bipolar disorder is a mood-stabilizing drug such as lithium. Anticonvulsant medications and antidepressants may be prescribed as well. Before the advent of such treatments, bipolar disorder was not usually considered a disabling condition. According to a 2007 review study, as many as 85% of bipolar patients in the first half of the 20th century regained complete functioning and returned to work. Now, only about 33% of patients avoid disability.[65] No conclusions from this study can yet be drawn, but clearly, more research is needed to tease out the factors behind the dramatic surge in disability among bipolar patients.

Hear people with bipolar disorder discuss their condition: www.webmd.com/bipolar-disorder/bipolar-tv/default.htm.

Anxiety Disorders

Anxiety disorders cover a wide range of conditions characterized by persistent feelings of fear, dread, and worry. They are the most common mental health problems among American adults, affecting over 40 million people each year.[39] Anxiety disorders frequently occur in conjunction with depressive disorders or substance abuse problems, and anxiety—ranging from nervousness to panic attacks—is a common side effect of many antidepressant medications.[39]

Generalized Anxiety Disorder (GAD)

People who suffer from **generalized anxiety disorder (GAD)** feel chronic anxiety, exaggerated worry, and pessimism, even when there is little or nothing to provoke it or they know they are overreacting. People with GAD develop a continuous cycle of worrying that can be difficult to break. They worry about common things and even when the concerns are valid, they worry to excess. GAD is diagnosed when this excessive worry lasts at least 6 months. Physical symptoms that often accompany the anxiety include fatigue, headaches, muscle tension, muscle aches, difficulty swallowing, trembling, and nausea. GAD affects about 6.8 million adult Americans and about twice as many women as men.[39] It usually develops gradually, with the highest risk of onset between childhood and middle age. It is often accompanied by depression, other anxiety disorders, or substance abuse.

Panic Attacks and Panic Disorder

Panic attacks are sudden feelings of terror that strike without warning. Symptoms include chest pain, shortness of breath, dizziness, weakness, and nausea. Panic attacks usually induce a sense of unreality and fears of impending doom, losing control, or dying, even though there is no rational reason for the person to believe something bad might happen. Panic attacks usually go away on their own in less than 10 minutes, and are sometimes much shorter. Although people experiencing panic attacks often truly fear that they might die, panic attacks will not kill you.

Many people have just one panic attack and never have another, but those experiencing repeated panic attacks may have **panic disorder.** Panic disorder affects about 6 million adults in the United States and is twice as common in women as men.[66] It often begins in late adolescence or early adulthood, and the susceptibility appears to be inherited.

A debilitating symptom of panic disorder is the dread of the next panic attack. People with panic disorder may begin to fear or avoid places where they have suffered a panic attack in the past, which can progressively restrict their mobility and even make it difficult for them to seek and receive treatment. This avoidance causes about a third of the people who suffer from panic disorder to develop *agoraphobia,* the fear of being places where they cannot quickly leave or where they cannot quickly receive help should they have a panic attack. Agoraphobia can eventually leave victims virtually housebound.[66]

anxiety disorders A category of mental disorders characterized by persistent feelings of fear, dread, and worry.

generalized anxiety disorder (GAD) An anxiety disorder characterized by chronic worry and pessimism about everyday events that lasts at least 6 months and may be accompanied by physical symptoms.

panic attacks Episodes of sudden terror that strike without warning.

panic disorder A mental disorder characterized both by recurring panic attacks and the fear of a panic attack occurring.

social anxiety disorder (social phobia) An anxiety disorder characterized by an intense fear of being judged by others and of being humiliated by your own actions, which may be accompanied by physical symptoms.

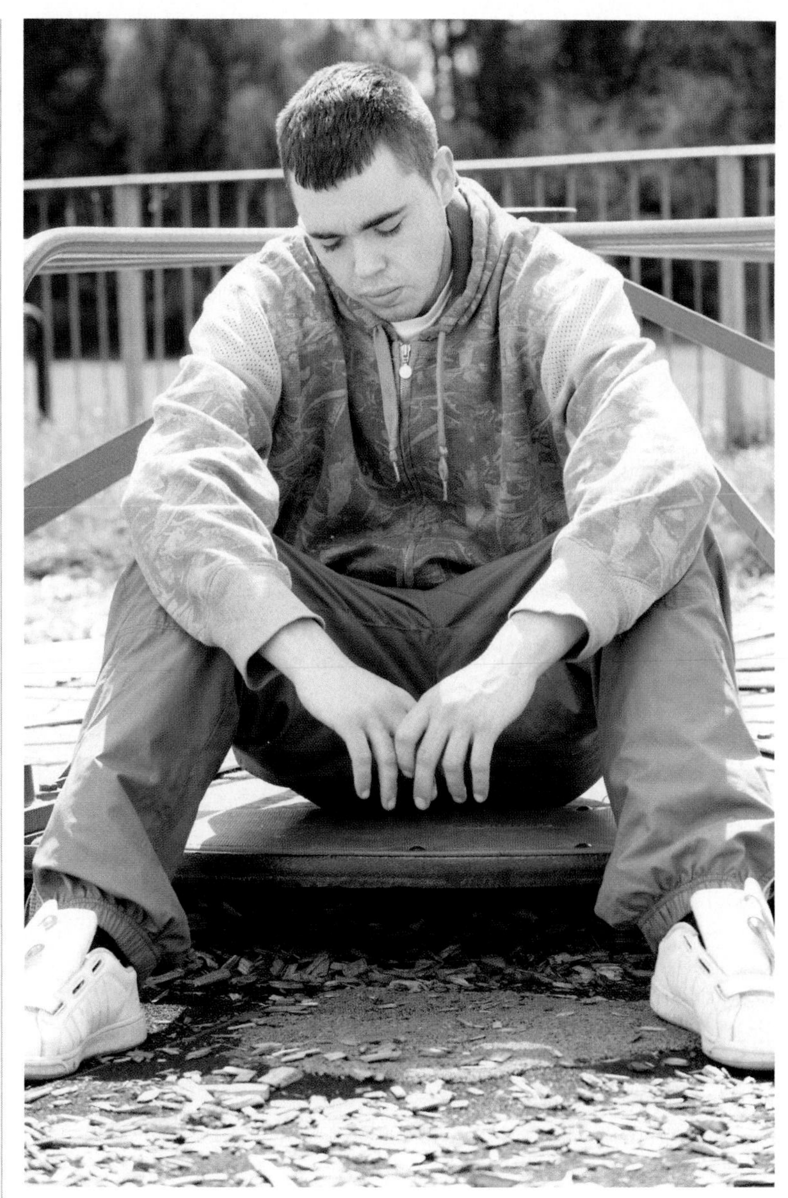

Social anxiety disorder can cause people to isolate themselves from others.

Social Anxiety Disorder

Social anxiety disorder, also called *social phobia,* typically involves an intense fear of being judged by others and of being humiliated by your own actions. It can be accompanied by physical symptoms such as sweating, blushing, increased heart rate, trembling, and stuttering. It may strike only in certain situations—for instance, speaking in public or eating in front of others—but in its most severe form a person might experience the symptoms any time he or she is around other people.[67] Social anxiety disorder affects about 15 million adults in the United States, and women and men are equally likely to develop it.[67]

This condition can be debilitating—leading people to avoid social situations even if doing so hurts them professionally or personally. In one survey of people with social anxiety disorder, 87% said their condition had a negative effect on personal relationships, 75% said it harmed their ability to perform normal daily activities, and 73% said it impaired their satisfaction with work.[68] Some sufferers try to self-medicate to reduce the anxiety, leading to drug and alcohol abuse.

In rare instances, people with social anxiety eventually blend their feelings of isolation and withdrawal with anger. The resulting mix, a phenomenon psychologists call *cynical shyness,* is more common in boys and men, and may be a factor in some episodes of violence at schools and other social environments.[69] If you experience social anxiety or isolation at a level that feels debilitating or makes you angry, seek professional help.

Phobias

Many people have an irrational fear of something—such as mice or spiders—that poses little or no actual danger. A **phobia** is similarly irrational, but so extreme as to be disabling. Phobias are common, and the usual age of onset is childhood to late adolescence. Women are twice as likely to suffer from phobias as men, and African Americans are more likely to suffer from phobias than Caucasians.[70] The American Psychiatric Association classifies simple phobias into five categories:[49]

- **Animal phobias.** Triggered by animals or insects, such as cats (ailurophobia) or spiders (arachnophobia).
- **Natural environment phobias.** Triggered by objects in the environment, such as heights (acrophobia) or water (hydrophobia).
- **Situational phobias.** Triggered by being in specific situations, such as on bridges (gephyrophobia) or in small confined spaces (claustrophobia) or in the dark (nyctophobia).
- **Blood, injection, or injury phobias.** Triggered by witnessing an invasive medical procedure, such as an injection (trypanophobia) or by witnessing an injury or blood.
- **Other phobias.** Triggered by some other stimulus, such as the number 13 (triskaidekaphobia) or clowns (coulrophobia).

Obsessive-Compulsive Disorder (OCD)

People with **obsessive-compulsive disorder (OCD)** have repeated and unwanted thoughts (obsessions), which cause them to develop rituals (compulsions) in an attempt to control the anxiety produced by these thoughts. The obsessions tend to be overblown or unrealistic worries, such as extreme concern about contamination by germs, fear of home intruders, or even fear of certain numbers, letters, or colors. The rituals provide brief relief from anxiety, even though the sufferer often knows they are meaningless.

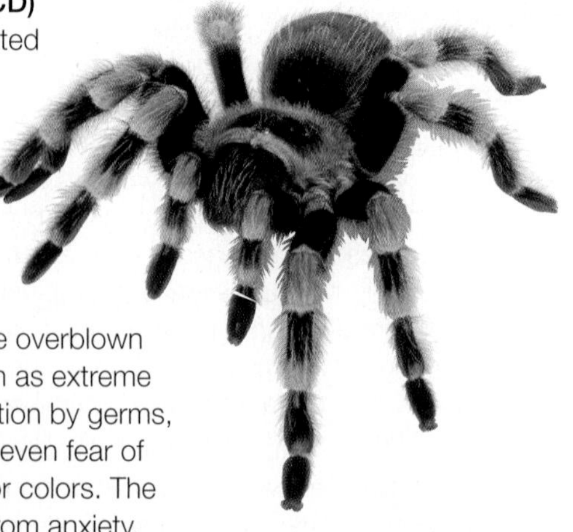

Fear of **spiders** is a common phobia.

In many cases, the rituals end up controlling the person's life. Although sufferers might be distressed, embarrassed, or inconvenienced by them, they cannot resist completing them. For example, a student obsessed with germs and sickness may develop hand-washing rituals that are so extensive that he is unable to leave his apartment to get to class on time. Other common rituals include the compulsion to repeatedly check things, touch things (in a certain order or a certain number of times), horde unnecessary items, or count things. Occurring equally in men and women, OCD affects 2.2 million adults in the United States.[39] First symptoms of OCD frequently appear in childhood or adolescence, and it is often diagnosed concurrently with eating disorders, other anxiety disorders, or depression.

Sufferers of OCD tell their stories: www.nytimes.com/interactive/2009/09/24/health/healthguide/TE_OCD.html?ref=health.

Post-Traumatic Stress Disorder (PTSD)

After a traumatic event, people sometimes feel recurrent fear, anger, and depression, a condition known as **post-traumatic stress disorder (PTSD).** Events that commonly cause PTSD are war, child abuse, natural disasters, automobile accidents, or being the victim of a violent crime. Currently, for example, some college campuses are offering veterans returning from military service in Afghanistan or Iraq specialized counseling services for PTSD.

People with PTSD often startle easily, feel numb emotionally, and can become irritable or even violent. They tend to obsessively relive the trauma in flashbacks or dreams, and will avoid places or experiences that might remind them of the traumatic event. PTSD can be accompanied by depression, other anxiety disorders, and substance abuse.

About 7.7 million adults in the United States experience PTSD each year, but it can strike children as well.[39] The condition strikes women more than men. Factors that increase the likelihood of developing PTSD are how intense the trauma was, how long

phobia An extreme, disabling, irrational fear of something that poses little or no actual danger.

obsessive-compulsive disorder (OCD) An anxiety disorder characterized by repeated and unwanted thoughts (obsessions) that lead to rituals (compulsions) in an attempt to control the anxiety.

post-traumatic stress disorder (PTSD) An anxiety disorder characterized by recurrent fear, anger, and depression occurring after a traumatic event.

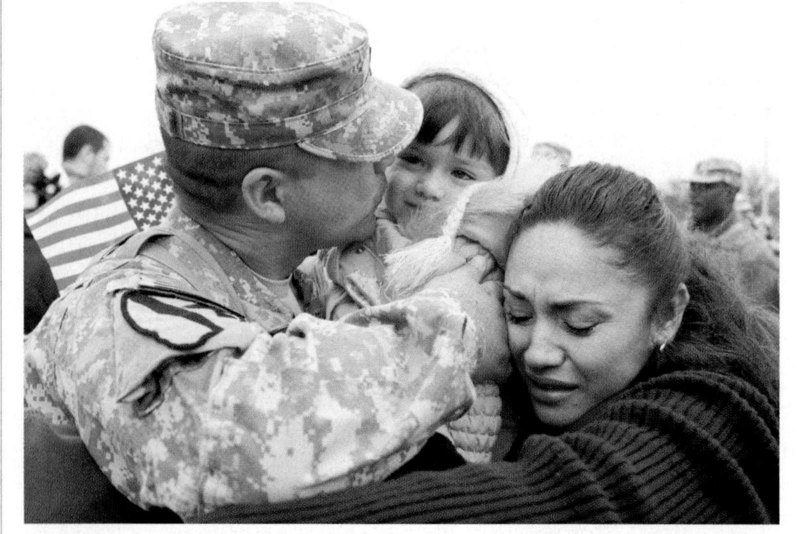

Soldiers returning home from war can often suffer from **PTSD.**

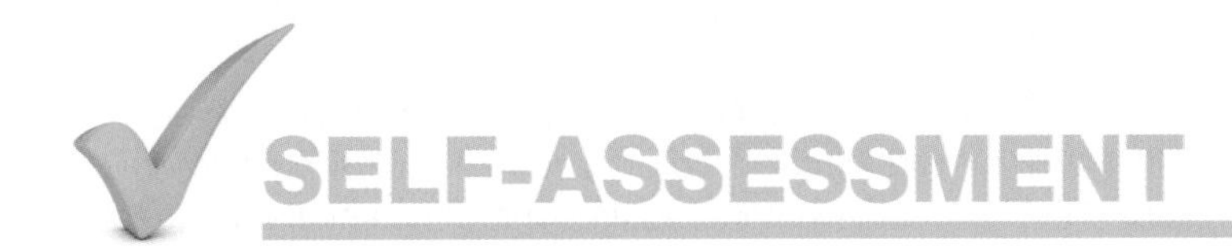

Anxiety Assessment

Instructions: How has each of these symptoms disturbed or worried you during the last seven days? Circle the most appropriate score relating to your state.

0 = Never 1 = A little 2 = Moderately 3 = A lot 4 = Extremely

	Symptom	Score
1.	Nervousness or shaking inside	0 1 2 3 4
2.	Nausea, stomach pain, or discomfort	0 1 2 3 4
3.	Feeling scared suddenly and without any reason	0 1 2 3 4
4.	Palpitations or feeling that your heart is beating faster	0 1 2 3 4
5.	Significant difficulty falling asleep	0 1 2 3 4
6.	Difficulty relaxing	0 1 2 3 4
7.	Tendency to startle easily	0 1 2 3 4
8.	Tendency to be easily irritable or bothered	0 1 2 3 4
9.	Inability to free yourself of obsessive thoughts	0 1 2 3 4
10.	Tendency to awaken early in the morning and not go back to sleep	0 1 2 3 4
11.	Feeling nervous when alone	0 1 2 3 4

HOW TO INTERPRET YOUR SCORE

If you indicated scores of 3 or 4 to 5 or 6 questions, your anxiety level is significant and you should consider different strategies such as better health practices, or adding relaxation techniques or physical exercise to your daily routine. If you indicated scores of 3 or 4 in all your answers, your level of anxiety is critical and you should consult your doctor.

Source: "Anxiety Self-assessment Questionnaire" used by permission of the Mental Illness Foundation, Montreal.

Take this self-assessment online at www.pearsonhighered.com/lynchelmore.

it lasted, how close to the event the victim was, whether the victim was injured or someone they were close to died, how in control of events the victim felt, and how much help or support the victim received after the event.[71]

Listen to soldiers talk about PTSD in their own words: www.youtube.com/watch?v=bsFg8wZul-4 and www.pbs.org/wgbh/pages/frontline/shows/heart/view.

Treating Anxiety Disorders

Cognitive-behavioral therapy (discussed shortly) is effective at teaching people with anxiety to recognize and redirect anxiety-producing thought patterns. One effective treatment, called *exposure therapy* or *systematic desensitization,* encourages patients to face their fears head-on. For instance, if a student with OCD fears dirt and germs, part of his therapy might involve getting his hands dirty and waiting progressively longer amounts of time before washing them. The therapist will help him work through his anxiety while his hands are dirty, and eventually his reaction will become less severe.

Anti-anxiety medications such as the benzodiazepines (Valium, Xanax, etc.) exert a calming effect that can be helpful in the short term; however, like other psychoactive medications, they trigger compensatory reactions in the brain that, as a result, make the person more vulnerable to anxiety—including severe generalized anxiety, panic attacks, and agoraphobia—in the long term.[72]

Other Disorders

The first edition of the APA's *Diagnostic and Statistical Manual of Mental Disorders* (DSM), published in 1952, included just 106 disorders. The current edition (DSM-IV-TR) includes 365, and more are expected for the upcoming fifth edition, to be released in 2013. What accounts for this more-than-tripling of diagnoses? Check out the **Myth or Fact?** box for a quick look at the debate over whether or not the APA is redefining normal. In this section, we discuss just two more of the 365 mental disorders now recognized by the APA. We chose attention disorders because they are common in college students, and schizophrenia because it is the most common psychotic disorder, and typically first appears during adolescence or young adulthood.

Attention Disorders

Attention disorders create difficulty with jobs that require sustained concentration, such as completing a single task over a long period of time or sitting still for extended periods. One study of children with attention disorders also found that they had difficulty forming social connections and durable friendships.[73] The most common form of attention disorder is **attention deficit hyperactivity disorder (ADHD),** which causes inattention, hyperactive behavior, fidgeting, and a tendency toward impulsive behavior.

The APA first identified ADHD as a disorder in 1980, and children diagnosed with ADHD became eligible for special educational services, paid for by federal funds, in 1991. Today the majority of diagnoses arise not because of problems noticed by parents, but because of teacher complaints.[74] National surveys estimate that almost 9% of children and teenagers have attention disorders.[75] Boys are more than twice as likely as girls to be diagnosed. Although attention disorders had been considered a disease of childhood, it is now thought that up to 60% of cases continue into adult life, and ADHD is diagnosed in about 4.5% of adults.[76] Among college students in the United States, 4.6% reported that they were diagnosed or treated for ADHD in the past year.[41]

College students with ADHD are at risk for poor academic performance.[77] They may also have problems at work and in personal relationships. They can have difficulty following directions, remembering information, and making deadlines; they may be chronically late, anxious, unorganized, or irritable. One study of adults with ADHD found that they could readily detect a problem, but preferred impulsive decisions over planning when trying to resolve it.[78] People with attention disorders are also at higher risk for tobacco use and substance abuse.

Options for treating attention disorders include cognitive-behavioral therapy and prescription medications. The medications typically prescribed to treat ADHD are stimulants such as methylphenidate (Ritalin or Concerta) or amphetamine/dextroamphetamine (Adderall). These drugs affect how the brain controls impulses and regulates attention.[79] Side effects include agitation, irritability, and anxiety, as well as insomnia, headache, nausea, stomachache, and loss of appetite significant enough that children taking the drugs long term commonly experience slowed growth. Also, as noted earlier, the FDA has warned that use of these drugs increases the risk for "adverse events" such as episodes of psychosis and mania.

attention disorders A category of mental disorders characterized by problems with mental focus.

attention deficit hyperactivity disorder (ADHD) A type of attention disorder characterized by inattention, hyperactive behavior, fidgeting, and a tendency toward impulsive behavior.

In 2009, a national survey found that 6.4% of college students use Adderall nonmedically; that is, without a prescription.[80] Nonmedical use of Ritalin and other ADHD drugs is estimated to be similar or even higher. Typically, students use these drugs to help them study longer; however, students also complain that the drugs take away their own coping skills and work ethic.[81] Moreover, the U.S. Department of Justice warns that these drugs have the same potential for abuse and addiction as illicit stimulants.[82]

schizophrenia A severe mental disorder characterized by inaccurate perceptions of reality, an altered sense of self, and radical changes in emotions, movements, and behaviors.

ADHD medications may improve social adjustment or academic performance for some children. A 2007 study found that children taking these medications were less likely to be held back a grade.[83] However, other studies suggest that academic benefits are not maintained over the long term.[79] A 2010 study following nearly 800 children for 12 months found that, although the use of prescription ADHD medications such as Ritalin prompted higher ratings of students' behavior from parents and teachers, the students' actual performances in reading and math were unimproved.[84] The researchers concluded that improving academic achievement requires more than simply increased focusing. It requires learning new skills and making creative leaps, abilities that may actually be impaired when the brain is exposed to stimulant drugs.

An unusual alternative treatment for ADHD has emerged in the last decade. At least two studies have shown increased levels of attention and decreased hyperactivity in students with ADHD who learn while sitting on stability balls (large fitness balls).[85]

Schizophrenia

Schizophrenia is a severe, chronic, and potentially disabling mental disorder that is characterized by *psychosis*, abnormal thinking and loss of contact with reality. It affects about 1% of adults in the United States, but it occurs in 10% of people who have a first-degree relative (parent or sibling) with the disorder.[39, 86] Although there is a genetic risk

MYTH OR FACT?

Is the American Psychiatric Association Making Us Sick?

Is Andy a gifted little firecracker—or does he have ADHD? Are you homesick since going off to college—or do you have separation anxiety disorder?

The number of mental disorders the American Psychiatric Association (APA) identifies in its *Diagnostic and Statistical Manual of Mental Disorders* (DSM) has more than tripled over the past 50 years as the criteria according to which psychiatrists identify a patient as sick have expanded. In the DSM-5, diagnostic boundaries are expected to broaden even further, by including preliminary versions of disorders, and by increasing the use of the term "spectrum," for signs and symptoms that don't quite fit the standard diagnosis.[1]

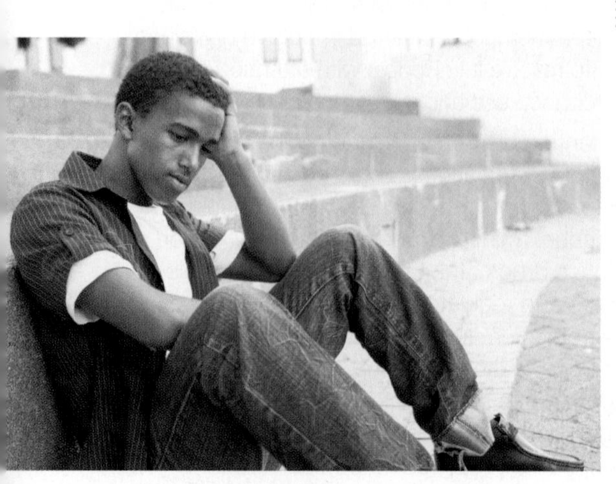

Is it just normal sadness . . . or a mental disorder?

How does the APA come up with its hundreds of diagnoses? Only the DSM authors know. The manual includes no citations of specific scientific studies to support its decisions. No wonder critics are asking whether or not the conditions it defines are valid mental disorders.[1, 2] "What I worry about most," said psychiatrist Allen Frances, emeritus professor at Duke University, "is that the revisions will medicalize normality and that millions of people will get psychiatric labels unnecessarily."[3]

As the DSM's diagnostic categories have expanded, so have the profits of the companies making the drugs to treat the new disorders. Does this coincidence simply reflect supply and demand—or does it suggest a potential conflict of interest? Should we be concerned that:

- Two researchers who are themselves working on the DSM-5 recently reported that 70% of DSM-5 task force members have direct financial ties to the pharmaceutical industry.[4]
- In 2006, the pharmaceutical industry provided 29% of the APA's $62.5 million in financing.[5]

Another major source of funding for the APA is the DSM itself, which, according to the APA's president, was developed to "facilitate diagnostic agreement" between clinicians, "given the need to match patients with the newly emerging pharmacologic treatments."[1] The retail price for the current edition of the DSM is $115. It has sold over a million copies.

References: **1.** "The Illusions of Psychiatry," by M. Angell, July 14, 2011, *The New York Review of Books*, pp. 20–22. **2.** "Distinguishing Between the Validity and Utility of Psychiatric Diagnoses," by R. Kendell & A. Jabloensky, January 2003, *American Journal of Psychiatry* 160, pp. 4–12. **3.** "Grief Could Join List of Disorders," by B. Carey, January 24, 2012, *The New York Times*, retrieved from http://www.nytimes.com/2012/01/25/health/depressions-criteria-may-be-changed-to-include-grieving.html?_r=1&ref=global-home. **4.** "Toward Credible Conflict of Interest Policies in Clinical Psychiatry," by L. Cosgrove, H. J. Bursztajn, D. J. Kupfer, & D. A. Regier, 2010, *Psychiatric Times, 26* (1). **5.** "Senate Investigations Spread to APA and ACCME," by A. Kaplan, 2008, *Psychiatric Times, 25* (10), retrieved from http://www.psychiatrictimes.com/display/article/10168/1290674.

for schizophrenia, researchers conclude that it is doubtful that genetics alone are sufficient to cause the disorder. Interactions between genetics, brain chemistry, and environment are thought to be necessary for the disease to develop.

People with schizophrenia often suffer from incorrect perceptions of reality, an altered sense of self, and radical changes in emotions, movements, and behaviors. They often have difficulty distinguishing what is real from what is imaginary, and have trouble functioning in society. Primary symptoms of schizophrenia include:[86]

- **Delusions.** False beliefs, such as thinking you possess unusual powers or believing that others are plotting against you.
- **Hallucinations.** False perceptions of reality, such as hearing or seeing things that are not there, most often voices.
- **Thought disorders.** Often called *disorganized thinking*—problems with thinking or speaking clearly or maintaining focus.
- **Movement disorders.** Agitated or repetitive body movements, or in some extreme cases becoming catatonic (immobile).
- **Reduction in professional and social functioning.** Social withdrawal, unpredictable behavior, poor hygiene, or paranoia can all impair social and professional function.
- **Inappropriate emotions.** Aloofness, a so-called "flat affect," or inappropriate or bizarre reactions to events.

Symptoms such as these usually appear in men in the late teens and early 20s and in women about a decade later. Research has shown that schizophrenia affects both sexes equally and occurs in similar rates in all ethnic groups.[86]

Although schizophrenia has a reputation of being incurable, both historic records and contemporary research studies have shown that many people do recover.[87, 88] Some even go on to successful, high-level jobs.

Suicide and Self-Injury

Attempting to cope with deep anguish, some people turn to self-injury or suicide.

Self-Injury

Self-injury occurs in the form of intentional, self-inflicted cuts, burns, or other injuries, without suicidal intent. Often performed in an effort to deal with overwhelming feelings, it provides the injurer with a moment of calm, but is usually followed by feelings of guilt and shame. Once largely hidden from public view, self-injury has become more prominent due to discussion of the practice on websites. One study of online self-injury discussions found hundreds of message boards and forums on the topic with thousands of members.[89] More than 5% of college students in the United States admit to performing self-injury in the past year, but the reliability of these statistics is questionable because most who do injure themselves conceal it.[41]

Self-injury often begins or occurs in adolescence. Although early research suggested that women were more likely than men to self-injure, more recent research has shown that rates are similar across sexes.[90] Therapy and medications can help self-injurers learn to deal with their difficult feelings more appropriately and stop their self-abuse. On the other hand, the use of certain medications, including some antidepressants and antipsychotics, is associated with an increased risk for self-injury.

Suicide

More than 32,000 people in the United States take their own lives every year, and for every death there are at least another eight attempted suicides.[91] College students are more likely than the general population to try to take their own lives, and suicide is the second leading cause of death on college campuses. More than 6% of students said they had seriously considered attempting suicide in the past year.[41] Although women attempt suicide two to three times more often than men, men are four times more likely to actually die by suicide, possibly because they choose more lethal means in their attempts.

Among college students, lesbian, gay, bisexual, and transgendered students have one of the highest risks for suicide. Factors contributing to this risk include verbal or physical harassment, discrimination, and lack of family or peer support and acceptance.[92]

Among ethnic groups, Native Americans and Alaska Natives have the highest overall suicide rates.[91] Caucasians are also at high risk.[91] Historically, African American teens and young adults have had lower suicide rates than their Caucasian counterparts, but their suicide rates have increased dramatically in recent decades. Now researchers predict that before the age of 17, 7% of African American females will attempt suicide.[93]

Another group that is at high risk for suicide is older adults. Caucasian males over the age of 85 actually have the highest suicide rate of any group in the United States.[91]

Causes and Warning Signs of Suicide

Several factors clearly play a role in driving up suicide risk. More than 90% of people who commit suicide in the United States have a diagnosable mental health or substance abuse problem.[39] In addition, financial problems, serious illness, and the loss of a loved one are frequently cited as catalysts. A family history of suicide, previous suicide attempts, having access to guns in the home, and a history of substance abuse also increase suicide risk. Ultimately, it seems that suicide becomes appealing to people when they feel hopeless about the direction of their life and helpless to change it.

Signs that a person may be considering suicide include:

- Statements that imply suicidal thoughts, such as "I don't have much to live for" or "You won't have to worry about me much longer"
- An inability to let go of grief
- A noticeable downturn in mood within the first few weeks of starting a new antidepressant medication
- Loss of interest in classes, work, hobbies, or spending time with friends and loved ones
- Expressions of self-hatred, excessive risk taking, or apathy toward one's own well-being
- Disregard for personal appearance
- Changes in sleep patterns or eating habits
- A preoccupation with thoughts or themes of death

Preventing Suicide

Don't assume that a person who talks of suicide is just having a bad day or seeking attention. Instead, let the person know you care and that you are there to help. Never be afraid to raise the subject. Offer to call a crisis hotline together, go to a counseling center, or head to the nearest emergency room. The National Suicide Prevention Lifeline is 1-800-273-TALK.

You can find suicide prevention help and resources at www.suicidepreventionlifeline.org.

STUDENT STORY

A Friend's Suicide

"Hi, I'm Kristina. In my senior year of high school one of my good girlfriends decided to take her own life. It was pretty devastating—emotionally, mentally, physically even. I don't think anyone expects, as a high-schooler, that one of their peers will commit suicide. At first I felt angry, and then it gradually hit me and I was very upset and cried all the time. I guess, after that all happened, the positive thing that came out of it was I had a closer relationship with my girlfriends and my family; we really watch out for each other and we say "I love you" more.

I just want people to know that nothing is bad enough to take your own life. Even if you feel like nothing's going right in your life, it doesn't mean that you can't turn those negative things into positive things. There are many problems that people have in their teenage years that they can't help, but they end up stronger people because of it."

1: Do you think that Kristina is right that young people don't expect one of their peers to commit suicide? Why or why not?

2: What do you think Kristina means about turning negative things into positive things? Have you ever turned a negative into a positive?

Do you have a story similar to Kristina's? Share your story at www.pearsonhighered.com/lynchelmore.

Getting Help for a Psychological Problem

If you or someone you know is ready to seek help for a psychological problem, you'll find many resources available.

Options on Campus and in Your Community

Most campuses offer a range of options to help address the mental and emotional pressures students face. These services may be provided for free or at low cost, or they may be covered by your insurance plan if you have one. Your campus health clinic or counseling center is a good place to start looking for help. No matter whom you consult initially, bear in mind that anxiety, depression, and other problems are common among college students and are not a sign of weakness or deficiency! What's more, seeking help is a sign of psychological health—it shows that you esteem yourself enough to reach out, and that you trust your community to respond effectively.

Maybe you're taking your health course remotely, or just don't feel comfortable accessing services on campus. No problem—you'll find many options for mental health services within your community. These include state and county services, which you can locate online or in your phone book, as well as community organizations. For example, look for your local chapter of Emotions Anonymous, a 12-step program for recovery from emotional distress and mental disorders that grew out of Alcoholics Anonymous and has been helping Americans for more than 50 years. And don't forget to check your local paper for calendar listings of meetings of other mental health support groups.

Clinical Options

Whether you begin at your campus health clinic, or by speaking to your primary health-care provider, it's important to be aware of the full range of your clinical options.

Types of Mental Health Professionals

The following are the types of licensed professionals who most commonly work with people experiencing psychological distress:

- **Counselors.** Counselors have a master's degree in counseling or social work and focus on talk therapy. Counselors may lead group, family, or individual therapy sessions, as well as recommend services available within your community.
- **Psychologists.** Psychologists have a doctoral degree and provide talk therapy. Many have particular specialties, and they may lead group, family, or individual therapy sessions.
- **Psychiatrists.** Psychiatrists have a medical degree and usually focus on the medical aspects of psychological issues. They can prescribe medication and may have admitting privileges at local hospitals. Psychiatrists and psychologists often work together to provide a person a full range of care.

See **Consumer Corner: Choosing a Therapist Who's Right for You** for information about what to discuss before picking a therapist.

Once you have found a mental health professional, the real work begins. Your treatment can succeed only if you are open and honest about your thoughts, emotions, and what is going on in your life. Therapy can sometimes bring up sad or uncomfortable feelings, but that isn't necessarily a bad thing—it can be a sign that you are working through issues. However, if at any point something happens in therapy that you don't like, say so. Therapists should be eager to work with you to resolve any problems that come up.

Types of Therapy

The type of therapy you choose should depend on your specific condition and your preferences. Some people benefit from a combination of several types of therapy.

Cognitive-Behavioral Therapy. According to the National Association of Cognitive-Behavioral Therapists, **cognitive-behavioral therapy (CBT)** is a form of psychotherapy that emphasizes the role of thinking (cognition) in how we feel and what we do. There are many approaches to CBT, but all are based on the idea that our *thoughts* cause our feelings and behaviors, not external things, like people, situations, and events. The benefit of this fact is that when we can change the way we think, we end up feeling and acting better

cognitive-behavioral therapy (CBT) A form of psychotherapy that emphasizes the role of thinking (cognition) in how we feel and what we do.

behavior therapy A type of therapy that focuses on changing a patient's behavior and thereby achieving psychological health.

psychodynamic therapy A type of therapy that focuses on the unconscious sources for a patient's behavior and psychological state.

positive psychology A new field of psychology that focuses on increasing psychological strengths and improving happiness, rather than on psychological problems.

even if our situation does not change.[94]

One premise of CBT is that consistent dysfunctional thinking, sometimes called *cognitive distortion,* results in unwanted feelings and behaviors. See **Practical Strategies for Change: Spotting Destructive Thoughts** for tips on how to notice cognitive distortions that you may have.

In CBT, the therapist and patient work collaboratively to identify distorted, negative thinking and replace it with more positive, reinforcing thinking. Cognitive therapy is usually short term and focused, and is most effective in treating mood and anxiety disorders. Over the last two decades, CBT has also come to be recognized as an effective form of therapy for patients with schizophrenia.[95]

Behavior Therapy. Either under the umbrella of CBT or alone, **behavior therapy** focuses on changing learned behaviors as efficiently and effectively as possible. The core idea behind behavior therapy is that, once our behavior changes, our thoughts, feelings, attitudes, and moods will follow. Common behavioral therapy techniques include exposure therapy, which is gradual exposure to an anxiety-provoking situation paired with relaxation techniques; positive reinforcement, which encourages desired behaviors; and aversion therapy, or negative reinforcement that discourages unwanted behaviors. Behavioral therapy is often used for anxiety and attention disorders.

Psychodynamic Therapy. Also called *psychoanalysis*, **psychodynamic therapy** is founded on the idea that there are unconscious sources for a person's behavior and psychological state. Together, patient and therapist unearth unresolved conflicts buried in the unconscious, then talk through these conflicts in order to understand them and to change the ways in which they affect the patient today. In doing this, the relationship between the patient and therapist becomes highly important, often exposing the interpersonal problems in the patient's life. For example, if a patient tends to doubt others' caring, he or she may accuse the therapist of maintaining an uncaring attitude. Psychodynamic therapy can take time, sometimes 2 years or more, although contemporary psychodynamic therapy can be considerably briefer.

Research supports the effectiveness of psychodynamic therapy for a variety of disorders.[96] In addition, the evidence indicates that the benefits of psychodynamic treatment extend beyond relieving the initial distress to fostering inner resources that allow patients to lead freer and more fulfilling lives.

Positive Psychology. Positive psychology is an emerging field that focuses on increasing psychological strengths and improving happiness, rather than dwelling on psychological problems. This type of therapy aims to nurture in patients traits such as kindness, originality, humor, optimism, generosity, and gratitude. In positive psychology, you perform a variety of activities—such as noting three good things that happen to you each day—with the goal of increasing your happiness.[97]

On iTunes, search for Live Happy, an iPhone application that can walk you through positive psychology activities.

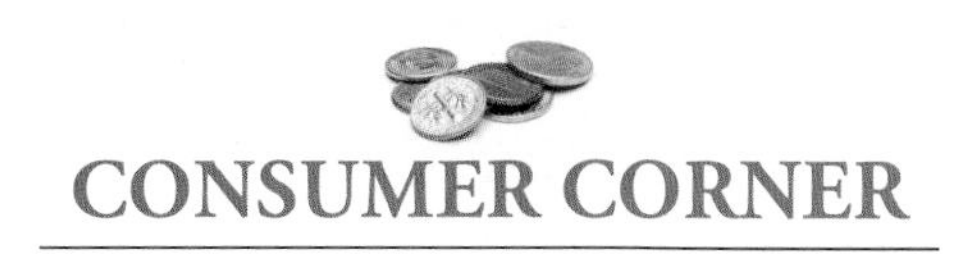

CONSUMER CORNER

Choosing a Therapist Who's Right for You

Therapy can help people with a variety of issues, but it's important to find a therapist with whom you feel comfortable and who is qualified to address your needs. Key points that you should address in your first discussion with a potential therapist are:

- Cost. Make sure you understand what the costs are and how they will be covered—whether it's low- or no-cost campus mental health care, outside care covered by an insurance plan, or paid directly out of your own pocket. If you are paying for care yourself, therapists will sometimes offer a sliding scale for fees, so be sure to ask.
- The therapist's credentials, education, and approach to therapy
- Areas of specialization that the therapist has or that you would prefer—for example, specializations in bipolar disorder, childhood trauma, cognitive therapy, and so on
- An overview of the problems you are experiencing and your goals for therapy
- The experience the therapist has in helping people with similar problems
- Whether or not you are taking or are interested in taking antidepressants or other medication. Keep in mind that psychologists and counselors cannot prescribe medication.
- Frequency and length of therapy sessions

The information that you get from this preliminary conversation, as well as your overall impression of the therapist, will help you determine whether you would like to undertake therapy with that person. Don't be afraid to have an initial consultation with a few different therapists or to switch to someone else if, after a few sessions, you don't feel comfortable.

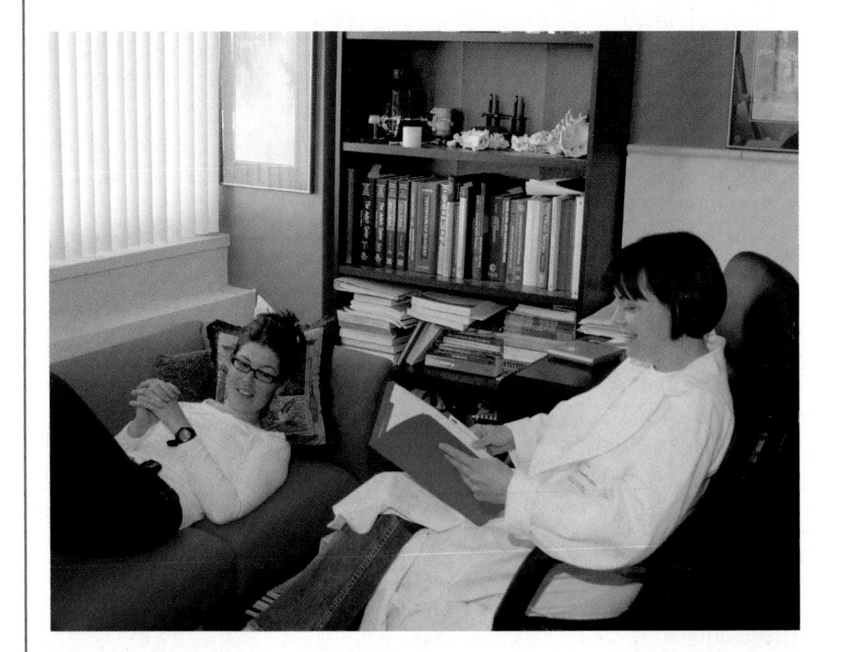

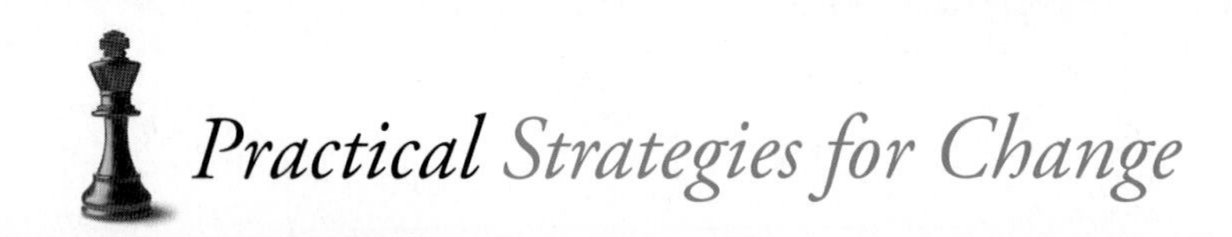

Practical Strategies for Change

Spotting Destructive Thoughts

Do you ever find yourself thinking thoughts like, "I *never* get things right!" or "I'm such a failure!"? If so, these cognitive distortions may be the sources of a bad mood or even a serious depression. Cognitive therapy can help you learn to challenge them. Here are some thought patterns to watch out for:

- **All-or-nothing thinking.** In all-or-nothing thinking there is no middle ground. You think of situations or yourself as either perfect or a complete failure.
- **Overgeneralization.** You make a general conclusion based on a single event or experience from the past. You see one negative event as a never-ending pattern of defeat.
- **Mental filter.** You dwell excessively on a single negative detail, although everything else is positive, so that your whole outlook is darkened.
- **Disqualifying the positive.** You reject positive experiences because they "don't count" for one reason or another.
- **Jumping to conclusions.** Without any definite facts to support it, you assume that other people are thinking or feeling negatively toward you. Or you predict that a situation will turn out badly and feel convinced that it is an already-established fact.
- **Magnification (catastrophizing) or minimization.** You exaggerate the importance of something minor (such as a poor grade on a quiz), predicting that it will trigger a whole chain of negative events. Or you minimize a significant positive event (such as acing the final exam), predicting that "it won't make any difference."
- **Emotional reasoning.** You assume that your negative emotions necessarily reflect the way things really are: "I feel it, so it must be true."
- **Should statements.** You tell yourself what you "should" do, and if you don't perform, you feel guilty. This can also be applied to other people; if they don't live up to the should statement, you can feel angry, frustrated, or resentful.
- **Labeling and mislabeling.** Instead of thinking of something in a balanced way, you attach labels to yourself or others, such as "I'm a loser," or "He's no good." Mislabeling involves describing an event with highly colored or emotionally loaded language.
- **Personalization.** You think that everything people do or say is in reaction to you; you think you are the cause of a negative external event that, in reality, you had nothing to do with.

Source: Adapted from *The Feeling Good Handbook,* by D. D. Burns, 1989, New York: William Morrow and Company, Inc.

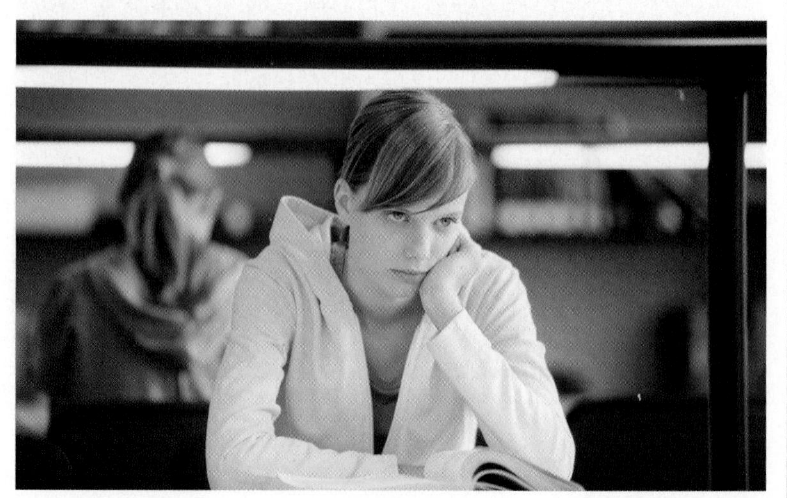

Other Clinical Options

One of the most commonly prescribed clinical options is, of course, pharmacologic therapy, which we have discussed with each specific disorder. In addition, although you might associate it with horror films, electroconvulsive therapy (ECT) is still sometimes used for severely ill patients who are not responsive to counseling or drug treatment. Formerly called *electroshock therapy*, ECT is administered by devices that transmit a jolt of electricity that induces seizures in the anesthetized patient. No one knows precisely how ECT produces therapeutic effects.

The FDA classifies ECT machines as high-risk devices because of the potential for significant adverse effects; most commonly, these are memory loss and cognitive impairment that may last for several months.[98] Some studies suggest that these effects may, in at least a percentage of patients, become permanent, although more rigorous research is needed. Despite the ongoing controversy over ECT, some psychiatrists support its use in patients with resistant suicidal depression and other severe mental disorders.

Complementary and Alternative Therapies

In addition, there is at least some scientific evidence that an herb called St. John's wort (*Hypericum perforatum*) may be effective in relieving mild to moderate depression.[99] However, St. John's wort may prompt side effects ranging from headache to anxiety, and can interfere with other medications. If you're considering using it, discuss it with your primary health-care provider first.

Massage therapy also appears to be effective in relieving anxiety and depression. Although massage should not be used to replace standard health care, it can be beneficial to many patients.[100]

Change Yourself, Change Your World

There are many steps you can take independently, among friends, and on campus to promote psychological well-being. Let's start with you.

Personal Choices

If you're feeling the need for a little psychological TLC, look no further. This section provides tips for self-care, building self-esteem and optimism, reaching out, and chilling out.

Take Care of Yourself

When you're experiencing mental or emotional distress, the basic tasks of daily life can feel overwhelming. Yet at such times self-care becomes more important than ever. If you're feeling on edge, be sure to:

- **Eat well.** Don't skip meals or binge on junk food. Calming your mind and emotions will be easier if your body isn't nutritionally stressed.
- **Get the right amount of sleep.** A regular schedule that includes 7–9 hours of quality sleep every night is important to both your physical and mental well-being. Despite your busy schedule as a college student, make sleep a priority. (See Chapter 4.) If you're depressed and find yourself sleeping in, know that the very act of getting out of bed can be an instant boost. Once you're up, open the curtains and windows, as letting in light and air will help improve your mood.
- **Get some exercise.** As noted earlier, exercise releases body chemicals that boost mood. Even a half-hour walk is likely to improve your

mood, clear your head, and make you feel better. Daytime exercise will also help make you tired and make it easier to sleep.

- **Set realistic goals.** Don't expect yourself to function at your regular level. Set smaller goals, and break big jobs up into small ones.
- **Take steps to build your self-esteem.** Cognitive-behavioral theory recognizes that there are things you can do to change the way you think and the way you act that will, as a result, change the way you feel. For suggestions, see the **Practical Strategies for Change: Building Self-Esteem.**

Learn Optimism

As with self-esteem, people tend to develop an optimistic view of life at a young age from their families and caregivers. But psychologist Martin Seligman assures us that we can learn optimism at any age. See **Practical Strategies for Change: Building Optimism** on page 52 for tips.

Reach Out

We discussed earlier how social support contributes to psychological health. Yet feelings of anxiety and despair can often cause you to prefer to be alone. If so, it's important to recognize a desire for isolation as a symptom of your distress. Defy it—and reach out. Remind yourself that mental and emotional concerns are common. Just as you would want a friend who's hurting to confide in you, your friends want to help. Talk to someone you trust, or if you'd prefer to confide in a professional, visit your campus counseling center. They can recommend therapists, or help you locate a support group that's right for you. Support groups are often free or low cost, and are usually led by a trained professional who can steer the group's interactions in positive ways.

Find online support at one of these websites: www.patientslikeme.com/mood/community; www.dailystrength.org; www.wellsphere.com/communities.

Chill Out

Psychological health also thrives when you withdraw your thoughts from the chaos of everyday life and spend at least a few minutes in stillness. For many people, stillness is initially uncomfortable—worries and other challenging thoughts can arise all too quickly. This is where a practice of prayer or meditation can help.

Prayer can take the form of repetition of a familiar passage, a dialogue with a higher power, or simply listening. One way some people approach prayer is by asking, "What is the Divine Mind knowing about me right now?" . . . and then listening for an answer. You can also use prayer to express gratitude, offer blessings to loved ones, grant or receive forgiveness, seek spiritual insights, or ask for guidance on how to conduct different aspects of your daily life. For many people, prayer brings comfort and clarity, decreases loneliness, and boosts the individual's ability to cope with challenges.

Prayer can have powerful effects on the body. For instance, prayer triggers the *relaxation response,* a state of relaxation defined by slowed metabolism, reduced blood pressure, slower breathing, decreased heart rate, and less active brain waves.[101] Evidence also suggests that prayer is associated with positive health outcomes in sick people.[102]

Another form of quiet contemplation practiced by both religious and non-religious people is meditation. Meditation can have different intended purposes, such as reaching higher states of consciousness, developing creativity and self-awareness, or simply achieving a more relaxed and peaceful state of mind.[103] For some, the practice of meditation is as simple as sitting quietly and focusing attention on a single idea, word, or symbol, or on their breath. Others find meditative contemplation in nature. This might mean a solitary walk through the park or getting up early to watch the sun rise.

Don't know how to meditate? Try one of these tools: www.mayoclinic.com/health/meditation/MM00623 or http://health.howstuffworks.com/wellness/stress-management/how-to-relieve-stress-in-daily-life2.htm.

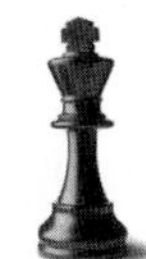

Practical Strategies for Change

Building Self-Esteem

- **Practice positive "self-talk."** If you criticize yourself in your head, stop. Instead, make a habit of complimenting yourself, or repeating positive affirmations.
- **Pat yourself on the back.** Notice when something you've done turns out well, and take a moment to congratulate yourself.
- **Listen to yourself.** What do you really want, need, and value? If you want others to listen to you, you need to understand and respect your own thoughts and feelings first.
- **Stretch your abilities.** Decide to learn something new, whether it's a school subject that seems intimidating or a sport you've never tried. Give yourself time to learn your new skill piece by piece, and then watch your talents grow.
- **Tackle your "to do" list.** Think about tasks you've been putting off, like calling a relative with whom you haven't spoken for a while or cleaning out your closet. Get a couple of them done each week. You'll be reminded of how much you can accomplish, and feel less distracted by loose ends.
- **Schedule some fun.** In your drive to finish your "to do" list, make sure you leave time in your schedule for fun. Don't wait for others to invite you to a party or a film—invite them first. If money is tight, suggest hitting the bike paths or hiking trails and get the added feel-good benefit of exercise.
- **Serve others.** There is no simpler, or more generous, way to build self-esteem than doing something nice for someone else. You'll both benefit.

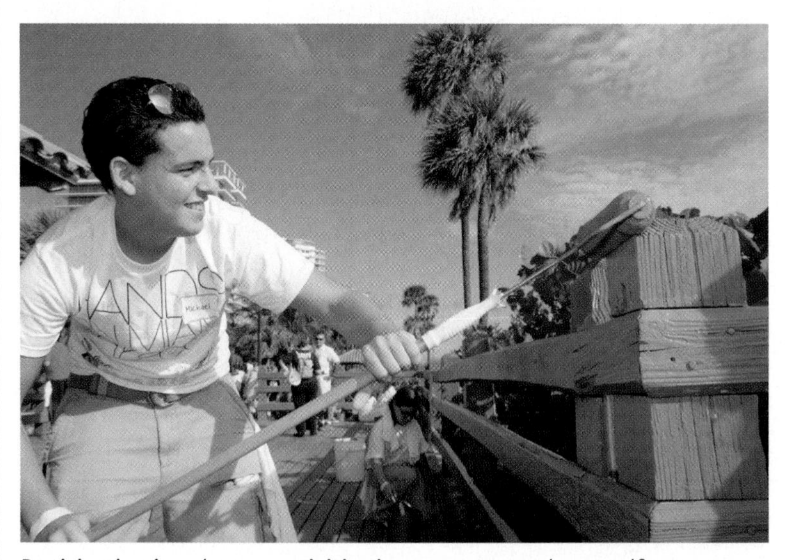

Participating in volunteer activities is a great way to boost self-esteem.

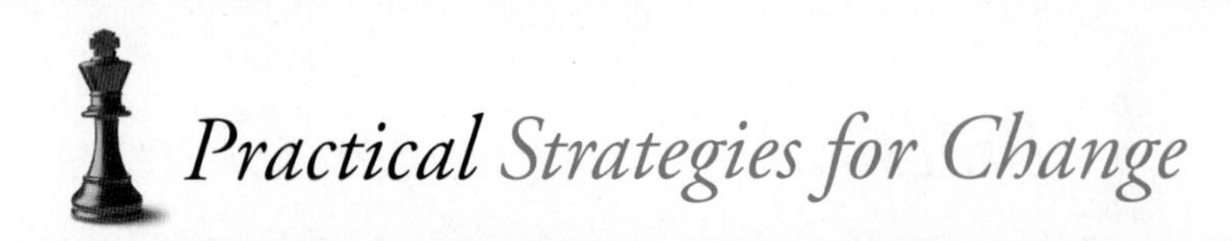

Practical Strategies for Change

Building Optimism

- **Notice when things go right.** When something works out for the better, take note. Recognizing when things go well will show you the likelihood of positive outcomes.
- **Learn from mistakes.** Everybody fails to reach a goal at some point. That doesn't mean that failure will happen again next time. Learn from what happened, and decide what you'll do differently in the future.
- **Challenge negative thoughts.** Are you really that hopeless at something? Is there truly no way to fix a problem? Chances are that things are not as bad as they seem.
- **Avoid absolutes.** Thinking about yourself or the challenges you face in black-and-white terms usually isn't helpful or realistic. Few things in life are all good or all bad.
- **Avoid doom scenarios.** Don't assume that because you flunked the test, you'll fail the course, won't get into grad school, and your life will be ruined. Instead, cut the film with a "but": "Okay, I flunked this one test, but . . . I can talk to the instructor about ways to make up some points."
- **Give yourself time.** When you are first hit with a disappointment, it's not always easy to step back and modify your thoughts. Take time to feel what you feel. Talk with friends, exercise, get some sleep. Then go back to these tips, and practice, practice, practice.

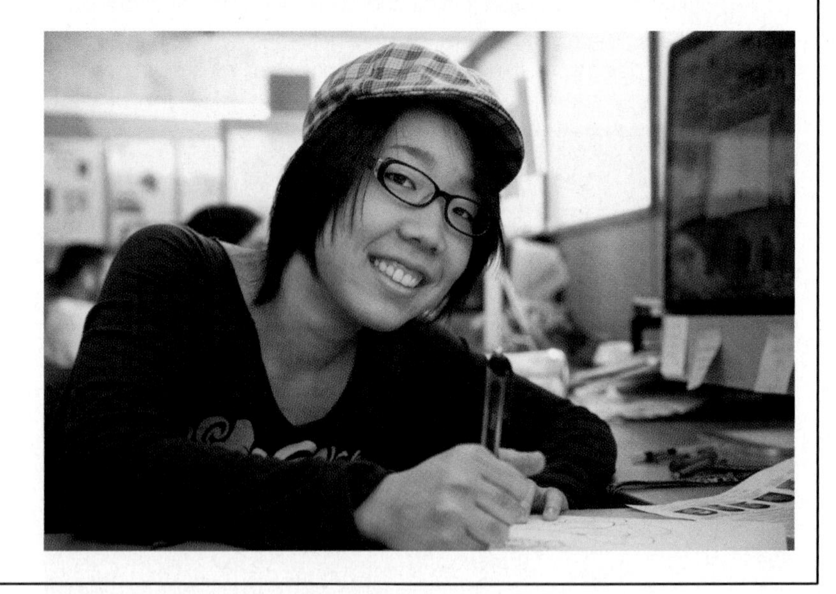

Helping a Friend

Earlier, we discussed what to do if you're concerned that a friend may be contemplating suicide. But how do you support a friend who's just generally down, or getting overwhelmed by anxiety, anger, or low self-esteem?

The first step is to get informed. Find out about what's going on—did your friend's arms get scratched when she tried to pet a neighbor's cat, as she claims, or is she cutting herself? Is your friend holing up in his dorm room because he's trying to finish a project, or is he depressed? Check your observations against those of mutual friends. If you agree there may be more going on than your friend is admitting to, then you may need to—gently but firmly—confront the person.

That's where the next step comes in: Listen, without judging. Acknowledge that your friend's pain is real for him or her. Don't dismiss it with assertions such as, "But your parents seem so understanding!" Such comments might only cause your friend to lose trust in you. On the other hand, if your friend refuses to say what's up, accept that, and simply affirm that you'll be there if needed.

Don't put pressure on yourself to fix things. Offer your support, and if it seems appropriate, offer to set up an appointment for your friend at your campus counseling center . . . and even to go along.

Finally, be the change you wish to see in your friend. That is, trust that maintaining your own balance will help your friend realize his or her own capacity to navigate life's challenges successfully.

Campus Advocacy

What steps can you take to increase psychological health on your campus and decrease the stigma associated with psychological distress? Active Minds is a student-founded and student-led organization working to change the conversation about mental health on college campuses. The organization works to increase students' awareness of mental health issues, provide information and resources regarding mental health and mental disorders, encourage students to seek help as soon as it is needed, and serve as a liaison between students and the mental health community. Currently, nearly 350 U.S. colleges and universities have chapters of Active Minds.

To find out if your college has an Active Minds chapter, click on the U.S. map at www.activeminds.org/index.php?option=com_content&task=view&id=27&Itemid=56. If your campus isn't listed, click on Start a New Chapter and find out how to set one up!

The National Alliance on Mental Illness (NAMI) is an organization founded in 1979 to improve the lives of individuals and families affected by mental disorders. One of its initiatives is NAMI on Campus, student-led clubs that provide support, education, and advocacy. The mission of NAMI on Campus is to increase mental health services on campus and eliminate the stigma that students with mental disorders face.

If you're not the organizational type, you can still promote psychological health on campus just by maintaining an accepting, nonjudgmental attitude. You can also step out of your comfort zone to reach out to those you suspect might be in need. Especially if you've successfully overcome a psychological challenge yourself, or even if you're "just getting by," consider volunteering as a member of a peer support group. Contact your campus counseling center to find out what peer counseling opportunities may be available for you.

Watch videos of real students discussing their psychological health at www.pearsonhighered.com/lynchelmore.

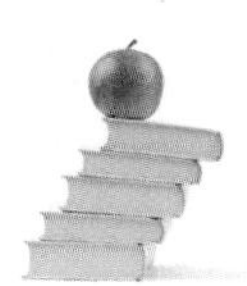

Choosing to Change Worksheet

To complete this workshop online, visit www.pearsonhighered.com/lynchelmore.

Part I. Building the Qualities of Psychological Health

Psychological health is the dimension of health and wellness that encompasses both mental and emotional components. One tool frequently used to assess psychological health is the Ryff Scales of Psychological Well-Being. The tool identifies six key facets: self-acceptance, positive relations with others, autonomy, environmental mastery, purpose in life, and personal growth. (See Figure 2.1 on page 29.) With this in mind, think about one facet of your psychological health that is important to you and needs improvement. Write this down in Step 1.

Step 1: Identifying a Facet of Psychological Health to Improve. ______________________________ is a facet of my psychological health that is important to me and needs improvement.

Which of the following statements best describes your readiness to improve this facet of your psychological health?

____________ I do not intend to work on this facet in the next 6 months. (Precontemplation)

____________ I might work on this facet in the next 6 months. (Contemplation)

____________ I am prepared to work on this facet in the next month. (Preparation)

____________ I have been working on this facet for less than 6 months but need to do more. (Action)

____________ I have been working on this facet for more than 6 months, and want to maintain it. (Maintenance)

Step 2: Making a Plan to Improve Psychological Health. Keeping your current stage of behavior change in mind, describe what you might do or think about as a "next step" to improve that quality of psychological health. You can use the strategies and tips presented in this chapter for ideas. Also list your timeline for making your next step.

____

____

____

____

Step 3: Overcoming Challenges to Psychological Health. In our daily lives we sometimes experience challenging situations that can put our psychological health to the test. What techniques can you use to counter roadblocks to developing your psychological health to the fullest? Again, you can refer to the information provided in this chapter.

____

____

____

____

Part II. Reducing Cognitive Distortions and Increasing Positive Thinking

Far too often we engage in negative self-talk and destructive thinking patterns. If you have thoughts that consistently weigh you down, work through the following steps to unravel that harmful pattern of thinking.

Step 1: Identifying Cognitive Distortions. Take a look at the types of cognitive distortions discussed in Practical Strategies for Change: Spotting Destructive Thoughts on page 50. Do any of these thinking patterns sound familiar to you? Write down any negative thoughts you have, and list which category each fits into.

Thoughts ______________________________ Categories ______________________________

____

____

____

Step 2: Disputing Your Negative Thoughts. Pick one of these thoughts to focus on. Do the facts of your current situation back up your negative perception? Write down all the facts that go against your current negative interpretation.

Thought: ____

Facts that go against the negative interpretation: ______________________________

____

____

Step 3: Reframing Your Experiences. Can you think of something that has happened in the past—no matter how small—that goes against the negative self-talk you're experiencing? Write it down.

Example: I received a good grade on my last test, so although I did poorly on this test, I know I can do well at school.

____

____

____

Step 4: Changing Your Perspective. Imagine that a friend or a family member was thinking these things. What would you say to cheer that person up? Would things seem so bad if they weren't happening to you?

____

____

____

Step 5: Creating a More Optimistic Viewpoint. Taking into account the evidence above that goes against your negative self-talk, can you think about the situation in a more optimistic way? Write down your new, more positive interpretation, and repeat it to yourself whenever your negative thought pops up.

Example: Instead of thinking "I received a bad grade on this test; I'm going to flunk out of school!" you could think "I did poorly on this test, but I've done well on tests before. Now I know to create a study plan and attend review sessions before the next test."

____

____

____

____

Chapter Summary

- Psychological health encompasses both mental and emotional health.
- Six facets of psychological health are self-acceptance, positive relations with others, autonomy, environmental mastery, a sense of purpose in life, and ongoing personal growth.
- Emotional intelligence enables you to process information of an emotional nature and use it to guide your thoughts, actions, and reactions.
- Optimism is the psychological tendency to have a positive interpretation of life's events.
- Psychological health is influenced by complex genetic factors interacting with aspects of our environment.
- Maslow's hierarchy of needs models the theory that people experience higher and higher levels of psychological health as they meet and master ever-higher levels of innate needs via successful interactions with their environment.
- Erikson's theory of developmental stages proposed that, to achieve peak psychological health, we must tackle and master specific developmental tasks that present themselves at each stage of life.
- Religion and spirituality can contribute to psychological health. Spiritual well-being is said to rest upon three pillars: a strong personal value system, connectedness and community in relationships, and a meaningful purpose in life.
- Everyone faces psychological challenges. Common concerns, such as shyness, loneliness, anger, and bad moods can often be addressed through rethinking and thoughtful self-care.
- Sometimes psychological issues become more serious mental disorders. College, with its pressures, is a high-risk time for mental health concerns.
- The United States has the highest rate of mental disorders in the world, and disability due to mental disorders has increased significantly over the past several decades.
- The chemical imbalance theory of mental illness arose in the 1950s; however, the American Psychiatric Association acknowledges that the causes of mental disorders are unknown, and contemporary research efforts are exploring interactions between genes, physiological control systems, and environmental factors.
- Depressive disorders and bipolar disorder are mood disorders. Depression is a serious concern for many students. Although women experience depressive disorders at higher rates than men, depressed men are more likely to suffer physical effects. Depression is considered one of the most treatable mental disorders, and many people recover spontaneously even without treatment.
- A variety of forms of psychotherapy are successful in treating depression, and regular exercise can help. Antidepressant medications, typically SSRIs, are often prescribed; however, they can prompt side effects ranging from mild to severe and recent studies have challenged their effectiveness.
- Bipolar disorder is increasing in the United States in both prevalence and severity, including among children. Research is ongoing to try to determine the factors behind these trends.
- Other mental disorders include anxiety disorders such as panic disorders and phobias, attention disorders such as ADHD, and schizophrenia.
- Self-injury is the act of cutting, burning, bruising, or otherwise injuring yourself in an effort to deal with negative or overwhelming feelings.
- Suicide is an attempt to relieve overwhelming distress, not a plea for attention, and should be taken seriously. Two to three times as many women attempt suicide as men, although four times as many men actually die from suicide.
- The most common options in psychotherapy include cognitive-behavioral therapy (CBT), behavior therapy, psychodynamic therapy, and positive psychology. Some therapists use a combined approach.
- Self-care can be a good place to start if you are experiencing psychological distress. Self-care includes eating well, getting the right amount of sleep, exercising, setting realistic goals, and taking practical "thought and action" steps to build your self-esteem.
- A desire to isolate yourself is a common symptom of psychological distress, and reaching out is an important coping strategy.
- Many people find that prayer or meditation can be helpful ways to chill out and induce the relaxation response.
- There are many ways to promote psychological well-being on campus, from joining an organization such as Active Minds to volunteering to become a peer counselor.

Test Your Knowledge

1. A core facet of psychological health is
   a. having a romantic relationship.
   b. achieving a fixed state of wellness.
   c. passivity.
   d. environmental mastery.

2. In Maslow's hierarchy of needs pyramid
   a. basic survival needs must be met first.
   b. all of our needs can be met simultaneously.
   c. emotional needs matter relatively little.
   d. self-actualization is the first step.

3. Erikson suggests that an identity crisis
   a. signifies an impending catastrophe.
   b. is characteristic of the period of adolescence.
   c. means that the individual has not established autonomy.
   d. threatens psychological health.

4. Social support is
   a. defined in terms of both quantity and quality of relationships.
   b. characterized by emotional concern rather than provision of goods and services.
   c. synonymous with assertiveness.
   d. more helpful for male college students than for female college students.

5. Values, relationships, and purpose are three pillars of
   a. religiosity.
   b. spirituality.
   c. generativity.
   d. ego integrity.

56. Posternak, M. A., & Miller, I. (2001). Untreated short-term course of major depression: A meta-analysis of outcomes from studies using wait-list control groups. *Journal of Affective Disorders, 66*, 139–146.

57. Ioannidis, J. P. A. (2008). Effectiveness of antidepressants: An evidence myth constructed from a thousand randomized trials? *Philosophy, Ethics, and Humanities in Medicine* 2008, 3:14

58. Kirsch, I. (2011). *The emperor's new drugs: Exploding the antidepressant myth*. New York: Basic Books.

59. Bridge, J. A., Iyengar, S., Salary, C. B., Barbe, R. P., Birmaher, B., Pincus, H.A. & Brent, D. A. (2007). Clinical response and risk for reported suicidal ideation and suicide attempts in pediatric antidepressant treatment, a meta-analysis of randomized controlled trials. *Journal of the American Medical Association, 297* (15), 1683–1696.

60. Kadison, R. (2005, September 15). Getting an edge: Use of stimulants and antidepressants in college. *New England Journal of Medicine, 353*, 1089–1091.

61. Harvard Medical School. (2011). Exercise and depression. In: *Understanding Depression*. Cambridge: Harvard Health Publications. Retrieved from http://www.health.harvard.edu/newsweek/Exercise-and-Depression-report-excerpt.htm.

62. Baethge, C. (2005). Substance abuse in first-episode bipolar I disorder. *American Journal of Psychiatry*, *162*, 1008–1010.

63. National Institute of Mental Health. (2009). *Bipolar disorder.* Retrieved from http://www.nimh.nih.gov/health/publications/bipolar-disorder/index.shtml.

64. U.S. Food and Drug Administration (FDA). (2006, March 3). Psychiatric adverse events in clinical trials of drugs for attention deficit hyperactivity disorder (ADHD). Center for Drug Evaluation and Research: DO60163. Retrieved from http://www.fda.gov/ohrms/dockets/ac/06/briefing/2006-4210b_10_01_Mosholder.pdf.

65. Huxley, N., & Baldessarini, R. (2007). Disability and its treatment in bipolar disorder patients. *Bipolar Disorders*, *9*, 183–196.

66. National Institute of Mental Health. (2009). *Panic disorder.* Retrieved from http://www.nimh.nih.gov/health/publications/anxiety-disorders/panic-disorder.shtml.

67. National Institute of Mental Health. (2009). *Social phobia (social anxiety disorder).* Retrieved from http://www.nimh.nih.gov/health/topics/social-phobia-social-anxiety-disorder/index.shtml.

68. Anxiety Disorders Association of America. (2007). *The effects of social anxiety disorder on personal relationships: Survey results.* 1–5.

69. Carducci, B. J., & Nethery, K. T. (2007, August). *High school shooters as cynically shy: Content analysis and characteristic features.* Poster session presented at the 115th annual convention of the American Psychological Association, San Francisco, CA.

70. U.S. Department of Health and Human Services, U.S. Public Health Service. (2001). *Mental health: Culture, race, and ethnicity;* a supplement to *Mental health: A report of the surgeon general.* Rockville, MD: U.S. Department of Health and Human Services, Substance Abuse and Mental Health Services Administration, Center for Mental Health Services. Retrieved from http://www.surgeongeneral.gov/library/mentalhealth/cre/sma-01-3613.pdf.

71. U.S. Department of Veterans Affairs, National Center for PTSD. (2009). *What is PTSD?* Retrieved from http://www.ptsd.va.gov/public/pages/what-is-ptsd.asp.

72. Pelissolo, A., Maniere, F., Boutges, B., Allouche, M., Richard-Berthe, C., & Corruble, E. (2007, January–February). Anxiety and depressive disorders in 4,425 long-term benzodiazepine users in general practice. *Encephale, 33* (1), 32–38.

73. Hoza, B., Mrug, S., Gerdes, A., Hinshaw, S., Bukowski, W., Gold, J., & Eugene, A. L. (2005). What aspects of peer relationships are impaired in children with attention deficit hyperactivity disorder? *Journal of Consulting and Clinical Psychology, 73* (3), 411–423.

74. Mayes, R., Bagwell, C., & Erkulwater, J. (2008). ADHD and the rise in stimulant use among children. *Harvard Review of Psychiatry, 16* (3), 151–166.

75. Waring, M. E., & Lapane, K. L. (2008). Overweight in children and adolescents in relation to attention deficit hyperactivity disorder: Results from a national sample. *Pediatrics, 112* (1), e1–e6.

76. Gentile, J. P., Atiq, R., & Gillig, P. M. (2006). Adult ADHD: Diagnosis, differential diagnosis, and medication management. *Psychiatry, 3* (8), 24–30.

77. DuPaul, G. J., & Weyandt, L. L. (2004, August). *College students with ADHD: What do we know and where do we go from here?* Paper presented at the annual meeting of Children and Adults with Attention Deficit Hyperactivity Disorder, Nashville, TN. Retrieved from http://www.allacademic.com/meta/p116618_index.html.

78. Price, M. (2007). Adults with ADHD see a problem, and then lose control. *Monitor on Psychology, 38* (11), 12.

79. WebMD. (2010, April 12). Stimulants for attention deficit hyperactivity disorder. Retrieved from http://www.webmd.com/add-adhd/stimulants-for-attention-deficit-hyperactivity-disorder.

80. Substance Abuse and Mental Health Services Administration. (2009, May/June). Adderall and college students. *SAMHSA News*, *17* (3). Retrieved from http://www.samhsa.gov/samhsanewsletter/volume_17_number_3/adderall.aspx.

81. Trudeau, M. (2001, February 5). More students turning illegally to "smart" drugs. National Public Radio. Retrieved from http://www.npr.org/templates/story/story.php?storyId=100254163.

82. Drug Enforcement Administration, U.S. Department of Justice. (1995). Methylphenidate: A background paper. *NCJRS (National Criminal Justice Reference System) Abstract,* NCJ 166349. Retrieved from http://www.ncjrs.gov/App/publications/abstract.aspx?ID=163349.

83. Barbaresi, W. J., Katusic, S. K., Colligan, R. C., Weaver, A. L., and Jacobsen, S. J. (2007). Modifiers of long-term school outcomes for children with attention-deficit/hyperactivity disorder: Does treatment with stimulant medication make a difference? Results from a Population-Based Study *Journal of Developmental & Behavioral Pediatrics,* 28(4): 274–287.

84. Epstein, J. N., Langberg, J. M., Lichtenstein, P. K., Altaye, M., Brinkman, W. B., House, K., & Stark, L. J. (2010, February). Attention deficit hyperactivity disorder outcomes for children treated in community-based pediatric settings. *Archives of Pediatrics and Adolescent Medicine, 164*, 160–165.

85. Fedewa, A. L., & Erwin, H. E. (2011, July/August). Stability balls and students with attention and hyperactivity concerns: Implications for on-task and in-seat behavior. *American Journal of Occupational Therapy, 65* (4), 393–399.

86. National Institute of Mental Health. (2009). *Schizophrenia.* Retrieved from http://www.nimh.nih.gov/health/publications/schizophrenia/index.shtml.

87. Kruger, A. (2000). Schizophrenia: Recovery and hope. *Psychiatric Rehabilitation Journal, 24* (1), 29-37.

88. McGuire, P.A. (2000). New hope for people with schizophrenia. *Monitor on Psychology 31*. (2), 24.

89. Whitlock, J., Powers, J., & Eckenrode, J. (2006). The virtual cutting edge: The Internet and adolescent self-injury. *Developmental Psychology, 42* (3), 407–417.

90. Young, R., van Beinum, M., Sweeting, H., & West, P. (2007). Young people who self-harm. *British Journal of Psychiatry, 191,* 44–49.

91. National Institute of Mental Health. (2009). *Suicide prevention in the U.S.: Statistics and prevention.* Retrieved from http://www.nimh.gov/health/publications/suicide-in-the-us-statistics-and-prevention.shtml.

92. Ohio State University. (2006). Suicide prevention for LGBT college students. Suicide Prevention Resource Center. Retrieved from http://suicideprevention.osu.edu/attachments/GLBTstudents-suicideprevention.pdf.

93. Baser, R. S., Neighbors, H. W., Caldwell, C. H., & Jackson, J. (2009). 12-month and lifetime prevalence of suicide attempts among black adolescents in the National Survey of American Life. *Journal of the American Academy of Child and Adolescent Psychiatry, 48* (3), 271–282.

94. National Association of Cognitive-Behavioral Therapists. (2010). What is cognitive-behavioral therapy? Retrieved from http://www.nacbt.org/whatiscbt.htm#.

95. Pilling, S., Bebbington, P., Kuipers, E., et al. (2002). Psychological treatment in schizophrenia: I. Meta-analysis of family intervention and cognitive behaviour therapy. *Psychol Med, 32*, 763–782.

96. Shedler, J. (2010, February–March). The efficacy of psychodynamic psychotherapy. *American Psychologist*, *65* (2), 98–109.

97. Seligman, M. E. P., Steen, T. A., Park, N., & Peterson, C. (2005). Positive psychology progress. *American Psychologist, 60* (5), 410–421.

98. Lowry, F. (2011, February 2). FDA panel wants electroconvulsive therapy to retain high-risk class III status. *Medscape Medical News*. Retrieved from http://www.medscape.com/viewarticle/736697.

99. National Center for Complementary and Alternative Medicine. (2010, July). *Herbs at a glance: St. John's wort*. Retrieved from http://nccam.nih.gov/health/stjohnswort/D269_Herbs.pdf.

100. National Center for Complementary and Alternative Medicine. (2010, August). *Backgrounder: Massage therapy*. Retrieved from http://nccam.nih.gov/health/massage/D327.pdf.

101. Koenig, H. G., Idler, E., Kasl, S., et al. (1999). Religion, spirituality, and medicine: A rebuttal to skeptics. *International Journal of Psychiatry in Medicine, 29* (2), 123–131.

102. Jantos, M., & Kiat, H. (2007). Prayer as medicine: How much have we learned? *Medical Journal of Australia, 186* (10), 851–853.

103. Mayo Clinic. (2009). *Meditation: Take a stress-reduction break wherever you are.* Retrieved from http://www.mayoclinic.com/health/meditation/HQ01070.

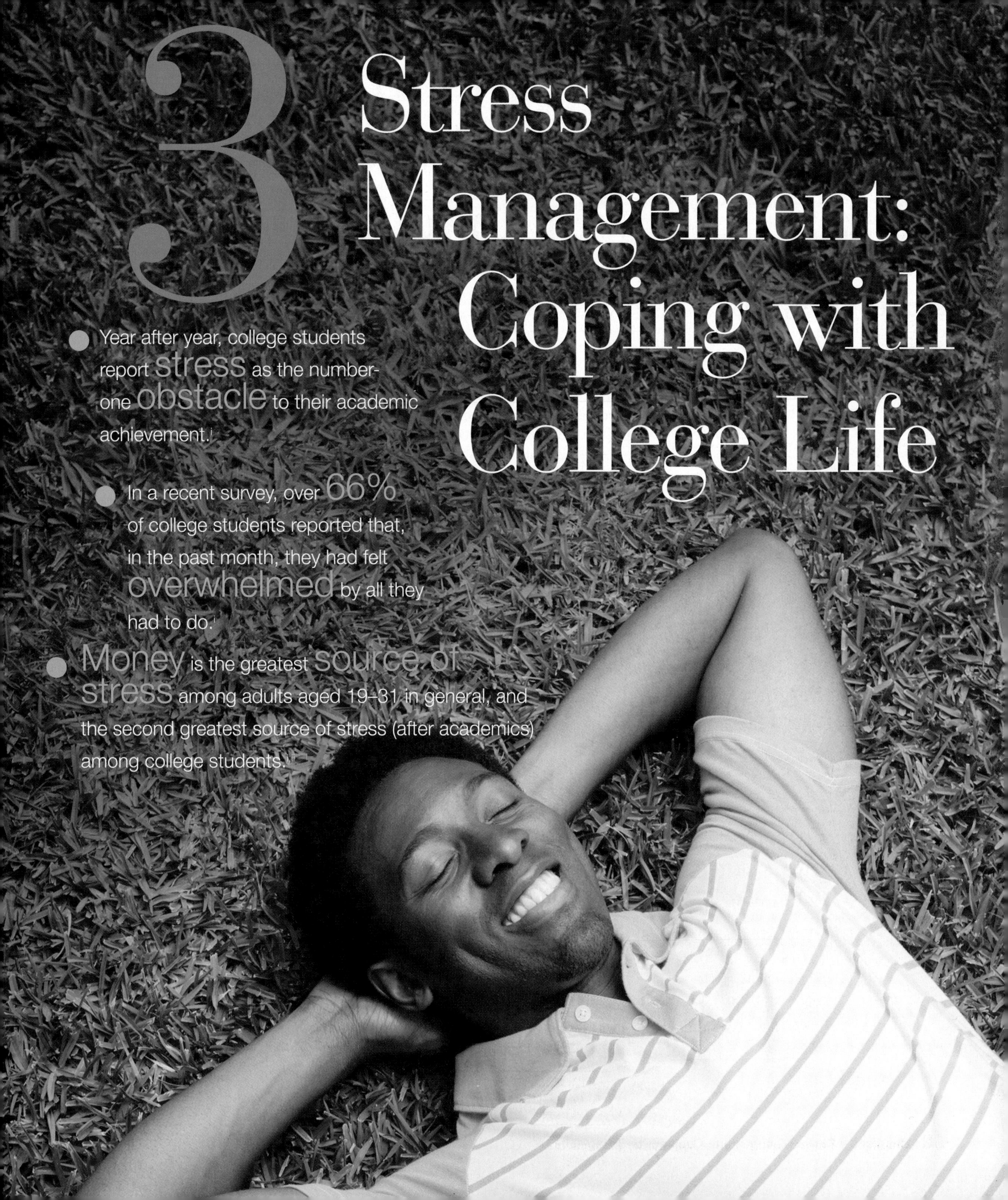

3 Stress Management: Coping with College Life

- Year after year, college students report stress as the number-one obstacle to their academic achievement.[i]
- In a recent survey, over 66% of college students reported that, in the past month, they had felt overwhelmed by all they had to do.[i]
- Money is the greatest source of stress among adults aged 19–31 in general, and the second greatest source of stress (after academics) among college students.[ii,iii]

LEARNING OBJECTIVES

DISTINGUISH between *stress, eustress,* and *distress.*

DESCRIBE the body's stress response.

EXPLAIN why chronic, excessive stress is harmful.

IDENTIFY factors that influence an individual's response to stress.

DISCUSS common sources of stress.

DESCRIBE strategies for effectively managing stress.

CREATE a personalized plan for stress management.

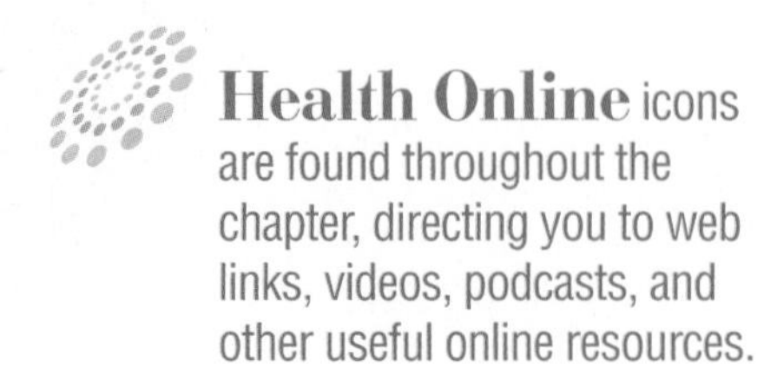
Health Online icons are found throughout the chapter, directing you to web links, videos, podcasts, and other useful online resources.

Three-fourths of Americans are living with a moderate to high level of stress.[1]

In a recent nationwide survey conducted by the American Psychological Association, respondents listed tight finances, work pressures, and family responsibilities as their biggest sources of stress. Unfortunately, many said they felt unable or unwilling to do anything to manage their stress load, whereas others admitted to using unhealthful coping mechanisms, such as smoking, drinking, overeating, gambling, or compulsive shopping.[1]

As a student, you've got some of the same reasons to feel stressed out—and more! Assignments, exams, relationships, and concerns about your future can all add to the pressure as you navigate your college years. But take heart: though you may not always be able to control the sources of stress in your life, this chapter identifies choices you can make today to begin to manage your stress. And doing this can have a profoundly beneficial effect on your health. To begin, let's examine what we mean by *stress*.

What Is Stress?

A young scientist named Hans Selye first brought the concept of stress to the public's attention in the 1930s: He defined *stress* as the body's response to any demand for change. No matter how different the demand for change might appear—a new job, a decision to quit smoking, infection with a virus, a loved one's death—Selye observed that it would prompt a characteristic response from the body that he called stress.[2]

In the decades since his initial discoveries, Selye and other stress researchers have identified both psychological and physiological components of stress. Acknowledging this research, we define **stress** as the collective psychobiological state that develops in response to a disruptive, unexpected, or exciting stimulus. We use the term **stressor** to refer to any physical or psychological condition, event, or factor that causes stress.

We usually think of stress as unpleasant, but not all stressors are negative. Positive events—such as going on a first date, or winning the lottery—can also be stressful. Selye coined the term **eustress** (*eu* means "good") to characterize stress resulting from positive stressors. He called stress resulting from negative stressors **distress.**[2] Think about how you feel when your favorite sports team comes from behind to win. Then think about what happens when you realize you've lost your wallet. The likely differences in your feelings—excitement in the case of eustress, panic in the case of distress—are actually derived from the same physiologic mechanisms.

stress The collective psychobiological state that develops in response to a disruptive, unexpected, or exciting stimulus.

stressor Any physical or psychological condition, event, or factor that causes positive or negative stress.

eustress Stress resulting from positive stressors.

distress Stress resulting from negative stressors.

Chronic eustress leads to well-being and chronic distress leads to unfavorable health outcomes. This video explains their different effects on the brain: www.sciencentral.com/articles/view.php3?type=article&article_id=218392038.

> *"We usually think of stress as unpleasant, but not all stressors are negative."*

Another fundamental characteristic of stress is that it involves our perception—which is often shaped by past experiences and learning. For example, imagine that, as a kid, you were bitten by a snake. Years later, you're out for a hike when you see a snake crossing the path ahead. Your heart starts to beat wildly and you freeze in fear. Another hiker noticing the same snake might experience no stress whatever, recognizing it as just a common garter snake. Notice that it is the *perception* of a threat, not the *reality,* that produces distress. In the same way, your response to an upcoming exam is influenced by your perception of the event as either a normal part of college life or as a threat to your well-being. This means that one strategy in defusing your stress response is to change your perceptions toward the stressor. But before we discuss this technique as well as other techniques for stress management, it's important to understand exactly what the stress response is.

The Body's Stress Response

The human body has a remarkable ability to respond to change in a way that enables it to maintain its internal conditions within a narrow, stable range.

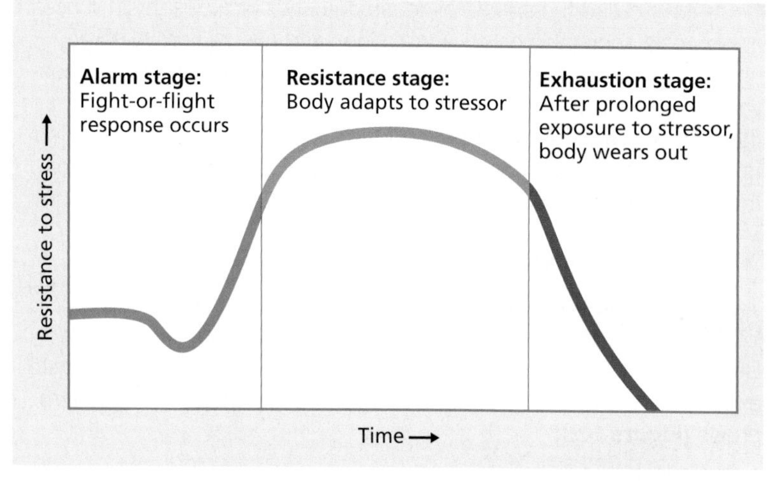
Alarm stage:
Fight-or-flight response occurs
Resistance stage:
Body adapts to stressor
Exhaustion stage:
After prolonged exposure to stressor, body wears out
Resistance to stress →
Time →

Figure 3.1 The general adaptation syndrome. The general adaptation syndrome, developed by Hans Selye, identifies three phases in our response to stress.

In 1932, American physiologist Walter B. Cannon named this ability **homeostasis,** from the Greek word *homios* meaning "similar," and *stasis,* indicating a "stance." For example, let's say you eat a large, sweet dessert. As you digest it, a load of sugar surges into your bloodstream. In response, homeostatic control mechanisms spring into action to bring your blood sugar level back into a healthful range.

homeostasis A physiologic ability to maintain the body's internal conditions within a normal, healthful range, usually achieved via hormonal and neurological mechanisms.

general adaptation syndrome (GAS) Theory explaining the stress response as a series of three phases (alarm, resistance, exhaustion) with characteristic physiologic events.

Like eating a super-sweet dessert, experiencing a stressor—whether a quarrel with your partner or a bounced check—triggers a characteristic homeostatic response. One of the best-known explanations of this response is the **general adaptation syndrome (GAS),** developed by Hans Selye **(Figure 3.1).**

SPOTLIGHT

Science Discovers Stress

The science of stress studies began by accident. In the 1930s, Hans Selye, a young Hungarian-born endocrinologist, was immersed in a study of hormones at McGill University in Montreal. Selye injected lab rats with a variety of hormones and observed their responses. He found that regardless of which hormone he used, the rats all seemed to demonstrate the same basic physical reactions each time, including enlargement of the adrenal cortex; atrophy of the thymus, spleen, and lymph nodes; and stomach ulcers. This led Selye to wonder if he could be observing something broader than merely the rats' responses to specific hormone injections. Were the rats reacting to something more general—to some other "external pressure" he was applying?

Selye decided to find out, using the simplest and cheapest method he could find. He set the hormones aside, and looked for a different external pressure to apply to the rats. He found inspiration in the frigid weather outside the walls of his laboratory. He placed a group of rats in a box and left them outside on his windowsill overnight. The next morning, the unhappy rats behaved in much the same way as those that had previously been injected with hormones. The rats' overall behavior, Selye surmised, had much more to do with external pressures—introduced hormones, freezing weather—than any one specific substance or force. In short, the rats' response reflected *stress.*

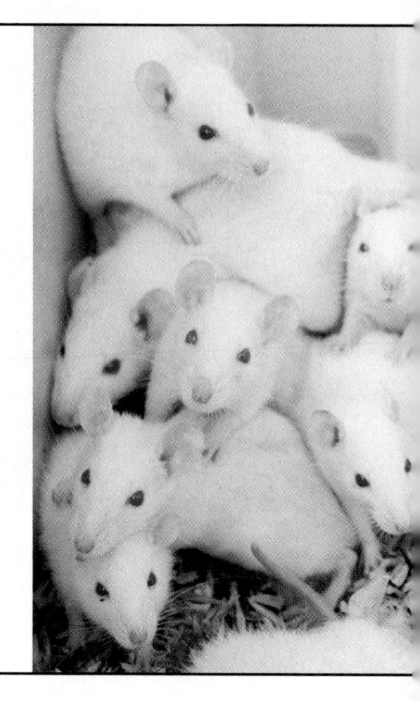

Commonly called the *stress response,* the GAS includes three phases: alarm, resistance (also called adaptation), and exhaustion. All three phases are not inevitable; instead, it's only when the alarm phase continues without successful resistance that exhaustion typically occurs. In the decades since Selye introduced the GAS, further research has led to refinements in our understanding of the phases and physiology of the stress response, as noted in the following discussion.

Alarm Phase: The Fight-or-Flight Response

Imagine you are walking to your car late at night in a poorly lit parking lot. Suddenly and without warning, you feel a hand on your shoulder. Before you realize it's just a friend sneaking up on you, you are likely to experience the following physical reactions characteristic of the alarm phase **(Figure 3.2):**

- Increased heart rate
- Trembling
- Sweating
- Rapid breathing

What's going on? Your brain, perceiving a threat, has activated your sympathetic nervous system (SNS), a part of your nervous system that operates without your conscious awareness. Within seconds, the SNS releases a neurotransmitter—a chemical that helps transmit nerve signals. The particular neurotransmitter that the SNS releases under stress is called *noradrenaline,* and the signals it helps transmit affect the body dramatically. For instance, noradrenaline directly increases your heart rate and the speed and depth of your breathing, explaining two of the reactions just mentioned. It also causes the following:

- Your blood pressure increases to support swift action.
- Your digestive system slows as blood diverts to the large muscles in your arms and legs, giving you more strength for fighting, running, or defending yourself.
- Your liver releases its stores of a simple sugar called *glucose* into your bloodstream, to fuel physical action if necessary.
- Your pupils dilate, sharpening your vision.
- Your circulatory system, anticipating injury, starts producing blood-clotting factor.
- Tiny hairs stand on end all over your body, a reflection of your heightened state of alarm.
- Your *adrenal glands,* two small organs sitting on top of your kidneys, are stimulated to produce a chemical similar to noradrenaline, called *adrenaline,* which sustains the above reactions.

Within about fifteen minutes, a second, hormonal, response begins. **Hormones** are chemicals released by glands into the bloodstream, which transports them to their target organs elsewhere in the body. When hormones reach their target, they act in a way that regulates its activity. Whereas nervous system responses are nearly instantaneous, hormonal responses require some "travel time." The second wave of the alarm phase begins when a region of your brain called the *hypothalamus* signals the nearby *pituitary gland* to release a hormone called ACTH. This travels through your bloodstream to the adrenal glands, where it stimulates the release of an important stress hormone called **cortisol.** The flood of cortisol further increases the amount of glucose in the bloodstream, allowing a sustained response to the threat. It also speeds up the breakdown of the body's nutrient compounds—carbohydrates, fats, and proteins. These actions ensure a supply of fuel to the muscles, should you need to run a long distance to escape a real assailant.

Like homeostasis, this complex set of reactions was first described by Walter B. Cannon, who named it the **fight-or-flight response.** Cannon theorized that it evolved as a survival mechanism to help early humans fight an enemy or escape from a predator; probably our ancestors could not have survived in their dangerous "eat-or-be-eaten" world without it. Even today, your fight-or-flight response temporarily boosts your strength and stamina to enable you to fight off a would-be assailant or flee a smoke-filled building.

Despite its continued usefulness in our modern world, the fight-or-flight response can also be unhelpful or even harmful. Most of our day-to-day stressors are not the extreme physical threats that our ancestors faced. Yet fight-or-flight kicks in *any* time you face a stressor—even when that stressor is mostly emotional or psychological, such as frustration at being

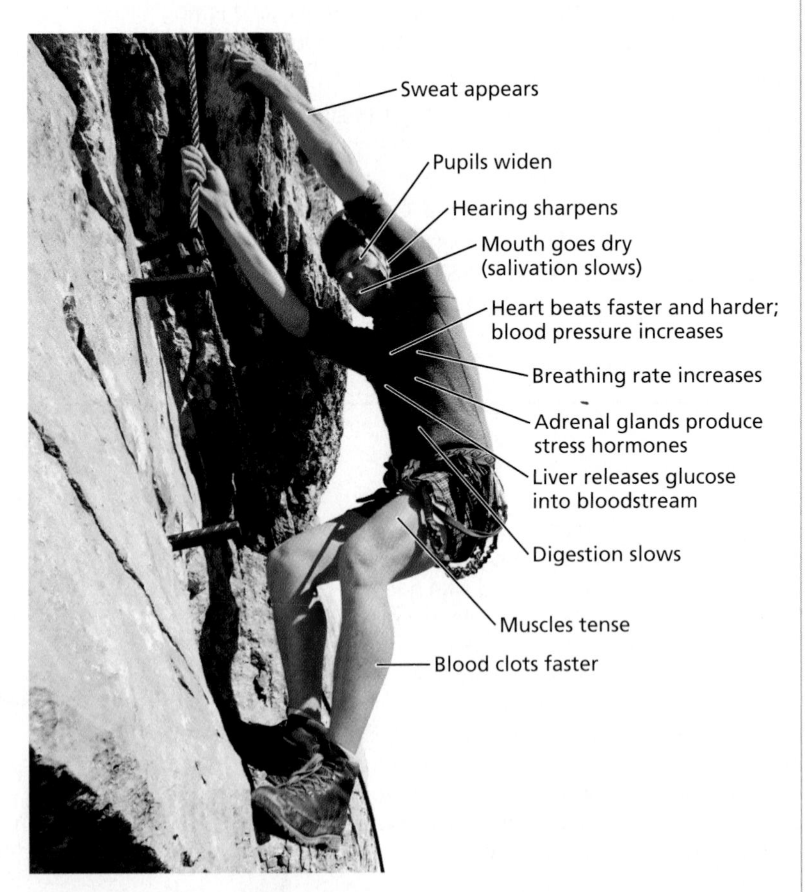

Sweat appears
Pupils widen
Hearing sharpens
Mouth goes dry (salivation slows)
Heart beats faster and harder; blood pressure increases
Breathing rate increases
Adrenal glands produce stress hormones
Liver releases glucose into bloodstream
Digestion slows
Muscles tense
Blood clots faster

Figure 3.2 **The fight-or-flight response.** The alarm phase is characterized by the fight-or-flight response, a set of physical reactions that prepares you to deal with a perceived threat.

hormone Chemical secreted by a gland and transported through the bloodstream to a distant target organ, the activity of which it then regulates.

cortisol Adrenal gland hormone that is secreted at high levels during the stress response.

fight-or-flight response A set of physiological reactions to a stressor designed to enable the body to stand and fight or to flee.

stuck behind a slow driver on the highway, or worry at finding yourself unprepared for mid-term exams. If you experience fight-or-flight too often, or find yourself unable to resist it successfully, then in a sense you remain perpetually in the alarm phase. Such "high-alert" living can take a powerful toll on your body and your health.

Resistance Phase

As a stressor continues, the body mobilizes homeostatic mechanisms that make it more resistant to the stressor. For example, the first time you hike a strenuous trail, you're likely to experience significant physical distress. But if you were to hike that trail twice weekly, you'd soon adapt to its demands and it would no longer set off the alarm phase.

Even with stressors that aren't primarily physical, you can develop strategies that increase your level of resistance and help you adapt. For instance, if you're a college freshman, you might feel stress hormones pouring into your bloodstream as you sit down to take your first mid-term exam. But over time, repetition helps you perceive the situation as more familiar (and thus less like a "change"). Moreover, you learn that, when you study thoroughly, you do well. Building this "track record" of success also helps calm your nerves. Finally, over time, you may learn a set of stretches, breathing techniques, or motivational phrases to keep you relaxed during exams. As a result of your growing familiarity with the situation, your confidence in your preparation, and your use of coping mechanisms, the jolt of stress you feel as you walk toward the exam room is likely to actually improve your performance by keeping you alert and focused. That's right: A little stress actually helps you do better.

This phenomenon was first identified in 1908 by psychologists Robert Yerkes and John Dodson. According to the Yerkes-Dodson law, performance improves with moderate physiological or mental arousal—which today we call stress. Similarly, in 1982, cardiologist Peter Nixon described a **human function curve** according to which a manageable degree of stress improves a performance . . . but too much stress leads to illness **(Figure 3.3).**[3]

Exhaustion Phase and Allostatic Overload

When the degree of stress is not manageable—when stressors are severe and persistent—the homeostatic mechanisms that formerly helped you adapt become depleted. Both Selye and Nixon recognized that, at this point, your body enters an exhaustion phase and, as a result, you experience stress-related disease and **burnout.**

Recently, some researchers introduced the term **allostatic overload** to describe the exhaustion phase. The prefix *allo-* means "variability," so an allostatic overload is a harmful state resulting from excessive change.[4] But whether we call it exhaustion or allostatic overload, the result of chronic, excessive stress is always a failure of homeostasis, which is inevitably manifested as disease.[5] If multiple commitments keep cutting into your time for study and sleep, your stress is likely to increase well

human function curve A model of the effect of stress on performance by which a moderate degree of stress improves performance. As stress increases, performance decreases and burnout becomes likely.

burnout Phenomenon in which increased feelings of stress and decreased feelings of accomplishment lead to frustration, exhaustion, lack of motivation, and disengagement.

allostatic overload A harmful state that develops as a consequence of chronic, excessive stress.

STUDENT STORY

Balancing School and Family

"Hi, I'm David. As a nontraditional student, some of the things that stress me out are maybe a little bit different than what other students go through. I own a house. I have to pay a mortgage, bills, and taxes. I have to put food on my kids' table, clothing on their backs, and spend time with my wife. These things really stress me out! And on top of all of that, I'm a full-time college student.

One of the ways that I balance being a family man and college student is to try to keep both worlds separate. I know that when I go to school, that's what I need to concentrate on. I try to do all my homework and everything else at school. And when I go home, I try to leave the school behind. Sometimes the two blend together, but that's a good thing, I think."

1: Identify at least three stressors that David is dealing with. Are these stressors caused by *eustress* or *distress*?

2: How well do you think David is managing his stress load? What negative health effects could he experience if he was unable to manage stress?

Do you have a story similar to David's? Share your story at www.pearsonhighered.com/lynchelmore.

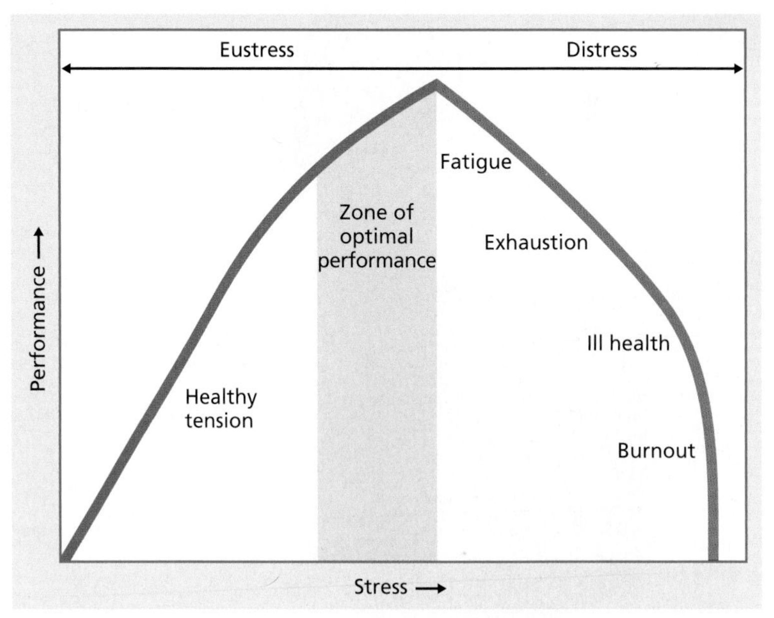

Figure 3.3 The human function curve. As long as you feel adequately prepared for a stressful event, a moderate degree of stress can actually improve your performance. But as stress becomes increasingly persistent and severe, performance deteriorates. Eventually, a person experiences illness or burnout.

Source: Adapted from Nixon, P. G. (1976). The human function curve. With special reference to cardiovascular disorders: part I. *Practitioner, 217* (1301), 765–770.

beyond the point of optimal performance. If it stays elevated for long, you may experience burnout and illness.

Check out this tutorial that explains the body's stress response, health effects of stress, and how to manage stress: www.nlm.nih.gov/medlineplus/tutorials/managingstress/htm/index.htm

Health Effects of Chronic Stress

Even short-term stress causes physical and psychological symptoms. While the specific effects vary from person to person, physical symptoms commonly include: fatigue, lying awake at night, headache, upset stomach, muscle tension, change in appetite, change in sex drive, teeth grinding, dizziness, feeling a tightness in the chest, change in menstrual cycle (in women), and erectile dysfunction (in men). Psychological symptoms of stress include feeling angry or irritable, lacking interest or motivation in daily activities, feeling anxious or nervous, and feeling sad or depressed.[1] Such symptoms can be disturbing even if you experience them only occasionally. But if your stress keeps getting more intense, your risk for serious health problems will increase along with it **(Figure 3.4).**

Effects on the Cardiovascular System

Release of stress hormones causes the heart to work harder and faster, raising blood pressure. Over time, high blood pressure can damage blood vessels and internal organs, greatly increasing the risk of a heart attack or stroke. Stress can also promote cardiovascular disease indirectly by prompting unhealthful coping mechanisms. For example, many people who are stressed out respond by overeating, smoking, abusing alcohol, or spending hours being sedentary, "zoned out" in front of a computer or TV. All of these behaviors increase the risk for chronic diseases, including heart disease and stroke.[1]

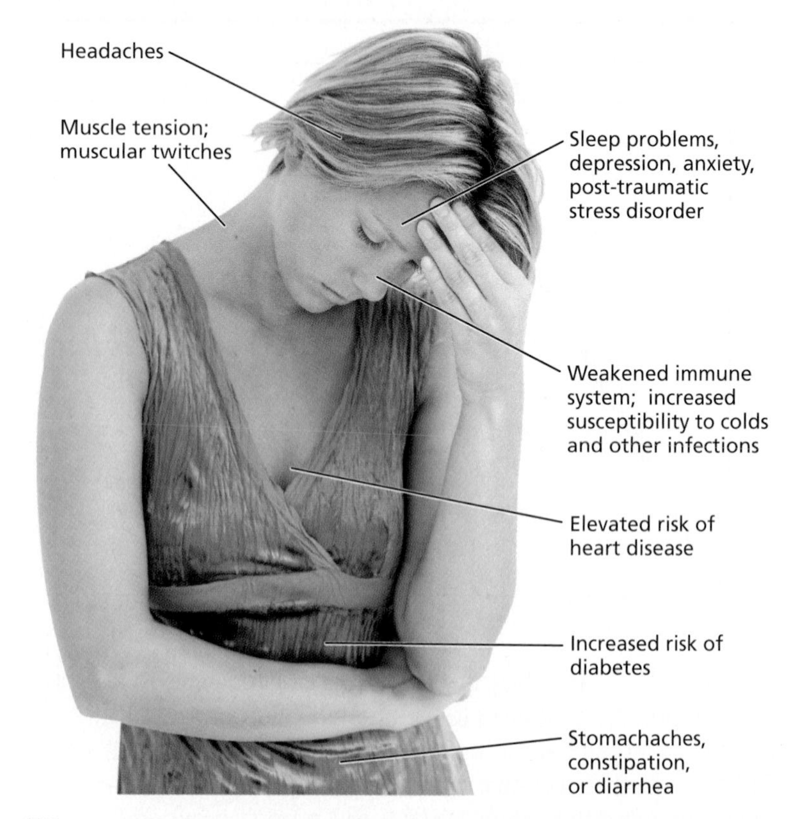

Figure 3.4 **Health effects of long-term stress.** Chronic stress can have long-term health effects, ranging from sleep problems to increased risk for a variety of diseases.

> *"Both children and adults who are overweight or obese report that they experience more stress, as compared to people of normal weight."*

Effects on the Digestive System

When the fight-or-flight response directs blood away from the stomach and intestines, the digestive system performs less effectively. This can result in stomachache, constipation, or diarrhea. Stress is also known to aggravate irritable bowel syndrome (IBS), a disorder characterized by painful abdominal cramps, bloating, gas, and either diarrhea or constipation. It can also worsen the symptoms of ulcerative colitis, a condition in which the lining of the colon becomes ulcerated and inflamed. Stress hormones can also affect the body's ability to regulate blood sugar levels, which may increase the risk of diabetes. You might be wondering whether or not stress can trigger the formation of ulcers. Check out the nearby **Myth or Fact?** box to find the answer.

Effects on Weight

Stress can reduce a person's appetite, or cause an upset stomach or other symptoms that cause a person to avoid eating. But for many, stress induces a longing for sweets, chips, or other "comfort foods" high in calories. Both children and adults can experience weight gain if they attempt to cope with stress by overeating. Moreover, researchers have long acknowledged an "income–body weight gradient" by which economic stressors provoke metabolic changes that are associated with increased weight.[6]

In addition, both children and adults who are overweight or obese report that they experience more stress, compared with people of normal weight.[1] Children who are overweight are more likely than normal-weight children to report that they worry a great deal about things in their lives, and that their parent worries or is stressed. They are also more likely to be victims of teasing and bullying. Similarly, a much greater percentage of obese adults (29%) than normal-weight adults (20%) report experiencing a very high degree of stress. Obese adults are also much more likely to report physical and emotional symptoms of stress, such as fatigue, irritability, anger, and sadness.[1]

Effects on the Immune System

Do you always seem to get sick during finals week? At the end of the term, a quarter or semester's worth of stress may weaken your body's ability to fight off infections. Why?

Psychoneuroimmunology (PNI) is the study of interactions among psychological processes, the nervous system, hormones, and the immune system.[7] PNI researchers have identified a relationship between stress and alterations in the immune system—the group of cells and tissues that work together to defend your body against microorganisms, tumor cells, and other threats. Recall that, when acute stress activates the fight-or-flight response, your hypothalamus triggers the release of cortisol. In the short term, this enables you to effectively respond to stressors; however, long-term overproduction of cortisol can suppress the immune system. It does this by actually causing immune cells to decrease and reducing the inflammatory response—a critical aspect of the body's defenses against infection and injury. This can in turn reduce your ability to fight off infection.[8] In addition, the fear, tension, anxiety, or depression that accompany stress may increase heart rate or blood pressure, which can compromise your immune system further.

psychoneuroimmunology (PNI) The study of interactions among psychological processes, the nervous system, hormones, and the immune system.

Intriguingly, short-term stress caused by relatively minor events such as academic exams can cause temporary increases in white blood cell counts, a sign that the immune system has been activated to ward off a threat.[9] Such demands on the immune system, if frequent, may leave you vulnerable to colds, trigger a recurrence of cold sores, promote asthma attacks, and increase your risk of developing other diseases.

Moreover, some research suggests that the effect of stress on immune function can increase the development of certain cancers associated with viruses, such as lymphomas. In addition, recent research suggests that the release of stress hormones into the blood can directly impair important processes in cells that help protect against the formation of cancer, such as DNA repair and the regulation of cell growth.[10]

Effects on the Nervous System

Stress is known to trigger two types of headaches. Tension headaches are mild to moderate headaches that typically feel like a constriction around the head. They can last from a few minutes to several hours. Migraines are much more severe and can be accompanied by nausea and vomiting as well as sensitivity to sound and light. They can last from hours to days. Stress can also increase chronic pain conditions such as lower back pain, fibromyalgia, and other pain disorders.

Effects on Sleep

Adequate sleep is essential to conserve body energy, grow, repair, and restore your body's cells and tissues, maintain your immune system, and organize and synthesize new learning and memories. Unfortunately, many college students are not experiencing these benefits of adequate sleep: A national survey found that over 1 in 20 college students had been diagnosed with or treated for a sleep disorder in the past year.[11] Although illness and disability, alcohol and other drug use, and many other factors can interfere with sleep, stress is one of the most common culprits.[12] (Sleep is discussed fully in Chapter 4.)

Effects on Mind and Mental Health

Stress disturbs our day-to-day mental functioning and increases our risk for a variety of mental health problems.

MYTH OR FACT?
Can Stress Give You an Ulcer?

You've got a huge set of lab problems to solve for class, and you're way behind on getting it done. After a quick dinner of extremely cold, old pizza, you head for the library. Your stomach is killing you—again.

Yes, the pizza was kind of nasty. But you still can't help but wonder if all the pressure this term is giving you an ulcer.

Ulcers are lesions in the lining of the stomach or small intestine that can cause pain, bloating, and nausea. But though all the stress you face could indeed be making you feel terrible, it probably isn't directly causing an ulcer. Researchers have found that most ulcers are caused by bacteria called *Helicobacter pylori*. Those ulcers not triggered by bacterial infection are often due to the overuse of painkillers, such as aspirin or ibuprofen, or to alcohol abuse. Smokers also have an increased risk of ulcers, and their ulcers are especially resistant to healing.

Although researchers no longer believe that stress directly causes ulcers, studies have shown that chronic stress can increase stomach acid production, disrupt immune system activity, and make the symptoms of an ulcer worse. If you suffer from ongoing stomach pain, visit your campus health center or personal doctor.

References: **1.** Mayo Clinic. (2009). Peptic ulcer: Causes. Retrieved from http://www.mayoclinic.com/health/peptic-ulcer/DS00242/DSECTION=causes. **2.** Merck Manual. (2006). Peptic ulcer. Retrieved from http://www.merckmanuals.com/home/sec09/ch121/ch121c.html.

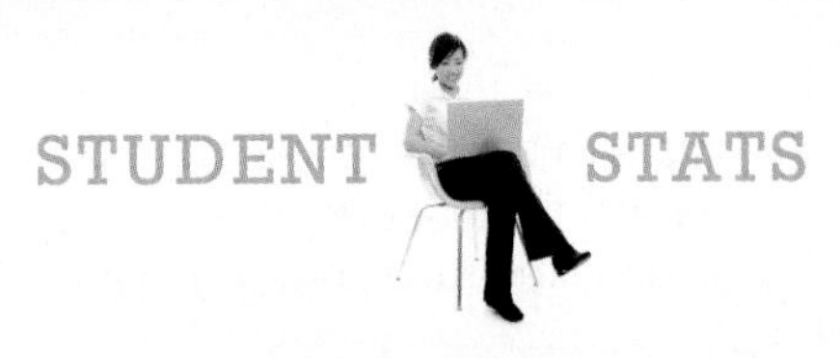

Top 10 Impediments to Academic Performance

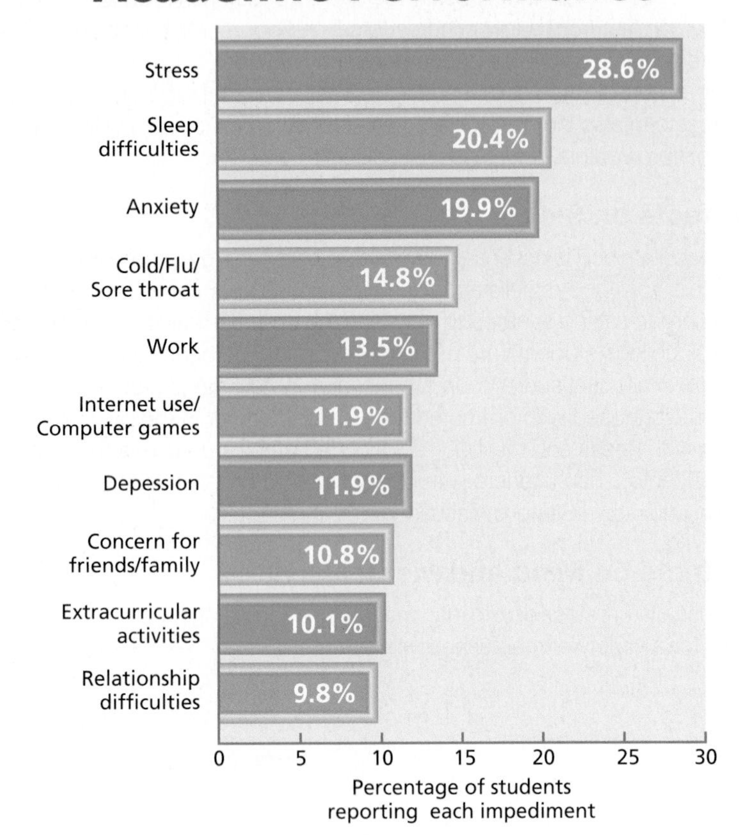

Data from American College Health Association. (2012). American College Health Association-National College Health Assessment II: Reference Group Executive Summary, Fall 2011. Linthicum, MD: American College Health Association. Retrieved from http://www.achancha.org/.

Learning and Memory

In a 2010 survey, college students rated stress as the number-one impediment to their academic performance.[11] It's not surprising, as studies have shown that excessive anxiety about grades, exams, papers, and deadlines can actually prevent you from being successful in college.[13] What's the link between stress and grades? Studies point to various factors, including the negative effect on brain cells when their receptors are flooded by stress hormones. For instance, a 2008 study demonstrated that stress lasting as little as a few hours can impair brain-cell communication in brain regions associated with learning and memory.[14]

Psychological Health Problems

Chronic stress is an important risk factor for many mental health problems. For example, over the past 20 years, research has increasingly suggested the existence of a complex and reciprocal relationship between stress and depression.[15] Not only does stress increase your risk for depression, but depression, in turn, increases your susceptibility to the kinds of stressful events that are at least partly influenced by the individual.[15] In other words, people experiencing severe long-term stress may develop depression, only to have their condition create more stress in their lives.[16]

Anxiety is a normal response to stressful situations; however, stress itself may also contribute to the development of anxiety disorders. For example, some researchers theorize that an inappropriate activation of the fight-or-flight response may at least partly explain the experience of a **panic attack,** a sudden episode of intense fear.[17] In addition, **post-traumatic stress disorder (PTSD)** can develop when people are exposed to very traumatic forms of stress, such as violence, deadly natural disasters, or combat. People with PTSD often relive the trauma, experiencing the intense stress of the original event again and again. Unfortunately, stress and these psychological health challenges can form a vicious cycle in which one feeds the other, complicating treatment. (For more information on psychological health, see Chapter 2.)

As a college student, you're bound to feel some degree of stress. So how do you know whether a few signs and symptoms you might be experiencing are normal—or increase your risk for illness? Check out the nearby **Practical Strategies for Health: Recognizing the Signs of Stress Overload.**

panic attack A sudden experience of intense fear, often involving feelings of dread or doom, loss of control, or impending death.

post-traumatic stress disorder (PTSD) A psychological disorder characterized by a person's repeatedly reliving (through nightmares or recollection) past traumatic or extremely stressful events.

personality type A set of behavioral tendencies.

What Influences Our Stress Response

We said earlier that our perception influences whether or not we experience an event as a stressor. But even two people who perceive the same stressor can have very different responses to it. For instance, let's say that Quillen and Jeb experience a last-place finish in an important relay race. Quillen is disappointed, but perceives the loss as just one event in an otherwise solid track season. That evening, he phones his dad to talk about it. Together, they discuss factors that might have been involved, and how Quillen can prepare better for next week's meet. As a result, he's able to get a good night's sleep and looks forward to getting back on the track to put his new strategies into practice. In contrast, Jeb perceives the defeat as one more piece of evidence that he just doesn't measure up. He lies awake that night dwelling on the loss, reliving every mistake, and wondering whether he should even remain on the team. What's going on here? Stress researchers believe that personality, sociocultural factors, and past experiences all play a role in how we perceive and respond to stress.

The Role of Personality Types

Are you an introvert or an extrovert? Left-brain or right-brain type? A **personality type** is a set of behavioral tendencies. For instance, if you tend to analyze situations, someone might refer to you as a left-brain type, as opposed to a right-brain type who leaps to creative solutions. Although many researchers see such distinctions as too broad to help us make predictions about the behavior of individual human beings, they may be useful in helping us to explore aspects of the stress response.

In 1959, cardiologists Meyer Friedman and Ray Rosenman identified a relationship between heart disease and what they referred to as *type A* behavior.[18] Their theory caught the public imagination, and soon researchers were studying potential type A links to a wide variety of stress-related diseases. Friedman identifies three basic characteristics of the type A personality:[18]

- The person is impatient, almost chronically irritated and exasperated, and has a low tolerance for mistakes, whether their own or those of others.
- The person exhibits a free-floating hostility; that is, almost anything can provoke a hostile response.
- The person has low self-esteem. Those who interact with the person are not likely to observe this directly; however, the person's competitive, achievement-oriented behavior may be an outward attempt to compensate for low self-esteem.

In contrast, people with a *type B* personality are typically characterized as patient, tolerant, and friendly, with a realistic sense of self-esteem that may even manifest as humility. These people are thought to have a lower risk of disorders related to stress.

Recently, some researchers have posited the existence of two additional personality types: *Type C* people are said to be stoical and internalize stress; therefore, they are thought to be at increased risk for immune disorders, including cancer.[19] *Type D* people are described as responding to stressful situations either with resignation or withdrawal, whether from a job or from academic pursuits.[20]

In thinking about these various personality types, it's important to recognize that there is a great deal of debate among researchers as to whether or not they have any real validity. Although they may be useful in theory, they cannot explain the complexity of human personality or behavior.

The Role of Personality Traits

In contrast to personality types, traits are individual qualities. Some stress researchers have linked certain personality traits to an improved ability to adapt to stress. Primary among these are optimism, hardiness, and resiliency.[21]

Optimism

Optimism can be defined as an expectation of a positive outcome in most situations. People who are optimistic are more likely to see stressors as transient and specific, and therefore within their power to change and control. At the same time, they are less likely to view stressors as a consequence of internal faults; like Quillen in our example of the relay race, they avoid blaming themselves and instead focus on positive change. (For more on optimism, see Chapter 2.)

Practical Strategies for Health

Recognizing the Signs of Stress Overload

It's important to be able to recognize the warning signs of too much stress before they add up to a serious health problem. Although many people find the following symptoms common, keep in mind that stress affects different individuals in different ways. You may have less typical signs of stress, but they still merit the same attention.

Emotional warning signs include:

- Anxiety
- Sleep disruption
- Anger and agitation
- Trouble concentrating
- Unproductive worry
- Frequent mood swings
- Depression

Physical warning signs include:

- Stooped posture
- Sweaty palms
- Chronic fatigue
- Weight loss or weight gain
- Migraine or tension headaches
- Neck aches
- Digestive problems
- Frequent infections
- Physical symptoms that your doctor can't attribute to another condition

Behavioral warning signs include:

- Overreacting to problems or difficult situations
- Increased use of alcohol, tobacco, or drugs
- Unusually impulsive behavior
- Withdrawing from relationships or contact with others
- Feeling "burned out" on school or work
- Frequent bouts of crying
- Feelings of anxiety or panic

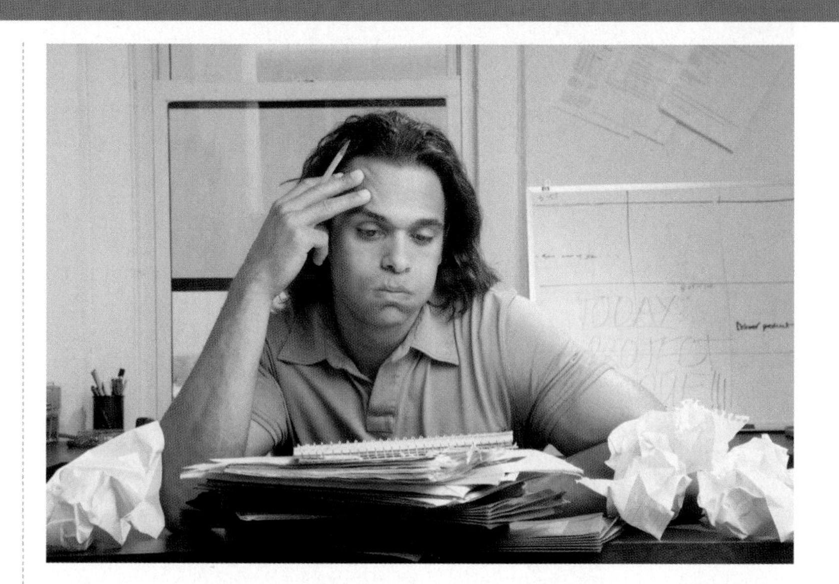

If you are experiencing the warning signs of stress overload, be proactive and seek the solutions that are right for you. Use the stress management techniques outlined in this chapter to help you manage your stress load. Also, consult your college health center, which may offer classes, workshops, or individual and group counseling to further help you cope with stress.

Hardiness

Why do some people experience significant stress, yet stay upbeat and healthy? In exploring this question, social psychologist Suzanne Kobasa identified a quality she called *hardiness* as important in enabling a person to successfully navigate the resistance phase of stress.[22] To Kobasa, hardiness is an ability to respond to the challenges of life and turn them into opportunities for growth. It includes three dimensions:[22]

- **Commitment.** The person is involved in and dedicated to relationships and ideals. Rather than feeling isolated and estranged from life, the person finds truth, value, and importance in life events, and sees adverse situations as meaningful and interesting. Committed people have a fundamental sense of worth and purpose.
- **Self-efficacy (belief in your ability to change things) and internal locus of control.** How much control a person perceives they have over any stressor will influence how difficult the stressor will be for him or her to cope with. There are two types of control, internal or external, and these can either intensify or reduce a stressor. The person with a high internal locus of control has a deep sense that he or she is capable of taking action to improve a stressful situation. That is, the person sees a relationship between his or her own efforts and external events. As a result, the person works to modify stressors to make them more manageable.
- **Challenge.** Essentially a positive attitude toward change, challenge allows the person to see adverse events not as threats to security but as opportunities for growth. The person expects and accepts mistakes and setbacks, and considers what can be learned from such experiences.

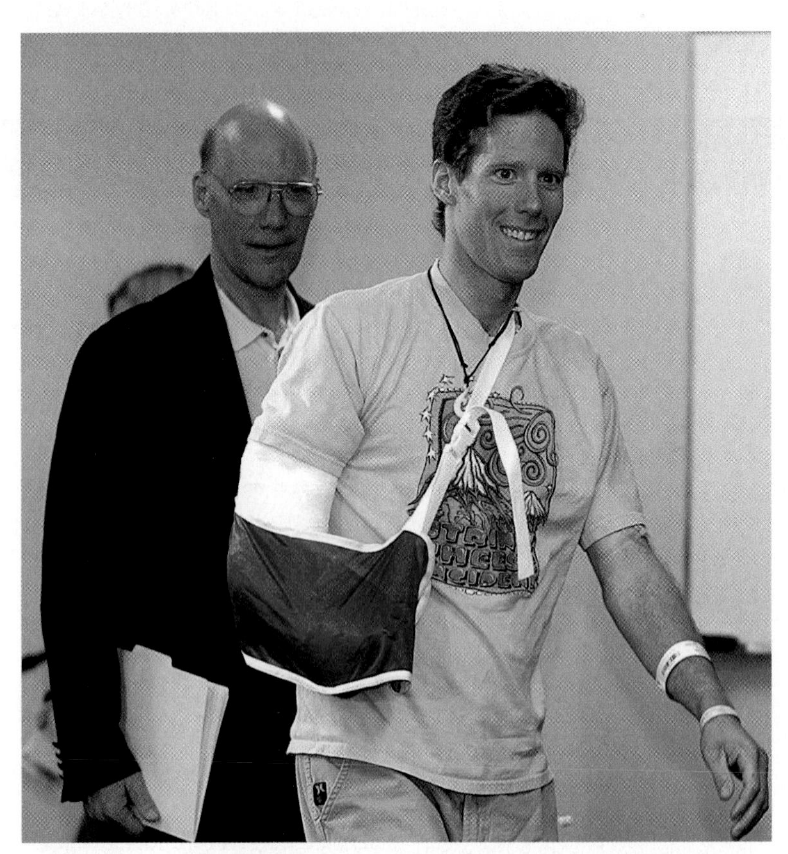

Hiker **Aron Ralston** saved himself from probable death by amputating his own arm with a pocket knife after it was crushed under a falling boulder. His ability to withstand such extreme stress likely derives in part from psychological **hardiness.** His story is the basis for the movie *127 Hours.*

Resiliency

In the years following Hurricane Katrina, news articles often described the people of New Orleans as resilient. What does this really mean? Resiliency is a property demonstrated by some physical and even biological materials that can spring back, recovering their former size and shape, after a change. For instance, after each pulse of blood from the heartbeat momentarily expands them, healthy arteries spring back to their normal size. In human beings, *resiliency* is an ability to experience success and satisfaction following trauma or other stressors. Resilient people are typically both optimistic and hardy, with an internal locus of control.[21] From an evolutionary perspective, resiliency is an innate capacity to adapt to changes in the environment, and thus to survive.

Although personality traits might seem fixed, by examining your thought patterns and behaviors, you can foster in yourself optimism, hardiness, and resiliency. Cognitive-behavioral therapy can help with this process. Other strategies for changing your thinking are discussed later in this chapter.

Sociocultural Factors

Every culture and community has its own set of typical stressors, as well as its own set of factors that influence an individual's response to those stressors. For instance, consider the values of independence versus interdependence: Many American teens experience family and cultural pressure throughout high school to distinguish themselves intellectually, athletically, and/or artistically so that they can get into a top university that will prepare them for a prestigious career. Other teens—for instance, those raised in closely knit immigrant enclaves, or in farming, fishing, mining, or logging towns—may feel pressure to set aside personal ambitions and maintain close ties to their community. Notice that these competing values prompt dramatically different stressors. But in addition, they influence the individual's response to stress. Studies suggest that people living in interdependent cultures resist and adapt to stressors more effectively than do people in independent cultures.[23] Other culturally influenced pairs that may influence our stress response include spirituality versus materialism, emotion versus reason, and the belief in the influence of fate versus the exercise of free will.

Our choice of coping mechanisms can also be influenced by culture. For instance, maybe you and your high school friends used to treat yourself to pizza and sodas after a rough day at school, but nowadays you bust your stress with a long swim in the fitness center's pool.

Our mental, material, and social resources also influence our perception of stress and our ability to cope with it. We are more likely to perceive a pop quiz as a threat if we've come to class unprepared. Similarly, an unexpected tuition hike will be more stressful for students on a tight budget. And having relatives and friends we can turn to for emotional support, encouragement, and advice can significantly reduce stress: In our earlier example, Quillen's stress level declined after he'd strategized with his dad.

Gender, age, and even geography also influence what we perceive as stressors and how we cope. See the **Diversity & Health** box for more information.

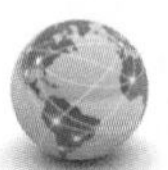

DIVERSITY & HEALTH

Stress Through the Lenses of Gender, Age, and Geography

In 2010, the American Psychological Association conducted a national survey of how Americans perceived the stress in their lives. Among the survey's findings:

Overall

- 51% of Americans rate their stress level as moderate, and 24% of respondents rate their stress level as high—that is, an 8, 9, or 10 on a 10-point scale.

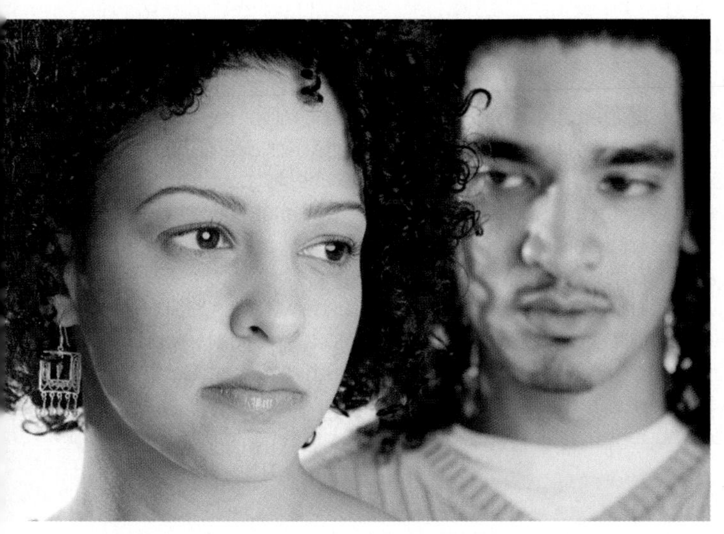

Women, in general, report higher levels of stress than men.

Gender

- Overall, women and men report similar levels of stress, but women are more likely than men to report having a great deal of stress.
- A greater percentage of women than men cited the economy, money, family health problems, and housing costs as significant stressors. Men are more likely to report work as a source of stress.
- Significantly more women than men reported experiencing headaches, an upset stomach, and emotional symptoms due to stress.

Age

- Whereas older adults report lower stress levels than the average, college-age adults report the highest stress levels of any age group.
- College-age students are also more likely than any other group to report physical symptoms of stress, such as headaches and fatigue, and emotional symptoms, such as irritation and anger.

Geography

- Regardless of where they live, Americans report experiencing comparable average levels of stress. Still, those living in the East are more likely than those living in other parts of the country to report having little or no stress.
- Americans living in the West reported the highest levels of stress related to work, the economy, and housing costs.
- People living in the Midwest are the most likely to report that they have eaten too much or eaten unhealthful foods in response to stress.
- Those living in the West are more likely to report that they exercise several times a week, compared to those living in other parts of the country. They are also more likely to say that exercising gives them energy and makes them happy.

Data from American Psychological Association. (2010, November 9). Stress in America. Retrieved from http://www.apa.org/news/press/releases/stress/national-report.pdf.

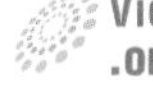

View the results of the complete Stress in America survey at www.apa.org/news/press/releases/stress/national-report.pdf.

Past Experiences

Remember the example of the snake on the trail? Past traumas can increase our tendency to perceive events as stressors. The opposite is true of past successes: job interviews, oral presentations, competitions, and exams all become easier to face over time if we build a "track record" of success.

Common Stressors

You have assignments to complete, tests to take, and papers to write. You may be juggling school and work, or facing loans and credit card debt. If you're in your first or second year of college, newer to the pressures of undergraduate academics, you may be experiencing more schoolwork stress than juniors or seniors.[24] Meanwhile, seniors close to getting their diploma need to grapple with the question of what to do after graduation.

As we've mentioned, any event that triggers your stress response is called a *stressor*. In today's world, many stressors are psychological, emotional, or biological. A looming deadline, angry parents, or a nasty case of food poisoning all count as potential stressors with the ability to throw your body into a state of heightened alarm. Some stressors come and go fairly quickly, such as getting called on in class or taking a big exam. Others may have effects that linger much longer, such as a bad breakup, a disabling injury, or the death of someone you love. And some stressors, such as childhood abuse, can continue to haunt a person's emotions and psyche long after the actual event itself has passed.[8]

> *"Past traumas can increase our tendency to perceive events as stressors. The opposite is true of past successes."*

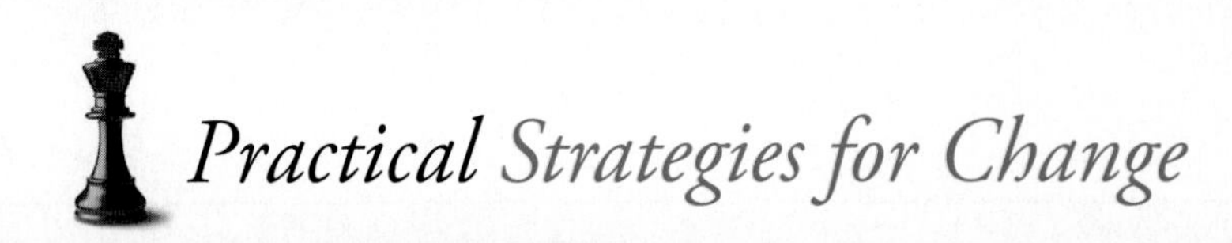

Practical Strategies for Change

Coping with Financial Stress

Even during the best of financial times, money is usually among the top five stressors reported by students. Financial concerns become even more of a stressor as parents lose jobs or as student work becomes less available and scholarship and loan dollars dry up.

Following are some strategies for coping with financial stress:

- Get a realistic handle on your finances. How much money do you have coming in from your parents, your job, and/or financial aid? How much money does it take to pay your rent, groceries, books and tuition, clothing, transportation, entertainment, and other day-to-day expenses? Try a (free) online budget tracker, such as **www.kiplinger.com/tools/budget,** which makes it easy for you to input information and identify where in your budget you can cut back.
- If you are carrying any credit card debt, develop a plan for paying it off. Reserve a set amount of money each month for paying off debt, and *stick to it*. You will feel less stress just by having a plan in place, versus doing nothing and watching your debt mount.
- If you've been completely reliant on your parents for financial support, consider taking on a part-time job—no matter how small. If there are no jobs to be found, get entrepreneurial! Consider your skills and advertise your services—for example, tutoring, babysitting, lawn mowing, car washing, general repairs, moving, housecleaning—you get the picture.
- Take an honest look at your current lifestyle. Do you pay for cable/premium TV or a cell phone plus a land line? How much money do you spend each month on eating out, expensive coffee drinks, or designer clothing? Distinguish luxuries from true necessities and *pare back*. Cancel any subscriptions or services you don't really need. Use public transportation instead of paying for gas and parking. Cut back on the number of times you eat out each month. You'd be surprised at how all of the "little things" can add up to quite a sizeable chunk of change.
- Talk to a financial aid advisor to make sure you've explored all the aid options available to you. Know exactly how much money you will need to pay off when you graduate. Only take on loans that you feel certain you will be able to pay back.

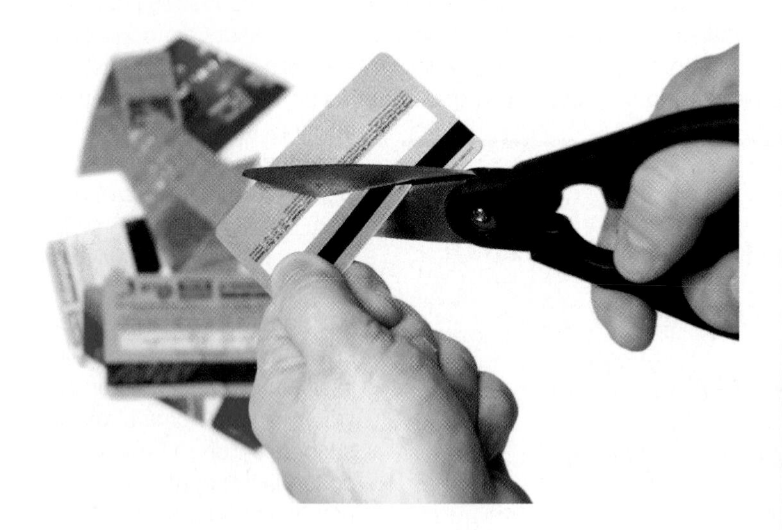

Academic Pressure

College represents a great opportunity—and a big responsibility. To graduate, get good internships, and land a fantastic job, you need to perform. No wonder students report that academics are their number-one stressor.[11] But as we noted earlier, studies have shown that too much anxiety about academics can actually reduce your success.[13] Later in this chapter, we offer tips on improving your test-taking skills.

Financial Stressors

College students rate financial concerns as second only to academics as a source of stress. Perhaps one of your parents is out of a job, and you are starting to worry about how you will pay for tuition next quarter—not to mention your student loans after you graduate. Maybe you already have a car loan, dental bills, and credit card debt. **Practical Strategies for Change: Coping with Financial Stress** provides some tips for relieving money-related stress.

Daily Hassles

Most of the stressors we encounter occur on a daily basis and are known as daily hassles. Our perception of these every day, minor, stressors, strongly influences how difficult we find them to be. For example, the school registration office says they can't find the check you sent to cover your tuition this term, even though your bank says the check has been cashed. You've completely gone over your limit of cell phone minutes for the month, and you can't find the research material you need for a class paper because your Internet connection has crashed. These problems may sound small, but daily hassles can add up to a significant source of stress. Complete the **Self-Assessment: Negative Event Scale for University Students** to rate daily hassles often encountered by college students and gauge the stress load in your own life.

Discrimination

Research over many years has established an association between experiences of discrimination and increased stress.[25, 26] Unfair treatment based on gender, age, weight, race, sexual orientation, or any other factor qualifies as discrimination. Among college students, this can manifest in varied ways. For example, a disabled student filling out a rental application for an off-campus apartment might be asked for a higher security deposit, or a student who is obese might be snubbed by peers. In one study, members of minority groups perceived discrimination or isolation to be a significant source of stress on campus.[27]

Social Stressors

Strong, supportive social networks can help carry you through tough times. Researchers have discovered, for instance, that the perceived emotional support college students experience using a social networking site like Facebook can lower their stress levels.[28] Social interactions that aren't supportive, on the other hand, increase stress; an untrue or unkind posting on a Facebook page, for example, can produce mild to overwhelming stress. And spending too much time online can promote social isolation, thereby limiting resources for coping with stress.

Job-Related Stressors

Show up to work on time, excel at your job to get that raise—and try not to think about all the school assignments you have hanging over your head at the same time! Many college students work to ease the

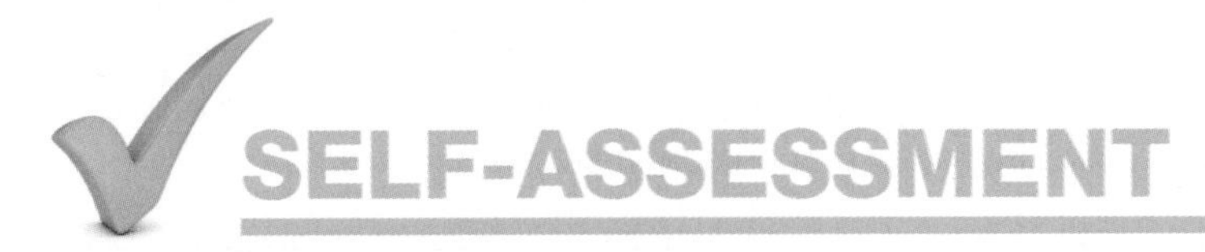

Take this self-assessment online at www.pearsonhighered.com/lynchelmore.

Negative Event Scale for University Students

You are asked to think about the negative events (hassles) that you have **experienced in the last month.** Negative daily events are the small day-to-day happenings that lead people to feel hassled. From such events people can feel distressed, upset, guilty, or scared. Negative events can also lead to people feeling hostile, irritable, nervous, afraid, ashamed, or frustrated.

Below are a list of items that can be negative events. **Please remember that it is important that you:**

- circle one number for **each item even if there was no hassle**
- consider each item with only **the last month in mind.**

How much of a hassle was this negative event?

0 = Did not occur
1 = Event occurred but there was no hassle
2 = Event occurred and a little of a hassle
3 = Event occurred and somewhat of a hassle
4 = Event occurred and a lot of a hassle
5 = Event occurred and an extreme hassle

In the last month:

Problems with Friends

1. Negative feedback from your friend/s 0 1 2 3 4 5
2. Negative communication with friend/s 0 1 2 3 4 5
3. Conflict with friend/s 0 1 2 3 4 5
4. Disagreement (including arguments) with friend/s 0 1 2 3 4 5

Problems with your Spouse/Partner (boy/girl friend)

5. Negative communication with your spouse/partner (boy/girl friend) 0 1 2 3 4 5
6. Conflict with spouse/partner (boy/girl friend) 0 1 2 3 4 5
7. Disagreement (including arguments) with spouse/partner (boy/ girl friend) 0 1 2 3 4 5
8. Rejection by your spouse/partner (boy girl friend) 0 1 2 3 4 5
9. Your spouse/partner (boy/girl friend) let you down 0 1 2 3 4 5

Work Problems

10. The nature of your job/work (if employed) 0 1 2 3 4 5
11. Your work load 0 1 2 3 4 5
12. Meeting deadlines or goals on the job 0 1 2 3 4 5
13. Use of your skills at work 0 1 2 3 4 5

Money Problems

14. Not enough money for necessities (e.g., food, clothing, housing, health care, taxes, insurance, etc.) 0 1 2 3 4 5
15. Not enough money for education 0 1 2 3 4 5
16. Not enough money for emergencies 0 1 2 3 4 5
17. Not enough money for extras (e.g., entertainment, recreation, vacations, etc.) 0 1 2 3 4 5

Problems with Children

18. Negative communication with your child(ren) 0 1 2 3 4 5
19. Conflict with your child(ren) 0 1 2 3 4 5
20. Disagreement (including arguments) with your child(ren) 0 1 2 3 4 5

Course Problems

21. Your study load 0 1 2 3 4 5
22. Study/course deadlines 0 1 2 3 4 5
23. Time pressures 0 1 2 3 4 5
24. Problems getting assignments/essays finished 0 1 2 3 4 5

Problems with Teachers/Lecturers

25. Negative communication with teacher/s, lecturer/s 0 1 2 3 4 5
26. Negative feedback from teacher/s, lecturer/s 0 1 2 3 4 5
27. Conflict with teacher/s, lecturer/s 0 1 2 3 4 5
28. Disagreement (including arguments) with your teacher/s, lecturer/s 0 1 2 3 4 5

Problems with Parents or Parents-in-law

29. Negative communication with your parents or parents-in-law 0 1 2 3 4 5
30. Conflict with your parents or parents-in-law 0 1 2 3 4 5
31. Disagreement (including arguments) with parents or parents-in-law 0 1 2 3 4 5
32. Negative feedback from your parents or parents-in-law 0 1 2 3 4 5

Problems with Other Students

33. Negative communication with other student/s 0 1 2 3 4 5
34. Conflict with other student/s 0 1 2 3 4 5
35. Disagreement (including arguments) with other student/s 0 1 2 3 4 5
36. Doing things with other student/s 0 1 2 3 4 5

Problems with Relative/s

37. Negative communication with relative/s 0 1 2 3 4 5
38. Conflict with relative/s 0 1 2 3 4 5
39. Disagreement (including arguments) with relative/s 0 1 2 3 4 5
40. Doing things with relative/s 0 1 2 3 4 5

Health Problems

41. Your health 0 1 2 3 4 5
42. Your physical abilities 0 1 2 3 4 5
43. Your medical care 0 1 2 3 4 5
44. Getting sick (e.g., flu, colds) 0 1 2 3 4 5

Problems with your Work Supervisor/Employer

45. Negative feedback from your supervisor/employer 0 1 2 3 4 5
46. Negative communication with your supervisor/employer 0 1 2 3 4 5
47. Conflict with your supervisor/employer 0 1 2 3 4 5
48. Disagreement (including arguments) with your supervisor/employer 0 1 2 3 4 5

Hassles Getting a Job

49. Finding a job (e.g., interviews, placements) 0 1 2 3 4 5
50. Finding work 0 1 2 3 4 5
51. Problems with finding a job 0 1 2 3 4 5
52. Employment problems (e.g., finding, losing a job) 0 1 2 3 4 5

Academic Limitations

53. Not getting the marks (results) you expected 0 1 2 3 4 5
54. Your academic ability not as good as you thought 0 1 2 3 4 5
55. Not understanding some subjects 0 1 2 3 4 5

Course Interest

56. Course not relevant to your future career 0 1 2 3 4 5
57. Your course is boring 0 1 2 3 4 5

HOW TO INTERPRET YOUR SCORE

Any negative events for which you score a 4 or 5 would be considered significant stressors. You can use the **Choosing to Change Worksheet** at the end of the chapter to help you modify your perceptions of these stressors and reduce the amount of hassle you feel. You can also use tips provided in the Change Yourself, Change Your World section of the chapter to manage your responses to these negative events.

Source: "Negative Event Scale for University Students," Author: Darryl Maybery, in *Negative Event Scale for University Students.*

Handling School Stress

STUDENT STORY

"Hi, I'm Jessica. The biggest source of stress in my life would probably be school and just the pressure to succeed in the future. My family doesn't really put pressure on me but I think I put a lot of pressure on myself, just based on the economy and based on the amount of money I feel I need to make to give myself a good future.

To minimize stress, exercise really is important to me. I don't do it as often as I would like but the days I do it, it does make me feel a lot better. I, unfortunately, relieve stress in other ways like drinking, like a lot of college students do. Not in any dangerous sense or any excess, maybe once a week at most. And, you know, I stress in typical other ways like crying, too."

1: Jessica uses several methods to manage stress. Which are more healthy and which are less so? What advice would you give Jessica about how to handle her stress?

2: Jessica mentions the economy as a source of stress. Does the economy affect your stress levels? If so, what can you do to address that now and in the future? Do you track your spending? How much of what you spend money on is true essentials (versus luxuries)?

Do you have a story similar to Jessica's? Share your story at www.pearsonhighered.com/lynchelmore.

financial pressure of school, but jobs increase academic stress because they inevitably cut into your time for classwork. Plus any job comes with its own stressors, from the necessity of learning new skills to meeting the demands of managers, colleagues, and clients.

Major Life Events

Traumas such as a bad breakup or a death in the family are obvious stressors. So are life-threatening events like natural disasters, motor vehicle accidents, or military service in regions experiencing combat. But as we noted earlier in the chapter, positive, exhilarating events such as starting college, graduating, or getting married can also bring heavy doses of stress. These major life event stressors are relatively rare; most of the stressors we encounter are daily hassles. In 1967, psychiatrists Thomas Holmes and Richard Rahe published what has come to be known as Holmes and Rahe's Social Readjustment Rating Scale (SRRS), an inventory of 43 stressful life events that can increase the risk of illness.[29] The scale assigns "life change units" from 1–100 for each stressful event, such as the death of a spouse (100 units), divorce (73 units), imprisonment (63 units), death of a close family member (63 units), personal injury or illness (53 units), marriage (50 units), and job loss (47 units). The scale also includes more minor stressors, such as Christmas (12 units), a change in sleeping habits (16 units), and a change in living conditions (25 units). According to this scale, the higher the number of "life change units" that a person accumulates over a given year, the greater that person's risk of illness.

Test your own stress levels with an abridged version of the SRRS scale at: www.mindtools.com/pages/article/newTCS_82.htm.

Environmental Stressors

Environmental stressors are factors in your living or working environments that you find disruptive. Examples of environmental stressors include poor air quality, pollution, toxic chemicals, and bad weather—as well as living in an unsafe neighborhood, having an annoying roommate, and dealing with a long commute. Digital technologies (such as cell phones or other mobile handheld devices) that beep at you every few minutes to alert you to text messages or voicemails can also be a source of environmental stress. In fact, all kinds of noise, from loud music to traffic sounds to people talking in the room next to yours—can be a significant source of stress for college students.

Internal Stressors

In an era when fewer of our stressors are physical, our worries, critical thoughts, and the demands we place on ourselves represent some of our most constant stressors. One study of university honors students, for example, found that those highly critical of themselves were more prone to feelings of stress, depression, and hopelessness.[30]

Do you find yourself overreacting to small problems? Do you view every task as critical when many of them really aren't? Are you often imagining horrific consequences for your actions that will probably, in reality, never come to pass? Do you procrastinate? These are all examples of situations you have the power to control or minimize, and thereby reduce your stress level.

To be sure, at some point in our lives, we all face stressors inflicted on us by events beyond our control. But often, many of us suffer from stress brought about by our own thoughts and actions. The good news

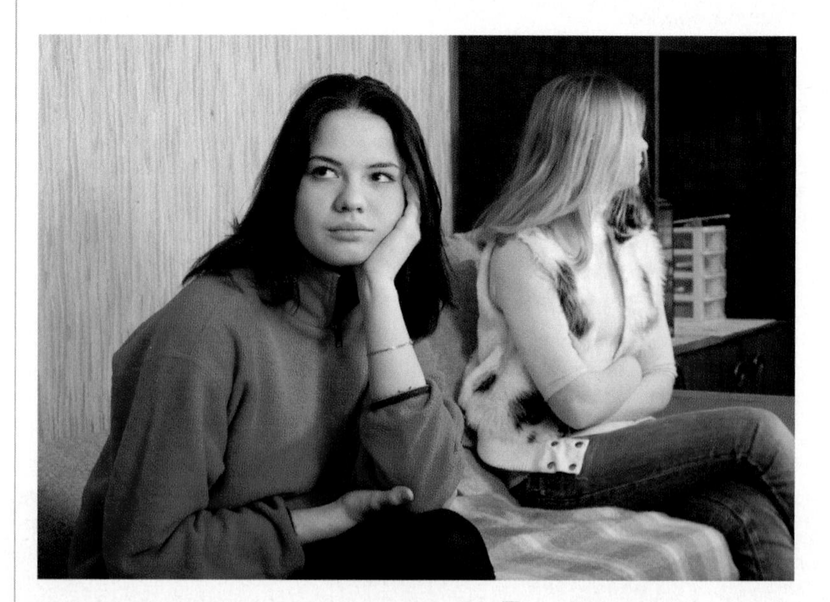

Stress comes from many sources. **Roommate troubles,** for example, can be a common source of stress for college students.

is that if we are the creators of our own stress, we can also find ways to lessen and manage that stress, as we will discuss shortly.

Getting Help for Managing Stress

Sometimes we face stress that feels truly overwhelming. If you find yourself having trouble managing stress on your own, trained professionals can help.

Clinical Options

A sensible first step is to visit your primary health-care provider or your student health center. In addition to the self-care strategies discussed in the next section of this chapter, these care providers may recommend counseling, medications, or biofeedback.

- **Counseling.** Talking with a mental health professional, either in group therapy or an individual setting, can help you manage the stressors in your life and reframe how you confront them. For example, cognitive behavioral therapy can help you learn how to identify and confront negative thoughts and responses, and replace them with positive ones. If cost is a concern, be aware that you may be eligible for free or low-cost group or individual counseling through your student health center.
- **Medications.** If you are experiencing a serious stress-related condition such as severe depression, panic attacks, or PTSD, a doctor may recommend a prescription drug, such as an antidepressant or anti-anxiety medication, to help you get your symptoms under control. Whereas some of these medications can also help you get a better night's sleep, others may interfere with sleep. A class of anti-anxiety medications called the benzodiazepines (such as Valium, Ativan, etc.) can be addictive and may have unpleasant side effects such as drowsiness, impaired balance, memory problems, and even depression and returned anxiety after the medication has worn off; therefore, they should be used only on a short-term basis.
- **Biofeedback.** In biofeedback, a device monitors your physiological stress responses, alerting you to stress symptoms such as increased heart rate or a rise in skin temperature. With guidance from a practitioner, biofeedback can help you become more aware of when your body exhibits signs of a stress response. You would then take steps to reduce that response, such as using prescribed breathing techniques, repeating an affirmation, and so on.

Complementary and Alternative Therapies

Many herbal supplement and vitamin companies sell products that promise to reduce stress or ease its symptoms. Before you try any of these products, however, talk to your health-care provider. Some supplements can react negatively with other medications you may be taking, increasing or reducing their effect, or even prompting harmful interactions.

Also ask whether the supplement you're considering has proven benefits, and whether it is associated with any harmful effects. For example, the herb kava, a member of the pepper family, is used to reduce anxiety, and some studies do support its effectiveness for anxiety management.[31] However, the U.S. Food and Drug Administration has issued a warning that using kava can result in liver damage, including hepatitis and liver failure.

Acupuncture has shown some promise in treating PTSD. Part of traditional Chinese medicine, acupuncture uses extremely fine needles to stimulate certain points on the body. In one study, acupuncture was as effective as cognitive-behavioral therapy in reducing the anxiety, depression, and other symptoms of PTSD.[32] Whether this therapy is effective for other stress-related disorders isn't yet clear.

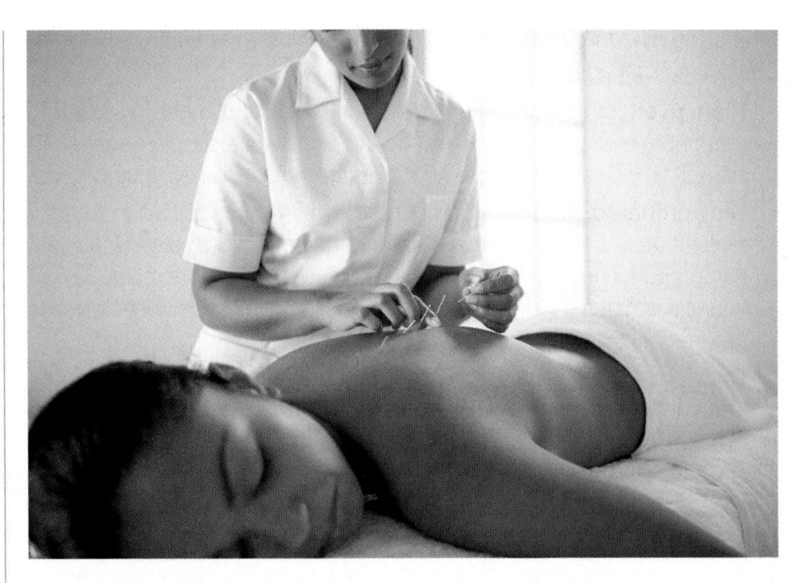

Complementary and alternative therapies like **acupuncture** may help you manage stress, but check with your doctor first.

Change Yourself, Change Your World

Stress doesn't have to escalate beyond your control. There's a lot you can do to relax, step back from stressful situations, and face your challenges with renewed energy and confidence. Some of these techniques involve making changes to your lifestyle and cultivating habits that strengthen your resilience and energy. Others give you ways to reframe situations in your mind, gain perspective about your stressors, and switch off your internal alarms. You can also get to work combating stressors you or other students might face on your campus.

Personal Choices

Several studies of college students show that with a few changes, life on campus can be more fun, and less stressful. These changes, though, take some effort and time.[33, 34] You can't expect to eliminate stress overnight. But by making changes to your daily routine, giving yourself opportunities to relax, and thinking about stress in useful ways, you can reduce and better manage the stressors in your life.

Manage Your Time Effectively

For many students, a 24-hour day seems about 10 hours too short. You may feel like you can't cram your classes, studying, assignments, job, friends, significant others, hobbies, physical activity, chores, and even basic survival needs (remember eating and sleeping?) into a typical day. If this describes you, take heart. Better time management can result in better stress management. The **Choosing to Change Worksheet** at the end of this chapter offers one way to evaluate where your time goes. The following are additional strategies you can employ for better time management:

- **Plan, even just a little.** Use a daily scheduler or planner to remind you of big events and track your to-do list. Even a simple paper-based scheduler can keep important tasks from sneaking up on you.
- **Stay prepared.** When you find out the dates of big assignments and tests at the start of the term, make note of them in your planner so you can prepare ahead of time. Read assignments before class, and review your class notes shortly after class ends. Both strategies will help you get more out of class, and make big study sessions a lot easier.
- **Break down big jobs.** Remember that a forest consists of individual trees. When a task feels overwhelming, write down all the steps required to get it done, and then tackle them one at a time.
- **Hate it? Do it first.** If you can get the task you like the least out of the way, everything that follows will feel much easier.
- **Leave time for surprises.** Your car breaks down, and you need a couple of hours to get it to the shop, for example. If every hour of your schedule is always booked, you won't have room to deal with the unexpected turns life takes.
- **Reward yourself.** Been wrestling with a challenging assignment for an hour? Take a break. Finish a paper early for a change? Let your laundry slide, and watch a movie. And leave time in your schedule to relax. If you are working hard in college, you've more than earned a reward.

Get Adequate, Restful Sleep

As we discussed earlier, sleep is a naturally restorative process that is essential for healthy physical and psychological functioning. (For information on how to get a better night's sleep, see Chapter 4.)

Live a Healthier Lifestyle

You can go a long way toward reducing your stress level by practicing the following basic wellness habits:

- **Eat well.** Food and stress have a reciprocal relationship. On the one hand, a nutritious diet allows your body to function smoothly and helps keep your stress responses in balance. On the other hand, chronic stress can lead to unhealthful eating habits. When they are stressed, many people turn to foods with sugar to increase their energy level. Sugar may satisfy in the short term, but after an hour or two, it actually leaves you with less energy and craving more food. People under stress may also turn to caffeine to help them keep going, but too much caffeine can cause sleep problems and add to the physiological effects of stress.[35] Weight gain is also associated with the too-busy-to-exercise lives of those with chronic stress.
- **Exercise.** Exercise, especially activities such as walking, cycling, weight training, or running that work your large muscles and build sustained strength, is an effective stress-reducer.[36] Scientists theorize that physical activity allows the body to complete the fight-or-flight response by actually doing what it has been prepared to do. After all, whether you are running around a track or running from a bear, you are still "fleeing" and thereby helping your body return to balance. As little as 20 minutes a day can help.[37] Moreover, even one exercise session can generate post-exercise euphoria that can last anywhere from 90 to 120 minutes.[38] For tips on exercising for stress management, see **Practical Strategies for Change: Exercising for Stress Management.**
- **Avoid caffeine, alcohol, tobacco, or other drugs.** Coffee and energy drinks might seem like harmless substances that keep you going. Likewise, drinking, smoking, and recreational drugs can seem to offer a brief vacation from stress. But numerous studies have shown that too much caffeine can cause physical symptoms such as jitteriness, and that the long-term health risks of smoking, drugs, or excess drinking far outweigh the few moments of relief they offer. If you find yourself drawn to potentially addictive substances to relieve stress, seek help from your doctor or from a health professional at your student health center.
- **Take time for hobbies and leisure.** It probably feels like you have no time at all right now for hiking, dance class, mountain biking, scrapbooking, or helping design t-shirts for friends' bands. But even small amounts of time spent away from school and work will reduce your stress and give you new energy to face the main tasks at hand. Breaks can also improve learning, giving you time to consider the material you've been studying in new ways. Research backs up this common-sense advice—one study of undergraduates found that those who valued their leisure time enjoyed better health and mental well-being.[39]
- **Keep a journal.** Make time to record what's going on in your life and how you feel about it. Keeping a journal may seem like a low priority amid all your schoolwork, but it has actually been linked to improved moods and higher GPAs.[40] If you don't feel like toting around a traditional diary, online blogs and personal web pages (with privacy controls) are also good ways to keep a journal.

Ask for Help

Ask your professors for help. Find out their office hours and visit them in person to get help on material you don't understand, or to voice your concerns. They might be able to offer you helpful advice about how to approach assignments or prepare for exams. If your stress should start to feel overwhelming, make an appointment at your campus health center to speak to a counselor.

Call your family and make time for your friends, especially old friends from high school who may now be far away. They know you well, and can help you keep the stress in your life in perspective. At the same time, building a new network of college friends through your dorm life or social clubs will let you find and give support in a group that knows the pressures you face firsthand.

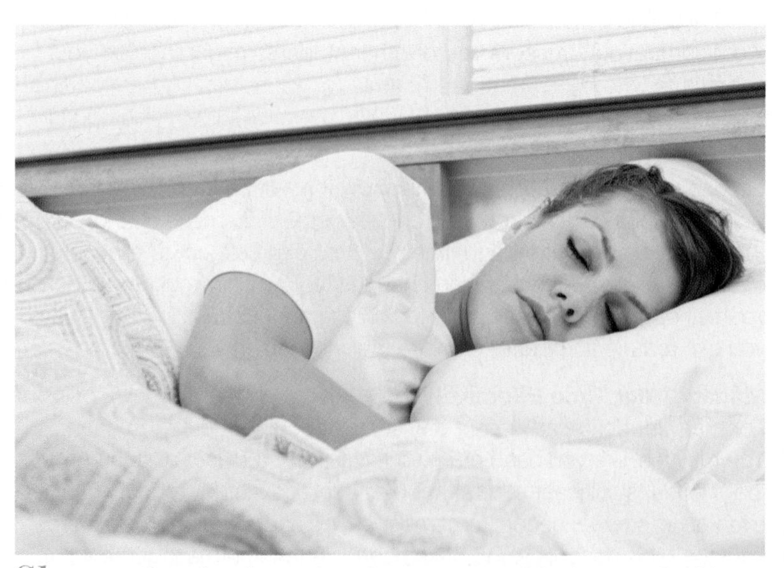

Sleep can refresh and revive you, and help you feel less stressed.

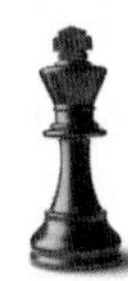

Practical Strategies for Change

Exercising for Stress Management

Having trouble getting moving? Consider the following tips:

- Think of exercise as "recess"—not as a chore, but as a chance to break up an otherwise routine day with a fun, active, recreational activity.
- Vary your exercise activity. You might go swimming one day and bicycling another day. This way, you will have more options to choose from depending on your mood, the free time you have available, and the weather report on any given day.
- Pick activities you genuinely enjoy. If you hate jogging but love to dance, by all means, dance!
- Remember that any activity that gets your body moving can ease stress. If you're not into sports, consider walking around campus just for fun, walking your dog, or even walking in a shopping center. Any physical activity is better than none!
- Consider exercise classes such as yoga or tai chi that focus on breathing and relaxation.
- Enlist a friend as an exercise partner. You can keep each other encouraged and have more fun while you exercise.
- Make exercise a regular part of your schedule. Prioritize it the same way you would prioritize your schoolwork or a job.
- Exercise releases endorphins in the body, which makes you feel good. So the next time you find yourself resisting the thought of getting up and moving, remind yourself of how great you will feel afterward!

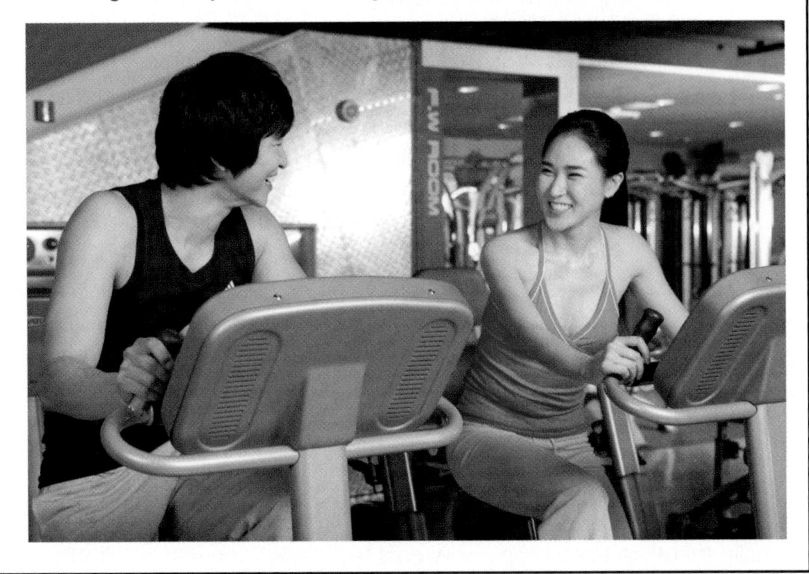

Communicate your feelings. For instance, let your roommates know that you have a big test in the morning and need them to wear headphones when the TV is on. Talk with supportive friends and family about the pressures you face and how they can help you cope. One study of university students found that those who talked about their stressors and sought support suffered less depression from academic stress.[41]

Improve Your Test-Taking Skills

The following steps can help get you ready for success *before* your next test.

> *"Recording your activities and thoughts has actually been linked to improved moods for students and higher GPAs."*

- **Learn test-taking skills.** Many colleges offer courses on test-taking skills. Sign up for one!
- **Learn about the test ahead of time.** Find out what topics the test will cover and what format it will be in. If your instructor provides practice tests or preparation materials, use them.
- **Schedule your study time.** Study over a series of days or weeks; avoid cramming at the last minute or pulling an "all nighter."
- **Talk with your instructor.** Tell your instructor in advance if you experience test anxiety. He or she may be able to offer suggestions or help.
- **Prepare yourself mentally.** Think positively. In the days leading up to the test, visualize yourself calmly taking the test and knowing the answers.
- **Prepare yourself physically.** Get enough sleep the night before.

When test day arrives, get up early so that you avoid having to rush. Before the test, eat a light meal so you are not hungry. Once you're in the testing room, choose a seat in a place that seems comfortable for you—for instance, near a window so you can get some fresh air, or away from a classmate whose mannerisms you find distracting. Avoid talking to other students right before the test. Doing so might cause you to feel confused or reduce your confidence. During the test, follow these strategies:

- **Read the directions carefully.**
- **Answer the easy questions first.** This will give you confidence and allow you to budget your remaining time on the more difficult questions.
- **If you get stuck, move on.** You can turn back to the question later.
- **Stay calm.** If you find yourself getting anxious: (1) Relax. Remind yourself that you are in control and are well-prepared for this test. (2) Take slow, deep breaths. (3) Concentrate on the questions, not on your fear. (4) Remind yourself that some anxiety is natural.
- **Even if you don't know the final answer, show your work.** Graders may give you partial credit.
- **Don't be alarmed if other students turn in their tests before you.** They might have left several questions unanswered. Use all the time you need.
- **When you have finished, check your work.** However, do not second-guess yourself or change an answer unless you have remembered more-accurate information.

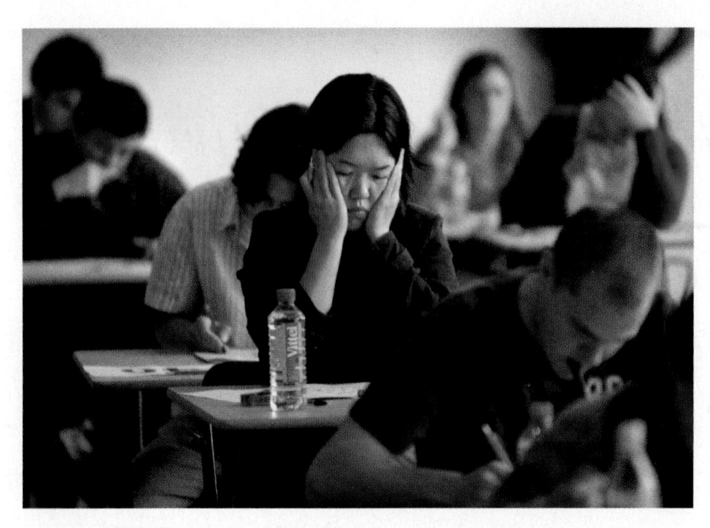

Stress less when preparing for and taking exams.

What if you've finished the test, and then start to stress out about your grade? Try these three post-test strategies:

- **Focus on the positive.** Think about all the things you did right either before or during the test.
- **Evaluate your test preparation.** Which strategies were helpful and which were not? Did you neglect anything? For instance, perhaps you were distracted because your mouth was dry during the test, and wished you had brought a bottle of water or some mints.
- **Develop a plan for your next test.** Base your new plan on what worked and didn't work for this test.

Elicit Your Relaxation Response

Recall that the stress response begins with activation of the sympathetic nervous system, which increases your heart rate, breathing rate, and metabolism, and generally prepares your body for fighting or flight. Fortunately, the stress response can be soothed by activation of your parasympathetic nervous system (PNS), which reduces your heart rate, quiets your breathing, slows your metabolism, and generally prepares you for rest. Moreover, you can actively promote these changes, collectively called your **relaxation response,** to slow yourself down, quiet your mind, and greatly reduce your stress.

relaxation response A set of physiological responses—including decreased heart rate, respiratory rate, and metabolism—regulated by the peripheral nervous system and inductive of rest; can be activated through relaxation techniques.

To elicit your relaxation response, try the following technique taught at the Benson-Henry Institute for Mind-Body Medicine at Massachusetts General Hospital, which includes two fundamental steps: (1) Repetition of a word, sound, phrase, prayer, or muscular activity; (2) Passive disregard of everyday thoughts that inevitably come to mind, and the return to your repetition.[42]

1. Pick a focus word, short phrase, or prayer that is firmly rooted in your belief system, such as "one," "peace," "love," "The Lord is my shepherd," or "shalom."
2. Sit quietly in a comfortable position.
3. Close your eyes.
4. Relax your muscles, progressing from your feet to your calves, thighs, abdomen, shoulders, neck, and head.
5. Breathe slowly and naturally, and as you do, say your focus word, sound, phrase, or prayer silently to yourself as you exhale.
6. Assume a passive attitude. Don't worry about how well you're doing. When other thoughts come to mind, simply say to yourself, "Oh well," and gently return to your repetition.
7. Continue for 10 to 20 minutes.
8. Do not stand immediately. Continue sitting quietly for a minute or so, allowing other thoughts to return. Then open your eyes and sit for another minute before rising.
9. Practice the technique once or twice daily. Good times to do so are before breakfast and before dinner.

Regular elicitation of the relaxation response has been scientifically proven to be an effective treatment for a wide range of stress-related disorders. In fact, to the extent that any disease is caused or made worse by stress, the relaxation response can help.[42]

Loosen Tight Muscles

For centuries, people have practiced a variety of techniques to stretch and relax tense or tired muscles. These include the following:

- *Progressive muscle relaxation (PMR).* This technique helps you relax each major muscle group in your body, one by one, adding up to a powerful reduction in physical tension. Start by choosing one part of your body, such as your left foot. Inhale as you flex and tense it. Then exhale as you relax it. Repeat this once or twice. Then move on to your left leg and repeat the same process. Slowly move through all the major muscle groups of your body, deliberately tensing and relaxing each one, until your whole body relaxes.
- *Yoga.* Fundamental to the ancient Indian healing system called *ayurveda,* yoga is a mind-body practice that includes three main components: physical postures called *asanas*—such as the mountain pose or the cat stretch—lengthen the muscles, improving physical fitness, strength, flexibility, and posture.[43] At the same time, a breathing technique called *pranayama* and a form of contemplation called *dhyana* reduce heart rate and blood pressure, and increase lung capacity. There is growing evidence to suggest that yoga not only relaxes your muscles, but also enhances stress-coping mechanisms and improves the individual's mood and sense of well-being.[43]
- *Massage.* A professional massage therapist uses pressure, stretching, friction, heat, cold, and other forms of manipulation to stimulate skin and muscles and relieve tension. Some studies have shown that massage can be helpful in reducing anxiety, decreasing pain, relieving sports-related soreness, and boosting the immune system.[44] Check with your campus wellness or recreation center to see if it offers reduced-price massages on campus.

Explore Other Tension Relievers

Finally, there are three simple, low-cost techniques you can do almost anywhere to bust your stress.

Breathe deeply. Research suggests that the following breathing exercise can reduce stress:[45]

- Take a slow, deep breath, drawing the breath in through the nose with your mouth closed, and then exhaling through the mouth. Inhaling and exhaling should take about 6 seconds each.
- Rest one hand gently on your abdomen and continue drawing long, slow, deep breaths.
- Notice that, while you are breathing deeply, your chest wall expands and contracts. At the

This university website offers instructions about how to perform various mind and body relaxation techniques: www.uhs.uga.edu/stress/relax.html

same time, your hand on your upper abdomen should move outward—away from your core—as your chest fills with air, and back in again as you empty your lungs. This happens in part because your diaphragm, a muscle that lies somewhat horizontally along the floor of your chest cavity, drops downward as you breathe in, then springs back upward as you breathe out.

- Throughout this exercise, your shoulders should remain stationary. Rising and falling shoulders mean your breathing is high and shallow. If this is happening, just focus on expanding your rib cage outward with each inspiration, and feeling it relax back inward with each exhalation.
- Once you've achieved a slow, steady breathing rate, continue this exercise for several minutes.

Listen to music. Taking a break can be as close as your MP3 player. Music therapy has been used in clinical settings for many years to control acute and chronic pain, relax tense muscles, reduce fatigue, relieve depression, and increase feelings of comfort.[46] It does this in part by helping to induce the body's relaxation response—but not all music has the desired effect! In one study, college students overwhelmingly preferred low-volume music over medium or loud music for relaxation, and researchers also noted that a soft volume was more effective at reducing heart rate.[47] Another study showed that slow, classical music can be effective at lowering blood pressure after a stressful situation.[48]

Visualize peace. Stressed out by your surroundings? Imagine you are somewhere you find relaxing. Close your eyes and visualize yourself lying on a beach, resting under a tree on a warm day, or napping on your favorite couch. If you're nervous about an upcoming event, such as giving a presentation in front of a class, imagine yourself giving the talk and getting a standing ovation at the end. Athletes often use visualization techniques to handle the pressures of competitive events.

Change Your Thinking

Changing the way you think about the stressors in your life can help hold stress at bay. To keep your everyday stressors from turning into mountains of tension, consider the following:

- **Rewrite internal messages.** How do you talk to yourself? When you have a test coming up, do you tell yourself you can ace it with consistent study ahead of time? Or do you tell yourself that you'll probably fail, so why bother studying? If you tend to tell yourself negative messages, first identify them, then restate them as positive, solution-oriented, constructive messages.
- **Set realistic expectations.** College brings new challenges—and a whole new level of competition. Do you feel disappointed if you don't ace every single course you take? Or do you give yourself permission to feel that your best effort is reward enough? Regardless of how ambitious you are, be honest with yourself and try to set realistic goals in order to keep your stress level manageable.
- **Build your self-esteem.** Increasing your self-worth through positive affirmations and self-talk, replaying compliments in your head, and the other self-esteem boosting tips we discussed in the psychological health chapter can help you build the inner strength and confidence to handle stressful situations when they come along.
- **Be proactive.** Do you have a professor who enjoys pop quizzes, and does this make you think about skipping class some days? Unfortunately, avoidance is a poor strategy for stress management. Studies have found that trying to avoid stressful scenes ahead of time will only worsen your stress later.[49] If you have a class with a professor who likes surprises, be prepared by keeping up with your studies. A little planning now will mean less stress later on.
- **Tackle problems head-on.** When confronted by a difficult task or situation, do you believe in your ability to find a creative, effective solution? Or do you automatically assume you'll fail from the start? Strong problem-solving skills are closely linked to better health and fewer feelings of stress in college students.[50] If a problem seems overwhelming, try breaking it into pieces and tackling one bit at a time. Ask your professors, classmates, and friends for help. Taking active steps to solve a problem can reduce your feelings of stress, whereas doing nothing but worrying has the opposite effect.
- **Have a sense of humor.** A little laughter can go a long way toward reducing stress. Laughter increases your intake of oxygen, improves your circulation, relaxes your muscles, and reduces tension. So read some cartoons, or watch some funny YouTube videos, or talk to your most hilarious friend. Humor can help you get a better

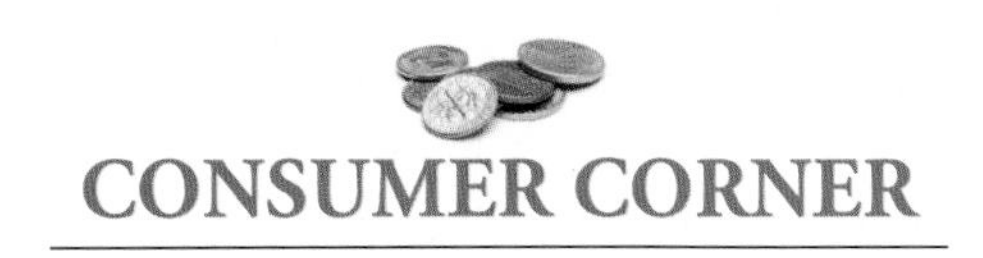

CONSUMER CORNER

Can Video Games Help Reduce Stress?

Can playing video games help relieve stress? The answer depends on the type of game. Some games involve exercise and movement—and as you've learned in this chapter, physical activity is a proven stress reducer. Other games require calm, focused concentration, a type of activity that also helps many people reduce stress. In one study, people suffering from PTSD (post-traumatic stress disorder) experienced fewer symptoms if they played a relatively quiet, systematic video game such as Tetris for 30 minutes a week.[1] On the other hand, studies have shown that games that simulate violence may actually increase players' levels of stress by triggering the body's fight-or-flight response.[2]

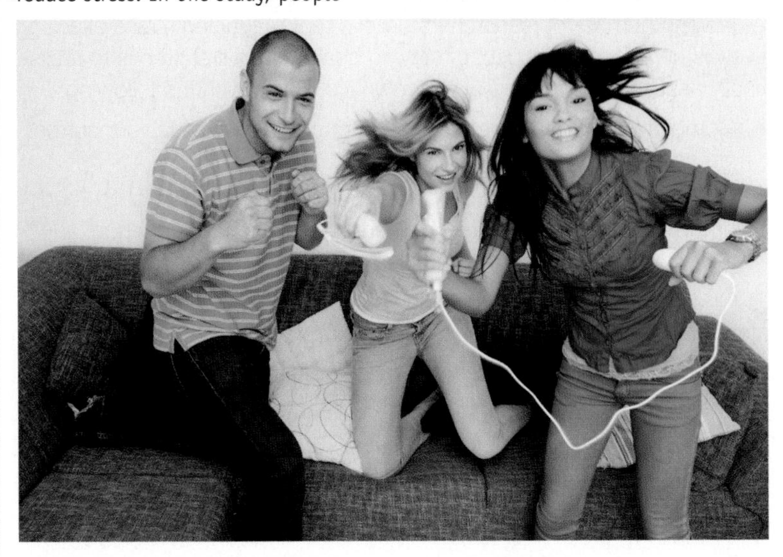

References: **1.** Holmes, E. A., James, E. L., Coode-Bate, T., & Deeprose, C. (2009). Can playing the computer game "Tetris" reduce the build-up of flashbacks for trauma? A proposal from cognitive science. *PLoS ONE, 4* (1), e4153, doi:10.1371/journal.pone.0004153. **2.** Sharm, R., Kera, S., Mohan, A., Gupta, S., & Ray, R. (2006). Assessment of computer games as a psychological stressor. *Indian Journal of Physiology and Pharmacology, 50* (4), 367–374.

perspective on which stressors are really important and which ones are overblown.

- **Take the long view.** Are most of the stressors in your life right now going to matter to you in a few years? Cultivating patience and a sense of what matters in the long term can help you keep problems in perspective.
- **Accept that you cannot control everything.** Being able to accept that you can't control everything—and being adaptable to less-than-ideal situations—can make a big difference in how well you deal with stress. For instance, if you play team sports, consciously acknowledge that the final score or season ranking isn't up to you alone. One area in which lack of control can be particularly stressful is social networking. If someone leaves a hurtful comment on your blog, you can simply delete it. But if negative comments about you start circulating on friends' social networking sites, much as you might want to refute them, it's better not to respond. Such comments are often made to provoke conflict, so just make sure your own postings reflect your integrity, and trust that time and silence will deflate the situation.

Create a Personalized Stress Management Plan

A growing number of researchers believe that managing stress effectively is an important aspect of staying healthy. The first step is to realistically assess the stressors in your own life. Begin with the following:

- Complete the **Self-Assessment** on page 71 to assess your current stressors.
- Complete the **Choosing to Change Worksheet** found at the end of this chapter to evaluate your readiness for behavior change, and take steps to reduce the controllable stressors.

Once you have done everything you can to minimize the controllable stressors in your life, it's time to think about how you can better respond to (and manage) the stress that remains. Review the section on strategies for managing stress. Which techniques seem like the best fit for your life and personality? Select the options you find the most comfortable and natural for you. Keep the following guidelines in mind:

- Remember that not all stress is harmful. You may find one of your classes tough, for example, but intellectually fun and challenging. Focus on changing your response to stressors that leave you exhausted, irritable, anxious, or sick.
- If the stress management technique that you pick requires adjustments to your schedule, take action to make room for it. For example, if you've resolved to shake some of that stress through more exercise, prioritize time for workouts into your schedule.
- Decide how long you will try the stress management technique to see if it is working. Remember that managing stress is a long-term commitment. Tackle your stressors little by little, rather than trying to eliminate all of your stress at once.

This video from Dartmouth College provides tips for students on how to incorporate stress management into their lives: www.dartmouth.edu/~acskills/videos/video_sm.html.

Campus Advocacy

When you feel stressed out on campus, look around and you'll realize very quickly that you aren't alone. Talk to your friends, classmates, and roommates about how you are feeling. Many student organizations and student health centers also offer support groups where you can vent about stress, hear what others are going through, and swap suggestions for coping. Find out what's happening on your campus, and get involved! Here's a sample of what you might find:

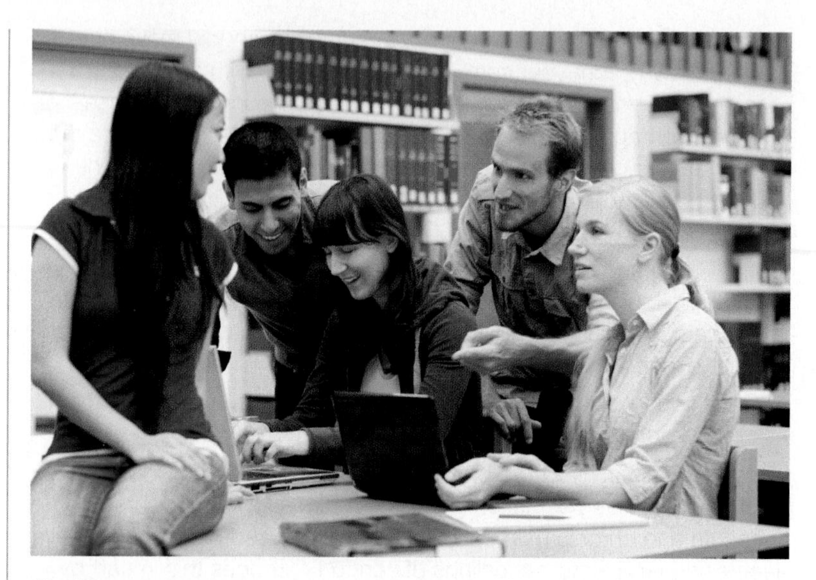

College brings many opportunities for stress, but with effective stress management, it can be a time of great growth and fun as well.

- *Transitioning.* Many researchers believe that the first year of college is the toughest.[51] Making the transition from home to campus can be easier if students have access to stress-management information and supportive services. A new campaign aims to give students exactly that. Called *The Transition Year,* it's jointly sponsored by the American Psychiatric Association and the Jed Foundation, a nonprofit established in 2000 by Donna and Phil Saltow, who lost their son Jed to suicide.[51] The campaign includes a website that offers tools and links to help students navigate all kinds of issues, from homework to dorm life. One of the links introduces students to Active Minds, a mental health advocacy group now operating on over 100 college campuses. Check out the foundation's website at **www.transitionyear.org.**
- *Debt.* Some campus financial aid departments are sponsoring informational websites and free crash courses to help students avoid or reduce their credit card debt. Some even offer short-term, emergency loans to help students pay off their high-interest consumer debt and get on a manageable payment plan. If your campus doesn't offer such a service, contact your local consumer credit counseling agency and suggest that it offer its services on your campus. For a list of approved consumer credit counseling agencies by state and district, see **www.justice.gov/ust/eo/bapcpa/ccde/cc_approved.htm.**
- *Grades.* Most colleges and universities have academic advising offices where students can go to get help with academic challenges. Many also have peer tutoring services. Don't hesitate to take advantage of these services—it's more effective to use them as soon as you realize there's a problem. In contrast, if you excel academically, consider sharing your talents. Helping others can reduce your own stress and increase your happiness.[52]

Watch videos of real students discussing stress management at www.pearsonhighered.com/lynchelmore.

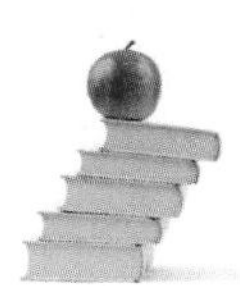

Choosing to Change Worksheet

Complete this worksheet online at **www.pearsonhighered.com/lynchelmore.**

You have acquired extensive information from this chapter about stressors and how to manage them. You had the opportunity to make observations about whether or not your perceptions toward negative events in your life may be contributing to making you feel distressed by completing the **Negative Event Scale for University Students** self-assessment on page 71.

Directions: Fill in your stage of change in Step 1 and complete the remaining steps with your stage of change in mind.

Step 1: Your Stage of Behavior Change. Please check one of the following statements that best describes your readiness to change your perceptions to stressors.

_____________ I do not intend to change my perception of stressors in the next 6 months. (Precontemplation)

_____________ I might change my perception of stressors in the next 6 months. (Contemplation)

_____________ I am prepared to change my perception of stressors in the next month. (Preparation)

_____________ I have been changing my perception of stressors for less than 6 months ago. (Action)

_____________ I have been changing my perception of stressors for more than 6 months ago. (Maintenance)

Step 2: Recognizing Chronic Stress. It is important to identify the warning signs of chronic stress to assess whether or not your health may be at risk. The following table lists some of the common warning signs and symptoms of stress overload. Check whether or not you have experienced any of these within the last month.

Recognizing Warning Signs and Symptoms of Stress Overload

Emotional	Yes	No	Physical	Yes	No	Behavioral	Yes	No
Anxiety			Stooped posture			Overreacting to problems or difficult situations		
Sleep disruption			Sweaty palms			Increased use of alcohol, tobacco, or other drugs		
Anger and agitation			Chronic fatigue			Unusually impulsive behavior		
Trouble concentrating			Weight loss or weight gain			Feeling "burned out" on school or work		
Unproductive worry			Migraine or tension headaches			Withdrawing from relationships or contact with others		
Frequent mood swings			Neck aches			Feelings of anxiety or panic		
Depression			Digestive problems			Frequent bouts of crying		
			Asthma attacks					
			Physical symptoms that your doctor can't attribute to another condition					

The more signs and symptoms you notice, the closer you may be to allostatic overload or excessive stress. Be mindful that the signs and symptoms of stress can also be caused by other psychological and physiological medical problems. If you're experiencing any of the warning signs of stress over time, it's important to see a health care professional for a full evaluation.

Step 3: Identifying Stressors. What were your top five stressors based on your completion of the **Negative Event Scale for University Students** self-assessment on page 71? Choose those that you scored as a 4 (a lot of a hassle) or 5 (an extreme hassle).

My top 5 stressors	How much of a hassle was this stressor? (4 or 5)
1.	
2.	
3.	
4.	
5.	

Now that you successfully completed Steps 2 and 3 you can begin to take action about changing the way you think about the primary stressors in your life and reduce or eliminate stress induced symptoms by completing Steps 4 & 5.

Step 4: Choosing Stress Management Techniques. For each of the stressors listed in Step 3 write down a stress management technique from the Change Yourself, Change Your World section of the chapter that can reduce this stressor. On a scale of 1–5 (1 being the lowest and 5 the highest), what is your confidence in your ability to implement the stress management technique the next time you experienced the stressor?

Stressor	Stress management technique	How confident are you in your ability to employ this technique?				
		Low confidence (1)				High confidence (5)
1.		1	2	3	4	5
2.		1	2	3	4	5
3.		1	2	3	4	5
4.		1	2	3	4	5
5.		1	2	3	4	5

Step 5: Using Effective Time Management to Reduce Daily Hassles. Things such as being stuck in a long line at the grocery store or dealing with the daily time pressures from classes or study deadlines add up. You can reduce some of your daily stress, and handle the hassles in your life more effectively, by rethinking how you use your time. Start by taking a closer look at your schedule. Using the following chart, fill in your activities every day for a week.

Time	Monday	Tuesday	Wednesday	Thursday	Friday	Saturday	Sunday
5:00 a.m.							
6:00 a.m.							
7:00 a.m.							
8:00 a.m.							
9:00 a.m.							
10:00 a.m.							
11:00 a.m.							
12:00 p.m.							

Time	Monday	Tuesday	Wednesday	Thursday	Friday	Saturday	Sunday
1:00 p.m.							
2:00 p.m.							
3:00 p.m.							
4:00 p.m.							
5:00 p.m.							
6:00 p.m.							
7:00 p.m.							
8:00 p.m.							
9:00 p.m.							
10:00 p.m.							
11:00 p.m.							
12:00 a.m.							
12 a.m.–5 a.m.							

Now, examine the chart and consider the following: Which tasks are most important to your goals in school and in your personal life? Which tasks are needed to keep you healthy, such as eating, sleeping, and making time to relax? Which tasks are unnecessary time-busters—that is, activities that eat away at your time, or waste it (be honest). Decide how you can kick a time-buster or two out of your schedule. Mark these areas with red pencil, and see how much more time you have for important tasks.

Chapter Summary

- Stress is the collective psychobiological state that develops in response to a disruptive, unexpected, or exciting stimulus. Eustress is stress resulting from positive stressors; distress is stress resulting from negative stressors.
- The general adaptation syndrome (GAS) is a theory developed by Hans Seyle that attempts to explain the biology of the stress response. It consists of three phases: alarm, resistance, and exhaustion.
- The fight-or-flight response is characteristic of the alarm phase of the GAS. It includes an instantaneous set of reactions prompted by the sympathetic nervous system's release of noradrenaline. These reactions temporarily boost strength and stamina to prepare the body to deal with a stressor. This is followed by a hormonal response, including the secretion of cortisol, that sustains the initial nervous system reactions.
- During the resistance phase, the body mobilizes homeostatic mechanisms that help it adapt to the stressor.
- According to the human function curve, a manageable degree of stress actually improves performance, but excessive, persistent stress results in exhaustion and burnout.
- Chronic stress can increase your risk of heart disease and stroke, result in digestive problems, promote weight gain, weaken your immune system, trigger headaches, disturb your sleep, and compromise learning, memory, and mental health.
- Researchers debate the role of various personality types in our response to stress. However, the traits of optimism, hardiness, and resiliency have been demonstrated to enhance our ability to cope with stress.
- Culturally influenced values, such as independence versus interdependence, influence the types of stressors we encounter as well as our response to stress. Our mental, material, and social resources, such as gender, age, geography, and our past experiences, also influence the stress response.
- Clinical options for managing stress include counseling, medications, and biofeedback.
- Personal strategies for reducing stress include managing your time effectively; getting enough sleep; eating well; exercising; avoiding caffeine, alcohol, tobacco, and other drugs; taking time for hobbies; and keeping a journal. You should also ask for help when you need it.
- Other practical steps for stress management include improving your test-taking skills, eliciting your relaxation response, trying progressive muscle relaxation, yoga, or massage to loosen tight muscles, practicing deep breathing, listening to music, and using visualization techniques. It's also important to restructure your thoughts in a more positive way.
- Creating a personal stress-management plan can help you realistically assess and get control of the stressors in your life.
- Opportunities abound on campus to take action to reduce your own stress level and help other students as well. Getting involved should even help you to reduce your own level of stress and increase your happiness.

Test Your Knowledge

1. The stress that results from positive experiences (such as graduating from college or getting married) is called
   a. eustress.
   b. distress.
   c. variable stress.
   d. allostasis.

2. In the "alarm" stage of the general adaptation syndrome
   a. the adrenal glands release cortisol.
   b. the stomach releases glucose.
   c. the heart rate slows.
   d. all of the above are correct.

3. The fight-or-flight response
   a. is characteristic of the resistance phase.
   b. is regulated by the nervous system and hormones.
   c. is a sign of allostatic overload.
   d. includes all of the above.

4. The effects of chronic stress can include
   a. increased risk of heart disease.
   b. stomachache, constipation, or diarrhea.
   c. a weakened immune system.
   d. all of the above.

5. Type A behavior is characterized by
   a. burnout.
   b. low self-esteem.
   c. passivity.
   d. all of the above.

6. Worries, critical thoughts, and the demands we place upon ourselves are examples of
   a. environmental stressors.
   b. internal stressors.
   c. social stressors.
   d. post-traumatic stress disorder.

7. Keeping a journal
   a. has been found to increase GPA.
   b. can be an effective way to reduce stress.
   c. can improve mood.
   d. can contribute to all of the above.

8. A clinical technique by which a device monitors the subject's physiologic stress responses is known as
   a. acupuncture.
   b. visualization.
   c. biofeedback.
   d. cognitive therapy.

9. Progressive muscle relaxation involves
   a. systematically contracting and relaxing muscle groups.
   b. taking naps of longer and longer lengths.
   c. stretching your muscles a little more each day.
   d. quietly focusing on relaxing only your body's tiniest muscles.

10. Music for relaxation should be
   a. soft but lively.
   b. loud and lively.
   c. soft, slow, and gentle.
   d. medium-volume, slow, and instrumental, without lyrics.

Get Critical

What happened:

On October 13, 2010, 33 Chilean miners who had been trapped more than 2,000 feet underground for 69 days were pulled out of the earth. As people around the world watched, the miners, once thought dead, emerged one by one. All but one—a miner suffering from pneumonia—were found to be in "more than satisfactory health." In the days following their rescue, many observers marveled that the miners had not simply managed to survive their ordeal, but had transformed it into a triumph.

How did they do it? During their first 17 days before contact with rescuers above, the miners met their physical needs by rationing their food, establishing a duct for potable water, and setting up a chemical toilet. They exerted what control they could over their confined living space by creating areas for eating, sleeping, and praying, and they chose unique roles for each miner according to his skills. They also mutually supported and encouraged one another.

Once they were discovered, the rescue team kept them busy with a variety of important tasks: transmitting information about the conditions underground; providing input on certain decisions; establishing and maintaining lighting that mimicked day/night; clearing away debris; and keeping themselves fit with obligatory exercise. Rescuers also provided the miners with supplies to keep them physically and emotionally healthy. They even sent down a video showing the birth of one of the miner's daughters, whose mother named her Esperanza, meaning "Hope."

What do you think?

1. Which phase of the stress response were the miners most likely to have experienced in the initial moments after the mine collapsed? What physical signs and symptoms did the miners probably experience during this phase?
2. As the miners' time underground expanded from days to weeks to months, what environmental, social, and internal stressors did they face?
3. How did they resist these stressors so successfully? Identify several resources the miners already had in place, as well as new coping techniques that they developed independently or that their rescuers initiated.

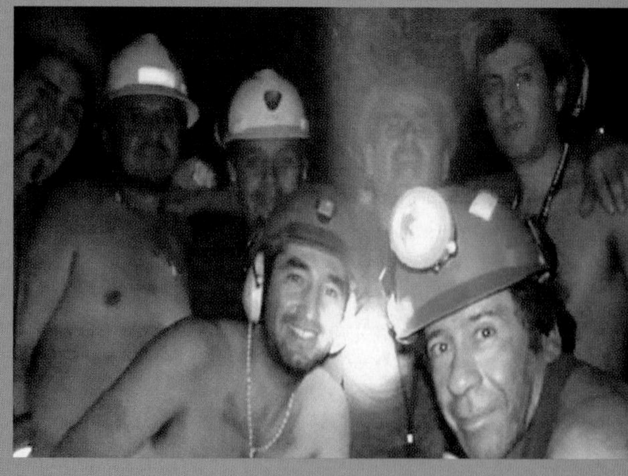

Get Connected

Mobile Tips!

Scan this QR code with your mobile device to access additional stress management tips. Or, via your mobile device, go to **http://mobiletips.pearsoncmg.com** and navigate to Chapter 3.

Health Online **Visit the following websites for further information about the topics in this chapter:**

- Study Guides and Strategies: My Daily Schedule
  www.studygs.net/schedule
- Stress and Health
  www.nlm.nih.gov/medlineplus/stress.html
- Managing Stress
  www.nlm.nih.gov/medlineplus/tutorials/managingstress/htm/index.htm
- Stress Management Techniques
  www.mindtools.com/pages/main/newMN_TCS.htm
- Budget Worksheet for College Students
  http://financialplan.about.com/od/moneyandcollegestudents/l/blcollbudget.htm
- Mint.com Online Money Manager
  www.mint.com

Website links are subject to change. To access updated Web links, please visit ***www.pearsonhighered.com/lynchelmore***.

References

i. American College Health Association. (2012). *American College Health Association National College Health Assessment (ACHA-NCHA II) reference group data report, Fall 2011.* Retrieved from http://www.acha-ncha.org/docs/ACHA-NCHA_Reference_Group_Report_Fall2011.pdf

ii. American Psychological Association. (2010, November 9). *Stress in America findings.* Retrieved from http://www.apa.org/news/press/releases/stress/national-report.pdf

1. American Psychological Association. (2010, November 9). *Stress in America findings*. Retrieved from http://www.apa.org/news/press/releases/stress/national-report.pdf

2. Selye, H. (1980). *Selye's guide to stress research* (Vol. 1). New York: Van Nostrand Reinhold.

3. Nixon, P. G. (1982). The human function curve—a paradigm for our times. *Activitas Nervosa Superior,* Suppl 3 (pt 1), 130–133.

4. McEwen, B. S. (2005, September). Stressed or stressed out: What is the difference? *Journal of Psychiatry and Neuroscience, 30* (5), 315–318.

5. Day, T. A. (2005, December). Defining stress as a prelude to mapping its neurocircuitry: no help from allostasis. *Progress in Neuro-Psychopharmacology and Biological Psychiatry, 29* (8),1195–1200.

6. Smith, T. G., Stoddard, C., & Barnes, M. G. (2009). Why the poor get fat: weight gain and economic insecurity. *Forum for Health Economics & Policy*, *12* (2) (Obesity), Article 5.

7. Friedman, H., Herman, T. W., & Friedman, A. L., Eds. (1995). *Psychoneuroimmunology, stress, and infection*. Florida: CRC Press.

8. Segerstrom, S. C., & Miller, G. E. (2004). Psychological stress and the human immune system: A meta-analytic study of 30 years of inquiry. *Psychological Bulletin, 130* (4), 601–630.

9. Nemade, R., Reiss, N. S., & Dombeck, M. (2007, July 20). Biology of depression. *Psychoneuroimmunology.* Retrieved from http://www.mentalhelp.net

10. Antoni, M. H., Lutgendorf, S. K., Cole, S. W., Dhabhar, F. S., Sephton, S. E., McDonald, P. G. . . . Sood, A. K. (2006). The influence of bio-behavioural factors on tumour biology: Pathways and mechanisms. *Nature Reviews Cancer, 6* (3), 240–248.

11. American College Health Association. (2012). *American College Health Association National College Health Assessment (ACHA-NCHA II) reference group data report, Fall 2011.* Retrieved from http://www.acha-ncha.org/docs/ACHA-NCHA_Reference_Group_Report_Fall2011.pdf

12. American Academy of Sleep Medicine. (2008). Insomnia. Retrieved from http://www.aasmnet.org/Resources/FactSheets/Insomnia.pdf

13. Murff, S. H. (2005, Sept./Oct.). The impact of stress on academic success in college students. *The Association of Black Nursing Faculty Journal*, 102–104.

14. Chen, Y., Dubé, C. M., Rice, C. J., & Baram, T. Z. (2008, March 12). Rapid loss of dendritic spines after stress involves derangement of spine dynamics by corticotropin-releasing hormone. *Journal of Neuroscience, 28*, (11) 2903–2918.

15. Liu, R. T., & Alloy, L. B. (2010, July). Stress generation in depression: A systematic review of the empirical literature and recommendations for future study. *Clinical Psychology Review, 30* (5), 582–593.

16. Joiner, Jr., T. E., Wingate, L. R., Gencoz, T., & Gencoz, F. (2005). Stress generation in depression: Three studies on its resilience, possible mechanism, and symptom specificity. *Journal of Social and Clinical Psychology, 24*(2), 236–253.

17. Mayo Foundation. (2010). Panic attacks and panic disorder. Retrieved from http://www.mayoclinic.com/health/panic-attacks/DS00338

18. Friedman, M. (1996). *Type A behavior: Its diagnosis and treatment*. New York: Plenum Press (pp. ix, 3, 4).

19. Blatný M., & Adam, Z. (2008, June). Type C personality (cancer personality): Current view and implications for future research. *Vnitr Lek., 54* (6), 638–645.

20. Polman, R., Borkoles, E., & Nicholls, A. R. (2010, September). Type D personality, stress, and symptoms of burnout: The influence of avoidance coping and social support. *Br J Health Psychol., 15* (3), 681–696.

21. Bissonette, M. (1998, August). Optimism, hardiness, and resiliency: A review of the literature. *The Child and Family Partnership Project*. Retrieved from http://www.reachinginreachingout.com/documents/Optimism%20Hardiness%20and%20Resiliency.pdf

22. Kobasa, S. (1982). The hardy personality: Toward a social psychology of stress and health. In G. S. Sanders & J. Suls (Eds.), *Social psychology of health and illness* (pp. 3–12). Hillsdale, NJ: Lawrence Erlbaum Associates.

23. Jobson, L., & O'Kearney, R. T. (2009, May). Impact of cultural differences in self on cognitive appraisals in posttraumatic stress disorder. *Behav Cogn Psychother., 37* (3), 249–266.

24. Misra, R., McKean, M., West, S., & Russo, T. (2000). Academic stress of college students: Comparison of student and faculty perceptions. *College Student Journal, 34* (2), 236–246.

25. Dawson, B. A. (2009, February). Discriminiation, stress, and acculturation among dominican immigrant women. *Hispanic Journal of Behavioral Sciences*, *31* (1), 96–111.

26. Sellers, R. M., Caldwell, C. H., Schmeelk-Cone, K. H., & Zimmerman, M. A. (2003, September). Racial identity, racial discrimination, perceived stress, and psychological distress among African American young adults. *J Health Soc Behav*., *44* (3), 302–317.

27. King, K. (2005). Why is discrimination stressful? The mediating role of cognitive appraisal. *Cultural Diversity and Ethnic Minority Psychology, 11* (3), 202–212.

28. Wright, K. B., Craig, E. A., Cunningham, C. B. & Igiel, M. (2007). Emotional support and perceived stress among college students using facebook.com: An exploration of the relationship between source perceptions and emotional support. Paper presented at the NCA 93rd Annual Convention, Chicago, IL.

29. Holmes, T. H., & Rahe, R. H. (1967). The social readjustment rating scale. *Journal of Psychosomatic Research, 11,* 213–218.

30. Rice, K. G., Leever, B. A., Christopher, J., & Porter, J. D. (2006). Perfectionism, stress, and social (dis)connection: A short-term study of hopelessness, depression, and academic adjustment among honors students. *Journal of Counseling Psychology, 33* (4), 524–534.

31. National Center for Complementary and Alternative Medicine. (2010, July). Kava. Retrieved from http://www.nccam.nih.gov/health/kava/

32. National Center for Complementary and Alternative Medicine. (2010, May 12). Acupuncture may help symptoms of posttraumatic stress disorder. Retrieved from http://www.nccam.nih.gov/research/results/spotlight/092107.htm

33. Deckro, G. R., Ballinger, K. M., Hoyt, M., Wilcher, M., Dusek, J., Myers, P., et al. (2002). The evaluation of a mind/body intervention to reduce psychological distress and perceived stress in college students. *Journal of American College Health, 50* (6), 281–287.

LEARNING OBJECTIVES

DESCRIBE the stages of a full night's sleep.

IDENTIFY the benefits of ample sleep and the risks of sleep deprivation.

DISCUSS a variety of factors that influence sleep.

DEFINE and describe insomnia, sleep apnea, and parasomnias.

DISCUSS the clinical diagnosis and treatment of sleep disorders.

IDENTIFY strategies for improving the quantity and quality of your sleep.

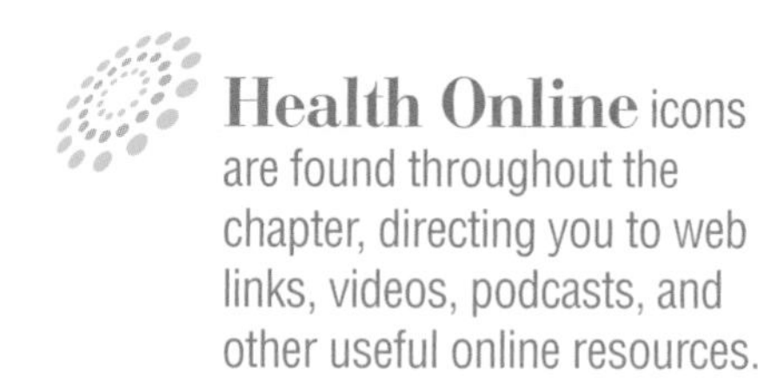
Health Online icons are found throughout the chapter, directing you to web links, videos, podcasts, and other useful online resources.

Troubled sleep. Few experiences in life can match its power to hijack your health and

drive you to despair. In a recent survey of over 1,000 college students, more than 60% said they suffer from troubled sleep.[1] These students also reported higher rates of physical and psychological problems than students getting ample sleep. What makes college students vulnerable to troubled sleep? And if you're among the sleep deprived, what can you do about it? Before we address these questions, let's define the strange phenomenon we call sleep.

What Is Sleep?

Until the middle of the 20th century, sleep was thought to be a state of "global shutdown" prompted by darkness, silence, and other reductions in stimulation from the environment. Then, experiments using a medical device called an **electroencephalograph (EEG)** revealed that sleep is induced by distinctive patterns of nerve cell communication involving several brain regions. Researchers also learned that, during sleep, all major organs continue to function, and that some activities of your brain and your endocrine glands actually increase. As a result, we now recognize **sleep** as a physiologically prompted, dynamic, and readily reversible state of reduced consciousness essential to human survival.

Regions and Rhythms of Sleep

Sleep is generated and maintained by structures in all three primary regions of your brain. These include the following **(Figure 4.1)**.

The Brain Stem

The *brain stem* is the lowest part of your brain. It connects to your spinal cord, and sends signals from your spinal cord to higher regions of your brain. Running through the core of the brain stem is a group of nerve cells called the *reticular activating system (RAS)* that helps regulate sleep. Active signaling of the RAS keeps you awake, whereas inactivity induces sleep.[2] Another region of the brain stem, called the *pons*, sends signals upward to initiate REM sleep—a stage of dreaming sleep discussed shortly—and sends signals downward to the spinal cord to paralyze your muscles so that you won't act out your dreams!

The Diencephalon

The *diencephalon*, the region above the brain stem, contains two structures especially important in sleep. These are the *hypothalamus* and the *pineal gland*, both of which help regulate your body's **circadian rhythm**—its distinctive 24-hour pattern of wakefulness and sleep.

electroencephalograph (EEG) Device that monitors the electrical activity of different regions of the cerebral cortex of the brain using electrodes placed on or in the scalp; a tracing of brain activity is called an *electroencephalogram*.

sleep A physiologically prompted, dynamic, and readily reversible state of reduced consciousness essential to human survival.

circadian rhythm Pattern of physical, emotional, and behavioral changes that follows a roughly 24-hour cycle in accordance with the hours of darkness and light in the individual's environment.

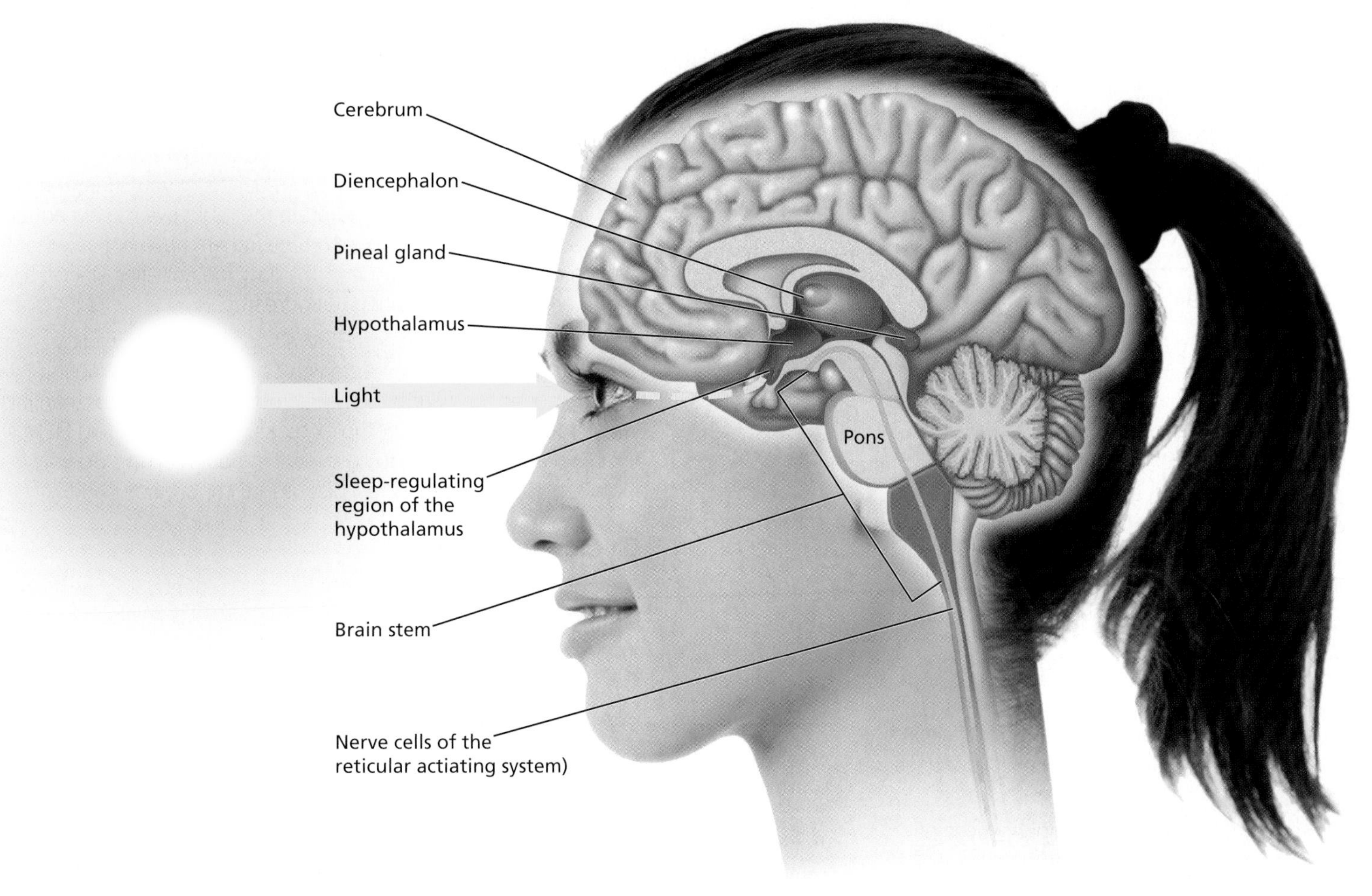

Figure 4.1 **Brain regions and structures involved in sleep.**

The hypothalamus contains a distinct region of tissue that functions as your "body clock," synchronizing with changing patterns of darkness and light in your environment to prompt you to feel sleepy and to wake up. The same region also regulates other body functions according to these changes in darkness and light—for instance, your body temperature and the release of certain hormones.

Meanwhile, the pineal gland responds to changing levels of darkness and light by altering its production of a hormone called *melatonin.* As dusk begins to fall, melatonin secretion begins to rise. Eventually, levels increase enough to make you sleepy.

Jet lag is thought to occur in part because, when you travel across time zones, you're subjected to a sudden change in the habitual pattern of darkness and light. Most people need 2 or 3 days to "reset" their circadian rhythm according to the dark–light cycle in the new location.

The Cerebrum

The *cerebrum* consists of two large masses of tissue located immediately beneath your skull. The cerebrum's outermost "bark," called the *cerebral cortex*, is the thinking area of your brain. When it's time to solve an equation or write a short story, your cerebral cortex goes into action. It even stays active during sleep! Patterns of electrical activity generated by the cerebral cortex distinguish each of the different stages of sleep identified next.

Stages of Sleep

Have you ever been sitting in an afternoon class, trying to stay alert, when suddenly your whole body jerked and startled as if you were about to fall off a cliff? Such an experience is characteristic of a drowsy state in which your body begins to relax. If you were to look at an EEG tracing of your brain waves during this time, you'd see alpha waves: These are slightly broader and slower than the waves of someone who's wide awake. The jerking sensation may be accompanied by sleep-induced hallucinations—for instance, hearing someone say your name. Of course, if you're nodding off in class, this might not be a hallucination, but your instructor calling on you! Fortunately, you're easily roused from drowsiness, and may even be able to answer your instructor's question.

Drowsiness represents a change from full alertness, but it is not a stage of true sleep. Decades ago, sleep researchers studying EEG recordings began to distinguish five stages of true sleep **(Figure 4.2).** They grouped these into two primary types characterized by the absence or presence of a key physiologic sign: *rapid eye movement (REM)*, a hallmark of dreaming sleep.

non-REM (NREM) sleep Type of restful sleep during which the rapid eye movement characteristic of dreaming does not typically occur.

During Non-REM Sleep, You Rest

Rapid eye movement does not occur during **non-REM (NREM) sleep.** Instead of dreaming, you rest. NREM sleep is also called *slow-wave sleep* because

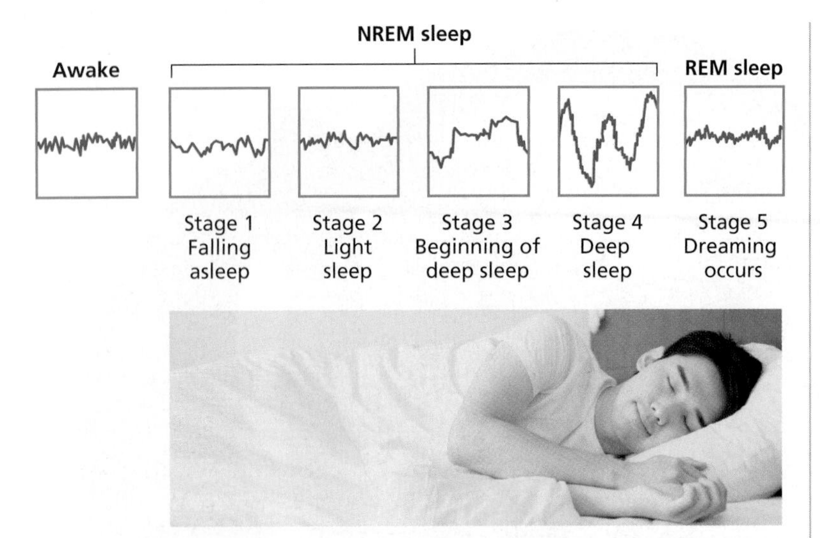

Figure 4.2 Characteristic brain waves for each stage of sleep. Drowsiness is followed by four stages of NREM sleep and a fifth stage of REM sleep. As the night goes on, the sleeper spends less time in deep sleep and more time in REM sleep.

it's characterized by broader, slower EEG waves. The four stages of NREM sleep are as follows (see Figure 4.2):

Stage 1. You're drifting off. The alpha waves of drowsiness are replaced by slower theta waves. Your muscles may twitch, and you are easily aroused. This light stage of sleep typically lasts just a few minutes.

Stage 2. You're truly—but lightly—asleep. Your body temperature cools. Your breathing rate and pulse slow. You are less easily aroused. This stage of sleep may initially last about 15 minutes, but over the course of a night, you spend more time in this stage than in any other.

Stages 3 and 4. These stages of NREM sleep—which some researchers consider a single stage—are often referred to as *delta sleep* because they are characterized by tall, slow brain waves called delta waves. In stage 3, delta waves are just beginning to appear, and you are falling into deep sleep. By stage 4, more than half of the brain waves are delta waves. Your breathing rate and pulse slow even more, and your blood pressure drops. You are sleeping deeply and are very difficult to rouse. Talking and sleepwalking, though uncommon, typically occur in this stage. Also during stage 4 sleep, the pituitary gland (located in the brain near the hypothalamus) releases *growth hormone*, which among other functions is important in the repair of wear and tear on body tissues. You may spend half an hour or more in stage 4 early in the night, but the longer you sleep, the less deep sleep you get.

During REM Sleep, You Dream

The fifth stage of sleep, **REM sleep,** is prompted by signals from the pons in the brain stem. The pons also inhibits the release of neurotransmitters necessary for muscle movement; as noted earlier, this protective mechanism means you're not able to act out your dreams. When this mechanism fails, the sleeper experiences a rare and potentially dangerous sleep disorder called *REM behavior disorder*.

Although the pons inhibits movements of most of your body's muscles, three groups remain active: your respiratory muscles allow you to continue to breathe; the tiny muscles of your inner ear still function; and your eye muscles generate the rapid eye movements that give this sleep stage its name.[3] Sleep researchers have noticed that these darting eye movements appear to follow the activities sleepers later say they were engaging in during their dreams.

Brain wave activity during REM sleep is characterized by the presence of beta waves—the same waves present during much of waking. Moreover, the brain's oxygen consumption is higher than it is even when you're performing complex tasks. In general during REM sleep, the brain appears to be doing everything but resting.[3] So why do we experience REM sleep? We'll discuss its importance shortly.

REM sleep Type of wakeful sleep during which rapid eye movement and dreaming occur.

To view a tutorial covering the stages of sleep and other aspects of sleep, visit www.nlm.nih.gov/medlineplus/tutorials/sleepdisorders/htm/index.htm.

Cycles of Sleep

A graph of brain activity during a full night's sleep looks as if it's plotting an 8-hour earthquake! After you first fall asleep, you progress through each of the four stages of NREM sleep. After 20–40 minutes in deep sleep, you cycle back to stages 3 and 2 before entering into a short phase of REM sleep. However, as the night continues, the duration of NREM sleep decreases, whereas the duration of REM sleep increases. After about 4 hours of sleep, stage 4 sleep all but disappears and the sleeper cycles back quickly into longer and longer periods of REM. Most researchers believe that 7–8 hours of sleep allow for adequate REM sleep. This is especially important during your college years because REM is thought to increase the capacity to learn new material, consolidate memories, and improve creativity—as we discuss in detail shortly.

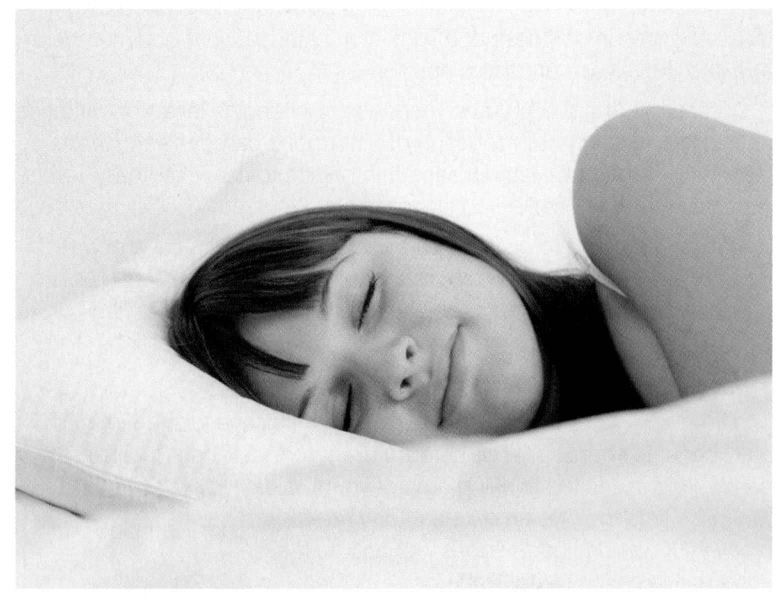

During **REM sleep**, you dream.

Sleep: How Much Is Enough?

Sleep experts report that most adults need 7–9 hours of sleep each night to feel alert and well rested.[4] Any amount less than 7 hours is referred to as *short sleep*, whereas any amount more than 9 hours is considered *long sleep*.

Many college students develop a **sleep debt,** an accumulated amount of sleep loss prompted by short sleep. While it may sound logical to reduce sleep debt by sleeping late on weekends, this may disrupt your sleep schedule and bring on insomnia. What about napping? Certainly a short nap—10 to 20 minutes in the early afternoon—can be refreshing. But longer or later naps can disturb your nighttime sleep.[5] Sleep experts agree that the best way to make up sleep debt is gradually, by getting just a little extra sleep each night.

sleep debt An accumulated amount of sleep loss that develops when the amount of sleep you routinely obtain is less than the amount you need.

Research on Short and Long Sleep

How do sleep researchers come up with their numbers? Do they simply ask people how much they sleep, and assume that the average must be the amount most people need? Not at all! Researchers conduct two types of studies to determine sleep needs. In one type, they compare the number of hours of sleep patients report—when they visit their physician, for example—and the age at which patients eventually die. Such studies have consistently linked short sleep with an increased risk for premature death.[6] On average, people who sleep at least 7 hours a night experience greater longevity.

The second method for determining sleep needs is to conduct sleep-lab experiments. In one type of study, participants who normally sleep 7–8 hours are tested for their performance on specific tasks—often computerized activities requiring quick decision-making. They're then allowed to sleep for only 6 hours a night—or less—for a period of several days or weeks, during which time they again perform the same tasks. Researchers compare their performances. Over many years, such studies have shown significant losses in performance among subjects getting less than 7 hours of sleep.[6] Some studies even show significant losses with exactly 7 hours of sleep![7] One researcher explained that the impairment doesn't show up after a single night, but appears consistently within five to seven nights of 7 hours of sleep a night. Thus, if you're shortchanging your sleep, what you gain in time you lose in performance. Moreover, study subjects don't appear to be aware of their impairment: They report that sleepiness is not affecting them even as their performance scores plummet.[7]

What about long sleep? Does it reduce or improve performance? We don't really know for sure, as people don't tend to sustain long sleep even when given the opportunity. For instance, in one study, researchers encouraged college students to "sleep as much as possible" over several weeks. The participants increased their average sleep time from 7.5 hours to nearly 10 hours for the first week, but then "settled in" at an average of 8.5 hours a night. This increased sleep was associated with improved alertness and reaction time.[8] Several other studies have also shown that a moderate increase in sleep duration (to more than 8 hours) improves not only alertness and performance, but also mood.[6]

Short Sleep: The American Way?

A national poll conducted in 2009 found that 30% of American adults experience short sleep every night of the week. As shown in **Figure 4.3,** 1 in 5 American adults experiences *very* short sleep—less than 6 hours—on weeknights. Moreover, the *average* number of hours American adults sleep on weeknights is 6.7—which also qualifies as short sleep. Intriguingly, even on weekends, the average creeps up only to 7.1 hours, barely edging into the range considered ample sleep.[9]

Although this might surprise you, Americans of college age (19 to 29) actually get more sleep than average. Only 23% experience short sleep, and most sleep about 7 hours, typically from midnight until about 7:00 a.m.[10] That said, no comparable data exists for young adults actually attending college, and a large national survey of college students found that the majority feel sleepy at least a few days of every week.[11] See the **Student Stats** box for more detail on sleepiness in college students.

Are *you* getting ample sleep? The American Academy of Sleep Medicine offers seven signs that you're sleep deprived. These include the following:[4]

1. You're dependent on an alarm clock. If you're getting enough sleep, then you should be able to wake up without a morning alarm.
2. You're drowsy when you're driving. Drifting off at the wheel is a sure sign that you're not getting enough sleep. It's also dangerous and often deadly.
3. You're attached to the coffee pot. A cup of coffee to start your day is fine, but you shouldn't have to drink coffee all day to stay alert.
4. You're making mistakes. It's harder to focus and concentrate when you're tired.
5. You're forgetful. Sleep deprivation impairs memory.
6. You're cranky. Being tired can make you feel depressed, anxious, and frustrated.
7. You're getting sick frequently. A sleep-deprived immune system is not as effective at fighting illness.

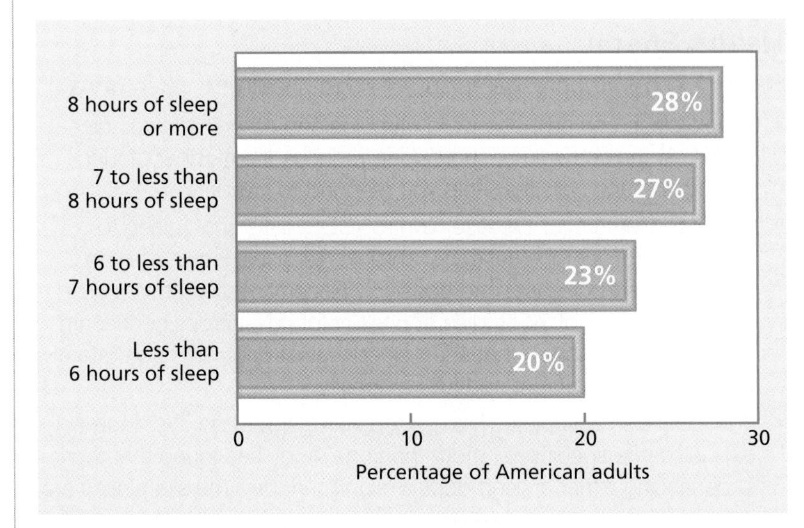

Figure 4.3 Sleep in America. Only 28% of American adults get 8 or more hours of sleep a night.

Source: Data from the *2009 Sleep in America Poll: Health and Safety*, by the National Sleep Foundation.

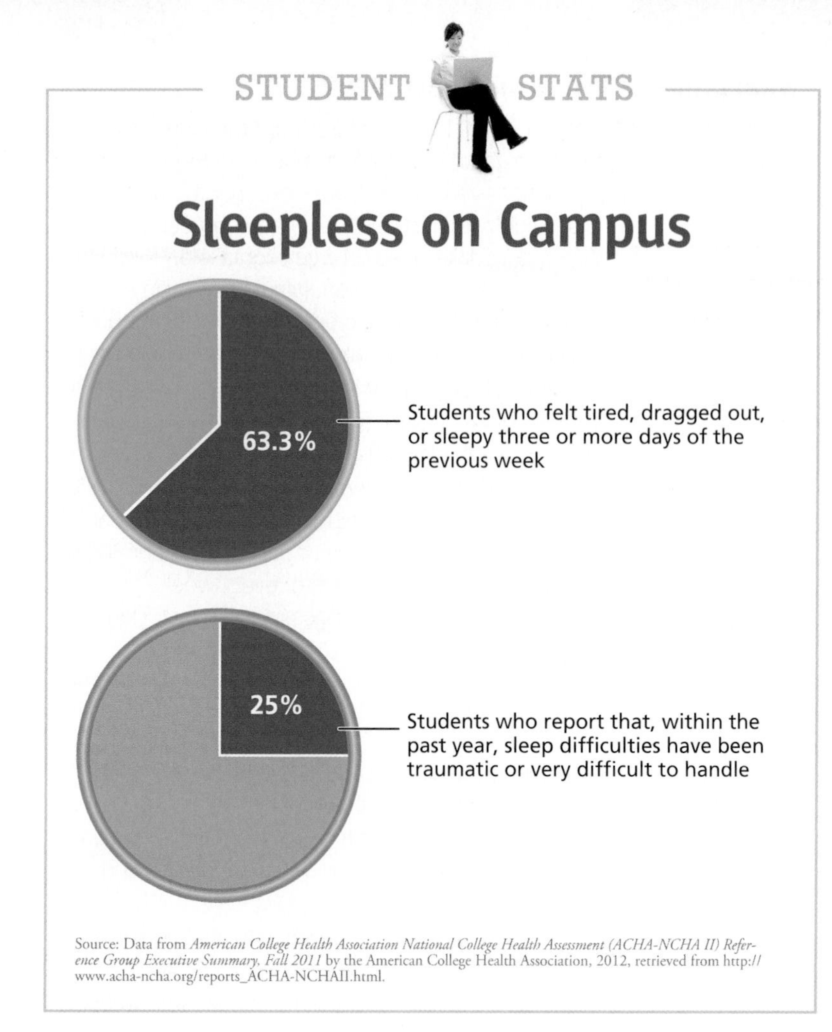

STUDENT STATS
Sleepless on Campus
63.3%
Students who felt tired, dragged out, or sleepy three or more days of the previous week
25%
Students who report that, within the past year, sleep difficulties have been traumatic or very difficult to handle

Source: Data from *American College Health Association National College Health Assessment (ACHA-NCHA II) Reference Group Executive Summary. Fall 2011* by the American College Health Association, 2012, retrieved from http://www.acha-ncha.org/reports_ACHA-NCHAII.html.

Why Is Ample Sleep Important?

The link between ample sleep and increased longevity and functioning has been recognized for decades. More recently, researchers have been uncovering additional benefits of ample sleep—and some serious risks of short sleep.

Health Effects

Sleep influences your physical and psychological health in a variety of ways:

- Ample sleep can help you ward off colds and other infectious diseases. At the same time, short sleep reduces the number of functioning immune cells that help you respond to invaders.[12]
- The U.S. Centers for Disease Control (CDC) links short sleep to an increased risk for a variety of chronic diseases, including type 2 diabetes, heart disease, and obesity.[13] Recently, researchers conducting a review of 36 studies of obesity found—across continents, ethnicities, and ages—that short sleep was strongly and consistently associated with current and future obesity.[14]
- The CDC also associates short sleep with depression.[13] Among college students specifically, more than one study has found that those experiencing either a sleep debt or significant daytime sleepiness are at increased risk for depression.[15, 16] Excessive sleeping, technically called *hypersomnia*, is also associated with depression. Another study has found that physical aggression and thoughts of suicide are increased in college students experiencing poor-quality sleep.[17]

Effects on Academic Performance

Sleep is closely related to college students' capacity for learning. Studies have consistently associated short sleep with impaired learning, and ample sleep with improved academic performance.[18, 19] Some researchers are linking these observations to effects of sleep on an area at the very front of the cerebral cortex (called the *prefrontal cortex*) that is associated with complex thinking and decision-making.[19]

In light of this, it's not surprising that college students experiencing insomnia and other sleep concerns are significantly overrepresented among students in academic jeopardy (GPA less than 2.0).[20] More specifically, college students who report pulling all-nighters to help them get their work done have, on average, lower GPAs than those who don't.[21]

On the other hand, students who report good sleep are more likely to succeed academically.[22] Why? One factor is that ample sleep after studying dramatically improves recall.[23] During REM sleep, the brain transfers short-term memories from a temporary holding region to a long-term storage site at the sides of the cerebral cortex (called the *temporal lobes*). This process is known as *memory consolidation*. Because you build up most of your REM sleep only after you've been asleep for 6 hours, short sleep means you won't be able to consolidate memories as effectively.[24] REM sleep also allows the brain to replenish its stores of certain neurotransmitters that participate in memory, learning, performance, and problem-solving.[24]

Some studies have even found that you continue to work on problems during your sleep! In one such study, participants in a sleep lab played a challenging game, after which they drifted off to sleep. When they were awakened, 75% reported experiencing visual images of the game, suggesting that they were continuing to work out their strategy while they slept.[25]

Risk for Traumatic Injury

Drowsy driving is involved in 1 out of every 6 fatal motor vehicle accidents in the United States, resulting in more than 1,500 American deaths each year.[26] In a national poll, more than one-third of adults admitted to having fallen asleep behind the wheel at least once in the past year.[9] Short sleep is also associated with other kinds of traumatic injury, including work-related injuries, athletic injuries, and recreational injuries.[27] Remember, if you're drowsy, you're within seconds of falling asleep. And if you're driving drowsy, you may be within seconds of a potentially fatal crash.

What Factors Influence Sleep?

The last time you lay awake at 3:00 a.m., did you think about the reasons? Maybe you blamed the energy drink you had while you were studying, or the hot weather, or anxiety about an upcoming exam. Or maybe, if you often have trouble sleeping, you wondered if it's just the way you are. Though no one can say for sure what keeps you awake on any particular night, overall researchers have identified factors that most commonly influence sleep.

This video explains the importance of sleep to the teenage brain: http://today.msnbc.msn.com/id/26184891/vp/42579523#42579523.

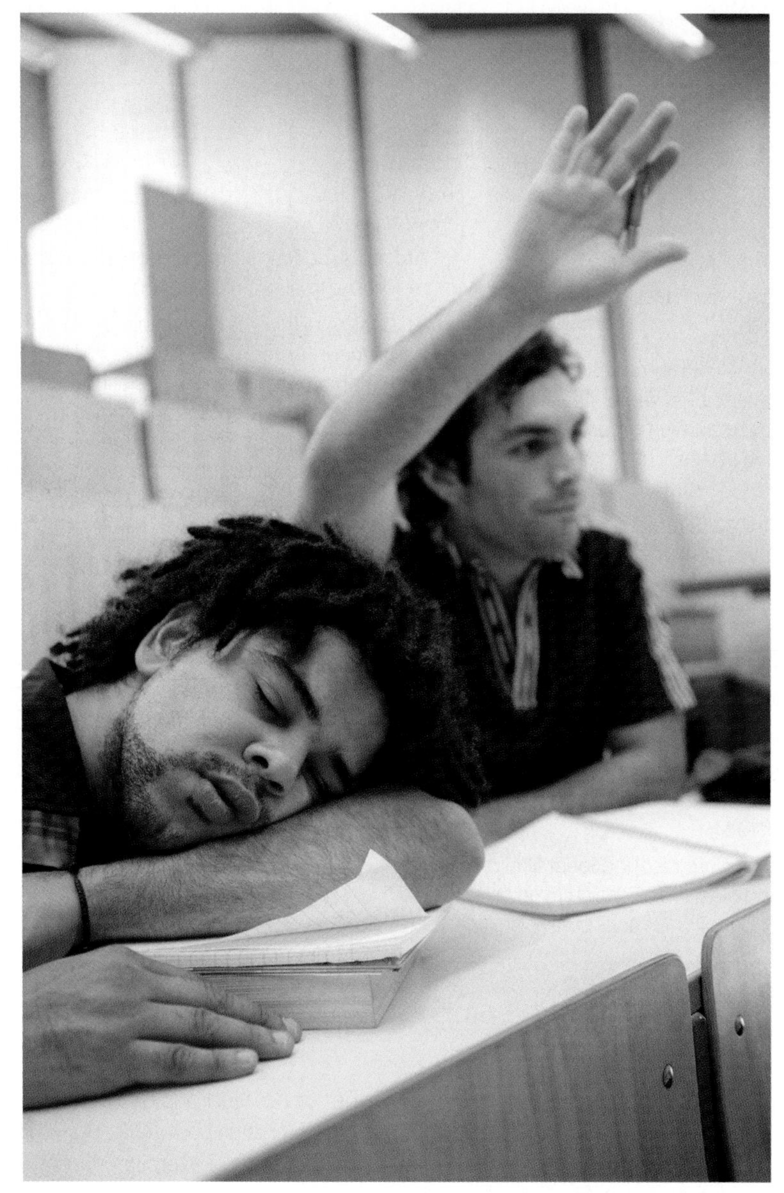

Short sleep has farther-reaching academic impacts than just falling asleep in class.

Biology and Genetics

Over many years, twin studies conducted in different countries have all shown a genetic influence on sleep patterns.[28] Nonetheless, environmental and behavioral factors are considered more important. Similarly, while gender and ethnic differences in sleep patterns exist, they are thought to be due to factors such as socioeconomic differences and discrimination.[29] For more on sleep differences across genders and ethnicities, see the **Diversity & Health** box.

Poor health commonly disrupts sleep, especially when it's accompanied by pain, impaired breathing, fever, or other distressing symptoms. A medical condition called sleep apnea, discussed shortly, causes frequent waking and restless sleep. In women, both pregnancy and the hormonal shifts of the normal menstrual cycle can contribute. Not only physical, but psychological conditions, including both depression and anxiety, commonly disturb sleep. Unfortunately, some medications for these disorders, including antidepressants and drugs for asthma and high blood pressure, can also interfere with sleep.

Individual Behaviors

If you're having trouble sleeping, any of the following factors may be contributing:

- **Presleep use of technology.** In a recent national survey, 95% of respondents said that they often use technology—a cell phone, computer, TV, or video games—in the bedroom during the hour before bedtime.[10] If you're part of this majority, you might be interested to know that researchers see two problems with your behavior: First, use of such devices can be "alerting" and provoke anxiety, making it difficult to disengage and fall asleep. Second, the screens of these devices emit light, and focusing on them just before trying to sleep can shift your circadian rhythm.[10] So in the hour before bedtime, choose an activity that will help you unwind, like reading a calming book—and not on your iPad or Kindle!
- **Hunger.** Food stays in your stomach about 2 to 4 hours before it is released a little at a time into the small intestine.[30] You should stay upright during this time. If you lie down, the acid your stomach naturally produces to help break down the food can seep backward into the lower portion of your esophagus, irritating its lining and giving you the sensation commonly known as heartburn. Gastroesophageal reflux disease (GERD), the technical name for persistent heartburn, commonly provokes sleepless nights.[31] But although you should definitely avoid eating a full meal before going to bed, you should also avoid trying to sleep if you are physically hungry. So go for a light snack. Some experts recommend a banana and a small glass of milk—a snack that not only takes away your hunger pangs but also provides amino acids, carbohydrates, and minerals in combinations that are thought to be relaxing.
- **Spicy foods.** Do spicy foods really keep you awake? Although you might think this is just a myth, several studies over the years suggest it's true. A classic study involving young, healthy males found that on nights when the participants had Tabasco sauce and mustard with their evening meals, it took longer for them to fall asleep and their sleep was more fitful throughout the first sleep cycle. Indigestion was not thought to be the culprit. Instead, the researchers believe that the spices elevated the participants' body temperature enough to disturb the nervous and hormonal mechanisms that normally initiate sleep.[32]
- **Smoking.** Many people believe that a smoke before sleep is relaxing, but the exact opposite is true: Nicotine, the psychoactive drug in tobacco, is a stimulant. Moreover, the adverse physical effects of smoking, including the so-called "smoker's cough," can disrupt sleep throughout the night. Finally, smoking in bed can be dangerous! Falling asleep with a lit cigarette can start a fire and every year, almost 1,000 Americans are killed in residential fires caused by smoking.[33] Bottom line: If you smoke, stop. (For more information, see Chapter 10.)
- **Caffeine.** The stimulant most commonly associated with sleep troubles is caffeine. But both the amount and the timing of intake matters. Studies suggest that the amount of caffeine in as many as 4 cups of coffee or 8 cups of tea per day confers little health risk.[34]

DIVERSITY & HEALTH

Sleep Through the Lens of Sex and Ethnicity

The National Sleep Foundation has been conducting a *Sleep in America* poll annually for the past decade. The subject of the 2007 poll was women and sleep, and the 2010 poll was on ethnicity and sleep. Here are key findings:

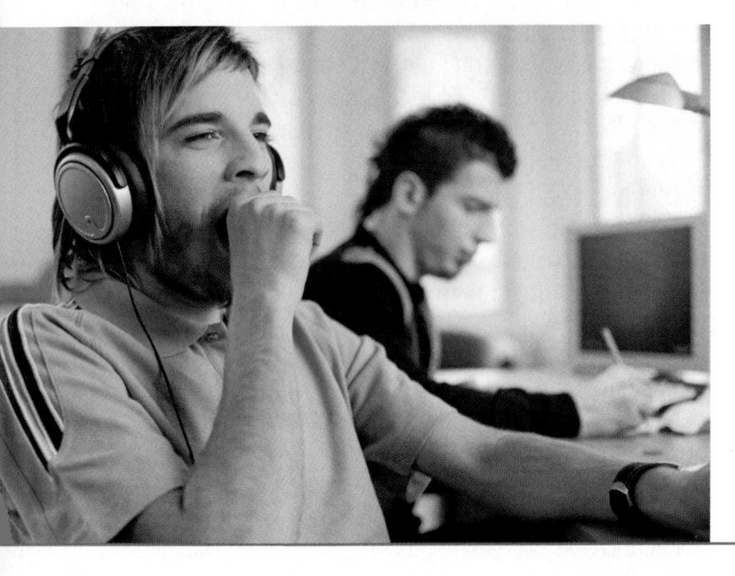

Sex

Overall, American men sleep better than American women:

- Men are about 11% more likely than women to say they get more sleep than they need, whereas women are about 11% more likely to say they get less sleep than they need.
- Men are about 13% more likely than women to have their sleep needs met both on weekdays and weekends.

Ethnicity

Overall, Asian Americans have fewer sleep problems than any other ethnic group:

- Asian Americans are the ethnic group most likely to say that they had a good night's sleep at least a few nights or more a week (84%).
- Asian Americans are also the least likely to report using sleep medication (5%). In contrast, 13% of Caucasians, 9% of African Americans, and 8% of Hispanics report using sleep medication.
- At least one-third of Hispanics (38%) and African Americans (33%) report that financial, employment, relationship, and/or health-related concerns disturb their sleep at least a few nights a week. These concerns disturbed the sleep of 28% of Caucasians and 25% of Asian Americans.
- African Americans report getting the lowest amount of sleep each night—at least half an hour less than the amount of sleep reported by other ethnic groups.
- Intriguingly, Caucasians are much more likely (14%) than any other ethnic group (2% each) to say they usually sleep with a pet!

Source: Sleep in America, by the National Sleep Foundation, 2010 and 2007, retrieved from www.sleepfoundation.org.

However, your body gets rid of caffeine only slowly, taking about 5 to 7 hours, on average, to eliminate *half* of it. Even after 8 to 10 hours, 25% of the caffeine is still present.[35] This means that, if you plan to get to bed at 11:00 p.m., you might be okay enjoying coffee or a cola at lunch, but not afterward.

- **Stimulant medications.** In 2009, 1.3 million Americans abused prescription stimulants, usually Ritalin, Adderall, and other drugs developed for people with attention disorders.[36] Abuse of these drugs on college campuses is an increasing concern among public health experts because of the drugs' potential for addiction, adverse effects on students' creativity, and relationship to sleep problems—which in turn reduce learning. In one study involving nearly 500 college students, those who reported stimulant abuse also reported lower sleep quality and greater sleep disturbance. Moreover, although the primary reason these students gave for abusing stimulants was to improve their concentration and academic performance, the students reporting high GPAs were actually the least likely to abuse stimulants.[37]
- **Alcohol.** Because alcohol is a sedative—a drug that promotes calm and drowsiness—drinking before bedtime can help you fall asleep. The problem is what happens a few hours later: In the second sleep cycle, the drowsiness wears off.[38] As a result, you are likely to awaken from periods of REM sleep and find it difficult to return to sleep.

Incidentally, if you're wondering whether or not vigorous exercise close to bedtime can disturb your sleep, the jury is still out. Although many health-care experts still advise against nighttime exercise, recent studies have not found that it disturbs sleep.[39]

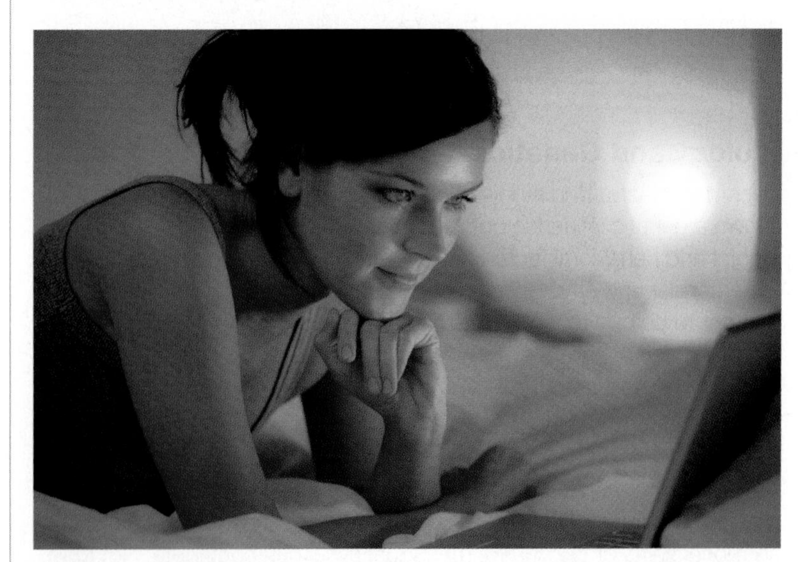

Using a laptop in bed can make it harder to get to sleep.

Factors in the Environment

Nearly any sensory disturbance in your environment—noise in the dorm hallway, prickly bedding, a sagging mattress, or a bedroom that's too hot or too bright—can disturb your sleep. So can a disturbance in your schedule—a shift in your work hours, travel, or transitioning from summer back into the academic year.

Other external stressors that commonly disrupt sleep are financial problems, academic concerns, relationship conflicts, and feelings of being overwhelmed—that there just aren't enough hours in a day for all you have to do. In a study of more than 1,100 college students, more than half stated that emotional and academic stress negatively impacted their sleep.[1] Unfortunately, the connection between stress and sleep is reciprocal: Stress affects the quality and duration of your sleep, and poor sleep reduces your ability to manage stress. Moreover, stressing out about your inability to sleep can actually reinforce your sleep problem!

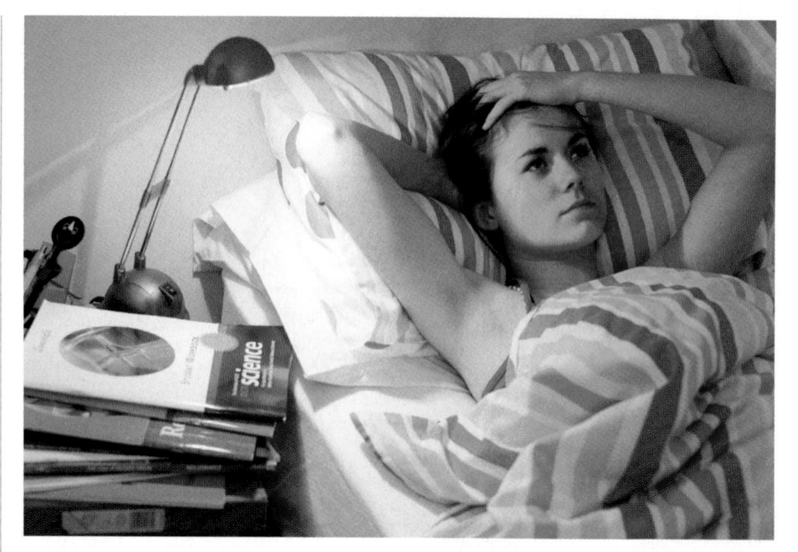

Insomnia can sometimes be caused by **stress.**

Sleep Disorders

In a recent, large-scale study, 27% of students at a public university were found to be at risk for at least one sleep disorder.[20] The American Academy of Sleep Medicine identifies 81 such disorders![40] Here, we discuss only the most common.

Insomnia

Insomnia—a term that literally means "no sleep"—is a condition characterized by difficulty falling or staying asleep, a pattern of waking too early, or poor-quality sleep. Although 30% of American adults occasionally suffer from insomnia in any given year, about 10% experience chronic insomnia; that is, insomnia that lasts for more than a month.[41]

There are two types of insomnia. *Secondary insomnia* is by far the most common, and is due to a behavior such as substance abuse or another medical disorder such as heart disease. *Primary insomnia* occurs in only about 20% of people with insomnia, and almost always develops as a result of stress. Before diagnosing primary insomnia, a physician will conduct an interview and a series of tests to rule out behaviors (such as alcohol or caffeine intake) and medical disorders that could be causing secondary insomnia. Treatment of insomnia and other sleep problems is discussed shortly.

Snoring

If you've ever been kept awake by someone's **snoring,** you know how irritating the sound can be. It occurs when breathing is obstructed during sleep. As many as half of all Americans snore at least occasionally.[42] Alcohol consumption, overweight, and colds and allergies all contribute to narrowing of your airways and can result in snoring. Occasional, light snoring is nothing to be concerned about; however, if your snoring is chronic, is loud enough to waken your roommate, or you wake up in the middle of the night feeling as if you are choking, you may have sleep apnea.

For tips on reducing snoring, go to: www.mayoclinic.com/health/snoring/DS00297/DSECTION=lifestyle-and-home-remedies.

Sleep Apnea

Sleep apnea (AP-nee-ah) is a disorder in which one or more pauses in breathing occur during sleep. These breathing pauses can last from a few seconds to minutes. They often occur 5 to 30 times an hour.[43] Typically, normal breathing then starts again, sometimes with a loud snort or choking sound.

Although it can develop at any age, sleep apnea becomes more common as you get older. At least 1 in 10 people over age 65 has sleep apnea. It is more common in men, in people who are overweight, and in people who smoke.[43]

As you can imagine, sleep apnea significantly disrupts sleep, jerking the person out of deep sleep and into light sleep, or even waking the person up. This results in overall poor-quality sleep. The pauses in breathing also increase the person's risk for a heart attack or stroke, and the poor sleep can lead to daytime drowsiness that sets the stage for traumatic injury. Any of these can be deadly: A comprehensive, long-term study found that Americans with sleep apnea have a threefold greater risk of premature death than those without the disorder.[44]

Types of Sleep Apnea

There are two types of sleep apnea. In *obstructive sleep apnea*, the airway collapses or becomes blocked during sleep **(Figure 4.4).** When the sleeper tries to breathe, any air that squeezes past the blockage can cause loud snoring. Breathing pauses may occur, and choking or gasping may follow the pauses. In *central sleep apnea*, which is less common, the area of the brain that controls breathing doesn't send the correct signals to the respiratory muscles. As a result, breathing stops for brief periods. Snoring doesn't typically happen with central sleep apnea.[43]

Diagnosis of Sleep Apnea

To check for sleep apnea, a physician would look for structural abnormalities—such as excessive tissue—in the back of the mouth and throat. The physician might also order a *polysomnogram*, a test conducted in a sleep lab that records brain wave activity, breathing, and other signs while the patient

insomnia Condition characterized by difficulty falling or staying asleep, a pattern of waking too early, or poor-quality sleep.

snoring A ragged, hoarse sound that occurs during sleep when breathing is obstructed.

sleep apnea Disorder in which one or more pauses in breathing occur during sleep.

sleeps. Alternatively, the physician may suggest testing at home using a sleep monitor.

Treatment of Sleep Apnea

For mild cases of sleep apnea, taking care of contributing factors may solve the problem. For example, the patient may need to lose weight, quit smoking, avoid all alcohol, or use nasal decongestants. Patients are also advised to sleep on their side.

For moderate cases, an orthodontist can fit the patient with a plastic mouthpiece that adjusts the lower jaw and tongue to keep the airways open during sleep. Or the patient can sleep with a CPAP machine. *CPAP* stands for *continuous positive airway pressure:* Through a mask that fits over the sleeper's nose and mouth, the device sends air into the sleeper's throat at a pressure just high enough to keep the airways open (see Figure 4.4c).

In cases of severe sleep apnea, surgery to widen the breathing passages may be necessary. It usually involves shrinking, stiffening, or removing excess tissue in the mouth and throat or resetting the lower jaw.

To watch a video on factors involved in sleep apnea and solutions for treatment, see http://abcnews.go.com/health/sleep/video/sleep-apnea-solutions-10511936.

Narcolepsy

Narcolepsy is a disorder in which the brain fails to regulate sleep–wake cycles normally. Patients sleep a normal amount, but cannot control the timing of their sleep. During the day, they may experience sudden attacks of sleepiness combined with a loss of muscle tone and sometimes hallucinations and brief paralysis. The disorder is also associated with insomnia. Although the precise cause of narcolepsy is still unknown, genetic, biological, and environmental factors all may play a part.[45]

Treatment for narcolepsy includes the use of certain medications, such as stimulants and antidepressants, to control sleep–wake cycles. Behavioral therapies are also important, and include scheduling regular naps, avoiding heavy meals, and avoiding alcohol.

Parasomnias

The prefix *para-* can mean both "along with" and "abnormal," so a **parasomnia** is a condition in which unusual events accompany sleep. The most common example is nightmares, frightening dreams that wake you up from REM sleep. About 75% of children and at least 50% of adults occasionally experience nightmares. They are not considered a sleep disorder unless they become chronic, in which case they may cause short sleep because the person fears falling asleep. Psychotherapy is the usual treatment.[46]

Sleep Terrors

Sleep terrors (also called *night terrors*) are similar to nightmares in that they involve either dreams or feelings of intense fear. However, nightmares tend to occur during one of the later cycles of REM sleep, toward morning,

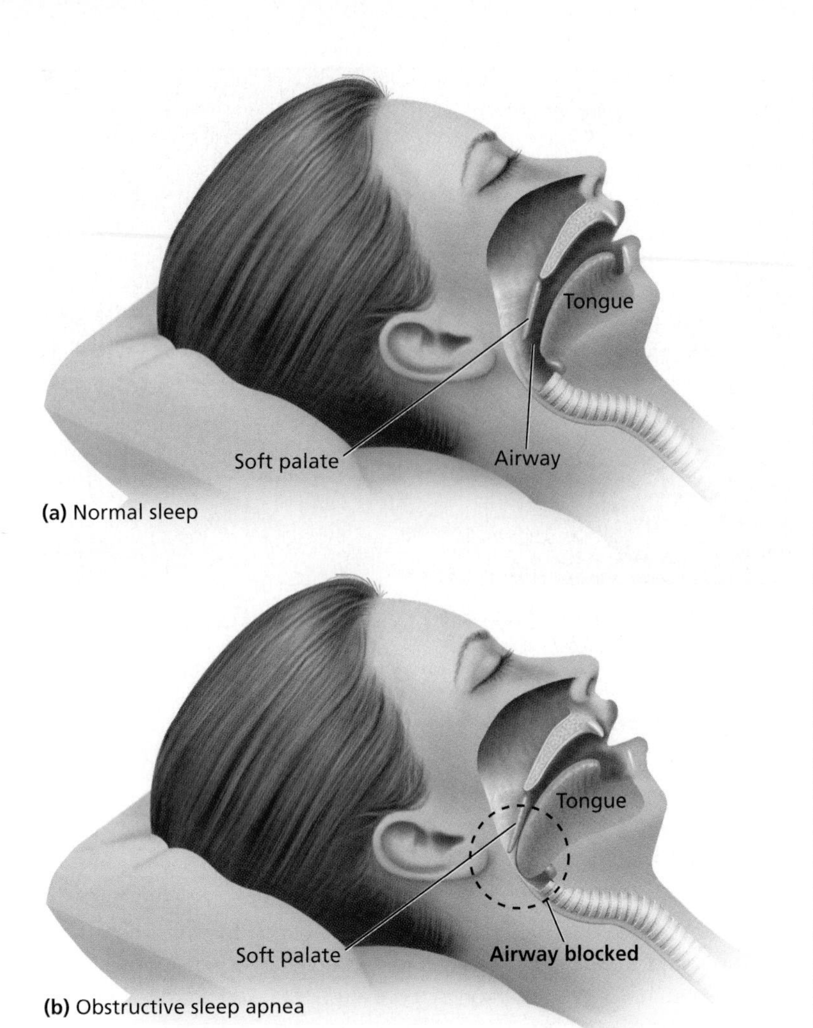

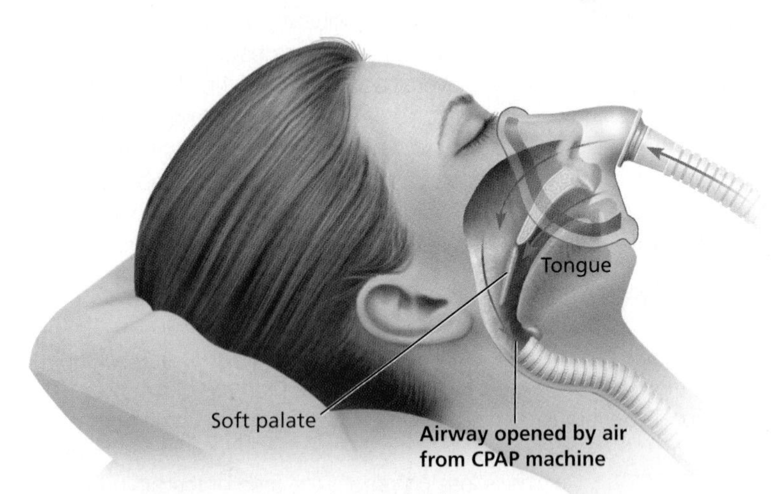

(c) Treatment of sleep apnea with CPAP machine

Figure 4.4 Obstructive sleep apnea. a) During normal sleep, the airways at the back of the mouth and throat remain open. **b)** In obstructive sleep apnea, tissues at the back of the mouth and throat are collapsed, blocking the airways. **c)** CPAP generates a wave of air that continuously presses against the sleeper's tissues, keeping the airways open.

narcolepsy A disorder in which the brain fails to regulate sleep–wake cycles normally.

parasomnia Condition in which unusual events accompany sleep.

sleep terror Parasomnia characterized by the appearance of awakening in terror during a stage of NREM sleep.

Sleep Apnea

STUDENT STORY

"Hi, I'm Remy. I was diagnosed with sleep apnea about 6 months ago. I had been feeling really tired every day, even though I thought I was getting enough sleep, and there were a few times when I almost fell asleep when I was driving. I went to the doctor and at first he wasn't sure what was wrong but when I told him that my roommate says I snore really badly, he organized for me to get a sleep apnea testing kit to take home with me. Now I sleep every night with a CPAP machine. It's a little weird to get used to, but it's worth it to not feel so tired."

1: Untreated sleep apnea increases Remy's risk for which physical problems? How might it affect his schoolwork?

2: Does Remy have obstructive sleep apnea or central sleep apnea? How can you tell? What's the difference between the two?

Do you have a story similar to Remy's? Share your story at www.pearsonhighered.com/lynchelmore.

whereas sleep terrors typically occur during one of the first NREM periods of the night. To observers, the sleeper appears to awaken from a dream screaming and often thrashing; however, the sleeper is not awake, and the episode may persist for 10 minutes or more despite attempts at arousal, such as calling or shaking. Often the terror subsides on its own and the person drifts back into restful sleep. If the person does wake up, he or she is usually very confused. Sleep terrors are much less common than nightmares, occurring mostly in children between 3 and 10 years of age.

Sleepwalking

Sleepwalking occurs during stages 3 and 4 of NREM sleep, usually early in the night. Although it can occur at any age, it is most common in childhood. Episodes can be as short as several seconds and as long as 30 minutes. The person rises out of bed, eyes open, but with a blank look, and typically begins walking or another activity such as dressing or going to the bathroom. If the person talks, the words make no sense. Because injury during sleepwalking is common, the sleeper should be gently guided back to bed or awakened. Sleepwalking is generally not serious and needs no treatment.[47]

Sleep Bruxism

If you ever awaken with a sore jaw, it's possible that you may have been clenching or grinding your teeth during sleep—a behavior called **sleep bruxism.** It can also cause earache, headache, and damage to your tooth enamel and the soft tissues of your mouth. Although the cause of sleep bruxism is not known, possible factors include stress, substance abuse (especially stimulants, including nicotine), and misalignment. If you suspect you're grinding your teeth at night, a first step is to see your dentist, who may prescribe a mouth guard or refer you to other specialists.[48]

Nocturnal Eating

Sleep and hunger are both fundamental physiological drives regulated by the hypothalamus and other regions involved in circadian rhythms.[49] When the coordination of these two drives is impaired, a **nocturnal eating disorder** can occur. Although two such disorders are recognized, they have more similarities than differences. In *night-eating syndrome*, a person awakens from sleep and eats a significant amount of food before returning to sleep.[30] In *sleep-related eating disorder*, the person typically reports that they are half asleep or even fully asleep while they eat. In both conditions, more than one eating episode may occur each night, and sufferers are at increased risk for obesity. Both conditions are more common in women than men, and depression, insomnia, and daytime eating disorders are typically seen in people with either diagnosis.[49] Treatment usually involves psychotherapy and medication.

sleepwalking Parasomnia in which a person walks or performs another complex activity while still asleep.

sleep bruxism Clenching or grinding the teeth during sleep.

nocturnal eating disorder Condition characterized by significant food consumption at night, and typically accompanied by depression, insomnia, and a daytime eating disorder.

REM behavior disorder (RBD) Parasomnia characterized by failure of inhibition of muscle movement during REM sleep.

REM Behavior Disorder

Recall that, normally, a region of the brain stem called the pons inhibits almost all muscle movement during REM sleep. In **REM behavior disorder (RBD),** this inhibition fails to occur, and the sleeper acts his

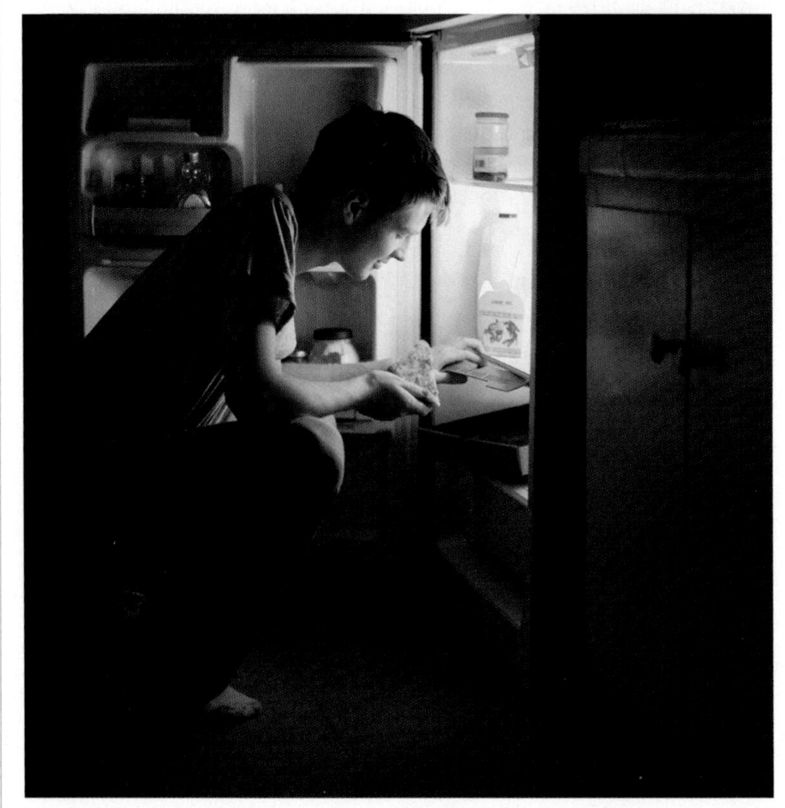

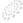

Those who suffer from a **nocturnal eating disorder** can be at risk for obesity.

dreams, sometimes with punching, kicking, or jumping. RBD is a rare parasomnia, occurring in less than 1% of the population, almost always in males. It's typically treated with medications, and the patient must also avoid alcohol.[50]

Restless Legs Syndrome
Although it might not sound like a sleep disorder, **restless legs syndrome (RLS)** only comes on when a person is inactive, so it commonly disrupts sleep. RLS causes a strong urge to move the legs, accompanied by creeping, burning, itching, or otherwise unpleasant feelings in the legs—and sometimes in the arms. Getting up and walking, or stretching or massaging the legs, can help. Although no one knows the precise causes of RLS, both alcohol and tobacco can trigger episodes, so both should be avoided. Some cases appear to be associated with iron deficiency, in which case an iron supplement may be prescribed. People with RLS may find that vigorous physical activity during the day reduces their symptoms at night.[51]

restless legs syndrome (RLS)
Nervous system disorder characterized by a strong urge to move the legs, accompanied by creeping, burning, or other unpleasant sensations.

This video by Harvard Medical School follows NBA star Shaquille O'Neal as he undergoes a sleep study and receives treatment for sleep apnea: www.youtube.com/watch?v=4JkiWvWn2aU&feature=related.

Getting Help for a Sleep Disorder

Fortunately, both campus health services and the medical community have become increasingly aware of the importance of addressing sleep problems early and aggressively, and effective help is available.

Campus and Community Support

Administrators and health-care providers on campuses across the United States are beginning to wake up to the need for programs and services to address sleep deprivation among their students.[52] Many campuses have delayed the start of the academic day, rescheduling all 8:00 a.m. classes to 9:00 a.m. or later. Some are instituting quiet hours and noise ordinances in dorms. Some are offering seminars, workshops, and extended programs to teach students the importance of sleep and strategies to improve their sleep. In a study of one such program, the Sleep Treatment and Education Program for Students (STEPS), participants reported significantly improved sleep quality.[53] So if you're having trouble sleeping, stop off at your campus health center. Chances are, the staff there will be able to help.

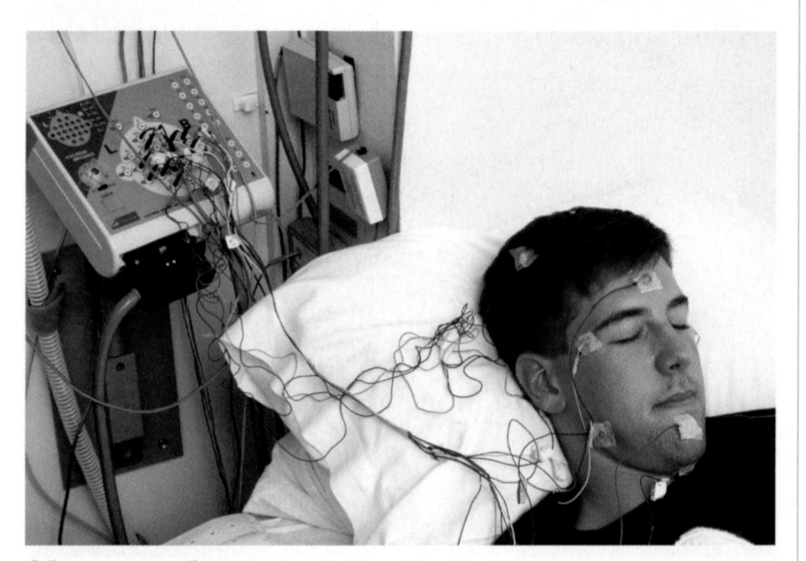

Sleep studies can determine the source of sleep problems.

Clinical Diagnosis and Treatment

If sleep problems persist beyond one month, it's time to see your doctor. Usually, a primary care provider is able to diagnose and treat sleep disorders following an interview and certain lab tests, but in some cases, referral to a sleep clinic may be necessary.

Sleep Studies
Sleep studies are tests conducted while you sleep—usually in a sleep lab within a hospital or at a specialized sleep clinic. Prior to the test, electrodes (small metal discs) are attached to your scalp and body. While you sleep, these send feedback to a device that records data such as your brain waves, eye movements, heart rate, and snoring. A soft belt around your torso records your breathing rate, and a clip on one fingertip records the level of oxygen in your blood. Although these devices may feel unusual, they do not cause pain.

The results of a sleep study may reveal, for example, blocked airflow or limb muscle movement. Typically, a sleep specialist reviews the findings and recommends appropriate treatment.

Medications
Twenty-five percent of Americans take some type of medication every year to help them sleep.[54] However, the American Academy of Sleep Medicine recommends that you avoid sleeping pills if possible, and suggests that physicians prescribe them for no more than 3 weeks.[55] This is in part because some types of sleep medications—benzodiazepines such as Valium—are highly addictive, and even the newer drugs—the so-called "z-drugs" such as Ambien—are habit forming, with some studies showing an addictive potential similar to that of the older drugs.[56, 57]

In addition, the z-drugs are associated with side effects that can be distressing or even dangerous. For example, the uncommon but severe side effects of Ambien include confusion, memory loss, hallucinations, new or worsening depression, thoughts of suicide, agitation, aggressive behavior, and anxiety. Rarely, after taking Ambien, people have gotten out of bed and sleepwalked, prepared and eaten food, made phone calls, and even driven their car while not fully awake. Often the person does not recall these events in the morning.

What about over-the-counter sleep aids? Are they effective—and safe? See the **Consumer Corner** for answers.

Cognitive-Behavioral Therapy
Several studies of college students have supported the effectiveness of cognitive-behavioral interventions in changing the thought patterns and behaviors that may be contributing to troubled sleep.[58] Techniques may include muscle relaxation, deep breathing, changes to your sleep routine, and psychotherapy to help you identify and cope with the anxieties or other thoughts that disturb your sleep. In one study, students learned a "worry control" procedure consisting of identifying worries keeping them awake, then writing down possible solutions to the worries. The study found that the procedure significantly reduced the time it took for students to fall asleep.[59]

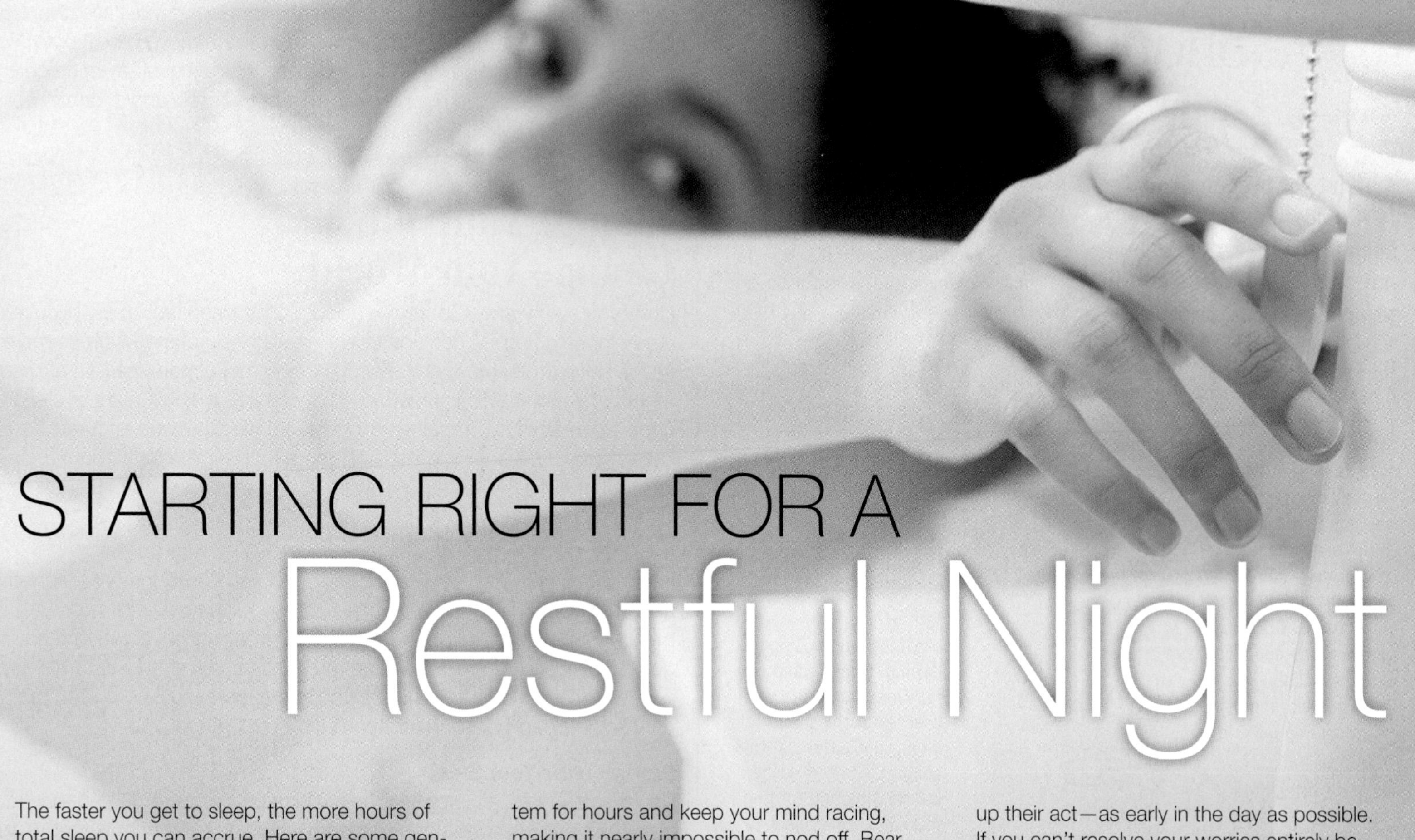

STARTING RIGHT FOR A Restful Night

The faster you get to sleep, the more hours of total sleep you can accrue. Here are some general tips for getting off to sleep more quickly:

- **Think of your bedroom as your "sleep cave."** Make it as dark as possible, using room-darkening shades if necessary to block out streetlights.
- **Aim for a warm bed in a cool room.** Many people find it difficult to fall asleep in a hot, stuffy room. In winter, turn down the thermostat a few degrees—to 65ºF or below—and put an extra blanket on the bed. In summer, use air conditioning or fans to cool the room as much as possible. And make sure the room has adequate ventilation. If appropriate, crack open a window.
- **Keep it quiet.** Many campuses are instituting quiet hours in dorms. But if you can't control noise in your building or out on the street, at least try to block it out with white noise, either by using the white-noise setting on your clock radio, or by downloading a free audio "soundscape" clip to play on your MP3 player. And, of course, there are always ear plugs.
- **Cut caffeine.** Avoid caffeinated drinks after lunchtime, as caffeine can stay in your system for hours and keep your mind racing, making it nearly impossible to nod off. Bear in mind that some energy drinks contain as much caffeine as a similar amount of brewed coffee. Moreover, bottled teas, iced-tea mixes, premium brands of coffee ice cream, hot cocoa, and chocolate all contain caffeine.
- **Watch your food intake.** Although a small snack before bed can help make you sleepy, avoid large meals, which can prompt heartburn. Also avoid spicy foods, which can raise your body temperature enough to cause you to lie awake.
- **Hit the gym earlier in the day.** Although vigorous exercise within a few hours of bedtime hasn't been proven to disturb sleep, you may still want to opt for more gentle exercise, such as yoga or *t'ai chi,* in the evening hours to prepare you for sleep.
- **Get adequate exposure to natural light throughout the day.** This helps provide your brain with stimuli that will help keep your body clock in sync with the environment. As a result, you'll find it easier to nod off.
- **Set stressors aside until morning.** Try to deal with stressors—anything from paying your bills to asking your roommates to clean up their act—as early in the day as possible. If you can't resolve your worries entirely before bedtime, at least try to set them aside—for instance, by writing them down along with two strategies for addressing them the next day. Sleep is your chance to rest and recover.
- **Don't work in bed.** If you read, study, or work on your laptop in bed, you may associate your bed with these activities instead of as a place for rest. Try to reserve your bed only for sleep.
- **Give yourself time to wind down.** You'll get a better night's sleep if you take some time to step away from your laptop, turn off the TV, and relax before you settle in to bed.
- **Don't stare at the ceiling.** If you've gone to bed and can't fall asleep within 20 minutes, get up and do something relaxing until you feel sleepy again and can head back to bed.

Sources: Sleep Hygiene Tips, by the Centers for Disease Control and Prevention, 2007, retrieved October 2009, from http://www.cdc.gov/sleep/hygiene.htm; *Sleep Hygiene—The Healthy Habits of Good Sleep,* by the American Academy of Sleep Medicine, October 2009, retrieved from http://www.sleepeducation.com/Hygiene.aspx; *Sleep Tips for Students,* by the American Academy of Sleep Medicine, 2007, retrieved October 2009 from http://www.sleepeducation.com/Topic.aspx?id=53; *Sleep Hygiene,* by the National Sleep Foundation, August 2011, retrieved from http://www.sleepfoundation.org/article/ask-the-expert/sleep-hygiene.

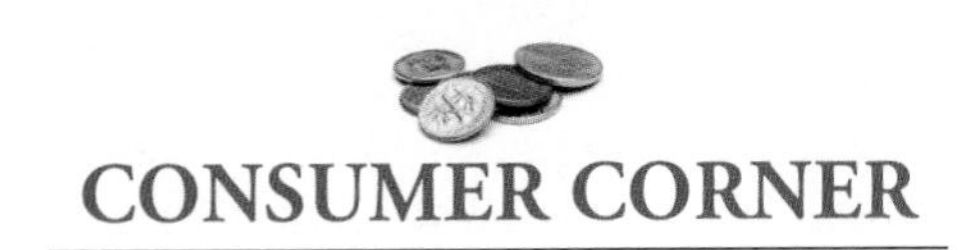

CONSUMER CORNER

Should You Try OTC Sleep Aids?

A variety of over-the-counter (OTC) sleep remedies have been available for decades, but do they work, and are they safe? The most popular OTC sleep drugs are antihistamines. That's right: Their active ingredient is the same thing you might take for hay fever or an allergic skin rash. That's because the same drug that blocks the release of histamine in allergic reactions also causes drowsiness—which is why you're not supposed to drive or operate any type of machinery when you're taking allergy medications. OTC antihistamines for sleep include Excedrin PM, Tylenol PM, Sominex, and others, including generic brands.

Sleep experts agree that these drugs are moderately effective and safe for an occasional sleepless night.[1] However, you build up tolerance quickly, so the more often you take them, the less effective they become. Moreover, they're notorious for leaving you feeling groggy and tired when you wake up—not exactly the best start for your hectic day. And, because they're identical to antihistamines sold for hay fever, they dry out your nose and mouth.[1, 2] In general, the long-term safety and effectiveness of OTC antihistamine sleep remedies has not been well studied, and many authorities recommend against their use, even in the short term.[2-4]

So if you're having trouble sleeping, what should you do? First, make sure you've tried all of the sleep-hygiene suggestions in this chapter. Then, if you're still tossing and turning, make an appointment to see your doctor.

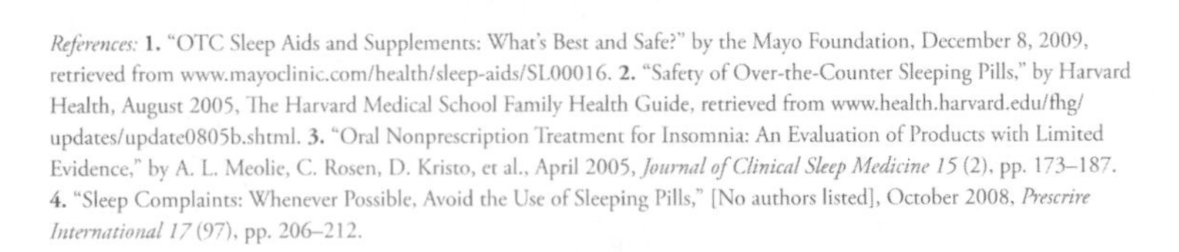

References: **1.** "OTC Sleep Aids and Supplements: What's Best and Safe?" by the Mayo Foundation, December 8, 2009, retrieved from www.mayoclinic.com/health/sleep-aids/SL00016. **2.** "Safety of Over-the-Counter Sleeping Pills," by Harvard Health, August 2005, The Harvard Medical School Family Health Guide, retrieved from www.health.harvard.edu/fhg/updates/update0805b.shtml. **3.** "Oral Nonprescription Treatment for Insomnia: An Evaluation of Products with Limited Evidence," by A. L. Meolie, C. Rosen, D. Kristo, et al., April 2005, *Journal of Clinical Sleep Medicine 15* (2), pp. 173–187. **4.** "Sleep Complaints: Whenever Possible, Avoid the Use of Sleeping Pills," [No authors listed], October 2008, *Prescrire International 17* (97), pp. 206–212.

Complementary and Alternative Therapies

Although over a million Americans use complementary and alternative therapies for sleep problems each year, the research into their effectiveness is limited. Both chamomile and valerian—two herbs commonly used for insomnia—are safe to use in moderation, but neither has been proven in clinical trials to be effective for sleep problems.[60] The evidence is somewhat stronger for melatonin supplements, which are typically used by travelers to ward off jet lag: Studies suggest that melatonin may be able to help elderly people with insomnia fall asleep a few minutes faster, and may also relieve jet lag. However, side effects have been reported, and more research is needed.[60]

In contrast, various forms of physical activity do appear to help reduce sleep problems. In one review study of 12 clinical trials involving patients with insomnia, cognitive-behavioral therapy was found most effective. However, both yoga and *t'ai chi* (a slow, meditative movement therapy from China) also significantly improved sleep.[61] Another study of college students found improvement in sleep with both *t'ai chi* and a form of body exercise called Pilates.[62]

Change Yourself, Change Your World

Have you ever woken up from a good night's sleep feeling as if you're ready for anything? When you're well-rested, you manage stress more easily, solve problems more effectively, and make more realistic assessments of yourself and your world. In one study, a single night of sleep deprivation seriously impaired subjects' abilities to make accurate assessments of risks versus benefits and effective decisions about their well-being.[63]

Personal Choices

In college, sleep may feel like the last thing you can fit into your schedule. But investing in sufficient, regular sleep will pay off with improvements in your academic performance and your health. If you're ready to give your sleep the time and attention it merits, a first step is to identify where you're starting from. Once you know that, you'll be able to recognize the sleep-boosting strategies that are right for you.

Self-Monitor Your Sleep

Earlier in this chapter, we listed seven signs that you're sleep deprived. If one or more of those signs applies to you, then you might want to ask yourself some questions about the quality and quantity of your sleep. Take the **Self-Assessment** to find some answers.

Improve Your Ability to Fall Asleep and Stay Asleep

Sleep experts recognize two tasks required for a good night's sleep. First, you have to be able to fall asleep! You can increase your success in this task, technically called *sleep initiation*, by paying attention to certain aspects of your **sleep hygiene**—the behaviors and environmental factors that together influence the quantity and quality of your sleep. The material on page 97 identifies several steps to help get you off to sleep.

Some people drift off to sleep quite easily only to waken again in a few minutes—or in the middle of the night—unable to get back to sleep. Other people sleep 5 or 6 hours, but still wake too early to be fully rested. Sleep experts consider such problems of *sleep maintenance* a form of insomnia. If they characterize your nights, here are some aspects of your sleep hygiene that just might be contributing to the problem.

Are you haphazard about the time you get to bed and the time you wake up—shifting your sleep schedule according to the tasks of the day? If so, this one bad habit could be the sole cause of your sleep problem. To solve it, set a regular sleep–wake schedule and stick to it. It might sound challenging, but going to bed and getting up at roughly the same time every day is the

sleep hygiene The behaviors and environmental factors that together influence the quantity and quality of sleep.

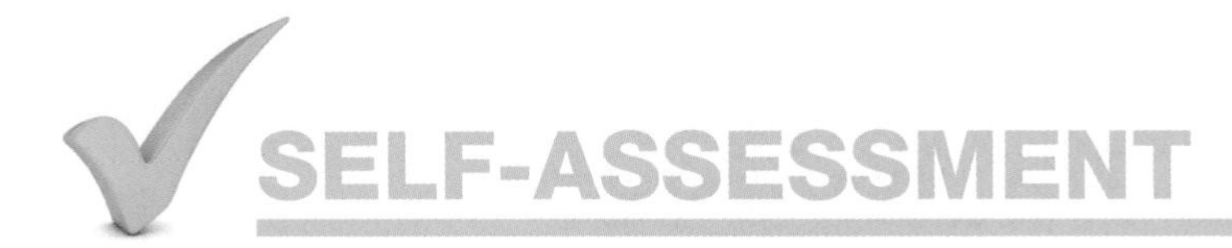

SELF-ASSESSMENT

How likely are you to doze off or fall asleep in the following situations, in contrast to feeling just tired? This refers to your usual way of life in recent times. Even if you have not done some of these things recently, try to gauge how they would have affected you. Use the following scale to choose the most appropriate number for each situation:

0 = no chance of dozing
1 = slight chance of dozing
2 = moderate chance of dozing
3 = high chance of dozing

Situation	Chance of Dozing
1. Sitting and reading	0 1 2 3
2. Watching TV	0 1 2 3
3. Sitting inactive in a public place (e.g., a theater or a meeting)	0 1 2 3
4. As a passenger in a car for an hour without a break	0 1 2 3
5. Lying down to rest in the afternoon when circumstances permit	0 1 2 3
6. Sitting and talking with someone	0 1 2 3
7. Sitting quietly after a lunch without alcohol	0 1 2 3
8. In a car, while stopped for a few minutes in traffic	0 1 2 3

Total Score: ____________

HOW TO INTERPRET YOUR SCORE

1–6: Congratulations, you are getting enough sleep!
7–8: Your score is average
9 and up: Seek the advice of a sleep specialist without delay

Source: Johns, M. W. (1991). A new method for measuring daytime sleepiness: The Epworth sleepiness scale. *Sleep* 14(6):540-545. This copyrighted material is used with permission granted by the Associated Professional Sleep Societies—March 2012. Unauthorized copying, printing or distribution of this material is strictly prohibited.

Take this self-assessment online at www.pearsonhighered.com/lynchelmore.

most important step you can take to help your body get into a regular sleep pattern.[64] If you're sure you're carrying a sleep debt and long to sleep in next weekend, set your alarm for no more than one hour later than your usual wake-up time. Paying back sleep debt gradually will help your body get back to a healthful sleep–wake cycle and maintain it all week long.

Try not to nap. You may feel like crashing in the afternoon, but you'll cut into your sleep that night. If you do need to nap, keep it as short as possible—10 to 20 minutes is ideal—and do it before 3 p.m.

Avoid alcohol for at least 6 hours before bedtime. A drink might seem relaxing, but when the sedative effect wears off—typically a few hours after you nod off—you're likely to wake up unable to get back to sleep. Watch your intake of other fluids, too. If you drink too much of any fluid right before bedtime, you'll almost certainly wake up in the middle of the night needing to use the bathroom. When you do, you might find it difficult to get back to sleep.

We all know that it's hard to get to sleep on a hot night, but did you know that elevated temperatures can also disrupt sleep maintenance? Researchers have found that when people can't dissipate their body heat, they're likely to suffer from "hyper-arousal"—waking up too easily.[65] So if possible, keep your room temperature between 60°F and 65°F.

Finally, make an all-out effort to avoid all-nighters, which leave you exhausted the next day and throw off your normal sleep cycle. Plan study time in advance to make all-nighters unnecessary.

Campus Advocacy

Some colleges are addressing sleep deprivation among their students by organizing 30-minute "nap-in" sessions every day during finals week. You can participate by bringing your own mat and pillow to the nap-in location—or organize your own nap-in for your dorm!

If your campus housing doesn't have an established policy for "quiet hours," get together with your floor mates and establish one for yourselves. Arm yourself with information on the real benefits of ample sleep—including higher grades!—and collaborate to determine a "quiet zone" and "quiet hours" that can meet everyone's needs.

You can also promote restful sleep in your apartment or dorm in little ways. If you're on the phone at midnight, keep your voice down. Wear headphones when you listen to TV or music at night, and if you need to be out in the hallways, avoid turning on all the overhead lights. Rely on the building's safety lights, or use a flashlight.

Watch videos of real students discussing their sleep at www.pearsonhighered.com/lynchelmore.

STUDENT STORY

Setting a Sleep Schedule

"Hi, I'm Rachel. When I was a freshman, I had major sleep issues. I would stay up all night long watching TV and I wouldn't think twice about going to sleep at 4 o'clock, waking up for class at 10, take a 2-hour nap in the afternoon, and then do it all over again. But it really takes a toll on your routine and your habits.

My sophomore year, especially with living off campus, it was a lot more important to be able to wake up on time and catch the bus to get to school. I had to learn how to control my sleep schedule and also how to not spend so much time napping. I really had to force myself to stick to a solid routine and get in bed and turn everything off at a decent hour, like midnight. And also, to always make sure I get 8 hours of sleep because it really does make a huge difference just to get the recommended amount of sleep. You feel amazing during the day and it's so much easier to get all the work done."

1: One of the reasons Rachel needed to set a sleep schedule was to catch the bus in the morning. What reasons do you have to set a sleep schedule?

2: Rachel suggests getting into bed and turning off all your gadgets as a way to get more sleep. What other tactics can help you get to bed at a decent hour?

Do you have a story similar to Rachel's? Share your story at www.pearsonhighered.com/lynchelmore.

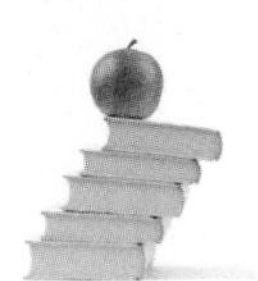

Choosing to Change Worksheet

To complete this worksheet online, visit www.pearsonhighered.com/lynchelmore.

In this chapter you learned about the importance of healthy sleep. To improve your sleep, follow the steps below.

Directions: Fill in your stage of change in Step 1 and complete Step 2 with your stage of change in mind. Then complete Steps 3, 4, or 5, depending on which ones apply to your stage of change.

Step 1: Your Stage of Behavior Change. Please check one of the following statements that best describes your readiness to obtain a good quality and quantity of sleep.

_____________ I do not intend to increase the quality or quantity of my sleep in the next 6 months. (Precontemplation)

_____________ I might increase the quality or quantity of my sleep in the next 6 months. (Contemplation)

_____________ I am prepared to increase the quality or quantity of my sleep in the next month. (Preparation)

_____________ I have been increasing my quality or quantity of sleep for less than 6 months. (Action)

_____________ I have been increasing my quality or quantity of sleep for more than 6 months. (Maintenance)

Step 2: Keep a Sleep Diary. A sleep diary is a useful tool for identifying sleep disorders and sleeping problems and pinpointing daytime and nighttime habits that may be contributing to your sleep struggles. Fill in the following chart for up to 7 days.

	Answer these Questions	Example	Monday	Tuesday	Wednesday	Thursday	Friday	Saturday	Sunday
Complete in the morning	Time I went to bed last night: Time I woke up this morning: Number of hours I slept last night:	11 p.m. 7 a.m. 8							
	Number of awakenings and total time awake last night:	5 times 2 hours							
	How long I took to fall asleep last night:	30 mins.							
	Medications taken last night:	None							
	How awake I felt when I got up this morning: 1 – Wide awake 2 – Awake but a little tired 3 – Sleepy	2							
Complete in the evening	Number of caffeinated drinks and time I had them today:	1 drink at 8 a.m.							
	Number of alcoholic drinks and time I had them today:	1 drink at 9 p.m.							
	Naptimes and lengths of naps today:	3:30 p.m. 45 mins.							
	Exercise times and lengths today:	None							
	How sleepy I felt during the day today: 1 – So sleepy I had to struggle to stay awake during much of the day 2 – Somewhat tired 3 – Fairly alert 4 – Wide awake	1							

Source: Your Guide to Healthy Sleep, by the National Heart, Lung, and Blood Institute, 2011. NIH Publication No. 11-5271. Available at http://www.nhlbi.nih.gov/health/public/sleep/healthy_sleep.htm.

After filling in the sleep diary, do you notice any habits, such as drinking alcohol or caffeine, taking medications, exercise, or napping, that could be negatively impacting your sleep?

____

____

Step 3: Precontemplation or Contemplation Stages. Answer the questions below to move toward improving your sleep patterns.

What are some reasons to improve your sleeping habits?______________________

____

What is holding you back from improving your sleeping habits?______________________

____

How can you overcome these obstacles to improving your sleep?______________________

____

Fill out the table in Step 4, below. Your confidence may be low for all strategies, but pick the one you feel may be the most helpful. How might you begin to implement that strategy?

____

____

Step 4: Preparation and Action Stages. The tips for getting to sleep more quickly provided on page 97 are listed below. On a scale of 1–5 (1 being the lowest and 5 the highest), rate your confidence in your ability to implement each strategy.

Practical Strategy	How confident are you in your ability to employ this technique? Low confidence				High confidence
1. Think of your bedroom as your "sleep cave."	1	2	3	4	5
2. Aim for a warm bed in a cool room.	1	2	3	4	5
3. Keep it quiet.	1	2	3	4	5
4. Cut caffeine.	1	2	3	4	5
5. Watch your food intake.	1	2	3	4	5
6. Hit the gym earlier in the day.	1	2	3	4	5
7. Get adequate exposure to natural light throughout the day.	1	2	3	4	5
8. Set stressors aside until morning.	1	2	3	4	5
9. Don't work in bed.	1	2	3	4	5
10. Give yourself time to wind down.	1	2	3	4	5
11. Don't stare at the ceiling.	1	2	3	4	5
12. Other	1	2	3	4	5

Select one strategy that you feel highly confident in implementing and set a start date. Start date:

____

Tell someone what you plan to do. Being accountable to others motivates you and also offers you the support and encouragement of others. Who did you tell?______________________

Step 5: Action and Maintenance Stages. For 3 days, keep track of your sleep quality and quantity. Evaluate your sleep and explain whether or not you plan to modify your plan to improve your sleep.

____

____

____

Chapter Summary

- Sleep is a physiologically prompted, dynamic, and readily reversible state of reduced consciousness essential to human survival.
- All three regions of the brain are involved in sleep. In the diencephalon, the hypothalamus and the pineal gland together help regulate your body's circadian rhythm.
- REM stands for rapid eye movement, a characteristic of dreaming sleep. A full night of sleep includes several cycles of non-REM and REM sleep.
- Most adults need 7–9 hours of sleep each night to feel alert and well rested. Any amount less than 7 hours is referred to as short sleep, whereas any amount more than 9 hours is considered long sleep.
- College students are prone to sleep debt, a condition that develops when you routinely get short sleep.
- Ample sleep is associated with increased longevity and increased cognitive functioning. Short sleep reduces the immune response, increases the risk for chronic disease and depression, and impairs complex thinking and decision-making.
- Drowsy driving is a major cause of death in automobile accidents and drowsiness is involved in other traumatic injuries each year.
- Although genetics appears to exert some influence on sleep patterns, environmental and behavioral factors are thought to be more important.
- Stress is a primary cause of troubled sleep.
- Insomnia is characterized by difficulty falling or staying asleep, a pattern of waking too early, or poor-quality sleep. Primary insomnia occurs in only about 20% of people with insomnia, and almost always develops as a result of stress. Secondary insomnia is caused by behaviors or an underlying medical condition.
- Although occasional snoring is common and not considered a disorder, sleep apnea is a potentially life-threatening disorder in which one or more pauses in breathing occur during sleep.
- In narcolepsy, the person is not able to regulate the timing of sleep appropriately, and may fall asleep frequently during activities of daily living.
- Parasomnias are conditions in which sleep is accompanied by an unusual event. Parasomnias include sleep terrors, sleepwalking, sleep bruxism, nocturnal eating, REM behavior disorder, and restless legs syndrome.
- Diagnosis of sleep disorders may require a sleep study conducted overnight in a sleep lab.
- Over-the-counter and prescription sleep remedies should be avoided if possible, and never used for longer than 3 weeks.
- Cognitive-behavioral therapy has been found effective in the treatment of troubled sleep.
- You can improve the quality and quantity of your sleep by adhering to recommended behaviors and environmental factors that influence your ability to initiate and maintain sleep.

Test Your Knowledge

1. The pineal gland responds to changing levels of darkness and light by changing its level of production of a hormone called
   a. growth hormone.
   b. insulin.
   c. melatonin.
   d. adrenaline.

2. Which of the following statements about REM sleep is true?
   a. REM sleep is the deepest stage of sleep, also called delta sleep.
   b. As the night continues, the duration of REM sleep increases.
   c. As the night continues, REM sleep entirely ceases.
   d. It is extremely difficult to waken someone from REM sleep.

3. Which of the following statements about short sleep is true?
   a. Short sleep is any amount of total nightly sleep below 7 hours.
   b. Half of all American adults experience short sleep every night.
   c. Short sleep is another name for stage 1 of non-REM sleep.
   d. Short sleep is associated with increased longevity.

4. Daytime drowsiness and difficulty concentrating are classic signs of
   a. long sleep.
   b. sleep deprivation.
   c. hypersomnia.
   d. sleep bruxism.

5. The stimulant most commonly associated with sleep problems is
   a. nicotine.
   b. alcohol.
   c. cocaine.
   d. caffeine.

6. Secondary insomnia is
   a. far less common than primary insomnia.
   b. almost always due to stress.
   c. prompted by an underlying medical disorder.
   d. treated with a CPAP machine.

7. Obstructive sleep apnea
   a. is the medical name for snoring.
   b. is typically diagnosed in underweight women.
   c. is less common than central sleep apnea.
   d. increases the risk for a heart attack, stroke, or traumatic injury.

8. REM behavior disorder is
   a. characterized by movements suggesting that the sleeper is acting out a dream.
   b. one of the most common types of parasomnia.
   c. likely to occur in the first sleep cycle of the night.
   d. accompanied by an unpleasant feeling in the legs.

9. As a first step in addressing sleep problems, health experts recommend
   a. herbal sleep remedies containing either chamomile or valerian.
   b. prescription sleep medications.
   c. vigorous exercise 1–2 hours before bedtime.
   d. assessing and altering aspects of your sleep hygiene.

10. The most important strategy for improving your sleep maintenance is
   a. taking a late-afternoon nap of no more than 10–20 minutes daily.
   b. setting and keeping a regular sleep–wake schedule.
   c. drinking a small glass of water just before bed.
   d. maintaining a bedroom temperature of at least 68°F.

Get Critical

What happened:

In the middle of a January night in 2011, college student Kelly Davis left her Milwaukee apartment without a coat, got into her car, and went for a drive—in her sleep. Earlier that evening, she had taken the prescription sleep medication Ambien. Police pulled her over for swerving and hitting a curb and charged her with driving while intoxicated. Davis pleaded not guilty. Her attorney explained that she was "involuntarily intoxicated" and was not acting of her own free will. Although she faced up to $1,000 in fines, Davis had much to be thankful for: Ambien has frequently been cited in motor vehicle accidents, falls, and other types of traumatic injury resulting in death.

What do you think?

- **In your view, is Davis guilty of driving while intoxicated?**
- **Should Ambien's manufacturer be held responsible for driving violations, injuries, and fatalities involving patients taking the drug, even if the majority use it without incident?**
- **If you were experiencing persistent insomnia, and had tried changing aspects of your sleep hygiene without success would you consider trying Ambien or a similar drug? If so, what precautions would you take to avoid its adverse effects?**

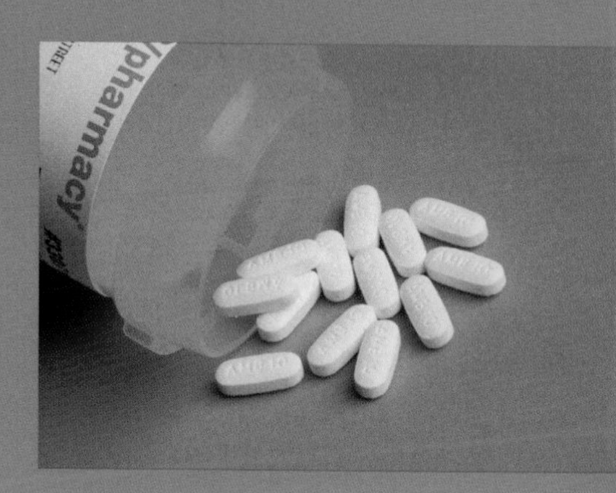

Get Connected

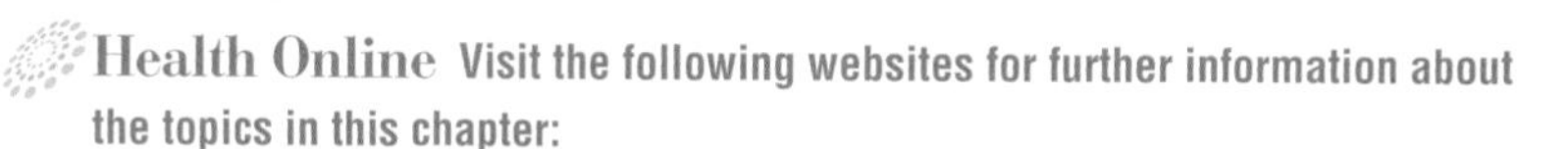

Mobile Tips!

Scan this QR code with your mobile device to access additional sleep tips. Or, via your mobile device, go to **http://mobiletips.pearsoncmg.com** and navigate to Chapter 4.

Health Online **Visit the following websites for further information about the topics in this chapter:**

- National Sleep Foundation
  www.sleepfoundation.org
- American Academy of Sleep Medicine's Consumer Information Site
  http://yoursleep.aasmnet.org
- Sleep Disorders
  www.nlm.nih.gov/medlineplus/tutorials/sleepdisorders/htm/index.htm
- Stanford University's Center for Sleep and Dreams's Sleep Guide
  www.end-your-sleep-deprivation.com/sleep-essentials.html#essentials

Website links are subject to change. To access updated Web links, please visit ***www.pearsonhighered.com/lynchelmore.***

References

i. National Sleep Foundation. (2011, March 7). 2011 Sleep in America poll: Communications technology in the bedroom. Retrieved from http://www.sleepfoundation.org/sites/default/files/sleepinamericapoll/SIAP_2011_Summary_of_Findings.pdf.

1. Lund, H. G., Reider, B. D., Whiting, A. B., & Prichard, J. R. (2009). Sleep patterns and predictors of disturbed sleep in a large population of college students. *Journal of Adolescent Health, 46* (2), 124–132.

2. Silverthorn, D. (2010). *Human physiology: An integrated approach*, 5th ed. San Francisco: Benjamin Cummings.

3. Bear, M. F., Connors, B. W., & Paradiso, M. A. (2007). *Neuroscience: Exploring the brain*, 3rd ed. Baltimore: Lippincott Williams & Wilkins, p. 596.

4. American Academy of Sleep Medicine. (2008, December 31). Seven signs you need sleep. Retrieved from http://yoursleep.aasmnet.org/Topic.aspx?id=89.

5. Mayo Foundation. (2008, October 8). Go ahead—catch a short nap. Retrieved from http://www.mayoclinic.org/news2008-mchi/5027.html.

6. Bonnet, M. H., & Arand, D. L. (2010). How much sleep do adults need? White paper, National Sleep Foundation. Retrieved from http://www.sleepfoundation.org/article/white-papers/how-much-sleep-do-adults-need.

7. Jones, M. (2011, April 15). How little sleep can you get away with? *The New York Times*. Retrieved from http://www.nytimes.com/2011/04/17/magazine/mag-17Sleep-t.html?scp=1&sq=maggie%20jones%20april%202011&st=cse.

8. Kamdar, B., Kaplan, K., Kezirian, E., & Dement, W. (2004). The impact of extended sleep on daytime alertness, vigilance, and mood. *Sleep Medicine, 5*, 441–448.

9. National Sleep Foundation. (2009, March 2). 2009 Sleep in America poll: Health and safety. Retrieved from http://www.sleepfoundation.org/sites/default/files/2009%20Sleep%20in%20America%20SOF%20EMBARGOED.pdf.

10. National Sleep Foundation. (2011, March 7). 2011 Sleep in America poll: Communications technology in the bedroom. Retrieved from http://www.sleepfoundation.org/sites/default/files/sleepinamericapoll/SIAP_2011_Summary_of_Findings.pdf.

11. American College Health Association. (2012). American College Health Association National College Health Assessment (ACHA-NCHA II) reference group executive summary, Fall 2011. Retrieved from http://www.acha-ncha.org/reports_ACHA-NCHAII.html.

12. Mann, D. (2011). Can better sleep mean catching fewer colds? WebMD. Retrieved from http://www.webmd.com/sleep-disorders/excessive-sleepiness-10/immune-system-lack-of-sleep.

13. Centers for Disease Control. (2011, January 27). *Sleep and sleep disorders*. Retrieved from http://www.cdc.gov/sleep/index.htm.

14. Patel, S. R., & Hu, F. B. (2008). Short sleep duration and weight gain: A systematic review. *Obesity, 16* (3), 643–653.

15. Regestein, Q., Natarajan, V., Pavlova, M., Kawasaki, S., Gleason, R., & Koff, E. (2010). Sleep debt and depression in female college students. *Psychiatry Research*, *176* (1), 34–39.

16. Brooks, P. R., Girgenti, A. A., & Mills, M. J. (2009). Sleep patterns and symptoms of depression in college students. *College Student Journal*, *43* (2), 464–472.

17. Vail-Smith, K., Felts, W., & Becker, C. (2009). Relationship between sleep quality and health risk behaviors in undergraduate college students. *College Student Journal*, *43* (3), 924–930.

18. Gilbert, S. P., & Weaver, C. C. (2010). Sleep quality and academic performance in university students: A wake-up call for college psychologists. *Journal of College Student Psychotherapy, 24* (4), 295–306.

19. Curcio, G., Ferrara, M., & De Dennaro, L. (2006). Sleep loss, learning capacity and academic performance. *Sleep Medicine, 10* (5), 323–337.

20. Gaultney, J. F. (2010, September–October). The prevalence of sleep disorders in college students: Impact on academic performance. *Journal of Am Coll Health*, *59* (2), 91–97.

21. Thacher, P. V. (2008). University students and the "all nighter": Correlates and patterns of students' engagement in a single night of total sleep deprivation. *Behavioral Sleep Medicine*, *6* (1), 16–31.

22. Becker, C. M., Adams, T., Orr, C., & Quilter, L. (2008). Correlates of quality sleep and academic performance. *Health Educator, 40* (2), 82–89.

23. American Academy of Sleep Medicine. (2011, January 7). Sleep: Nature's study aid. *Sleep Education*. Retrieved from http://yoursleep.aasmnet.org/Article.aspx?id=2030.

24. Greer, M. (2004, July). Strengthen your brain by resting it. American Psychological Association. *Monitor, 35* (7), 60.

25. Carpenter, S. (2001, October). Research confirms the virtues of "sleeping on it." American Psychological Association. *Monitor*, *32* (9), 49.

26. National Sleep Foundation. (2011, July 27). Drowsy driving prevention week highlights prevalent and preventable accidents. Retrieved from http://drowsydriving.org/2010/11/drowsy-driving-prevention-week®-highlights-prevalent-and-preventable-accidents.

27. Lee-Chiong, T. (2006). *Sleep: A comprehensive handbook*. Hoboken, NJ: Wiley-Liss, 205.

28. Watson, N. F., Goldberg, J., Arguelles, L., & Buchwald, D. (2006). Genetic and environmental influences on insomnia, daytime sleepiness, and obesity in twins. *SLEEP*, *29* (5), 645–649.

29. Roberts R. E., Roberts, C. R., & Chan, W. (2006). Ethnic differences in symptoms of insomnia among adolescents. *SLEEP, 29* (3), 359–365.

30. Thompson, J., and Manore, M. (2012). *Nutrition: An applied approach*, 3rd ed. San Francisco: Benjamin Cummings, 85.

31. Orr, W. C., et al. (2007, February). Acidic and non-acidic reflux during sleep under conditions of powerful acid suppression. *Chest, 131*, 460–465.

32. Edwards, S. J., Montgomery, I. M., Colquhoun, E. Q., Jordan, J. E., & Clark, M. G. (1992, September). Spicy meals disturb sleep: An effect of thermoregulation? *International Journal of Psychophysiology*, *13* (2), 97–100.

33. U.S. Fire Administration. (2010, September 23). *Smoking and fire safety*. Retrieved from http://www.usfa.dhs.gov/citizens/home_fire_prev/smoking.shtm.

34. Ruxton, C. H. S. (2008). The impact of caffeine on mood, cognitive function, performance and hydration: A review of benefits and risks. British Nutrition Foundation. *Nutrition Bulletin, 33*, 15–25.

35. WedMD Medical Reference. (2011, February 27). *Caffeine myths and facts*. Retrieved from http://www.webmd.com/balance/caffeine-myths-and-facts.

36. Substance Abuse and Mental Health Services Administration, Office of Applied Studies. (2010, September). *Results from the 2009 national survey on drug use and health: Volume I: Summary of national findings*. Retrieved from http://oas.samhsa.gov/nsduh/2k9nsduh/2k9ResultsP.pdf.

37. Clegg-Kraynok, M. M., McBean, A. L., & Montgomery-Downs, H. E. (2011). Sleep quality and characteristics of college students who use prescription psychostimulants nonmedically. *Sleep Medicine, 12*, 598–602.

38. Roehrs, T., and Roth, T. (2008, July). *Sleep, sleepiness, and alcohol use*. National Institute on Alcohol Abuse and Alcoholism. Retrieved from http://pubs.niaaa.nih.gov/publications/arh25-2/101-109.htm.

39. Myllymaki, T., Kyrolainen, H., Savolainen, K., et al. (2011, March). Effects of vigorous late-night exercise on sleep quality and cardiac autonomic activity. *J Sleep Res*, *20* (1, Part 2), 146–153.

40. American Academy of Sleep Medicine. (2010). *Sleep disorders*. Retrieved from http://yoursleep.aasmnet.org/Disorders.aspx.

41. National Institutes of Health. (2009, March). *Insomnia*. Retrieved from http://www.nhlbi.nih.gov/health/dci/Diseases/inso/inso_whatis.html.

42. Mayo Foundation. (2010, May 25). *Snoring*. Retrieved from http://www.mayoclinic.com/health/snoring/DS00297.

43. National Institutes of Health. (2009, March). *Sleep apnea*. Retrieved from http://www.nhlbi.nih.gov/health/dci/Diseases/SleepApnea.html.

44. Young, T., Finn, L., Peppard, P., Szklo-Coxe, M., Austin, D., Nieto, F. J., Stubbs, R., and Hla, K. M. (2008). Sleep disordered breathing and mortality: Eighteen-year follow-up of the Wisconsin sleep cohort. *SLEEP*, *31* (8), 1071–1078.

45. National Sleep Foundation. (2011). *Narcolepsy and sleep*. Retrieved from http://www.sleepfoundation.org/article/sleep-related-problems/narcolepsy-and-sleep.

46. Townsend, D. R. (2005, October 21). *Nightmares*. American Academy of Sleep Medicine. Retrieved from http://yoursleep.aasmnet.org/Disorder.aspx?id=37.

47. National Library of Medicine. (2009, June 20). *Sleepwalking*. MedlinePlus. Retrieved from http://www.nlm.nih.gov/medlineplus/ency/article/000808.htm.

48. Mayo Foundation. (2011, May 19). *Sleep bruxism*. Retrieved from http://www.mayoclinic.com/print/bruxism/DS00337.

49. Winkelman, J. W. (2006). Sleep-related eating disorder and night-eating syndrome: Sleep disorders, eating disorders, or both? *SLEEP, 29* (7), 876–877.

50. Schutte-Rodin, S. L. (2005, October 21). REM sleep behavior disorder. *American Academy of Sleep Medicine*. Retrieved from http://yoursleep.aasmnet.org/Disorder.aspx?id=29.

51. National Institutes of Health. (2010, November). *Restless legs syndrome*. Retrieved from http://www.nhlbi.nih.gov/health/dci/Diseases/rls/rls_WhatIs.html.

52. Austin, E. (2008). Addressing sleep deprivation in college students. *American Journal for Nurse Practitioners*, *12* (6), 34.

53. Brown, F. C., Buboltz, W. C., & Soper, B. (2006). Development and evaluation of the sleep treatment and education program for students (STEPS). *Journal of American College Health, 54* (4), 231–237.

54. National Sleep Foundation. (2011). *Sleep aids and insomnia*. Retrieved from http://www.sleepfoundation.org/article/sleep-related-problems/sleep-aids-and-insomnia.

55. American Academy of Sleep Medicine. (2011). Sleep hygiene: The healthy habits of good sleep. Retrieved from http://yoursleep.aasmnet.org/Hygiene.aspx.

56. WebMD. (2005, June 1). Addictive sleep medications remain popular. Retrieved from http://www.webmd.com/sleep-disorders/news/20050601/addictive-sleep-medications-remain-popular.

57. [No authors listed.] (2008, October). Sleep complaints: Whenever possible, avoid the use of sleeping pills. *Prescrire International, 17* (97), 206–212.

58. Kloss, J. D., Nash, C. O., Horse, S. E., & Taylor, D. J. (2011). The delivery of behavioral sleep medicine to college students. *Journal of Adolescent Health, 48* (6), 553–561.

59. Carney, C. E., & Waters, W. F. (2006). Effects of a structured problem-solving procedure on pre-sleep cognitive arousal in college students with insomnia. *Behavioral Sleep Medicine, 4* (1), 13–28.

60. National Center for Complementary and Alternative Medicine. (2010, December). Sleep disorders and CAM: What the science says. Retrieved from http://nccam.nih.gov/health/providers/digest/sleepdisorders-science.htm.

61. Kozasa, E. H., Hachul, H., Monson, C., Pinto, L., Jr., Garcia, M. C., de Araujo Moraes Mello, L. E., & Tufik, S. (2010, December). Mind–body interventions for the treatment of insomnia: A review. *Revista Brasileira de Psiquiatria*, *32* (4), 437–443.

62. Caldwell, K., Harrison, M., Adams, M., & Triplett, N. (2009). Effect of Pilates and taiji quan training on self-efficacy, sleep quality, mood, and physical performance of college students. *Journal of Bodywork and Movement Therapies, 13* (2), 155–163.

63. Harmon, K. (2011, March 8). Short on sleep, the brain optimistically favors long odds. *Scientific American*.

64. National Sleep Foundation. (2011). *Sleep hygiene*. Retrieved from http://www.sleepfoundation.org/article/ask-the-expert/sleep-hygiene.

65. Lack, L. C., Gradisar, M., Van Someren, E. J., Wright, H. R., & Lushington, K. (2008, August). The relationship between insomnia and body temperatures. *Sleep Medicine Reviews,12* (4), 307–317.

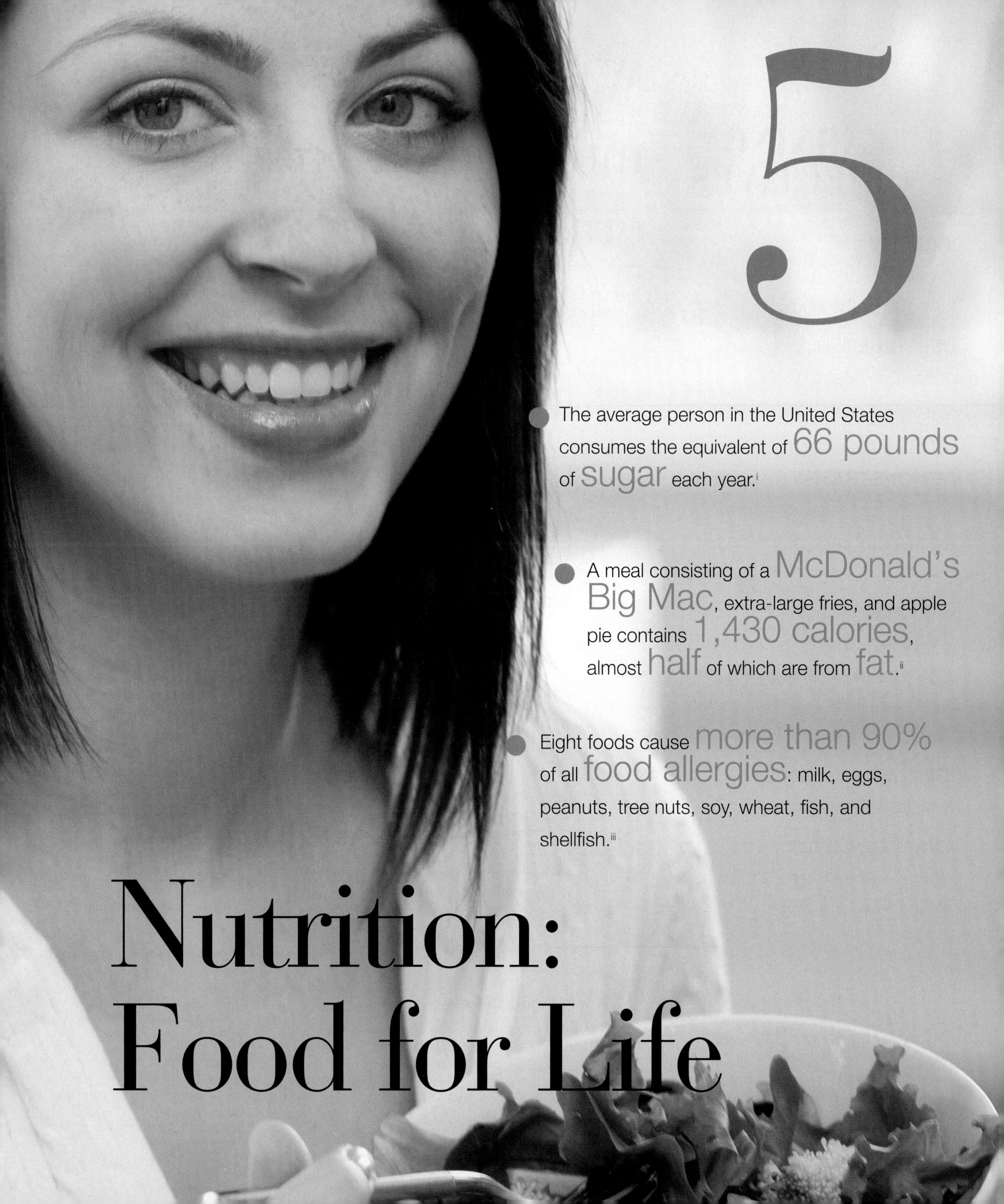

5

- The average person in the United States consumes the equivalent of 66 pounds of sugar each year.[i]
- A meal consisting of a McDonald's Big Mac, extra-large fries, and apple pie contains 1,430 calories, almost half of which are from fat.[ii]
- Eight foods cause more than 90% of all food allergies: milk, eggs, peanuts, tree nuts, soy, wheat, fish, and shellfish.[iii]

Nutrition: Food for Life

LEARNING OBJECTIVES

IDENTIFY the six classes of nutrients and explain their functions in the body.

DESCRIBE the importance of fiber, phytochemicals, antioxidants, and probiotics in foods.

DEMONSTRATE how to use MyPlate and other government resources to design a healthful diet.

EXPLAIN how nutrition guidelines can vary according to a person's age, gender, activity level, and dietary preferences or needs.

IDENTIFY strategies for handling food safely.

ANALYZE your current diet and create a personalized plan for improving your nutrition.

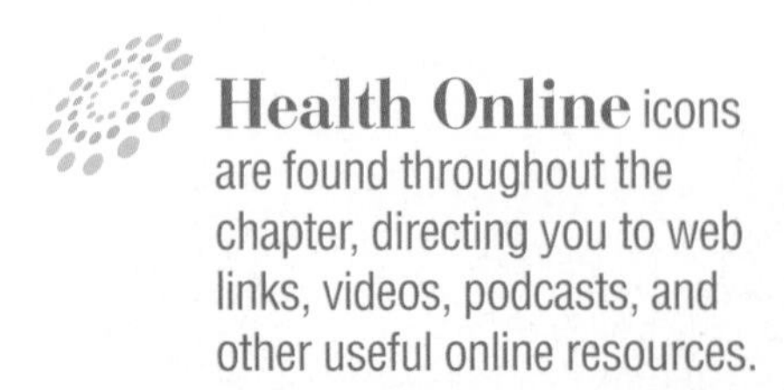
Health Online icons are found throughout the chapter, directing you to web links, videos, podcasts, and other useful online resources.

Why is orange juice more nutritious than orange soda?

Why does a baked potato beat French fries? Why is fat from a fish better than fat from a cow? In short, what foods should you limit, and what foods should you favor? Most importantly, why does it matter?

The science of **nutrition** examines how the foods you eat affect your body and health. A nutritious **diet** provides you with energy, helps you stay healthy, and allows you to function at your best. Diets lacking in nutrition can drain your energy and decrease your sense of well-being, as well as increase your risk for developing chronic health problems such as high blood pressure, heart disease, type 2 diabetes, and obesity. Whether you're in line at the deli or your dining hall, knowing the basic principles of good nutrition can help you make choices that will benefit your health for a lifetime.

What Are Nutrients?

Your body relies on food to provide chemical compounds called **nutrients.** In a process called digestion, the food you eat is broken down into nutrients that are small enough to be absorbed into your bloodstream **(Figure 5.1).** Once in your body, nutrients work together to provide energy; support growth, repair, and maintenance of body tissues; and regulate body functions.

Six major classes of nutrients are found in food:

- Carbohydrates
- Fats (more appropriately called *lipids*)
- Proteins
- Vitamins
- Minerals
- Water

Within these six classes are about 45 specific nutrients that your body is unable to make or can't make in needed quantities to support health. These are called **essential nutrients.** You must obtain essential nutrients from food, beverages, and/or supplements.

Nutrients your body needs in relatively large quantities are called *macronutrients* (*macro* means "large"). These are carbohydrates, fats, proteins, and water. Nutrients you need in relatively small quantities are called *micronutrients* (*micro* means "small"). These are vitamins and minerals.

Energy and Calories

Three of the four macronutrients—carbohydrates, fats, and proteins—are also known as *energy-yielding nutrients* because they provide you with the energy you need to move, to think, and simply to survive. Whether you're running a marathon or sound asleep, your body is expending energy, which it obtains by breaking down

nutrition The scientific study of food and its physiological functions.

diet The food you regularly consume.

nutrients Chemical substances in food that you need for energy, growth, and survival.

essential nutrients Nutrients you must obtain from food or supplements because your body either cannot produce them or cannot make them in sufficient quantities to maintain health.

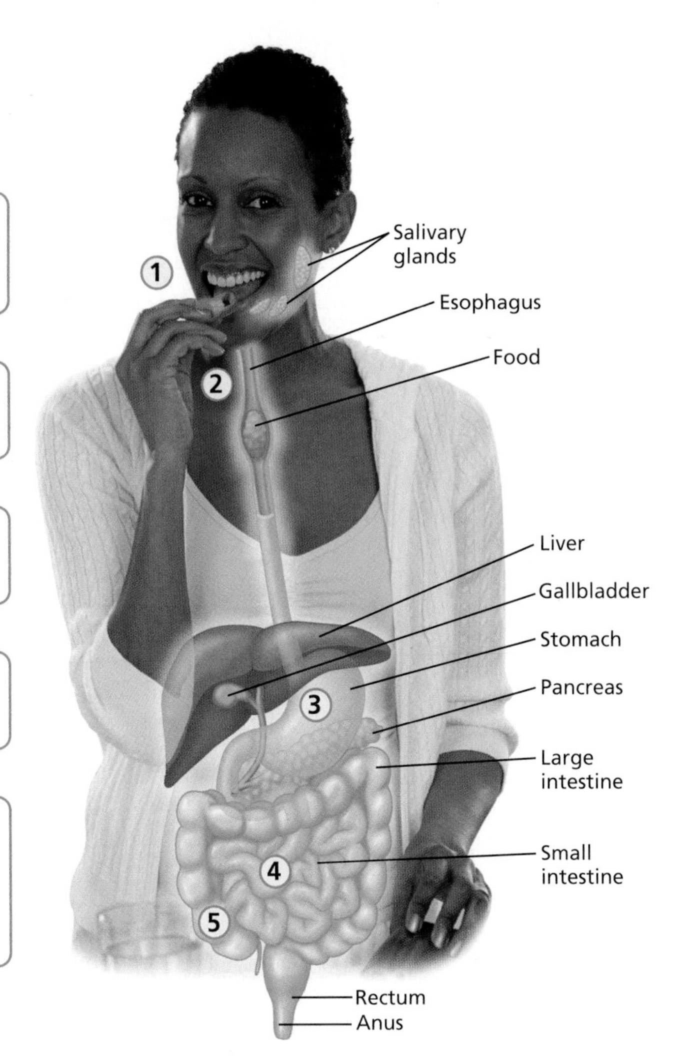

1 Digestion begins in the mouth. Chewing mixes saliva with food and begins to break it down.
2 The food travels from the mouth to the stomach through the esophagus.
3 The stomach mixes food with chemicals that break it down further.
4 Most digestion and absorption occurs in the small intestine.
5 Water, vitamins, and some minerals are absorbed in the large intestine. The remaining wastes are passed out of the body in stool.
Salivary glands
Esophagus
Food
Liver
Gallbladder
Stomach
Pancreas
Large intestine
Small intestine
Rectum
Anus

Figure 5.1 The digestive process. Digestion is the process of breaking food down into nutrients that can be used by the body for energy.

Source: Adapted from Thompson, J., & Manore, M. (2012). *Nutrition: An Applied Approach* (3rd ed.). San Francisco, CA: Pearson Education.

the carbohydrates, fats, and proteins in the foods you eat. Although vitamins, minerals, and water assist this process, they don't supply you with energy.

If you've ever thought that you felt warmer after eating a meal, you weren't imagining it! Scientists determine the amount of energy that a food provides by measuring how much heat it generates. They calculate that heat in units called *kilocalories*. Specifically, 1 kilocalorie is an amount of heat that raises the temperature of 1 kilogram (about 2.2 pounds) of water by 1 degree Celsius.

Although food scientists use the term *kilocalorie*, you're probably more familiar with the simpler term **calorie,** which is used in the media, on food labels, and in everyday conversation. We use the term *calorie* throughout this text as well.

The energy-yielding nutrients differ in their calorie content. Carbohydrates and proteins each provide 4 calories per gram. (A gram is a very small amount; for instance, a standard packet of sugar contains about 3 grams.) Fats provide 9 calories per gram—more than twice the amount in carbohydrates or proteins. Alcohol is not a nutrient because it doesn't provide any substance you need to grow or survive. However, alcohol does provide energy, 7 calories per gram, which explains why consuming alcohol regularly can pack on the pounds. Regardless of their source, calories consumed in excess of energy needs are converted to fat and stored in the body.

Although vitamins and minerals provide no energy, they serve as components of body structures and help regulate many of your body functions. In addition, many vitamins and minerals are essential to **metabolism,** the process by which your body breaks down foods into molecules small enough to absorb, and then converts those molecules into energy.

Water is calorie free, so it doesn't supply you with energy. Still, water is the medium in which the body's chemical reactions occur—including the metabolic reactions that convert nutrient molecules into energy.

People vary in how many calories they need to eat each day to meet their energy needs, yet avoid gaining weight. Children and people over age 50 need fewer calories than young and middle-aged adults, and women, on average, need fewer than men. And because vigorous activity burns more calories than sitting still, athletes need many more

calorie Common term for *kilocalorie*. The amount of energy required to raise the temperature of 1 kilogram of water by 1 degree Celsius.

metabolism The sum of all chemical reactions occurring in body cells that break large molecules down into smaller molecules.

calories than people who spend hours every day watching TV, surfing the Internet, and, yes, sitting in the library studying.

How many calories do *you* need each day? Find out in seconds using this simple tool: www.cancer.org/healthy/toolsandcalculators/calculators/app/calorie-counter-calculator.

Carbohydrates

Carbohydrates are compounds that contain three common elements: carbon, hydrogen, and oxygen. Plants manufacture carbohydrates using energy from the sun, and we derive the carbohydrates in our diets predominantly from plant foods. Milk and other dairy products are the exception, but even the carbohydrates in these foods come from the plants that the cow, goat, or sheep consumed.

Carbohydrates are sometimes called the body's universal energy source because most body cells, especially during high-intensity activities, prefer carbohydrates for energy. Some body cells, including those in your brain, can use only carbohydrates for fuel.

There are two categories of carbohydrates: *simple carbohydrates* and *complex carbohydrates*. Both are composed of the same basic building blocks: sugar molecules, whose names usually end in "ose."

carbohydrates A macronutrient class composed of carbon, hydrogen, and oxygen, that is the body's universal energy source.

simple carbohydrates The most basic unit of carbohydrates, consisting of one or two sugar molecules.

complex carbohydrates Contain chains of multiple sugar molecules; commonly called *starches* but also come in two non-starch forms: *glycogen* and *fiber*.

fiber A nondigestible complex carbohydrate that aids in digestion.

Simple Carbohydrates

Simple carbohydrates are constructed from just one or two sugar molecules. That means they are easily digested. We commonly refer to simple carbohydrates as *sugars*, and six are important in nutrition: glucose, fructose (fruit sugar), galactose, maltose (malt sugar), sucrose (table sugar), and lactose (milk sugar). Of these, the most important is glucose. It is the most abundant sugar in foods and in our bodies, and it is our most important energy source.

Sugars provide much of the sweetness found naturally in fruits, some vegetables, honey, and milk. They are also added to soft drinks and other beverages, desserts, and even some peanut butters, soups, and other foods you might not normally think of as sweet. In fact, studies indicate that adults in the United States consume an average of 22.5 teaspoons of added sugars a day.[1]

As it breaks down, absorbs, burns, or stores the simple carbohydrates you eat, your body is unable to distinguish between those that came naturally from whole foods and those that were added to foods as sweeteners. The fructose present in an orange is the same, chemically, as the fructose in the high-fructose corn syrup (HFCS) that is used to sweeten orange soda. This doesn't mean, however, that drinking fresh-squeezed orange juice is the same as drinking orange soda! Foods with naturally occurring sugars contain many vitamins, minerals, and other substances that promote health. Foods high in added sugars generally provide empty calories and few, if any, health-promoting benefits.

Speaking of empty calories, you may have seen news stories blaming HFCS for America's obesity epidemic. But is HFCS different from any other type of sugar? Check out the **Myth or Fact?** discussion for some answers.

> *"Some body cells, including those in your brain, can use only carbohydrates for fuel."*

Complex Carbohydrates

Complex carbohydrates are made up of long chains of multiple sugar molecules; therefore, they take longer to digest. Commonly called *starches*, they are found in a variety of plants, especially grains (barley, oats, rice, rye, wheat, etc.), legumes (dried beans, lentils, and peas), other vegetables, and many fruits. Processed foods made from grains, such as breads, pasta, and breakfast cereals, also are good sources of starches.

There are two non-starch forms of complex carbohydrate. *Glycogen* is a storage form of glucose in animal tissues, including the liver and muscles. We consume very little glycogen from meat, however, because it typically breaks down when an animal is slaughtered. **Fiber** is a tough (fibrous) complex carbohydrate that gives structure to plants. Although it's not a nutrient, because it's nondigestible, it's a very important component of a healthy diet. Let's see why.

Facts About Fiber

Whereas starch is readily digested and its components absorbed, fiber passes through the intestinal tract undigested. Nevertheless, it has many health benefits:

- **Weight control.** Fiber gives plant foods their substance, so it can make you feel full before you've consumed lots of calories. In this way, a high-fiber diet can help you avoid weight gain.
- **Bowel health.** Fiber helps promote bowel regularity because, as it moves through your large intestine, it provides bulk for feces. Because it absorbs water along the way, it also softens feces, making stools easier to pass. A diet rich in fiber can help you to avoid hemorrhoids, constipation, and other digestive problems.
- **Heart health.** No doubt you've heard of cholesterol, an oily substance that can clog your blood vessels and increase your risk for heart disease. A diet rich in fiber can help lower the level of cholesterol in your blood. It's thought that this happens because fiber binds to bile, a cholesterol-containing substance that your liver makes. When fiber is excreted from your body in feces, bile—and its cholesterol load—is excreted along with it. This leaves less cholesterol in your bloodstream.
- **Blood glucose control.** Finally, by slowing the transit of foods through your intestinal tract, fiber promotes a more gradual absorption of their nutrients, including glucose, into your bloodstream. This can help prevent wide fluctuations in glucose levels in your blood, which is important in managing diabetes.

For all these reasons, it's recommended that you maintain a high-fiber diet. Men need 38 grams of fiber per day, and women need 25 grams per day. For men and women 50 years or older, the recommendations are 30 and 21 grams, respectively.[2] Remember we said that fiber absorbs water, so a high-fiber diet should be accompanied by plenty of fluids to keep the fiber moving along the intestinal tract.

Fiber is plentiful in legumes and other vegetables, many fruits, nuts, and seeds, as well as whole grains. But what exactly qualifies as a whole grain food?

whole grains Unrefined grains that contain bran, germ, and endosperm.

Choose Whole Grains

Unrefined grains, or **whole grains,** include three parts—bran, germ, and endosperm—and generally can be sprouted (**Figure 5.2** on page 110). Common examples are whole wheat, rolled or whole oats, hulled barley, popcorn, brown rice, rye, millet, and quinoa. Whole grains are especially nutritious because the bran and germ provide valuable vitamins, minerals, and fiber. Like any fiber-rich food, whole grains are bulky, and the body digests them slowly, allowing people to feel full sooner and for a longer time. As a result, people who eat a diet rich in whole grains tend to consume fewer calories. And because

MYTH OR FACT?

Does High-Fructose Corn Syrup Deserve Its Bad Rap?

Corn refiners produce high-fructose corn syrup (HFCS) by converting cornstarch into a syrup that, by the end of the process, contains 55% fructose. The USDA reports that 90% of this so-called HFCS-55 is sold to the beverage industry, where it is used in the production of soft drinks, sweetened juices, and other sweet drinks.

A 42% fructose version is also used in beverages, as well as in sweetened breakfast cereals, baked goods, candies, and many other processed foods.[1] Beverage and food manufacturers have embraced HFCS because it is much less expensive than sucrose (table sugar typically made from sugar cane). As a result, since it was introduced into the American diet in 1970, our consumption of HFCS has jumped more than 1,000% while our consumption of sucrose has steadily declined.[2]

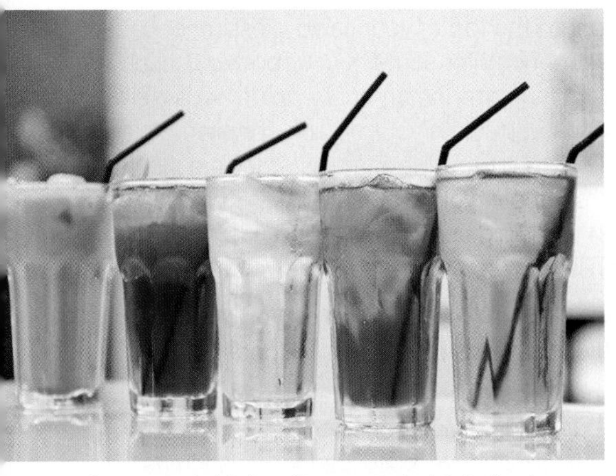

Sweetened drinks often contain high-fructose corn syrup.

Meanwhile, our average body weight has soared. For example, in 1970, just 4% of Americans aged 18 to 19 were obese. In 2008, the obesity rate in this group was nearly 18%.[3] Among adults aged 20 and older, the rate is much higher: Nearly 34% are obese. So it's not surprising that some researchers have begun to ask whether or not our increased consumption of HFCS is contributing to America's expanding waistline.

One of the concerns about HFCS is the fact that our bodies metabolize fructose differently from sucrose. Many studies have shown that, as a result of the unique way our bodies process it, consuming fructose doesn't cause us to feel satiated (full). This means that, even after we've downed a couple of cans of orange soda—and taken in 358 calories—we're likely to continue eating. In contrast, if we had a beverage sweetened with sucrose, we would have felt a certain level of satiation . . . and consumed fewer calories overall.[4]

Another concern relates to stored fat: some researchers contend that we're more likely to store body fat when we consume an excess of fructose than when we consume too much sucrose. Supporting this claim is a recent study that found that rats fed HFCS gain more weight and body fat than rats fed the same amounts of sucrose.[2]

Not all nutrition experts agree. They point out that the research findings are mixed: Some studies have found little difference in weight gain between high-fructose and high-sucrose diets.[5] They also theorize that our weight gain has resulted from an overall increase in calorie consumption and a decrease in our level of physical activity, and that the precise ingredients in soft drinks, cookies, and other foods matter very little.

The bottom line? More research into the precise health effects of HFCS is needed. Meanwhile, consider these tips from the Mayo Clinic to cut back on your intake of all refined sugars:[5]

- Avoid sweetened sodas. Drink water, skim milk, 100% fruit juices, diet soda, or other healthful beverages instead.
- Choose breakfast cereals carefully. Skip the frosted Os, squares, and flakes. Oatmeal is an excellent choice.
- Eat fewer processed foods, especially pastries and packaged meals.
- Snack on vegetables, fruit, low-fat cheese and yogurt, and whole grain pretzels instead of candy and cookies.

References: **1.** "Sugar and Sweeteners: Background," by the Economic Research Service, August 6, 2009, Briefing Room, United States Department of Agriculture, retrieved from http://www.ers.usda.gov/briefing/sugar/background.htm. **2.** "High-Fructose Corn Syrup Causes Characteristics of Obesity in Rats: Increased Body Weight, Body Fat and Triglyceride Levels," by M. E. Bocarsly, E. S. Powell, N. M. Avena, & B. G. Hoebel, 2010, *Pharmacol Biochem Behav*, doi:10.1016/j.pbb.2010.02.012. **3.** "Obesity Among Children and Adolescents 2–19 Years of Age, by Selected Characteristics," by the Centers for Disease Control and Prevention, 2010, retrieved from http://www.cdc.gov/nchs/data/hus/2010/072.pdf. **4.** "The Role of High-Fructose Corn Syrup in Metabolic Syndrome and Hypertension," by L. Ferder, M. D. Ferder, & F. Inserra, 2010, *Current Hypertension Report, 12*, pp. 105–112. **5.** "High-Fructose Corn Syrup: What Are the Health Concerns?" by J. K. Nelson, October 23, 2010, the Mayo Foundation, retrieved from http://www.mayoclinic.com/health/high-fructose-corn-syrup/AN01588/METHOD=print.

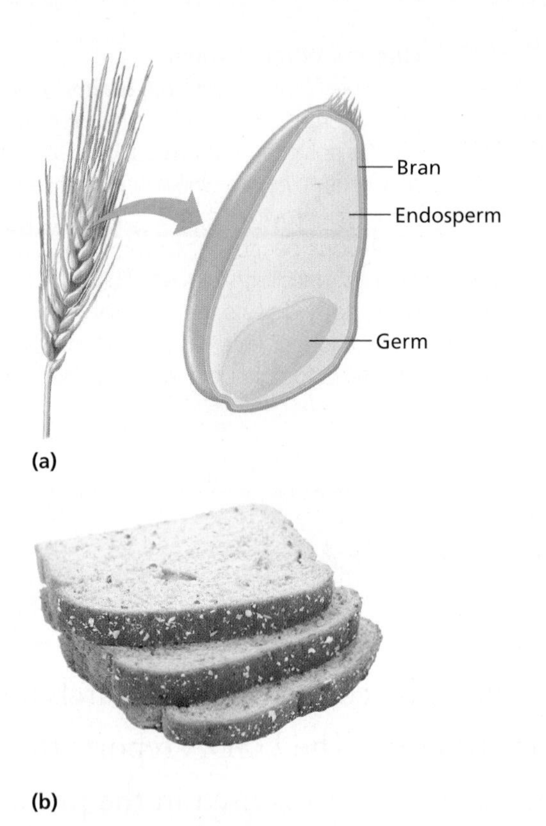

Figure 5.2 **Whole grains.** (a) A whole grain includes the bran, endosperm, and germ. (b) Whole wheat bread is an excellent source of whole grain.

nutrients from whole grains enter the bloodstream at a slow, steady pace, the body is able to use the energy they provide more efficiently.

In contrast, refined grains are stripped of their bran and germ during processing. Only the starchy endosperm is retained. By removing fiber and many nutrients, refinement makes grain-based foods less nutritious. Examples are white bread, white rice, crackers, and most baked goods such as cookies and pastries. Despite having fewer nutrients, these products usually retain all the calories of their unrefined counterparts.

Many refined carbohydrates, including white bread, are "enriched" after processing, meaning that some of the lost nutrients such as iron and some B vitamins are replaced. However, many other important nutrients are not replaced, nor is the fiber.

Most people in the United States eat less than one serving of whole grains a day.[3, 4] If you're among them, you may be missing out on essential nutrients and fiber, while overconsuming calories. So the next time you're debating between the plain bagel or the whole grain toast, go for the whole grain.

Does Glycemic Index Matter?

The **glycemic index** refers to the potential of foods to raise the level of the simple sugar glucose in your bloodstream. When you eat foods with a high glycemic index, they're quickly broken down into glucose, which then flows rapidly from your intestinal tract into your bloodstream. Your pancreas detects this excessive blood glucose and, in response, releases a flood of insulin, a hormone that acts to get the glucose out of your blood and into your cells. This stresses your pancreas and may contribute to the development of type 2 diabetes as well as cardiovascular disease. (See Chapter 11.) Moreover, that surge in insulin prompts a dramatic clearing of glucose out of your bloodstream, leaving you feeling hungry again very quickly. This may lead to overeating and weight gain.

glycemic index Value indicating the potential of a food to raise blood glucose.

For an online list of the glycemic index of over 100 foods, go to: www.health.harvard.edu/newsweek/Glycemic_index_and_glycemic_load_for_100_foods.htm.

In contrast, when you eat low-glycemic-index foods, glucose seeps more slowly into your bloodstream, and your pancreas releases a smaller amount of insulin to move it into your cells. As a result, your blood glucose level falls gradually, and you feel satiated (full) much longer.[5]

Foods with a high glycemic index include white bread, pastries, white rice, sweetened soft drinks, and candies. A few healthful foods—like carrots!—have a high glycemic index; however, because we eat them in small amounts, their overall effect on blood glucose is minimal. Foods with a low glycemic index include legumes and most other vegetables, and most foods made with whole grains.[4]

Recommended Carbohydrate Intake

Glucose is such a critical fuel source that, if you don't get enough in your diet, your body will make it by breaking down proteins in your blood and other tissues, including your muscles! So to spare your body from having to break down your tissues for energy, it's important to eat enough carbohydrates every day. But what's enough?

Adults 19 years of age or older should consume an absolute minimum of 130 grams of carbohydrates each day.[2] This amount—which you'd get from eating about 3 slices of whole wheat bread—is estimated to supply adequate fuel to your brain. But you also need carbohydrates to fuel physical activity, and they're an excellent source of other nutrients, as well as fiber. For these reasons, nutrition experts recommend that you consume about half (45–65%) of your total daily calories as carbohydrates. Focus on getting the majority of your carbohydrates from whole grains, fruits, and legumes and other vegetables. **Practical Strategies for Health: Choosing Complex Carbohydrates** shows you how.

Fats

Fats are one type of a huge group of compounds called *lipids* that are found throughout nature. Like carbohydrates, lipids are made up of carbon, hydrogen, and oxygen. But these elements are arranged in very different ways that give lipids their key characteristic: They are not soluble in water. Olive oil will float to the top of your salad dressing because it's a lipid. This insolubility is required for some of your body's tissues and chemicals to function, so in moderate amounts, lipids are essential to your health. They cushion and insulate your organs, for example, and they enable your body to absorb fat-soluble vitamins. They are also the most concentrated energy source in your diet, supplying 9 calories per gram. In fact, lipids supply your body with energy both while you are active and while you sleep.

Fats Are One of Three Types of Food Lipids

Three types of lipids are present in foods.

Phospholipids. The least common dietary lipids are phospholipids. They are found only in peanuts, egg yolk, and a few processed foods such as salad dressing. Phospholipids are made up of lipid molecules attached to a compound called phosphate. They're important to your health because,

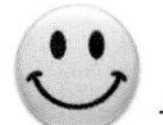 *Practical Strategies for Health*

Choosing Complex Carbohydrates

A diet high in complex carbohydrates provides a wide variety of essential nutrients. It's also rich in fiber, a non-nutrient substance that keeps your digestive tract running smoothly. Maintaining a high-complex-carbohydrate diet also reduces your risk of obesity, heart disease, and type 2 diabetes. So how can you choose more complex carbohydrates? Here are some tips:

- Start your day with whole grain cereal and a piece of fresh fruit.
- Switch to whole grain bread for morning toast and lunchtime sandwiches.
- Choose vegetarian chili or a bean burrito for lunch.
- Instead of a side of French fries or potato chips, choose a small salad, carrot sticks, or slices of sweet red pepper.
- For an afternoon snack, mix dried fruits with nuts, sunflower seeds, and pieces of whole grain cereal.
- If dinner includes rice, pasta, pizza crust, or tortillas, choose whole grain versions.
- Include a side of beans, peas, or lentils with dinner, along with a leafy green vegetable, sweet potato, or vegetable soup.
- For an evening snack, choose popcorn, popcorn cakes, a whole grain toaster pastry, low-fat oatmeal cookies, or a bowl of whole grain cereal with milk.

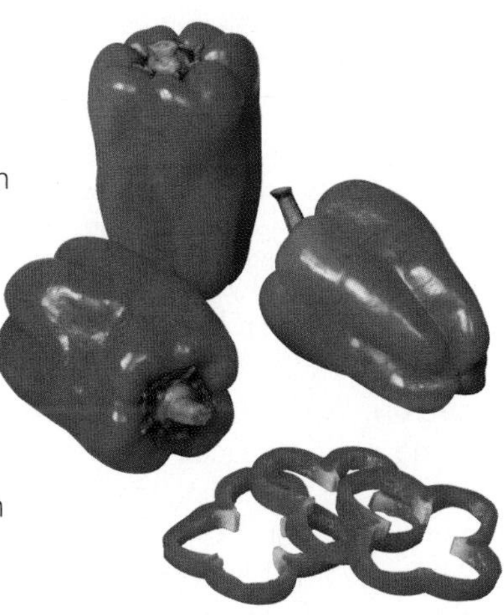

among other things, they're a key component of the cell membrane—the flexible "wall" that keeps the contents of your cells in place. But if you don't like peanuts or eggs—no problem! Your body can make phospholipids from other substances, so you don't need to consume them.

Cholesterol. *Sterols* are ring-shaped lipids found in both plant- and animal-based foods. Plant sterols are not very well absorbed by the body, but are thought to have an important health benefit: They appear to block the absorption of **cholesterol,** the animal sterol most common in the American diet. Cholesterol is found in animal-based foods such as meats, eggs, shellfish, butter, lard, and whole milk. As we mentioned earlier, you want to block the absorption of dietary cholesterol because, as it circulates in your bloodstream, it can accumulate along the lining of your blood vessels, increasing your risk for a heart attack or stroke. Still, some cholesterol is absolutely essential for your survival because, like phospholipids, it's a component of cell membranes. Your body also needs cholesterol to make reproductive hormones and other important compounds. But even though cholesterol is critical to your health, you don't have to consume it! That's because the liver can make all the cholesterol you need, using components from the breakdown of fats, the third type of food lipid.

Fats. The lipid found most abundantly in your diet, **fats** are present in a wide variety of plant and animal foods. Food scientists refer to dietary fats as *triglycerides*, because they are made up of three fatty acid chains (*tri-* means "three") attached to a compound called glycerol (a type of alcohol). Depending on the structure of the fatty acid chains, one of three different types of fats is formed: saturated, monounsaturated, or polyunsaturated. As we explain next, each type has different characteristics and different effects on your health.

cholesterol An animal sterol found in the fatty part of animal-based foods such as meat and whole milk.

fats (triglycerides) Lipids made up of three fatty acid chains attached to a molecule of glycerol; the most common types of food lipid.

saturated fats Fats that typically are solid at room temperature; generally found in animal products, dairy products, and tropical oils.

unsaturated fats (oils) Fats that typically are liquid at room temperature; generally come from plant sources.

Saturated Fats

Saturated fats got their name because their fatty acid chains are "saturated" with hydrogen. This makes them solid at room temperature, and stable; that is, they aren't easily altered, and they tend to have a long shelf life.

A diet high in saturated fats is associated with an increased risk for cardiovascular disease.[6] So what foods should you avoid? Saturated fats generally are found in animal products such as meat, cream, whole milk, cheese, lard, and butter. Red meats tend to have more saturated fat than poultry or fish, and fried meats have more than meats that are broiled, grilled, or baked. Processed foods, including pastries, chips, French fries, prepared meals, mayonnaise, and some sauces and dressings, are often loaded with saturated fat. Palm, palm kernel, and coconut oils, although derived from plants, also are highly saturated.

Unsaturated Fats

Unsaturated fats got their name because their fatty acid chains have one or more areas that are not "saturated" with hydrogen. This makes them more flexible, and they are typically liquid at room temperature. In fact, we commonly refer to them as *oils*. These are heart-healthy fats that generally come from plant sources. The two types of unsaturated fats are monounsaturated and polyunsaturated.

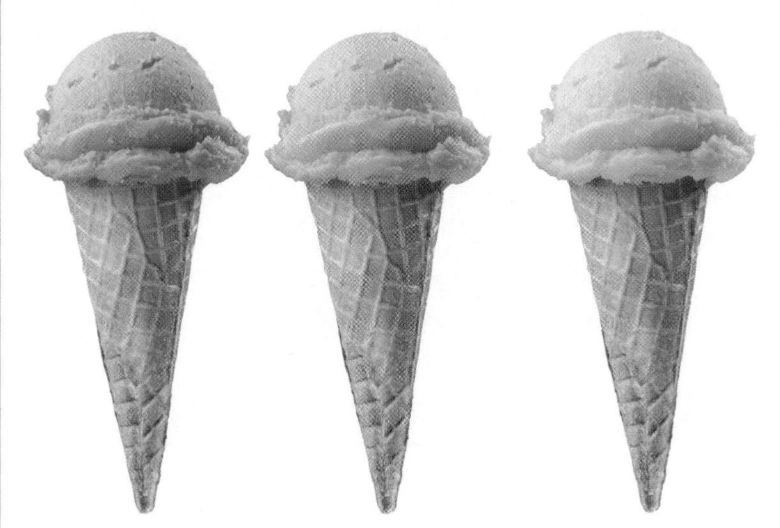

Ice cream, unfortunately, is loaded with saturated fat.

Monounsaturated Fats. *Mono-* means "one," and monounsaturated fats have fatty acid chains with one unsaturated region. Consuming monounsaturated fats triggers less total cholesterol production in your body, and when replacing saturated fats, reduces your risk for cardiovascular disease and may help protect you against some cancers.[7] Sources of monounsaturated fats include canola oil, olive oil, peanut oil, nuts, avocado, and sesame seeds.

essential fatty acids (EFAs) Polyunsaturated fatty acids that cannot be synthesized by the body but are essential to body functioning.

trans fat A type of fat that is produced when liquid fat (oil) is turned into solid fat during food processing.

Polyunsaturated Fats. *Poly-* means "many," and polyunsaturated fats have fatty acid chains with two or more unsaturated regions. They tend to help your body get rid of newly formed cholesterol, thereby lowering your blood cholesterol level and reducing deposits in blood vessel walls.[5] Sources of polyunsaturated fats include corn oil, soybean oil, safflower oil, non-hydrogenated margarines, salad dressings, mayonnaise, nuts, and seeds.

Essential Fatty Acids. Two polyunsaturated fats have been getting a lot of media attention lately. These are *omega-6 fatty acid* and *omega-3 fatty acid*. Both are essential to your body's functioning and are thought to provide some protection against heart disease. As they cannot be assembled by your body and must be obtained from your diet or from supplements, they are also known as the **essential fatty acids (EFAs).**

Most people in the United States get plenty of omega-6 fatty acids from plant oils, seeds, and nuts. However, most people need to increase significantly their consumption of omega-3 fatty acids, which are found in fatty fish (like salmon and mackerel), walnuts, flaxseed, canola oil, and dark green, leafy vegetables. Two types of long-chain omega-3 fatty acids found in fish, EPA and DHA, are thought to be particularly effective in reducing your risk for cardiovascular disease. Eating fish twice a week (a total of 8 ounces) provides an appropriate level of EPA and DHA for most adults.[8] If you never eat fish, ask your doctor for advice about taking a fish-oil supplement.

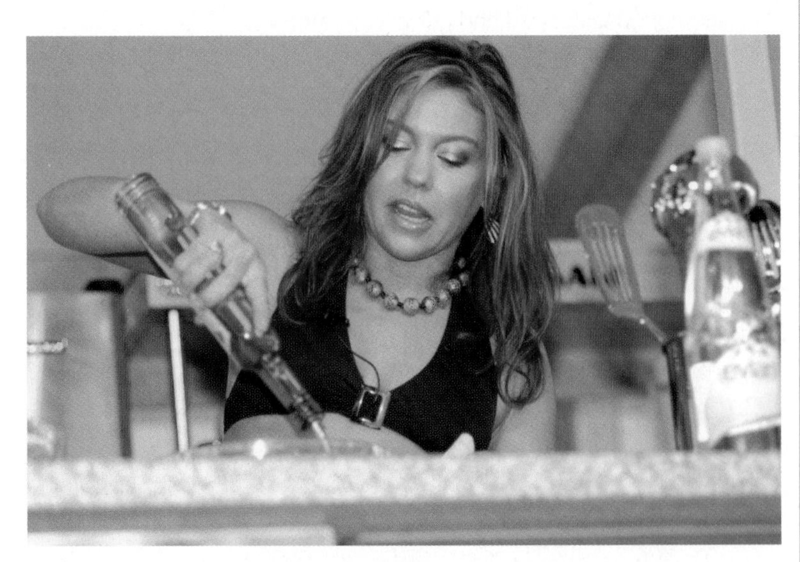

Celebrity cook **Rachael Ray** popularized the use of "EVOO": extra-virgin olive oil, a monounsaturated fat.

Avoid *Trans* Fats

So far, we've been discussing fats that occur naturally in foods. Now let's turn our attention to a particularly harmful form of fat that occurs almost exclusively in processed foods.

During food processing, an unsaturated fat such as corn oil may undergo a chemical process called *hydrogenation.* To "hydrogenate" means to saturate with hydrogen, so, as you've probably guessed, hydrogenation changes oils into more stable, saturated, solid fats that are less likely to spoil. The greater the degree of hydrogenation, the more solid the fat becomes. For instance, corn oil can be hydrogenated to various degrees, forming a liquid (squeeze bottle), soft tub, or stick margarine.

Hydrogenation creates a unique type of fatty acid chain called a ***trans* fat** that is worse for blood cholesterol levels than saturated fats! *Trans* fats also prompt inflammation, an immune system response that has been implicated in heart disease, stroke, diabetes, and other chronic conditions.[9] Even small amounts of *trans* fats—anything greater than 2 grams per 2,000 calories—can have harmful health effects.[10] The average person in the United States eats about 6 grams of *trans* fats a day. For every 2% increase of calories from *trans* fats daily, the risk of heart disease increases by 23%.[9]

Most *trans* fats in your diet come from vegetable shortenings, some margarines, commercially prepared baked goods, snack foods, processed foods, and other foods made with or fried in partially hydrogenated oils. A small amount of *trans* fat also occurs naturally in beef, lamb, and dairy products. You can find out the *trans* fat content of any packaged food by reading the label. However, foods containing half a gram of *trans* fat or less per serving can claim to be "*trans* fat free," so look for the words "hydrogenated" or "partially hydrogenated vegetable oil" in the ingredients list. If they're present, the food contains *trans* fats.[6]

Recommended Fat Intake

Dietary recommendations for fats have changed in recent years, shifting the emphasis from lowering total fat to limiting saturated and *trans* fats. Current recommendations suggest carefully replacing the saturated fats with monounsaturated and polyunsaturated fats and enjoying them in moderation.[11] Here are some specific recommendations:

- In general, fats should make up between 20% and 35% of your total calories to meet daily energy and nutrition needs while minimizing your risk for chronic disease.
- *Trans* fat intake should be kept to an absolute minimum.
- Saturated fats should be less than 7% of calories, or less than 16 grams (about 140 calories) for someone consuming 2,000 calories per day.
- Omega-6 fatty acid intake should be about 14 to 17 grams per day for men and about 11 to 12 grams per day for women.
- Omega-3 fatty acid intake should be about 1.6 grams per day for men and about 1.1 grams per day for women. Eating 8 ounces of fish per week is recommended to meet your needs for EPA and DHA.

Because most college students don't monitor their diets closely every day, a good habit is to choose unsaturated fats over saturated

Practical Strategies for Health

Choosing Healthful Fats

To choose healthful fats, start by sorting the good guys from the bad. Make it a standard practice to pick foods with zero *trans* fats, and replace saturated fats with unsaturated fats. Consume small amounts of vegetable oils, walnuts, flaxseed, leafy green vegetables, and/or fish daily to meet your essential fatty acid needs. Here are some additional tips:

- Instead of butter or a margarine made with hydrogenated oils, spread your toast with a non-*trans* fat margarine or peanut, almond, cashew, or walnut butter.
- If you normally eat two eggs for breakfast, discard the yolk from one. Do the same when making egg dishes such as quiches or casseroles, and in baking.
- Make low-fat foods a priority at each meal. Choose whole grain foods, legumes, fruits, vegetables, non-fat or low-fat dairy products, lean red meats (rump, round, loin, and flank), skinless poultry, and fish.
- Trim all visible fat from red meat and poultry. Instead of choosing fried meats, poultry, or fish, choose baked or broiled. Finally, remove the skin from poultry before eating it.
- Skip the French fries. Opt for a baked potato or side salad instead.
- Make sure that any cookies or other baked goods you buy are *trans* fat free.
- Instead of ice cream, which is high in saturated fat, choose ice milk, sorbet, or low-fat or non-fat frozen yogurt.
- When the munchies hit, go for air-popped popcorn, pretzels, rice cakes, or dried fruit instead of potato chips.

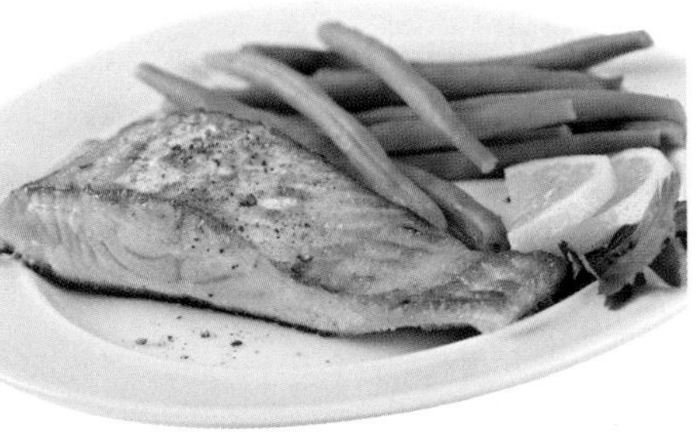

and *trans* fats whenever possible. You can do this by adopting the habits described in **Practical Strategies for Health: Choosing Healthful Fats.**

Proteins

Dietary **protein** is a macronutrient available from both plant and animal sources. Although it's one of the energy nutrients, protein is used for fuel only if your body does not have adequate amounts of carbohydrate and fat to burn. Assuming you're well nourished, your body uses the protein you eat to build biological compounds, cells, and tissues.

The Role of Amino Acids

Some misconceptions surround the roles of protein in the diet and in the body. For instance, people who associate meat with protein and protein with strength may eat lots of meat to build their muscles. This is unnecessary: Whenever you consume proteins, whether they come from meats or plants, your body breaks them apart into their component building blocks, which are nitrogen-containing compounds known as **amino acids.** Once absorbed through the intestinal tract, amino acids enter the bloodstream and become part of the amino acid pool. Just as you might go to an auto parts store to buy an air filter or some spark plugs for your car, your body cells draw from the amino acid pool the precise amino acids they need to build or repair a wide variety of body proteins. These include:

- **Antibodies,** which protect you from disease
- **Enzymes,** which speed up chemical reactions
- **Hormones,** which regulate body temperature, use of nutrients, and many other body functions
- **Transport proteins,** which help carry substances into and out of cells
- **Buffers,** which help maintain a healthy balance of acids and bases in your blood

Of course, your body also uses the amino acids from dietary proteins to grow, repair, and maintain body tissues. In short, you consume dietary protein primarily to maintain your stock of amino acids for your body cells to generate whatever proteins they need.

protein A macronutrient that helps build many body parts, including muscle, bone, skin, and blood; a key component of enzymes, hormones, transport proteins, and antibodies.

amino acids The building blocks of protein; 20 common amino acids are found in food.

Complete and Incomplete Proteins

Although all of the 20 amino acids your body needs are available in foods, you don't have to consume them all. That's because your body can produce ample amounts of 11 of them independently. The other nine are called *essential amino acids* because your body either cannot make them or cannot make sufficient quantities to maintain your health. Thus, you need to consume these amino acids in your diet.

Dietary proteins are considered *complete proteins* if they supply all nine essential amino acids in adequate amounts. In contrast, *incomplete proteins* are lacking one or more of the essential amino acids. Meat, fish, poultry, dairy products, soy, and quinoa provide complete proteins. Most plant sources provide incomplete proteins. However, combinations of plant proteins—peanut butter on whole grain bread, for instance, or brown rice with lentils or beans—can complement each other in such a way that the essential amino acids missing from one are supplied by the other. The combination yields complete proteins (**Figure 5.3** on page 114). Incidentally, foods with complementary amino acids don't have to be consumed at the same meal. People following a plant-based diet simply need to consume a variety of plant proteins throughout the day.

Recommended Protein Intake

For good health, experts recommend that adults consume between 10% and 35% of their calories as protein. Staying within this range can provide adequate protein and other nutrients while reducing the risk for chronic diseases such as type 2 diabetes, heart disease, and cancer. When an individual's protein intake falls above or below this range, the risk for development of these chronic diseases appears to increase.[2]

How much protein do *you* need? Healthy adults typically need 0.36 grams of protein per pound (0.8 grams per kilogram) of body weight, equaling 54 grams per day for a 150-pound person. Athletes can require up to twice as much protein, depending

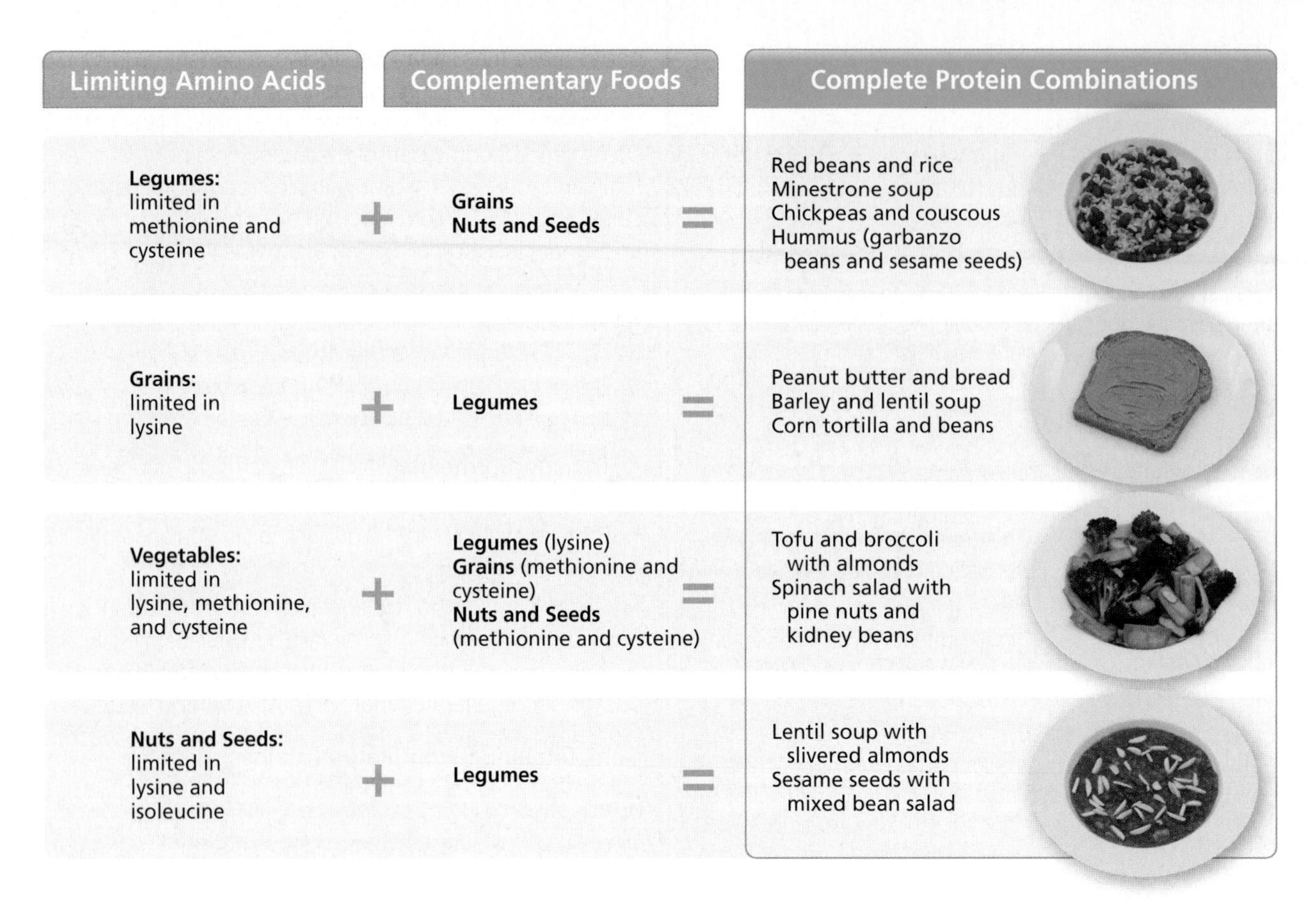

Limiting Amino Acids
Complementary Foods
Complete Protein Combinations
Legumes: limited in methionine and cysteine
+
Grains
Nuts and Seeds
=
Red beans and rice
Minestrone soup
Chickpeas and couscous
Hummus (garbanzo beans and sesame seeds)
Grains: limited in lysine
+
Legumes
=
Peanut butter and bread
Barley and lentil soup
Corn tortilla and beans
Vegetables: limited in lysine, methionine, and cysteine
+
Legumes (lysine)
Grains (methionine and cysteine)
Nuts and Seeds (methionine and cysteine)
=
Tofu and broccoli with almonds
Spinach salad with pine nuts and kidney beans
Nuts and Seeds: limited in lysine and isoleucine
+
Legumes
=
Lentil soup with slivered almonds
Sesame seeds with mixed bean salad

Figure 5.3 Complementary food combinations. These dishes provide complete protein.

Source: Adapted from *Nutrition for Life* (3rd ed.), Fig. 5.4, by J. Thompson & M. Manore, 2013, San Francisco, CA: Pearson Education.

Table 5.1: Key Facts About Vitamins

	Type	Vitamin	Functions	Food Sources
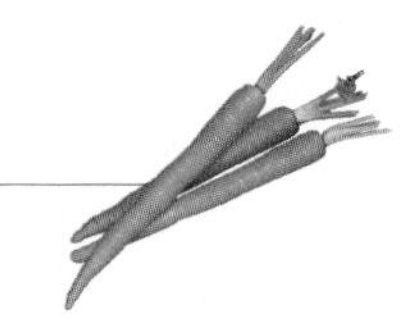	*Fat soluble*	A	Required for vision, cell differentiation, reproduction; contributes to healthy bones and a healthy immune system	Beef, chicken liver, egg yolk, milk, spinach, carrots, mango, apricots, cantaloupe, pumpkin, yams
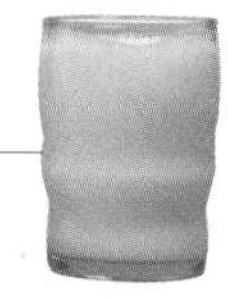	*Fat soluble*	D	Regulates blood calcium levels; maintains bone health; assists in cell differentiation	Canned salmon and mackerel, fortified milk or orange juice, fortified cereals
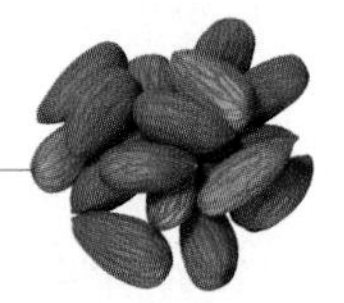	*Fat soluble*	E	Protects white blood cells, enhances immune function, improves absorption of vitamin A; protects cell membranes, fatty acids, and vitamin A from oxidation	Sunflower seeds, almonds, vegetable oils, fortified cereals
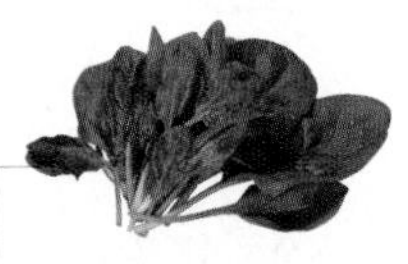	*Fat soluble*	K	Needed for the production of proteins that assist in blood clotting and maintenance of healthy bone	Kale, spinach, turnip greens, brussels sprouts
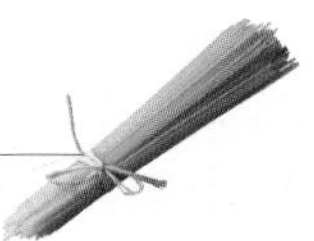	*Water soluble*	B_1 (Thiamin)	Needed for carbohydrate and amino acid metabolism	Pork, fortified cereals, enriched rice and pasta, peas, tuna, beans
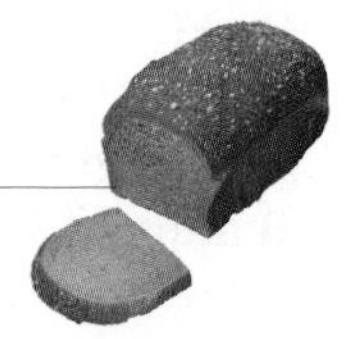	*Water soluble*	B_2 (Riboflavin)	Needed for carbohydrate and fat metabolism	Beef liver, shrimp, dairy products, fortified cereals, enriched breads and grains
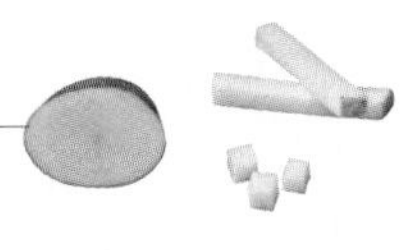	*Water soluble*	B_6	Needed for carbohydrate and amino acid metabolism; synthesis of blood cells	Chickpeas (garbanzo beans), red meat/fish/poultry, fortified cereals, potatoes

on the requirements of their sport. Athlete or not, few people in the United States suffer from protein deficiencies. Protein makes up between 12% and 18% of most Americans' diets.[12] Don't fall for the myth that consuming excessive protein—whether from foods or expensive supplements—will help you build muscle. Any protein you consume beyond your body's needs is stored as fat.

vitamins Compounds, with no energy value of their own, needed by the body in small amounts for normal growth and function.

Unfortunately, many animal sources of protein are high in cholesterol and saturated fat. Follow these tips to go lean with protein:[13]

- Choose lean cuts of meats such as rump, round, loin, and flank. Better yet, choose poultry (remove the skin). Best of all, choose fish.
- Avoid fried meats, as this cooking method adds fat. Choose baked, broiled, or grilled.
- For a lunchtime sandwich, choose turkey, roast beef, canned tuna or salmon, or peanut butter. Avoid deli meats like bologna or salami, which are high in saturated fat and sodium.
- Vary your protein sources by consuming vegetarian meals several times a week. Choose legumes, soy products such as tofu dogs and burgers, nuts, and seeds.
- Don't forget eggs: On average, one egg a day doesn't increase your risk for heart disease, and only the yolk contains cholesterol and saturated fat, so make an omelet with one whole egg and two egg whites.
- Choose a small portion of nuts or seeds as a snack, on salads, or in main dishes to replace meat or poultry.

Vitamins

Vitamins are carbon-containing compounds required in small amounts to regulate body processes such as blood-cell production, nerve function, digestion, and skin and bone maintenance. They also help chemical reactions take place. For example, although not an energy nutrient, vitamins do help your body to break down carbohydrates, fats, and proteins for energy.

Humans need 13 vitamins. Four of these—vitamins A, D, E, and K—are *fat soluble*, meaning they dissolve in fat and can be stored in your body's fatty tissues. Because your body can store them, consuming the fat-soluble vitamins two to three times a week is adequate. Nine vitamins—vitamin C and the eight B-complex vitamins (thiamin, riboflavin, niacin, pantothenic acid, B_6, biotin, folic acid, and B_{12}) are *water soluble*. They dissolve in water, and excesses are generally excreted from the body in urine. Your body can store vitamin B_{12} in the liver, but you cannot store any of the other water-soluble vitamins. Thus, it's important that you consume adequate amounts daily.

Sources of Vitamins

Selected vitamins are listed in **Table 5.1,** along with their food sources. As you can see, many vitamins are abundant in fruits, vegetables, and whole grains. Others are more plentiful in animal-based foods. Vitamin B_{12} is available naturally only from animal foods, so strict vegetarians have to get it from supplements or from eating processed foods to which B_{12} has been added, such as fortified soy or nut milks or breakfast cereals. In fact, food manufacturers often add or replace many different vitamins during processing, providing more dietary sources for meeting needs.

One vitamin with a unique source is vitamin D, which has many functions in your body, but is best known for its role in calcium regulation and bone health. Your body is able to manufacture vitamin D from a cholesterol compound in your skin if you have adequate exposure to sunlight. For most people, this means about 5 to 30 minutes between the hours of 10 a.m. to 3 p.m. twice a week, on bare arms and legs,

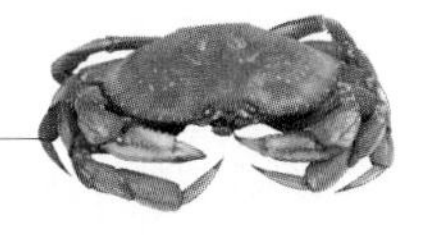

Water soluble

Vitamin: B_{12}

Functions: Assists with formation of blood; required for healthy nervous system

Food Sources: Shellfish, red meat/fish/poultry, dairy products, fortified cereals

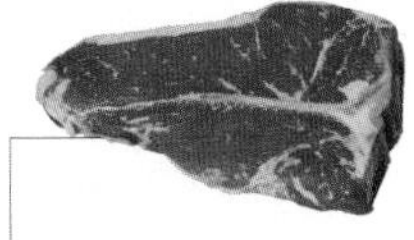

Water soluble

Vitamin: Niacin

Functions: Needed for carbohydrate and fat metabolism; assists in DNA replication and repair; assists in cell differentiation

Food Sources: Beef liver, red meat/fish/poultry, fortified cereals, enriched breads and grains, canned tomato products

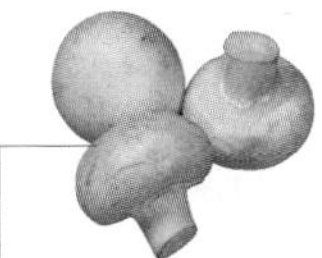

Water soluble

Vitamin: Pantothenic acid

Functions: Assists with fat metabolism

Food Sources: Red meat/fish/poultry, mushrooms, fortified cereals, egg yolk

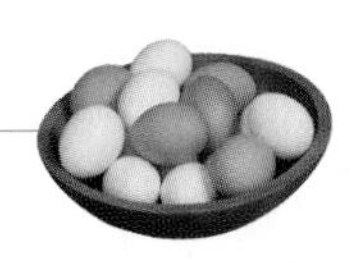

Water soluble

Vitamin: Biotin

Functions: Involved in carbohydrate, fat, and protein metabolism

Food Sources: Nuts, egg yolk

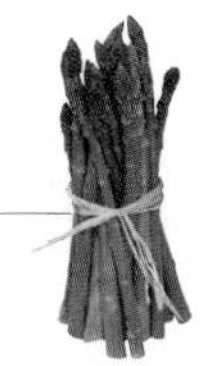

Water soluble

Vitamin: Folate (Folic acid)

Functions: Needed for amino acid metabolism and DNA synthesis

Food Sources: Fortified cereals, enriched breads and grains, legumes (lentils, chickpeas, pinto beans), spinach, romaine lettuce, asparagus, liver

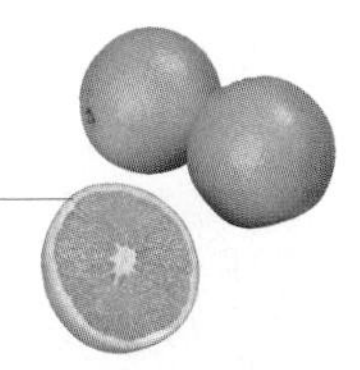

Water soluble

Vitamin: C

Functions: Antioxidant; enhances immune function; assists in synthesis of important compounds; enhances iron absorption

Food Sources: Sweet peppers, citrus fruits and juices, broccoli, strawberries, kiwi fruit

Source: Adapted from *Nutrition: An Applied Approach* (3rd ed.), by J. Thompson & M. Manore, 2012, San Francisco, CA: Pearson Education.

> *"The likelihood of consuming too much of any vitamin from food is remote. However, excesses of vitamins from supplements—especially high-potency single-vitamin products—can reach toxic levels."*

without sunscreen.[14] If you cannot get this much average sun exposure each week—for instance, during the winter in a cold climate, or year-round if you live in an area with heavy smog, then you need to make sure you consume enough vitamin D either in foods such as oily fish and fortified milks, or in supplements.

Vitamin Deficiencies and Toxicities
Because vitamins are readily available from the U.S. food supply, deficiencies among people in the United States are rare. However, there are exceptions. For example, people with dark skin need longer sun exposure to synthesize vitamin D, and consistently have lower levels of vitamin D in their blood than people with light skin. As noted earlier, people who avoid all animal-based foods, including milk and eggs, are at increased risk for vitamin B_{12} deficiency. Finally, a deficiency of folate may develop in people who don't consume dark green vegetables, legumes, or fortified commercial breads and breakfast cereals. Women who don't get adequate folate in their diet before and after becoming pregnant are at increased risk for giving birth to a newborn with a neural tube defect, a serious and sometimes fatal birth defect in which the spinal cord fails to close properly. The critical period for healthy development of the neural tube is the first 4 weeks after conception, typically before a woman even realizes she is pregnant. For this reason, all women of childbearing age, whether or not they intend to become pregnant, are advised to consume 400 micrograms of folic acid daily either from a supplement or from fortified foods.[15]

The likelihood of consuming too much of any vitamin from food is remote. However, excesses of vitamins from supplements—especially high-potency single-vitamin products—can reach toxic levels, causing side effects such as nausea, diarrhea, vomiting, skin rash, numbness of hands and feet, nosebleeds, hair loss, and pain. Toxicity involving vitamin A or D can even cause organ damage. For this reason, single-vitamin supplementation is recommended only for certain populations at high risk for deficiency. In contrast, a general multivitamin/mineral supplement is often prescribed as "insurance" for children and teens, pregnant women, the elderly, people with serious illness, and patients recovering from surgery.

For more detailed information on specific vitamins and minerals, visit Oregon State University's Micronutrient Information Center at http://lpi.oregonstate.edu/infocenter/vitamins.html.

minerals Elements, with no energy value of their own, that regulate body processes and provide structure; constituents of all cells.

Minerals

Minerals are elements that originate in the Earth and cannot be made by living organisms. They also cannot be broken down. Plants obtain minerals from the soil, and most of the minerals in your diet come directly from plants or indirectly from animal sources. Minerals also may be present in the water you drink.

Your body relies on more than a dozen essential minerals each day to regulate body processes and provide structure. Minerals adjust fluid balance, aid in muscle contraction and nerve transmission, help release energy, and provide structure for bones and teeth.

The *major minerals* are those your body needs in amounts greater than 100 milligrams daily. These include sodium, potassium, chloride, calcium, phosphorus, sulfur, and magnesium. You need *trace minerals* in much smaller amounts, typically less than 10 milligrams daily. The trace minerals include iron, fluoride, iodine, selenium, zinc, copper, manganese, and chromium. **Table 5.2** provides more information about selected minerals.

A varied and balanced diet provides most people with all the minerals they need in adequate amounts—not too low or too high. Single-mineral supplements are not recommended for most healthy people and should be used only under medical supervision. Iron, calcium, and fluoride are single minerals commonly prescribed:

- **Iron.** A trace mineral, iron enables blood to transport oxygen throughout your body. Iron needs are heightened during pregnancy, and most pregnant women are advised to take supplemental iron. Some iron is lost in the menstrual flow, so women who experi-

Vitamins and minerals are abundant in fruits and vegetables.

ence excessive menstrual bleeding may need supplemental iron. And because your body absorbs the form of iron found in meat, poultry, and fish better than the form in plant foods, menstruating women who eat a vegetarian diet may also benefit from iron supplementation.

- **Calcium.** The major mineral calcium is the primary component of bone, and both growing children and older adults may need supplemental calcium to maintain healthy bones. For more about the nutrients essential to bone health, see the **Spotlight** on page 118.
- **Fluoride.** A trace mineral, fluoride is important for the development and health of teeth and bone. Many municipal water systems now add fluoride to public drinking water, and fluoride is a common ingredient in toothpastes and mouthwashes. However, pediatricians may prescribe fluoride drops for infants and toddlers who do not drink fluoridated water. People who drink only bottled water may also need supplemental fluoride.

One major mineral commonly found to excess in the American diet is sodium. Although the recommended intake is about one teaspoon of salt per day, most Americans are thought to consume much more, largely through processed foods, from canned goods to frozen meals, snack foods, and condiments. This is a concern because some Americans are sodium sensitive, and high blood pressure is more common in these people if they consume a high-sodium diet. (See Chapter 11 for more information on high blood pressure.)

Water

You may be able to survive for weeks or even months without food, but you can live for only a few days without water. **Water** is dispersed throughout your body and is vital to nutrient digestion, absorption, and transportation. It serves as a lubricant, regulates body temperature, reduces fluid retention, helps prevent constipation, provides moisture to skin and other tissues, carries wastes out of the body, is the medium in which most chemical reactions take place, and contributes to a feeling of fullness when consumed with a meal.

water A liquid composed of hydrogen and oxygen that is necessary for life.

Sources of Water

Nearly all foods contain water. Many fruits and vegetables are more than 75% water, and even meats and grain-based foods contain water. On average, foods provide about 20% of an adult's total water intake. Beverages provide the remaining 81% of total water intake. Let's take a look at some commonly consumed beverages:[16]

- **Bottled water.** Plain drinking water hydrates your body and does not contribute calories that can lead to weight gain. Although it may be convenient, bottled water is typically no safer or more healthful than plain tap water, and its bottling and packaging takes a greater toll on the environment than filling your own reusable bottle from the faucet.
- **Sports beverages.** Traditional sports drinks provide water, some minerals, and a source of carbohydrate. They can help athletes and manual laborers avoid fluid imbalances during strenuous physical activity lasting an hour or longer. However, people who exercise for less than an hour don't benefit from drinking sports drinks as compared with plain water.
- **Milk and milk substitutes.** Low-fat and skim milk are healthful beverage choices, providing protein, calcium, and phosphorus, as well as vitamin D and often vitamin A. A variety of plant-based milks—including soy milk, rice milk, and almond and other nut milks—are also good sources of plant protein and are typically fortified with the same vitamins and minerals.

Table 5.2: Key Facts About Selected Minerals

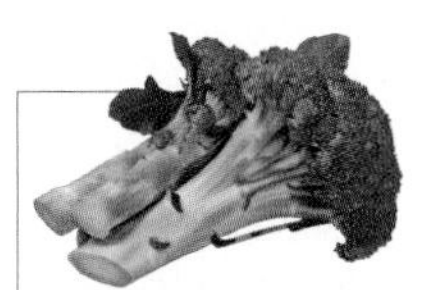

Mineral: Calcium

Functions: Primary component of bone; needed for acid-base balance, transmission of nerve impulses, and muscle contraction

Food Sources: Dairy products, fortified juices, fish with bones (such as sardines or salmon), broccoli, kale, collard greens

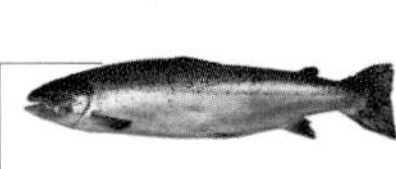

Mineral: Iron

Functions: Helps transport oxygen in blood cells; assists many functional systems

Food Sources: Clams, chicken, turkey, fish, ham

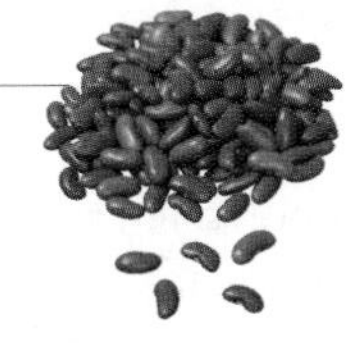

Mineral: Magnesium

Functions: Component of bone; aids in muscle contraction; assists many functional systems

Food Sources: Oysters, beef, pork, chicken, turkey, tuna, lobster, shrimp, salmon, milk, yogurt, whole grain cereals, almonds, walnuts, sunflower seeds, beans

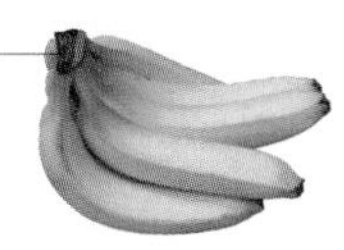

Mineral: Potassium

Functions: Needed for fluid balance, transmission of nerve impulses, and muscle contraction

Food Sources: Fruits (bananas, oranges, grapefruit, plums), vegetables (spinach, beans)

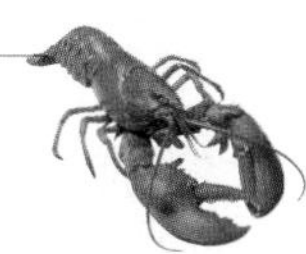

Mineral: Zinc

Functions: Assists many functional systems; aids in immunity, growth, sexual maturation, and gene regulation

Food Sources: Red meat, poultry, seafood (oysters, tuna, lobster)

Source: Adapted from *Nutrition: An Applied Approach* (3rd ed.), by J. Thompson & M. Manore, 2012. San Francisco, CA: Pearson Education.

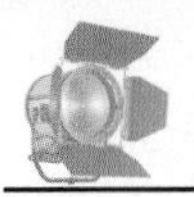

SPOTLIGHT

Feeding Your Bones

Osteoporosis is a disease characterized by brittle bones and decreased bone mass. You probably think of osteoporosis as a disease of the elderly, but even young adults can start to develop this disorder if they fail to properly nourish their bones.

Calcium is the main component of the mineral crystals that make up healthy bone. As you age from childhood to adulthood, your bones are not only lengthening, they're increasing in density. They do this by depositing calcium-containing crystals on a protein "scaffold" in the bone interior. If you don't consume enough calcium during these critical years, the supply will run short, and your bones won't be able to increase their density. From age 9 to 18, you should consume at least 1,300 milligrams of calcium a day. If you consider that an 8-ounce glass of milk contains about 300 milligrams of calcium, you can easily see that this level of daily calcium intake can be challenging to meet. After the age of 18, the requirement drops to 1,000 milligrams per day. Calcium is available in dairy foods such as milk, yogurt, and cheese; in green, leafy vegetables; and in fortified tofu, soy milk, rice milk, and juices.

Vitamin D is another important nutrient for bone health. Your body can absorb only a small fraction of the calcium you consume if your level of vitamin D is inadequate. Recall that you synthesize vitamin D in your skin if you have adequate exposure to sunlight. If you do not spend much time in the sun, you will need to obtain vitamin D through your diet or supplements. Food sources of vitamin D include fatty fish, and milk and other fortified foods.

What else can you do to keep your bones strong? Stay active. Any weight-bearing activity, from jogging to carrying textbooks up a flight of stairs, places positive stress on your skeleton and encourages your bones to increase their density.

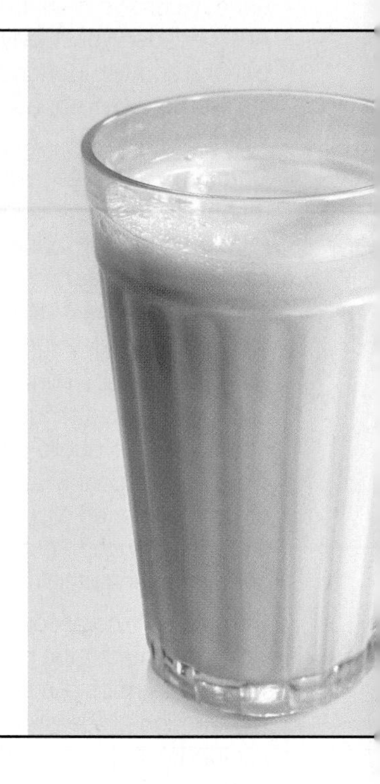

- **Beverages containing caffeine.** Coffee, tea, and hot cocoa all provide caffeine, a stimulant that can interfere with sleep. (See Chapter 4.) However, they can be healthful beverage choices if consumed in moderation, earlier in the day. Energy drinks vary greatly in their caffeine content, but on average contain as much as a strong cup of brewed coffee—about 150 milligrams.[17] Many contain far more, from 200 to as much as 500 milligrams per serving. Most also contain guarana, another source of caffeine, as well as sugar—providing from about 60 to 200 calories per can. And whereas coffee is usually hot and must be sipped slowly, you can chug an energy drink, dumping a load of caffeine and sugar into your bloodstream. Sure, this produces a jolt that can get you to your 9 a.m. class, but it also leaves you vulnerable to a mid-morning crash.

Think you already know all there is to learn about caffeine? Take this test from Consumer Reports and find out! www.consumerreports.org/cro/food/beverages/coffee-tea/test-your-caffeine-iq/index.htm.

Recommended Water Intake

You lose water every day through sweat, urine, and feces. You also experience water losses you've probably never noticed, from evaporation off your skin and from exhalation of breath from your lungs. Moreover, when you're feverish, or suffering from a runny nose, coughing, diarrhea, or vomiting, you lose more water. This explains why doctors advise you to drink plenty of fluids when you're sick.

Despite these losses, you can maintain a healthy level of hydration by consuming a wide variety of foods and beverages, including plain water. Although recommendations for intake of water as a beverage specifically have not been established, most adult women can maintain an adequate water intake by drinking 9 cups (2.2 liters) of beverages daily and men by drinking 13 cups (3 liters) of beverages daily.[18] If you are physically active or live in a very hot climate, you may require more total water.

If you don't drink enough water, you can become dehydrated. In otherwise healthy adults, this can cause minor symptoms such as thirst, headache, diminished appetite, and an overall uncomfortable feeling. Normally, these symptoms would prompt you to drink and restore fluid balance. But dehydration can become serious—even life-threatening—in infants, the elderly, people suffering from burns, and athletes and laborers engaged in vigorous physical activity in a hot climate. In these populations, prompt and adequate fluid replacement, sometimes via an intravenous infusion, is critical.

Other Healthful Substances in Foods

Today, people are increasingly interested in consuming *functional foods*; that is, foods that confer some kind of health benefit in addition to the benefits provided by their basic nutrients. For example, researchers are studying non-nutrient substances in food that may improve your body's gastrointestinal functioning, boost your immunity, slow memory loss, delay aging, or prevent heart disease or cancer. Although many such non-nutrient substances are currently under investigation, we'll limit our discussion to those you're most likely to hear about in the news or in food advertisements—these are phytochemicals, antioxidants, and probiotics.

phytochemicals Naturally occurring plant substances thought to have disease-preventing and health-promoting properties.

Phytochemicals

Phytochemicals are naturally occurring chemicals in plants (*phyto* means "plant") that may have health benefits, but are not considered essential nutrients.[19] Sources of phytochemicals include fruits,

abundant plant protein, plant oils, complex carbohydrates, and micronutrients (not to mention fiber and antioxidant phytochemicals) for a relatively low number of calories **(Figure 5.6a).**

Notice that our peanut butter sandwich is also very low in saturated fat, has no cholesterol, and although it has a few grams of natural sugar, contains no added sugars. In other words, it is free of **empty calories.** These are calories from solid fats and/or added sugars that provide few or no nutrients. The USDA recommends that you limit the empty calories you eat. Examples of foods loaded with empty calories are cookies **(Figure 5.6b),** cakes, doughnuts, candies, alcohol, soft drinks, sausages, hot dogs, bacon, and ribs.

empty calories Calories from solid fats, alcohol, and/or added sugars that provide few or no nutrients.

(a) Nutrient dense

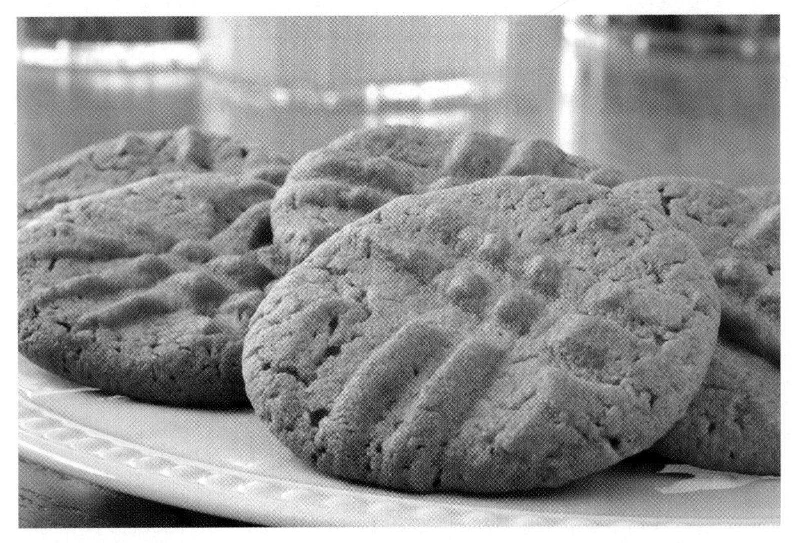

(b) Empty calories

Figure 5.6 Nutrient density versus empty calories. You have only a limited number of calories to "spend" each day. (a) A nutrient-dense snack such as a peanut butter sandwich on whole wheat bread buys you plenty of healthful nutrients at a relatively low calorie cost. (b) A snack such as peanut butter cookies does provide healthful plant oils and protein from the peanut butter, but it's very high in solid fats (butter) and added sugars, both of which cost you lots of empty calories. So overall, it's a poor choice.

How Much of Each Group Do You Need?

Now that you know what the five food groups are, you might be wondering *how much* of each food group you should eat. There's no one-size-fits-all answer: The amounts you need are determined according to your age, gender, height, current weight, and activity level. To learn your unique needs, log onto **www.choosemyplate.gov** and click on "Get a personalized plan." Fill out the information requested, and in seconds you'll learn not only how much of each food group you need, but also how many calories you should consume daily, including your allotment of empty calories. The program will also let you know if you're currently underweight or overweight, and offer advice for moving toward a healthier weight.

When your plan appears, you'll notice that the recommended daily intakes of vegetables, fruits, and dairy are given in cups. For example, 1 cup of carrot juice, orange juice, or milk qualifies as a cup, as does 1 cup of sliced carrots, orange wedges, or yogurt. In a few cases, however, a cup is not a cup! Lettuce and other leafy green vegetables are high-volume items: 2 cups is equivalent to a 1-cup serving. In contrast, dried fruits are dense, so ½ cup counts as a 1-cup serving. And what about cheese? Two cups of cottage cheese, 1½ ounces of hard cheese, and ⅓ cup of shredded cheese all count as 1-cup servings.

Recommended amounts of grains and protein foods are given in ounces and *ounce-equivalents*, which, as their name implies, are serving sizes that are equivalent to an ounce. For instance, an egg, 3 cups of popcorn, ½ cup of cooked pasta, and ½ ounce of sunflower seeds all qualify as ounce-equivalents. For more examples, see **Figure 5.7.**

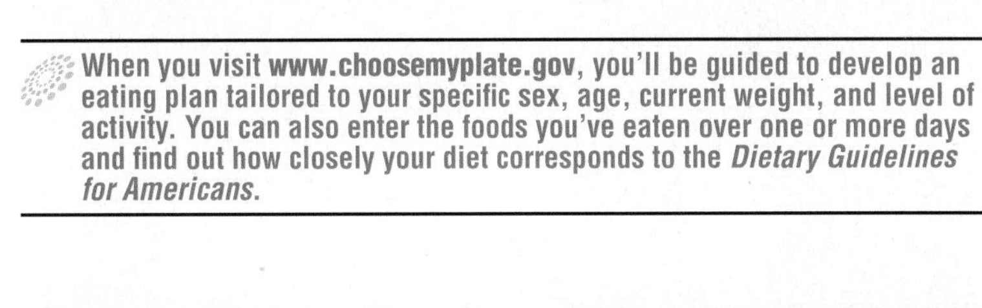
When you visit www.choosemyplate.gov, you'll be guided to develop an eating plan tailored to your specific sex, age, current weight, and level of activity. You can also enter the foods you've eaten over one or more days and find out how closely your diet corresponds to the *Dietary Guidelines for Americans*.

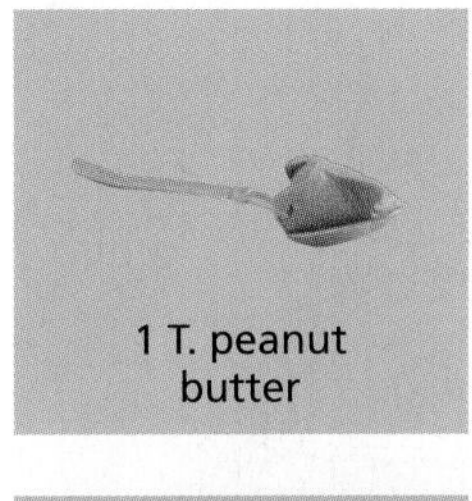

1 T. peanut butter

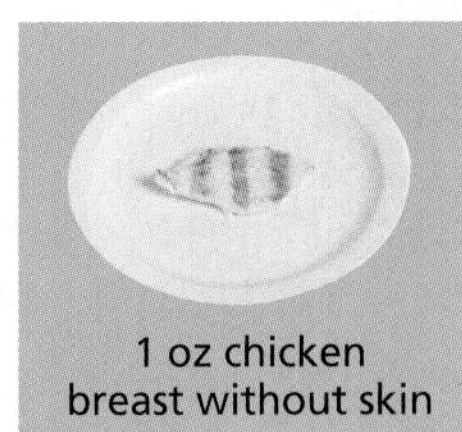

1 oz chicken breast without skin

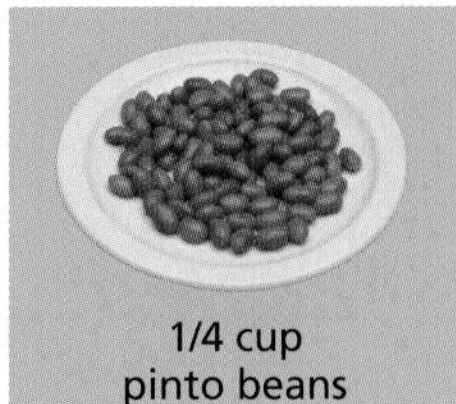

1/4 cup pinto beans

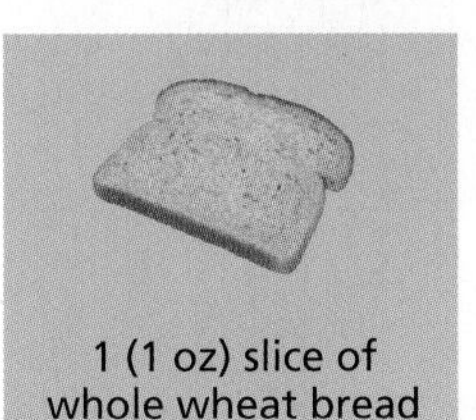

1 (1 oz) slice of whole wheat bread

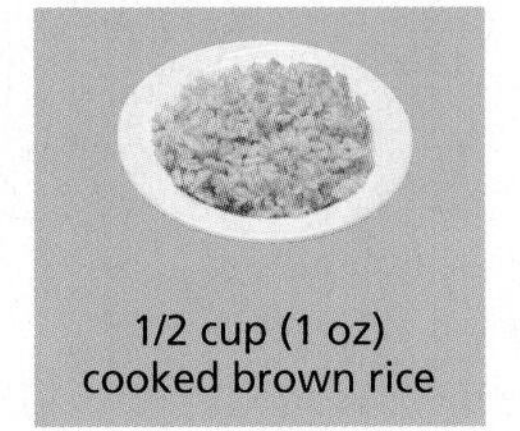

1/2 cup (1 oz) cooked brown rice

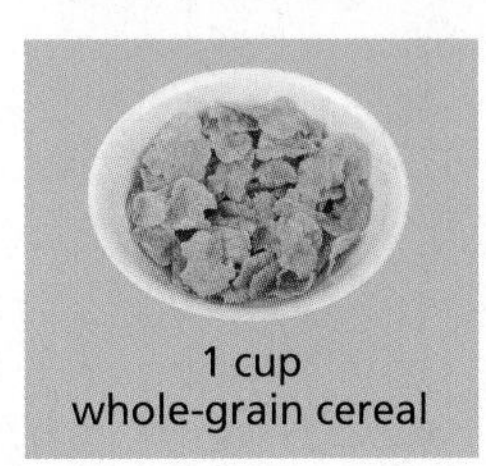

1 cup whole-grain cereal

Figure 5.7 What's an "ounce-equivalent"? Here are sample 1 "ounce-equivalent" servings of various meats, beans, and grains.

How Do Nutrition Guidelines Vary for Different Groups?

The *Dietary Guidelines for Americans* provide expert advice relevant to most population groups. However, because of their age, gender, level of physical activity, or diet preferences, some people may have special dietary needs.

Nutrition Needs Change Over Time

Although everyone needs the same nutrients, people of different ages may need different amounts. Here are key ways the DRIs differ throughout the life cycle:[2]

- To promote optimal bone density, children and teens aged 9 to 18 actually need more calcium (1,300 mg/day) than adults do (1,000 mg/day). In fact, calcium needs are never higher, even during pregnancy. This age group also needs more phosphorus (1,250 mg/day) than adults do (700 mg/day).
- After age 50, the calcium recommendation bumps up again, to 1,200 mg/day. The phosphorus requirement remains the same as for middle-aged adults. Older adults also need to consume more vitamin B_6 and vitamin D. They have slightly decreased needs for iron and fiber. Why the differences? One reason is that physical changes with aging affect how your body digests food, absorbs nutrients, and excretes wastes. Moreover, many mature adults have a reduced ability to absorb naturally occurring vitamin B_{12}, but are able to absorb the synthetic form. For this reason, although the recommended amount of B_{12} intake doesn't change, the source does: Older adults are encouraged to eat foods with added vitamin B_{12} or take the vitamin as a supplement.

With a little effort, Americans can consume adequate nutrients throughout the life span. Fruits, vegetables, whole grains, and low-fat or fat-free dairy products should be the focus of everyone's diet.

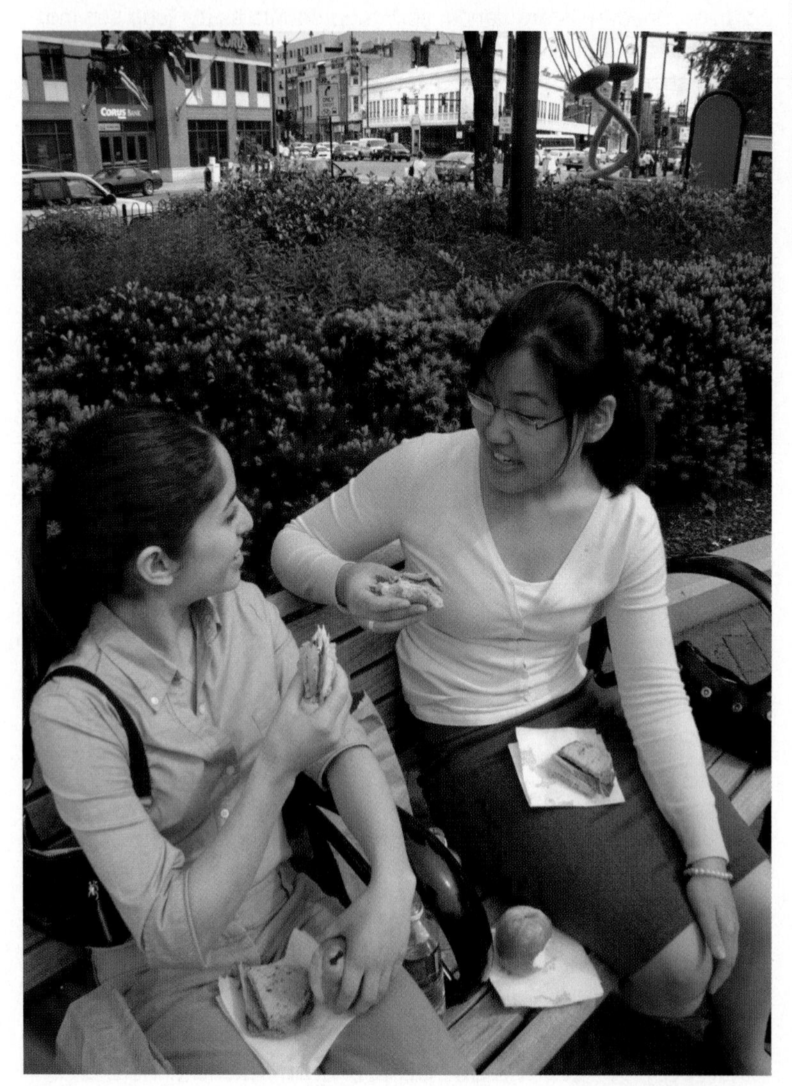

Especially for women, nutrition needs **change** over time.

STUDENT STORY

Why I'm Vegetarian

"Hi, I'm Nidya. I am a vegetarian and I decided to become one basically because of my cousin. She's also a vegetarian and she showed me a PETA video that showed how they treated animals when they kill them for food. So I guess ever since then I've been kind of traumatized and I stopped eating meat. That was about two years ago.

In my household, since my family is Mexican, there's meat every day. So instead I eat a lot of beans and rice and fish and also vegetables, fruits, and salads, so I usually get all my nutrients."

1: What type of vegetarian is Nidya, as her diet includes fish?

2: Is Nidya eating any complementary proteins? If so, what are they?

3: What are the benefits and drawbacks of Nidya's diet?

 **Do you have a story similar to Nidya's? Share your story at www.pearsonhighered.com/lynchelmore.**

Nutrition Needs Differ for Men and Women

Men and women have slightly different nutrient needs. Because most men are larger, taller, and have more muscle mass (lean muscle tissue) than most women, they require more calories. Eating more means it's easier for men to obtain the nutrients they need even if their food choices aren't the wisest.

Unless men shift their physical activity level, their nutrition needs don't change much over a lifetime. That's not true for women. Complexities of the reproductive system, hormone shifts, pregnancy, and breast-feeding all affect nutrition needs. During childbearing years, women's nutrition requirements for iron and folic acid increase. Iron, found mostly in the blood, is lost during menstruation and is used by the developing fetus during pregnancy. Folic acid helps to make new cells and DNA, the blueprint of the body. Adequate amounts are critical just prior to and in the first few weeks after conception, to reduce the risk of fetal spinal cord defects. And later in life, with the onset of menopause and depletion of the hormone estrogen, women's needs for calcium and vitamin D to ward off osteoporosis become greater. However, this recommendation increases for older males, too.

Athletes May Have Increased Nutrition Needs

Whether you train for competitive sports, work out for the health benefits, or are physically active for fun, nutrition is fundamental to peak physical performance. Athletes require the same nutrients as non-athletes, but need to pay more attention to meeting energy needs and consuming fluids.[27]

An athlete's diet should provide enough carbohydrates (45–65% of calories) and fats (10–35% of calories) for weight maintenance and energy production. Athletes also need adequate protein to build, repair, and maintain body tissues, though the precise recommendations vary according to the intensity, frequency, and duration of activity. Note that eating extra protein will not make muscles larger! Like anyone else, athletes should consume fruits and vegetables in meals and as snacks to gain essential vitamins and minerals, phytochemicals, and fiber. A multivitamin/mineral supplement may be appropriate if an athlete is dieting or is ill or recovering from injury.

Fluids, especially water, are important to health and athletic performance. Dehydration of as little as 2% can keep even the finest athletes from performing their best. Drink plenty of fluids before exercise or competition, and about eight ounces (1 cup) every 15 minutes during vigorous exercise in a hot climate to replace losses from sweat. For moderate exercise in a cooler climate, fluid needs are lower.

Athletes should be counseled regarding the appropriate use of ergogenic aids (performance enhancers). Most are a waste of money and some are dangerous. Such products should only be used after careful evaluation for safety, effectiveness, strength, and legality.

Vegetarians Have Unique Nutrition Concerns

For years, people have chosen vegetarianism for religious, personal, health, ethical, environmental, or economic reasons. Today, **vegetarian** eating styles are gaining more attention among consumers, health professionals, environmentalists, restaurant owners, and the food industry. See **Diversity & Health: Vegetarian Diets** on page 128 for more details.

The MyPlate site provides some tips and resources for vegetarians: www.choosemyplate.gov/healthy-eating-tips/tips-for-vegetarian.html.

Is Our Food Supply Safe?

In early 2009, a nationwide outbreak of foodborne illness caused by contaminated peanut products killed 9 people in the United States and sickened over 700 more.[28] In response to this and other outbreaks, the U.S. House of Representatives passed legislation in July 2009 that would require more frequent inspections of food processing plants and would give the FDA greater authority to order the recall of tainted food. In September 2009, a new national website, **www.foodsafety.gov**, was launched to provide Americans with a "gateway" to food safety tips, news, alerts, recalls, and instructions for reporting food poisonings and other food problems. Then, in 2011, the U.S. Congress passed into law the Food Safety Modernization Act, which included new requirements for food manufacturers and importers to improve food safety measures, and new enforcement tools for the FDA.[29] These measures are important in reducing the estimated 48 million cases of foodborne illness that occur in the United States each year.[30]

vegetarian A person who avoids some or all foods from animal sources: red meat, poultry, seafood, eggs, and dairy products.

foodborne illness (food poisoning) Illness caused by pathogenic microorganisms consumed through food or beverages.

Foodborne Illness

Foodborne illness, which most people call *food poisoning,* generally refers to illnesses caused by microbes consumed in food or beverages, or by the toxins that certain microbes secrete into food that has not been properly preserved or stored. In otherwise healthy adults, foodborne illness often resolves in a few days without treatment. However, infants and toddlers, pregnant women and their fetuses, the elderly, and those with weakened immune systems, such as people with HIV infection, cancer, or diabetes, are more at risk for severe complications and death.

Pathogens Involved in Foodborne Illness

Pathogens are disease-causing agents (*patho-* indicates "disease"). Viruses and bacteria are the two types of microbial pathogens most commonly responsible for foodborne illness.

Norovirus. The culprit responsible for the most cases, by far, of foodborne illness, hospitalization, and death is norovirus **(Figure 5.8).**[31] This highly contagious virus is transmitted from person to person in places like restaurants, hotels, daycare centers, cruise ships, at catered events, and, yes, on many college campuses. Infection causes stomach cramps, vomiting, and diarrhea. Although most people recover within a couple of days, severe illness is not uncommon, especially in the vulnerable populations mentioned earlier.

Salmonella. The microbe responsible for most bacterial foodborne illnesses—an estimated 1.4 million cases annually in the United States—is *Salmonella.* Although there are more than 2,000 different

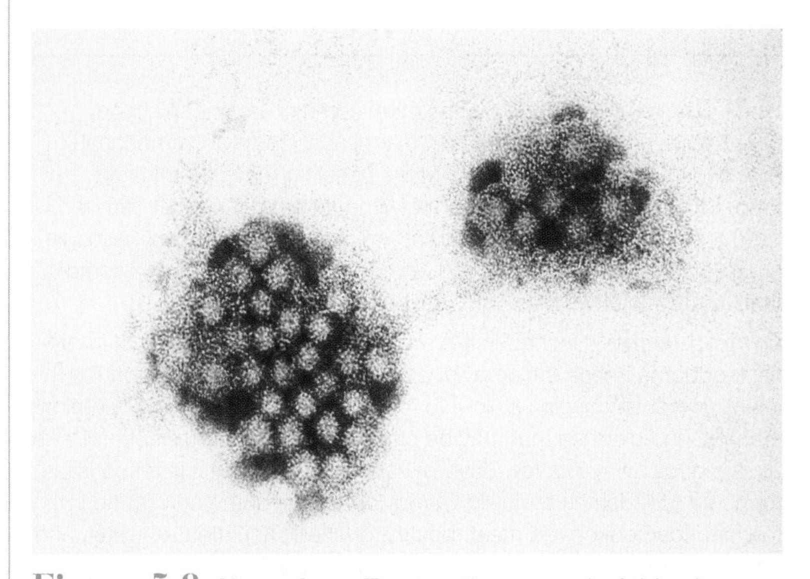

Figure 5.8 **Norovirus.** To stop the spread of this virus, wash your hands after using the bathroom and before preparing food and eating.

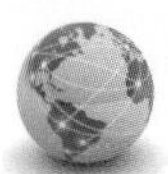

DIVERSITY & HEALTH

Vegetarian Diets

What does it mean to be a vegetarian? For some it's an eating style, for others a lifestyle. In its broadest description, vegetarian means avoiding foods from animal sources. But the term has many subcategories:

- The strictest vegetarians are *vegans.* They consume nothing derived from an animal—no meat, poultry, seafood, eggs, milk, cheese, or other dairy products, and typically no gelatin or honey. Many vegans also avoid products made from or tested on animals.
- More moderate vegetarians are *lacto-ovo-vegetarians.* They avoid meat, poultry, and seafood but will consume dairy products and eggs.
- *Pesco-vegetarians* avoid red meat and poultry but will eat seafood (*pesce* means "fish"), dairy products, and eggs.
- *Semivegetarians* (also called *flexitarians*) may avoid only red meat, or may eat animal-based foods only once or twice a week.

Can vegetarians get enough protein without consuming red meat, poultry, or seafood? Yes, they can. Except for fruit, every edible plant contains protein—grains, vegetables, legumes, nuts, and seeds. When meals and snacks contain a variety of plant-based foods and caloric intake is sufficient to meet energy needs, protein needs can be met easily.

Vegetarians who consume dairy products and eggs don't have different nutrient needs from their nonvegetarian counterparts. But for vegans, nutrition requires special attention. They may not get enough vitamin B_{12}, which is available only from animal sources or fortified foods or supplements. Other nutrients of concern include riboflavin, vitamin D, vitamin A, calcium, iron, and zinc. Even so, planned wisely, a vegan diet can provide adequate nutrients for overall good health.

Although health experts don't necessarily recommend that everyone become a vegetarian, they are increasingly suggesting that you adopt a plant-based diet, in which many or most of the meals you consume are vegetarian. Why? Vegetarian diets tend to be lower in saturated fat and cholesterol, and higher in carbohydrates, fiber, magnesium, folate, potassium, and antioxidant phytochemicals than the typical American diet. Studies show that such diets can reduce your risk for obesity as well as several chronic diseases and some forms of cancer.[1] For example, a recent analysis of thousands of studies, conducted by the American Institute for Cancer Research, found that a combination of physical activity and a plant-based diet could prevent one-third of cancer cases in the United States.[2]

What steps can you take to move toward a plant-based diet? Here are some tips from the USDA:[3]

- Build meals around legumes or other vegetables and whole grains. Think lentil soup with barley, a bean burrito on a whole grain tortilla, or mixed vegetables over whole wheat pasta.
- Experiment with veggie versions of your favorite foods: veggie burgers, hot dogs, subs, pizza, lasagna, quiche, tacos, lo mein, sushi, chili, or spaghetti with marinara sauce or pesto.
- Add vegetarian meat substitutes to soups and stews to boost protein without adding saturated fat or cholesterol. These include tempeh (cultured soybeans with a chewy texture), tofu, or wheat gluten (seitan).
- Most importantly, have confidence that a nonmeat meal—whether breakfast granola with fruit and yogurt, a veggie sandwich at lunch, or cheese tortellini and salad for dinner—will provide you with all the protein, and abundant vitamins, minerals, fiber, and phytochemicals, that your body needs.

References: **1.** "Position of the American Dietetic Association: Vegetarian Diets," by W. J. Craig & A. R. Mangels, 2009, *Journal of the American Dietetic Association, 109*, pp. 1266–1282. **2.** "Evidence Shows Activity and Plant-Based Diet Lowers Cancer Risk, Even Later in Life," by the American Institute for Cancer Research, March 9, 2011, retrieved from http://www.aicr.org/press/press-releases/Evidence-Shows-Activity-and-Plant-Based-Diet-Lowers-Cancer-Risk-Even-Later-in-Life.html. **3.** "Tips and Resources: Vegetarian Diets," by the U.S. Department of Agriculture, August 9, 2011, retrieved from http://www.choosemyplate.gov/tipsresources/vegetarian_diets.html.

types, *Salmonella enteritidis* is the most common culprit. Infection, called *salmonellosis*, causes fever, diarrhea, abdominal cramps, nausea, and vomiting within 8 to 72 hours of eating the contaminated food. Salmonellosis usually resolves without treatment, but it can be life-threatening in vulnerable populations. Any raw food of animal origin, such as meat, poultry, dairy products, eggs, and seafood, and some fruits and vegetables may carry *Salmonella* bacteria.[32]

Campylobacter. Second in line among the common causes of bacterial foodborne illness is *Campylobacter*. Symptoms of *Campylobacter* infection typically begin within 2 to 4 days, and include fever, abdominal cramps, and diarrhea that may be bloody. Like salmonellosis, the illness usually goes away in a few days without treatment, but it is responsible for about 124 deaths annually. *Campylobacter* is commonly found in raw or undercooked red meat, poultry, or shellfish, untreated water, and unpasteurized milk.[33]

Escherichia coli. Most types of *Escherichia coli* (*E. coli*) are harmless. Of concern to human health are a small number that produce a dangerous toxin, called *Shiga toxin*. Of these, the strain associated with most cases of *E. coli* illness in the United States is *E. coli O157:H7*. However, in the spring of 2011, a different Shiga toxin–producing strain, *E. coli O104:H4*, caused nearly 900 cases of illness and 32 deaths. Shiga toxin attacks the intestinal tract (causing vomiting and bloody diarrhea), the kidneys (causing kidney failure), and sometimes the nervous system. Symptoms can begin as soon as 1 day after ingesting the contaminated food, or can be delayed for as long as 10 days. *E. coli* lives in human and animal feces, and may contaminate water, unpasteurized milk and juices, undercooked meats, and even raw fruits and vegetables.[34]

Clostridium botulinum. Although responsible for fewer cases of foodborne illness than any of the previous three bacterial pathogens, *Clostridium botulinum* produces a nerve toxin that is one of the most deadly substances known. A potentially fatal poisoning, called *botulism*, can develop after ingesting even a microscopic amount of contaminated food. For this reason, if you suspect that a food may be contaminated, you should never taste it. Botulism is commonly linked to improperly canned foods, homemade salsa, honey, and baked potatoes sealed in aluminum foil. If you're shopping for groceries and see a dented or bulging can, bring it to the store manager.

Other Pathogenic Microbes. Many other viruses and bacteria, as well as microscopic worms and other parasites, and nonliving protein particles called *prions* can contaminate food. Prions in the nervous tissue of infected cows cause *bovine spongiform encephalitis*, commonly called "mad cow disease." Humans who consume the contaminated tissue are at risk for a variant form of this disease, called *variant Creutzfeldt-Jakob disease (vCJD)*, which causes progressive loss of nervous system functioning and eventually death. A total of 217 patients worldwide have been diagnosed with vCJD, and three of these cases occurred in the United States.[35]

Reducing Your Risk for Foodborne Illness

Generally, pathogenic microbes spread easily and rapidly, requiring only nourishment, moisture, a favorable temperature, and time to multiply. Animal protein foods—red meat, poultry, eggs, and seafood—are common hosts for foodborne pathogens; however, almost any food, including fruits, vegetables, juices, canned foods, and even frozen foods, can harbor microbes. So, of course, can unwashed hands, as well as sponges, dish towels, cutting boards, and kitchen utensils.

So what can you do to keep food safe? Check out these steps:[36]

1. **Clean.** Wash your hands, kitchen items, and fruits and veggies. Here's how:
   - Wash your hands for at least 20 seconds with soap and running water. Do it before you eat any meal or snack, as well as before, during, and after preparing food. Also wash your hands after using the bathroom, changing diapers, or touching garbage or animal waste, caring for someone who is sick, coughing, sneezing, or blowing your nose.
   - Wash utensils and small cutting boards with hot soapy water after each use. To clean surfaces and larger cutting boards that won't fit in the sink, mix 1 teaspoon of bleach with 1 quart of water, flood the surface, and let it sit for 10 minutes before rinsing with clean water and allowing to air dry.
   - Before you cut or peel them, wash fruits and vegetables. If they're delicate, rinse them under running water. You can scrub firm produce, such as carrots or apples, under running water with a clean produce brush.
2. **Separate.** Use different cutting boards for bread, produce, and raw meats, poultry, and seafood. At the grocery store, keep meats, poultry, and seafood separate from all other foods in your shopping cart, and wrap these foods in plastic bags so that they don't drip onto your other foods. Keep them wrapped in your fridge, or if you don't plan to use them for a few days, freeze them. Keep eggs in their packaging, and put them in the main compartment of the fridge where they'll stay cooler, not in the door.
3. **Cook.** The bacteria that cause food poisoning multiply quickest in the **danger zone** between 40°F and 140°F. So when cooking and storing foods, it's essential to avoid their remaining within this zone. See **Table 5.5** for safe minimum cooking temperatures for various types of meats, poultry, seafood, and egg dishes. Always use a food thermometer to make sure the meat is cooked to a temperature that is safe for eating.
4. **Chill.** Bacteria can reproduce—and secrete their toxins—in foods left at room temperature within 2 hours. On a hot day, that time can be as short as an hour! So always refrigerate foods, including leftovers, within 2 hours at a temperature between 40°F and 32°F. And thaw foods in the refrigerator, not on the counter. Set your freezer at 0°F and, if the power goes out, keep it closed. When power is restored, check the freezer thermometer: If it reads 40°F or below, the food is safe to prepare or refreeze. Foods in the refrigerator should be discarded if the power was out longer than 4 hours.

If you're not sure whether a food has been prepared, served, and/or stored safely, don't risk it. Heed the advice, "When in doubt, throw it out!"

danger zone Range of temperatures between 40° and 140° Fahrenheit at which bacteria responsible for foodborne illness thrive.

Table 5.5: Safe Minimum Cooking Temperatures

Category	Food	Temperature (°F)	Rest Time
Ground Meat and Meat Mixtures	Beef, pork, veal, lamb	160	None
	Turkey, chicken	165	None
Fresh Beef, Veal, Lamb	Steaks, roasts, chops	145	3 minutes
Poultry	Chicken and turkey, whole	165	None
	Poultry breasts, roasts	165	None
	Poultry thighs, legs, wings	165	None
	Duck and goose	165	None
	Stuffing (cooked alone or in bird)	165	None
Pork and Ham	Fresh pork	145	3 minutes
	Fresh ham (raw)	145	3 minutes
	Precooked ham (to reheat)	140	None
Eggs and Egg Dishes	Eggs	Cook until yolk and white are firm.	None
	Egg dishes	160	None
Leftovers and Casseroles	Leftovers	165	None
	Casseroles	165	None
Seafood	Fin fish	145 or cook until flesh is opaque and separates easily with a fork.	None
	Shrimp, lobster, and crabs	Cook until flesh is pearly and opaque.	None
	Clams, oysters, and mussels	Cook until shells open during cooking.	None
	Scallops	Cook until flesh is milky white or opaque and firm.	None

Source: Data from *Safe Minimum Cooking Temperatures*, by FoodSafety.gov, available at http://www.foodsafety.gov/keep/charts/mintemp.html.

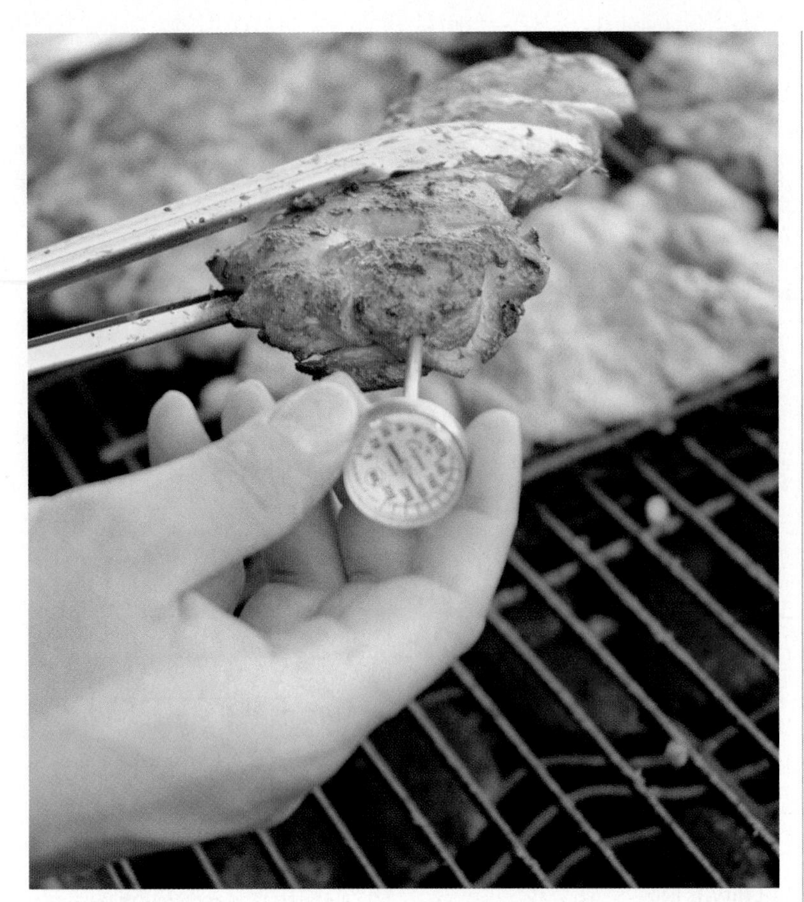

Food thermometers help you know your food is out of the danger zone.

Food Allergies and Intolerances

Another food safety concern for millions of people in the United States is food allergies. Although allergies to pollen, grass, or other environmental sources typically cause discomfort during spring and fall, food allergies know no season. Although the precise incidence in the United States is not known, the FDA estimates that millions of Americans have allergic reactions to foods each year.[37, 38]

food allergy An adverse reaction of the body's immune system to a food or food component.

food intolerance An adverse food reaction that doesn't involve the immune system.

food additive A substance added to foods during processing to improve color, texture, flavor, aroma, nutrition content, or shelf life.

persistent organic pollutants (POPs) Industrial chemicals that resist degradation, can persist in the air, soil, and water for decades, and tend to bioaccumulate.

Broadly speaking, we can describe a **food allergy** as an adverse reaction of the body's immune system to a food or food component, usually a dietary protein. The body's immune system recognizes a food allergen as foreign and, in an attempt to combat the invasion, produces symptoms of inflammation. These may include swelling of the lips or throat, digestive upset, skin hives or rashes, and breathing problems. The most severe response, called *anaphylaxis,* includes most of these symptoms within minutes of exposure to the allergen. If not treated quickly, it can progress to anaphylactic shock, in which the cardiovascular and respiratory systems become overwhelmed. Without immediate treatment, anaphylactic shock is usually fatal.

Eight foods cause more than 90% of all food allergies: milk, eggs, peanuts, tree nuts (such as almonds, Brazil nuts, cashews, hazelnuts, pine nuts, and walnuts), soy, wheat, fish, and shellfish (such as lobster, crab, and shrimp).[37] The FDA requires that food labels clearly identify the presence of any of these eight allergens. The only known "treatment" for food allergies is avoidance of the offending food; however, some medical researchers have had success with a program of progressive introduction of the food into the patient's diet—under close supervision.

An adverse food reaction that doesn't involve the immune system is known as a **food intolerance.** This type of reaction generally develops within a half hour to a couple of days after eating the offending food. The most common example is *lactose intolerance,* an inability to properly digest the milk sugar lactose. Symptoms, which occur within about 30 minutes of consuming dairy products, include abdominal bloating, painful intestinal cramps, and diarrhea. Food intolerances have also been reported to wheat and to gluten, a protein present in wheat, rye, and barley. Gluten intolerance should not be confused with celiac disease, an immune system disorder in which consumption of gluten prompts inflammation and destruction of the lining of the small intestine. (See Chapter 13.) Finally, many people believe that they have an intolerance to certain preservatives, flavor enhancers, and other food additives.

Food Additives

Food additives are substances that manufacturers add to foods to preserve, blend, flavor, color, or thicken them, or to add or replace essential nutrients. Of the more than 3,000 substances intentionally added to food, the most common are spices and other flavorings and sweeteners. Preservatives are also common additives, and help ensure the availability of safe, convenient, and affordable foods year-round.[39]

For decades, consumers have been questioning whether food additives are safe. All food additives must be approved by the FDA, which also regulates the types of foods in which additives can be used and the maximum amounts to be used. If new evidence suggests that an additive already in use may be unsafe, federal authorities can stop its use or conduct further studies to determine its continued safety.[38]

If you are concerned about food additives, read the ingredients list on food labels. Food additives usually are the long, unfamiliar names in the list. Another way to detect food additives is by the length of the ingredients list. Generally, the longer the list, the more additives a food contains.

Food Residues

Food residues are contaminants that are not naturally part of the food, but remain in the food despite cleaning and processing. Two residues of concern to consumers are persistent organic pollutants and pesticides.

Persistent Organic Pollutants

Many different chemicals are released into the air, soil, and water as a result of industry, agriculture, automobile emissions, and improper waste disposal. Some of these chemicals, called **persistent organic pollutants (POPs),** resist degradation by natural forces and,

pesticides A chemical used to kill pests, including agricultural chemicals used to help protect crops from weeds, insects, fungus, slugs and snails, birds, and mammals.

once they get into the environment, can persist for decades. Plants grown in contaminated soil or with contaminated water can absorb the POP, and then you ingest it when you eat the plant. The plant can also pass it on to food animals that feed on it. Fish and land animals can also absorb POPs directly into their tissues or ingest them when they eat other contaminated animals. The larger the fish or land animal, the more likely it is that this process, called *bioaccumulation*, has produced a high level of POPs in the animal's tissues.

Because they can travel on wind and in water, POPs have been found all over the globe, including in remote, pristine locations such as the Arctic.[40] They've also been found in virtually all categories of foods. And it is estimated that all animals, including humans, have at least some measure of POPs in their tissues, including in human breast milk. Their presence is of particular concern during fetal and childhood development, because they are associated with an increased risk for preterm birth, and for neurological and developmental disorders.

Mercury is an especially potent POP. Fish is a great source of protein and essential fatty acids, but nearly all fish contains at least some traces of mercury, and the mercury levels in some kinds of fish can be harmful, especially for pregnant women and young children.[41] Federal, state, and local governments monitor water quality and issue advisories about the level of mercury in fish. As a general guideline, the U.S. Environmental Protection Agency (EPA) advises that you avoid eating shark, swordfish, king mackerel, or tilefish, as these have high levels of mercury. Albacore (white) tuna has more mercury than light tuna, so you should limit consumption of albacore tuna to no more than 6 ounces (one average meal) a week.

The Monterey Bay Aquarium has a handy guide for making safe and sustainable seafood choices at www.montereybayaquarium.org/cr/cr_seafoodwatch/sfw_recommendations.aspx?c=ln. Smartphone apps are also available.

Pesticides

Pesticides are any bait, liquid, powder, or spray used in the field, in storage areas, or in homes and gardens to kill pests. In conventional farming, pesticides are used to help protect crops from weeds, insects, fungus, slugs and snails, and birds and mammals. Before the EPA began tightly regulating pesticide use, many—including the notorious DDT—were used indiscriminately and still persist in the environment as POPs. Today, the EPA approves pesticides for use only if they have minimal impact on the environment. Nevertheless, many pesticides still in use are toxic and do leave residues on foods. When these residues are not effectively removed, they can build up in the body's tissues and cause health problems, including nerve damage, endocrine disorders (which affect the production and release of body hormones), and cancer.[42] Considering the health effects of pesticides, are organic foods better? See **Consumer Corner: Are Organic Foods Better?** to find out.

The National Pesticide Information Center provides the following tips to reduce your exposure to pesticides:[43]

- Wash all fresh fruits and vegetables thoroughly under running water. Scrub firm fruits and vegetables like melons and potatoes.

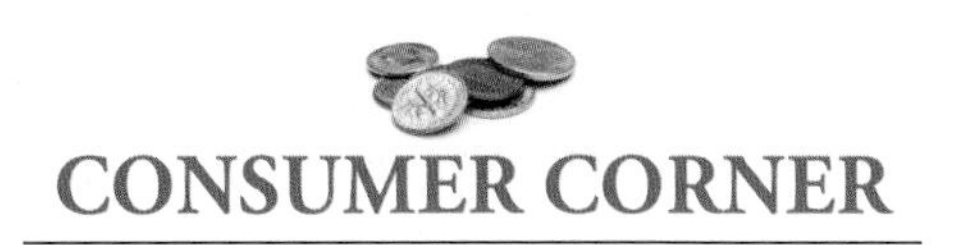

CONSUMER CORNER

Are Organic Foods Better?

You're at the deli, waiting for your sandwich, so you go to the cooler to look for a beverage. You spy a bottle of apple juice with an enticing label showing an apple orchard and the words "100% organic" beside an organic seal. You're about to select it when you notice beside it a bottle of a commercial brand of apple juice, apparently not organic, costing about $1 less. Which should you buy?

Organic foods are grown without the use of synthetic pesticides. Red meat, poultry, eggs, and dairy products that are certified organic come from animals fed only organic feed and not given growth hormones or antibiotics. To earn the USDA organic seal, a food must contain 95% organically produced ingredients by weight, excluding water and salt. Farms must be certified as organic by the USDA, and any companies that handle the food after it leaves the farm must also be certified.

Does this mean that organic foods are safer choices than foods grown with pesticides? That depends. If a conventionally grown fruit or vegetable can be thoroughly scrubbed or peeled, or if it tends to have a low pesticide residue anyway, then its safety is probably comparable to that of organically grown versions. Foods that don't tend to absorb pesticides include onions, corn, peas, broccoli, asparagus, tomatoes, and eggplant. Foods that have tended to show a high level of pesticides include peaches, nectarines, apples, strawberries, cherries, imported grapes, celery, sweet bell peppers, and carrots, among others.[1]

Are organic foods more nutritious? To date, research does not support this. Keep in mind that the term "organic" refers only to how food has been farmed and produced. It is not synonymous with "nutritionally better for you." As a consumer, it is up to you to weigh the pros and cons of organic versus conventional produce and then decide for yourself what is right for you.

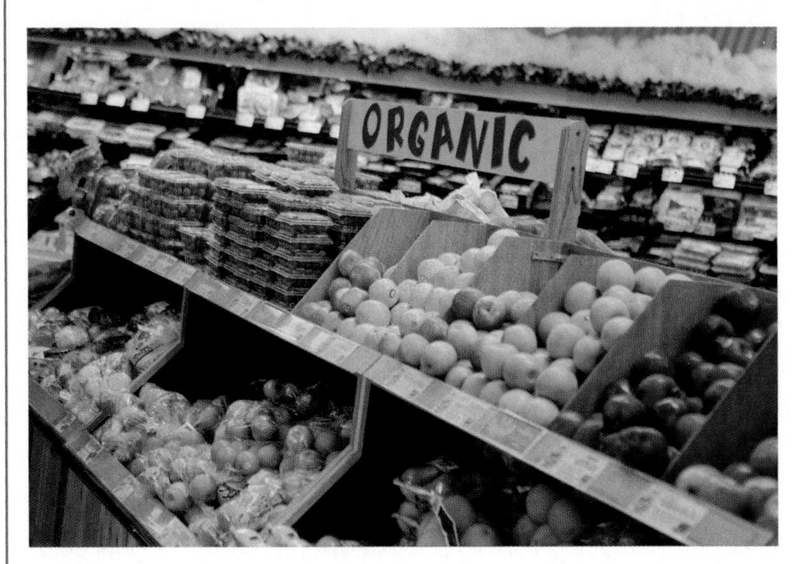

Reference: 1. "Shopper's Guide to Pesticides," by the Environmental Working Group, based on USDA food consumption data 1994–1996, retrieved from http://www.foodnews.org/walletguide.php.

- After washing, peel fruits and vegetables whenever possible. Discard the outer leaves of leafy vegetables such as cabbage and lettuce.
- Trim the fat from meat and remove the skin from poultry and fish because some pesticide residues collect in the fat.
- Eat a variety of foods from various sources, as this can reduce the risk of exposure to a single pesticide.

genetic modification Altering a plant's or animal's genetic material in order to produce desirable traits such as resistance to pests, poor soil tolerance, or lower fat.

Genetically Modified Foods

Scientists create genetically modified fruits and vegetables by altering the genetic material inside the cells of plants, then cultivating their seeds for agricultural production. For example, the process is used to produce food plants that resist heat or pests, tolerate poor soils, or have a higher yield. **Genetic modification** is also used on animals, to produce meat or poultry products with lower fat, for instance.

Supporters of genetically modified foods say that their use increases agricultural productivity, decreases the level of pesticides used, and can improve nutrient content. Opponents express concern about environmental hazards, such as loss of biodiversity, or unintended transfer of modified genes to other crops when pollen is spread on the wind or by bees or birds. The debate continues to this day.

For more information on genetically modified foods, check out this special report from PBS's *Nova/Frontline:* www.pbs.org/wgbh/harvest.

Change Yourself, Change Your World

Armed with the information in this chapter, you're ready to improve your own diet, advocate for healthier food choices on campus, and take action to improve the safety of your community's food supply.

Personal Choices

Maintaining a healthy diet is easier than you might believe. Start by visiting **www.choosemyplate.gov** for a step-by-step guide to healthful eating and physical activity that's tailored to your age, gender, height, current weight, lifestyle, and calorie needs. Then choose "Analyze my diet" to find out how well a day's or week's food choices are meeting your needs. What food groups should you eat more of? What do you need to decrease? Are you eating too many calories overall, or too few? For a quick assessment of your diet, see the **Self-Assessment** on the next page.

Once you've identified your dietary drawbacks, you're ready to create a practical plan for improving your nutritional health. The **Choosing to Change Worksheet** at the end of this chapter will help you generate a plan that fits your food preferences, your goals—your life! But even with a plan in place, how do you put it into action? Follow the suggestions ahead.

Think Smart When Making Choices

You understand the reasons why it's better to choose a black bean burger on whole grain bread over a hamburger on a white bun, but have you persuaded yourself to do so when you're choosing lunch in the dining hall—today? By adopting a smart thinking style, you'll find it easier not just to understand the *Dietary Guidelines for Americans*, but to embrace them. Here are some strategies:

- **Be realistic.** Make small changes consistently over time—they often work better than giant leaps. If your fruit intake is low, try adding a serving to one of your meals each day or as a snack. You don't have to add fruits to all meals right away. Or if you need to increase your calcium intake, start replacing soda with milk every day at lunch, or choose a cup of yogurt every day as your afternoon snack.
- **Be sensible.** Enjoy food, but in moderation. Pay attention to portion sizes and try to minimize your intake of empty calories. Remember that if you're physically active, you can consume more calories than if you are sedentary. Plan a diet that makes sense for your energy needs.
- **Be adventurous.** Expand your tastes to include a variety of fruits, legumes and other vegetables, and whole grains. Have fun trying a new healthful food once a week.
- **Be flexible.** If you happen to overeat for one meal, let it go. Get back on track the next meal. Overindulging for one meal, one occasion, or one day does not make you unhealthy or overweight. Don't let yourself get stressed out about it.
- **Be active.** You don't need to run 10 miles a day. You just need to be physically active. Consistently choose the stairs instead of the elevator or escalator. Park farther away from a building rather than circling the parking lot until the space closest to the building becomes available. Walk over to your friends' dorm room rather than calling them on your cell phone. Every step counts—just get moving. (For more tips, see Chapter 6.)

Eat Smart When Eating Out

If you're like most college students, you get a lot of your meals from the campus dining hall, food kiosks, restaurants, or fast food outlets. But you can still make smart choices when you're eating out. For instance, compare these two fast food meals:

- A McDonald's Big Mac, extra-large fries, and an apple pie contain about 1,430 calories, a whopping 47% of which come from fat.
- A McDonald's Premium Grilled Chicken Classic Sandwich, side salad, and a package of apple slices contains 385 calories and 20% of its energy as fat.

"Make small changes consistently over time—they often work better than giant leaps."

SELF-ASSESSMENT

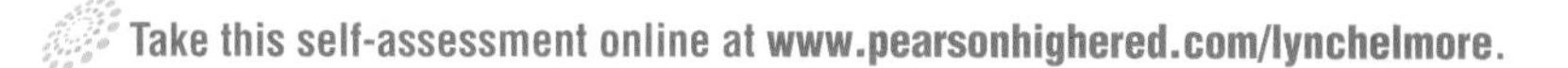
Take this self-assessment online at www.pearsonhighered.com/lynchelmore.

The following 13 descriptions of healthy eating behaviors are based on the 2010 *Dietary Guidelines for Americans* recommendations regarding the foods and nutrients all Americans should increase or reduce. Next to each statement, check how often each applies to you.

1. I eat a variety of vegetables, especially dark green, red, and orange vegetables and beans and peas.
   ☐ Always ☐ Sometimes ☐ Never
2. I consume at least half of all grains as whole grains and/or increase whole grain intake by replacing refined grains with whole grains.
   ☐ Always ☐ Sometimes ☐ Never
3. I consume fat-free or low-fat milk and milk products, such as milk, yogurt, cheese, or fortified soy beverages.
   ☐ Always ☐ Sometimes ☐ Never
4. I choose a variety of protein foods, which include seafood, lean meat and poultry, eggs, beans and peas, soy products, and unsalted nuts and seeds.
   ☐ Always ☐ Sometimes ☐ Never
5. I increase the amount and variety of seafood consumed by choosing seafood in place of some meat and poultry.
   ☐ Always ☐ Sometimes ☐ Never
6. I replace protein foods that are higher in solid fats with choices that are lower in solid fats and calories and/or are sources of oils. (The fats in meat, poultry, and eggs are considered solid fats, while the fats in seafood, nuts, and seeds are considered oils.) Meat and poultry should be consumed in lean forms to decrease intake of solid fats.
   ☐ Always ☐ Sometimes ☐ Never
7. I use oils to replace solid fats where possible.
   ☐ Always ☐ Sometimes ☐ Never
8. I choose foods that provide more potassium, dietary fiber, calcium, and vitamin D, which are nutrients of concern in American diets. These foods include vegetables, fruits, whole grains, and milk and milk products.
   ☐ Always ☐ Sometimes ☐ Never
9. I choose and prepare foods with little salt and consume less than 2,300 milligrams (mg) of sodium per day.
   ☐ Always ☐ Sometimes ☐ Never
10. I consume less than 7 percent of calories from saturated fats by replacing them with monounsaturated and polyunsaturated fatty acids.
   ☐ Always ☐ Sometimes ☐ Never
11. I keep *trans* fatty acid consumption as low as possible by limiting foods that contain synthetic sources of *trans* fats, such as partially hydrogenated oils, and by limiting other solid fats.
   ☐ Always ☐ Sometimes ☐ Never
12. I limit the consumption of foods that contain refined grains, especially refined grain foods that contain solid fats, added sugars, and sodium.
   ☐ Always ☐ Sometimes ☐ Never
13. If I consume alcohol, I consume it in moderation—up to one drink per day for women and two drinks per day for men—and only because I am of legal drinking age.
   ☐ Always ☐ Sometimes ☐ Never

HOW TO INTERPRET YOUR SCORE:

The more "Always" responses, the better. Focus on improving the eating behaviors for which you selected "Never" or "Sometimes." The Choosing to Change Worksheet at the end of the chapter will assist you in improving these areas.

As you can see, small choices you make every day can make a big difference in your nutrition, weight, and health. For some tips for eating at fast food restaurants, see **Practical Strategies for Change: Eating Right While on the Run** on page 134.

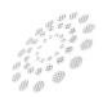
This site compares serving sizes, calories, saturated fat, *trans* fat, and sodium content for several popular fast foods: www.acaloriecounter.com/fast-food.php.

Shop Smart When Money's Tight

You might believe that it costs more to eat right, but in fact, some of the cheapest foods in your supermarket are also among the most healthful. Here are some smart choices:

- **Legumes.** Dried beans, peas, and lentils are a must-have staple. They're least expensive sold in bulk or in plastic packages, but if you don't have the hour or two it can take to cook them yourself, stock up on canned beans. Canned black beans, for instance, cost less than 50 cents per serving, and provide 7 grams of protein, 7 grams of fiber, calcium, and iron.
- **Canned tuna.** Skip the albacore, which is more expensive and has more mercury. Choose light tuna in water. A small can provides two servings, each of which should cost you less than 75 cents, while providing 12 grams of protein and about 250 milligrams of omega-3 fatty acids.

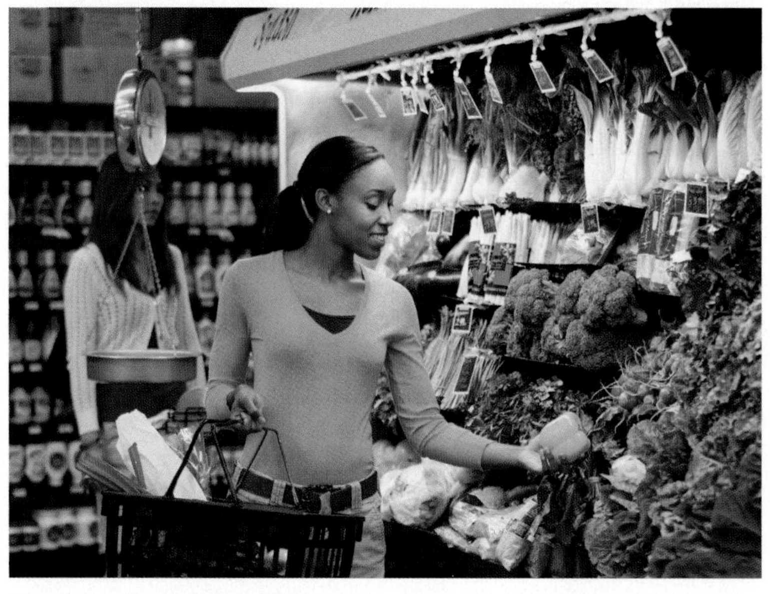

Eating healthfully doesn't have to break the bank.

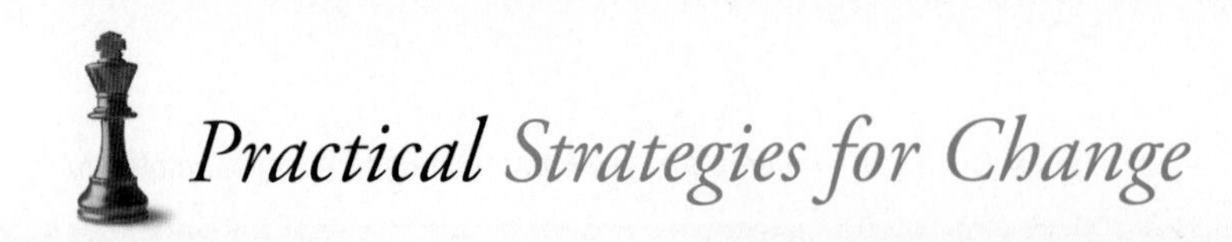

Practical Strategies for Change

Eating Right While on the Run

You're a college student, right? So almost by definition, you eat lots of your meals on the run. Fortunately, healthful choices are available, even from fast food restaurants. Here are some tips:

- Order a vegetarian version of popular fast foods, such as burgers, pizzas, tacos, burritos, or subs.
- When ordering meat, choose chicken, turkey, or fish instead of beef or pork.
- Order your burger or sub without cheese.
- Don't super-size it! Instead, order the smallest size of burger or sandwich available, or cut it in half and share it with a friend.
- Order a side salad instead of a side of fries.
- If you crave fries, order the smallest serving size.
- Order a carton of low-fat or skim milk, a bottle of water, or a diet soda instead of a regular soda or a milkshake.
- Skip dessert or order a piece of fruit instead. Watch out for those "yogurt parfaits" now offered at many fast food restaurants. They're typically loaded with saturated fat, added sugars, and calories.
- Monitor your sensations of fullness as you eat, and stop as soon as you're satisfied.

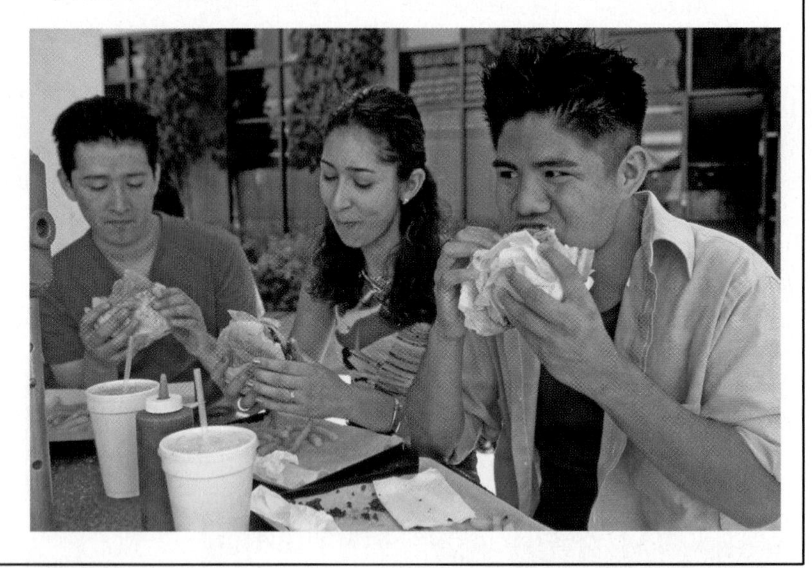

- **Lean meats, poultry, and fish.** Instead of building meals around large portions of low-quality, high-fat meats, fill most of your plate with veggies and grains, accompanied by a small portion of high-quality lean meat, poultry, or fish. You'll save money and reduce your intake of saturated fat and cholesterol, not to mention calories.
- **Whole grains.** Choose brown rice, old-fashioned or quick oats, whole grain pasta, and whole wheat bread. These foods are all inexpensive—especially if you choose the store brand—and are loaded with nutrients and fiber.
- **Frozen vegetables.** These are just as nutritious as fresh vegetables, but much less expensive. Plus they're quick to prepare: All you have to do is open the package, pour the amount you want into a bowl with a tablespoon of water, and microwave it.
- **Frozen fruits.** These are also inexpensive. Make smoothies by blending them with low-fat yogurt and half a banana.
- **Non-fat dry milk.** This is a quick source of all the nutrients in liquid milk, at about half the cost, with no refrigeration required.

The bottom line? Stay on the pathway to good health every day. Make smart food choices, watch portion sizes, and find your balance between food and activity. Over time, these little changes can have an enormous impact on your health and well-being.

Campus Advocacy

Whenever you make a food choice, you're promoting that food. So whether you're buying frozen blueberries in your supermarket, or ordering the bean burrito at your favorite Mexican hangout, you're sending the message that consumers value healthful foods and that it's profitable to offer them. On the other hand, when you avoid choosing foods with empty calories, you limit their profitability and discourage their production.

On campus, make friends with the staff at your dining hall. Provide feedback—positive and negative—about the nutritional quality of the selections offered, and ask for more plant-based meals. Find out where the food they serve comes from—is produce locally grown when possible, and what food safety measures are in place? Check out the vending machines on campus, too. Do they offer nutritious snacks, or junk? Water and 100% juices, or sodas? Who decides what's sold, and how can you improve the choices?

And while you're advocating for more healthful food choices for yourself and other students, don't forget those less fortunate. One way to help is to join a branch of the National Student Campaign Against Hunger and Homelessness. For more than 25 years, this organization has fought hunger and homelessness by educating, engaging, and training college students to directly meet individuals' immediate needs while advocating for long-term systemic solutions. In 2011, for instance, members raised funds for Oxfam America's famine-relief efforts in Somalia, while also sponsoring local awareness and education events, holding fundraisers, volunteering with shelters, and advocating for anti-poverty programs. For a list of participating colleges and universities, go to www.studentsagainsthunger.org/participating-schools. If you find out that your campus doesn't have a branch, start one yourself!

Watch videos of real students discussing their nutrition at www.pearsonhighered.com/lynchelmore.

http://www.acha-ncha.org/reports_ACHA-NCHAII.html.

22. U.S. Department of Agriculture, Agricultural Research Service. (2010, May). Oxygen radical absorbance capacity (ORAC) of selected foods, release 2. Nutrient Data Laboratory Home Page. Retrieved from http://www.ars.usda.gov/nutrientdata/orac.

23. Doron, S., & Gorbach, S. L. (2006). Probiotics: Their role in the treatment and prevention of diseases. *Expert Review of Anti-Infective Therapy*, *4* (2), 261–275.

24. U.S. Food and Drug Administration. (2011, March 11). How to understand and use the Nutrition Facts label. Retrieved from http://www.fda.gov/food/labelingnutrition consumerinformation/ucm078889.htm.

25. U.S. Food and Drug Administration. (2011, August 1). *Food labeling guide*. Retrieved from http://www.fda.gov/Food/GuidanceComplianceRegulatoryInformation/GuidanceDocuments/FoodLabelingNutrition/FoodLabelingGuide/ucm064908.htm#health.

26. U.S. Department of Agriculture. (2011, June 4). Food groups. Retrieved from http://www.choosemyplate.gov/foodgroups/index.html.

27. Rodriguez, N., DiMarco, N., & Langley, S. (2009). Position of the American Dietetic Association, Dietitians of Canada, and the American College of Sports Medicine: Nutrition and athletic performance. *Journal of the American Dietetic Association, 109* (31), 509–527.

28. Centers for Disease Control and Prevention (CDC). (2009, March 17). Investigation update: Outbreak of *Salmonella typhimurium* infections, 2008–2009. Retrieved from http://www.cdc.gov/salmonella/typhimurium/update.html.

29. Hamburg, M. A. (2011, January 3). Food Safety Modernization Act: Putting the focus on prevention. Available at http://www.whitehouse.gov/blog/2011/01/03/food-safety-modernization-act-putting-focus-prevention.

30. Centers for Disease Control and Prevention. (2010, December 15). CDC reports 1 in 6 get sick from foodborne illnesses each year. Retrieved from http://www.cdc.gov/media/pressrel/2010/r101215.html.

31. Hall, A. J. (2011, March 22). Norovirus in the news. FoodSafety.gov. Available at http://www.foodsafety.gov/blog/norovirus.html.

32. U.S. Department of Agriculture, Food Safety and Inspection Service. (2011, May 25). Fact sheets: *Salmonella* questions and answers. Retrieved from http://www.fsis.usda.gov/factsheets/salmonella_questions_&_answers/index.asp.

33. U.S. Department of Agriculture, Food Safety and Inspection Service. (2011, May 23). Fact sheets: *Campylobacter* questions and answers. Retrieved from http://www.fsis.usda.gov/factsheets/Campylobacter_Questions_and_Answers/index.asp.

34. Centers for Disease Control and Prevention. (2011, July 8). *Escherichia coli O157:H7* and other Shiga toxin-producing *Escherichia coli* (STEC). Retrieved from http://www.cdc.gov/nczved/divisions/dfbmd/diseases/ecoli_o157h7/#whysick.

35. Centers for Disease Control and Prevention. (2010, August 23). Variant Creutzfeldt-Jakob disease. Retrieved from http://www.cdc.gov/ncidod/dvrd/vcjd/factsheet_nvcjd.htm.

36. U.S. Department of Health & Human Services. (2011). Check your steps. Retrieved from http://www.foodsafety.gov/keep/basics/index.html.

37. *New York Times*. (2010, May 16). The squishy science of food allergies. Retrieved from http://roomfordebate.blogs.nytimes.com/2010/05/16/the-squishy-science-of-food-allergies.

38. U.S. Food and Drug Administration. (2011, January 27). Food allergies: What you need to know. Retrieved from http://www.fda.gov/food/resourcesforyou/consumers/ucm079311.htm.

39. U.S. Food and Drug Administration. (2011, May 23). Food ingredients and colors. Retrieved from http://www.fda.gov/Food/FoodIngredientsPackaging/ucm094211.htm.

40. U.S. Environmental Protection Agency. (2002, March). The foundation for global action on persistent organic pollutants: A United States perspective. Retrieved from http://www.epa.gov/ncea/pdfs/pops/POPsa.pdf.

41. U.S. Environmental Protection Agency. (2011, July 18). What you need to know about mercury in fish and shellfish. Retrieved from http://water.epa.gov/scitech/swguidance/fishshellfish/outreach/advice_index.cfm.

42. U.S. Environmental Protection Agency. (2011, April 6). Pesticides: Human health issues. Retrieved from http://www.epa.gov/opp00001/health/human.htm.

43. National Pesticide Information Center. (2011, March 30). Minimizing pesticide residues in food. Retrieved from http://npic.orst.edu/health/foodprac.html.

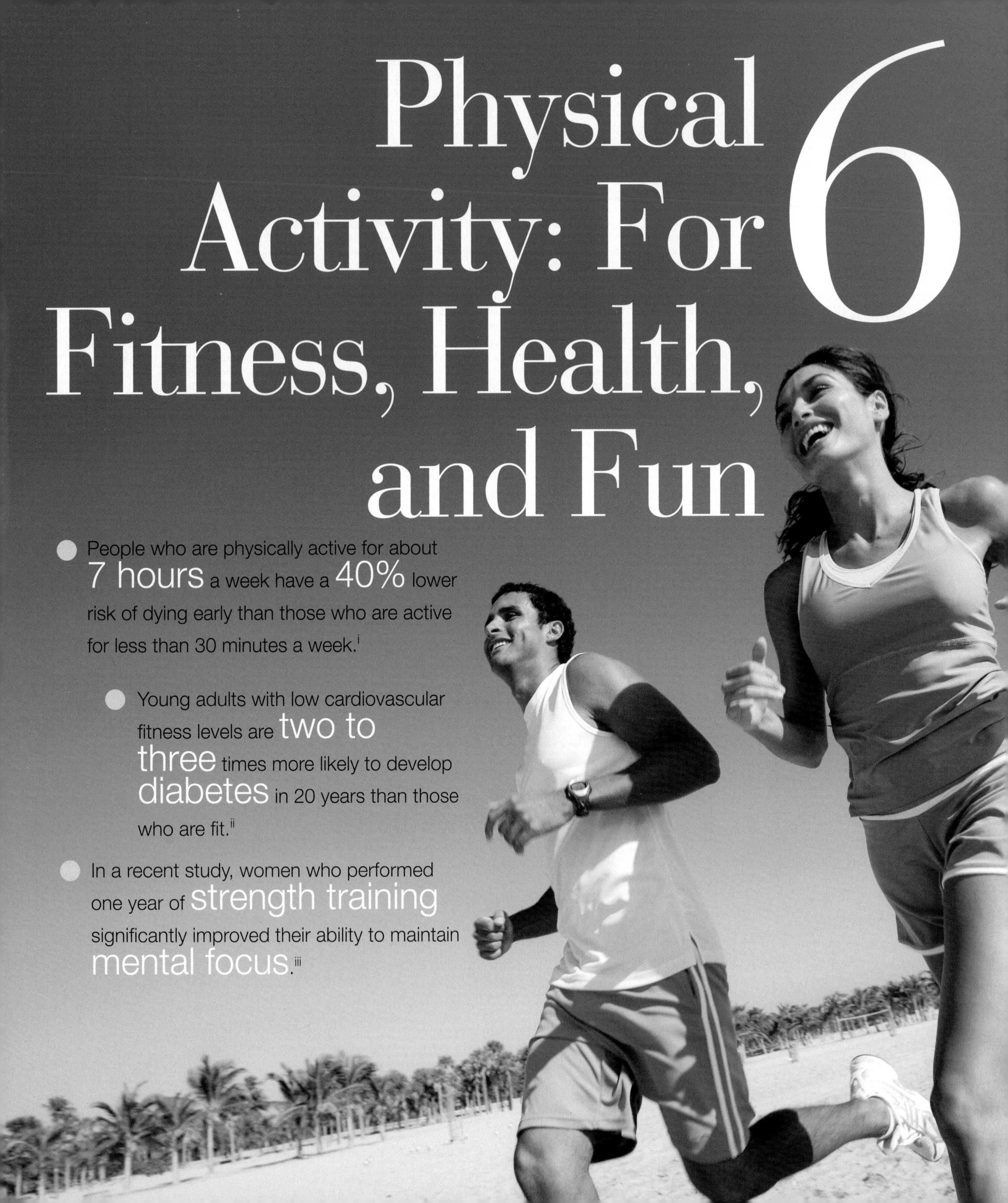

6 Physical Activity: For Fitness, Health, and Fun

- People who are physically active for about **7 hours** a week have a **40%** lower risk of dying early than those who are active for less than 30 minutes a week.[i]
- Young adults with low cardiovascular fitness levels are **two to three** times more likely to develop **diabetes** in 20 years than those who are fit.[ii]
- In a recent study, women who performed one year of **strength training** significantly improved their ability to maintain **mental focus**.[iii]

LEARNING OBJECTIVES

IDENTIFY the five components of health-related physical fitness.

EXPLAIN the health benefits of physical activity.

IDENTIFY the principles of fitness training.

DESIGN an effective, personalized fitness program.

DISCUSS how to exercise safely.

IDENTIFY strategies for overcoming obstacles and for maintaining a long-term fitness program.

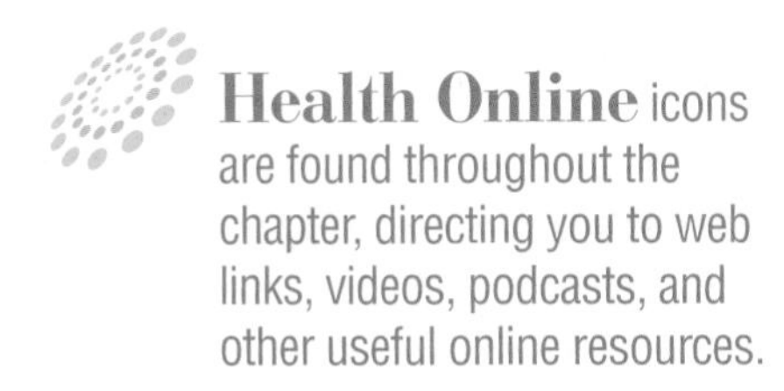
Health Online icons are found throughout the chapter, directing you to web links, videos, podcasts, and other useful online resources.

As a society, we are out of shape.

Many of our daily activities no longer require significant physical effort, and busy schedules cut into our time for exercise—an especially critical problem for students, who often see their physical activity levels decline in college. Even when we do have time for recreation, hours that could be spent getting exercise or playing sports are instead too often spent in the car, in front of the TV, or on the computer. The result: Americans are experiencing more long-term health problems, such as overweight and obesity, diabetes, cardiovascular disease, and even reduced mental health.

The good news is that in recent years the percentage of people in the United States who report getting at least some regular physical activity has grown from 43% to 46.7% among women and from 48% to 49.7% among men, a small but hopeful sign that more people are aware of the benefits of fitness.[1] And if given the chance to be more active, our bodies thrive. Even small changes in physical activity levels can make a significant difference in your fitness and health, both in school now and in the years ahead.

What Is Physical Fitness?

Most of us equate fitness with appearance. We assume that those of us with trim builds or visible muscles are more fit, while those of us with a bit of a belly or flabby triceps are less fit. But physical fitness is not that simplistic. **Physical fitness** is the ability to perform moderate to vigorous levels of activity, and to respond to physical demands without excessive fatigue. Physical fitness can be built up through physical activity or exercise. **Physical activity** is bodily movement that substantially increases energy expenditure. Taking the stairs instead of the elevator, biking to class instead of driving, gardening, and walking the dog all count as types of physical activity. **Exercise** is physical activity that is carried out in a planned and structured format. Any type of activity will provide health benefits, but optimal physical fitness can only be achieved through regular exercise. Team sports, aerobics classes, brisk walks, and working out at the gym all count as exercise.

There are two types of physical fitness: **skills-related fitness** and **health-related fitness.** In this chapter, we will focus on health-related fitness. The five key components of health-related fitness are cardiorespiratory fitness, muscular strength, muscular endurance, flexibility, and body composition.

Cardiorespiratory Fitness

Put together "cardio" for heart and "respiratory" for breath, and you've got a good idea of what this component of fitness covers. **Cardiorespiratory fitness** refers to the ability of your heart and lungs to effectively deliver oxygen to your muscles during prolonged physical activity. Experts agree that cardiorespiratory fitness should be the foundation upon which all the other areas of fitness are built. It is the component that is the best indicator of overall physical fitness and in addition it helps lower your risk of chronic disease and premature death.[2] You can boost your cardiorespiratory fitness by

physical fitness The ability to perform moderate to vigorous levels of activity and to respond to physical demands without excessive fatigue.

physical activity Bodily movement that substantially increases energy expenditure.

exercise A type of physical activity that is planned and structured.

skills-related fitness The capacity to perform specific physical skills related to a sport or other physically demanding activity.

health-related fitness The ability to perform activities of daily living with vigor.

cardiorespiratory fitness The ability of your heart and lungs to effectively deliver oxygen to your muscles during prolonged physical activity.

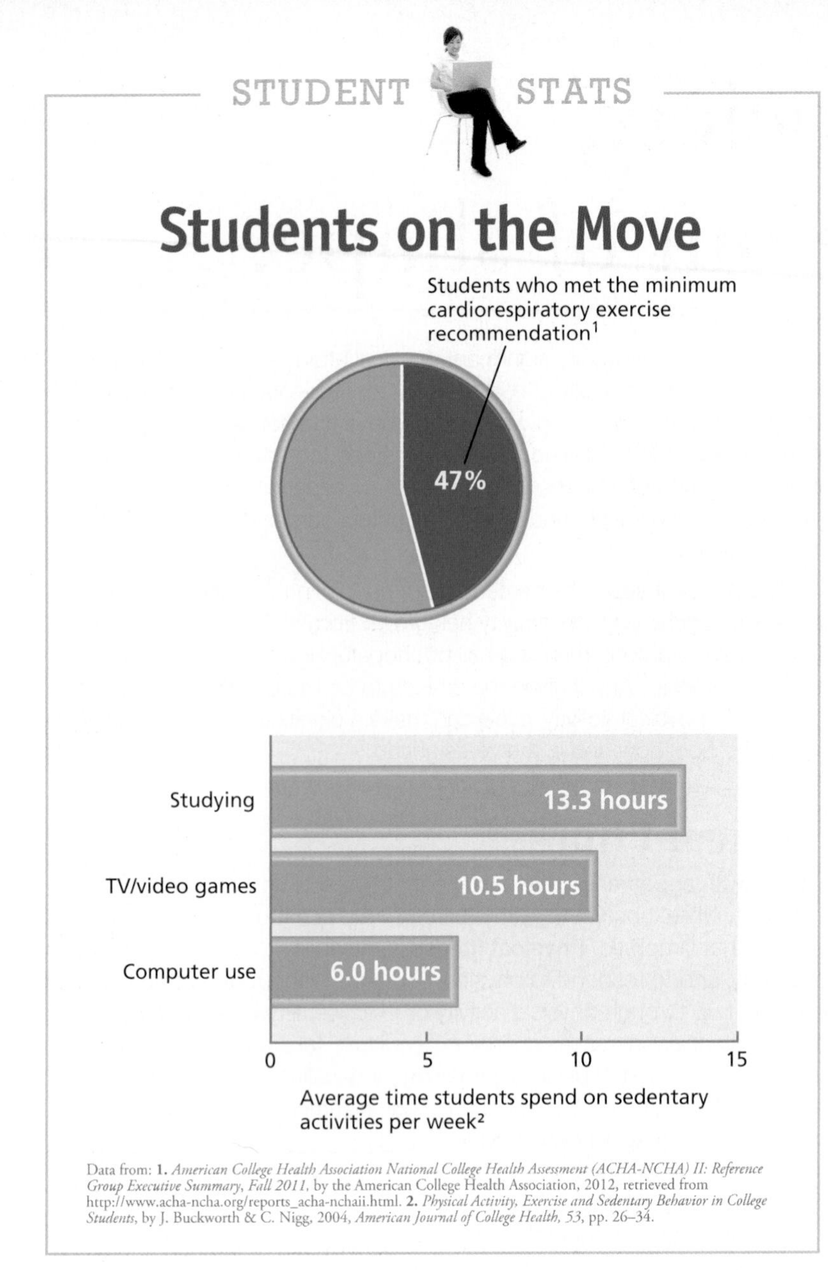

Data from: 1. *American College Health Association National College Health Assessment (ACHA-NCHA) II: Reference Group Executive Summary, Fall 2011*, by the American College Health Association, 2012, retrieved from http://www.acha-ncha.org/reports_acha-nchaii.html. 2. *Physical Activity, Exercise and Sedentary Behavior in College Students*, by J. Buckworth & C. Nigg, 2004, *American Journal of College Health, 53*, pp. 26–34.

any continuous, rhythmic exercise that works your large muscle groups and increases your heart rate, such as brisk walking, swimming, or cycling.

Muscular Strength

Muscular strength is the maximum force your muscles can apply in a single effort of lifting, pushing, or pressing. Building stronger muscles will help keep your skeleton properly aligned, aid balance, protect your back, boost your athletic performance, and increase your metabolic rate. Building muscular strength also results in much higher bone mineral density and stronger bones.[3] You can build muscular strength by performing strength training exercises using machines, free weights, resistance bands, or simply the weight of your own body (as in push-ups, for example).

Muscular Endurance

Muscular endurance is the capacity of your muscles to repeatedly exert force, or to maintain force, over a period of time without tiring. Muscular endurance is measured in two ways: *static muscular endurance,* or how long you can hold a force that is motionless, and *dynamic muscular endurance,* or how long you can sustain a force in motion. A sustained sit-up, where you contract your abdominal muscles and do not move until they fatigue, is an example of static muscle endurance. Repeated sit-ups, done until you can't contract your abdominals any more, rely on dynamic muscle endurance. Muscular endurance is important for posture and for performing activities over an extended time. Muscular endurance can be improved by gradually increasing the duration that your muscles work in each bout of resistance exercises, such as slowly increasing the number of push-ups you perform each time you exercise.

Flexibility

Flexibility refers to the ability of your joints to move through their full ranges of motion, such as how far you can bend your trunk from side to side or how far you can bend forward from the hips toward your toes. Flexibility does not only pertain to the movement of muscle, but also depends on connective tissues such as your ligaments and tendons. Benefits of flexibility include the relief of muscle tension, reduction of joint pain, reduction of back pain, and improved posture. Flexibility can be improved through stretching exercises and activities such as yoga, Pilates, and tai chi.

Body Composition

Body composition refers to the relative proportions of fat tissue and lean tissue (such as muscle and connective tissues) in your body. A low ratio of fat to lean tissue is optimal. As we'll discuss in Chapter 7, many of us carry more body fat than is healthful. Excessive body fat, especially in the abdominal area, increases the risk of three of the four leading causes of death in the United States: heart disease, cancer, and stroke. It is also related to other serious conditions, including osteoarthritis, diabetes, hypertension (high blood pressure), and sleep apnea. The newest research indicates that even if you are healthy in other ways, having too much body fat will still negatively impact your health.[4] Body composition affects your level of fitness, but the reverse is also true—as you become more physically fit, your body composition will usually improve.

What Are the Benefits of Physical Activity?

Physical activity is one of the best things you can do for yourself. It benefits every aspect of your health, at every stage of your life. Some of these benefits are purely physical, such as a stronger heart and healthier lungs. But physical activity can also put you in a better mood and help you to manage stress. Physical activity lowers your risk of premature death, and as you age it will help postpone physical decline and many of the diseases that can reduce quality of life in your later years.

muscular strength The maximum force your muscles can apply in a single maximum effort of lifting, pushing, or pressing.

muscular endurance The capacity of muscles to repeatedly exert force, or to maintain a force, over a period of time.

flexibility The ability of joints to move through their full ranges of motion.

body composition The relative proportions of the body's lean tissue and fat tissue.

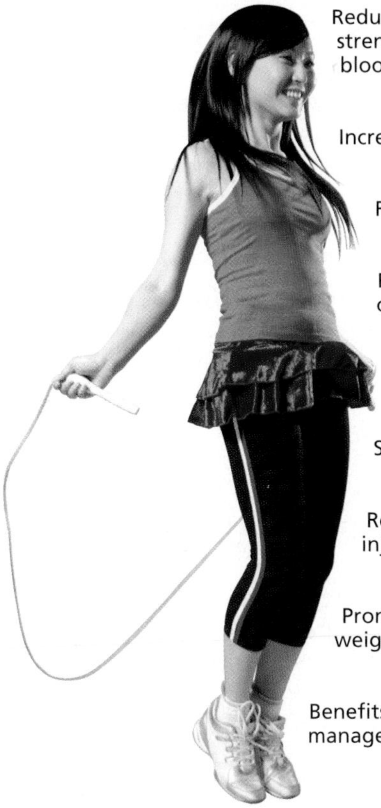

Reduces risk of heart disease, strengthens heart, reduces risk of high blood pressure

Increases lung efficiency and capacity

Reduces risk of type 2 diabetes

Reduces risk of colorectal, breast, and ovarian cancers

Strengthens immune system

Strengthens bones

Reduces risk of bone, muscle, and joint injuries

Promotes healthful body composition and weight management

Benefits psychological health and stress management

Figure 6.1 Health benefits of physical activity.

Figure 6.1 summarizes the major benefits of physical activity; we'll discuss each one next.

Stronger Heart and Lungs

As the organs that pump your blood and deliver oxygen throughout your body, your heart, lungs, and entire circulatory system literally keep you going. By increasing your body's demand for oxygen, physical activity pushes these systems to work harder, which helps keep them strong and efficient, even as you age. As your body adapts to physical activity, your heart becomes stronger and pumps a greater volume of blood with each beat. Your lungs become able to inhale more air and absorb more oxygen. Physical activity also appears to help stabilize the parts of your brain that control the function of these vital systems.[5]

Participating in physical activity and exercise can cut your risk of cardiovascular disease in half through its positive effect on several major risk factors: It lowers LDL (bad) cholesterol, raises HDL (good) cholesterol, helps prevent or control diabetes, and helps you lose excess weight.[6] In addition, because physical activity keeps your blood vessels healthier, it lowers your risk of high blood pressure.

The stronger your heart and lungs, the longer you're likely to live. One study followed more than 20,000 men who weren't overweight, but had differing levels of cardiorespiratory fitness.[7] The researchers found that just being thin isn't enough to protect your health—fitness is also key. In the 8-year-long study, thin men with low rates of cardiorespiratory fitness were twice as likely to die from any cause as thin men with higher rates of cardiorespiratory fitness. Those greater risks included a higher risk of dying from heart disease. (See Chapter 11 for a more detailed discussion of heart disease.)

Management and Prevention of Type 2 Diabetes

Exercise can control your blood glucose level and blood pressure, help you lose weight and maintain weight loss, and improve your body's ability to use insulin, all of which help control or prevent type 2 diabetes. If you have type 2 diabetes, any daily physical activity is helpful. If you are at risk for the disease, even as little as 30 minutes of exercise a day 5 days a week can help lower your risk.[8] When combined with a healthful diet, exercise proves more powerful than prescription medication in lowering type 2 diabetes risk. A federal health study of people at high risk for diabetes showed that daily exercise and a healthful diet lowered risk by 58%, compared with a 31% reduction in risk for a common prescription diabetes drug.[8, 9, 10] (We'll discuss diabetes in more detail in Chapter 11.)

Reduced Risk of Some Cancers

Inactivity is one of the most significant risk factors for cancer that you can control. Physical activity lowers the long-term risks of developing colorectal cancer in men and women and breast and ovarian cancers in women.[11, 12] One long-term study of more than 110,000 women found that those who performed at least 5 hours of moderate to strenuous exercise a week cut their risk of breast cancer by at least half.[13] Activity appears to help in part by controlling weight, a risk factor for certain cancers. It may also help by regulating certain hormones that are factors in some types of cancers and by encouraging your body to process and remove substances—including potential toxins that might cause cancer—more quickly.

Increased Immune Function

Do you want to lower your risk of getting sick during the next cold and flu season? Physical activity can help you fend off common illnesses by boosting your immune system. In one study, 60–90% of active individuals felt that they experienced fewer colds than their sedentary counterparts.[14] Scientists still aren't entirely sure how physical activity helps build immunity, but exercise's role in flushing impurities from the body, along with regulating hormones related to immune function, may play a part.[15] (For more information on infectious diseases and immunity, see Chapter 13.)

Stronger Bones

Physical activity builds and protects your bones.[16] Weight-bearing exercise such as walking, running, or lifting weights makes your bones denser and stronger. Non–weight-bearing exercise, such as swimming, is healthful in other ways but does not strengthen bones. Bone strength helps protect your skeleton from injury, so it is important for everyone, but it is especially important for those at risk for **osteoporosis,** a serious condition that mostly affects older adults, in which reduced bone mineral density causes the bones to become weak and brittle. Although many college-age students don't think they need to worry about osteoporosis, bone density peaks during early adulthood, so this is precisely the time to build the bone strength that could prevent the disease's onset later.

osteoporosis A condition in which reduced bone mineral density causes the bones to become weak and brittle.

Reduced Risk of Injury

The stronger bones, muscles, tendons, and ligaments that result from physical activity can help protect you from injury. A strong back, for example, is much less likely to get strained and sore the next time you lift boxes while moving to a new dorm or apartment. Strong muscles can help you keep your balance and avoid falls, and strong joint-supporting muscles can help reduce the risk of a variety of injuries, including sprains, tendinitis, runner's knee, and shin splints.

Healthful Weight Management

Physical activity helps you lose and control weight in more ways than one. Not only does it burn calories, but it also boosts your metabolism, so your body uses more calories. This boost in metabolism occurs both during and after workouts. Consistent exercise can slowly lower your overall percentage of body fat and help build and maintain muscle, whereas if you try to lose weight by dieting alone, you risk burning muscle mass along with body fat. Having more muscle also increases your metabolism and helps you maintain your weight long-term. (We'll look more closely at metabolism and weight loss in Chapter 7.)

Benefits to Psychological Health, Stress Management, and Sleep

When people say they work out to "blow off steam," they are describing the effect physical activity has on their stress levels. Physical activity reduces stress and anxiety, and also helps boost concentration. These benefits appear to hold true no matter what type of physical activity you enjoy. Some may go for a long hike to help reduce stress and recharge; other people might prefer a spin class, 30 minutes on the rock wall at a climbing gym, or a pickup game of hoops. Any activity can help, especially if you participate in it regularly. In one study of the Chinese movement and meditation discipline called *qigong*, participants saw a significant decrease in stress, anxiety, and fatigue.[17]

Certain studies have shown that exercise can be just as effective in relieving depression as antidepressant medication.[18] And the latest research concludes that exercise can prevent depression in the first place.[19] Any type of physical activity is considered helpful, but in one study of college women with signs of depression, vigorous-intensity exercise classes led to the most significant decrease in symptoms.[20] (You can learn more about depression and its treatments in Chapter 2.)

In addition, active lifestyles may help you be more focused during the day and more tranquil at night. Physical activity may be associated with higher levels of alertness and mental ability, including the ability to learn and achieve academically.[5, 21] Exercise also keeps your mind sharp as you age. Physical activity reduces the risk of dementia and Alzheimer's disease in later life.[22] A physically active lifestyle may also be beneficial when bedtime rolls around: A daily routine that includes at least moderate levels of exercise has been associated with improved sleep quality.[23] In one study, those who were least active initially saw the greatest improvements to their sleep as a result of exercise.[24]

overload Increasing the stress placed on your body through exercise, which results in an improved fitness level.

progressive overload Gradually overloading the body over time in order to avoid injury.

FITT Exercise variables that can be modified in order to accomplish progressive overload: frequency, intensity, time, and type.

Principles of Fitness Training

Participating in regular exercise and physical activity is one of the most healthful habits you can maintain throughout your life, and you'll receive the greatest benefits if you approach your exercise routine in a systematic way. In order to design an effective fitness program, you should first understand the basic principles of fitness training: *overload, specificity, reversibility,* and *individuality.*

Overload

Whatever your fitness capabilities, improving means pushing yourself to the next level. That increased demand on the body, be it a longer walk, a heavier weight, or a deeper stretch, is the **overload** principle in action. The overload principle requires that you increase the stress placed on your body, creating a greater demand than your body is accustomed to meeting. This forces your body to adapt and become more fit. In other words, you improve fitness by exercising beyond your comfort zone.

For overload to work effectively, new stresses should be steady and gradual. This requires **progressive overload,** or increasing the demands on your body gradually over time to avoid injury. If you push yourself too intensely too quickly, your efforts may be set back by injuries that can take weeks or months to heal. You can achieve progressive overload safely by modifying and personalizing one or more of the exercise variables collectively known as **FITT.**

This acronym stands for four important dimensions of progressive overload that work together to build fitness: frequency, intensity, time, and type:

- **Frequency** encompasses how often you exercise. This dimension refers to number of times you engage in a particular physical activity each week. Your frequency may vary with the type of exercise you are undertaking, as well as personal factors that help determine safe exercise frequencies for you. A frequency of 3 to 5 days a week is typically recommended for activities that strengthen your heart and lungs, such as walking or cycling. For many people, optimal strength training means a frequency of 2 to 3 days per week, and improved flexibility often means a frequency of at least 3 days a week or more, as well.
- **Intensity** refers to the level of effort at which you exercise. For cardiorespiratory fitness, intensity is usually measured in terms of how fast you get your heart beating (your heart rate). For muscular strength and endurance training, intensity depends on the amount of resistance and number of repetitions. For flexibility, intensity is measured by the depth of the stretch. Although intensity matters, it is best increased slowly. Attempts to quickly increase your level of intensity in a particular activity may greatly increase your risk of injury.
- **Time** measures the duration of your exercise. Breezing through your workout won't bring you much benefit. The amount of time you spend on a particular exercise is crucial to progressive over-

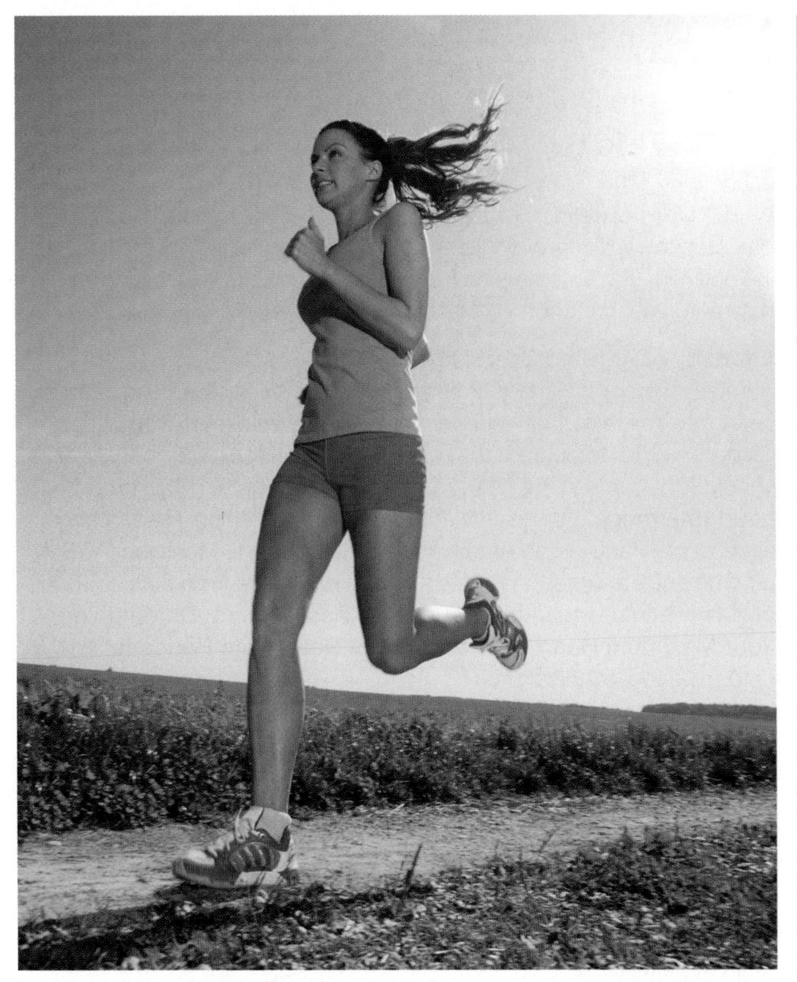

Using the FITT principle will help you achieve progressive overload.

load and improving your fitness. Effective exercise durations are often closely tied to the type of activity at hand. Workouts that strengthen your lungs and heart often require at least 20 minutes of continuous activity, while an effective stretch often takes about 30 to 60 seconds.

- **Type** refers to the sort of activity you engage in. As you'll learn later in this chapter, each area of fitness requires targeted activities that engage a particular part of your body, from your heart and lungs to your muscles or connective tissues. Whereas rowing is an overall workout, for example, this type of exercise delivers its greatest benefits to your heart and lungs. Stretching, on the other hand, benefits connective tissues and flexibility.

Exercise type is closely linked to the principle of specificity, which we'll look at next. (To see the FITT principle applied to various types of workouts, see **Table 6.1**.)

Specificity

The **specificity** principle means that in order to improve a specific component of fitness, you must perform exercises designed to address that component in a deliberate, targeted way. Many exercises will improve some components of fitness but not others. Cycling, for example, is great for cardiorespiratory fitness, but doesn't build upper body strength or increase your flexibility. You should take into account the principle of specificity when deciding which activities you choose to perform. You'll learn more about the links between specific activities and fitness goals later in this chapter.

specificity The principle that a fitness component is improved only by exercises that address that component.

reversibility The principle that fitness levels decline when the demand placed on the body is decreased.

individuality The principle that individuals will respond to fitness training in their own unique ways.

Table 6.1: **The FITT Principle in Action**

FITT Dimensions	Cardiorespiratory Exercise	Strength Training	Flexibility
Frequency	3 to 5 times per week	2 to 3 times per week	At least 2 to 3 days per week, preferably more
Intensity	60 to 85 percent of personal maximum heart rate	8 to 12 repetitions, or until the point of muscle fatigue	Tension (not pain), followed by feeling of release of tension
Time	At least 20 minutes or more (continuous)	As needed to work out safely	30 to 60 seconds
Type	Running, hiking, walking, swimming, rowing, stair climbing, vigorous dancing	Weight machines, free weights, resistance bands	Stretching

Source: Data from *Physical Activity and Public Health: Updated Recommendation for Adults from the American College of Sports Medicine and the American Heart Association,* by W. L. Haskell, I. M. Lee, R. R. Pate, K. E. Powell, S. N. Blair, B. A. Franklin, . . . A. Bauman, 2007, *Medicine & Science in Sports & Exercise, 39* pp. 1423–1434.

Reversibility

Your personal level of fitness can easily go up—or down. The **reversibility** principle states that your fitness level will decline if you don't maintain your physical activity. Just as your body adapts to overload to increase your fitness, if you stop or reduce your exercise routine your body will adapt to the reduced demand and your fitness will suffer. Fitness declines can happen quickly, sometimes in as little as 10 days.[25] Therefore, it is important to maintain a consistent exercise routine to avoid reversing your fitness gains. Even if you can't take on a new round of progressive overload and increased physical stress at a particular time, maintaining your current workout will help keep your level of fitness from declining.

Individuality

The principle of **individuality** means that you will respond to the demands you place on your body in your own unique way. We each react differently to specific exercises, with some people gaining more benefit from a particular exercise than others. These individual responses are shaped, in part, by genetics. Men's muscles, for example, may "bulk up" differently than women's during a strength training program. Identifying the exercises best suited to you is a key part of designing an effective fitness program. Whatever your individual needs and responses, however, one overarching principle applies to all of us—we can all benefit from exercise.

Cardiorespiratory Fitness

STUDENT STORY

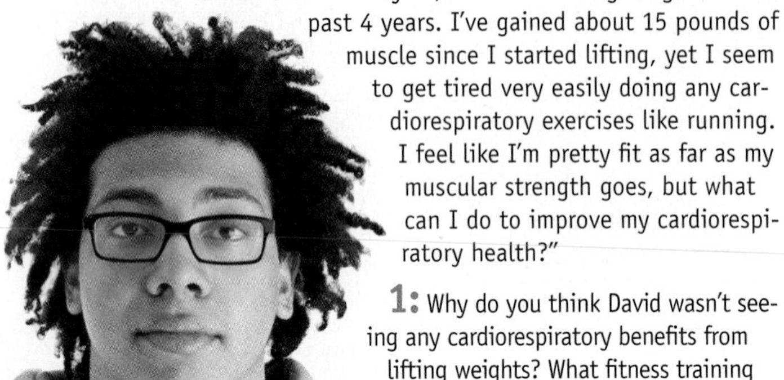

"Hi, I'm David. One day I'd like to become a personal trainer. In order to stay fit, I've been lifting weights for the past 4 years. I've gained about 15 pounds of muscle since I started lifting, yet I seem to get tired very easily doing any cardiorespiratory exercises like running. I feel like I'm pretty fit as far as my muscular strength goes, but what can I do to improve my cardiorespiratory health?"

1: Why do you think David wasn't seeing any cardiorespiratory benefits from lifting weights? What fitness training principle applies to his situation?

2: What types of exercises could David do to build cardiorespiratory fitness?

Do you have a story similar to David's? Share your story at www.pearsonhighered.com/lynchelmore.

What Types of Physical Activity Should You Consider?

Any type of regular, sustained physical activity is beneficial, especially if you have been inactive for a while. However, in order to increase your overall health and fitness, you should look into activities that increase your cardiorespiratory fitness, muscular strength and endurance, and flexibility. Whatever activities you choose, be sure they are ones you truly enjoy, which will help you stick with them over the long term.

Aerobic Exercise

You can build cardiorespiratory fitness through **aerobic exercise,** which is any prolonged physical activity that raises your heart rate and works the large muscle groups. Aerobic exercise makes your heart, lungs, and entire circulatory system stronger by requiring them to work harder to deliver adequate oxygen to your muscles.

Types of Aerobic Exercise

There are numerous forms of popular aerobic exercise, including:

- Running and jogging
- Hiking or brisk walking for extended periods of time
- Cycling and "spinning" (a structured workout on a stationary bicycle)
- Swimming
- Rowing
- Cardio classes, including aerobic dance and step aerobics training
- Vigorous martial arts, such as karate or cardio kickboxing
- Jumping rope
- Stair climbing

The types of aerobic exercise you choose, however, represent just one step toward improved fitness. As the FITT principle discussed earlier outlined, you'll also need to consider other factors, including just how hard you work out.

Intensity of Aerobic Exercise

Aerobic intensity is usually measured by heart rate because increased heart rate indicates that your cardiorespiratory system is working harder. In order to achieve the maximum cardiorespiratory benefit, you should aim to raise your heart rate so that it falls within your **target heart rate range.** For healthy adults who are not entirely sedentary or exceptionally active, the American College of Sports Medicine (ACSM) recommends a target heart rate range of anywhere from 64% to 91% of your maximum heart rate.[26] See **Self-Assessment: Determining Your Maximum Heart Rate and Target Heart Rate Range** for how to determine these indicators.

Aerobic exercises are often categorized as lifestyle/light-intensity, moderate-intensity, or vigorous-intensity activities. According to the Centers for Disease Control and Prevention, light-intensity activity gets you moving but raises your heart rate to less than 50% of your maximum heart rate; moderate-intensity activities will raise your heart rate to 50–70% of your maximum heart rate; and vigorous-intensity activities raise your heart rate to 70–85% of your maximum heart rate.[27] **Table 6.2** shows the examples and benefits of these three categories of aerobic activities.

The best way to begin an aerobic exercise program is to start by performing exercises at intensities near the low end of your target heart rate range, or even lower if you have not exercised in a while. Start with a minimum of 10 minutes of activity at a time, more if you are able. Slowly increase the duration of your exercise by 5–10 minutes every 1–2 weeks for the first 4–6 weeks of your program.[26] After that, you can build fitness by gradually increasing the duration, frequency, or intensity of exercises. Always be sure to warm up before and cool down after an

aerobic exercise Prolonged physical activity that raises the heart rate and works the large muscle groups.

target heart rate range The heart rate range to aim for during exercise. A target heart rate range of 64–91% of your maximum heart rate is recommended.

> *"Simple changes, such as doing some errands on foot instead of in the car, can quickly add up to significant aerobic exercise."*

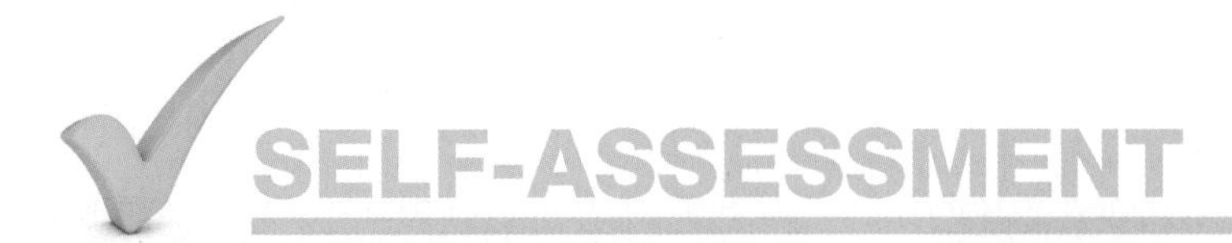

Take this self-assessment online at www.pearsonhighered.com/lynchelmore.

Determining Your Maximum Heart Rate and Target Heart Rate Range

During aerobic exercise, the rate at which your heart is working lets you know if you are exercising effectively. You will gain the most cardiorespiratory benefit if you exercise within your target heart rate range.

MAXIMUM HEART RATE

To start, you need to know your maximum heart rate. The American College of Sports Medicine (ACSM) has found the most accurate way to determine your maximum heart rate is through the following equation:[1]

206.9 − (0.67 × age) = maximum heart rate

Step 1: ____________ × 0.67 = ____________
(your age)

Step 2: 206.9 − ____________ = ____________ = maximum heart rate
(answer from Step 1)

TARGET HEART RATE RANGE

You can narrow down the ACSM's target heart rate range of 64–91% of your maximum heart rate based on your current activity level.[2]

- If you perform only minimal physical activity right now, aim for a target heart rate of about 64–74% of your maximum heart rate. Use the following formulas to determine your target heart rate range:
  Low end of target heart rate range: ____________ × 0.64 = ____________
  (maximum heart rate)
  High end of target heart rate range: ____________ × 0.74 = ____________
  (maximum heart rate)
- If you perform sporadic physical activity right now, aim for a target heart rate of about 74–84% of your maximum heart rate. Use the following formulas to determine your target heart rate range:
  Low end of target heart rate range: ____________ × 0.74 = ____________
  (maximum heart rate)
  High end of target heart rate range: ____________ × 0.84 = ____________
  (maximum heart rate)
- If you perform regular physical activity right now, aim for a target heart rate of about 80–91% of your maximum heart rate. Use the following formulas to determine your target heart rate range:
  Low end of target heart rate range: ____________ × 0.80 = ____________
  (maximum heart rate)
  High end of target heart rate range: ____________ × 0.91 = ____________
  (maximum heart rate)

MEASURING YOUR HEART RATE

While you exercise, take your pulse by placing your first two fingers (not your thumb) on the side of your neck next to your windpipe. Using a clock or watch, take your pulse for 6 seconds and then multiply that number by 10. The result will be your number of heartbeats per minute, which is your heart rate.

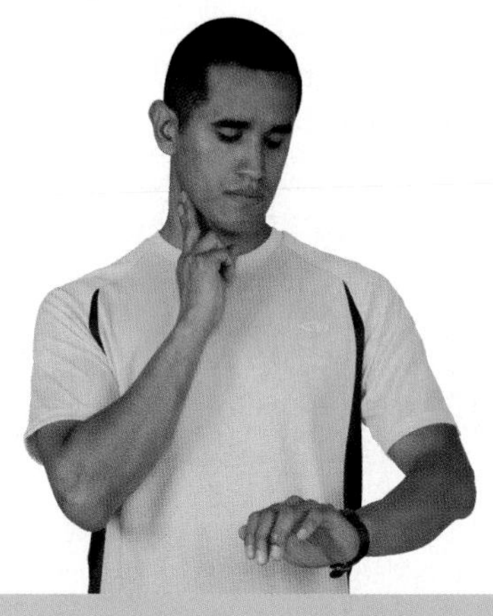

HOW TO INTERPRET YOUR SCORE

- Some cardiorespiratory equipment in gyms, such as stair climbers, offer real-time heart rate calculators, but you can easily track your heart rate using the measurement method above.
- If your heart rate is below your target heart rate range, increase your intensity until you are in your target range; if your heart rate is above your target heart rate range, reduce your intensity.
- There are several methods for calculating maximum heart rate and target heart rate ranges. The formula presented above is the ACSM's most accurate method; some organizations or online calculators may calculate your target heart rate range differently.

References: 1. *ACSM's Guidelines for Exercise Testing and Prescription* (8th edition, p. 155), by the American College of Sports Medicine, 2010, Baltimore, MD: Wolters Kluwer/Lippincott Williams & Wilkins. 2. Ibid., pp. 166–167.

aerobic session, and to follow other safety precautions for exercise. See pages 158–163 for more about warming up, cooling down, and safety.

Incorporating Aerobic Exercise into Your Daily Life

Dedicated time for aerobic exercise is important, but building cardiorespiratory fitness doesn't hinge on lots of time at the gym. Even engaging in activity for as little as 10 minutes can be an effective way to get more exercise into your life. Simple changes, such as doing some errands on foot instead of in the car, can quickly add up to significant aerobic exercise.

Walking. Consider using your feet to get to class or go to the store. If you don't have time for a long walk, try breaking your time on foot into shorter stretches that fit into your daily routine. One study that compared women who walked briskly for longer single stretches (one 30-minute walk per day) or shorter multiple ones (three 10-minute walks per day), for example, found that both groups of women achieved similar and significant improvements in fitness and decreased levels of body fat.[28] In another study of young men, 10 three-minute brisk walks per day were as effective at lowering resting blood pressure and levels of fats in the blood after meals as one longer walk.[29]

Taking the Stairs. Opting for the stairs over the escalator or elevator on a regular basis can make a real difference. In one study at a university hospital where workers frequently had to move between floors, employees who were relatively inactive were encouraged to take the stairs more often. Over the 6-month study, the group logged the equivalent of about 20 flights of stairs per day, a significant increase over their typical four flights of stairs per day. After 3 months, participants had improved their aerobic capacity and decreased their waist circumference, weight, body fat, blood pressure levels, and blood cholesterol.[30]

Cycling. When you need to travel longer distances, walking isn't always practical. But riding your bike can be a time-saving alternative that is equally healthful. Cycling is great aerobic exercise, as well as a quick (and parking ticket–free!) way to get around many college and university campuses. If safety concerns keep you off your bike, remember that regular use of a helmet and a little defensive riding go a long way toward keeping you safe. In one study that estimated the costs and risks of switching from a car to a bike for short trips, the 3 to 14 months of life expectancy gained far outweighed the estimated 5 to

Table 6.2: Physical Activity Intensities

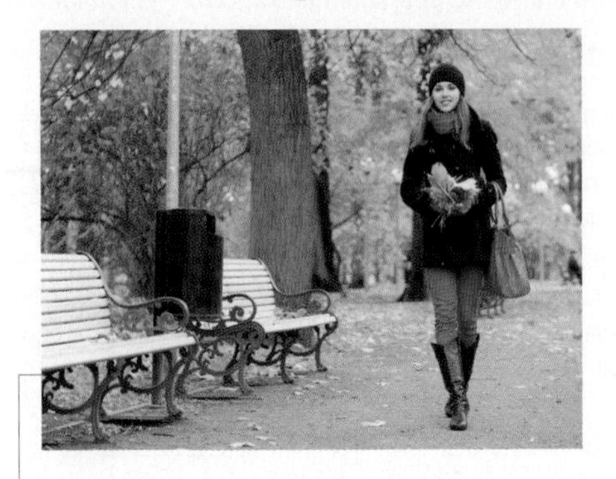	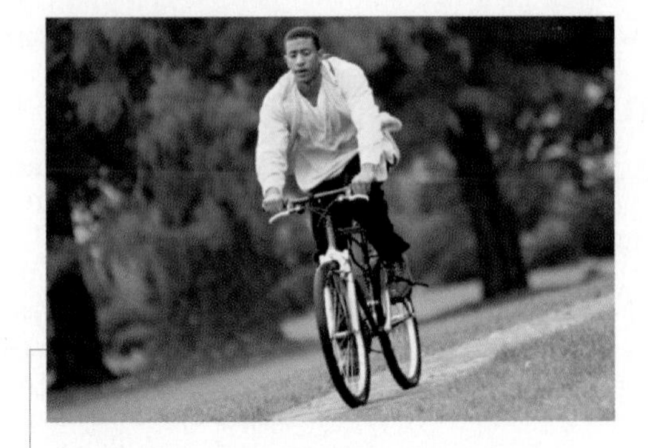	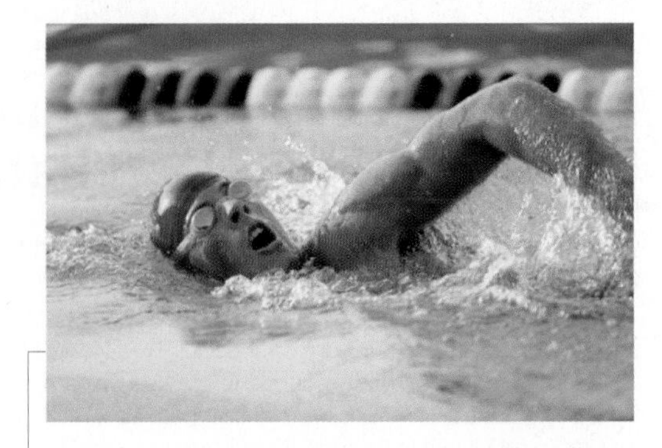
Activity Intensity Level: Lifestyle/light **Heart Rate Range:** Less than 50% maximum heart rate **Examples:** Light yard work and housework, leisurely walking, self-care and bathing, light stretching, light occupational activity **Health Benefits:** A moderate increase in health and wellness in those who are completely sedentary; reduced risk of some chronic diseases	**Activity Intensity Level:** Moderate **Heart Rate Range:** 50–70% maximum heart rate **Examples:** Walking 3–4.5 miles per hour on a level surface, resistance training, hiking, climbing stairs, dancing, doubles tennis, using a manual wheelchair, recreational swimming, water aerobics, moderate yard work and housework **Health Benefits:** Increased cardiorespiratory endurance, lower body fat levels, improved blood cholesterol and pressure, better blood sugar management, decreased risk of disease, increased overall physical fitness	**Activity Intensity Level:** Vigorous **Heart Rate Range:** 70–85% maximum heart rate **Examples:** Jogging, running, basketball, soccer, circuit training, backpacking, aerobics classes, competitive sports, swimming laps, martial arts, singles tennis, heavy yard work or housework, hard physical labor/construction, bicycling 10 miles per hour or faster up steep terrain **Health Benefits:** Increased overall physical fitness, decreased risk of disease, further improvements in overall strength and muscular endurance

Data from **1.** *Physical Activity for Everyone: Target Heart Rate and Estimated Maximum Heart Rate,* by the Centers for Disease Control and Prevention, 2009, retrieved from http://www.cdc.gov/physicalactivity/everyone/measuring/heartrate.html. **2.** *Get Fit, Stay Well!* (2nd edition, brief edition, fig. 2.1, p. 33, by J. Hopson, R. Donatelle, & T. Littrell, 2013, San Francisco: Pearson Benjamin Cummings.

9 days lost to traffic accidents.[31] For more information on safe cycling, see Chapter 20.

Other Types of Aerobic Exercise. No matter what kind of activity you prefer, you are almost certain to find some kind of aerobic exercise you enjoy. If you like being outside, go beyond walking and running to hiking, swimming, or games like Ultimate Frisbee or soccer. If you prefer indoor exercise, try an elliptical trainer, a Zumba class, or an aerobic workout DVD at home. It's easy to make aerobic exercise fun if you find activities that are so enjoyable that the time—and your workout—flies by.

Exercise for Muscular Strength and Endurance

Not all full-body exercises increase cardiorespiratory fitness. Short, intense activities, such as sprint running, sprint swimming, or heavy weight lifting, usually require more oxygen than the body can take in and deliver quickly. As a result, the muscles develop an oxygen deficit and you tire in a short amount of time. However, these **anaerobic exercises** increase your body's ability to deliver short bursts of energy and build muscular strength.

Many people think building muscle means increasing the amount of weight you can lift—in other words, building strength. But endurance is also an important component of muscular fitness. Strength allows you to lift that heavy box when you move to your next apartment, but muscular endurance will let you carry it all the way out to the moving truck without straining your shoulders or wrenching your back.

In order to build muscle, the muscle must work against some form of resistance—this is called *resistance training* or *strength training*. There are several ways to create resistance that your muscles can work against: free weights (such as dumbbells or barbells), weight machines, resistance bands, or even using your own body weight. You can perform a variety of different exercises with free weights, resistance bands, and your own body weight, whereas weight machines are usually designed for only one or two specific exercises. Weight machines, however, promote correct movement and safe lifting and allow you to easily change the amount of resistance or pinpoint specific muscles.

Isometric versus Isotonic

You can do several different types of exercises while your muscles work against resistance. In **isometric exercise,** the muscle contracts but there is no visible movement. This is accomplished by working against some immovable form of resistance such as your body's own muscle (pressing the palms together) or a structural item (pushing against a door frame). It is most helpful to hold isometric contractions for 6–8 seconds and to perform each exercise 5–10 times. During **isotonic exercise,** muscle force is able to cause movement. The tension in the muscle remains unchanged, but the muscle length changes. Performing a biceps curl with a free weight, walking up stairs, and punching a punching bag are examples of isotonic exercises.

anaerobic exercise Short, intense exercise that causes an oxygen deficit in the muscles.

isometric exercise Exercise where the muscle contracts but the body does not move.

isotonic exercise Exercise where the muscle contraction causes body movement.

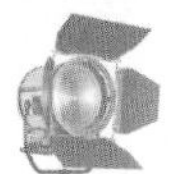

SPOTLIGHT

Core Concerns: Why You Should Strengthen Your Core

Your core muscles run the entire length of your torso, stabilizing the spine, pelvis, and shoulders. They also provide a solid foundation for movement of the arms and legs and make it possible for you to stand upright, move on two feet, balance, and shift movement in any direction. Standing upright and walking around on two feet is not easy on your body. A strong core distributes the stresses of bearing your weight and protects the back.

Weak core muscles can compromise the appropriate curvature of your spine, often resulting in low back pain and other injuries. The greatest benefit of core strength is increased functional fitness—the fitness that is essential to both daily living and regular activities. Core strength can be built through exercises such as abdominal curls, planks, back extensions, Pilates, and any other exercises that work core muscles.

Watch a video about core training at www.webmd.com/fitness-exercise/video/core-strengthening-tips.

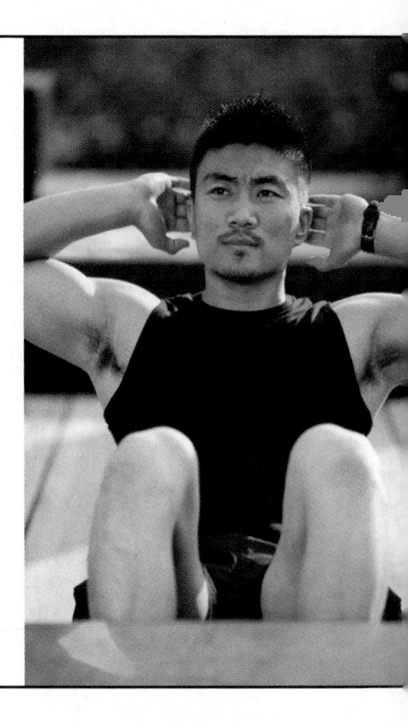

Repetitions and Sets

When developing your resistance training program, you should decide on the numbers of sets and repetitions that you will do for each exercise. **Repetitions** are the number of times you perform the exercise continuously. **Sets** are separate groups of repetitions. The numbers of sets and repetitions to do depends on whether you are trying to build strength or endurance. Strength develops best when you do a few repetitions (approximately 8–12) with heavier weights or more resistance. Endurance develops best when you do more repetitions (approximately 15–25) with lighter weights or less resistance. Increase the amount of resistance once you can easily perform the desired number of repetitions.

Training Tips

When participating in a resistance training program, be sure to follow these guidelines:

- Use proper technique when performing weightlifting exercises. See **Practical Strategies for Health: Safe Weight Lifting** on page 152.
- Because resistance exercises are specific to the particular muscles they are designed for, be sure to include exercises for all the major muscle groups.
- Rest for 2–3 minutes between sets. If you are building muscular endurance you can slightly shorten the time between sets.[26]
- Vary your resistance training routine from time to time to lessen the risk of injury and keep your workouts from getting dull. You'll also want to revisit your program as you get stronger. Finally, you may need different levels or types of resistance training to preserve fitness and muscle mass as you get older.

Keep a log of your workouts so you can be sure to allow each muscle group adequate recovery time. Try these online logs: www.tweetyourhealth.com, www.wellsphere.com, www.sparkpeople.com, https://www.supertracker.usda.gov/physicalactivitytracker.aspx.

repetitions The number of times you perform an exercise repeatedly.

sets Separate groups of repetitions.

recovery The period necessary for the body to recover from exercise demands and adapt to higher levels of fitness.

static flexibility The ability to reach and hold a stretch at one endpoint of a joint's range of motion.

dynamic flexibility The ability to move quickly and fluidly through a joint's entire range of motion with little resistance.

static stretching Gradually lengthening a muscle to an elongated position and sustaining that position.

Figure 6.2 on pages 150–151 shows examples of some simple resistance exercises you can perform.

Recovery

Once you've begun a resistance program, be sure to allow overloaded muscle at least 48 hours for repair and **recovery** before another exercise bout. However, because muscles begin to atrophy after about 96 hours, don't let too much time pass without another training session. If different muscle groups are worked on different days (for example, lower body versus upper body), it is acceptable to perform resistance exercise on consecutive days as long as each muscle group receives the recommended 48 hours of recovery time.

Exercises for Improving Flexibility

There are two major types of flexibility. **Static flexibility** is the ability to reach and hold a stretch at one endpoint of a joint's range of motion. **Dynamic flexibility** is the ability to move quickly and fluidly through a joint's entire range of motion with little resistance. Static flexibility determines whether a martial artist can reach her leg as high as her opponent's head, but it is dynamic flexibility that would enable her to kick her leg that high in one fast, fluid motion. Flexibility can vary a lot among individuals, but everyone can increase his or her flexibility through consistent stretching exercises.

Stretching

Stretching applies gentle, elongating force to both a muscle and its connective tissue. **Static stretching,** the most common form of stretching, involves a gradual stretch and then hold of the stretched position for a certain amount of time. Static stretching

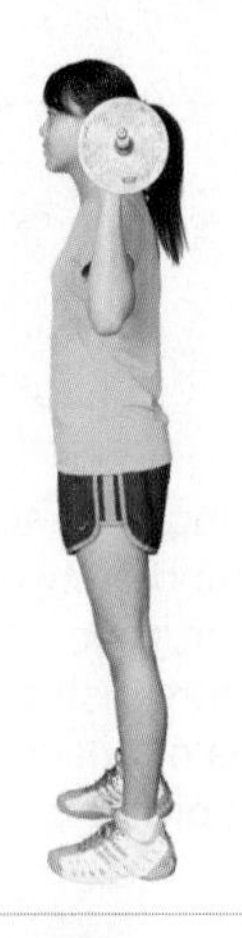

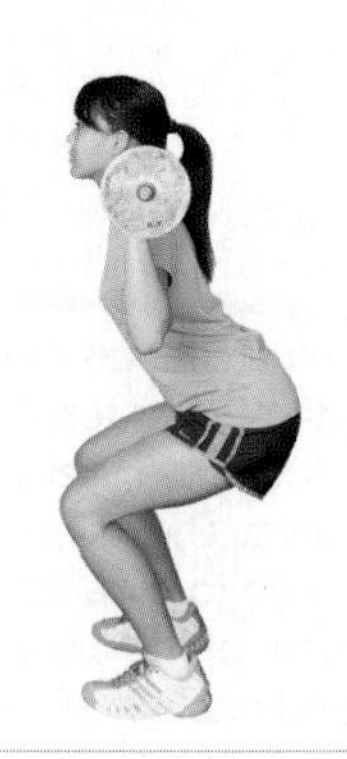

(a) Squat
Stand with feet shoulder-width apart, toes pointing forward, hips and shoulders aligned, abdominals pulled in. Bend your knees and lower until you have between a 45- and 90-degree angle. Keep your knees behind the front of your toes. Contract your abdominals while coming up.

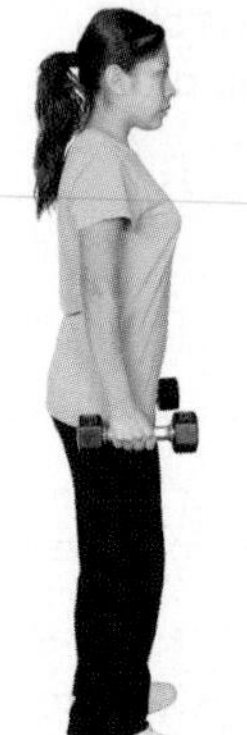

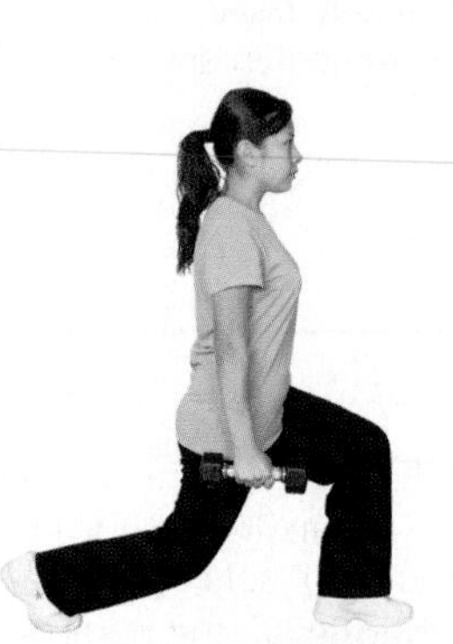

(b) Lunge
Stand with feet shoulder-width apart. As you step forward, keep your front knee in line with your ankle; make sure the front knee does not extend over your toes. Distribute your weight evenly between the front and back leg.

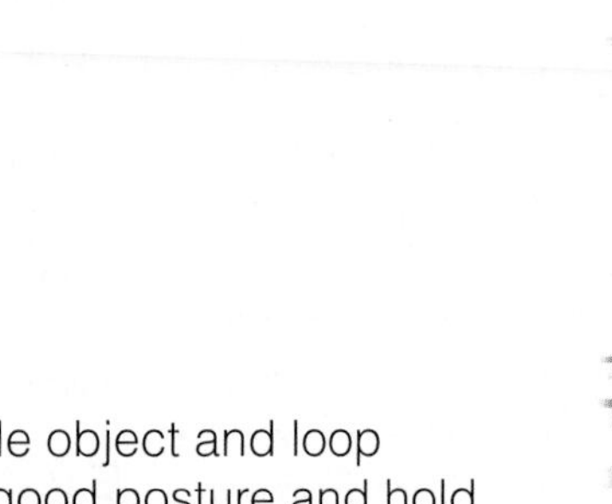

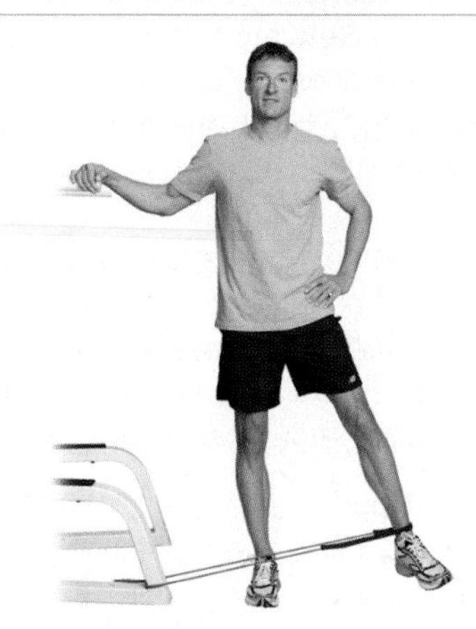

(c) Hip Abduction
Connect a resistance band to a stable object and loop around your outside leg. Stand with good posture and hold onto something stable. Slowly extend your leg out and return.

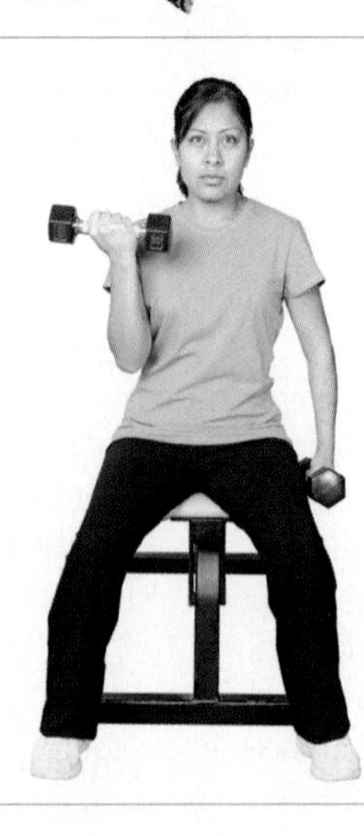

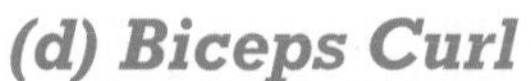

(d) Biceps Curl
Sit on a bench or chair with a dumbbell in each hand. Sit with good posture (ears and shoulders over hips and abdominals contracted) and your feet planted on the ground for balance. Lift one dumbbell up to your shoulder, turning your palm toward your shoulder as you lift. Slowly lower the dumbbell to the starting position as you lift the dumbbell in your other hand.

Figure 6.2 **Simple resistance exercises.** Be sure to perform exercises equally on both sides.

(e) Curl-up

Lie on a mat with your arms by your sides, palms down, elbows straight, and fingers extended. Bend your knees at about 90-degrees. Curl your head and upper back upward, reaching your arms forward, then curl back down so that your upper back and shoulders touch the mat. During the entire curl-up, your feet and buttocks should stay on the mat.

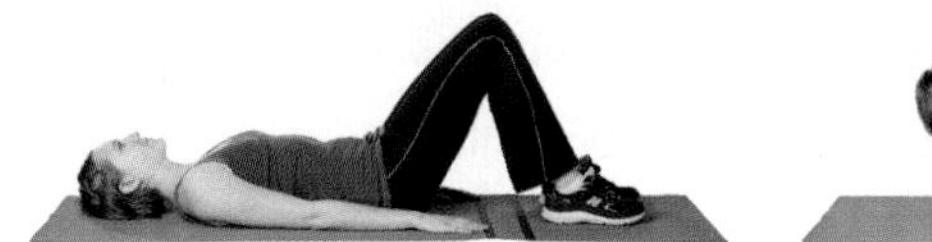
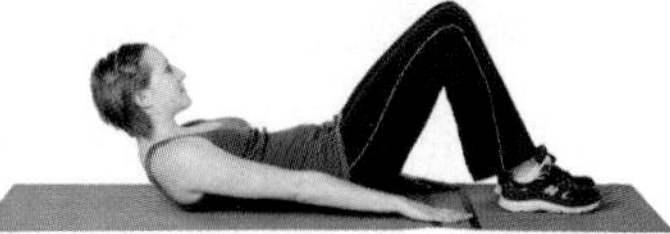

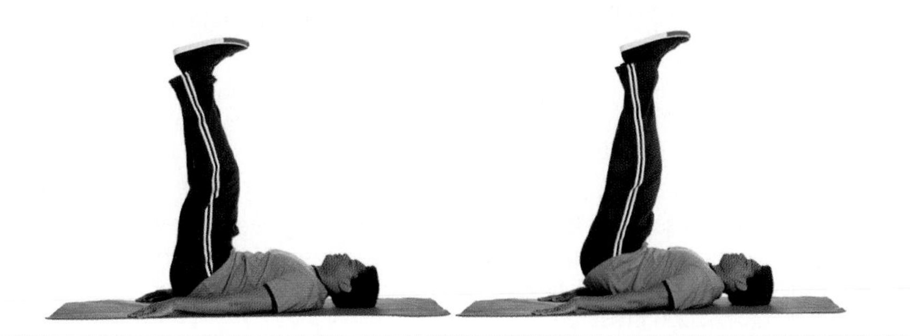

(f) Reverse Curl

Lie on your back and place your hands near your hips. Lift your legs to 90-degrees from the floor. Your knees may be bent or straight. Contract your abdominals, pulling them in, while you lift your hips off the floor. Slowly return hips to floor. Be careful not to rock back and forth.

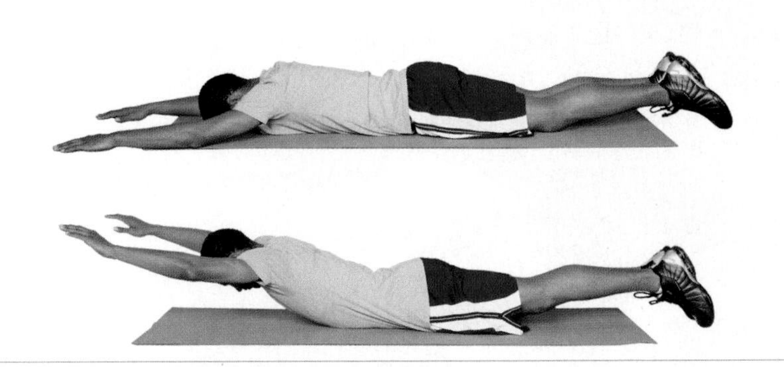

(g) Back Extension

Start lying on your stomach with your arms and legs extended, forehead on the floor. Lift and further extend your arms and legs using your back muscles. Hold for 3–5 seconds and slowly lower back down.

(h) Plank

Support yourself in plank position (from the forearms or hands) by contracting your trunk muscles so that your neck, back, and hips are completely straight. Hold for 5–60 seconds, increasing time as you become stronger. Your forearms should be slightly wider than your shoulders.

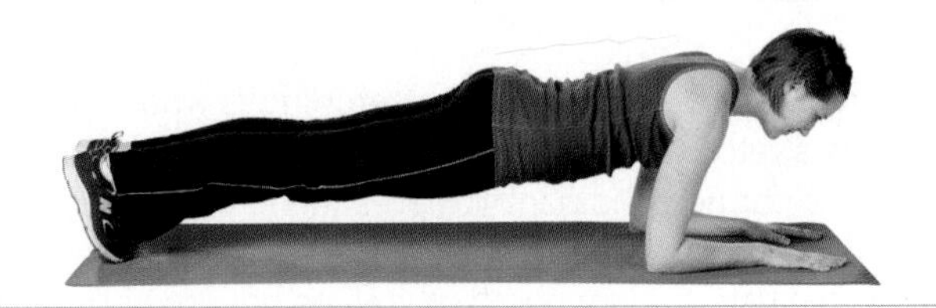

(i) Modified Push-Ups

Support yourself in push-up position as shown by contracting your trunk muscles. Place hands slightly wider than your shoulders. Keep your neck, back, and hips completely straight; do not let your trunk sag in the middle or raise your hips. Slowly lower your body down toward the floor, being careful to keep a straight body position. Your elbows will press out and back as you lower to a 90-degree elbow joint. Press yourself back up to start position.

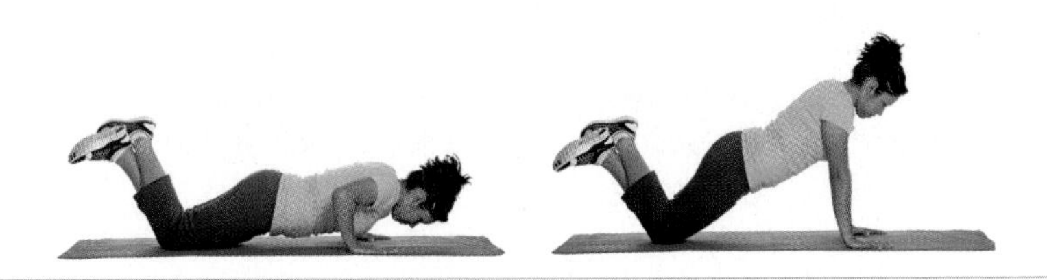

Practical Strategies for Health

Safe Weight Lifting

- If you are just beginning to use weights, make an appointment with a fitness specialist who can teach you the proper techniques that reduce the risk of injury and maximize the benefits you receive.
- Always warm up before weight lifting.
- Take your time and lift mindfully.
- Breathe out as you lift the weight and in as you release the weight—don't hold your breath, as that can cause dangerous increases in blood pressure.
- Focus on the muscle you're trying to work. Feel the effort in the muscle, not in the joint.
- Equally train opposing muscle groups, such as the lower back and abdomen or the biceps and triceps.
- Use only the amount of weights that your body can handle without having to cheat by using other muscles or momentum.
- When using free weights, always have a partner who can check your form and "spot" for you.

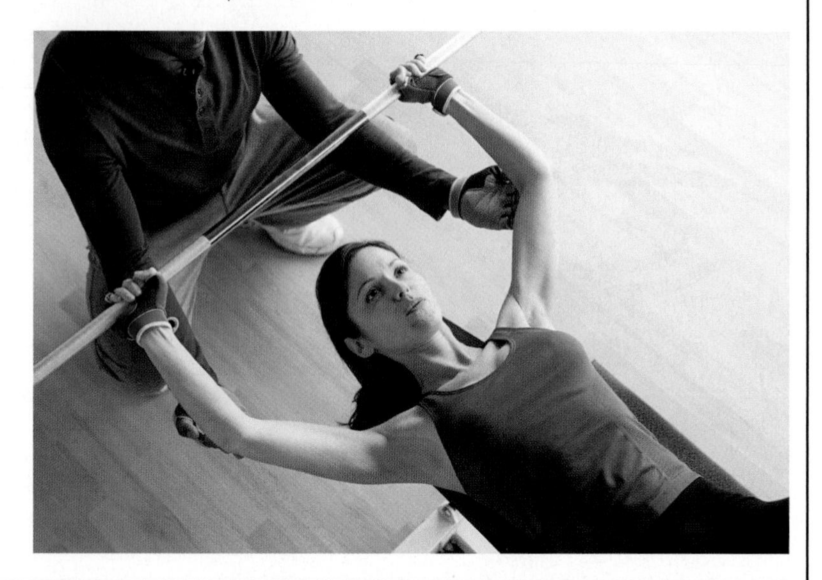

can be either active or passive. **Active stretching** is where you apply the force for the stretch. **Passive stretching,** on the other hand, is performed with a partner who gently applies the force to the stretch. Passive stretching may provide a more intense flexibility workout but also increases the risk of injury because you are not controlling the stretch yourself. **Ballistic stretching** focuses on the use of dynamic repetitive bouncing movements to stretch a muscle beyond its normal range of motion. If ballistic stretching is performed improperly, it can increase the risk of injury, so it is best for recreational exercisers to avoid this form of stretching.[32] **Dynamic stretching,** or slow movement stretching, incorporates movements performed in a controlled manner that mimic a specific sport or exercise and are often included during the warm-up or in preparation for a sports event. An example in soccer would be gently swinging a leg back and forth as if to kick an imaginary ball.

Flexibility varies for each joint, and flexibility exercises are specific to the joint they're designed for, so when creating a flexibility program, be sure to stretch all the major muscle and joint areas of the body (neck, shoulders, upper and lower back, pelvis, hips, and legs). Also, stretching cold muscles is not a good idea. Instead, warm up muscles by walking or jogging or some other low-intensity activity for at least 5 minutes prior to stretching, or stretch at the end of your workout. The following tips will help you create a flexibility program for yourself:[33]

- Hold static stretches for 10–30 seconds.
- Perform 2 to 4 repetitions of each stretch, accumulating 60 seconds per stretch.
- Stretch at least 2 to 3 days per week.
- Stretch until your muscle feels tight or until there is slight discomfort.
- Do not hold your breath while stretching. Try to relax and breathe deeply.
- Do not lock your joints while stretching.

Holistic Flexibility Programs

In addition to regular stretching exercises, there are several other types of mind- and whole body–centered activities that increase flexibility. These types of activities are also sometimes referred to as *neuromotor exercise*, or workouts designed to improve balance and agility. Three of the most popular are yoga, Pilates, and tai chi:

- **Yoga.** Yoga moves you through a set of carefully constructed poses designed to increase flexibility and strengthen your body. Yoga also focuses on mood and thought, using techniques such as breathing exercises to encourage reduced stress and anxiety. Many people start yoga in a class setting, gradually developing their own personal yoga practices.
- **Pilates.** Pilates combines stretching and resistance exercises to create a sequence of precise, controlled movements that focuses on flexibility, joint mobility, and core strength. Many movements in Pilates are performed on an exercise mat, but some require a machine called a Reformer, which can be found at many gyms. Because Pilates movements are so precise, it is recommended to begin Pilates in a group or private class rather than on your own.
- **Tai chi.** Tai chi is a Chinese practice designed to work the entire body gently through a series of quiet, fluid motions. The discipline also focuses on your energy, referred to in Chinese as "chi" (sometimes spelled "qi") or life force. The practice aims to keep a participant's body and chi in balance, requiring a focus on mood and thought.

You can find classes for yoga, Pilates, tai chi, and other flexibility-improving programs through private studios, community centers, and campus wellness centers. **Figure 6.3** on pages 153–154 shows simple flexibility exercises you can easily perform on your own as well.

Visit the iTunes store and search for podcasts on topics like running, action sports, yoga, or activities in the great outdoors.

active stretching A type of static stretching where you gently apply force to your body to create a stretch.

passive stretching Stretching performed with a partner who increases the intensity of the stretch by gently applying pressure to your body as it stretches.

ballistic stretching Performing rhythmic bouncing movements in a stretch to increase the intensity of the stretch.

dynamic stretching A type of slow movement stretching in which activities from a workout or sport are mimicked in a controlled manner, often to help "warm up" for a game or event.

been linked to many high-profile controversies among professional athletes. Androstenedione is illegal for sale or use in the United States, and its side effects include breast development and impotence in men, abnormal periods and facial hair in women, and liver disease and blood clots.

- **Ephedra.** Typically used to boost energy and promote weight loss, ephedra has such serious adverse effects that the U.S. Food and Drug Administration has banned its sale in the United States. Research has not shown ephedra to be effective in boosting energy or athletic performance, and its side effects include high blood pressure, irregular heartbeat, stroke, gastrointestinal distress, and psychological problems.[48]

Change Yourself, Change Your World

Improved fitness is as much a public health goal as it is a personal one. Some of the factors that contribute to one's level of fitness reflect individual choice—whether to drive or cycle, watch TV or go outside, spend time online or spend time at the gym. But the communities in which we live also play a key role. Getting fit starts with you, but through the choices you make, you have the potential to help improve the lives of those around you as well.

Personal Choices

In the busy life of a student, scheduling regular exercise may seem daunting. But if you set goals, find activities you enjoy, think about how you will overcome obstacles, and periodically reassess your progress, you'll be able to stay motivated, have fun, and enjoy the benefits of fitness.

Set Realistic Goals

One of the most important aspects of a fitness program is working at an intensity and rate that makes sense for you. Trying to reach too high a level of strength or stamina too quickly can be dangerous and discouraging. It is important to realistically assess your current fitness level (see the **Self-Assessment** on the next page) in order to set fitness goals that are appropriate. Fitness goals can be based on a specific activity-related improvement you want to make, such as cycling 40% farther than you currently can; a health-related goal you may have, such as reducing your blood pressure or increasing your energy; or a social or lifestyle desire, like preparing for a backpacking trip with your friends. Make sure your goals are easily measurable, so you can clearly tell when you've met one.

"One key to sticking with exercise is to schedule in exercise as you would a job or a class. If you have a set time devoted to exercise, you will be more likely to stick with it."

Write down your goals and track your progress toward them. It is helpful to break down long-term goals into smaller short-term goals, and build toward your larger goal over time. For example, if your goal is to meet the *Physical Activity Guidelines for Americans*' recommended aerobic activity levels, but you haven't worked out in years, you should begin with smaller goals. Your goals could look like this:

Goal: Perform 150 minutes of moderate-intensity activity each week.

Subgoal 1: Perform 30 minutes of brisk walking twice a week for 2–3 weeks.

Subgoal 2: Add to the walking program by attending a 45-minute low-impact cardio class once a week.

Subgoal 3: After 1 month to 6 weeks of the walking and cardio class program, add 45 minutes of working out on the stationary bike at the gym each week. 150 minutes of activity attained!

If you don't make a particular goal you have set, don't get discouraged. Take that chance to reevaluate your goal and possibly break it down into smaller subgoals.

Take this self-assessment for a quick idea of how fit you are: www.nhs.uk/Tools/Pages/Fitness.aspx.

Find Activities You Enjoy

To exercise on a regular basis, focus on physical activities you naturally enjoy. Ask yourself which of those activities will help you reach the fitness goals you have set for yourself, which ones you are most likely to stick with, which ones will fit most easily into your schedule, and which ones you can afford. Don't be afraid to mix it up—a wide range of activities can bring you all the benefits of fitness and will stave off boredom. If you can only afford to take tennis lessons twice a month, combine that with free aerobics classes at school and resistance exercises you can perform at home.

Schedule Time

One key to sticking with exercise is to schedule in exercise as you would a job or a class. If you have a set time devoted to exercise, you will be more likely to stick with it. See Step 3 of the **Choosing to Change Worksheet** at the end of this chapter for a schedule where you can plan activity.

Team Up!

Find a friend or family member with similar fitness goals and make plans to work out together on a regular basis. You'll not only enjoy the company and extra motivation to stay on track, but may achieve greater health benefits. One study found that people with regular workout partners, especially workout partners who'd received a significant amount of fitness training and coaching, lost more weight compared with those who trained alone.[49]

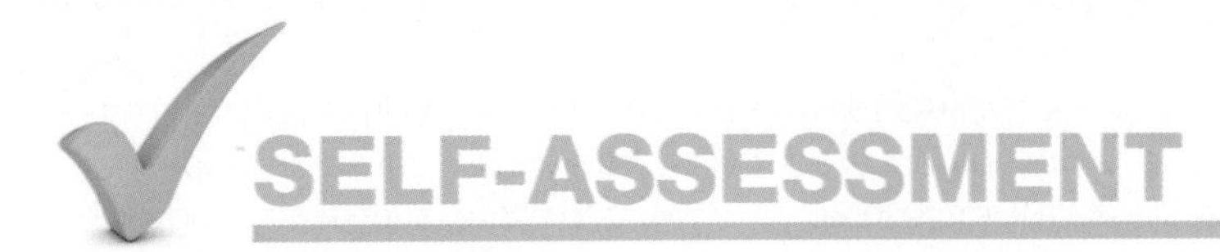

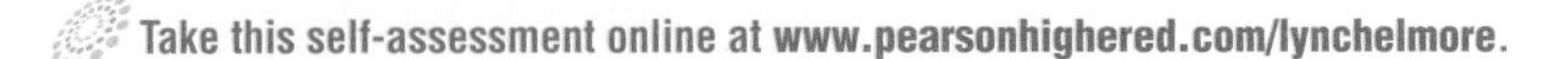

Fitness Testing at Home

The following home fitness tests are designed to quickly gauge a person's general fitness level with minimal equipment. When performing the tests, wear loose, comfortable clothes and comfortable athletic shoes for walking. Do each test with plenty of rest between so that you are fully recovered. Do a warm-up first. A general warm-up procedure for your testing is to walk briskly for 5 to 10 minutes. The tests are listed in recommended order.

1. **Push-Up Test: Assesses upper body muscular endurance.** Assume the standard position for a push-up, with the body rigid and straight, toes tucked under and hands about shoulder-width apart and straight under the shoulders. Lower the body until the elbows reach 90 degrees. Return to the starting position with arms fully extended. Complete as many pushups as you can in 1 minute, or until failure without any break in proper form. Record your number _______.
2. **Crunches or Sit Up Test: Assesses core strength and stability.** Lie on a carpeted floor or an exercise mat. Assume the starting position for a crunch with bent knees at approximately right angles, feet flat on the floor, and hands resting on your thighs. Slide your hands along your thighs until your fingers touch the top of your knees while keeping your lower back on the floor. Return to the starting position. Do not pull with your neck or head. Complete as many crunches as you can in 1 minute, or until failure without any break in proper form. Record your number _______.
3. **Chair Squat Test: Assesses lower body muscular endurance.** Stand in front of a chair with your feet at shoulder width apart, facing away from it. Place your hands on your hips. Squat down as if you are going to take a seat in the chair. Lightly touch the chair with your buttocks before standing back up. Keep your weight in your heels and do not let your knees shoot past your toes. Select a chair size that allows your knees to rest at 90 degrees when you are sitting. Complete as many squats as you can in 1 minute, or until failure without any break in proper form. Record your number _______.
4. **Sit-and-Reach Test: Assesses hamstring and lower back flexibility and upper back flexibility.** You'll need a yardstick and masking tape to perform this assessment. Put the yardstick on the floor and place a 12-inch piece of tape perpendicular across the yardstick at the 15-inch mark. Sit with your legs on either side of the yardstick with your heels on the piece of masking tape. The zero end of the yardstick should be closest to your body. Keeping your legs extended straight in front of you, your knees straight but not locked, and your feet slightly apart, reach forward with both hands, bending at hips. At the point of your greatest reach, hold for a couple of seconds, and measure how far your fingertips on the yardstick have touched. If you can touch your toes, your reach is 15 inches. If you can touch 2 inches past your toes, your reach is 17 inches. Record your number _______.
5. **One-Mile Walk Test: Assesses cardiorespiratory fitness.** Find a flat measured track or a flat street near your home. Make sure you know how far you need to walk to reach 1 mile. Walk the mile as fast as you can, keeping a steady pace without feeling strained. At the end of the mile, record your time in minutes and seconds: _______ minutes _______ seconds.

HOW TO INTERPRET YOUR SCORES

Use the results as a benchmark for future testing. Set fitness goals based on what you've learned. For example, you may want to set a goal of being able to touch your toes if you currently cannot. The Choosing to Change Worksheet at the end of the chapter will assist you in setting goals. You may want to track your progress by taking these assessments again after you have participated in a fitness program for 4 weeks and then again after 8 weeks.

Overcome Obstacles

You can probably come up with a long list of reasons for why you do not already have a regular fitness routine. Here are some common obstacles and solutions for overcoming them:

- **I don't have time.** Remember that only 30 minutes of moderate exercise a day can improve or maintain your fitness and that time can be broken down into 10-minute sessions. Substituting exercise for TV or computer time, even just a little, is a good place to start. If you don't have time to make it to a gym, find activities you can do at home, such as walking, jogging, jumping rope, lifting free weights, or doing exercise videos. Another tactic is to combine exercise with social time: Get a buddy to exercise with you, or sign up for a recreational team with friends.
- **I have kids, so I *really* have no time.** If you are both a student and a parent, you face a tough time crunch when it comes to exercise. One study comparing students who were parents with those who weren't found that only 16% of parent-students performed enough physical activity, compared with 50% of other students.[50] If you have children, get exercise by actively playing with them. Some gyms also offer free or inexpensive child care, or you can trade babysitting with a friend and use that time for exercise.
- **I don't know how.** If you feel like a klutz at the gym, start by walking or running on your own. If you don't know how to play a particular sport, take a class. Consider working with a personal trainer, who will build your skills with lots of one-on-one attention. Many campus wellness centers offer low-cost personal training and classes.
- **I don't want to go to the gym.** If working out on the machines isn't your thing, try alternative exercises, like joining a dodgeball or kickball team, rock climbing, snowboarding, Ultimate Frisbee, golf, or even using video games designed for fitness, like the Wii Fit™.
- **I'm embarrassed about how I look.** If you aren't ready to hit the campus pool in a bathing suit, start with activities where you'll be comfortable in sweat pants and a T-shirt. Also, seek out exercise environments in which you feel comfortable and supported (for example, a fitness center designed for women only, or a class designed for weight loss).
- **I don't have anywhere to exercise.** If your neighborhood and campus don't make it easy to be active, find a space in your community that does, such as a community recreation center. Remember, too, that you can exercise in the comfort of your own living room with an exercise video.
- **I don't have the money.** If you can't afford a gym membership, choose exercises that require no more than a good pair of shoes, such as walking or running. Or, purchase low-cost equipment like exercise bands, exercise balls, dumbbells, or a jump rope. Your campus or community recreation center may have free or low-cost gyms or classes. See **Consumer Corner: No-Cost Exercise Equipment** on page 166 for tips on how to create equipment from everyday items.

Safe Exercise for Special Populations

Exercise can do everyone good. If you have health concerns, the key is to modify your fitness program to reduce risk and maximize the benefits you receive. The following measures can help.

Asthma

- If prescribed, use pre-exercise asthma inhalers before beginning exercise.
- Extend your warm-up and cool-down to help your lungs prepare for and recover from exercise.
- Check for environmental irritants that could promote an asthma attack, such as a recently mowed lawn, high pollen counts, or high levels of air pollution, and consider exercising indoors at those times. If exercising in cold weather, cover your mouth and nose with a scarf or mask.
- Try swimming. The warm, moist environment is soothing, and swimming helps build cardiorespiratory endurance.
- If you begin to cough, wheeze, have difficulty breathing, or have tightness in your chest, halt exercise and use your inhaler or other prescribed medication.

Pregnancy

- Avoid contact sports or activities that may cause trauma or a fall. Walking and swimming are great low-impact options, but you can also dance, run, or hike.
- You can still perform resistance exercises. Focus on muscular endurance exercises rather than strengthening exercises.
- Halt exercise if you experience vaginal bleeding, dizziness, headache, chest pain, calf pain or swelling, preterm labor, or decreased fetal movement.
- After the first trimester, avoid exercises in which you lie on your back; they can reduce blood flow to the uterus.

Obesity

- Start by focusing on low-intensity aerobic activity, and gradually increase duration. At the beginning of your program, the frequency and duration of the activity is more important than the intensity.
- Aim for exercising 4 or 5 days a week for 30 to 60 minutes. If you haven't been exercising, these sessions can be broken up into three 10-minute sessions, with gradual increases in duration.
- Engage in activity that puts minimal stress on the joints, such as walking, swimming or water exercises, and cycling.
- Be especially careful about heat exhaustion. Wearing light clothing will allow for better heat exchange while exercising.
- Be sure to drink fluids frequently before, during, and after exercise.
- Slow down or stop if you experience chest pains, shortness of breath, palpitations, nausea, pain in the neck or jaw, or major muscle or joint pain.

High Blood Pressure

- If you have high blood pressure, it's critical that you design your exercise program in consultation with your health-care provider. A typical program will begin with 20 to 30 minutes of gentle cardiorespiratory exercise every other day, and will increase in frequency, intensity, and duration as you gain strength and fitness.
- If you'd like to follow a strength training program, you'll need to practice extra caution, as some weight lifting can cause a temporary jump in blood pressure. Don't hold your breath when lifting weights. Try lifting lighter weights for more repetitions, rather than lifting a heavy weight just a few times. Stop your session if you become dizzy, lose your breath, or experience chest pain. Talk to your doctor before beginning a strength training program.
- Start your workout slowly and be sure to cool down afterward. Stop your exercise session and seek medical attention right away if you experience any warning signs of high blood pressure complications, such as dizziness, chest pain, or shortness of breath.

Diabetes

- Monitor your blood glucose before and after exercise, especially when beginning or modifying your exercise program.
- Wear a diabetes ID bracelet during exercise.
- Carry a snack if you will be active for a few hours.
- If you begin to feel shaky, anxious, or suddenly begin to sweat more, halt exercise and consume a fast-acting carbohydrate.
- Make sure to wear well-fitting shoes and check your feet for blisters or sores before and after exercise.

Older Adults

- Improved balance is an especially important fitness goal for older adults, who are at greater risk of injury from falls. Try to do balance training, such as heel walking and sideways walking, at least three times a week. Many senior centers offer balance training. Regular *tai chi* can also help improve balance.
- Even if you have a chronic condition, such as arthritis, regular exercise is beneficial to your overall health and may also help improve or manage your condition. Talk to your doctor about an exercise program that's right for you.
- If you can't manage a longer workout, remember that shorter episodes of exercise done several times a day can also be beneficial.

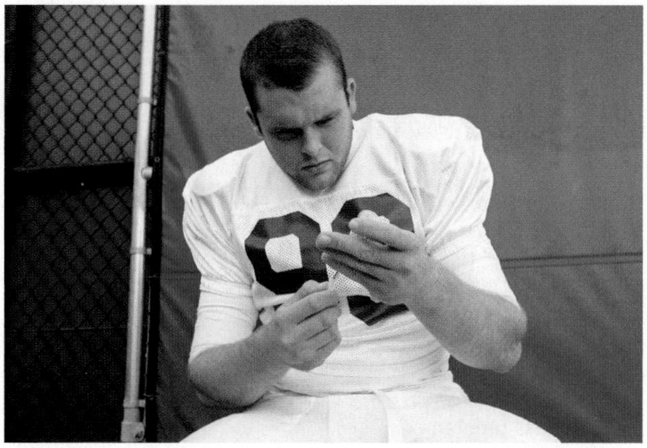

This college football player with diabetes is preparing an insulin injection for himself.

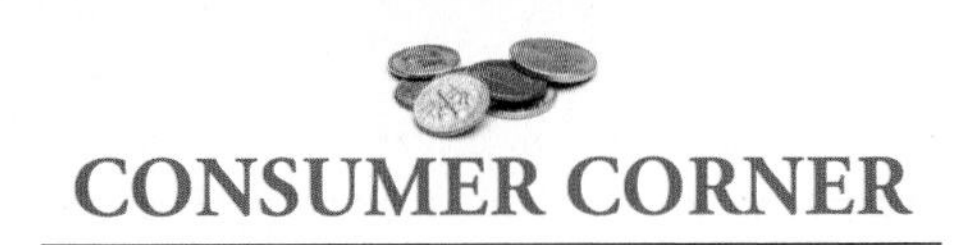

CONSUMER CORNER

No-Cost Exercise Equipment

Don't have the money to join a gym or buy a home exercise machine? Try improvising equipment from ordinary household items.

- **Canned goods.** Use canned goods in place of free weights when doing arm and shoulder exercises.
- **Milk or water jugs.** Fill empty jugs with water or sand and secure the tops with duct tape. You can weigh the jugs on a scale to see how much you're lifting, and adjust the weight as you get stronger by adding more water or sand.
- **Stairs.** Are there stairs in your home or building? Try using them for calf raises, or walk up and down them for the original "stair master." Or, use the bottom stair as a step platform and choreograph a step routine.
- **Step stools.** A low, sturdy step stool can become a step platform as well.
- **Door jambs.** Stand in the middle of an open doorway and press against each side with your hands for an isometric arm workout.

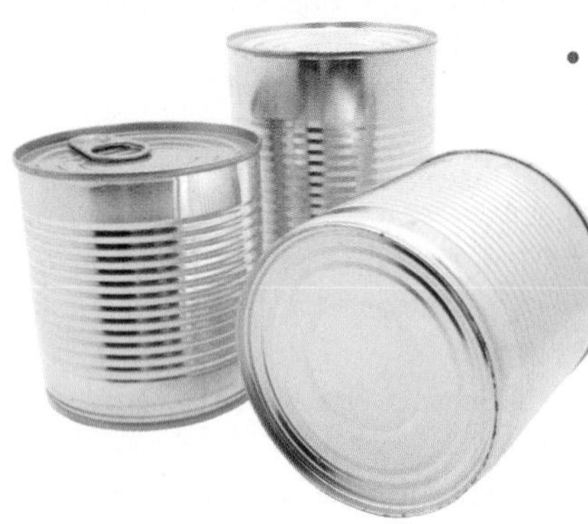

Source: Adapted from *Fitness for Less: 4 Low-Cost Ways to Shape Up*, by the MayoClinic.com, 2008, retrieved from http://www.mayoclinic.com/health/fitness/HQ00694_D.

- **I live in a place with bad weather.** If snow, frequent rain, or high heat and humidity make exercising outside tough, look for indoor options. Consider exercise videos and free weights at home. Find a gym. If you just want to walk, check the hours at your local shopping mall. Some malls now open their doors in the early morning, long before the shops open, to give walkers a comfortable place to stroll.

Assess Your Progress

Every 4 to 6 weeks, look back and assess how far you've come. Periodically evaluating your progress can be highly motivating. Look back on all the exercise you've done, think about the positive effects on how you feel or how fit you are becoming, and evaluate how close you are to the goals you set. At the beginning of an exercise program you may want to assess your progress even more often.

Campus Advocacy

Through your own fitness efforts, you'll also learn a key fact firsthand: Your surrounding community has a direct effect on physical activity. Do your campus and community have sidewalks, pathways, and trails that make walking safe and easy? What about bike lanes and bike paths? Are there accessible, affordable sports facilities, gyms, and pools? Are at least a few stores, coffee shops, and restaurants accessible by foot or bike, or are they all marooned in distant shopping centers ringed by parking lots?

All across the country, citizens of all ages have worked together to start creating communities that make physical activity an easier part of everyday life. Look around your campus and surrounding community, and see if any of the following types of projects need a leader or more support. Any one of these three projects is a great place to start:

- Walkability: One of the best ways to assess pedestrian ease and safety is to take a walk with a child, or at least through the eyes of a child, as a child's perspective helps you assess pedestrian safety in a very direct way. Did you have room to walk safely, away from cars and traffic? Was it easy to cross streets? Did drivers behave well? Was your route enjoyable? If you and your younger companion were left stressed by the experience of dodging traffic or trying to find a pleasant path, get involved in community efforts to put people on foot. Go to **WalkingInfo.org** (**www.walkinginfo.org/library/details.cfm?id=12**) for ideas on fixing problems.

STUDENT STORY

Adapting Exercise to My Needs

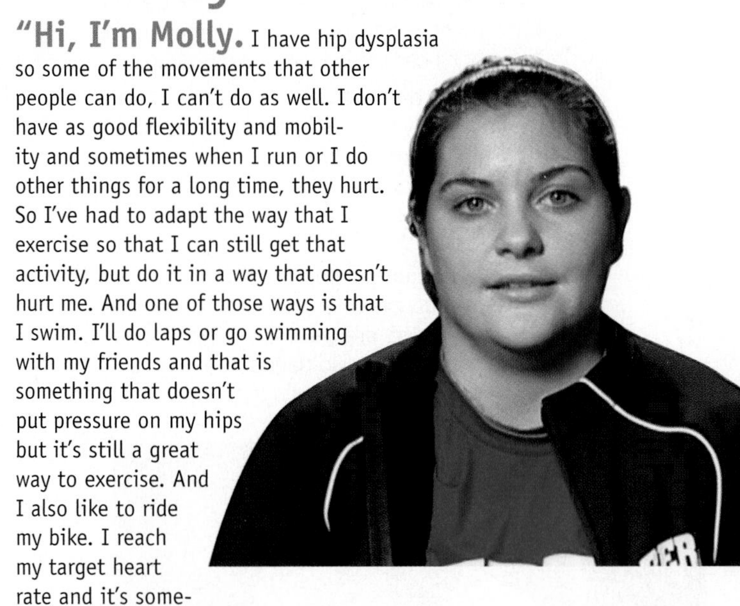

"Hi, I'm Molly. I have hip dysplasia so some of the movements that other people can do, I can't do as well. I don't have as good flexibility and mobility and sometimes when I run or I do other things for a long time, they hurt. So I've had to adapt the way that I exercise so that I can still get that activity, but do it in a way that doesn't hurt me. And one of those ways is that I swim. I'll do laps or go swimming with my friends and that is something that doesn't put pressure on my hips but it's still a great way to exercise. And I also like to ride my bike. I reach my target heart rate and it's something that I can do just as well as anyone else."

1: Molly figured out how to structure an exercise program around her needs. Do you have any needs—physical or otherwise—that you want to structure your exercise around? How will you go about doing that?

2: Exercising with friends and varying your exercise activities, as Molly does, can help you stay motivated. What else will help you stay motivated with your fitness program?

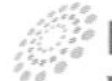

Do you have a story similar to Molly's? Share your story at www.pearsonhighered.com/lynchelmore.

- Start or join a bicycle club: You don't have to aspire to the Tour de France to have fun riding with a group. Across the country, bicycle clubs meet regularly to cycle local streets, raise awareness of the rights and needs of cyclists, and advocate for community improvements that make cycling safer and easier. Visit the League of American Bicyclists for ideas on starting a club (**www.bikeleague.org/action/creategroup**). If your campus doesn't provide incentives for cyclists, such as reduced tuition or other fees for students who bring a bike rather than a car to campus, start advocating for them.
- Find fitness improvement projects in your community and share their stories to help inspire others and drive change. Students at the University of North Carolina did just that through a campus television and video effort looking at programs to create more physically active communities in their state. See their work at **www.unctv.org/ncnow/fitcommunity/index.html**.

Watch videos of real students discussing physical activity and fitness at www.pearsonhighered.com/lynchelmore.

Choosing to Change Worksheet

To complete this worksheet online, visit www.pearsonhighered.com/lynchelmore.

In this chapter you have learned about the importance of physical fitness. To improve your overall fitness, follow the steps below.

Directions: Fill in your stage of behavior change in Step 1 and complete the rest of the worksheet with your stage of change in mind.

Step 1: Your Stage of Behavior Change. Please check one of the following statements that best describes your readiness to improve your overall fitness.

____ I do not intend to improve my overall fitness in the next 6 months. (Precontemplation)

____ I might improve my overall fitness in the next 6 months. (Contemplation)

____ I am prepared to improve my overall fitness in the next month. (Preparation)

____ I have been improving my overall fitness for less than 6 months. (Action)

____ I have been improving my overall fitness for more than 6 months. (Maintenance)

In order to create and maintain a fitness program you should set goals, find activities you enjoy, schedule time, overcome obstacles, and assess your progress.

Step 2: Creating and Maintaining a Fitness Program.

1. What are your fitness goals? Do you want to run 5 miles? Touch your toes? Bench press a specific weight? Something else? Make sure the goals are specific, focused, and easily measurable, and set a realistic timeline for your goal. If your goal is large, break it down into smaller subgoals.

Goal:____ Timeline:____

Subgoal 1:____________________________________ Timeline:____

Subgoal 2:____________________________________ Timeline:____

Subgoal 3:____________________________________ Timeline:____

2. What activities do you enjoy that could help you meet your fitness goals? Think about activities that you honestly like, that you have relatively easy access to, and that you can afford. Write down all the activities that meet these criteria. Remember, participating in more than one type of activity will help you combat boredom.

____

____

3. Think about times in your week when you can perform a minimum of 10 minutes of exercise. Factor in travel to and from your workout location. Write down all the times when exercise is possible.

____

____

4. What obstacles might you face in adhering to a fitness program and what could you do to combat them? See pages 164–166 for tips.

Obstacle	**How to Overcome**

5. Once you have been working out for a few weeks, take some time to reflect on how your workout has affected you. Write down the improvements you see and feel.

Physical improvements:

Mental improvements:

Step 3: Scheduling Time for Fitness. How do you find time to get enough exercise? One of the best ways is to write it down in a schedule as you would for any other commitment. Fill out the table below to create an exercise schedule for yourself.

Type of Activity	Monday	Tuesday	Wednesday	Thursday	Friday	Saturday	Sunday	Recommended Minimum Amount
Aerobic Exercise								150 minutes moderate intensity OR 75 minutes vigorous intensity OR Equivalent combination of both
Resistance Training								2 days per week in sets of 8–12 reps
Flexibility Exercise								2–3 days per week for at least 10–30 seconds per stretch

Chapter Summary

- Physical fitness is the ability to perform moderate- to vigorous-intensity physical activity and to be able to respond to physical demands without excessive fatigue.
- The five key components of health-related fitness are cardiorespiratory fitness, muscular strength, muscular endurance, flexibility, and body composition.
- Physical activity builds the health of your heart and lungs. It also lowers your risk of certain diseases, increases immunity, helps your bones stay strong, helps protect you from injury, helps you manage your weight, and helps you cope with stress and improve mental health.
- The principles of fitness training are overload, specificity, reversibility, and individuality.
- A well-rounded fitness program should include a mix of activities that build your cardiorespiratory fitness, work your muscles, and increase your flexibility.
- You need at least 150 minutes of moderate-intensity or 75 minutes of vigorous-intensity aerobic activity each week, or an equivalent mix of the two. You also need 2 to 3 days of resistance training and flexibility exercise per week. You may also want to consider 2 to 3 days of neuromotor exercise per week. Increased amounts of activity each week will promote greater health benefits and build endurance, strength, and flexibility.
- In addition to engaging in regular physical activity, limit sustained sitting, which has been found to be harmful and can even increase the risk of death. If you find yourself sitting for extended periods of time, get up and move around at least every 30 minutes.
- If you haven't exercised for a while, you can meet activity recommendations by starting slowly and looking for ways to build from there. If you already work out, you can meet or exceed recommendations by exercising longer, more often, or at a greater intensity. If you are overweight or obese, it is especially important to add activity to your life, focusing first on regular low-intensity aerobic activities.
- You can avoid injury while you exercise by taking some simple precautions, such as getting medical clearance, warming up and cooling down, getting instruction, wearing suitable clothes, eating right, staying hydrated, preparing for hot or cold weather, selecting facilities and equipment carefully, starting slowly, caring for your injuries, and being wary of performance-enhancing drugs.
- To maintain fitness habits, remember to set measurable goals, focus on activities you enjoy, schedule time, find ways around obstacles, and assess your progress.
- You may find that your workouts are more successful and enjoyable if you spend time with others. Team up with a friend to exercise, help start a fitness program on campus, or get involved in efforts to build more physical activity into your school's everyday life.

Test Your Knowledge

1. Which one of the following is NOT a component of physical fitness?
   a. cardiorespiratory fitness
   b. muscular strength
   c. flexibility
   d. balance

2. Muscular strength
   a. does not help your bones.
   b. is the same thing as muscular endurance.
   c. is important for performing extended activities.
   d. is the maximum force your muscles can apply in a single effort.

3. Body composition
   a. refers to your ratio of fat to lean tissue.
   b. only matters in weight loss.
   c. can be changed by physical activity.
   d. Choices a and c are both correct.

4. People who are overweight
   a. shouldn't exercise, because it can hurt their joints.
   b. should focus on flexibility rather than cardiovascular fitness.
   c. should begin a fitness program with light-intensity physical activity.
   d. don't need to exercise but should focus on their diets.

Get Critical

What happened:

When the 2011 lineup for major league baseball's Milwaukee Brewers was announced, most of the players on the roster were in their 20s. But in the high-pressure role of relief pitcher, one pitcher's age stood out at 41. Takashi Saito, who also goes by "Sammy," is originally from Japan, and didn't start pitching in the major leagues in the United States until he was 36. Saito had a successful 14-year career in Japanese baseball before being recruited to come play across the Pacific, and has said he won't let age stop him from making the most of his time in the major leagues. "I definitely wanted to be in those kind of pressure situations," Saito said in a media interview.[1] In the United States, he has pitched successfully for four major league teams, and despite being older than many other players, has even made the All-Stars.

What do you think?

- **Saito has been playing baseball for decades. What activities would you like to participate in throughout your life?**
- **Striving to play in the major leagues helped Saito stay motivated. What kinds of goals will help you stick with a fitness program for the long term?**

Reference: **1.** "Braves Add Saito to Rebuilt Bullpen," *Atlanta Journal-Constitution*, December 3, 2009, retrieved from http://www.ajc.com/sports/atlanta-braves/braves-add-saito-to-224709.html.

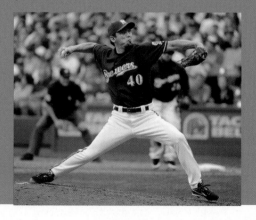

5. Students under a lot of stress
    a. shouldn't exercise, because it will just take time they don't have.
    b. can get stress relief from working out.
    c. are better off in the gym than working out on their own.
    d. won't be able to stick to an exercise program.

6. The principle of individuality means that
    a. you should only do one type of exercise during each workout.
    b. you need to do exercises in different orders each day to get the full benefit.
    c. you can improve only one component of fitness at a time.
    d. each individual adapts to exercise differently.

7. Aerobic exercise
    a. is not recommended for everyone.
    b. builds your cardiorespiratory fitness.
    c. requires expensive equipment, such as a mountain bike.
    d. can only be done in cardio classes.

8. If you were to find yourself getting really hot, nauseated, and faint during a workout, you should
    a. stop, find a cool spot, and drink water.
    b. keep going—this means you are getting a good workout.
    c. keep going if your friends or teammates are.
    d. stop and dial 9-1-1.

9. Sports drinks
    a. should only be used with light exercise.
    b. provide the vitamins you need to keep exercising.
    c. can be used during prolonged exercise.
    d. are always a good idea when working out.

10. To make exercise a habit, you should
    a. focus on physical activities that make you happy.
    b. do activities you don't like, because you need work in those areas.
    c. buy a lot of expensive equipment; it will motivate you to work out.
    d. work out at the highest possible intensity so you get fit quickly.

Get Connected

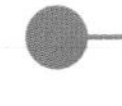

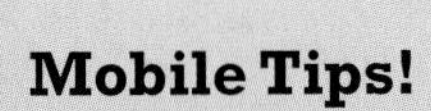

Mobile Tips!

Scan this QR code with your mobile device to access additional physical activity and exercise tips. Or, via your mobile device, go to **http://mobiletips.pearsoncmg.com** and navigate to Chapter 6.

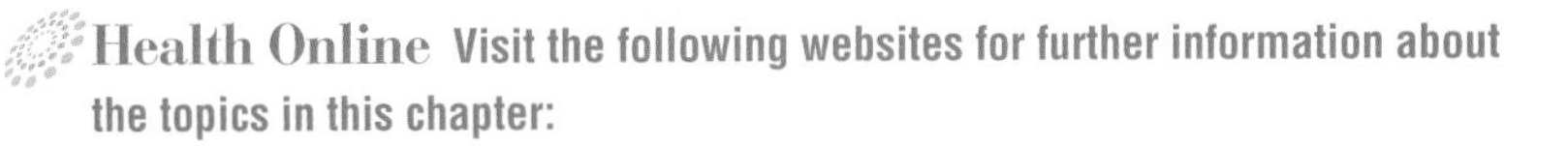

Health Online Visit the following websites for further information about the topics in this chapter:

- American College of Sports Medicine Public Resources
  www.acsm.org/access-public-information
- American Council on Exercise
  www.acefitness.org
- Start! Walking Program for Individuals, American Heart Association
  http://startwalkingnow.org
- President's Challenge Program: The Active Lifestyle Activity Log
  www.presidentschallenge.org/tools-resources/docs/PALA_log.pdf

Website links are subject to change. To access updated web links, please visit ***www.pearsonhighered.com/lynchelmore***.

References

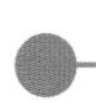

i. Centers for Disease Control and Prevention. (2008). *Physical activity for everyone: Physical activity and health.* Retrieved from http://www.cdc.gov/physicalactivity/everyone/health/index.html.

ii. Aerobically unfit young adults on road to diabetes in middle age. (2009, June 20). *ScienceDaily*. Retrieved from http://www.sciencedaily.com/releases/2009/06/090618124944.htm.

iii. Liu-Ambrose, T., Nagamatsu, L. S., Graf, P., Beattie, B. L., Ashe, M. C., & Handy, T. C. (2010). Resistance training and executive functions: A 12-month randomized controlled trial. *Archives of Internal Medicine, 170* (2), 170–178.

1. Centers for Disease Control and Prevention. (2007, November 23). Prevalence of regular physical activity among adults—United States, 2001 and 2005. *Morbidity and Mortality Weekly Report*. Retrieved from http://www.cdc.gov/mmwr/preview/mmwrhtml/mm5646a1.htm?s_cid=mm5646a1_e.

2. William, P. T. (2008). Vigorous exercise, fitness and incident hypertension, high cholesterol, and diabetes. *Medicine & Science in Sports & Exercise, 40* (6), 998–1006.

3. Bushman, B., & Clark-Young, J. (2005). *Action plan for menopause.* Indianapolis, IN: American College of Sports Medicine.

4. Ärnlöv, J., Ingelsson, E., Sundström, J., & Lind, L. (2010). Impact of body mass index and the metabolic syndrome on the risk of cardiovascular disease and death in middle-aged men. *Circulation, 121*, 230–236.

5. Mueller, P. (2007). Exercise training and sympathetic nervous system activity: Evidence for physical activity dependent neural plasticity. *Clinical and Experimental Pharmacology and Physiology, 34,* 377–384.

6. Centers for Disease Control and Prevention. (1999, November 17). *Physical activity and health: A report of the Surgeon General.* Retrieved from http://www.cdc.gov/nccdphp/sgr/sgr.htm.

7. Lee, C., Blair, S., & Jackson, A. (1999). Cardiorespiratory fitness, body composition, and all-cause and cardiovascular disease mortality in men. *American Journal of Clinical Nutrition, 69* (3), 373–380.

8. National Institutes of Health, National Institute of Diabetes and Digestive and Kidney Diseases. (2008, October). *Diabetes prevention program (DPP)* (NIH Publication No. 09-5099). Washington, DC: Government Printing Office.

9. Sigal, R., Kenny, G., Boulé, N., Wells, G., Prud'homme, D., Fortier, M., . . . Jaffey, J. (2007). Effects of aerobic training, resistance training, or both on glycemic control in type 2 diabetes. *American College of Physicians, 147* (6), 357–369.

10. Knowler, W., Barrett-Connor, E., Fowler, S., Hamman, R., Lachin, J., Walker, E., & Nathan, D. M. (2002). Reduction in the incidence of type 2 diabetes with lifestyle intervention or metformin. *New England Journal of Medicine, 346* (6), 393–403.

11. Slattery, M. L. (2004). Physical activity and colorectal cancer. *Sports Medicine, 34,* 239–252.

12. Clarke, C. A., Purdie, D. M., & Glaser, S. L. (2006). Population attributable risk of breast cancer in white women associated with immediately modifiable risk factors. *BMC Cancer, 6,* 170.

13. Dallal, C., Sullivan-Halley, J., Ross, R., Wang, Y., Deapen, D., Horn-Ross, P., . . . Bernstein, L. (2007). Long-term recreational physical activity and risk of invasive and in situ breast cancer: The California teachers study. *Archives of Internal Medicine, 167* (4), 408–415.

14. Nieman, D. C. (2000). Is infection risk linked to exercise workload? *Medicine & Science in Sports & Exercise, 32* (7 Suppl), S406–S411.

15. Medline Plus. (2008). *Exercise and immunity*. Retrieved from http://www.nlm.nih.gov/medlineplus/ency/article/007165.htm.

16. Ondrak, K., & Morgan, D. (2007). Physical activity, calcium intake and bone health in children and adolescents. *Sports Medicine, 37* (7), 587–600.

17. Johansson, M., Hassmén, P., & Jouper, J. (2008). Acute effects of qigong exercise on mood and anxiety. *International Journal of Stress Management, 15* (2), 199–207.

18. Blumenthal, J. A., Babyak, M. A., Doraiswamy, P. M., Watkins, L., Hoffman, B. M., Barbour, K. A., . . . Sherwood, A. (2007). Exercise and pharmacotherapy in the treatment of major depressive disorder. *Psychosomatic Medicine, 69,* 587–596.

19. Sui, X., Laditka, J. N., Church, T. S., Hardind, J. W., Chase, N., Davis, K., & Blaira, S. N. (2009). Prospective study of cardiorespiratory fitness and depressive symptoms in women and men. *Journal of Psychiatric Research, 43* (5), 546–552.

20. Balkin, R., Tietjen-Smith, T., Caldwell, C., & Shen, Y. (2007). The utilization of exercise to decrease depressive symptoms in young adult women. *ADULTSPAN Journal, 6* (1), 30–35.

21. Åberg, M. A. I., Pedersen, N. L., Torén, K., Svartengren, M., Bäckstrand, B., Johnsson, T., . . . Kuhn, H. G. (2009). Cardiovascular fitness is associated with cognition in young adulthood. *Proceedings of the National Academy of Sciences, 106,* 20906–20911.

22. Radak, Z., Hart, N., Sarga, L., Koltai, E., Atalay, M., Ohno, H., & Boldogh, I. (2010). Exercise plays a preventive role against Alzheimer's disease. *Journal of Alzheimer's Disease,* 10.3233/JAD-2010-091531.

23. King, A., Oman, R., Brassington, G., Bliwise, D., & Haskell, W. (2007). Moderate-intensity exercise and self-rated quality of sleep in older adults. A randomized controlled trial. *Journal of the American Medical Association, 277* (1), 32–37.

24. Buman, M., Hekler, E., Bliwise, D., & King, A. (2011). Moderators and mediators of exercise-induced objective sleep improvements in midlife and older adults with sleep complaints. *Health Psychology*, *30* (5), 579–587.

25. Jespersen J. G., Nedergaard A., Andersen L. L., Schjerling P., & Andersen J. L. (2009). Myostatin expression during human muscle hypertrophy and subsequent atrophy: Increased myostatin with detraining. *Scandinavian Journal of Medicine & Science in Sports.* Published online November 9, 2009.

26. American College of Sports Medicine. (2010). *ACSM's guidelines for exercise testing and prescription* (8th edition). Baltimore, MD: Wolters Kluwer/Lippincott Williams & Wilkins.

27. Centers for Disease Control and Prevention. (2009). *Physical activity for everyone: Target heart rate and estimated maximum heart rate*. Retrieved from http://www.cdc.gov/physicalactivity/everyone/measuring/heartrate.html.

28. Murphy, M., & Hardman, A. (1998). Training effects of short and long bouts of brisk walking in sedentary women. *Medicine & Science in Sports & Exercise, 30* (1), 152–157.

29. Miyashita, M., Burns, S., & Stensel, D. (2008). Accumulating short bouts of brisk walking reduces postprandial plasma triacylgylcerol concentrations and resting blood pressure in healthy young men. *American Journal of Clinical Nutrition, 88* (5), 1225–1231.

30. Meyer, P., Kayser, B., Kossovsky, M., Sigaud, P., Carhallo, D., Keller, P., . . . Mach, F. (2010). Stairs instead of elevators at workplace: Cardioprotective effects of a pragmatic intervention. *European Journal of Cardiovascular Prevention and Rehabilitation, 17* (5), 569–575.

31. de Hartog, J., Boogard, H., Nijland H., & Hoek, G. (2010). Do the health benefits of cycling outweigh the risks? *Environmental Health Perspectives, 118* (8), 1109–1116.

32. Smith, J. W. (2004). Flexibility basics: Physiology, research, and current guidelines. *ACSM's Certified News, 14* (3), 7–9.

33. Garber, C., Blissmer, B., Deschenes, M., Franklin, B., Lamonte, M., Lee, I., Nieman, D., & Swain, D. (2011.) Quantity and quality of exercise for developing and maintaining cardiorespiratory, musculoskeletal, and neuromotor fitness in apparently healthy adults: Guidance for prescribing exercise. *Medicine & Science in Sports & Exercise, 43* (7), 1334–1359.

34. Centers for Disease Control and Prevention. (2008). *Physical activity guidelines for Americans*. Retrieved from http://www.health.gov/paguidelines/default.aspx.

35. Ross, R., Dagnone, D., Jones, P. J. H., Smith, H., Paddags, A., Hudson, R., & Janssen, I. (2000). Reduction in obesity and related comorbid conditions after diet-induced weight loss or exercise-induced weight loss in men. *Annals of Internal Medicine, 133,* 92–103.

36. Patel, A., Bernstein, L., Deka, A., Feigelson, H., Campbell, P., Gapstur, S., Colditz, G., & Thun, M. (2010). Leisure time spent sitting in relation to total mortality in a prospective cohort of US adults. *American Journal of Epidemiology, 172*, 419–429.

37. Centers for Disease Control and Prevention. (2008). *Physical activity guidelines for Americans: Be active your way: A guide for adults* (ODPHP Publication No. U0037). Retrieved from http://www.health.gov/paguidelines/adultguide/default.aspx.

38. Mayo Clinic. (2010). Eating and exercise: 5 tips to maximize your workouts. Retrieved from http://www.mayoclinic.com/health/exercise/HQ00594_D.

39. American Dietetic Association. (2009). Position of the American Dietetic Association, Dietitians of Canada, and the American College of Sports Medicine: Nutrition and athletic performance. *Journal of the American Dietetic Association, 109* (3), 509–527.

40. Manore, M. M., Meyer, N. L., and Thompson, J. L. (2009). *Sports nutrition for health and performance,* 2nd ed. Champaign, IL: Human Kinetics.

41. Judelson, D., Maresh, C., Anderson, J., Armstrong, L., Casa, D., Kraemer, W., . . . Volek, J. (2007). Hydration and muscular performance: Does fluid balance affect strength, power, and high-intensity endurance? *Sports Medicine, 37* (10), 907–921.

42. American College of Sports Medicine. (n.d.). Selecting and effectively using a health/fitness facility. Retrieved from http://www.acsm.org/AM/Template.cfm?Section=Brochures2&Template=/CM/ContentDisplay.cfm&ContentID=1534.

43. Hampton, Tracy. (2006). Researchers address use of performance-enhancing drugs in nonelite athletes. *Journal of the American Medical Association, 295* (6), 607.

44. U.S. House of Representatives, U.S. Government Accountability Office, Committee on Oversight and Government Reform. (2007). *Federal efforts to prevent and reduce anabolic steroid abuse among teenagers*. Washington, DC: Government Printing Office.

45. Frederick, D., Sadehgi-Azar, L., Haselton, M., Buchanan, G., Peplau, L., Berezovskaya, A., . . . Lipinski, R. (2007). Desiring the muscular ideal: Men's body satisfaction in the United States, Ukraine, and Ghana. *Psychology of Men and Masculinity, 8* (2), 103–117.

46. MedlinePlus. (n.d.). *Creatine*. Retrieved from http://www.nlm.nih.gov/medlineplus/druginfo/natural/patient-creatine.html.

47. Liu, H., Bravata, D., Olkin, I., Friedlander, A., Liu, V., Roberts, B., . . . Hoffman, A. (2008). Systematic review: The effects of growth hormone on athletic performance. *Annals of Internal Medicine, 148* (10), 747–758.

48. National Center for Complementary and Alternative Medicine. (2009). *Consumer advisory: Ephedra.* Retrieved from http://nccam.nih.gov/news/alerts/ephedra/consumeradvisory.htm.

49. Kumanyika, S., Wadden, T., Shults, J., Fassbender, J., Brown, S., Bowman, M., . . . Wu, X. (2009). Trial of family and friend support for weight loss in African American adults. *Archives of Internal Medicine, 169* (19), 1795–1804.

50. Sabourin, S., & Irwin, J. (2008). Prevalence of sufficient physical activity among parents attending a university. *Journal of American College Health, 56* (6), 680–685.

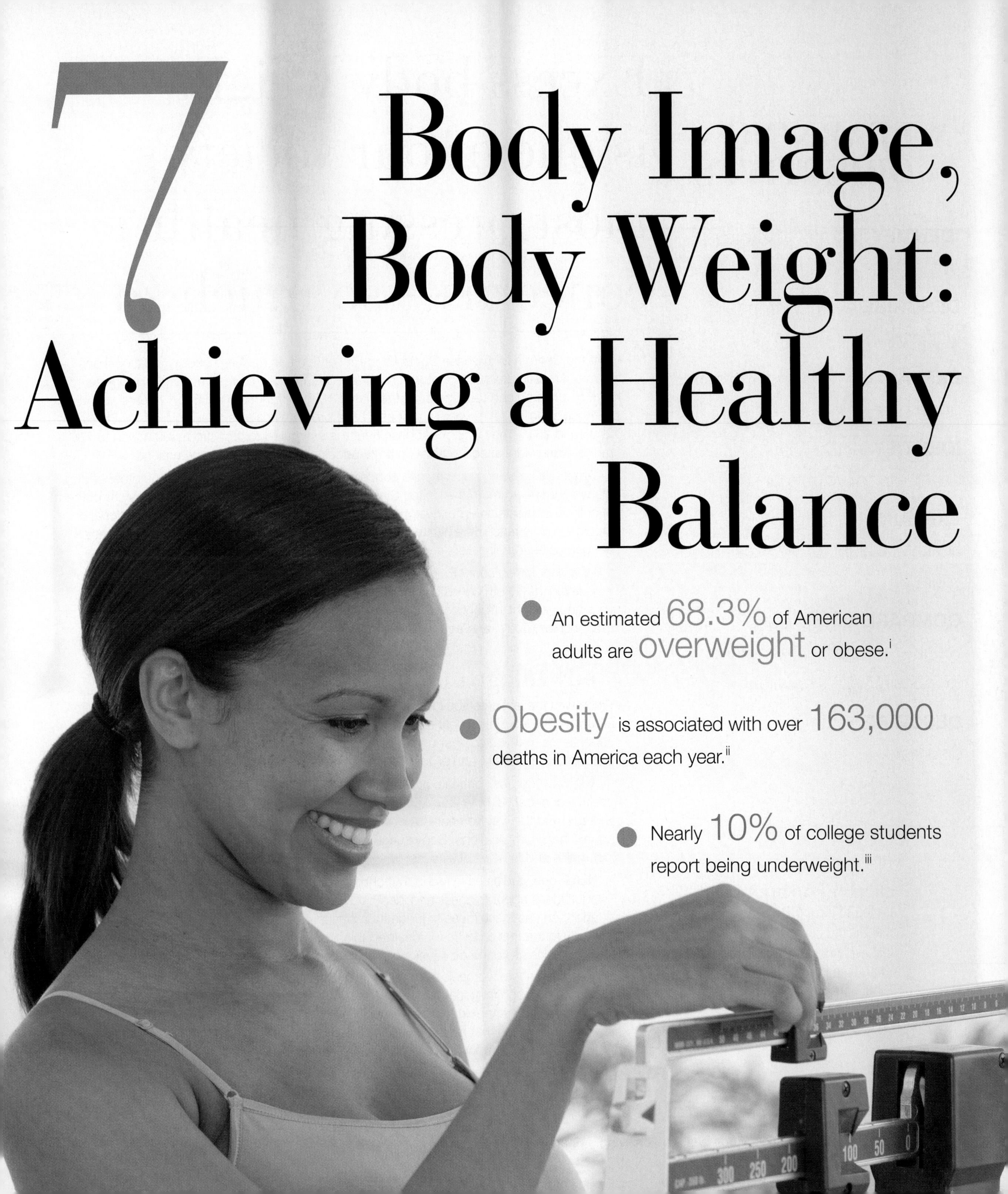

7 Body Image, Body Weight: Achieving a Healthy Balance

- An estimated 68.3% of American adults are overweight or obese.[i]
- Obesity is associated with over 163,000 deaths in America each year.[ii]
- Nearly 10% of college students report being underweight.[iii]

LEARNING OBJECTIVES

IDENTIFY important factors in body image and body weight.

DESCRIBE alarming trends in weight gain.

EXPLAIN the risks and costs of obesity.

IDENTIFY factors that contribute to weight gain.

EXPLAIN how to maintain a healthful weight for yourself and your community.

COMPARE and contrast weight-management programs for obesity and overweight.

DESCRIBE common eating disorders.

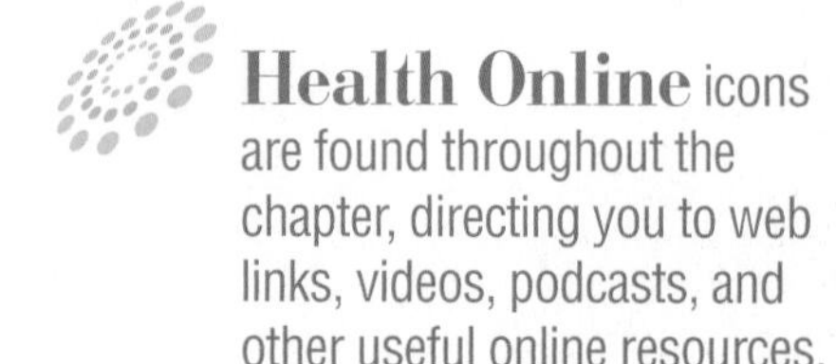
Health Online icons are found throughout the chapter, directing you to web links, videos, podcasts, and other useful online resources.

Excess body weight is one of our society's most pressing health concerns—so much so

that the Centers for Disease Control and Prevention has declared obesity a national epidemic. An estimated 68.3% of American adults over age 20 are **overweight** or **obese.**[1] Among children and teenagers, an estimated 19.6% of those aged 6 to 11 years and 18.1% of those aged 12 to 19 years are obese.[1] The problem is also spreading globally: Between 2005 and 2015, the number of obese adults is estimated to grow from 400 million to 700 million worldwide, affecting those in both industrialized and developing nations.[2]

Amid this pressing public health concern, others face difficult issues at the other end of the weight spectrum. In the United States, nearly 2 percent of adults and almost 10 percent of college students are underweight.[3,4] Some of these individuals may need nutritional or medical help in reaching a healthful weight, while others may be suffering from potentially dangerous eating disorders such as bulimia or anorexia nervosa.

Why should you care? Being overweight or underweight affects your life in a myriad of ways every day. Both conditions increase your risk of disease and early death. Moreover, your body weight influences your self-confidence and self-image, which in turn affects your relationships, goals, and activities—essentially all aspects of your life.

Body Image and Body Weight

When was the last time you looked at your body in a mirror and thought it could be more attractive? When did you last criticize yourself for your body shape or size? Did you use harsh terms that you'd never use to describe a friend? If you are like many of us, those self-criticisms come easily, and all too often.

The way you view, critique, and feel about your own body is called **body image.** Whether positive or negative, how you view your body can shape the way you feel, the way you treat yourself, and the way you eat—all of which have important health implications. Body image concerns affect males and females of all ages:

- Numerous studies have found that children absorb adult ideas about thinness and ideal body type, and then use these ideas to judge themselves. One study found that a desire for idealized thinness begins in girls as young as 6 years old.[5]
- Men often share women's self-criticisms of size and shape, although they may experience them more sharply at different points in their lives. One 20-year-long study found that men's dissatisfaction with their bodies went up with time and age. Women, while persistently displeased with their bodies, were often more critical when they were younger, and become more self-accepting as they grew older.[6]

overweight The condition of having a body weight that exceeds what is generally considered healthful for a particular height. A weight resulting in a BMI of 25 to 29.9.

obese A weight disorder in which excess accumulations of nonessential body fat result in increased risk of health problems. A weight resulting in a BMI of 30 or higher.

body image A person's perceptions, feelings, and critiques of his or her own body.

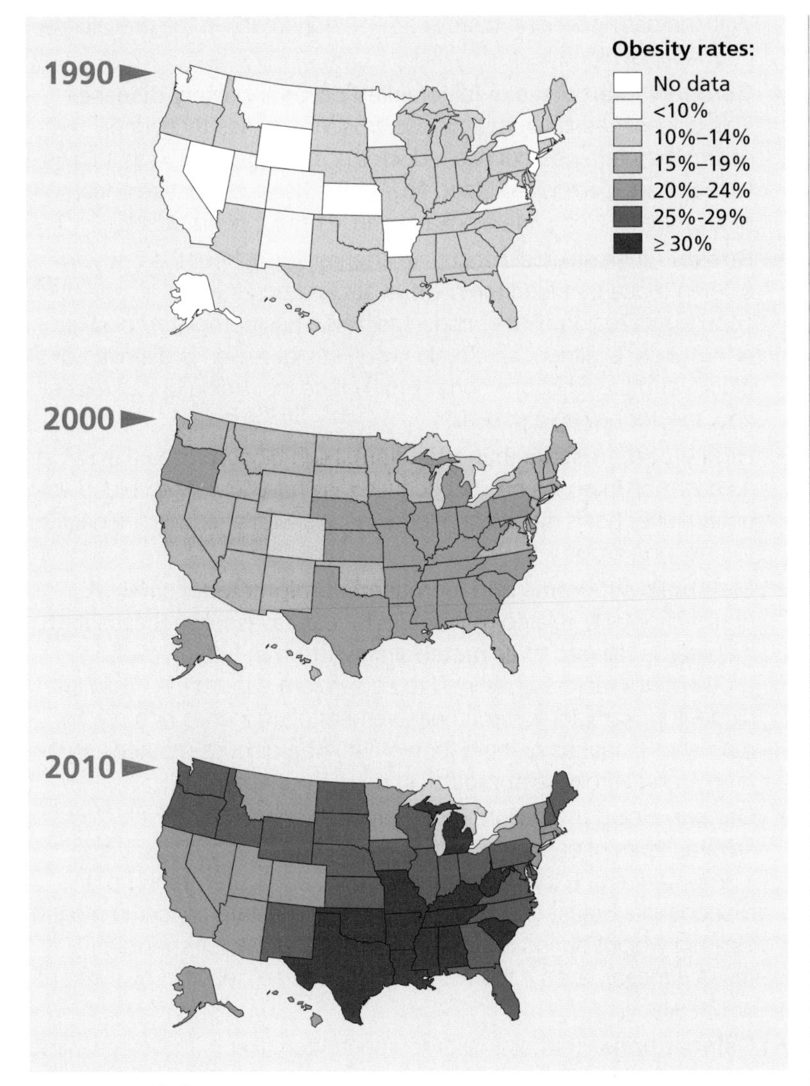

Figure 7.2 Obesity is increasing in the United States.
Data from *U.S. Obesity Trends 1985 to 2010*, by the Centers for Disease Control and Prevention, retrieved from http://www.cdc.gov/obesity/data/adult.html.

your first year. Most students, it turns out, don't gain weight so quickly. But avoiding early weight gain can be a challenge.

Most first-year students do gain some weight once they start college—usually about 7 to 8 pounds.[17] More importantly, this weight often doesn't disappear once the first year is over. Instead, many students gain a few more pounds every year of college. One study found that 23% of students were classified as overweight their first year, and that number grew to about 28% by their fourth year.[18] Male students experienced weight gain more often—about 35% of them qualified as overweight, compared with about 20% of female students. In another survey, about 50% of college students said they were trying to lose weight.[19]

What's the big culprit behind campus weight gain? While excess calories clearly contribute, a decline in physical activity also appears to be a major factor. Female students, for example, often find that their level of physical activity drops substantially in college.[20, 21] For all students, larger amounts of time spent being sedentary and smaller amounts of physical activity have been closely linked with excess weight.[18]

The problem is compounded by the fact that more students are starting college at heavier weights than ever before. About 17% of American adolescents between the ages of 12 and 19 are overweight, compared with 5% in 1970.[22] Another 17% carry enough extra pounds to put them at serious risk of becoming overweight.[22] For many, these problems start during early childhood, with about 14% of children between the ages of 2 and 5 qualifying as overweight.[22] As the number of overweight children climbs, so do cases of childhood diabetes and high blood pressure, conditions once mostly limited to adults. Overweight children are far more likely to carry extra pounds into adulthood.[10]

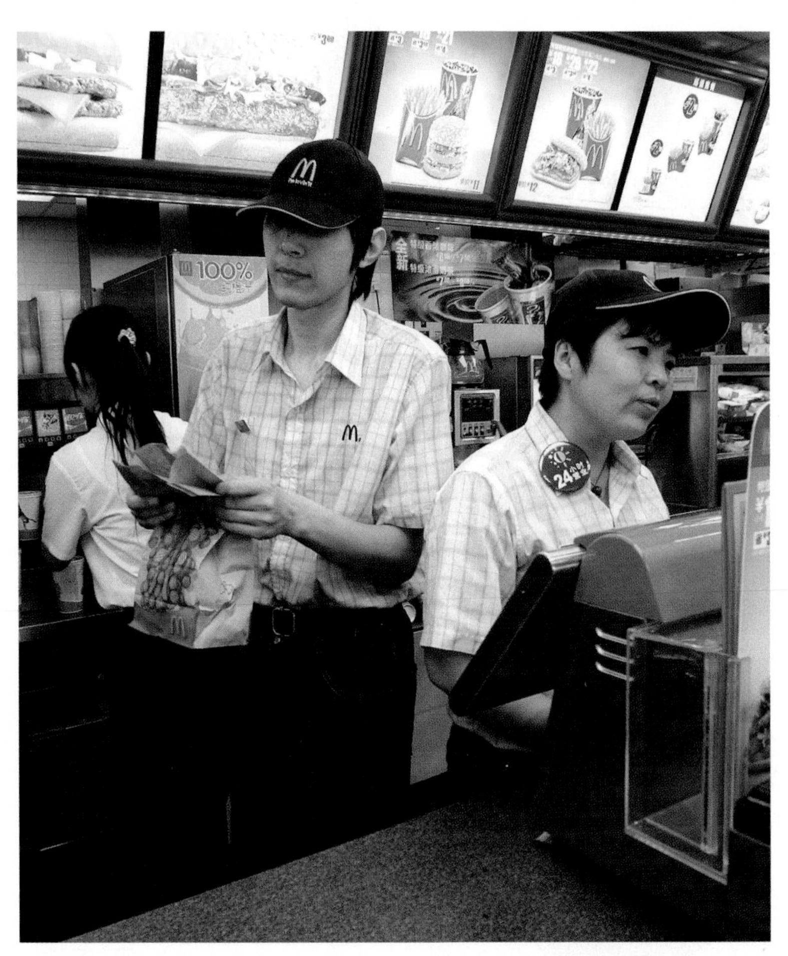

As developing countries adopt more Westernized diets, their rates of **overweight and obesity** are increasing.

Risks and Costs of Obesity

Because overweight and obesity are common, it is easy to underestimate the health risks they pose. You could be tempted to think: How bad can a few extra pounds be, when so many people you know carry some? But just because weight concerns are common doesn't make them any less serious.

Health Risks

Being overweight or obese is associated with many health problems, including:[23, 24]

- **Type 2 diabetes.** Type 2 diabetes is strongly associated with increased body weight. More than 85% of people with type 2 diabetes are overweight or obese.[24] Excess fat makes your cells resistant to

STUDENT STATS

Overweight, Obesity, and Dieting on Campus

22% Students who are overweight[1]

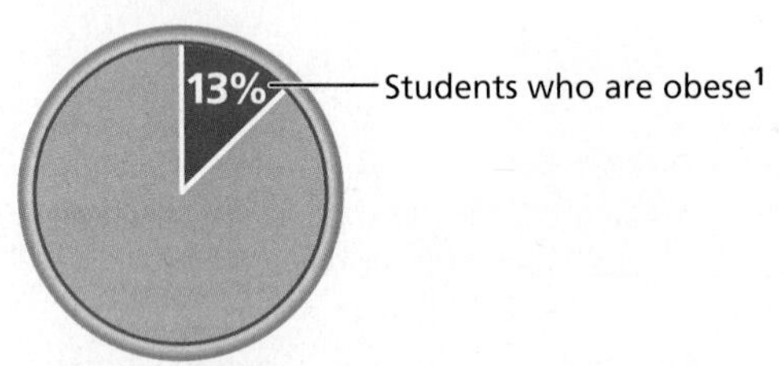

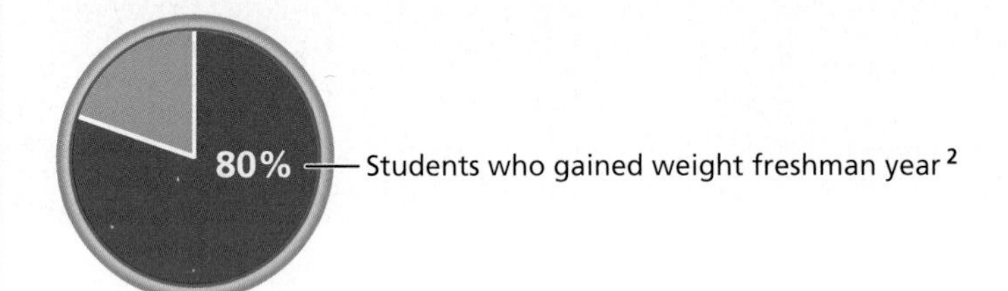

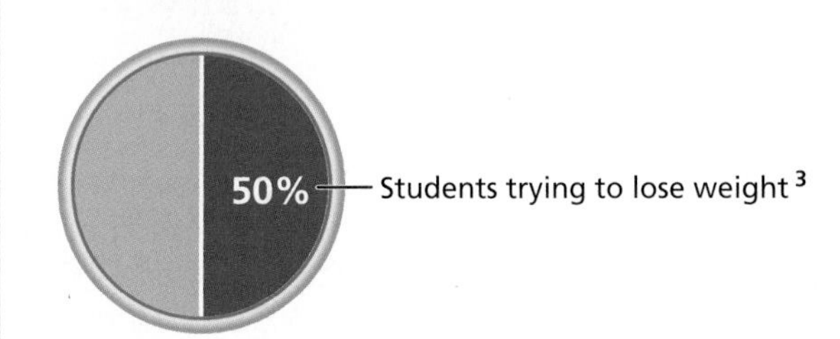

References: **1.** *American College Health Association National College Health Assessment II: Reference Group Executive Summary, Fall 2011,* by the American College Health Association, 2012. **2.** *College Freshman Stress and Weight Change: Differences by Gender,* by C. Economos, M. Hildebrandt, & R. Hyatt, 2008, *American Journal of Health Behaviors, 32*, pp. 16–25. **3.** *Weight Loss Practices and Body Weight Perceptions among US College Students,* by C. Wharton, T. Adams, & J. Hampl, 2008, *Journal of American College Health, 56*, pp. 579–584.

insulin, a hormone that allows glucose to be transported out of the bloodstream and into cells. When *insulin resistance* develops, glucose stays in the bloodstream, leaving cells depleted of energy and causing damage to blood vessels throughout the body.

- **Abnormal levels of blood lipids.** Obesity is associated with low blood levels of HDL cholesterol ("good" cholesterol) and high levels of LDL cholesterol ("bad" cholesterol) and triglycerides. Over time, abnormal blood lipids can contribute to *atherosclerosis*—an accumulation of deposits on the lining of blood vessels that narrows them and impedes blood flow. Atherosclerosis puts a person at risk for coronary heart disease and stroke. With increasing weight, there is a 9–18% increase in the prevalence of abnormal blood lipids.[25]
- **Coronary heart disease (also called coronary artery disease).** This disease results from atherosclerosis in arteries that supply the heart. The narrowed arteries reduce the amount of blood that flows to the heart. Diminished blood flow to the heart can cause chest pain (angina). Complete blockage can lead to a heart attack.
- **Stroke.** Atherosclerosis occurs in arteries throughout the body, including those that feed the brain. A stroke occurs when an artery supplying a region of the brain either becomes completely blocked or ruptures. In either case, brain tissue in that region is deprived of blood, and the functions controlled by it cease. Being obese raises your risk for having a stroke.
- **High blood pressure (hypertension).** High blood pressure is twice as common in obese adults because they have increased blood volume, higher heart rates, and blood vessels with a reduced capacity to transport blood.
- **Metabolic syndrome and increased cardiometabolic risk.** A group of obesity-related risk factors for cardiovascular disease and diabetes is referred to as **metabolic syndrome,** and an expanded group of risk factors is referred to as *cardiometabolic risk*. They include, for example, a waist measurement of 40 inches or more for men and 35 inches or more for women. (We discuss metabolic syndrome and cardiometabolic risk in detail in Chapter 11.)
- **Cancer.** Being overweight may increase your risk for developing several types of cancer, including colon, rectal, esophageal, and kidney cancers. Excess weight is also linked to uterine and postmenopausal breast cancer in women and prostate cancer in men. Gaining weight during adult life increases the risk for several of these cancers, even if the weight gain does not result in overweight or obesity.
- **Osteoarthritis.** This joint disorder most often affects the knees, hips, and lower back. Excess weight places extra pressure on these joints and wears away the cartilage that protects them, resulting in joint pain and stiffness. For every two-pound increase in weight, the risk for developing arthritis increases 9% to 13%.
- **Sleep apnea.** Sleep apnea causes a person to stop breathing for short periods during sleep. A person who has sleep apnea may suffer from daytime sleepiness, difficulty concentrating, and even heart failure. The risk for sleep apnea is higher for people who are overweight. A person who is overweight may have more fat stored around his or her neck, making the airway smaller, leading to breathing difficulty, loud snoring, or not breathing at all.
- **Gallbladder disease.** The gallbladder is a small sac that stores bile from the liver and secretes it into the small intestine to break apart dietary fats. Gallbladder disease includes inflammation or infection as well as the formation of gallstones (solid clusters formed mostly of cholesterol). Overweight people may produce excessive cholesterol and/or may have an enlarged gallbladder that may not work properly. The most common symptom is abdominal pain, especially after consuming fatty foods.
- **Fatty liver disease.** The level of stored fat often increases in the livers of overweight and obese people. When fat builds up in liver cells it can cause injury and inflammation leading to severe

metabolic syndrome A group of obesity-related factors that increase the risk of cardiovascular disease and diabetes, including large waistline, high triglycerides, low HDL cholesterol, high blood pressure, and high fasting blood glucose.

liver damage, cirrhosis (scar tissue that blocks proper blood flow to the liver), or even liver failure. Fatty liver disease is like alcoholic liver damage, but is not caused by alcohol and can occur in people who drink little or no alcohol.

- **Fertility problems.** Approximately 10% of women of childbearing age experience polycystic ovary syndrome (PCOS), which is the most common cause of female infertility.[26] Many women with PCOS are overweight or obese.
- **Pregnancy complications.** Pregnant women who are overweight or obese raise their risk of pregnancy complications for both themselves and their child. These women are more likely to develop insulin resistance, high blood glucose, and high blood pressure. The risks associated with surgery, anesthesia, and blood loss also are increased in obese pregnant women.

Excess weight is also linked to physical discomfort, social and emotional troubles, and (in the case of obesity) lower overall life expectancy. A long-term study conducted by Oxford University found that life expectancy of severely obese individuals may be reduced by 3 to 10 years.[27] **Figure 7.3** summarizes some of the major health risks associated with overweight and obesity.

Financial Burden of Obesity

Recently, a national group of financial experts responsible for assessing risks and associated health-care costs took a close look at obesity. Their findings were staggering. They estimated that overweight and obesity cost the United States and Canada about $300 billion a year in health-care costs and lost productivity, with $270 billion of that total belonging to the United States.[28] Another study found that some states spend up to $15 billion a year on obesity-related health care, with a significant portion of that cost paid for by the public.[29]

The individual costs are high as well—especially for women. In a study of the personal costs of obesity, researchers found that it costs an obese woman about $4,870 more per year to live in the United States compared with a woman of healthy weight, and an obese man about $2,646 per year.[30] Some of these costs are medical, such as for doctor's visits and medications. Others are work-related, pertaining to wages and missed work days. And some are personal, such as for transportation and life insurance premiums. Strikingly, the researchers found that obese women are less likely to earn the same wages as women of healthy weight—a factor that contributes to the greater costs for obese women. Obese men did not share the same wage discrepancy.

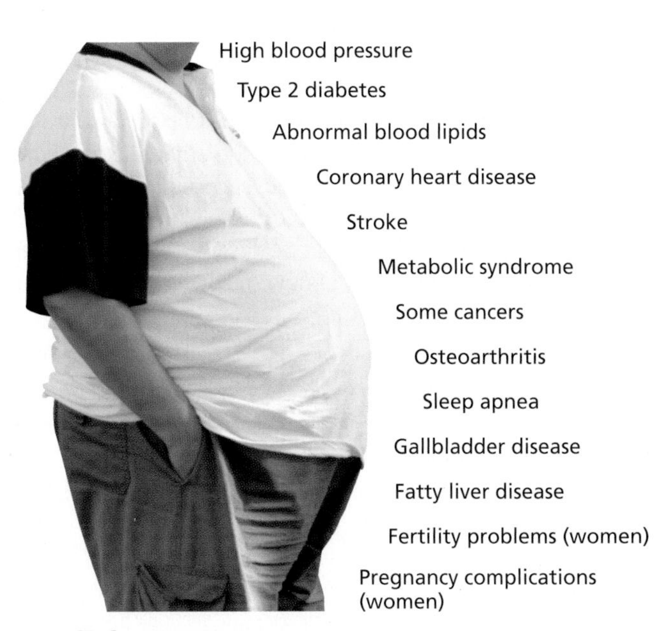

Figure 7.3 Major health risks associated with overweight and obesity.

energy balance The state achieved when energy consumed from food is equal to energy expended, maintaining body weight.

basal metabolic rate (BMR) The rate at which the body expends energy for only the basic functioning of vital organs.

Factors That Contribute to Weight Gain

Many of us watch the number on the bathroom scale rise or fall because of a simple concept: **energy balance.** The calories in the foods and beverages you consume are a form of "energy in." Your body uses this energy to perform all of its activities, from breathing and circulating your blood to studying and exercising. Think of these activities as "energy out." If, over time, the calories you consume match the calories you expend, then you are in energy balance and your weight will not change. If you take in fewer calories than you use, you'll lose weight. Take in more calories than you use, and you'll gain weight **(Figure 7.4).**

But while excess weight ultimately results from an energy intake in excess of energy used, other factors influence how that equation plays out in each of us individually. We discuss these factors in the next section, starting with those that are less controllable.

Biology and Genetics

Why does it seem as if some people can eat whatever they want all day long and not gain a pound, while others who monitor every mouthful just keep watching the scale go up? This is partly due to misperceptions and mistakes; for instance, people fail to count the sodas and chips they had while watching TV after dinner. But it also occurs because factors unique to us as individuals affect our energy needs.

Differences in Basal Metabolism

About two-thirds of the energy a person uses each day goes toward *basal metabolism*—that is, the body's maintenance of basic physiological processes (like keeping vital organs functioning) when at complete digestive, physical, and emotional rest. The remainder of energy a person uses is for food digestion and absorption, adjusting to environmental changes such as temperature, trauma, and stress, and engaging in physical activity.

The rate at which basal metabolism occurs in an individual is his or her **basal metabolic rate (BMR).** A similar measure of energy output, called *resting metabolic rate* (RMR), is measured when a person is awake and resting quietly. BMR and RMR may vary greatly from person to person and may vary for the same person with a change in circumstance or physical condition. In general, BMR and RMR are highest in people who are growing (children, adolescents, pregnant women), are tall (greater surface area = more heat loss = more calories burned), and have more lean body mass (physically fit people and males). These people generally use more energy per day.

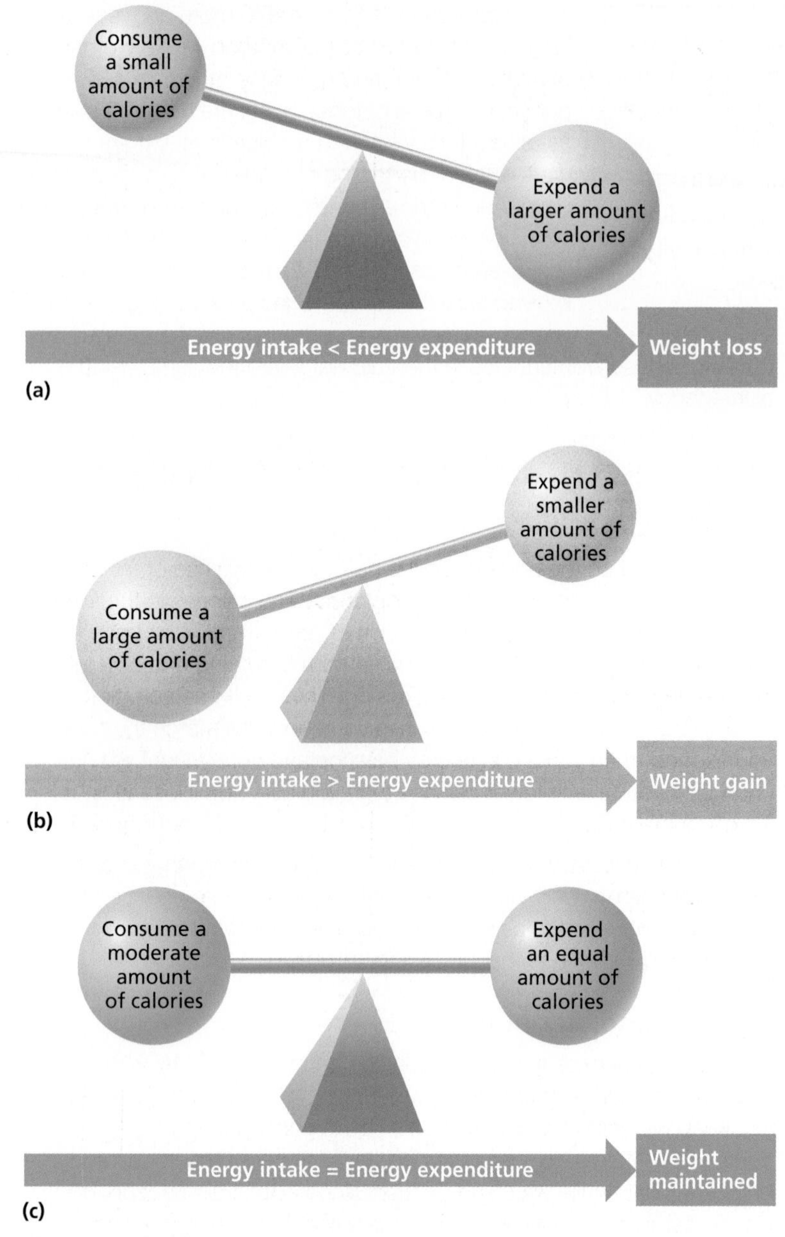

Figure 7.4 Energy balance. Energy balance is attained when the calories you consume equal the calories you expend.

Source: Thompson, J. and Manore, M., *Nutrition: An Applied Approach*, 2nd ed., p. 448, Fig. 11.6 © 2009. Reprinted by permission of Pearson Education, Inc.

Regular physical activity can build your muscles, a component of your lean body mass. If you increase your physical activity, you will burn more energy through exercise while increasing your BMR; together these factors can contribute greatly to weight loss.

Age

As people age, they tend to become less active and lose muscle mass. Because of this, BMR declines about 2% for each decade.[31] This reduced energy expenditure in turn reduces calorie needs. However, older adults who remain active can avoid gaining weight as they age, or gain weight in terms of muscle mass rather than body fat. Aerobics, strength training, and flexibility exercises are all recommended.

Sex and Gender Differences

Men and women each have unique factors that contribute to weight gain. Men may be more likely than women to consume high-calorie diets in response to social expectations. "Real men," according to the stereotype, eat ribs, not salad. In one study of college students, male students were less interested in making careful food choices and less inclined to scrutinize food labels. Some male students in the survey said more healthful eating was a female concern, not something men would focus on.[32] However, preventing weight gain is just as important in men as in women, if not more so. Men are more likely to store fat in their abdomens, which, as discussed earlier, confers greater health risks, such as heart disease.[33, 34]

Women, on the other hand, have unique health considerations that increase their risk of excess weight. Up to about age 10, energy needs for girls and boys are similar; then puberty triggers a change. When boys begin to develop more lean body mass, they need more calories. Their greater height and size demand more energy, too.[31] In contrast, female hormones play an important role in fat storage.[35] Women's bodies need adequate fat for the production of female reproductive hormones and women naturally keep body fat stores in reserve for pregnancy and breast-feeding. As evidence of that, it is not uncommon for women with inadequate body fat to cease menstruating. Because women tend to have a higher percentage of body fat than men, and body fat burns less energy than lean tissue, women, on average, need fewer calories than men do.

Life cycle factors also affect women's weight more drastically than men's. Pregnancy leads to necessary weight gain, and many women find that the extra pounds are difficult to lose afterward. Additionally, between puberty and menopause, women are more likely to store body fat in their hips and thighs, but after menopause, fat storage patterns begin to more closely resemble men's, with fat storage shifting to the abdominal area, increasing the risk of conditions such as heart disease.

Genetics

Overweight and obesity often run in families. If one or both of your parents are overweight or obese, your chances of being overweight increase. To be sure, some of this influence may be due more to habits than genes. Families tend to share eating and exercise patterns (whether the habits are healthful or unhealthful). However, studies have shown that genes, too, can affect the tendency to gain weight, how much fat a person stores, and where he or she carries excess weight. Scientists are also studying specific genes, such as a certain variation of a gene that is related to fat mass and obesity, known as FTO. FTO appears to increase a person's risk of obesity by 30% to 70%, depending on the specific variety of FTO and how many copies of that obesity-linked variation a person carries.[36]

Race and Ethnicity

Overweight and obesity disproportionately affect certain racial and ethnic groups. According to a study conducted by the Kaiser Family Foundation, overweight and obesity are problems for:[37]

- 73.7% of African Americans
- 72.2% of Native Americans/Alaskan Natives
- 69.1% of Hispanic Americans
- 64.9% of other racial or ethnic groups
- 62.8% of Caucasian Americans
- 42.1% of Asian Americans

The reasons for these disparities are complex. Factors may include cultural differences in diet and exercise, socioeconomic differences in patterns of food consumption, inequalities in access to nutritious food, and inequalities in access to education about nutrition and fitness. Other influences may arise from genetic differences. For more detail, see the **Diversity & Health** box for a discussion of theories behind one particular gene—dubbed the "thrifty gene"—that may affect weight-gain tendencies among people of different ancestries.

The disparities occur in more than just body weight. One study of *central obesity*, or excessive fat concentrated in the abdomen, found that while levels of abdominal fat have increased for Caucasian Americans, African Americans, and Mexican Americans since 1900, African American women have seen the largest shifts.[38] If patterns of central obesity increases continue, the researchers estimate that by 2020, about 71% of African American women would qualify as having central obesity and would be likely to face the increased health risks it confers.

Income and Education

A person's socioeconomic status and levels of education may also play a role in weight gain, although the effects and outcomes appear to vary between and within groups.[39] Among men, for example, rates of obesity are similar across income levels, although men at higher income levels are slightly more likely to be obese.[39] Among women, however, rates of obesity rise as income drops.[39]

Among men, national statistics show no significant trend between education level and obesity rates, but among women, obesity rates increase as education levels decrease.[39] National statistics also raise questions about making quick assumptions about obesity and income: The majority of obese adults and children do not qualify as "low income."[40] Since 1998, obesity rates have increased across all income levels.[39]

Health History

Certain health issues or medications may also trigger weight gain. Women, for example, may experience weight gain tied to hormones and reproductive issues, such as during and after pregnancy or menopause. As mentioned earlier, polycystic ovary syndrome, which is due to an imbalance of reproductive hormones, is also linked to excess weight.

In some cases, weight gain may also reflect hormonal imbalances triggered by an underactive thyroid. In this condition, called hypothyroidism, the thyroid gland fails to make enough thyroid hormone, leading to a variety of symptoms, including excess weight, fatigue, and being more sensitive to cold. If you have concerns about your thyroid, your doctor can check your thyroid hormone levels with a simple blood test.

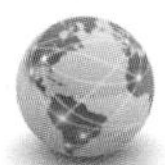

DIVERSITY & HEALTH

Overweight, Obesity, Ancestry, and the "Thrifty Gene"

While the reasons behind disproportionate rates of obesity among certain racial and ethnic groups are complex, researchers speculate that an ancient factor may be at work among some populations in our modern environment: a gene intended to prevent starvation.

This theory, centered around the idea of a "thrifty gene," is based on the fact that for thousands of years, certain populations, such as the native populations of the Americas, relied on hunting, fishing, and gathering for their food.[1] Access to food was seasonal and cyclical, swinging between times of plenty and times when food was scarce. To compensate, these populations developed a gene that allowed them to store fat easily when food was plentiful so as to prevent starvation later. Fast-forward to today, however, and the same gene overcompensates, encouraging fat storage even though the food supply is more reliable, encouraging weight gain and obesity among contemporary populations such as modern-day Native Americans, who have high rates of obesity and diabetes. Latinos, whose ancestors often include Native American peoples, may also be affected.

Although this theory is still under study, geneticists have identified a particular gene called PPARγ as one likely "thrifty gene."[2] This gene affects energy metabolism and fat storage, and a particular variant of the gene linked to an increased risk for obesity and type 2 diabetes has been found in some Native Americans strongly affected by weight concerns.[3] Further research will help determine if this gene variant is often found in other populations, and over time may help provide strategies for how to better address the effects of this ancient gene in today's society.

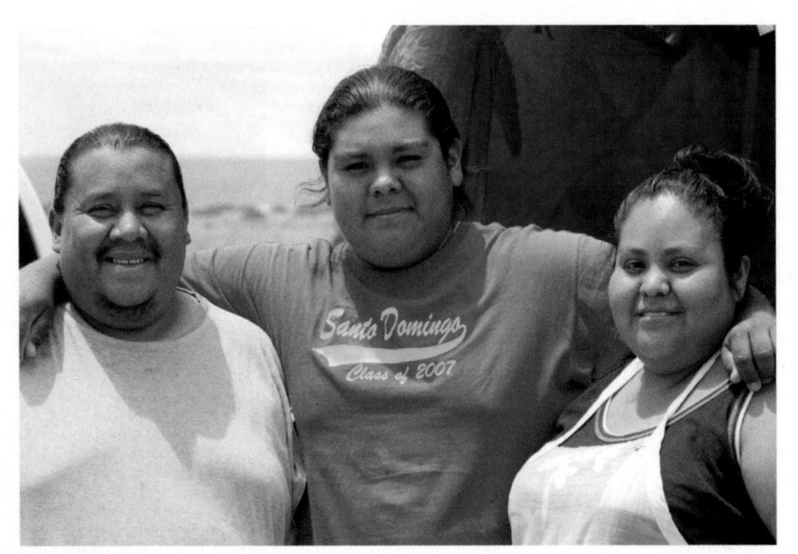

Does a "thrifty gene" promote weight gain in Native Americans and other groups?

References: **1.** "The Pima Indians: Obesity and Diabetes," by the National Institute of Diabetes and Digestive and Kidney Diseases, (date not provided), retrieved from http://diabetes.niddk.nih.gov/dm/pubs/pima/obesity/obesity.htm. **2.** "PPARγ, the Ultimate Thrify Gene," by J. Auwerx, 1999, *Diabetologia, 42*, pp. 1033–1049. **3.** "A Functional Variant in the Peroxisome Proliferator-Activated Receptor Gamma2 Promoter Is Associated with Predictors of Obesity and Type 2 Diabetes in Pima Indians," by Y. Muller, C. Bogardus, B. Beamer, A. Shulinder, & L. Baier, 2003, *Diabetes, 52*, pp. 1864–1871.

Psychosocial health may also play a role, although research in this area is still inconclusive. Researchers remain uncertain if there is a relationship between excess weight and psychological disorders like depression. There is no scientific evidence that overweight or obese people are any more or less likely to suffer from psychological disorders than people with a healthful weight. However, if you use food as a reward or to cope with negative emotions, you learn to eat for reasons other than satisfying hunger, making overeating and weight gain more likely.

Individual Behaviors

Although factors such as biology and genetics are an important consideration in an individual's weight, they cannot alone explain the dramatic surge in weight gain seen worldwide in recent decades. Personal choices related to diet and physical activity clearly have had a major effect.

Increased Calorie Consumption

The average American ate 1,950 pounds of food in 2003, an increase from 1,675 pounds in 1970—which translates to an estimated increase of 523 calories per day.[41] Many of these increased calories are in the form of fats and sugar.[42] Our diets are especially high in saturated fats (fried foods, fatty meats, cheeses, etc.) and added sugars (especially in soft drinks, candies, many breakfast cereals, and desserts). Americans also consume more than the recommended servings of grains—and mostly refined grains, in items like pasta, flour tortillas, and white bread, rather than high-fiber whole grains.

Large portion sizes and dining away from home also increase calorie intake. Across the board, portion sizes have ballooned. Servings of fast foods and soft drinks, for example, often are two to five times larger now than when they were introduced.[42] For example, in 1954 Burger King's hamburger was 2.8 ounces and 202 calories. In 2004 it had grown to 4.3 ounces and 310 calories.[42] A serving of McDonald's French fries weighed 2.4 ounces and contained 210 calories in 1955. By 2004 the fries had reached 7 ounces and 610 calories.[42] Bottled Coca-Cola contained 6.5 fluid ounces and 79 calories in 1916. By 2004 the standard container size for the beverage reached 16 fluid ounces and 194 calories.[42] While large portions may appeal to our lifestyles, tastes, and wallets, they contribute to excess weight and can harm our health.

Take the Portion Distortion Quiz to see how increasing portion sizes piles on the calories at http://hp2010.nhlbihin.net/portion.

Lack of Physical Activity

Today, did you spend more time on your feet, or more time sitting, likely staring at a screen? For a growing number of Americans, the answer falls on the more sedentary side. Fewer than one in three Americans gets the recommended minimum of 30 minutes of moderate activity a day, most days of the week. In fact, one-third of Americans over the age of 18 do not engage in any leisure-time physical activity at all, and that percentage climbs steadily with age.[43] About 25% of those between the ages of 18 and 24 get no leisure-time physical activity, and among those 65 or older, that number jumps to 49%.[44]

Many people work at jobs that require sitting in front of a computer rather than actively moving and using their muscles. In 1860, the average workweek was 70 hours of heavy physical labor, compared with 40 hours of sedentary work today. The least physically active groups are older adolescents and adults over 60 years old who spend about 60% of their waking time in sedentary pursuits.[44] According to the Nielsen Company's "Three Screen Report" (measuring television, computer, and cell phone usage), during the first 3 months of 2010, Americans watched a record 158 hours per month of television on average, viewing over 2 hours more TV per month than in the previous year.[45] Americans also spent 25 hours per month on the Internet, and almost another 7 hours watching video over the Internet on either their computer or a mobile phone.[45]

Coupled with the fact that Americans spend more than 100 hours a year commuting to work, little time is left in the day for physical

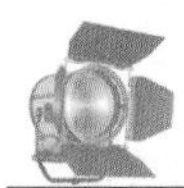
SPOTLIGHT

Michael Phelps's 12,000-Calorie Diet

At the height of his training for the Beijing Olympics, swimmer Michael Phelps consumed a 12,000-calorie-per-day diet, at least four to five times the recommended calorie intake for males his age. His breakfast consisted of three fried-egg sandwiches with cheese, lettuce, tomatoes, fried onions, and mayonnaise, one five-egg omelet, one bowl of grits, three slices of French toast topped with powdered sugar, and three chocolate-chip pancakes with syrup. His other meals were just as huge, and he consumed multiple energy drinks as well. And yet, the 14-time Gold medal winner didn't gain weight!

How did Phelps manage to eat so much and retain his athletic build? The secret is energy balance. Phelps expended so much energy during daily training sessions that all the excess calories went toward powering his laps, rather than being stored in his body as fat. In other words, he was using all the energy he was taking in, so he didn't gain weight. If Phelps hadn't eaten as much as he did, he would not have had the energy to train so intensely, and would not be the world-famous athlete he is today.

But don't count on consuming a diet like Phelps's just because you spend an extra hour at the gym! Use an online activity tracker, like the one at www.choosemyplate.gov/SuperTracker, to assess how many calories you're expending on exercise and adjust your diet accordingly.

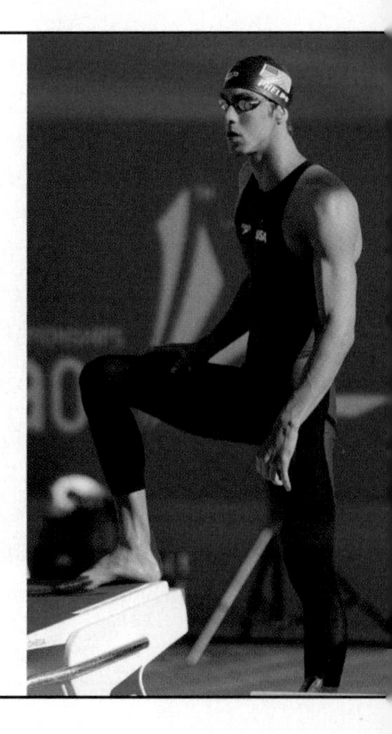

activity.[46] With less physical activity, lean body mass decreases and fat takes its place.

Social Factors

Although most people seem to appreciate the importance of a healthful diet and regular physical activity, many social factors in our everyday lives encourage behaviors that run counter to healthful weight management:

- Long work and school days, combined with commuting, leave many people little time for being physically active. One study of college students found that those with a drive time of 16 minutes or more were 64% more likely to be overweight or obese.[47]
- Most of us are stressed, and reach for food as comfort. One study found that the stresses of everyday life often trigger the urge to eat, with many people favoring less healthful food options.[48]
- Many of us also have little time to cook, turning instead to restaurants, where "super-sized" portions offer far more calories than we need.
- The fast food so many of us go for could be more aptly named "fat food." Most popular fast food choices are stuffed with calories and saturated fat.[49]
- Food ads promote brand-name, manufactured foods. These are often high in calories. When was the last time you saw a food ad for apples?

While these social factors affect all aspects of American society, they play an especially acute role for those facing the greatest economic challenges. In what researchers sometimes call the "food insecurity-obesity paradox," individuals and families of lower socioeconomic status are often at the greatest risk for obesity. A complex web of factors appears to underlie this paradox, including limited ability to access and purchase healthful foods, fewer opportunities for physical activity, and high levels of stress. Also influential are cycles of food deprivation and overeating, in which lack of food at some points leads to overeating and weight gain at others.[50] Many nutrition experts now push for food assistance programs that provide healthy nutrition choices and promote physical activity, rather than simply providing adequate calories.[51]

Physical Factors

Look at the built environment around you, and chances are you'll see a few features that demonstrate how we have literally helped construct the obesity epidemic. Health experts now describe many of our built areas as "obesogenic environments," meaning that they are spaces that promote obesity. Here are just a few examples:

- Many neighborhoods lack sidewalks, resulting in more driving and less walking. Protected bike routes are rare in many communities.
- In some neighborhoods, supermarkets are scarce, leaving residents to rely on smaller stores that rarely carry healthful choices such as fresh fruits and vegetables. In many such neighborhoods, fast food is often the most available restaurant option.
- Many of us don't have ready access to gyms, sports facilities, or other opportunities for physical activity and recreation. Paradoxically, those of us at the greatest risk for obesity often have the least access. Researchers have found that lower socioeconomic and high-minority areas had reduced access to recreational facilities, which in turn was associated with decreased physical activity and increased overweight or obese status.[52]

STUDENT STORY

Losing Weight

"Hi. My name is Josh. As a teenager, I often struggled with my weight. When I was 14 or 15 I was overweight, and I felt really down about myself and had low self-esteem. So, in an effort to lose weight and to get more healthy, I started looking for activities that I enjoyed and I found basketball and I found running. And through these activities, I started gradually losing weight, and I stuck to it. And so, if I could suggest anything for losing weight, I'd say find an activity that you like and which you can motivate yourself to do."

1: What side of the energy balance equation did Josh change to lose weight: energy in or energy out?

2: Do you think it really matters that Josh likes the activities he's doing, or will any activity work to lose weight?

3: What activities do you like that you could use to lose weight?

Do you have a story similar to Josh's? Share your story at www.pearsonhighered.com/lynchelmore.

Public Policy

Laws, regulations, and federally sponsored promotional programs around food also affect our nutritional environment, perhaps not always for the better. While state and federal public health officials now pour substantial money and attention into understanding and addressing the obesity epidemic, critics argue that other agencies create policies that make obesity more likely.

The United States Department of Agriculture, for example, is tasked with promoting and helping to find markets for the crops produced by U.S. farmers, ranchers, and dairy producers. One of the main crops produced in the United States, with the help of federal subsidies, is corn. You may think of corn as a vegetable for humans, but its primary use is as animal feed. One study analyzed nearly 500 food samples from fast food restaurants, and found that almost without exception, they were chemically derived from just one source: corn.[53] But corn is not just the main ingredient in fast food meals: It's used to make corn oil and corn-oil margarines, high-fructose corn syrup (HFCS), and thousands of processed foods containing these ingredients on your supermarket shelves, including baked goods, yogurts, peanut butter, soups, and spaghetti sauce. In fact, since the introduction of HFCS into the American food supply, our consumption of sweeteners has increased dramatically—from about 119 pounds per person in 1970 to 142 pounds per person in 2005.[54] Because the heavy federal subsidies paid to corn growers keep fast foods, HFCS-sweetened foods, and other high-calorie corn-based foods cheap, some nutrition experts blame federal policy for having a role in the obesity epidemic.

A similar debate exists for many other federally subsidized agricultural products. According to one group's research, more than 60% of recent agricultural subsidies have directly and indirectly supported meat and dairy production, while less than 1% have gone to fruits and vegetables.[55]

Add up all the above factors, and the recipe for our current epidemic of overweight and obesity becomes clear. We are surrounded by forces that undermine healthful weight management.

Change Yourself, Change Your World

For most people, the key to healthful weight loss lies in the ability to better control "energy in" and "energy out." If you want your body to use and reduce its fat stores, you need to make sure less energy is coming in and more energy is going out. This requires consistent work. Losing weight doesn't have to mean depriving yourself. But it does mean eating wisely and changing your lifestyle to be as physically active as possible.

Some of us practice successful weight management on our own. But many of us benefit from some support, whether that help comes from a friend, a trainer, a counselor, a formal program, or even a doctor.

Personal Choices

Did you grab a snack before sitting down to study this chapter? If so, what did you choose? Seemingly small decisions about what and how much you eat can support or undermine successful weight

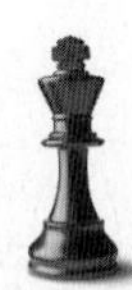

Practical Strategies for Change

Cutting Calories, Not Nutrition

You can reduce the total number of calories you eat while boosting your intake of healthful nutrients by following these basic guidelines:

- **Shop smart.** Never shop on an empty stomach! You'll make wiser purchases if you're not particularly hungry. Also, avoid buying high-calorie foods that you'll have difficulty eating in moderate amounts. And don't be fooled by "low-fat" foods. They may be just as high in calories as the regular versions, because manufacturers often make up for the fat with added carbohydrates.
- **Track your food intake.** Use a free online tracker, like the MyPlate SuperTracker (**www.supertracker.usda.gov**) or **www.sparkpeople.com**, to calculate the calories you are consuming and compare them with your MyPlate calorie intake recommendations.
- **Practice portion control.** Match the amount of food on your plate to your desired servings and calorie intake level. Try gauging the higher-calorie foods you tend to choose (such as red meats, fats, and sweets), cutting their portion sizes in half, and replacing the rest with lower-calorie options **(see Figure 7.5)**. Another strategy is to share your portion with a friend.
- **Fill your plate!** Low-calorie meals do not have to be skimpy. If you fill most of your plate with legumes and other vegetables alongside smaller portions of foods higher in calories, you can still have an ample, nutritious meal without busting your calorie count for the day.
- **Choose healthful fats.** Nuts, seeds, and most plant oils are excellent sources of healthful unsaturated fats. Salmon and other fish are good sources of essential fatty acids.
- **Eat whole foods as close to their natural state as possible.** Highly processed foods are more likely to contain empty calories. If you reach for an apple instead of a cup of sweetened applesauce, for example, you will avoid the calories that were added during the manufacturing process. You will also be consuming more fiber, which helps you feel full longer.
- **Don't skip meals.** This will only leave you overwhelmingly hungry later on. If you're often too rushed to eat breakfast, fix yourself a peanut butter and banana sandwich on whole grain bread before you go to bed, and grab it on your way out the door the next morning.
- **Avoid drastic measures.** Cutting your calorie intake in half may help you lose a few pounds for a week or two, but it's a losing strategy. That's because your BMR drops right along with your calorie cutting. At the same time, your feelings of hunger and deprivation make you crave food even more strongly. Sustained weight loss requires steady, gradual lifestyle change. Aiming to lose 10 percent of your body weight over a 6-month period is reasonable goal.

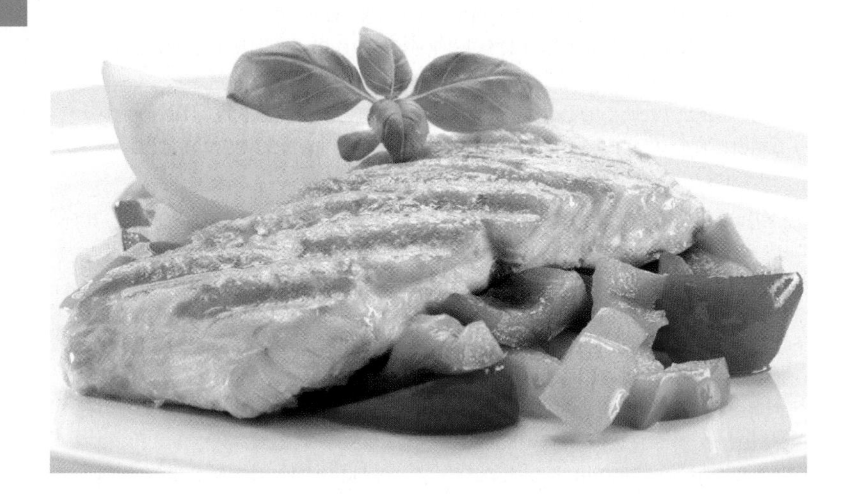

- **Drink water instead of sugary drinks filled with calories.** Approximately 20% of our total calorie consumption comes from what we drink.[1] Juices, "vitamin waters," soft drinks, and energy drinks are all extra sources of calories. If plain water gets a little dull, opt for sparkling water flavored with a wedge of lemon, lime, or orange, or make yourself a spritzer by adding a dash of juice to a glass of sparkling water.
- **Use artificial sweeteners in moderation.** Artificial sweeteners are low- or no-calorie sugar substitutes. Artificial sweeteners containing aspartame (for example, Equal and Nutrasweet) have been studied extensively and have been found to be safe in moderation.[2] However, people with phenylketonuria (PKU) should avoid aspartame because it contains phenylalanine, which their bodies cannot process.
- **Change one habit at a time.** Instead of trying to overhaul all of your eating habits at once, choose one meal or snack and make small changes little by little. At lunch, for example, opt for fruit instead of dessert. Give that new habit some time to "stick" before trying another change.

References: **1.** "Effects of Soft Drink Consumption on Nutrition and Health: A Systematic Review and Meta-Analysis," by L. R. Vartanian, M. B. Schwartz, M. K. D. Brownell. April 2007, *American Journal of Public Health, 97*, pp. 667–675. **2.** "Aspartame: Review of Safety," by Harriett H. Butchko, 2002, *Regulatory Toxicology and Pharmacology, 35*, pp. S1–S93, 200.

management. The nearby **Practical Strategies** box lists several helpful behaviors to practice.

hunger The physiological sensation caused by the lack of food.

appetite The psychological response to the sight, smell, thought, or taste of food that prompts or postpones eating.

satiety Physical fullness; the state in which there is no longer the desire to eat.

Can Dieting Work?

Hunger is the physiological sensation caused by a lack of food. Hunger is triggered in our brains, as a response to signals sent by the digestive tract and hormones circulating in our blood. Hunger is different from **appetite,** the psychological response to the sight, smell, thought, or taste of food that prompts or postpones eating. Appetite can prove helpful, stimulating you to eat before you get too hungry. It can also prove harmful, steering you toward too much food or toward tempting but unhealthful food choices. When we've eaten and relieved or prevented hunger, a feeling called **satiety** helps turn off the desire to eat more.

Given that both hunger and appetite compel us to eat, can dieting work? Weight-loss diets can be helpful for some people, especially those who like the support of a structured plan or program. However, dieting is a slow, steady process. You can't achieve healthful or permanent weight loss by starving yourself for a week. Diets also work best if they are accompanied by regular exercise. To keep the weight off, successful dieters must work to make their new eating and exercise habits into a way of life that they can sustain long term.

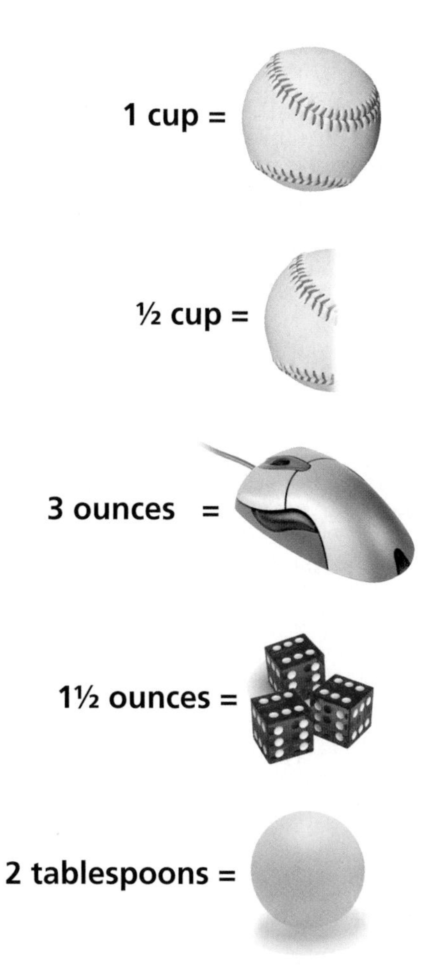

Figure 7.5 Estimating portion sizes. You can use common household items to estimate the portion sizes of your food.

Millions of Americans follow weight-loss diets **(Table 7.2)**. In a year-long study that compared four popular diets—Atkins, Ornish, The Zone, and Weight Watchers—roughly half the participants lost an average of 7 pounds and improved some of their health indicators, such as heart disease risk.[56] But in a pattern familiar to many dieters, the other half of the study's participants dropped out.

Three common dieting approaches are low-calorie diets, low-fat diets, and low-carbohydrate diets.

Low-Calorie Diets. Cutting 500 to 1,000 calories a day typically leads to a loss of 1 or 2 pounds a week. **Figure 7.6** shows a healthful way to reduce the calories in a daily diet.

But a low-calorie diet is rarely a simple matter of food math. Without a healthful eating plan in place, abruptly restricting one's daily calorie intake below recommended levels can be dangerous and deprive you of the energy you need for daily activities. You may find yourself withholding calories all day, only to lunge for a double cheeseburger at night. If you don't maintain a balanced diet while you cut calories, you will deplete your body of nutrients and possibly end up adding more calories along the way.

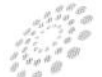 ***Frontline: Diet Wars*** **investigates popular diets and America's obesity problem. View this program online at www.pbs.org/wgbh/pages/frontline/shows/diet.**

Low-Fat Diets. Diets that focus on reducing daily fat intake are also common. Most aim to cut the dieter's total fat intake to about 25% of calories or less. Some of these diets are vegetarian, others vegan, and others allow lean meats, poultry, and fish. Long-term weight loss is a challenge with low-fat diets, because dieters find them difficult to follow and to maintain. That said, we can all benefit from following these general fat intake guidelines:

- **Cut *trans* fats from your diet.** *Trans* fats are created when manufacturers add hydrogen to vegetable oil—a process called hydrogenation. Consumption of *trans* fats reduces your "good cholesterol" (HDL) and raises your "bad cholesterol" (LDL), thereby increasing your risk of cardiovascular disease. Prepackaged snack and dessert foods (crackers, chips, cookies, cakes, pies, etc.) were once the largest sources of *trans* fat in our diet, although in recent years, due to the requirement to list *trans* fat content on food labels, food manufacturers have used less of them. However, labeling regulations allow any food product with 0.5 gram of *trans* fats or less per serving to claim zero grams of *trans* fats on the label. If you eat multiple servings of such foods, you may wind up consuming significant amounts of *trans* fats after all. Restaurant foods, such as French fries, may also contain *trans* fats, and do not carry labeling requirements.[57]
- **Consume more "good" fats.** Fats found in plant oils, nuts, seeds, and fish should make up the majority of fats in your diet.

Low-Carbohydrate Diets. First popularized by Dr. Robert Atkins, low-carbohydrate diets propose greatly reducing sugar and starch intake and increasing intake of lean protein. Several weight-loss studies have found that dieters tend to stick with low-carbohydrate approaches longer and lose slightly more weight—at first.[58, 59] The diuretic effect of a low-carbohydrate diet initially promotes loss of water, not body fat.

Table 7.2: **Popular Diets**

Name	Description	Foods to Eat	Foods to Avoid	Practicality	Analysis
Atkins Diet	Claims that eating too many carbohydrates causes obesity and other health problems. Emphasizes the consumption of protein and fat over carbohydrates.	Meat, fish, poultry, eggs, cheese, low-carb vegetables, butter, oil	Carbohydrates, specifically bread, pasta, most fruits and vegetables, milk, alcohol	Difficult to eat in restaurants because only plain protein sources and limited vegetables or salads are allowed. Difficult to maintain long term because of limited food choices.	The composition of a sample menu is 8% carbohydrate, 56% fat, and 35% protein. Initial weight loss is mostly water. Does not promote a positive attitude toward food groups. Eliminates virtually all carbohydrate foods. May encourage overly high-fat diets.
Eat Right for Your Type	Claims that blood type is the key to your immune system, which determines your diet and supplementation.	Varies based on blood type	Varies based on blood type	Promotes some foods, such as dairy and wheat, even if individuals experience intolerances for those foods, potentially leading to gastrointestinal discomfort and other health problems.	This diet has no scientific basis. People may use this diet to attempt to fight cancer, asthma, infections, diabetes, arthritis, hypertension, and infertility, but there is no evidence that it is effective.
Jenny Craig	This program's philosophy for successful weight loss is: (1) a healthful relationship with food, (2) an active lifestyle, and (3) a balanced approach to living. Dieters are required to have a 15-minute personal consultation weekly with Jenny Craig "counselors" (who lack formal nutrition/behavior training). A variety of online support tools are also available to strengthen dieters' motivation.	Promotes Jenny Craig-brand packaged meals, snacks, and supplements. Fruits, vegetables, and nonfat dairy foods are limited per Jenny Craig's 28-day menu planner. Vegetarian choices are available.	"Homemade" meals, commercial items (except those carrying the Jenny Craig label), sweets, and other foods that are not listed on Jenny Craig's 28-day menu planner	Eating packaged meals long term may be difficult and not realistic.	The targeted composition of the 1,200- to 1,500-calorie menus is 60% carbohydrate, 20% fat, and 20% protein. Packaged meals are not conducive for teaching dieters how to shop, cook, and eat their own healthful, calorie-controlled meals. After completing the program, dieters who resume their usual eating habits are likely to regain weight. The cost of purchasing required ready-made meals can be expensive for some dieters.
Slim-Fast	This program promotes Slim-Fast products as staples of breakfast and noon meals; evening meal is 500 calories and nutritionally balanced. Portion control, avoidance of sugary and fatty foods, and frequent water consumption are encouraged. Dieters are expected to track food intake, physical activity, and weight changes via online Slim-Fast tools.	Promotes 3–5 servings of fruits and vegetables daily. Promotes Slim-Fast products, vegetables, fruits, whole grains, salad, lean proteins, low-fat cheese, water, and other non-calorie beverages. Snacks of 120 calories or fewer are allowed.	Regular candy, cookies, and other sweets, fried or other high-fat foods, some dairy products and snack items	Buying meal-replacement products for breakfast and lunch becomes expensive over time.	The targeted composition of the 1,200- to 1,800-calorie menus is 63% carbohydrate, 15% fat, and 22% protein. The "sensible" evening meal is the most educational component of the plan because it teaches dieters about appropriate portions of a moderate-calorie meal. Dieters are expected to purchase Slim-Fast products for their breakfast and lunch meals. This requirement leads to dieters' "burnout" and limits individuals' ability to select healthful, traditional foods.
South Beach Diet	This diet advocates the intake of "good" fats and "good" carbohydrates for cardiac protection, improved nutrition, and the management of hunger, insulin resistance, and weight control. The diet is divided into three phases. Three meals plus two snacks are the eating pattern for all phases of the diet.	Mostly healthful foods are consumed. Lean proteins, some fruits, vegetables, and oils are the staples of this diet. Initially: seafood, chicken breast, lean meat, low-fat cheese, most vegetables, nuts, and oils are promoted. Later: whole grains, most fruits, low-fat milk or yogurt, and beans are promoted.	Refined carbohydrates and added sugars, fatty meats, full-fat cheese, refined grains, sweets, juice, potatoes	Phase I of the diet is restrictive and may be difficult to complete. Phase II includes more foods and Phase III is maintenance.	The composition of a sample menu from Phase I of the plan is 42% carbohydrate, 43% fat, and 15% protein. Research to support this diet is very limited. The two short-term studies that were completed had a small sample size and were funded by South Beach Diet affiliates.

Table 7.2: Popular Diets (continued)

Name	Description	Foods to Eat	Foods to Avoid	Practicality	Analysis
Volumetrics	The Volumetrics Eating Plan focuses on enhancing the feeling of fullness while simultaneously consuming fewer calories. The diet aims to maximize the amount of food available per calorie. Foods are assigned to one of four categories based on their energy (calorie) density. Category 1 foods can be enjoyed on a daily basis; Category 4 foods are portion controlled and consumed on an occasional basis.	Focuses on fiber-rich foods with high moisture content. Fruits, vegetables, whole grain pasta, rice, breads and cereals, soups, salads, low-fat poultry, seafood, meats, and dairy are promoted. Moderate amounts of sugar and alcohol are permitted, too.	No foods are forbidden, but limiting fatty foods like deep-fat-fried items, sweets, and fats added at the table is recommended. Limited amount of dry foods (crackers, popcorn, pretzels, etc.) due to their high caloric value and low satiety index.	The large amount of fiber-rich foods recommended for meals and snacks may cause gastrointestinal distress for some dieters.	The composition of the diet is ≥ 55% carbohydrate, 20% to 30% fat, and 15% to 35% protein. Fiber intake is 25 to 38 grams/day. This is a sensible and nutritionally balanced eating plan developed by a nutrition researcher.
Weight Watchers	A program that uses weekly meetings and weigh-ins for motivation and behavioral support for diet and exercise changes. Clients follow a point system that they can track online.	Theoretically, all foods are allowed. Fruits, vegetables, whole grains, lean protein, low-fat or nonfat dairy, and 2 teaspoons of healthful oils are staples of the program.	Although there are no "forbidden" foods, limiting intake of foods high in saturated and *trans* fats, sugar, and alcohol is emphasized.	Weekly Weight Watchers meetings have been shown to significantly strengthen participants' weight-loss successes. If a dieter is unable to attend weekly meetings, his or her results could be impacted. Once clients reach their target weights, they are allowed to attend meetings for free.	The composition of the diet plan is 50% to 60% carbohydrate, 25% fat, and 15% to 25% protein. No research supports the program's effectiveness, but its sensible advice is used and supported by millions, including nutrition experts.

Sources: Adapted from *Nutrition Action Healthletter*, January/February 2004, "Nutrition Fact Sheets: Fad Diets," by the Northwestern University Feinberg School of Medicine, January 2007, retrieved from http://www.feinberg.northwestern.edu/nutrition/fact-sheets.html, and "Top Diets Reviewed," by *Consumer Reports*, June 2007, retrieved from http://www.ConsumerReports.org.

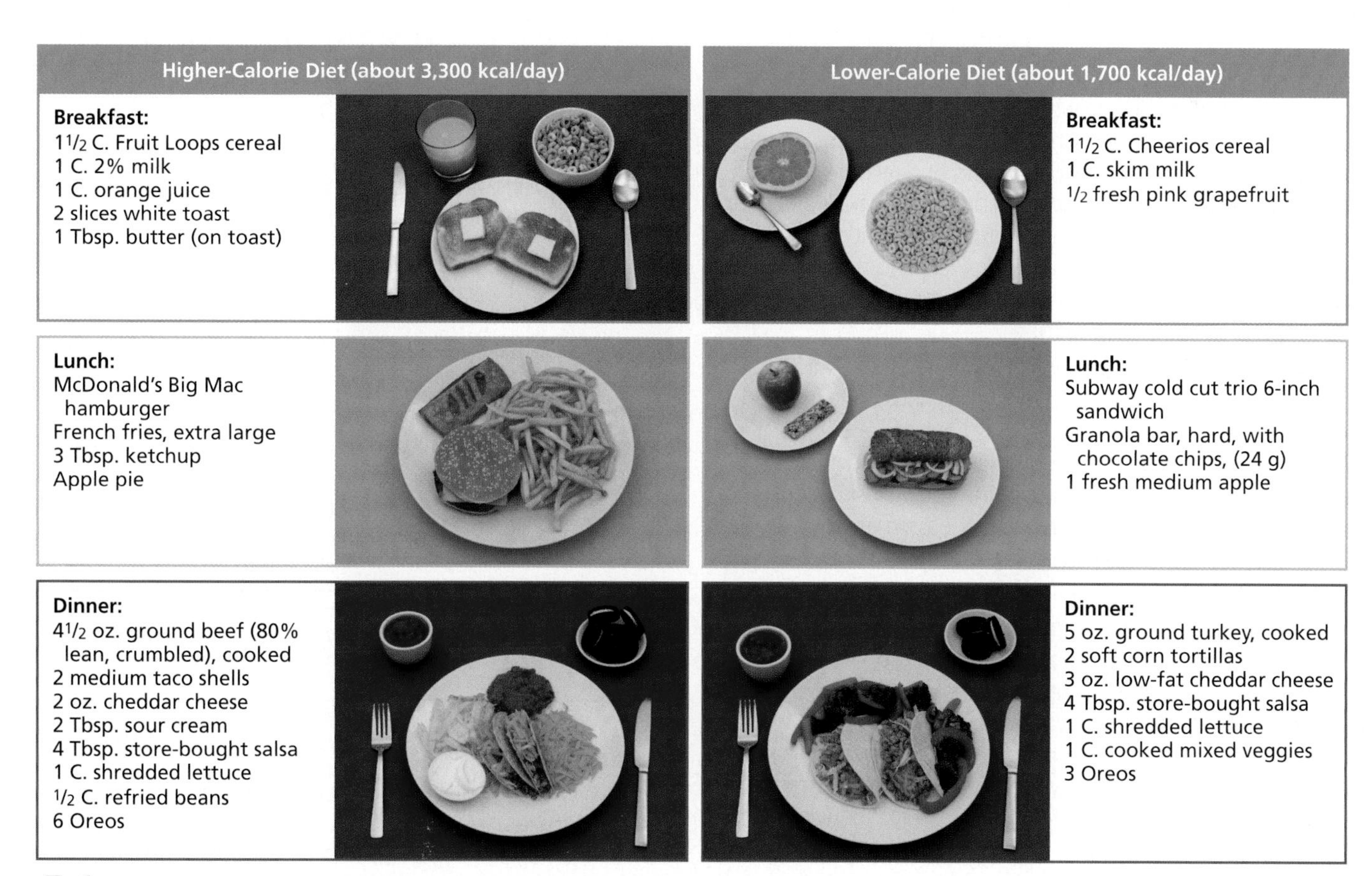

Figure 7.6 How to cut calories while maintaining a balanced diet. The meals on the right show healthful alternatives to the higher-calorie meals on the left.

Source: Thompson, J. and Manore, M., *Nutrition: An Applied Approach*, 2nd ed., p. 464, Fig. 11.10. © 2009. Reprinted by permission of Pearson Education, Inc.

For weight loss to be sustained, a person must follow the diet beyond the initial period to begin losing more body fat.

Most nutrition experts agree that Americans eat too many refined carbohydrates, especially from added sugars. But fiber-rich carbohydrates—including fruits, legumes and other vegetables, and whole grains—are nutritious foods that your body needs. Follow these guidelines:

- **Choose fiber-rich carbohydrates.** Carbohydrates found in whole grains, fruits, and vegetables are better options than refined carbohydrates found in white breads, cakes and other commercial baked goods, soft drinks, and candy.
- **Watch your total calories.** Consuming lots of protein and fat won't help you lose weight. Total calorie consumption is what matters. If you eat a McDonald's double cheeseburger without the bun, you may have cut carbohydrates, but you've still eaten nearly 400 calories. To lose weight, you need to consume fewer calories than you expend, regardless of the type of diet you are following.
- **When choosing protein-rich foods, look for leaner options.** Fish, skinless chicken breasts, or rump, round, flank, and loin cuts of meat are choices lower in saturated fats. Better yet, choose plant proteins, which provide healthful unsaturated fats, and are high in fiber and micronutrients.

What About Diet "Aids"?

Walk into most grocery or health food stores and you'll find a variety of foods, drinks, and pills all claiming to help you lose weight. But it's worth considering these products carefully before getting out your wallet.

Visit *Medline Plus* for reliable information about drugs and supplements at www.nlm.nih.gov/medlineplus/druginformation.html.

It's easy, for example, to find numerous high-protein energy bars or protein drinks that claim to help with weight loss. But many of these products are high in empty calories from added sugars. Unless you adjust your food intake for the additional calories an energy bar or protein drink contains, you might actually wind up adding more calories to your diet and sabotaging your weight-management efforts. In addition, high-protein food items are not necessarily helpful in weight loss; maintaining energy balance, rather than high levels of a particular nutrient, is the most important factor over the long term.

Diet pills claim to help with weight loss in a variety of ways, from tricking your body into thinking it's full to regulating hormones that affect your desire to eat. Although many diet pills have never been proven to work, manufacturers of these products do a booming business. In 2010, Americans spent $2.69 billion on over-the-counter diet aids, including pills and meal replacements such as low-calorie energy bars.[60] One study of college women at risk for eating disorders found that 32% reported having used a diet drug.[61]

Most over-the-counter diet pills are considered dietary supplements, a category that the FDA only minimally regulates.[62] They do not need to be proven safe by the manufacturer unless they include a new ingredient, and are not tested by the FDA until they have already gone on the market and problems are reported. In addition, because labeling requirements remain less strict for supplements, many supplement firms downplay the risk of side effects in packaging and advertising. So, buyer beware.

Here are just some of the problems that have surfaced in recent years with over-the-counter diet pills and supplements:

- In 2011, the FDA and FTC (Federal Trade Commission) started the process of removing over-the-counter weight-loss products containing a hormone called HCG from the market. The hormone, human chorionic gonadotropin, is FDA approved as an injectable prescription drug for the treatment of some medical conditions, but has no proven effect on weight loss. The two agencies sent warning letters to companies marketing HCG-based substances for weight loss and urged consumers to avoid such products.[63]
- In 2009, the FDA warned consumers to immediately stop using Hydroxycut diet supplements because they were linked to serious liver injury and disease.[64]
- From December 2008 to May 2009, the FDA recalled over 70 weight-loss supplements because they were found to illegally contain prescription-drug ingredients.
- Even though the FDA prohibited the sale of weight-loss supplements containing the ingredient ephedra more than a decade ago, pills claiming to contain ephedra still appear for sale on the Internet. The ingredient has been linked to thousands of cases of side effects that include tremors, insomnia, heart palpitations, and increased risk of heart attack and stroke.[65]

Only one pill has received full clearance from the FDA for sale as an over-the-counter weight-loss medication. Alli, a lower dose of the prescription weight-loss medication orlistat, was released to the public in 2007. The drug works by causing your body to excrete some of the fat that passes through your digestive tract, and is intended to help you lose about 5% of your body weight over time. But side effects, such as digestive discomfort and gas with oily spotting, can be unpleasant. Alli is also expensive, costing about $50 for a one-month supply of the pills.

See **Table 7.3** for a more detailed look at some commonly found supplements claiming to help with weight loss.

Get Physically Active

Physical activity does more than burn off calories and reduce body fat. While a particularly strenuous workout might leave you reaching for a snack, regular exercise over time appears to help reduce feelings of hunger and mediate appetite.[66] It also builds muscle, which burns more calories than fat tissue. Choose an activity you enjoy, whether it is dancing, skateboarding, or playing a favorite sport. If you make exercise fun, weight loss will be more enjoyable!

Keep in mind the basic exercise guidelines we discussed in Chapter 6. If you are trying to maintain weight loss or lose weight, aim for 60 to 90 minutes each day. At least two to three times a week, some of that exercise should focus on building muscle. If you have time for nothing else, try to build a little more walking into your daily routine.

There are lots of free online programs that can track your diet and physical activity, such as www.supertracker.usda.gov/physicalactivitytracker.aspx, www.sparkpeople.com, www.tweetyourhealth.com, and www.fitday.com.

Finding Help

If you've tried to lose weight, you may have discovered how difficult it can be to do it on your own. Fortunately, there are people and organizations that can give you the help and support you need.

Options on Campus. Start by visiting your campus health center. There, you may be able to sign up to join a weight-loss support group. If that's not your style, consider individual consultations. A nutritionist or dietitian

Table 7.3: Supplements Making Weight-Loss Claims

Product	Claim	Effectiveness	Side Effects
Alli — OTC version of prescription drug orlistat (Xenical)	Decreases absorption of dietary fat	Effective; but weight loss is even more modest than that with Xenical	Loose stools, oily spotting, frequent or hard-to-control bowel movements; reports of rare, but serious, liver injury
Bitter orange	Increases calories burned	Probably ineffective	Similar to ephedra: raised blood pressure and heart rate
Chitosan	Blocks absorption of dietary fat	Probably ineffective	Uncommon: upset stomach, nausea, gas, increased stool bulk, constipation
Chromium	Decreases appetite and increases calories burned	Probably ineffective	Uncommon: headache, insomnia, irritability, mood changes, cognitive dysfunction
Conjugated linoleic acid	Reduces body fat	Possibly effective	Upset stomach, nausea, loose stools
Green tea extract	Decreases appetite, and increases calorie and fat metabolism	Insufficient evidence to evaluate	Dizziness, insomnia, agitation, nausea, vomiting, bloating, gas, diarrhea
Guar gum	Blocks absorption of dietary fat and increases feeling of fullness	Possibly ineffective	Abdominal pain, gas, diarrhea
Hoodia	Decreases appetite	Insufficient evidence to evaluate	Insufficient information available

Source: Adapted from *Over-the-Counter Weight-Loss Pills: Do They Work?* by the Mayo Clinic, 2012, retrieved from http://www.mayoclinic.com/health/weight-loss/HQ01160

familiar with available food options at your school can help you make choices most convenient for your college routine. If you think you might have emotional or stress-related issues around eating, you can also talk to your campus health center about available psychotherapy options.

Also visit your campus fitness center. Many offer personal training and/or nutrition consultations; if you are a student, these services are often at a lower cost than you'll find at off-campus facilities.

Community-Based Programs. If you'd like more formal weight-loss assistance, consider joining a community-based or professional weight-loss program. Nonprofit groups such as Overeaters Anonymous or TOPS (Take Off Pounds Sensibly) provide supportive, nonjudgmental help in understanding and rethinking emotional responses to food. Overeaters Anonymous is a nonprofit network of support groups, in which members attend in-person meetings to help themselves and each other overcome compulsive overeating. TOPS, which focuses on many different aspects of weight loss, also centers around supportive in-person meetings to discuss everything from healthful eating to general wellness. Overeaters Anonymous is free of charge, while membership in TOPS involves an annual fee of about $30 a year and small monthly dues (usually $5 or less). If your campus doesn't have OA or TOPS chapters of its own, you'll likely find them in the surrounding community.

Your campus health center may also be able to help you enroll in a clinical weight-loss program in your community. These have proven effective at helping participants achieve and maintain weight loss through long-term behavior change. Sessions are usually held at a clinic or fitness facility. Participants first receive a health and risk assessment from a clinician, followed by a nutrition assessment and an evaluation from an exercise specialist. After personalized recommendations are compiled from these specialists, participants embark on an individualized weight-loss program, with frequent check-ins, exercise log-ins and review, group classes, and options for individual guidance and counseling.

Commercial groups such as Weight Watchers focus on a combination of online tools and group meetings as part of their program, and many campuses have their own Weight Watchers chapters. Many other commercial programs, such as Jenny Craig, are also widely available. But some base their weight-loss plans around purchasing prepared meals from the program, which can get expensive, especially on a student budget.

Take a small step toward achieving your target weight. Visit http://people.bu.edu/salge/52_small_steps/weight_loss/index.html for 52 tips on eating better, getting more active, and tracking your progress toward your goals.

If you're interested in joining a commercial weight-loss program, the Federal Trade Commission has a downloadable booklet, including a checklist, that can help you assess each plan: www.ftc.gov/bcp/edu/pubs/consumer/health/hea05.pdf.

To be successful, all such programs require sustained effort on the part of participants. But they can also pay off: In one such program tracked by researchers, participating men lost about 7% of their body weight and women lost about 5% over a 6-month period. The more participants attended regular exercise and counseling sessions, the greater their weight loss.[67]

What If You Want to Gain Weight?

If you want or need to gain weight for optimal health, you should consume more calories than you expend. As you do, use the following approaches:

- **Boost your calories, but in healthful ways.** Piling the cheese on your pizza isn't a good way to gain weight. Instead, reach for a diverse mix of foods, including 100% fruit juices, nuts and seeds, dried fruits, peanut butter, hummus, and meal replacement drinks and bars. Keep a supply of nut-based trail mix with you, and reach for that as a snack. **Table 7.4** lists a healthful 3,000-calorie-per-day diet that can be used to gain weight.
- **Eat smaller meals more frequently throughout the day.** If you don't have much of an appetite, try eating four or five smaller meals throughout the day, rather than two or three big ones.
- **Add calories to your favorite meals.** If you enjoy salad, for example, choose an olive oil dressing instead of a fat-free version. Add in some protein as well, such as diced chicken, cheese, avocado, tofu, or a handful of nuts. You also can add dry milk powder to mashed potatoes and meal replacement powders to milk and malt shakes.
- **Get regular exercise to build both appetite and muscle.** Participate in activities such as weight lifting to increase muscle mass and swimming to improve cardiovascular fitness.

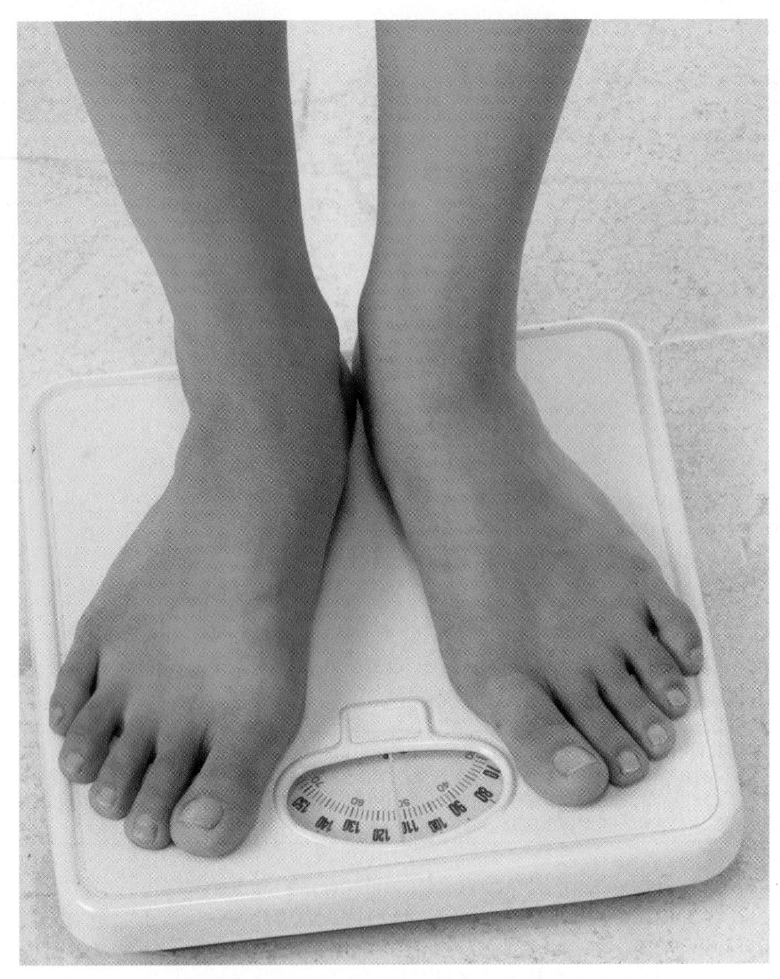

Talking to someone at your campus health center or joining a weight-loss program can be a **first step** to losing weight.

Table 7.4: Healthful Weight Gain: A Sample 3,000-Calorie Diet

Meal	Food
Breakfast	1 cup Grape Nuts 2 cup 2% milk 1 cup cranberry juice
Snack	6 Tbsp. raisins 1 cup orange juice
Lunch	8 oz. 2% milk 3 oz. tuna 2 tsp. mayonnaise 1 bun Lettuce, tomatoes, sprouts 2 oz. chips/snack food 1 cup whole baby carrots
Snack	Met-Rx fudge brownie bar 1 cup orange juice
Dinner	5 oz. chicken 1 cup instant mashed potatoes with 1/3 cup 2% dry milk powder 1 cup 2% milk 1 Tbsp. *trans* fat–free margarine 1 cup green beans Lettuce salad with vegetables 2 Tbsp. salad dressing
Snack	16 oz. water 16 animal crackers

How Do You Maintain a Healthful Weight?

Reaching or being at a healthful weight is only one piece of the puzzle. Once you've achieved your target weight, you have to maintain it.

Long-term weight management doesn't have to mean endless days of dull meals or counting calories. Instead, look at your food habits, your level of physical activity, and your feelings about eating, and choose options that make it easy and fun to keep your weight in balance. Keep in mind:

- **Your healthful weight is a range, not a fixed number.** Sometimes you may be at the lower end of that range, and sometimes at the upper end. If you find your weight creeping up, reduce your calorie intake a bit and exercise a little more. A flexible approach lets you manage your weight and still enjoy your life.
- **Find reasons to be active.** Often, we make excuses for not exercising. Try turning that habit around. Leave your car at the far end of the parking lot and walk. Take the stairs instead of the elevator. Turn off your laptop or TV for a couple of hours a week and join an intramural sports team instead. Look for part-time work that requires being on your feet, not sitting at a desk.
- **When choosing physical activity, aim for consistency over intensity.** A half-hour brisk walk every day will do more for you in the long run than a 2-hour intense workout done only on Saturdays. In one study of college students, those with four or more low-intensity workouts a week were twice as likely to have healthful BMIs.[68]
- **Snack smarter.** Replace higher-calorie snacks such as chips and energy bars with fruits and vegetables. If you crave something more substantial, reach for whole grains or nuts before you opt for candy or a muffin. Store snacks in cupboards rather than leaving them lying around in plain sight.
- **Don't be too hard on yourself.** If you have a few high-calorie days, don't tell yourself that you've blown your diet. Instead, follow up with a few days of lower-calorie choices.
- **Let food be one of life's pleasures.** If you're focused on weight maintenance, you can afford to indulge in some empty calories, as long as you make a point of eating healthfully for the rest of the day.

Helping a Friend

The motto of weight-loss support group Overeaters Anonymous is, "I put my hand in yours, and together we can do what we could never do alone."[69] Even professional groups like Weight Watchers depend on bonding between members to support weight loss. And social support doesn't have to be face to face. An analysis of 500,000 users of the calorie-tracking app MyFitnessPal revealed that the more friends users had, the more weight they lost. Moreover, people who gave friends access to their calorie counts lost 50% more weight than the average user.[70] If you want to help a friend shed pounds for good, try the following:

- Find non-food ways to celebrate successes together. Go to the movies, or catch a game. Find fun in something other than food.
- Don't coach—join in! Instead of suggesting your friend walk more often, arrange to walk to class together in the morning rather than drive.

- Cook a low-calorie meal together. Cooking for one isn't always practical. Prepping meals for and with friends is more cost-effective and fun.
- Let the slip-ups pass. If your friend couldn't pass up the doughnuts today, calling attention to the fact might only generate guilt and resentment. Instead, suggest your friend join you for an after-class workout.
- Don't tempt. Offering just a bite of something can open the door to breaking your friend's resolve. If your friend is enjoying a healthy meal, have something similar.
- Seek out a sport or activity you both enjoy. Hoops? Hiking? Zumba? Find something fun and share it regularly.

Campus Advocacy

College doesn't have to mean scary food in the dining hall and worrying about the "freshman 15." Get involved to help bring healthier options to your school that promote weight management and make it easier for you and your fellow students to avoid weight gain.

For inspiration, check out the Real Food Challenge (http://realfoodchallenge.org), a network of students working to improve the options students have at mealtime and bring better nutrition to campuses. This group, which has chapters at more than 360 colleges and universities so far, aims to "shift $1 billion of existing university food budgets away from industrial farms and junk food and towards local/community-based, fair, ecologically sound and humane food sources—what we call "real food"—by 2020." That's an ambitious goal, but the group provides support and training for campus chapters, and also has ways to start smaller, such as getting just one real food item into the menu at your dining hall. If your school doesn't have a chapter, start one, and if it does, get involved. Groups such as these show that students don't have to be at the mercy of the campus food service.

Maybe you make most of your own meals. If so, consider starting a cooking club with like-minded friends, where you share the meal-planning, shopping, cooking—and eating! Doing your own cooking doesn't have to take long, and by planning and preparing your own meals, you'll save money, and have more control over ingredients and calories.

If your campus doesn't offer safe walking and biking options, work with other students to lobby the administration and make these changes happen. (Check Chapter 6 for more ideas on how to increase access to physical activity on your campus.)

Although it's important to work toward a healthful campus environment, it's also essential to avoid judging yourself or your fellow students because of weight. If you find yourself struggling with such negative feelings, check your course catalog! Many colleges and universities now offer courses in so-called "Fat Studies," which prompt students to research issues such as how weight is perceived in different countries, and what our media obsession with thinness reveals about our values as a society. Or check out NAAFA, the National Association to Advance Fat Acceptance. Founded in 1969, NAAFA is a civil rights organization that works to end size-based discrimination. Find it at www.naafa.org.

Clinical Options for Obesity

In 2011, a national survey of college students found that 11 percent were obese. As you've learned in this chapter, obesity is a significant health risk. If your BMI is 30 or higher, your doctor may recommend medical treatment. These options range from psychotherapy to prescription drugs to weight-loss surgery.

Psychotherapy. Psychotherapy can be a vital component of both weight-loss and weight-management programs. This is especially true for people who turn to food to reduce stress or relieve depression. Others may have significant body image issues that are most effectively addressed with the help of a therapist. Psychologists have found that both individual and group therapy can be helpful in treating obesity and related issues such as shame or a distorted view of one's own body.[71]

Prescription Drugs. Prescription weight-loss medications include those approved by the U.S. Food and Drug Administration (FDA) for short-term use in weight loss, including diethylpropion, phendimetrazine, and phentermine, and three approved for long-term use, orlistat, lorcaserin, and Qsymia. Another medication, sibutramine (sold under the brand name Meridia) is no longer available in the United States, after concerns about increased risk of heart attack and stroke led the manufacturer to pull the drug from the U.S. market in 2010.[72] Each has side effects ranging from increased blood pressure, sleepiness, nervousness, dizziness, and headaches to cramping and explosive diarrhea. They are typically prescribed only for obesity, not more moderate cases of weight management.

These drugs help patients shed only a small percentage of body weight, and only when combined with changes in diet and exercise. They are usually prescribed to obese patients who are experiencing health problems due to their weight, and only for short periods of time. Although approved for long-term use, their effectiveness and safety has not been established for use beyond 2 years. In 2010, the FDA required a new safety warning label for orlistat to alert patients that a few people using the drug had suffered severe liver injury, and to watch for symptoms of liver trouble, such as yellow eyes or skin, when taking the drug.[73]

Surgery. A growing number of obese people—about 220,000 in 2009 alone—are opting for surgery to alter the sizes of their stomachs and reduce the amount of food they can ingest.[74] This type of surgery, called **bariatric surgery,** comprises several different types of procedures (**Table 7.5** on page 194). One subset of procedures, known as *gastric banding*, involves partitioning off part of the stomach with a removable band. The other subset, *gastric bypass*, involves permanently reducing the size of the stomach. After either type of procedure, the reshaped stomach can only hold a limited amount of food—sometimes as little as an ounce—resulting in greatly reduced calorie intake. In more extreme types of surgery, other portions of the digestive tract are also altered to limit calorie absorption.

Weight-loss surgery may be increasingly common, but it's not for everyone. Doctors only recommend weight-loss surgical procedures for people who:

- Have a BMI of 40 or more. That usually means you are about 100 pounds or more overweight.
- Have a lower BMI (between 35 and 40) but also have a dangerous obesity-related health condition, such as heart disease, type 2 diabetes, severe joint pain, or high cholesterol

bariatric surgery Weight-loss surgery using various procedures to modify the stomach or other sections of the gastrointestinal tract in order to reduce calorie intake or absorption.

Table 7.5: Weight-Loss Surgery

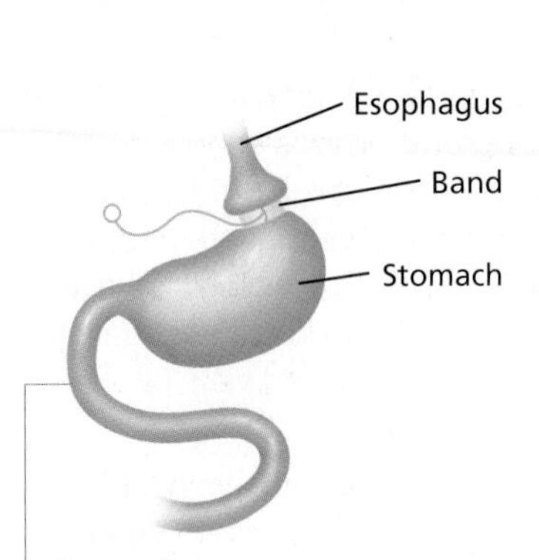

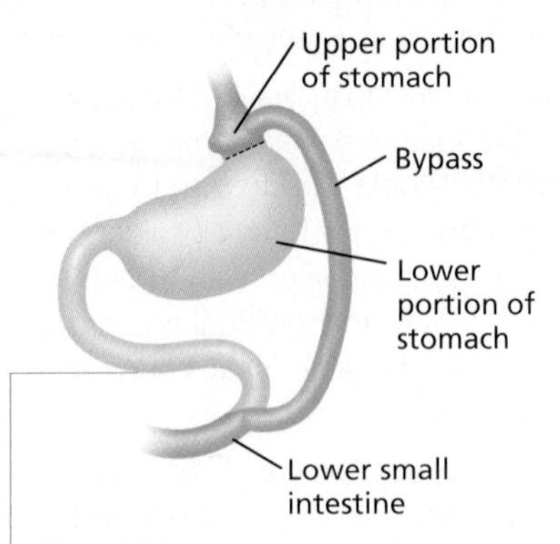

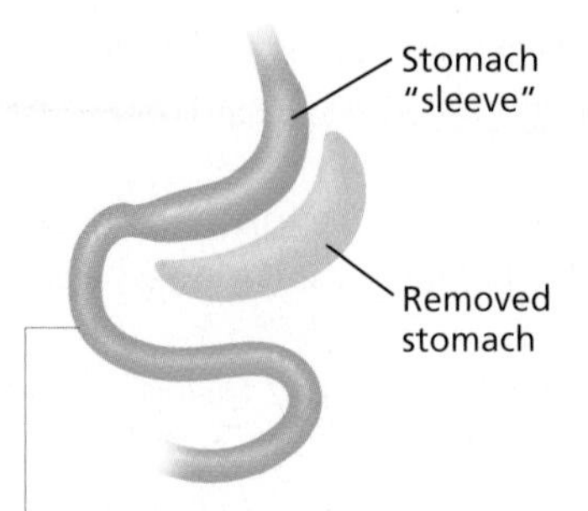

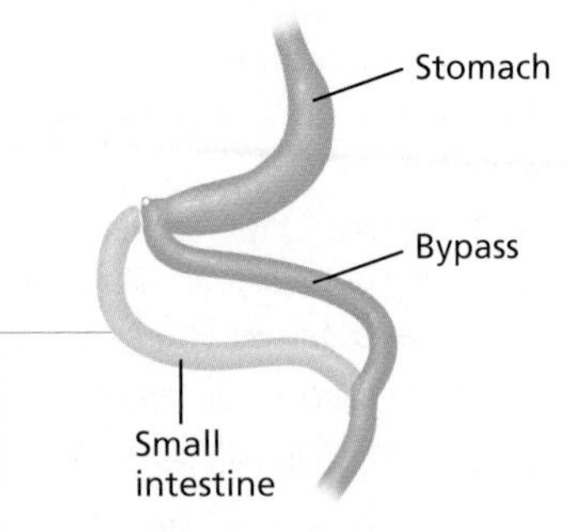

	Adjustable Gastric Band	Gastric Bypass Surgery	Vertical Sleeve Gastrectomy	Biliopancreatic Diversion
Description:	An inflatable band is used to squeeze the stomach and restrict food intake. The LAP-BAND is one type of adjustable gastric band.	The stomach is divided into two parts, and the upper portion is then connected to the lower portion of the smaller intestine, bypassing the lower stomach and upper small intestinal tissue (also called "Roux-en-Y gastric bypass")	About three-quarters of the stomach is removed, leaving a narrow "sleeve" of stomach that connects to the intestines	A more severe form of gastric bypass, in which much of the stomach is removed and more of the small intestine is bypassed
Pros:	Relatively less invasive; faster recovery; band is relatively easy to adjust or remove; intestines are not affected	Most common weight-loss surgery in the United States; weight loss and health improvements are often dramatic; weight reduction is often sustained over the long term	Often a safer choice for very obese or ill patients than more invasive procedures; intestines are not affected	Even faster and greater weight loss than with regular gastric bypass
Cons:	Band may slip out of place or leak; less dramatic weight loss and greater chance of eventual weight gain	Procedure is irreversible. Food may also be passed into the intestines before being properly digested, leading to nausea, a phenomenon called "dumping."	Irreversible; for many very obese or sick patients, further surgeries are often required later to facilitate further weight loss	An even greater risk of nutritional deficiencies than with regular gastric bypass; greater risk of "dumping"
Risks:	Vomiting, infection, small chance of life-threatening complications	Infection, blood clots, gallstones, risk of life-threatening complications. Because the intestines are affected, the body's ability to absorb nutrients is impaired. Patients are at risk for nutritional deficiencies for the rest of their lives.	Blood clots, infection, sleeve may leak	In addition to standard surgical risks, this is one of the more complicated and high-risk weight-loss surgeries. Risk of postsurgical hernia.

Data from *Bariatric Surgery for Severe Obesity*, by the Weight Control Information Network—NIH, 2011, retrieved from http://win.niddk.nih.gov/publications/gastric.htm; *JAMA Patient Page—Bariatric Surgery*, by J. Torpy, 2010, *Journal of the American Medical Association, 303*, p. 576; *Patient Information: Weight-Loss Surgery*, by M. Andrews, 2011, *UpToDate*, retrieved from http://www.uptodate.com/contents/patient-information-weight-loss-surgery?view=print.

- Have tried and failed to lose weight other ways
- Fully understand the risks, and realize that the surgery is just one step in making dramatic, long-term lifestyle changes to lose weight and keep it off. Weight-loss surgery doesn't give you the freedom to gorge on burgers and chocolate afterwards. It's part of a lifetime commitment to weight management.

In early 2011, the FDA also approved the use of a relatively less invasive gastric banding procedure, called LAP-BAND, in those with a BMI of 30 or higher who have at least one obesity-related condition.

Some patients see significant weight loss and other health improvements after undergoing these procedures, such as a significant reduction in blood glucose. But others eventually gain back the weight they lost. Others find they can no longer absorb certain nutrients properly, or experience chronic diarrhea or vomiting or other problems. Also, any major surgery involving an obese patient carries an unusually high risk for complications such as infection and the formation of blood clots. Overall, about 1 in 200 patients dies within 90 days following the surgery.[75]

Bariatric surgery has become more popular among obese teenagers looking for a way to lose weight and avoid the almost-certain onset of diseases such as diabetes. But leading medical experts advise proceeding cautiously before undergoing bariatric surgery at a young age. Even though about 1,000 U.S. teenagers a year are now undergoing such procedures, little is known about how the surgery will affect their health later in life.[76]

Some people opt for a different, less invasive type of surgery that focuses on targeted removal of body fat from specific parts of the body, such as the arms, thighs, or waist. This type of procedure, called *liposuction* or lipoplasty, is usually performed for cosmetic reasons and is not considered an effective treatment for obesity.[77] In recent years, a new version of the treatment that combines liposuction and laser technologies has grown in popularity. Proponents of laser liposuction say that the use of a laser to liquefy fat before it is removed makes the procedure more effective. Some doctors, however, caution that the procedure can be risky and can result in burns, and that more study is needed.[78]

Body Image and Eating Disorders

Have you ever thought about the fact that ads for junk foods like fried chicken or cheeseburgers are funding TV programs featuring actors so thin they look like they've never had a bite of either? For some people, contradictions like this contribute to the development of a distorted view of their body, or a dangerous relationship with food.[79] We'll start by looking at disorders related to body image.

Body Image Disorders

While many of us have concerns about our bodies and our appearance from time to time, some people experience worries about body image to such a strong degree that their thoughts and perceptions interfere with their happiness and daily life. Such body image disorders represent a form of chronic mental illness that often requires counseling or therapy to resolve.

Body Dysmorphic Disorder

In **body dysmorphic disorder,** a person can't stop thinking about a perceived flaw with his or her appearance. The prefix *dys-* means abnormal, and *morph-* refers to form—but the flaw is either minor or imagined. People with this disorder obsess over their appearance, and may seek out numerous products or cosmetic procedures to try to "fix" perceived flaws, only to remain anxious and unsatisfied.[80] Though this disorder can apply to any physical feature, it often centers on weight and body shape, and often starts during the teen years. Men and women experience the disorder in equal numbers.[81]

This condition can have serious effects, including depression, anxiety, social isolation, eating disorders, seeking out unnecessary cosmetic procedures or surgeries, and even suicidal thoughts. Treatment often centers on psychotherapy, although in some cases, antidepressant medications may also be recommended.

Social Physique Anxiety

Many of us get a little uncomfortable at the thought of appearing before others in shorts or a bathing suit, but for those with **social physique anxiety,** this concern is amplified to a degree that makes them extremely nervous and fearful of having their bodies judged by others. Psychologists have developed a 12-point scale to help understand the severity of this disorder, with people at the higher end of the scale more likely to experience consequences such as social isolation or extreme self-criticism.[82] While males and females may both experience this disorder, women and girls are more likely to have higher levels of social physique anxiety and lower levels of physical self-esteem than males.[83]

If you know someone who might have one of these body image disorders, encourage him or her to seek professional help. Your campus health center is often a good place to start.

Eating Disorders

Sometimes people let negative body image or other psychological factors steer them toward unhealthful eating behaviors. When these behaviors produce drastic weight changes and put health and even life at risk, they are called **eating disorders.** Teenage girls are most at risk for eating disorders, especially if they are preoccupied with being thin, experience social or family pressure to be thin, come from more affluent families, and have tendencies toward extreme self-control and perfectionism. But young men and athletes under pressure to adhere to a particular body shape are also vulnerable. According to national estimates, about 2.7 percent of 13- to 18-year-olds, including 3.8% of girls and 1.5% of boys, suffer from an eating disorder.[84]

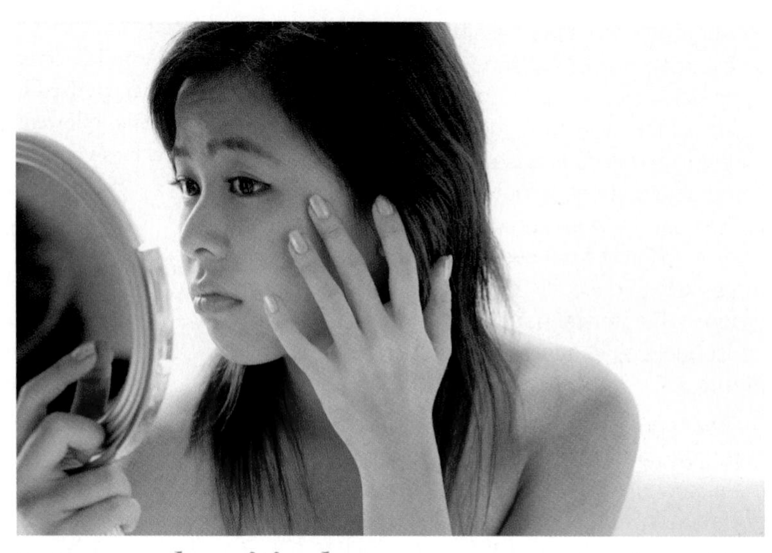

Being **overly critical** of your body can interfere with your happiness.

Three dangerous eating disorders are anorexia nervosa, bulimia nervosa, and binge eating disorder. Other eating and weight-related behaviors, while not yet classified by medical experts as full-blown eating disorders, can also have serious health effects; these include night-eating syndrome and the female athlete triad.

Anorexia Nervosa

People with **anorexia nervosa** see food as an enemy that must be controlled. They eat as little as possible, often setting up elaborate rituals and practices to control food intake. They have an extremely unhealthful body image, seeing themselves as fat even when they are dangerously underweight. In the United States, experts estimate that about 0.6% of the population suffers from anorexia, including about 0.9% of women and 0.3% of men.[85]

While the exact cause of anorexia nervosa is unknown, a variety of factors play a role in many cases. Psychological factors, such as a tendency toward obsessive-compulsive personality traits, may make it more possible for some people to focus intently on their weight and forgo food even when hungry. Environmental factors, such as the body image concerns and media influences discussed earlier, often play a part. Biological factors, such as genetics, may also be a contributing factor, but this aspect of anorexia is still being studied.[86]

Signs and symptoms of anorexia nervosa include:

- An intense fear of gaining weight or being overweight
- A highly distorted body image that continues to see fat where none exists
- A refusal to maintain a normal body weight
- A refusal to eat, or eating patterns that tightly restrict food intake

body dysmorphic disorder Mental disorder characterized by obsessive thoughts about a perceived flaw in appearance.

social physique anxiety Mental disorder characterized by extreme fear of having one's body judged by others.

eating disorders A group of mental disorders, including anorexia nervosa, bulimia nervosa, and binge eating disorder, that is characterized by physiological and psychological disturbances in appetite or food intake.

anorexia nervosa Mental disorder characterized by extremely low body weight, body image distortion, severe calorie restriction, and an obsessive fear of gaining weight.

Anorexia nervosa is classified as a serious mental disorder. Starvation leads to wasting: A body deprived of calories will begin to break down the proteins in muscle and other body tissues to use for energy. This can cause serious and sometimes irreparable damage throughout the body, especially to the heart muscle, and can prompt sudden death. People suffering from anorexia nervosa are 18 times more likely to die early than people in the same age group in the general population.[87] Other physical consequences of anorexia nervosa are illustrated in **Figure 7.7.**

Treatment for the disorder is key, although experts estimate that only about 34% of those with the disorder receive care.[86] The good news, though, is that once treatment is accessed, most patients do respond. In a national survey of over 9,000 adults, just 15.6% of people who had ever been diagnosed with anorexia still had a BMI below 18.5 (underweight) at the time of the survey.[88] The type and duration of treatment varies according to the severity of the illness. Patients with less severe cases often receive a blend of treatment and support services, such as psychiatric care, medications, nutritional counseling, and individual or group therapy, in outpatient settings that allow them to continue to live at home, even if receiving treatment daily. Patients with more severe cases, especially those whose life is at risk, may receive treatment in the hospital, where patient care, including nutritional support in the form of supervised feedings, can be more closely monitored.[89]

During and after treatment for anorexia nervosa, support from family and friends is key. Many treatment plans include family therapy to help loved ones find new ways to support the patient and each other, and avoid prior patterns of behavior that may have contributed to the condition. Patients also benefit from finding new ways to manage stress and reduce anxiety, helping themselves find the calm they need to better care for themselves physically and emotionally and sustain a new path toward a more healthful body image and relationship with food. Patients are also helped by disengaging from "pro-anorexia" websites and online forums where those with untreated anorexia nervosa discuss how they sustain their disorder or hide it from friends and family. To help in the ongoing effort to prevent and treat anorexia, several large blogging and social media platforms recently announced that they would start removing posts and websites that could promote anorexia and other eating disorders.[90]

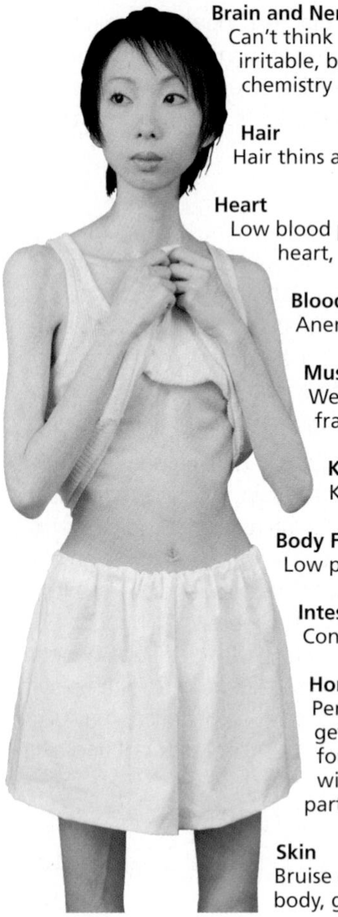

bulimia nervosa Mental disorder characterized by episodes of binge eating followed by a purge behavior such as vomiting, laxative abuse, or extreme exercise.

binge eating The rapid consumption of an excessive amount of food.

purging Behaviors, such as vomiting, laxative abuse, or overexercising, intended to reduce the calories absorbed by the body.

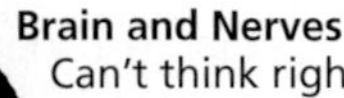

Brain and Nerves
Can't think right, fear of gaining weight, sad, moody, irritable, bad memory, fainting, changes in brain chemistry
Hair
Hair thins and gets brittle
Heart
Low blood pressure, slow heart rate, fluttering of the heart, palpitations, heart failure
Blood
Anemia and other blood problems
Muscles, Joints, and Bones
Weak muscles, swollen joints, bone loss, fractures, osteoporosis
Kidneys
Kidney stones, kidney failure
Body Fluids
Low potassium, magnesium, and sodium
Intestines
Constipation, bloating
Hormones
Periods stop, growth problems, trouble getting pregnant. If pregnant, higher risk for miscarriage having a C-section baby with low birthweight and post partum depression.
Skin
Bruise easily, dry skin, growth of fine hair all over body, get cold easily, yellow skin, nails get brittle

Figure 7.7 Major physical and health effects associated with anorexia.

Source: Adapted from *Anorexia Nervosa Fact Sheet,* by Womenshealth.gov, 2009, retrieved from http://www.womenshealth.gov/publications/our-publications/fact-sheet/anorexia-nervosa.cfm#top.

Bulimia Nervosa

This disorder is marked by an ongoing cycle of seeking large amounts of food and then trying to get rid of the calories consumed. People who have **bulimia nervosa** have elaborate food rituals that typically start with **binge eating,** the consumption of a large amount of food in a short amount of time. After a binge, bulimics then try to remove these calories from their bodies by **purging** through self-induced vomiting, heavy laxative use, fasting, or excessive exercise.

An estimated 0.3% of American adults develop bulimia nervosa in any given year, comprising about 1.5% of women and 0.5% of men.[91] Unlike anorexia nervosa, those suffering from bulimia nervosa often maintain a healthy or normal weight, but as in anorexia nervosa, bulimics are often intensely anxious about gaining weight and extremely critical of their own bodies. Many conduct bulimic behavior in secret, sometimes as often as several times each day.[92]

Bulimia nervosa carries serious health risks, including dental problems such as cavities and tooth enamel erosion, dehydration from vomiting and other forms of forced purging, stomach problems such as ulcers and even stomach rupture, and cardiac risks including irregular heartbeat and heart failure. Signs of bulimia nervosa include:

- Regular binge eating episodes, at a rate of at least two per week for several months
- Binges followed by purging, strict dieting, or excessive exercise to prevent weight gain
- Using self-induced vomiting or laxatives as part of purging
- An obsession with weight and body shape

As with anorexia nervosa, treatment for bulimia nervosa can be extremely effective. Bulimia treatments usually focus on a combination of medical, psychiatric, and psychosocial care tailored to the needs of the individual patient. Bulimics often receive nutritional guidance, as well as therapy aimed at understanding and changing binge-purge behavior.

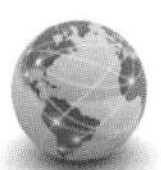

DIVERSITY & HEALTH

A Look at Eating Disorders in Men

An obsession with food and body shape. Excessive exercise or calorie restriction. Feelings of low self-esteem and a drive for perfection. It sounds like a classic eating disorder, right? The difference: The victim is male.

For years, eating disorders have been thought of as "women's diseases," and it is true that the majority of those who suffer from them have been female. However, national statistics indicate that 10% of those diagnosed with an eating disorder are male, and a recent Harvard study found an even higher prevalence: 25% of the people with anorexia or bulimia and 40% of the binge eaters were men.[1, 2] In addition, it is likely that the number of men with eating disorders is underdiagnosed, due to the still widespread perception among physicians and patients that eating disorders are a female concern.

Many of the factors that promote eating disorders are the same in both sexes, such as low self-esteem, depression, traumatic events or abuse in the past, or participation in a sport that values low body weight, such as gymnastics, running, or wrestling.[3] Unlike women, men who develop eating disorders are more likely to have actually been overweight in the past.[4] Men with eating disorders also tend to have higher levels of sexual anxiety than women with eating disorders.[5] There is some evidence that homosexual males may be more likely to develop eating disorders, although that could be due to higher levels of reporting among homosexual males than among heterosexual males.[6]

Men are also much more likely than women to develop *muscle dysmorphia*, an all-consuming belief that they are not muscular enough and an obsession with building muscle.[7] These men tend to be more concerned with their percent of muscle to body fat as opposed to their weight on the scale. Men with all types of eating disorders are more likely to purge calories through compulsive exercise than through vomiting or laxative abuse.[8]

A few high-profile men have spoken publicly about their battles with eating disorders, including actors Dennis Quaid and Billy Bob Thornton, and singer Elton John.[9] If you are a male and suspect you have an eating disorder, know that you are not alone—and seek help.

References: **1.** "Research on Males and Eating Disorders," by the National Eating Disorders Association, 2008, retrieved from www.nationaleatingdisorders.org. **2.** "The Prevalence and Correlates of Eating Disorders in the National Comorbidity Survey Replication," by J. H. Hudson, 2007, *Biological Psychiatry*, pp. 348–358. **3.** See note 1. **4.** "Eating Disorders in Males," by A. S. Robb, & M. J. Dadson, 2002, *Child and Adolescent Psychiatric Clinics of North America, 11*, pp. 201–218. **5–6.** See note 1. **7.** "Eating Disorders: How Are Men and Boys Affected?" by the National Institute of Mental Health, 2009, retrieved from www.nimh.nih.gov/health/publications/eating-disorders/how-are-men-and-boys-affected.shtml. **8.** "Eating Disorders in Men," by M. Tartakovsky, October 7, 2008, retrieved from http://psychcentral.com/blog/archives/2008/10/07/eating-disorder-in-men. **9.** "Eating Disorders: Not Just for Women," by S. G. Boodman, March 13, 2007, *The Washington Post*, p. HE01.

Some patients also benefit from antidepressant medications such as fluoxetine (Prozac), which is the only prescription drug approved by the FDA as a treatment for bulimia. These medications help some patients reduce depression and anxiety, as well as reduce binge-purge behavior and the chance of relapse.[93]

Binge Eating Disorder

Binge eaters may periodically consume thousands of calories in a matter of hours, do little to burn off those calories afterward, and then repeat a session of binge eating within a few days. As more binges lead to weight gain, many binge eaters say they begin to feel depressed, worried, and concerned about their ability to control their appetite. Those feelings lead many binge eaters to eat in private or try to hide their eating from others. About 2.8% of U.S. adults, including 3.5% of women and 2% of men, suffer from binge eating disorder.[94]

Signs of binge eating disorder include:

- Eating large amounts of food in a relatively short period of time, whether you are hungry or not, at least twice a week
- Eating until you feel overly full
- Eating large amounts of food alone
- Choosing to consume particular personal "comfort foods," such as certain types of cookies, ice cream, or other foods you find especially pleasurable, during these concentrated sessions of heavy eating

Treatment options for binge eating disorder are similar to those used to treat bulimia nervosa, and may include nutritional counseling, behavior therapy, and antidepressant medication.

Other Unhealthful Eating Behaviors

There are other unhealthful eating behaviors that do not qualify as full-blown eating disorders but still have serious effects on weight, mental health, and well-being. These behaviors are classified as **disordered eating,** a range of unhealthful eating habits in which food is used primarily to deal with emotional issues. Disordered eating is common on college campuses—in one poll, about 20% of students said they had experienced some kind of disordered eating.[95]

disordered eating A range of unhealthful eating behaviors used to deal with emotional issues that does not warrant a diagnosis of a specific eating disorder.

Night-Eating Syndrome

While it's common for many of us to occasionally visit the fridge after dinner, some people suffer from a regular pattern of night-time eating, disrupted

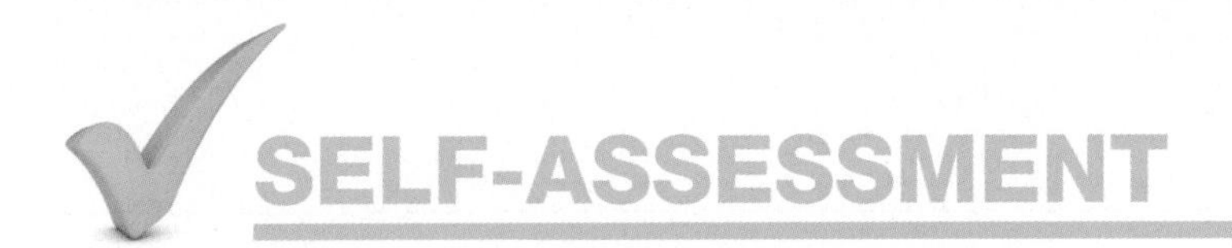

Could I Have an Eating Disorder?

To help find out, a doctor would ask you the following questions:

- Do you regularly eat large quantities of food, and continue eating long after you're full?
- Do you worry that you have lost control over how much you eat?
- Do you regularly avoid food, even when you're hungry?
- Do you have obsessive negative feelings about how your body looks?
- Do you feel extremely anxious about gaining weight?

HOW TO INTERPRET YOUR SCORE

Score 1 point for every "yes" answer. If you score 2 points or more, talk with a health professional.

Take this self-assessment online at www.pearsonhighered.com/lynchelmore.

sleep, and mood disorders that can add up to depression and weight gain. Those with night-eating syndrome often skip breakfast and eat little during the first part of the day. Then, beginning in the evening, food intake increases dramatically, often focusing on starchy or sugary foods. People with this syndrome may eat before going to bed, and then wake up several times during the night for more food.

While the syndrome isn't yet fully understood, researchers suspect that a range of sleep and health difficulties may play a role, leading the body to seek food and carbohydrates in an effort to better produce and regulate sleep-related hormones. Because of these variable underlying causes, the prevalence of night-eating syndrome varies widely—while experts estimate that about 1.5% of the general population suffers from the condition, a study of a group of psychiatric patients found that about 12% experienced night-eating syndrome.[96, 97] In another study of overweight and obese patients with serious mental illness, about 25% had the condition.[98]

Night-eating syndrome can be difficult to treat, but is sometimes addressed with hormonal supplements such as melatonin or antidepressant medications.[99]

Female Athlete Triad

This multifaceted disorder is more prevalent in female athletes participating in sports that require a lower body weight, such as gymnastics, diving, or distance running. Women and girls with this syndrome experience a trio of disorders: disordered eating (focusing on weight control and calorie restriction), amenorrhea (irregular or absent menstrual period), and osteoporosis (low bone density).[100] The combination of disordered eating and frequent high-intensity exercise leaves the body with inadequate energy to maintain fat stores and reproductive functioning. Low blood levels of the female reproductive hormone estrogen lead to cessation of menstrual periods, and loss of bone density. This in turn increases the athlete's risk for fractures. Depending on the athlete's age, the loss of bone density may be irreversible, resulting in a life-long increased risk for fractures. Because this disorder is difficult to treat, medical experts stress prevention, urging coaches, friends, and parents of female athletes to avoid excessive focus on an athlete's weight, watch for signs of the triad, and seek professional help if they suspect the disorder is present.[101]

Compulsive Overeating

Some people feel the need to eat constantly, even when they are full. They eat quickly, often snacking around the clock instead of sitting down to eat at set mealtimes. They are also often embarrassed about their eating and the weight gain it brings, and may find ways to eat in private whenever possible. Compulsive overeaters usually turn to food as a source of comfort against feelings of self-doubt and fears of failure or abandonment.

Signs of compulsive overeating include:

- Continuing to eat, whether you are hungry or not
- Eating quickly and often
- A pattern of failed dieting efforts, accompanied by worries about dieting again
- Using food as comfort or as a reward
- Thinking and talking about food throughout the day

Compulsive Exercise

Daily exercise may be something we should all aspire to, but for some people, exercise becomes an unhealthful obsession. Compulsive exercise, or working out excessively for hours a day to the exclusion of other activities, often accompanies disordered eating and body image disorders.

Signs that an exercise habit may be unhealthful include:[102]

- Your exercise is motivated primarily by a desire to control your weight, body shape, or appearance.
- Preoccupation with exercise leads you to skip other activities, miss work, or skip class.
- You never let yourself miss a workout, even if you are injured or ill.
- You are never satisfied with your fitness achievements.
- You become angry, anxious, or start feeling guilty if your workout routine is disturbed.
- Your food choices are centered around exercise—you only let yourself eat certain foods if you've worked out, or you deny yourself food if you haven't exercised.

Extreme Dieting

Extreme dieters don't just watch calories or exercise often. Dieting and weight loss become obsessions, causing them to calculate the calories in each bite of food and track every pound of weight lost or gained. As a result, extreme dieters can suffer health problems from excessive weight loss, such as weakness from diminished muscle mass. They are also at greater risk for developing anorexia nervosa.

Signs of extreme dieting include:

- A preoccupation with eating as a source of potential weight gain
- A preoccupation with burning off calories
- Misconceptions about food and exercise that fuel these preoccupations. Some extreme dieters may insist, for example, that a particular type of fruit is essential to weight loss, even if little evidence supports that claim.

- Frequent use of over-the-counter pills to try to control weight, including laxatives and diet pills

Getting Help for a Body Image or Eating Disorder

If you struggle with a negative body image or unhealthful eating behaviors, seek support and treatment from trained professionals. Many people who experience eating disorders and disordered eating also get a great deal of help from guided support groups. In these groups, you'll not only receive help in shifting your self-perceptions and habits, but get valuable advice from others who've been in your shoes.

If you have a serious eating disorder, you may first need medical treatment to stabilize your body and stop your health from deteriorating. Once your health is stabilized, your network of social and emotional support will be an essential part of reframing your views of yourself, food, and how your eating habits have defined your life so far.

If you think someone you know has an unhealthful eating or weight-control behavior:

- Locate support and treatment resources on campus or in your community.
- Once you know where to find help, have a compassionate, open conversation with the person you are concerned about. Try to listen and talk about your worries, rather than accuse or blame.
- Try not to talk with your friend or loved one about dieting, body size, or weight. Instead, focus on behaviors that worry you and how they might be unhealthful.
- Offer to direct the person to the treatment resources you've found, and offer to go along for support if desired.
- Know that one conversation may not go far. Keep trying. If you let your friend or loved one know that you are concerned, that person will know where to turn when he or she is ready to seek help.

STUDENT STORY

Eating Disorders

"Hi, my name is Viege. My freshman year in college I had a friend named Lisa, who suffered from an eating disorder. She would always starve herself to try to look like other people or starve herself to get a guy. To be honest with you, I really didn't take it seriously. I just told her that it's just a phase she was going through. Everything will be all right. And then, as I saw her getting skinnier and skinnier, I was like, hey, maybe you do need to get some help. And all she would say is, I'm not crazy. I just want to be beautiful. So I just let it go. And that was the biggest mistake I've ever made because a couple months later, Lisa was rushed to the hospital because she had something wrong with her heart.

So, if you do have a friend that's struggling with eating disorders, you should probably talk to them. You may not think of it as serious but it can be, even if they're young."

1: What do you think was wrong with Viege's friend's heart? What could have caused her to be hospitalized?

2: Do you think it's common for people to take eating disorders seriously? What would prompt you to talk to a friend about a possible eating disorder? Do you think it's your place to convince a friend to get help?

Do you have a story similar to Viege's? Share your story at www.pearsonhighered.com/lynchelmore.

Personal Choices: Develop a More Positive Body Image

While energy balance—calories in versus calories burned—is important, it's also critical to understand how you view your body and your health. Here are a few strategies for building a more positive body image to help yourself achieve and maintain a healthy weight and shape:

- Accept yourself for who you are. Beauty comes in many shapes and sizes. You don't have to look like a starved fashion model or amped-up bodybuilder to be happy.
- Pay attention to your fitness rather than your appearance. Build healthy habits that benefit both your mind and your body.
- Be kind to yourself. No one can look their healthiest or eat wisely all the time. Accept your setbacks as temporary obstacles, not personal failures.
- Know that the beauty and fitness industries are businesses designed to make money, not be health-care providers. Take corporate and mass media beauty and fitness advice with a large grain of salt.
- Remember that your worth is not defined by your appearance, and your health is not defined by the number on the scale.

"Remember that your worth is not defined by your appearance, and your health is not defined by the number on the scale."

Watch videos of real students discussing weight management and body image at www.pearsonhighered.com/lynchelmore.

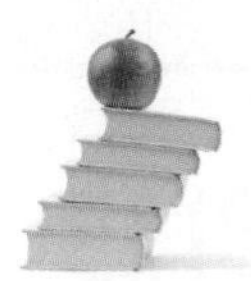

Choosing to Change Worksheet

To complete this worksheet online, visit **www.pearsonhighered.com/lynchelmore**.

What can you do to manage your weight? What is an appropriate goal for weight management? Follow the steps below to develop a weight-management plan.

Directions: Fill in your stage of behavior change in Step 1 and complete the rest of the worksheet with your stage of change in mind.

Step 1: Your Stage of Behavior Change. Please check one of the following statements that best describes your readiness to manage your weight.

_____________ I do not intend to change my body weight in the next 6 months. (Precontemplation)

_____________ I might change my body weight in the next 6 months. (Contemplation)

_____________ I am prepared to change my body weight in the next month. (Preparation)

_____________ I have been changing my body weight for less than 6 months. (Action)

_____________ I have been changing my body weight for more than 6 months. (Maintenance)

Step 2: Creating a Weight-Management Plan

1. What does your BMI and waist-to-hip ratio tell you about the effect of your weight on your health? How do you feel about your weight when you look in the mirror? Do you want to maintain your current weight? Gain weight? Lose weight? By how many pounds? Write down exactly what you want to accomplish with your weight-management plan.

BMI and waist-to-hip ratio: ____

Effect on health: ____

Weight-management goal: ____

2. Given your current stage of behavior change, what can you do next to accomplish your weight-management goal? Which side of the energy balance equation do you want to change: energy in or energy out? You can also modify both. Include a realistic timeline for your next step and list a reward for yourself once you have accomplished your next step.

Next step: ____

____

Timeline: ____

Reward: ____

3. Consider that a healthful prescription for weight loss is cutting 500 to 1,000 calories a day, through reduced calorie intake or increased exercise. This typically leads to a weight loss of 1 or 2 pounds a week. To gain weight, you would add a similar amount of calories daily. Now, consider the weight-management techniques introduced in this chapter. Which techniques can you try to better manage your weight? Keep in mind that you should not cut calories below your recommended MyPlate levels that you can find at **www.choosemyplate.gov**.

____

____

____

4. If you want to simply maintain your current weight, what will you do to ensure that your energy expenditure meets the energy you consume? Think about extended amounts of time when you might consistently consume more food (such as holiday breaks), or where you might be less active than usual (such as during finals). What steps can you take during those times to make sure you stay in energy balance?

____

____

Step 3: Promoting a Healthful Body Image

1. What are your current feelings about your body? When you think about your body, are you usually thinking about how it looks? How it feels? What it does for you? Write down your general thoughts.

____

____

2. What do you like about your body? Write down *at least* three things.

____

____

3. Are there factors that lead you to think negatively about your body (for example, images you see in the media, the opinions of friends or family, the presence of scars or injury, etc.)? If so, how could you combat those factors and improve your body image?

____

____

Chapter Summary

- Your weight affects your health, not just your appearance. Many of us, however, become preoccupied with body image when thinking about our weight.
- Health risks of excess weight include high blood pressure, type 2 diabetes, abnormal blood fats, coronary heart disease, stroke, cancer, osteoarthritis, sleep apnea, gallbladder disease, fatty liver disease, and fertility and pregnancy complications.
- Your weight is shaped by your energy balance, physical activity, basic energy needs, age, genes, gender, and environment. Ultimately, excess weight results from an imbalance of calories consumed and calories used.
- Excess body weight is a critical issue for college students. Decline in physical activity is often a major contributor to college weight gain.
- Overweight and obesity are serious and common health problems, not just in the United States, but around the world.
- BMI, waist circumference, and waist-to-hip ratio can give indicators of whether your weight will increase your risk for certain health conditions and diseases.
- To truly understand your weight and its effects on your health, you need to know your body composition, not just how much you weigh.
- Reaching a healthful lower weight requires consistent, long-term work on both eating habits and increasing physical activity. Short-term diets are often of limited help. Diet aids can be expensive, may not work, and may even be harmful.
- Medical options, including prescription drugs and bariatric surgery, may be beneficial for people who are extremely obese.
- To gain weight, boost your calories in healthful ways by eating nutritious foods like nuts, juices, peanut butter, and meal replacement bars. Also, eat more often and get exercise to stimulate appetite.
- Maintaining a healthful weight is most effective when you establish and consistently follow eating and exercise habits you enjoy, and use them to keep your weight within a healthful range.
- Societal contradictions that encourage weight gain while glorifying thinness lead many of us to have negative views of our own bodies. These body image issues contribute to disordered eating and eating disorders.
- Eating disorders are complicated psychiatric conditions that are affected by family, social dynamics, and feelings of self-worth. Eating disorders that carry significant health risks include anorexia nervosa, bulimia nervosa, and binge eating disorder.
- Disordered eating behaviors, while not qualifying as psychiatric disorders, are also unhealthful. These include night-eating syndrome, the female athlete triad, and compulsive overeating.
- While eating disorders and disordered eating can significantly harm a person's health, or even lead to death in some cases, the good news is that treatments are available, and are often effective. If you know someone who you think might have an eating-related disorder, help them find resources on campus for support and treatment.

Test Your Knowledge

1. Which of the following conditions is NOT related to obesity?
  a. polycystic ovary syndrome
  b. high blood pressure
  c. fatty liver disease
  d. low LDL levels

2. What percentage of 18- to 24-year-olds engage in no leisure-time physical activity?
  a. 75%
  b. 50%
  c. 25%
  d. 10%

3. When most students start college, how many pounds do they gain?
  a. 1 to 4
  b. 7 to 8
  c. 9 to 12
  d. 13 to 16

4. What is the healthful weight range for someone who is 5 feet 11 inches tall?
  a. 133 to 172 pounds
  b. 140 to 171 pounds
  c. 149 to 183 pounds
  d. 164 to 196 pounds

5. What is BMI?
  a. a ratio between your height and your weight, used to help assess health risks
  b. a measurement of how much fat you have
  c. a measurement of how much muscle you have
  d. a 100% reliable indicator of how healthy you are

6. What is the best approach to weight loss?
  a. Eat more protein and drink more water.
  b. Take in fewer calories and exercise more.
  c. Avoid foods containing carbohydrates.
  d. Take in more energy and eat less fat.

7. What term best describes our response to the sight, smell, thought, or taste of food?
  a. satiety
  b. craving
  c. hunger
  d. appetite

8. In order to maintain weight loss, you should
  a. eat as little as possible.
  b. stop working out; it makes you hungry.
  c. never allow yourself to have a high-calorie day.
  d. focus on eating fruits and vegetables.

9. Which of the following statements about body image is true?
  a. In body dysmorphic disorder, a person refuses to perceive a permanent physical flaw.
  b. Among college students, about 10 percent of males and 35 percent of females are dissatisfied with their body.
  c. Men and boys are more likely to have higher levels of social physique anxiety than women and girls.
  d. Women become more self-accepting of their bodies with age.

10. The risk for fractures is increased in women with
  a. bulimia nervosa.
  b. night-eating syndrome.
  c. the female athlete triad.
  d. compulsive overeating.

Get Critical

What happened:

The fashion world revolves around women's appearance, but top Chanel designer Karl Lagerfeld may have taken his opinion a little too far when he decided to comment on the physique of rising singing star Adele when he told a reporter "She is a little too fat, but she has a beautiful face and a divine voice."[1]

Adele's many fans responded angrily, wondering why Lagerfeld would use the body size standards of his industry to critique others who never saunter down a runway. But no one hit back more eloquently than Adele herself, saying "I've never wanted to look like models on the cover of magazines. I represent the majority of women and I'm very proud of that."[2] Lagerfeld later apologized.[3]

What do you think?

- **Does the entertainment industry support people of different physiques and sizes? If so, how? If not, why doesn't it?**
- **What effects do you think the body size standards favored by the fashion industry have on your standards of ideal body size, and your body image? Even if you know a model has had to severely restrict her eating to get down to runway size, do you think it still affects your idea of what beauty is?**
- **What could the worlds of fashion and entertainment do to represent and celebrate many people with many different body types?**

References: **1**. "Karl Lagerfeld on Adele, the Greek Crisis and M.I.A.'s Middle Finger," by *Metro World News*, February 8, 2012 (UPDATED). Retrieved from http://www.metro.us/newyork/life/article/1089980--karl-lagerfeld-on-lana-del-rey-the-greek-crisis-and-m-i-a-s-middle-finger. **2**. "Adele Hits Back at Karl Lagerfeld's 'Too Fat' Insult," by L. Potter, February 9, 2012, retrieved from http://www.marieclaire.co.uk/news/celebrity/534771/adele-hits-back-at-karl-lagerfeld-s-too-fat-insult.html#index=1. **3.** "EXCLUSIVE: Karl Lagerfeld: 'Adele, I am your biggest admirer'," by K. Hunt, February 8, 2012, retrieved from http://www.metro.us/newyork/entertainment/article/1092121.

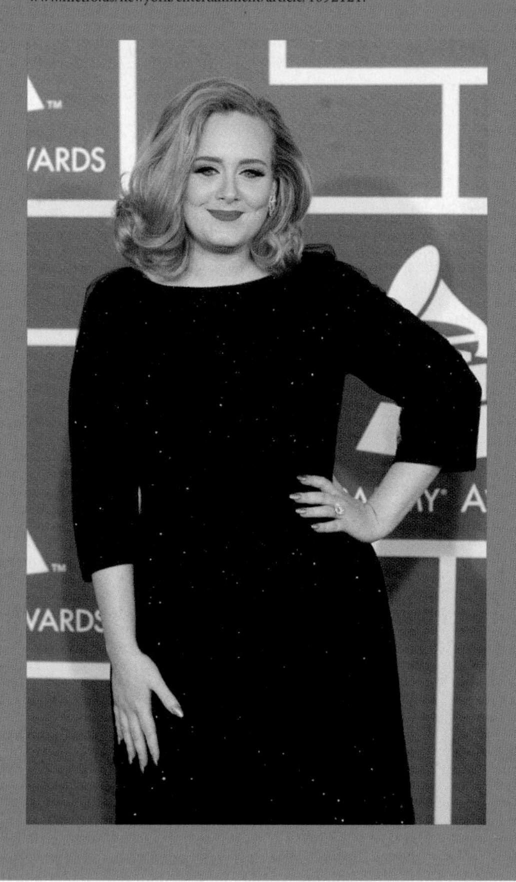

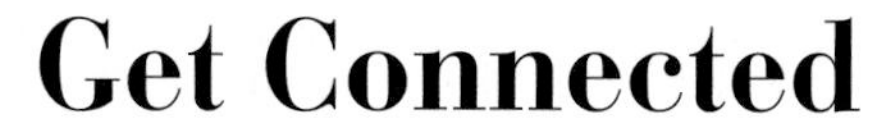

Get Connected

Mobile Tips!

Scan this QR code with your mobile device to access additional weight-management and body image tips. Or, via your mobile device, go to **http://mobiletips.pearsoncmg.com** and navigate to Chapter 7.

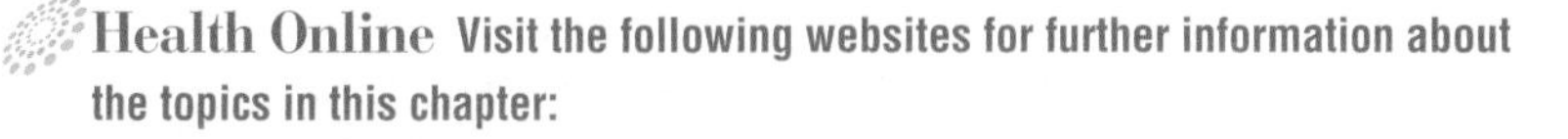

Health Online Visit the following websites for further information about the topics in this chapter:

- National Institute of Mental Health: Eating Disorders
  www.nimh.nih.gov/health/publications/eating-disorders/complete-index.shtml
- Academy of Nutrition and Dietetics
  www.eatright.org
- Centers for Disease Control and Prevention: Overweight and Obesity
  www.cdc.gov/obesity/index.html
- American College of Sports Medicine Exercise Guidelines
  www.acsm.org
- World Health Organization: Obesity
  www.who.int/topics/obesity/en
- Buddy Slim (find a weight-loss partner)
  www.buddyslim.com
- NEDA: Ten Steps to Positive Body Image
  www.nationaleatingdisorders.org/nedaDir/files/documents/handouts/TenSteps.pdf

Website links are subject to change. To access updated Web links, please visit ***www.pearsonhighered.com/lynchelmore.***

References

i. Centers for Disease Control/National Center for Health Statistics. (2011). *FastStats: Overweight prevalence.*

ii. National Institute of Diabetes and Digestive and Kidney Diseases. (2011). *Weight-control information network: Overweight and obesity statistics.*

iii. American College Health Association. (2012). *American College Health Association national college health assessment II: Reference group data report fall 2011.* Retrieved from http://www.acha-ncha.org/reports_acha-nchaii.html.

1. Centers for Disease Control/National Center for Health Statistics. (2011). *FastStats: Overweight prevalence.*

2. World Health Organization. (2009). *Obesity and overweight. Fact sheet number 311.*

3. Centers for Disease Control and Prevention. (2010). Health behaviors of adults: United States, 2005–2007. *Vital and Health Statistics, 10* (245).

4. American College Health Association. (2012). *American College Health Association national college health assessment II: Reference group data report fall 2011.*

5. Lowes, J., & Tiggemann, M. (2003). Body dissatisfaction, dieting awareness and the impact of parental influence in young children. *British Journal of Health Psychology, 8,* 135–147.

6. Keel, P., Baxter, M., Heatheron, T., & Joiner, T. (2007). A 20-year longitudinal study of body weight, dieting, and eating disorder symptoms. *Journal of Abnormal Psychology, 116* (2), 422–432.

7. Forrest, K., & Stuhldreher, W. (2007). Patterns and correlates of body image dissatisfaction and distortion among college students. *American Journal of Health Studies, 22* (1), 18–25.

8. Hawkins, N., Richards, P., Granley, H., & Stein, D. (2004). The impact of exposure to the thin-ideal media image on women. *Eating Disorders, 12* (1), 33–50.

9. Halliwell, E., Easun, A., & Harcourt, D. (2011). Body dissatisfaction: Can a short media literacy message reduce negative media exposure effects amongst adolescent girls? *British Journal of Health Psychology, 16* (2), 396–403.

10. Freedman, D., Kettel Khan, L., Serdula, M., Dietz, W., Srinivasan, S., Berenson, G. (2005). The relation of childhood BMI to adult adiposity: The Bogalusa heart study. *Pediatrics, 115* (1), 22–27.

11. Brooks, Y., Black, D., Coster, D., Blue, C., Abood, D., & Gretebeck, R. (2007). Body mass index and percentage of body fat as health indicators for young adults. *American Journal of Health Behaviors, 31* (6), 687–700.

12. Bray, G. (2006). Obesity: The disease. *Journal of Medicinal Chemistry, 49* (14), 4001–4007.

13. Nappo-Dattoma, L. (2007, July). Part I: Obesity and its threat to your patients' health. *Access,* 36–40.

14. Centers for Disease Control and Prevention (CDC). (2012). *Overweight and obesity: Adult obesity facts.*

15. Wang, Y., & Beydoun, M. (2007). The obesity epidemic in the United States—gender, age, socioeconomic, racial/ethnic, and geographic characteristics: A systematic review and meta-regression analysis. *Epidemiological Reviews, 29,* 6–28.

16. World Health Organization. (2004, April 19). *Diet, physical activity, and health: A report by the Secretariat.* (Electronic version.) Retrieved from http://www.who.int.

17. Economos, C. D., Hildebrandt, M. L., & Hyatt, R. R. (2008). College freshman stress and weight change: Differences by gender. *American Journal of Health Behavior, 32* (1), 16–25.

18. Nelson, T., Gortmaker, S., Subramanian, S., Cheung, S., & Wechsler, H. (2007). Disparities in overweight and obesity among US college students. *American Journal of Health Behaviors, 31* (4), 363–373.

19. Wharton, C., Adams, T., & Hampl, J. (2008). Weight loss practices and body weight perceptions among US college students. *Journal of American College Health, 56* (5), 579–584.

20. Jung, M., Bray, S., & Ginis, K. (2008). Behavior change and the "freshman 15": Tracking physical activity and dietary patterns in 1st-year university women. *Journal of American College Health, (56)* 5, 523–530.

21. Kasparek, D., Corwin, S., Valois, R., Sargent, R., & Morris, R. (2008). Selected health behaviors that influence freshman weight change. *Journal of American College Health, 56* (4), 437–444.

22. Ogden, C. L., Carroll, M. D., Curtin, L. R., McDowell, M. M., Tabak, C. J., & Flegal, F. (2006). Prevalence of overweight and obesity in the United States, 1999–2004. *Journal of the American Medical Association, 295* (13), 1549–1555.

23. Mayo Clinic. (2009). *Obesity.* Retrieved from http://www.mayoclinic.com/health/obesity/DS00314.

24. National Institute of Diabetes and Digestive and Kidney Diseases/National Institutes of Health. (2007). *Do you know the health risks of being overweight?* NIH Publication No. 07–4098.

25. Nguyen, N. T., Magno, C. P., Lane, K. T., Hinojosa, M. W., & Lane, J. S. (2008, December). Association of hypertension, diabetes, dyslipidemia, and metabolic syndrome with obesity: Findings from the National Health and Nutrition Examination Survey, 1999–2004. *Journal of the American College of Surgeons, 207* (6), 928–934.

26. U.S. Department of Health and Human Services, Office on Women's Health. (2010). *Polycystic ovary syndrome (PCOS) fact sheet.*

27. Olshansky, S. J., Passaro, D. J., Hershow, R. C., Layden, J., Carnes, B. A., Brody, J., . . . Ludwig, D. S. (2005). A potential decline in life expectancy in the United States in the 21st century. *New England Journal of Medicine, 352,* 1103–1110.

28. Finkelstein, E., Trogdon, J., Cohen, J., & Dietz, W. (2009). Annual medical spending attributable to obesity: Payer- and service-specific estimates. *Health Affairs, 28* (5), 822–831.

29. Trogdon, J., Finkelstein, E., Feagan, C., . . . Cohen, J. (2011, June 16). State- and payer-specific estimates of annual medical expenditures attributable to obesity. *Obesity,* doi: 10.1038/oby.2011.

30. Dor, A., Ferguson, C., Langwith, C., & Tan, E. (2010). A heavy burden: The individual costs of being overweight and obese in the United States. *The George Washington University School of Public Health and Health Services.*

31. Duyff, R. L. (2006). *American Dietetic Association complete food and nutrition guide* (p. 26). New York: John Wiley and Sons.

32. Levi, A., Chan, K., & Pence, D. (2006). Real men do not read food labels: The effects of masculinity and involvement on college students' food decisions. *Journal of American College Health, 55* (2), 91–98.

33. Power, M., & Schulkin, J. (2008). Sex differences in fat storage, fat metabolism, and the health risks from obesity: possible evolutionary origins. *British Journal of Nutrition, 99* (5), 931–940.

34. Coutinho, T., Goel, K., Corrêa de Sá, D., Kragelund, C., Kanaya, A., Zeller, M., . . . Lopez-Jimenez, F. (2011). Central obesity and survival in subjects with coronary artery disease: A systematic review of the literature and collaborative analysis with individual subject data. *Journal of the American College of Cardiology, 57,* 1877–1886.

35. Mayo Clinic. (2011). *Belly fat in women: Taking—and keeping—it off.* Retrieved from http://www.mayoclinic.com/health/belly-fat/WO00128/NSECTIONGROUP=2.

36. Frayling, T., Timpson N., Weedon, M., Zeggini, E., Freathy, R., Lindgren, C., . . . McCarthy, M. (2007). A common variant in the FTO gene is associated with body mass index and predisposes to childhood and

adult obesity. (Electronic version.) *Science 12.* Retrieved from http://www.sciencemag.org/cgi/content/abstract/1141634v1.

37. Kaiser Family Foundation. (2010). *Overweight and obesity rates for adults by race/ethnicity, 2010.* Retrieved from http://www.statehealthfacts.org.

38. Beydoun, M., & Wang, Y. (2009). Gender-ethnic disparity in BMI and waist circumference distribution shifts in US adults. *Obesity, 17* (1), 169–176.

39. Ogden, C., Lamb, M., Carroll, M., & Flegal, K. (2010). NCHS data brief: Obesity and socioeconomic status in adults: United States, 2005–2008.

40. Ogden, C., Lamb, M., Carroll, M., & Flegal, K. (2010). NCHS data brief: Obesity and socioeconomic status in children and adolescents: United States, 2005–2008.

41. Farah, H., & Buzby, J. (2005, November). U.S. food consumption up 16 percent since 1970. *U.S. Department of Agriculture: Amber Waves.*

42. Newman C. (2004, August). Why are we so fat? *National Geographic, 206* (2), 46–61.

43. National Center for Health Statistics, Health Indicators Warehouse. (2010). Leisure-time physical activity—none (percent). Retrieved from http://www.healthindicators.gov/Indicators/Noleisure-timephysicalactivity_1313/Profile/Data.

44. Matthews, C. E., Chen, K. Y., Freedson, P. S., Buchowski, M. S., Bettina, M., Beech, B. M., Pate, R. R., & Troiano, R. P. (2008). Amount of time spent in sedentary behaviors in the United States, 2003–2004. *American Journal of Epidemiology, 167* (7), 875–881.

45. The Nielsen Company. (2010). *What consumers watch: Nielsen's Q1 2010 three screen report.*

46. U.S. Census Bureau. (2005). *Americans spend more than 100 hours each year commuting to work, Census Bureau reports.* American Community Survey, 2005.

47. Moczulski, V., McMahan, S., Weiss, J., Beam, W., & Chandler, L. (2007). Commuting behaviors, obesity risk, and the built environment. *American Journal of Health Behaviors, 22* (1), 26–32.

48. O'Connor, D., Jones, F., Conner, M., & McMillan, B. (2008). Effects of daily hassles and eating styles on eating behavior. *Health Psychology, 27* (1), 20–31.

49. McDonald's. (2012). McDonald's USA nutrition facts for popular menu items. (Electronic version.) Retrieved from http://nutrition.mcdonalds.com/getnutrition/nutritionfacts.pdf.

50. Food Research and Action Center. (2011). *Food insecurity and obesity: Understanding the connections.* Retrieved from http://frac.org/pdf/frac_brief_understanding_the_connections.pdf.

51. Larson, N., & Story, M. (2011). Food insecurity and weight status among U.S. children and families: A review of the literature. *American Journal of Preventive Medicine, 40* (2), 166–173.

52. Gordon-Larsen, P., Nelson, M., Page, P., & Popkin, B. (2006). Inequality in the built environment underlies key health disparities in physical activity and obesity. *Pediatrics, 117* (2), 417–424.

53. Jahren, A. H., & Kraft, R. A. (2008). Carbon and nitrogen stable isotopes in fast food: Signatures of corn and confinement. *Proceedings of the National Academy of Sciences of the United States of America, 105* (46), 17855–17860.

54. Wells, H., & Buzby, J. (2008). High fructose corn syrup usage may be leveling off. *Amber Waves* (United States Department of Food and Agriculture).

55. Physicians Committee for Responsible Medicine. (2011). *USDA's new MyPlate icon at odds with federal subsidies for meat, dairy.* Retrieved from http://pcrm.org/media/news/usdas-new-myplate-icon-at-odds-with-federal.

56. Dansinger, M., Gleason, J., Griffith, J., Selker, H., & Schaefer, E. (2005). Comparison of the Atkins, Ornish, Weight Watchers, and Zone diets for weight loss and heart disease risk reduction. *Journal of the American Medical Association, 293* (1), 43–53.

57. Mayo Clinic. (2011). Trans *fat is double trouble for your heart health.* Retrieved from http://www.mayoclinic.com/health/trans-fat/CL00032.

58. Gardner, C., Kiazand, A., Alhassan, S., Kim, S., Stafford, R., Balise, R., Kraemer, H., & King, A. (2007). Comparison of the Atkins, Zone, Ornish, and LEARN diets for change in weight and related risk factors among overweight premenopausal women. *Journal of the American Medical Association, 297* (9), 969–977.

59. Yancy W., Olsen, M., Guyton, J., Bakst, R., Westman, E. (2004). A low-carbohydrate, ketogenic diet versus a low-fat diet to treat obesity and hyperlipidemia. *Annals of Internal Medicine, 140,* 769–777.

60. Marketdata Enterprises, Inc. (2011). *U.S. weight loss market worth $60.9 billion.* (Electronic version.) Retrieved from http://www.prweb.com/releases/2011/5/prweb8393658.htm.

61. Celio, C., Luce, K., Bryson, S., Winzelberg, A., Cunning, D., Rockwell, R., Celio Doyle, A., Wilfley, D., & Taylor, C. (2006). Use of diet pills and other dieting aids in a college population with high weight and shape concerns. *International Journal of Eating Disorders, 39* (6), 492–497.

62. Jordan, M., & Haywood, T. (2007). Evaluation of Internet websites marketing herbal weight-loss supplements to consumers. *Journal of Alternative and Complementary Medicine, 13* (9), 1035–1043.

63. U.S. Food and Drug Administration. (2011, December 6). *FDA, FTC act to remove "homeopathic" HCG weight loss products from the market.* FDA News Release.

64. U.S. Food and Drug Administration. (2009, May 1). *FDA warns consumers to stop using Hydroxycut products.* FDA News.

65. U.S. Food and Drug Administration. (2005). *FDA news release: FDA acts to seize ephedra-containing dietary supplements.* P05-94.

66. Elder, S., & Roberts, S. (2007). The effects of exercise on food intake and body fatness: A summary of published studies. *Nutrition Reviews, 65* (1), 1–19.

67. Graffagnino, C., Falko, J., La Londe, M., Schaumburg, J., Hyek, M., Shaffer, L., Snow, R., & Caulin-Glaser, T. (2006). Effect of a community-based weight management program on weight loss and cardiovascular disease risk factors. *Obesity, 14,* 280–288.

68. Kasparek, D., Corwin, S., Valois, R., Sargent, R., & Morris, R. (2008). Selected health behaviors that influence college freshman weight change. *Journal of the American College Health Association, 56* (4), 437–444.

69. Overeaters Anonymous. (2012). OA Program of Recovery. Retrieved from http://www.oa.org.

70. Thomas, O. (2011, February 9). Apps to share your pride at the gym. *The New York Times.*

71. Weiss, F. (2004). Group psychotherapy with obese disordered-eating adults with body-image disturbances: An integrated model. *American Journal of Psychotherapy, 58* (3), 281–303.

72. U.S. Food and Drug Administration. (2010.) *Meridia (sibutramine): Market withdrawal due to risk of serious cardiovascular events.*

73. U.S. Food and Drug Administration. (2010). *Questions and answers: Orlistat and severe liver injury.*

74. American Society for Metabolic and Bariatric Surgery. (2011). *Fact sheet: Metabolic and bariatric surgery.* Retrieved from http://asmbs.org/asmbs-press-kit.

75. Ebell, M. (2008). Predicting mortality risk in patients undergoing bariatric surgery. *American Family Physician, 77* (2), 220–221.

76. Ingelfinger, J. (2011). Bariatric surgery in adolescents. *New England Journal of Medicine, 365* (15), 1365–1367.

77. American Society of Plastic Surgeons. (2011). Liposuction procedure. Retrieved from http://www.plasticsurgery.org/cosmetic-procedures/liposuction.html.

78. Mann, D. (2010). Study shows technique removes fat and helps skin tightening; critics worry about burns. Retrieved from http://www.webmd.com/healthy-beauty/news/20100426/debate-on-laser-liposuction-to-remove-fat.

79. Carney, T., & Louw, J. (2006). Eating disordered behaviors and media exposure. *Social Psychiatry and Psychiatry Epidemiology, 41,* 957–966.

80. Haas, C., Champion, A., & Secor, D. (2008). Motivating factors for seeking cosmetic surgery: A synthesis of the literature. *Plastic Surgery Nursing, 4,* 177–182.

81. Mayo Clinic. (2010). *Body dysmorphic disorder.* Retrieved from http://www.mayoclinic.com/health/body-dysmorphic-disorder/DS00559.

82. Hart, E., Leary, M., & Rejeski, W. (1989). The measurement of social physique anxiety. *Journal of Sport Exercise Psychology, 11* (1), 94–104.

83. Hagger, M., & Stevenson, A. (2010). Social physique anxiety and physical self-esteem: Gender and age effects. *Psychology and Health, 25* (1), 89–110.

84. National Institute of Mental Health. (2011). *Eating disorders among children.*

85. National Institute of Mental Health. (Date of publication not reported.) *Eating disorders among adults—anorexia nervosa.*

86. Mayo Clinic. (2012). *Anorexia nervosa: Causes.* Retrieved from http://www.mayoclinic.com/health/anorexia/ds00606/dsection=causes.

87. Steinhausen, H. (2009). Outcomes of eating disorders. *Child and Adolescent Psychiatric Clinics of North America, 18,* 225–242.

88. Hudson, J. I., Hiripi, E., Pope, Jr., H. G., & Kessler, R. C. (2007). The prevalence and correlates of eating disorders in the National Comorbidity Survey replication. *Biological Psychiatry, 61* (3), 348–358.

89. U.S. Department of Health and Human Services, National Guideline Clearinghouse. (2011). *Practice guideline for the treatment of patients with eating disorders.*

90. Salahi, L. (2012, April 19). Internet crackdown on pro-anorexia sites. ABCNews.com. Retrieved from http://abcnews.go.com/Health/Wellness/internet-crackdown-pro-anorexia-sites/story?id=16158270.

91. National Institute of Mental Health. (Date of publication not reported.) *Eating disorders among adults—bulimia nervosa.*

92. National Institute of Mental Health. (2011). *Eating disorders: What are the different types of eating disorders?*

93. U.S. Department of Health and Human Services, Office on Women's Health. (2009). *Bulimia nervosa fact sheet.*

94. National Institute of Mental Health. (Date of publication not reported.) *Eating disorders among adults—binge eating disorder.*

95. Eating Disorders Review. (2006.). *In a recent poll, nearly 20 percent of students admit to disordered eating*. Retrieved from http://www.eatingdisordersreview.com/nl/nl_edr_17_6_9.html.

96. Rand, C., Macgregory, A., & Stunkard, A. (1997). The night eating syndrome in the general population and among postoperative obesity surgery patients. *International Journal of Eating Disorders, 22* (1), 65–69.

97. Lundgren, J., Allison, K., Crow, S., O'Reardon, J., Berg, K., Galbraith, J., Martino, N., & Stunkard, A. (2006). Prevalence of the night eating syndrome in a psychiatric population. *American Journal of Psychiatry, 163*, 156–158.

98. Lundgren, J., Rempfer, M., Brown, C., Goetz, J., & Hamera, E. (2010.) The prevalence of night eating syndrome and binge eating disorder among overweight and obese individuals with serious mental illness. *Psychiatry Research, 175* (3), 233–236.

99. O'Reardon, J., Peshek, A., & Allison, K. (2005.) Night eating syndrome: Diagnosis, epidemiology, and management. *CNS Drugs, 19* (12), 997–1008.

100. American College of Sports Medicine. (2011). *The female athlete triad.* Retrieved from http://www.acsm.org/docs/brochures/the-female-athlete-triad.pdf.

101. Hobart, J., & Smucker, D. (2000). The female athlete triad. *American Family Physician, 61* (11), 3357–3364.

102. Gerard Eberle, S. (2004). Compulsive exercise: Too much of a good thing? National Eating Disorders Association. Retrieved from http://uhs.berkeley.edu/edaw/cmpvexc.pdf.

8 Compulsive Behaviors and Psychoactive Drugs: Understanding Addiction

- About 2 million adults in the United States are addicted to gambling.[i]

- An estimated 8.7% of Americans currently use illicit drugs.[ii]

- College students tend to vastly overestimate how many of their peers use drugs.[iii]

LEARNING OBJECTIVES

IDENTIFY the characteristics of and risk factors for addiction.

DISCUSS common behavioral addictions.

DESCRIBE the prevalence of drug use among college students.

COMPARE AND CONTRAST the terms *drug misuse, drug abuse, addiction,* and *dependence.*

DESCRIBE the body's response to drugs.

IDENTIFY commonly abused drugs, describing their mechanisms, effects, and health risks.

EXPLAIN the costs and consequences of drug abuse.

DISCUSS the prevention and treatment of drug abuse.

DESCRIBE personal strategies for overcoming addictions and drug abuse.

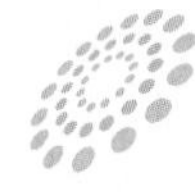

Health Online icons are found throughout the chapter, directing you to web links, videos, podcasts, and other useful online resources.

Senator resigns—checks into rehab!

Superstar's spending out of control! When addiction or abuse involves a celebrity, you hear about it. But what about the untold stories—the more than 30,000 drug-induced deaths in the United States each year, the 5% of female college students who have experienced a drug-related forcible sexual assault, the over 22 million Americans with substance abuse or dependence, or the 2 million Americans whose lives are ruined by addiction to gambling? [1–4] Chances are, you've witnessed one or more of these stories among your own family members or friends—or maybe the untold story is your own.

Even if your life hasn't been directly touched by addiction, you share the costs. These include the economic costs of health care, lost productivity, social services, and law enforcement for increased crime. They also include the social costs of broken families and ravaged communities.

What can you do about addictions and drug abuse? Change starts with knowledge—about the nature of addictions, how to avoid them, how to recover, and how to help a friend. Start here.

An Overview of Addiction

From time to time, we all do things for fun even though we know they might cause us trouble in the long term: We cut classes, eat that extra slice of pizza, or buy those concert tickets that we "really can't afford." Such behavior is normal—and reflects the fact that the pleasure centers in our brains evolved for short-term survival, not for the kind of long-term planning that leads to academic success, healthy weight maintenance, or financial security. But why do some people repeatedly engage in problematic behaviors that have long since stopped providing any real pleasure? Why, in short, do some people develop addictions? To explore this perplexing question, let's first take a look at what an addiction really is.

What Is Addiction?

The American Society of Addiction Medicine defines **addiction** as a chronic disease of brain reward, motivation, memory, and related circuitry. Dysfunction in these brain circuits is reflected in the individual pathologically pursuing reward and/or relief by substance use or other behaviors.[5]

Perhaps the most fundamental characteristic of addiction is craving. The person experiences an uncontrollable compulsion to engage in the behavior, and seeks it out even in the face of significant negative consequences.[6] Often, these negative consequences are entirely clear to loved ones, but the addict may have a diminished capacity to recognize the problems caused by his or her behavior.[5] Denial of both the negative consequences and the addiction itself is common.

Another characteristic of addiction is loss of pleasure. Although the person originally may have engaged in the activity for pleasurable recreation, he or she now derives very little satisfaction from it. Instead, the addict's motivation becomes an increasingly powerful compulsion to relieve the physical discomfort and emotional anguish experienced when abstaining. As a result, the person experiences an escalating loss of control over the act and comes to feel increasingly controlled by it.[7]

addiction A chronic, progressive disease of brain reward, motivation, memory, and related circuitry characterized by uncontrollable craving for a substance or behavior despite both negative consequences and diminishment or loss of pleasure associated with the activity.

Although this upward trend is alarming, the actual rates of current illicit drug use are lower for college graduates (6.3%) than for those who did not graduate from high school (10.8%) and high school graduates who did not attend college (8.5%).[3] However, college graduates are more likely to have experimented with illicit drugs at some point during their lifetime compared with adults without high school diplomas.

Interestingly, students tend to vastly overestimate the percentage of their peers who use drugs. For example, in a national survey conducted in 2011, students reported believing that almost 80% of their peers use marijuana, when only 14% of students reported actually using it.[25] The number of students who report using illicit drugs other than marijuana is even lower—less than 13%. So as you read on in this chapter, it's important to bear in mind that *not everyone is using drugs*—far from it.

View a video of young adults telling personal stories about their drug addictions at http://pact360.org/programs/youth360.

Why Do Some Students Use Illicit Drugs?

In the past, people believed that use of illicit drugs was due to moral failure, rebellion, or laziness. We now know that the problem is more complicated than that. Earlier, we explored some determinants of addiction. But why do people begin to use illicit drugs in the first place?

The National Institute on Drug Abuse (NIDA) identifies four main reasons that people use drugs:[8]

- **To feel good.** Some use drugs to seek pleasure, or to feel more powerful or self-confident. Some use drugs for increased energy, whereas others seek feelings of relaxation or sedation.
- **To relieve pain or escape from distress.** We noted earlier that some people begin to use drugs in an effort to "self-medicate"; that is, to relieve chronic pain or feelings of depression or anxiety. Stress can play a major role in initiating drug use, continuing it, or experiencing relapse.
- **To do better.** Many college students turn to drugs to try to improve their academic or athletic performance.
- **Curiosity or "because others are doing it."** Popular culture often glamorizes drugs: Think of how many "stoner" characters you see featured in movies, and how often you see actors, actresses, and rock stars smoking or drinking. The social pressure to experiment with drugs can be especially intense for college students living away from home, perhaps for the first time, and who form friendships with students who use drugs.

The Body's Response to Psychoactive Drugs

By definition, all psychoactive drugs **intoxicate** the brain, producing characteristic physical, psychological, and behavioral changes. Typically, the user experiences the onset, peak, and diminishment of these changes in rapid succession, sometimes within minutes and typically within a few hours. How quickly and to what extent intoxication occurs depends to some extent on the method of administration.

intoxicate To cause physical and psychological changes as a result of the consumption of psychoactive substances.

Methods of Administration

There are five basic ways that people self-administer drugs (**Table 8.1**):

- *Ingestion* is the process of swallowing and absorbing a drug through the digestive system. For example, pills and alcoholic beverages are both ingested. Ingestion is the slowest way for a chemical to reach the brain.
- *Injection* is the process of using a syringe to inject a drug into the skin (*subcutaneous injection*), muscle (*intramuscular injection*), or bloodstream (*intravenous injection*). Injecting a drug can expose a user to diseases, including HIV, hepatitis B and C, and other types of infection that can enter the body on a shared or otherwise dirty needle. Injecting a drug into a vein also sends it more quickly to the brain. As a result, the drug can deliver a quicker rush, but the high can also fade faster, often prompting the user to inject again. This pattern can increase the addictive power of a drug.
- *Inhalation* is the process of breathing a drug into the lungs through the mouth or nostril—that is, by sniffing or smoking it. Like injection, inhalation increases a drug's addictive potential because it speeds drugs into the bloodstream.
- *Mucosal absorption* is the absorption of a drug through the mucous membranes. Chewing tobacco is absorbed through the mucous membranes of the mouth. Cocaine that has been snorted is absorbed through the mucous membranes of the nose.
- *Topical administration* is application of a drug directly onto a body surface—typically the skin. A nicotine patch, which is applied directly to the skin's surface, is an example of topical administration.

Table 8.1: Common Methods of Drug Administration

Method	Description	Typical Drugs
Ingestion	Swallowing a drug and absorbing it through the digestive system	Alcoholic beverages, pills, LSD
Injection	Using a syringe to inject a drug directly into the skin, muscle, or bloodstream	Cocaine, methamphetamine, heroin
Inhalation	Breathing a drug into the lungs through the mouth or nostrils (snorting or smoking)	Marijuana, tobacco, cocaine (crack), inhalants such as paint thinner or glue
Mucosal absorption	Absorbing a drug through the mucous membranes	Chewing tobacco (absorbed through the membranes in the mouth); snorted cocaine (absorbed through the membranes in the nose)
Topical administration	Applying a drug directly onto a body surface, like the skin	Nicotine patch

Effects on the Brain

Once a drug enters the bloodstream, it is transported to body cells, including those of the brain. To understand its effects there, it helps to understand the fundamental structure and functions of the brain.

Weighing an average of just 3 pounds, your brain has a processing capacity far greater than any supercomputer yet invented. Every waking second, it's regulating your basic body functions like breathing and thirst; receiving signals from your eyes, ears, taste buds, and other sensory structures and interpreting them as experiences; determining and directing your responses; reasoning and solving problems; creating, storing, and retrieving memories; and shaping your emotions. Psychoactive drugs can alter many of these functions, as well as drive the craving that characterizes addiction. Brain areas affected by drug abuse include the following **(Figure 8.1)**:[8]

- The *brain stem* is the lowest portion of the brain. It connects the top of the spinal cord with the base of the *cerebrum* (the two brain hemispheres housed in the skull) and controls the basic functions most critical to sustaining life, such as heart rate, breathing, and sleeping.
- The *cerebral cortex* is the outermost "rind" of grey matter covering the cerebrum. It performs the highest functions of human consciousness, such as reasoning, language, and creativity.
- The *limbic system* is an "association area"—that is, a part of the brain involved in integration. It is buried deep within the cerebrum, and is critical to the formation and storage of memories. The limbic system also contains the brain's "reward circuit," which integrates a number of brain structures involved in your ability to feel pleasure. This reward circuit is activated, for example, by eating enjoyable food, working out, and using certain psychoactive drugs. The limbic system is also responsible for perception of other emotions besides pleasure, a fact that explains the mood-altering properties of many drugs.[8]

As you can imagine, the functions of the different brain regions depend on communication: the coding, transmitting, and receiving of messages back and forth among billions of nerve cells, called *neurons.* Every neuron in the brain receives and sends messages in the form of electrical impulses. Because adjacent neurons don't physically touch, when an impulse reaches the end of a transmitting neuron, it has to cross a gap, called a *synapse,* in order to reach the receiving neuron. (See Figure 2.4 in Chapter 2.) The release of chemicals called *neurotransmitters* into the synapse enables impulses to cross. Neurotransmitters attach to sites called *receptors* on the receiving neuron. When they do, they act somewhat like a key opening a lock, allowing the impulse to enter into the receiving cell.

Psychoactive drugs interfere with this delicate communication system, altering how neurons send, receive, and process information. For instance, some drugs mimic the effects of natural neurotransmitters, but the transmission of messages they prompt is abnormal. Other drugs directly or indirectly trigger a rush of one of the brain's neurotransmitters, particularly *dopamine.* Among other functions,

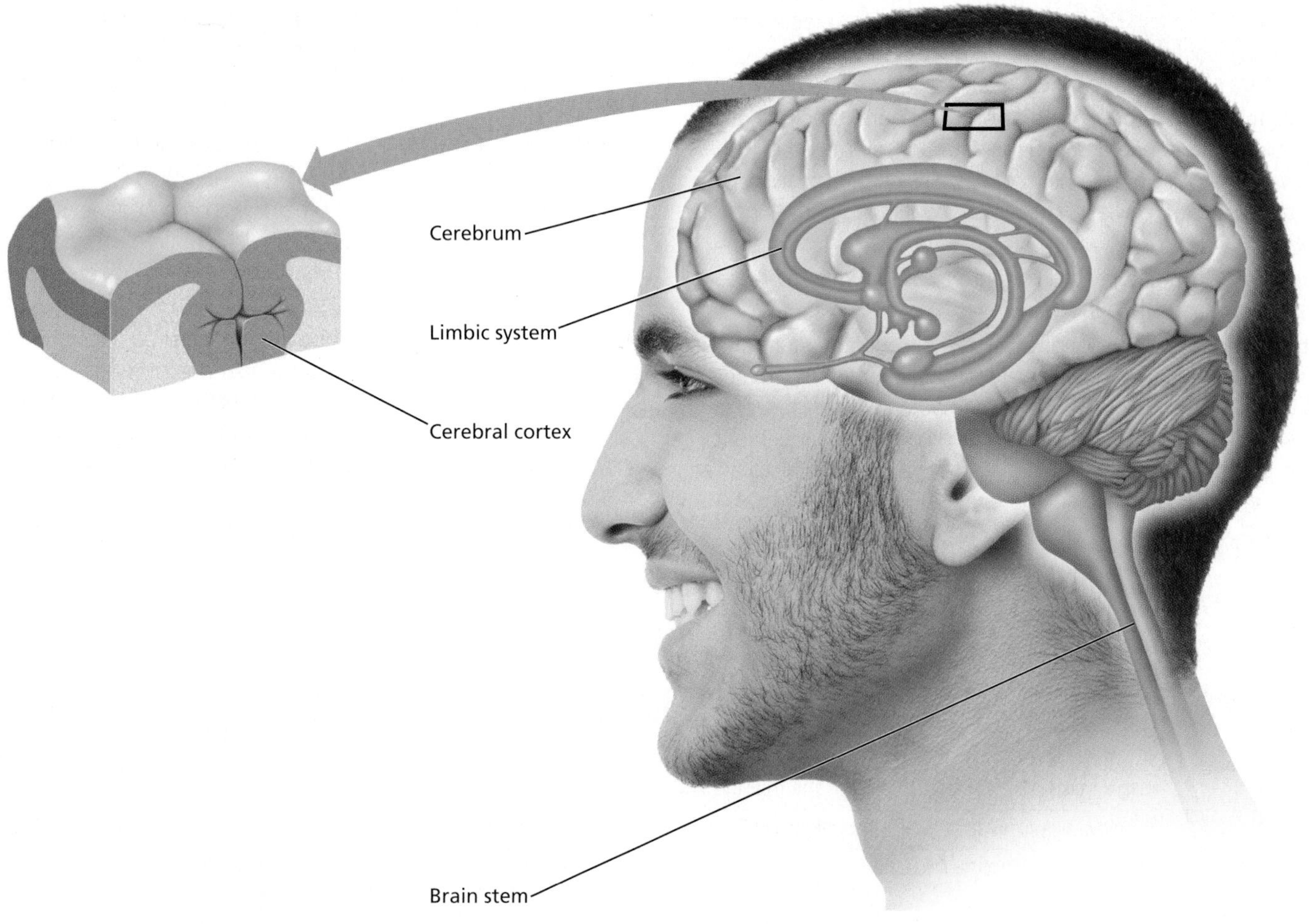

Figure 8.1 Brain regions affected by psychoactive drugs.

dopamine acts as the brain's "feel-good" chemical: It activates the reward circuit in the limbic system, stimulating feelings of pleasure and satisfaction. Users experience a sense of **euphoria** that primes their bodies to repeat the stimulation. Some drugs cause the release of as much as 10 times the amount of dopamine that a naturally pleasurable activity—such as eating—would produce.[8] The effect of this powerful reward strongly motivates people to use the drug again . . . and again. Eventually, however, the brain adapts to the drug and the excessive levels of dopamine it produces. As a result, when the drug is no longer externally supplied, users may feel "flat" or depressed, uninterested in things that formerly brought them pleasure.

euphoria A feeling of intense pleasure.

tolerance Reduced sensitivity to a drug so that increased amounts are needed to achieve the usual effect.

psychological dependence A mental attachment to a drug.

physical dependence The physical need for a drug.

withdrawal Physical symptoms that develop when a person stops using a drug.

Tolerance, Dependence, and Withdrawal

Prolonged or repeated use of chemical substances can actually alter the brain's structure and function. For example, the brain may begin to produce less dopamine (and other neurotransmitters) or reduce the number of receptors that can receive signals.[8] Eventually, the user develops **tolerance**, meaning that the brain has grown so accustomed to the drug that more of the drug is required to achieve the effect that a smaller amount previously had. Tolerance may also cause users to need to keep using a drug just to feel "normal."

This cycle of drug use and tolerance feeds drug addiction. Although people do have control over the choice of whether to initiate drug use, once they start, the pleasurable effects often compel them to keep using. **Psychological dependence** ("psychological addiction") means a mental attachment to a drug—the belief that a drug is needed to relieve stress, anxiety, or other feelings of mental discomfort. With **physical dependence**, the body requires the regular use of a substance in order to function. A physically dependent person also develops tolerance; therefore, larger and larger doses are needed to achieve a high, or even to feel normal. Both psychological dependence and physical dependence are characterized by an intense craving.

The American Psychiatric Association defines *substance dependence* as a pattern of substance use that leads to "significant impairment or distress" and that is characterized by at least three or more of the following within a one-year period:

- The development of tolerance to the substance
- Using the substance in larger quantities or over a longer period than intended
- Inability to cut down or control one's use of the substance
- Spending an inordinate amount of time on activities aimed at obtaining the substance, using the substance, or recovering from the substance's effects
- Sacrificing important social, occupational, or recreational activities due to the substance use
- Continuing use of the substance despite knowledge that the substance has either caused or is exacerbating a physical or psychological problem
- The experience of withdrawal symptoms

Withdrawal refers to the process and experience of ceasing to take a drug that has created a physical dependence. Withdrawal can make some common drugs extremely difficult to quit. Effects can include headaches, nausea and vomiting, sleep disturbances, and psychological symptoms, depending on the drug and degree of dependence.

"Prolonged or repeated use of chemical substances can actually alter the brain's structure and function."

Variations in Response

The response to psychoactive drugs can vary according to several factors:

- **Body size.** Someone who is heavyset may require a greater amount of a drug than someone who is thin to achieve a similar psychoactive effect.
- **Gender.** Women have a greater fat-to-muscle ratio and a lower amount of water in their bodies compared with men, both of which can influence how a drug affects their bodies.
- **Ethnicity.** Caucasians generally transform antipsychotic and anti-anxiety medications in the body more quickly than Asians, and show lower concentrations of these drugs in their bloodstream. As a result, they may use relatively higher doses of these drugs than Asians do.[26]
- **History of drug use.** An individual's history of drug use is an important factor, as long-term use can result in a tolerance to the drug that isn't seen in first-time users.
- **Interactions.** A drug's effect on the body can also change if it is combined with another drug. In *additive interactions,* the effect of one drug is combined with the effect of another. In *antagonistic interactions,* the effect of one drug is diminished when combined with another drug.

Distribution and Metabolism

How long a drug remains active in the body depends on several factors. The *distribution half-life* is the amount of time it takes a drug to move from general circulation to body tissues such as muscle and fat. This information is important for treating overdose patients and is used to estimate the amount of a chemical in a patient's circulation at a given time.[27]

The organs involved in metabolizing (breaking down and eliminating, or "clearing") drugs are the same organs that break down and eliminate nutritional waste. The liver metabolizes drug chemicals into substances that can be excreted by the bowels in stool and by the kidneys in urine. Some substances, like alcohol, are also excreted through the skin or expelled by the lungs. Elimination can also occur through exhaled breath, sweat, saliva, or in the breast milk of nursing mothers. With abuse, almost any psychoactive drug can cause tissue damage or death. The dosage level at which the drug becomes poisonous to the body and can cause temporary or permanent damage is referred to as **toxicity**.

toxicity The dosage level at which a drug becomes poisonous to the body.

opioids Drugs derived from opium or synthetic drugs that have similar sleep-inducing, pain-reducing effects.

Commonly Abused Drugs

Figure 8.2 summarizes the most commonly used illicit drugs in the United States. The following section discusses these and other commonly abused drugs.

Prescription and Over-the-Counter Medications

The use of prescription and over-the-counter (OTC) medications is increasing. A record 3.4 billion prescriptions were handed out in 2005—an increase of nearly 60% since 1995.[28] An estimated 81% of adults in the United States now take at least one prescription or OTC medication every week, and 27% take at least five.[29] Taken as directed, medications can restore and improve health and boost quality of life, but all carry risks, including unwanted side effects.

Misuse of Prescription Medications

Many people do not take prescription medications properly. An estimated half of all prescriptions dispensed each year in the United States are not taken according to directions, and fully 96% of patients fail to ask questions about how to use their medicine.[30] The four most common types of misuse are:

- Taking the incorrect dose
- Taking the medicine at the wrong time
- Forgetting to take a dose
- Failing to take all the medicine

For financial reasons, low-income populations (including many college students) sometimes put themselves at risk for disease complications by not purchasing and using as much of a medication as they have been advised to take. Some people start to feel better and mistakenly assume they do not need to finish their prescription. When the prescribed medication is an antibiotic, this practice can promote the reproduction of antibiotic-resistant bacteria, so-called "super germs" that can no longer be treated by current medications.

Abuse of Prescription Opioids

Prescription drug abuse is the fastest growing drug problem in the United States.[31] A national survey conducted by the American College Health Association found that 13.1% of college students reported using prescription drugs that were not prescribed to them.[25] Many of these non-sick college students are taking prescription drugs for their psychoactive effects.[32]

The most commonly abused prescription drugs are **opioids,** pain medications derived from the opium poppy *Papaver somniferum.* A milky fluid found in the unripe seedpods of its flower is drained and dried to produce *opium,* from which morphine, codeine, and other prescription opioids are derived. Morphine is often given to patients before or after surgery to alleviate severe pain, whereas codeine is used for milder analgesia (pain relief) or serious coughs. Other prescription opioids include hydrocodone (Vicodin) and oxycodone (marketed under the brand names OxyContin, Percodan, and Percocet). The most commonly abused nonprescription opioid, heroin, is discussed later in this chapter.

Drug	Numbers in millions
Illicit drugs	22.6
Marijuana	17.4
Prescription drugs (nonmedical use)	7.0
Cocaine	1.5
Hallucinogens	1.2
Inhalants	0.7
Heroin	0.2

Axis: 0, 5, 10, 15, 20, 25 — Numbers in millions

Figure 8.2 Illicit drug use in the United States. Marijuana and the nonmedical use of prescription drugs top the list of illicit drugs used in the United States.

Source: Data from *Results from the 2010 National Survey on Drug Use and Health: National Findings,* by the Substance Abuse and Mental Health Services Administration, 2011, retrieved from http://www.oas.samhsa.gov/NSDUH/2k10NSDUH/2k10Results.htm#Fig2-1. Data represents past-month use of illicit drugs among persons aged 12 or older in 2010.

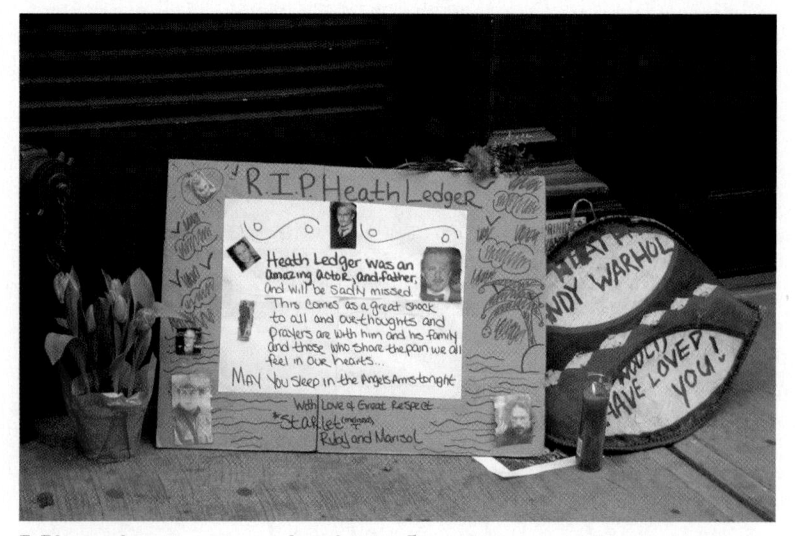
R.I.P Heath Ledger
Heath Ledger was an amazing actor, and father, and will be sadly missed
This comes as a great shock to all and our thoughts and prayers are with him and his family and those who share the pain we all feel in our hearts...
May you sleep in the Angels Arms tonight

Misusing prescription drugs—especially more than one—is dangerous. A lethal combination of prescription drugs caused the death of actor Heath Ledger.

Opioids attach to special receptors on body cells and block the transmission of pain signals to the brain. When taken as directed, prescription opioids can manage pain effectively. In too large a dose, however, they can cause respiratory depression or even death. The nonmedical use of prescription opioids is implicated in hundreds of thousands of emergency room visits annually, and is now increasingly the cause of overdose deaths.[32, 33] Other effects of opioids include euphoria, drowsiness, nausea, and constipation.

Long-term abuse of opioids can lead to physical dependence and withdrawal symptoms if use is suddenly stopped. Withdrawal symptoms include restlessness, insomnia, diarrhea, vomiting, and involuntary leg movements.

Over the past two decades, prescription opioid abuse has progressively overtaken heroin abuse: The milligram per person use of prescription opioids increased between 1997 and 2007 by more than 400%.[32] An estimated 5.2 million people in the United States over the age of 12 reported abusing a prescription pain reliever over the previous year, with people aged 18 to 25 most likely to do so.[34]

Literally tons of opioids are legally imported into the United States every year and medically prescribed. The drugs can enter the black market in a variety of ways. Some physicians unintentionally overprescribe or illegally prescribe or dispense opioids. Some patients "doctor shop," visiting multiple prescribers, sometimes in different states, in order to obtain opioids for personal use or trafficking. Over half of all Americans reporting prescription drug abuse stated that they had obtained the drugs "from a friend or relative for free," and that this source had obtained them from a physician.[3] Increasingly, however, a search for opioids is a factor in home burglaries.

Other Prescription Drug Abuse

The second most commonly abused prescription drugs are stimulants, including drugs traditionally prescribed for attention deficit hyperactivity disorder (ADHD) such as Ritalin and Adderall. In 2010, 1.1 million Americans abused prescription stimulants.[3] The average age at which this abuse began was 21, and the problem is increasing on campus (see **Consumer Corner: Are "Study Drugs" Smart—and Safe?**).

Other commonly abused prescription drugs include sedatives, antidepressants, and erectile dysfunction drugs. Again, many prescription drugs, including opioids and stimulants, have a high potential for addiction. And prescription drug abuse—especially when it involves combinations of drugs—can be fatal.

View an ABC News segment on the increasing misuse and abuse of prescription drugs at www.abcnews.go.com/Health/video?id=3571649.

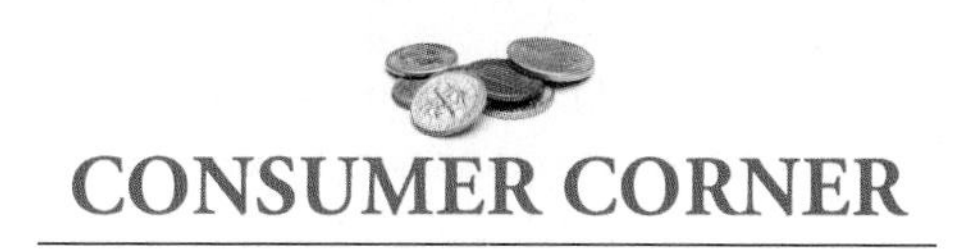

CONSUMER CORNER

Are "Study Drugs" Smart—and Safe?

In recent years, there has been an increase in college students' use of prescription medications such as Adderall, Ritalin, Concerta, and Provigil (drugs intended for the treatment of attention deficit hyperactivity disorders) as enhancement drugs to aid in concentration and study. Users believe these drugs help keep them alert and focused for extended periods of time, allowing them to study for much longer than without the drugs. Dr. Anjan Chatterjee, a University of Pennsylvania neurologist, coined the term "cosmetic neurology" to describe the practice of taking medications intended for specific medical conditions as cognitive enhancers.

The drugs work by increasing blood flow to the prefrontal cortex of the brain—a region involved in higher-level functions such as decision-making. In the same brain region, they also enhance levels of the neurotransmitters dopamine, serotonin, and norepinephrine. This increases the brain's ability to focus and decreases impulsivity and distraction.

Although these drugs can measurably increase concentration and motivation, serious disadvantages are associated with their use: First, by causing students to think more narrowly, they tend to stifle creativity—thinking outside the box. So students may be better able to process data, but less able to make meaningful connections with what they're studying. Then, there are the adverse physical effects: The drugs almost universally disrupt normal sleep patterns, and can also cause nervousness, headaches, decreased appetite, fever, and an increased or erratic heart rate. Sudden death from a heart attack can occur. Many users experience the same "binge-crash" phenomenon common with abuse of other types of stimulants, and psychosis is not uncommon. Some of the drugs are also highly addictive: In addition to craving, withdrawal symptoms can include exhaustion, panic attacks, depression, and insomnia. Adderall—sometimes referred to as "college crack"—has an FDA warning on its label cautioning that the drug has "a high potential for abuse" and can lead to dependence and addiction.

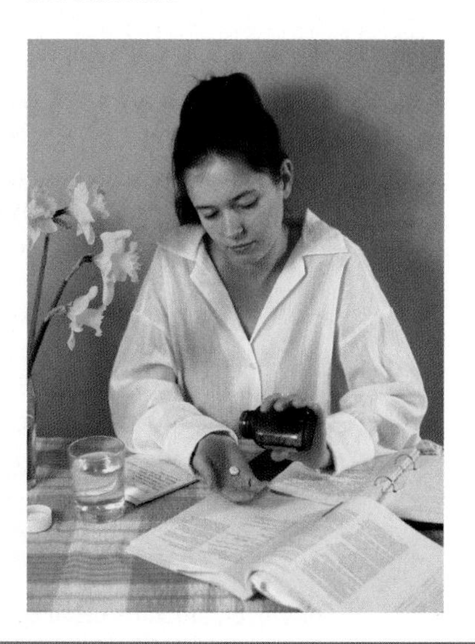

Over-the-Counter (OTC) Drugs

"Over-the-counter" drugs are medications available for purchase without a prescription. OTC drugs include aspirin, allergy pills, and cough or cold medications. There are now more than 700 OTC products available that contain ingredients that were available only by prescription three decades ago—some at greater dosage strength.[35]

OTC drugs pose many of the same challenges as prescription drugs. They need to be taken as directed and may interact with other medicines, herbal supplements, foods, or alcohol. Some OTC drugs are hazardous for people with certain medical conditions, such as asthma. Pregnant women should always check with a doctor before taking any OTC drug.

People tend to wrongly assume that if a little medicine is good, a lot must be better. Yet OTC medications are not meant to be taken in higher doses or for longer periods than is indicated on the label. If symptoms do not go away after a few days of using an OTC drug, it is time to see a doctor or nurse practitioner.

The U.S. Food and Drug Administration (FDA) cautions against the misuse of several common OTC pain relievers. For example, too much acetaminophen (a common pain-relief drug, sold as Tylenol among other brand names) can lead to serious liver damage. If ingested with alcohol or after a long night of drinking, the risk of liver problems increases. In a review of the key studies on acetaminophen and alcohol, government researchers found that as few as four or five "extra-strength" acetaminophen pills taken over the course of a day could damage the liver if alcohol was also consumed.[36] The OTC anti-inflammatory drug ibuprofen also has serious adverse effects if taken to excess or if taken with alcohol. These include diarrhea, nausea, and vomiting, ulcers, internal bleeding, rapid heartbeat, difficulty breathing, drowsiness, and even coma.

Cough and cold formulations can also be dangerous. In 2006 about 3.1 million Americans aged 12 to 25 (5.3%) had used an over-the-counter cough and cold medication to get high.[37] The cough suppressant dextromethorphan (DXM) is found in more than 140 OTC cough and cold medications. DXM is generally safe when taken in recommended doses but in large amounts can cause hallucinations, feelings of being detached from one's body, vomiting, diarrhea, and other dangerous side effects.

Marijuana

Marijuana is the most commonly used illegal drug in the United States.[3] According to the most recent National Survey on Drug Use and Health, 17.4 million Americans reported using marijuana in the past 30 days, representing about 6.9% of the population over the age of 12.[3]

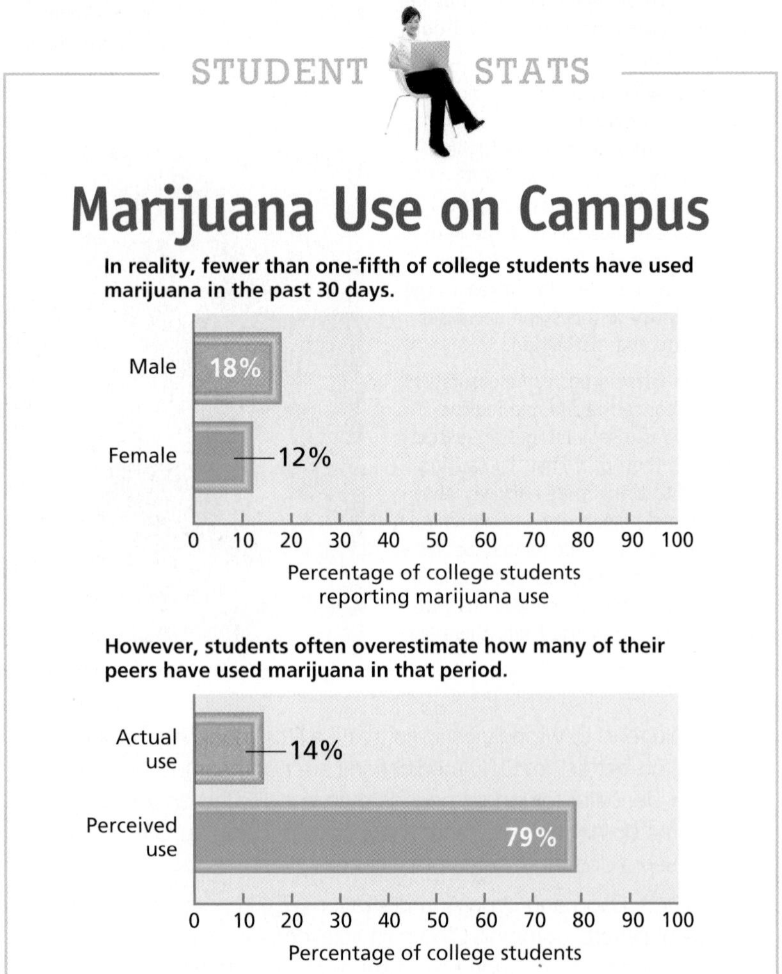

STUDENT STATS

Marijuana Use on Campus

In reality, fewer than one-fifth of college students have used marijuana in the past 30 days.

Male 18%

Female 12%

0 10 20 30 40 50 60 70 80 90 100

Percentage of college students reporting marijuana use

However, students often overestimate how many of their peers have used marijuana in that period.

Actual use 14%

Perceived use 79%

0 10 20 30 40 50 60 70 80 90 100

Percentage of college students

Source: Data from *American College Health Association National College Health Assessment (ACHA-NCHA II) Reference Group Executive Summary, Fall 2011* by the American College Health Association, 2012, retrieved from http://www.acha-ncha.org/reports_ACHA-NCHAII.html.

marijuana The most commonly used illegal drug in the United States; derived from the plant *Cannabis sativa.*

Marijuana (the plant *Cannabis sativa*) grows wild and is farmed in many parts of the world. "Pot"—a dry, shredded mix of flowers, stems, seeds, and leaves of the plant—is usually rolled and smoked as a cigarette (a "joint"), or by using a water pipe (a "bong") that passes the smoke through water to cool it. It is also sometimes mixed in food such as brownies, or brewed as a tea.

Short-Term Effects

Over the years, marijuana growers have bred the plant to contain increasingly higher percentages of its psychoactive ingredient, THC (tetrahydrocannabinol). When a person inhales THC in marijuana smoke, it takes just a few minutes to move from the lungs to the bloodstream to the brain. Ingesting marijuana from food is slower. In the brain, THC binds to cannabinoid receptors, initiating a series of cellular reactions that ultimately result in a surge of dopamine that causes users to experience a high. The heart beats faster (in some users, double the normal rate); the bronchi (large air passages in the lungs) become enlarged; and blood vessels in the eyes expand, reddening the whites of the eye. Other manifestations include dry mouth ("cotton mouth"), hunger, and sleepiness.

Users report that they like the drug because it makes them feel euphoric and because colors and sounds seem more intense. It can also make time seem to slow. Some report being relaxed by THC intoxication, and patients who use it say that, although it does not relieve pain, it helps them tolerate it. However, other short-term mental effects are less pleasant. They include impaired coordination, confusion, difficulty thinking, solving problems, learning, and remembering, and reduced reaction time; these effects can last for days or weeks in chronic users.[38] Moreover, THC has a well-documented effect of making users get "the munchies" (feel hungry), and weight gain is not uncommon with frequent use.

Long-Term Effects

Chronic marijuana use can have serious effects on mental and physical health **(Figure 8.3).** Indeed, opponents of medical marijuana use often cite these adverse effects in explaining their opposition.

A number of studies have shown an association between chronic use and increased rates of anxiety, depression, and schizophrenia; however, it is not clear whether marijuana use causes these disorders, exacerbates them, or reflects an attempt to self-medicate symptoms already present.[38] Long-term attention, learning, and memory have all been shown to be impaired in heavy, chronic marijuana users. Students who chronically use the drug make more errors and have more difficulty processing information than those who use it just once a month.[39]

Marijuana smoke contains more cancer-causing chemicals than tobacco smoke, and is similarly irritating to lung tissues. Thus, people who smoke marijuana can end up with many of the same respiratory problems associated with tobacco smokers. Problems may be heightened because pot smokers inhale deeply and hold the smoke in their lungs. Long-term health risks include daily cough and phlegm production, bronchitis and other lung infections, damage to the lung's lining cells, and *possibly* an increased risk of cancer of the respiratory tract and lungs.[38] Frequent and/or long-term marijuana use may also significantly increase a man's risk of developing the most aggressive type of testicular cancer.[40]

Can lead to addiction

Increases risk of chronic cough, bronchitis

Increases risk of schizophrenia in vulnerable individuals

May increase risk of anxiety and depression

Impairs attention, memory, and learning

Figure 8.3 Long-term effects of marijuana use. Smoking marijuana can cause health problems throughout the body.

Increasingly, research is finding that marijuana can be a hard habit to kick: Addiction develops in about 9% of all users, but in 25–50% of daily users,[38] attempts to quit result in irritability, anxiety, sleep problems, and craving. Admissions to drug treatment centers for help in overcoming marijuana addiction have more than doubled since the early 1990s.

Note that there is no safe way to purchase drugs "on the street"—including marijuana. Drugs purchased through illegal dealers can be laced or "cut" with other drugs and contain impurities. They may even be sold as one drug but actually contain a different drug. Those who purchase drugs illegally for recreational use are undertaking a very serious risk to their health.

What About "Medical Marijuana"?

Many people who smoke marijuana say that they do it to relieve nausea, vomiting, or chronic pain. Is this use of so-called "medical marijuana" legal?

The federal government regulates drugs through the Controlled Substances Act, which classifies marijuana as a Schedule I drug, meaning that the federal government views marijuana as highly addictive and having no medical value. Therefore, physicians are prohibited by federal law from prescribing marijuana, even if they practice medicine in one of the 15 states, along with the District of Columbia, where the use of marijuana as medicine is legal for people with serious illness. These states have an established protocol that physicians follow in order to ensure that their prescribing is in compliance with state law. Nonetheless, the federal Drug Enforcement Administration actively prosecutes anyone who cultivates, sells, or uses marijuana, including in states with medical marijuana laws. The DEA's position is that, no matter what the patient's medical condition, the clinical evidence is clear that smoked marijuana is harmful.[41]

On the other hand, a prescription drug containing synthetic THC is legal, approved by the U.S. Food and Drug Administration, and widely available to physicians to prescribe medically—for instance, to relieve nausea and vomiting in cancer patients. An important guarantee conferred by FDA approval is that the drug has been rigorously tested for safety, effectiveness, and purity. When thinking about medical marijuana, it's helpful to consider the fact that the FDA does not approve of any drugs that are delivered via smoking. There are many FDA-approved opiates available by prescription in pill form, for example, but smoking opium is not approved.

For more information on the health effects of marijuana, visit www.drugabuse.gov/publications/drugfacts/marijuana.

Stimulants

stimulants A class of drugs that stimulate the central nervous system, causing acceleration of mental and physical processes in the body.

Stimulants are a class of drugs that stimulate the function of the central nervous system, resulting in increased heart rate, higher blood pressure, and an elevated rate of mental function. Stimulants also elevate mood and increase feelings of happiness and well-being—explaining why they're commonly referred to as "uppers." Legal stimulants include nicotine, caffeine, and

STUDENT STORY

Tainted Drugs

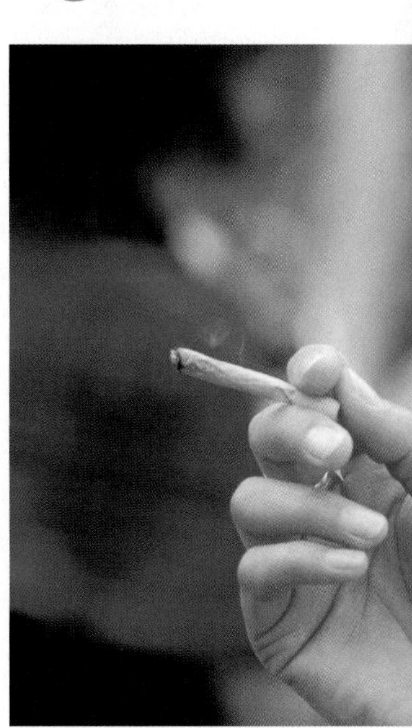

"Hi, I'm Andrea.* One Halloween, me and my friends were at a party and we got a call saying we had to pick up my friend's boyfriend. So we picked him up, and he had marijuana on him, which he offered to us. We smoked it, thinking it's her boyfriend, so it must be okay. Well, it ended up being laced with PCP and it was one of the worst things I've ever gone through. The day after that, when I woke up, I could not stop jittering. My chest felt like it was going to explode. It was a really bad experience and ultimately made me give up marijuana for good."

1: Was there any way Andrea could have known that the marijuana was laced with another drug?

2: If a friend offered you marijuana, how would you respond?

*Name changed at student's request

Do you have a story similar to Andrea's? Share it at www.pearsonhighered.com/lynchelmore.

certain medications when used as prescribed. Illegal stimulants include cocaine, amphetamines, and methamphetamine.

Caffeine

Caffeine is a central nervous system stimulant that, in its pure form, is a white crystalline powder that tastes very bitter. However, as a component in coffee, tea, soft drinks, energy drinks, and chocolate, it is the most popular psychoactive drug in the world. In the United States, 87% of adults consume some type of caffeine regularly, many for the boost in energy that comes with it.[42] **Table 8.2** lists the caffeine content in some commonly consumed foods and beverages, and it is also found in some prescription and OTC medications, including some headache remedies.

The effects of caffeine start in less than an hour after consumption. As the drug stimulates the body's central nervous system, users feel more alert and energetic. Caffeine can also put users in a better mood, improve their concentration, and even boost their athletic prowess and endurance.[43] However, while most people can safely drink two to four cups of coffee a day, excessive caffeine consumption can cause restlessness, anxiety, dehydration, and irritability. Caffeine can also trigger headaches and insomnia and lead to abnormal heart rhythms. Even relatively small amounts, such as a single cup of coffee, can significantly raise your blood pressure. Studies suggest that people who consume five or more cups of coffee per day may be at increased risk of heart disease.[44] Pregnant women who drink a cup and a half of coffee a day may double their risk of having a miscarriage.[45]

Caffeine is physically addictive. As with other types of drugs, regular users can suffer withdrawal symptoms if they suddenly go "cold turkey." Withdrawal usually lasts for 2 to 9 days and may include headaches, anxiety, fatigue, drowsiness, and depression.

caffeine A widely used stimulant found in coffee, tea, soft drinks, chocolate, and some medicines.

cocaine A potent and addictive stimulant derived from leaves of the coca shrub.

Table 8.2: Caffeine Content of Selected Foods and Beverages

Food/Beverage/Pill	Caffeine (milligrams)
Generic brewed coffee, 8 oz.	95–200
NoDoz, maximum strength, 1 tablet	200
Excedrin, extra strength, 2 tablets	130
Rockstar, 8 oz.	79–80
Red Bull, 8.4 oz.	76–80
Restaurant-style espresso, 1 oz.	40–75
Black tea, 8 oz.	14–61
Mountain Dew, 12 oz.	46–55
Coca-Cola Classic, 12 oz.	30–35
Generic decaffeinated brewed coffee, 8 oz.	2–12
Arizona iced tea, lemon flavored, 8 oz.	11
Hershey's kisses, 9 pieces	9

Source: Data from *Caffeine Content for Coffee, Tea, Soda and More*, by the Mayo Clinic, 2012, retrieved from http://www.mayoclinic.com/health/caffeine/AN01211.

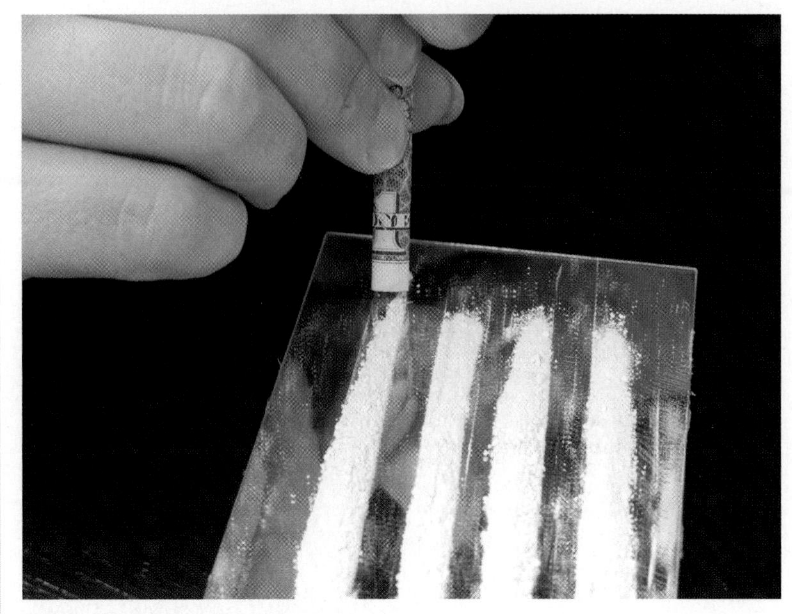

Cocaine use can result in heart damage, stroke, and sudden death.

Cocaine

Cocaine is derived from South American coca leaves, which people have ingested for thousands of years. "Coke" refers to cocaine in its fine white powder form. It is inhaled (snorted) or dissolved in water and injected intravenously. *Freebase cocaine* is a rocklike crystal that is heated so that its vapors can be smoked (inhaled). It is also known as "crack," which refers to the crackling sound that freebase makes when heated. Crack became extremely popular and a major drug of abuse in inner cities during the 1980s because it gives the user a high in less than 10 seconds and because it costs much less than powder cocaine.

Short-Term Effects. Cocaine is a strong central nervous system stimulant that triggers the release of dopamine. Almost immediately, cocaine use causes a rush of euphoria. These effects typically disappear within a few minutes or a few hours. To continue the euphoria, users must continue taking the drug.

Taken in small amounts, cocaine usually makes the user feel energetic and mentally alert. It can also temporarily reduce the need for food and sleep. Whereas some people find it helps them perform simple physical and mental tasks more quickly, others notice the opposite effect. Paranoia is also common.

Some of cocaine's more common side effects include loss of appetite, increased heart rate, increased blood pressure, and increased respiration. They also include chest pain, blurred vision, fever, and muscle spasms. Less commonly, cocaine use can cause abnormal heart rhythms, heart damage, strokes, abdominal pain and nausea, seizures, coma, and death.

Long-Term Effects. Continued use of cocaine often leads to tolerance, so that higher doses and more frequent binges are needed to derive the same level of pleasure. Repeated snorting of cocaine can lead to nosebleeds, a reduced sense of smell, and a chronically runny nose. Ingesting cocaine can reduce blood flow, which can cause severe bowel gangrene. Injection can trigger allergic reactions and put users at risk for blood-borne diseases such as HIV and hepatitis. Injections also leave puncture marks called "tracks" on the forearms or other sites of injection. Another hazard of the powder is that dealers often dilute it with cornstarch, talcum powder, or sugar, or with other stimulants such as amphetamines.

Mixing cocaine and alcohol is especially dangerous. Taken together, the two drugs are converted by the body into cocaethylene, which is more toxic than either drug alone, and can cause death.

Listen to a podcast about how a mechanism in the brain contributes to cocaine cravings in users: www.drugabuse.gov/news-events/podcasts/2008/07/researchers-identify-brain-mechanism-underlying-cocaine-cravings.

Amphetamines

Amphetamines have a chemical structure similar to certain neurotransmitters naturally produced by the body that regulate excitement and alertness. They exert their effects by increasing the concentration of certain neurotransmitters, such as dopamine, serotonin, and norepinephrine, in different regions of the brain. This increases the user's sense of alertness, decreases appetite and the need for sleep, and enhances physical performance. Amphetamines also induce feelings of well-being and euphoria.

The acute effects of amphetamines resemble those of cocaine. For 8 to 24 hours after the drug enters the body, breathing rate, heart rate, body temperature, and blood pressure increase. Users who are more experienced develop feelings of euphoria, decreased appetite, and a boost in alertness and energy. Adverse and potentially lethal changes can occur and may cause convulsions, chest pains, or stroke. Even healthy young athletes have suffered heart attacks after using amphetamines. Because amphetamines increase blood pressure and heart rate, long-term use can increase the risk of heart-related illness.

Addiction is common with amphetamine use, especially because their effect causes users to take them again and again to avoid the "down" they begin to feel as soon as the drug wears off. Eventually, users must take larger and larger amounts to get the same effect. People who abruptly stop taking amphetamines experience a variety of physical effects, including fatigue, irritability, and depression.

amphetamines Central nervous system stimulants that are chemically similar to the natural stimulants adrenaline and noradrenaline.

methamphetamine A highly addictive and dangerous stimulant that is chemically similar to amphetamine, but more potent and harmful.

Amphetamines are legally classified as Schedule II drugs, meaning that they have a high potential for abuse and addiction, but also have a recognized medical use. They are found in the prescription drugs for ADHD mentioned earlier, as well as in drugs used for certain rare sleep disorders and for chronic fatigue syndrome.

Methamphetamine

The highly addictive **methamphetamine** is a chemical similar to amphetamines, but it is much more potent, longer lasting, and more harmful to the central nervous system. Methamphetamine is prescribed medically for ADHD and extreme obesity; however, because of its high potential for abuse, it is legal only by a one-time, nonrefillable prescription. Most methamphetamine that is sold on the street is made by small illegal labs from household materials. It can be ingested, injected, smoked, or snorted. "Crystal meth" refers to methamphetamine in its clear, chunky crystal form. In 2010, there were about 353,000 users of methamphetamine in the United States.[3]

Short-Term Effects. Like amphetamines, methamphetamine exerts its effects by causing the brain to flood with dopamine, serotonin, and norepinephrine. However, its added "methyl" group allows it to cross into the brain more efficiently and to degrade more slowly than amphetamines. Smoking the drug causes an intense rush. Snorting it produces a longer high, which can last for more than a day.

Even small amounts of methamphetamine can have big effects on the body. Methamphetamine can cause a rapid or irregular heartbeat, boost blood pressure, and reduce appetite. Other side effects include irritability, anxiety, insomnia, confusion, and tremors. Users quickly develop tolerance, needing more of the drug to get the same high. But increasing the dose is very dangerous: High doses can elevate body temperature to lethal levels, as well as cause convulsions. Cardiovascular collapse and death are not uncommon.

View "before" and "after" images of people who became addicted to methamphetamine at www.facesofmeth.us/main.htm.

Long-Term Effects. Chronic methamphetamine use significantly changes how the brain functions. Long-term use can reduce motor speed and impair verbal learning.[46] Research also suggests that methamphetamine may alter areas of the brain associated with emotion and memory, which could account for many of the emotional and cognitive problems that have been observed in abusers.[46] Chronic abusers may also experience aggressiveness, anorexia, memory loss, hallucinations, and a paranoia that sometimes causes homicidal or suicidal thoughts. Some users hallucinate that bugs are crawling all over them and therefore scratch themselves repeatedly.

Over time, some methamphetamine users begin to develop what is known as "meth mouth"—severely stained teeth that appear to be rotting away or falling out. Methamphetamine can also damage tissues and blood vessels, promote acne, and slow down the healing of sores. Open sores, in fact, are a hallmark of methamphetamine use **(Figure 8.4).**

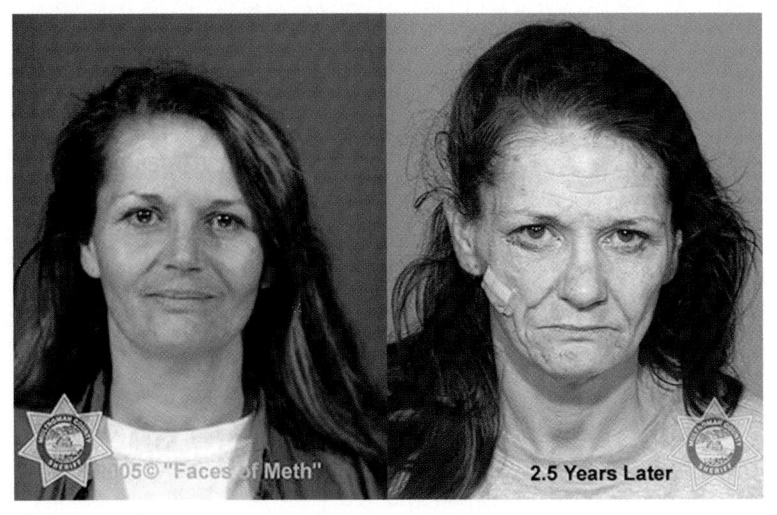

Figure 8.4 Methamphetamine. Methamphetamine use can take a dramatic physical toll.

Despite such serious side effects, users often find themselves hooked. The addiction is very difficult to treat, and for chronic users withdrawal includes physical symptoms such as depression, anxiety, fatigue, aggression, and paranoia, as well as intense craving for the drug.

Injecting methamphetamine increases risk of contracting HIV, hepatitis, and other infectious diseases commonly spread through dirty needles. In individuals who already have HIV, health and cognition can decline more rapidly from use of methamphetamine, compared with HIV-positive patients who do not use the drug.

Methamphetamine labs affect the environment, too. For every pound of the drug produced clandestinely, an estimated 5 to 6 pounds of hazardous waste is created.[47] The waste can leave farmland or forests unsafe and useless until thoroughly cleaned up by hazmat teams. Several states now require that prospective home buyers and tenants be informed about residences that once housed a "meth lab."

Hallucinogens

Hallucinogens are so named because, in addition to altering perceptions, thoughts, and mood, they cause hallucinations. That is, people who use hallucinogenic drugs often report seeing "real" things and hearing "real" sounds that others know do not exist. Some hallucinogens come from plants, like the button-shaped top of the mescal cactus that produces mescaline, and certain types of mushrooms. But other, manufactured hallucinogens can be more potent.

hallucinogens Drugs that alter perception and are capable of causing auditory and visual hallucinations.

LSD (lysergic acid diethylamide) A powerful hallucinogen manufactured from lysergic acid, a substance found in a fungus that grows on rye and other grains.

PCP (phencyclidine) A dangerous synthetic hallucinogen that reduces and distorts sensory input and can unpredictably cause both euphoria and dysphoria.

dissociative drug A medication that distorts perceptions of sight and sound and produces feelings of detachment from the environment and self.

psilocybin A hallucinogenic substance obtained from certain types of mushrooms that are indigenous to tropical regions of South America.

club drugs Illicit substances, including MDMA (ecstasy), GHB, and ketamine that are most commonly encountered at nightclubs and raves.

LSD

LSD (lysergic acid diethylamide) is one of the strongest mood-altering chemicals. Commonly known as "acid," it is derived from lysergic acid, which is found in a fungus called *ergot,* which grows on rye and other grains. Its hallucinogenic effects were discovered in 1943 when the scientist who first synthesized it accidentally swallowed some. LSD "trips" were heavily promoted in the 1960s as a means of enhancing creativity or experiencing spiritual insight, and the fad emerged again among teens in the 1990s.

Liquid LSD is commonly dried into blotter paper and ingested by holding the paper in the mouth. The effects are unpredictable, varying according to the amount taken, the user's personality, and the surroundings in which the drug is used. First effects are often felt within 30 to 90 minutes, as the user moves from one emotion to another or feels several emotions simultaneously. A heavy dose can cause delusions and visual hallucinations. Physical changes include dilated pupils; increased body temperature, heart rate, and blood pressure; sweating; sleeplessness; and tremors.

LSD is not addictive, but some users grow tolerant, needing progressively larger doses to reach a previous level of high. Sometimes LSD users have "bad trips" that are extremely disturbing, or experience "flashbacks," meaning they relive parts of a previous LSD experience long after the drug has worn off. Flashbacks may occur a few days or even a few years after actual use.

PCP

The street names for **PCP (phencyclidine)** include "angel dust," "killer weed," "embalming fluid," and "rocket fuel." As these names suggest, the drug can have volatile, bizarre, and fatal effects. Originally developed in the 1950s as an anesthetic, its medical use was discontinued because of many side effects. Today, street PCP comes from illegal labs, its color ranging from tan to brown and its consistency from powdery to gummy. Users usually apply it to a smokable, leafy material such as parsley, mint, or marijuana. Many people take in PCP unknowingly when someone else adds it to marijuana, LSD, or methamphetamine.

PCP is a **dissociative drug,** meaning it produces feelings of detachment or dissociation from a person's surroundings. Dissociative drugs act by changing the distribution of the neurotransmitter glutamate in the brain. Glutamate is responsible, in part, for a person's memory and perception of pain. While some users say PCP makes them feel stronger—or at least gives them the perception of strength, power, and invulnerability—others have very bad reactions, including confusion, agitation, and delirium. To date, no one knows why reactions vary so much. Other effects can include shallow breathing, flushing, sweating, numbness of the extremities, and poor muscular coordination. In adolescents, frequent use may interfere with hormones related to growth.

At high doses, the health risks become severe. Effects can range from nausea and vomiting to blurred vision and drooling. Seizures, coma, and death also occur. PCP is known for triggering violent behavior in people, and is associated with traumatic injury requiring emergency treatment. Suicides associated with PCP have also been reported. Symptoms such as memory loss, difficulties with speech, and depression can last for up to a year after taking PCP.

Psilocybin (Magic Mushrooms)

Psilocybin, also known as "magic mushrooms" or "shrooms," is popular at parties, clubs, and increasingly on college campuses. This hallucinogen is found in certain mushrooms, available fresh or dried, that are grown in South America, Mexico, and parts of the United States. The mushrooms are often brewed as a tea or eaten with foods that mask their bitter flavor.

Within 20 minutes of ingestion, users begin to notice changes, usually hallucinations and an inability to separate fantasy from reality. Panic attacks can also occur. The effects usually fade away after 6 hours. Psilocybin is not known to be addictive, and there seem to be no withdrawal effects. But serious risks include the onset of psychosis in susceptible users, and poisoning if another, deadlier mushroom (of which there are many) has been confused with the psilocybin mushroom.

"Club Drugs"

NIDA uses the term **club drugs** to refer to LSD and four other psychoactive substances: MDMA (ecstasy), GHB, Rohypnol, and ketamine. These four drugs were first popularized by young adults at all-night

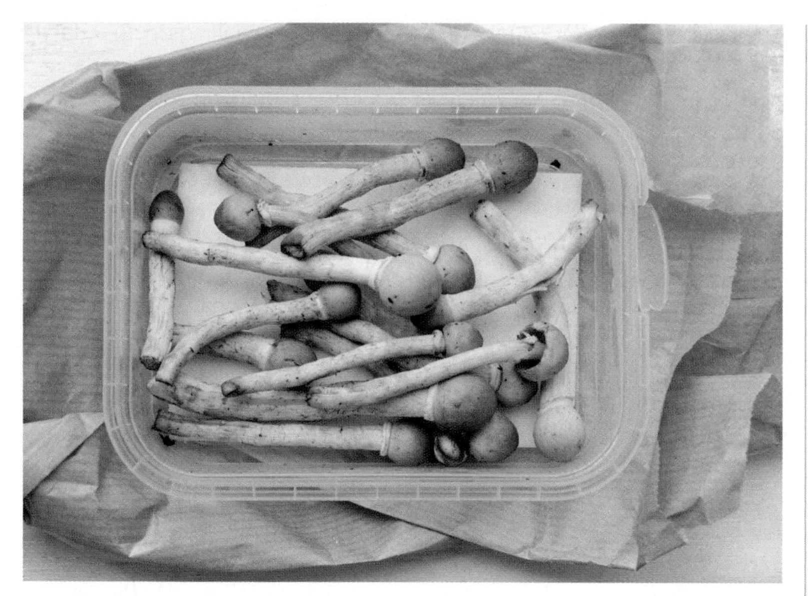

Psilocybin, also called "magic mushrooms," induces hallucinations and can cause psychosis in some users.

raves. They have begun to fall out of favor, but still attract some party-goers by their relatively low prices. More than 23,000 emergency room visits each year are a result of using club drugs.[33]

MDMA (Ecstasy)

Methylenedioxymethamphetamine (MDMA), commonly known as ecstasy, is a synthetic drug chemically similar to methamphetamine. Ecstasy is less popular now than it was during the heyday of raves, but it is still the drug of choice for some partygoers looking for mood enhancement and an energy boost. Ecstasy comes in tablets, often colorful round pills imprinted with smiley faces, peace signs, and hearts. It is also known as "E," "X," and "XTC."

Typically, an ingested tablet takes about 15 minutes to enter the bloodstream and reach the brain. Ecstasy produces feelings of self-confidence, peacefulness, empathy, and increased energy. About 45 minutes later, the user feels the peak of the high. Some users then "bump" (take another tablet). The effects of a single tablet can last for 3 to 6 hours.

Ecstasy's negative effects are similar to those of amphetamines and cocaine. Psychological effects include confusion, sleep problems, anxiety, drug craving, and paranoia. More distinctly physical effects can include nausea, blurred vision, chills, sweating, muscle tension, rapid eye movement, involuntary teeth clenching, faintness, and increases in heart rate and blood pressure. Because the stimulant effects enable users to dance for long periods of time, many have suffered dehydration and heatstroke. Heatstroke can lead to kidney, liver, or cardiovascular failure, and if left untreated is nearly always fatal.

Regular use can cause depression, anxiety, and memory problems that last for up to a week. Studies have shown that some regular users of MDMA have significant memory loss and that chronic users perform more poorly on cognitive tasks than non-users.[48]

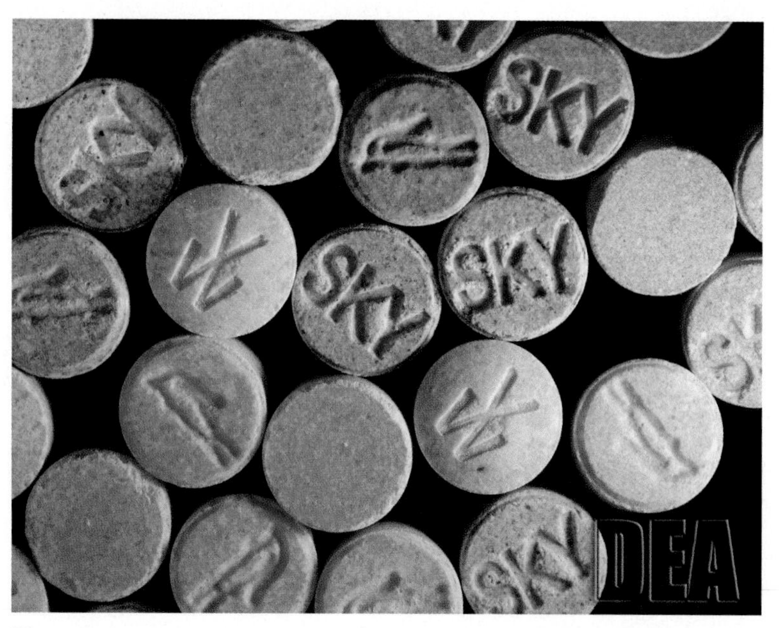

Ecstasy use can cause anxiety, confusion, and paranoia. Coupled with dehydration, it can also result in fatal organ failure.

View the documentary "Ecstasy Rising: The History of MDMA" at http://video.google.com/videoplay?docid=-1564288654365150131#.

GHB

For years, a central nervous system depressant nicknamed **GHB (gamma-hydroxybutyric acid)** was sold over the counter in health food stores throughout the United States. Bodybuilders used GHB to help reduce fat and build muscle. Today, however, GHB is a controlled substance and is often referred to as a "date rape drug" because perpetrators commonly slip it into drinks in order to make victims unconscious and vulnerable. People also ingest GHB for its euphoric effects and for the perception of increased libido and sociability. Ingested usually as a liquid (often with alcohol), GHB is generally colorless, tasteless, and odorless.

Low doses of GHB can cause drowsiness, dizziness, nausea, and vision problems; higher doses are associated with seizures, respiratory distress, and comas. GHB is addictive, and users who try to kick the habit often experience insomnia, anxiety, tremors, and sweating.

Rohypnol (Roofies)

Rohypnol is a drug that induces sedative effects similar to those of Valium. Used legally in Latin America and Europe as a short-term treatment for insomnia, at high doses it can cause unconsciousness. Rohypnol has never been approved for medical use in the United States. Doctors cannot prescribe it, and pharmacists cannot sell it.

Rohypnol can cause decreased blood pressure, drowsiness, visual disturbances, dizziness, and confusion. It can also cause partial amnesia, rendering users unable to remember certain events that they

MDMA (methylenedioxymethamphetamine) A synthetic drug, commonly called "ecstasy," that works as both a stimulant and a hallucinogen.

GHB (gamma-hydroxybutyric acid) A central nervous system depressant known as a "date rape drug" because of its use to impair potential victims of sexual assault.

Rohypnol A powerful sedative known as a "date rape drug" because of its use to impair potential victims of sexual assault.

experienced while under the influence of the drug. Like GHB, it is often called a "date rape drug" because it can be used to incapacitate unsuspecting victims. As a result, sexual assault victims may not be able to clearly recall the assault, the assailant, or the events surrounding the assault.

Because of increasing reports about the misuse of GHB and Rohypnol, Congress passed the Drug-Induced Rape Prevention and Punishment Act of 1996. This legislation increased the federal penalties for using any controlled substance to aid in a sexual assault.

Ketamine

Ketamine, commonly known as "special K," is a rapid-acting anesthetic most commonly used on animals. It is also snorted or swallowed by humans for an "out-of-body" or "near-death" experience known as a "K-Hole." Ketamine is odorless and tasteless, and so can be undetectable when added to beverages.

Ketamine is chemically similar to PCP. Like PCP, ketamine can cause a dreamlike state and hallucinations, but is less associated with confusion, irrationality, and violent behavior. But the risk isn't light. Low doses of ketamine often result in impaired attention, learning ability, and memory. In high doses, it can cause delirium, amnesia, high blood pressure, depression, and severe respiratory problems.

Inhalants

Psychoactive **inhalants** include more than 1,000 common household items, such as paint, glue, and felt-tip markers, which people sniff in order to get high. They are cheap, legal, and easy to buy.

Types of Inhalants

Examples of substances commonly used as inhalants include:

- **Solvents** (liquids in which chemicals are dissolved). Paint thinners or removers, gasoline, glue, dry-cleaning fluids, correction fluids, the ink in felt-tip pens, electronic contact cleaners
- **Aerosols** (particles of a liquid or solid that are suspended in a gas). Spray paints, hair or deodorant sprays, vegetable oil sprays, aerosol computer cleaning products, fabric protector sprays
- **Gases.** Butane lighters, propane tanks, whipped cream dispensers, refrigerant gases, ether, chloroform, halothane, nitrous oxide ("laughing gas")
- **Nitrites** (a type of chemical compound that includes the element nitrogen). Various products often bottled and labeled as "video head cleaner," "room odorizer," "leather cleaner," or "liquid aroma"

Short-Term Effects

Most psychoactive inhalants work somewhat like anesthetics, slowing down the body's functions. Inhalants can cause intoxication, usually for just a few minutes. By repeated sniffing, users extend the high for several hours. At first, inhalants make people feel slightly stimulated. After repeated inhalations, they can feel less inhibited but also less in control.

Health risks vary by type of inhalant. Some inhalants can lead to unconsciousness. Butane, propane, and the chemicals in aerosols have all been linked to what is known as "sudden sniffing death"—fatal heart failure within minutes of repeated inhalations. Some young users also cover their heads with a paper or plastic bag to inhale a higher concentration of chemical. This can backfire, as the practice can cause suffocation.

Long-Term Effects

Inhalant abuse often starts at an early age. According to a recent national survey, 28% of eighth-graders reported experimenting with inhalants.[49] Some adolescents turn to inhalants because they are easier to obtain than alcohol. But inhalants are much more dangerous: Long-term users risk brain damage, including neurological dysfunction, cognitive impairment, and both psychological and social problems. Chronic abuse of solvents specifically can also cause severe damage to the liver and kidneys. Other side effects include hearing loss, limb spasms, bone marrow damage, and blood oxygen depletion.

Depressants

Depressants (also known as "downers") include alcohol, barbiturates, and benzodiazepines. All are substances that depress the central nervous system and slow the brain's activity. The effect is a drowsy or calm feeling that can reduce feelings of anxiety or pain, and help induce sleep. Misuse of depressants can result in addiction, health problems, and even death.

Barbiturates and Benzodiazepines

Barbiturates are a type of central nervous system depressant often prescribed to induce sleep. They were extremely popular in the early 20th century, and have been used as sedatives, hypnotics, anesthetics, and anticonvulsants. Barbiturate sedation can range from mild and short term to severe and long term (inducing coma). Because of their side effects, potential for abuse, and safety concerns, fewer than 10% of all depressant prescriptions in the United States are for barbiturates.

Benzodiazepines are medications commonly prescribed to treat anxiety and panic attacks. They were first marketed in the 1960s and have become the depressant of choice in many medical practices. Considered safer and less addictive than barbiturates, they now account for about one in every five prescriptions for controlled substances.[50] They are most commonly used to sedate, induce sleep, relieve anxiety and muscle spasms, and help prevent seizures. More than a dozen benzodiazepines are approved for use in the United States, including lorazepam (Ativan), alprazolam (Xanax), diazepam (Valium), midazolam (Versed), and chlordiazepoxide (Librium).

Short-Term Effects

People who take benzodiazepines to get high experience reduced inhibition and impaired judgment. Small doses can induce calmness and muscle relaxation; larger doses can slur speech, impair judgment, and hinder motor coordination. Benzodiazepines are not usually prescribed for long-term use. Symptoms of chronic use include memory loss, irritability, and changes in alertness. Long-term use can cause amnesia, hostility, irritability, and disturbing dreams. Very high doses of benzodiazepines can lead to respiratory distress, coma, and death.

ketamine An anesthetic that can cause hallucinations and a dreamlike state; commonly known as "special K."

inhalants Chemical vapors that, when inhaled, produce mind-altering effects.

depressants Substances that depress the activity of the central nervous system and include barbiturates, benzodiazepines, and alcohol.

barbiturates A type of central nervous system depressant often prescribed to induce sleep.

benzodiazepines Medications commonly prescribed to treat anxiety and panic attacks.

Long-Term Effects

Long-term users can develop tolerance and physical dependence. Withdrawal can be dangerous. Because depressants work by slowing the brain's activity, abruptly ending long-term use can cause the brain to race out of control. Insomnia and anxiety—the same symptoms that may have prompted a person to use these drugs in the first place—are common. Long-term users may also experience tremors and weakness upon withdrawal. More severe withdrawal can include seizures and delirium. Hospitalization may be required to ease and get through withdrawal. Anyone who is dependent on barbiturates or benzodiazepines should seek medical treatment before giving them up, to reduce the risk of seizures and death.

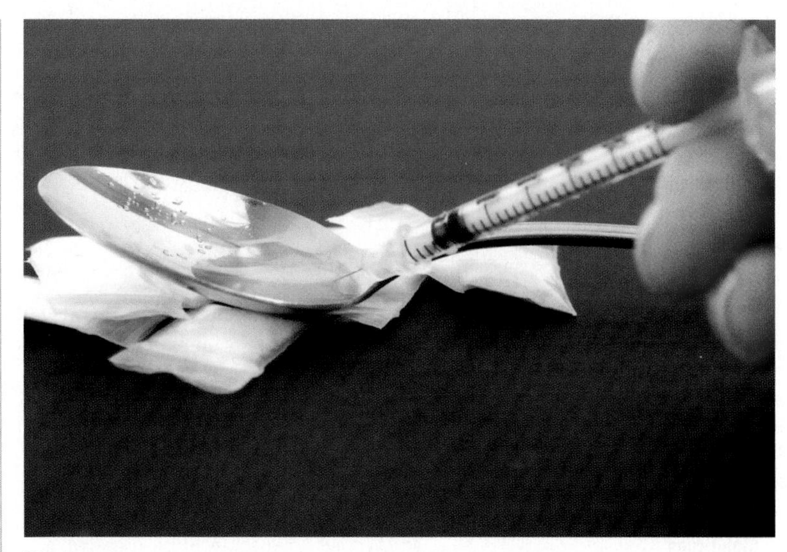

Heroin users can develop collapsed veins, infections, and liver disease.

Heroin

Earlier we discussed the growing epidemic of prescription opioid abuse. The most abused nonprescription opiate is **heroin,** a fast-acting, highly addictive, illegal drug. Heroin is typically sold as a white or brown powder, or as a sticky black substance known as "black tar heroin." Known on the street as "smack," "H," and "junk," heroin is usually injected directly into a vein, though it can also be smoked. About 200,000 people in the United States currently abuse heroin.[3]

heroin The most widely abused of opioids; typically sold as a white or brown powder or as a sticky black substance known as "black tar heroin."

Heroin is particularly addictive because it crosses into the brain quickly, producing an intense "rush" of pleasure accompanied by a sensation of heaviness, clouded mental functioning, and sometimes nausea, vomiting, and severe itching. Drowsiness typically follows, and heart function and breathing slow. These effects usually last several hours.[51]

Withdrawal symptoms, which may begin only a few hours after the last time the drug is taken, include craving, restlessness, muscle and bone pain, insomnia, diarrhea, vomiting, cold flashes, and involuntary leg movements. Although these symptoms typically subside after about a week, they persist in some people for many months.[51]

Heroin injection can lead to a variety of bacterial infections as well as hepatitis and HIV. Liver and kidney disease are not uncommon. Moreover, additives in the drug may clog blood vessels, cutting off the blood supply to regions of body tissues. Immune reactions to these contaminants can result in inflammation and joint pain.

Table 8.3 provides a summary of commonly abused drugs, their intoxication effects, and the health risks of using them.

Table 8.3: **Commonly Abused Drugs**

Category	Representative Drugs	Method of Administration	Intoxication Effects and Health Risks
Cannabis	Marijuana (street names: pot, dope, weed, grass, joint, reefer)	Inhaled or ingested	*Effects:* Psychoactive agent THC causes a sense of euphoria. Heart rate increases, bronchi enlarge, blood vessels expand. *Risks:* Addiction, impaired cognition, lung damage, increased cancer risk
Stimulants	Cocaine (street names: crack, rock, blow, C, coke, snow)	Inhaled or injected	*Effects:* Derived from coca leaves, this drug first produces feelings of increased energy and euphoria. Heart rate and blood pressure increase, appetite drops. *Risks:* Addiction, irritability, anxiety, paranoid or violent behavior, damage to heart, brain, and other vital organs
	Amphetamines (street names: speed, uppers, crank)	Inhaled, ingested, injected	*Effects:* This large, varied group of synthetic drugs improves mood and alertness. Heart rate and blood pressure increase. *Risks:* Addiction, restlessness, appetite suppression, hallucinations, erratic or violent behavior
	Methamphetamines (street names: meth, crystal, ice, glass, tina) *Shown at left*	Inhaled, ingested, injected	*Effects:* A common form of amphetamine, this highly addictive drug quickly produces a sense of euphoria followed by a dramatic drop in emotion and energy as the drug wears off. *Risks:* Addiction, appetite suppression, dental damage, brain damage, psychosis, paranoia, aggression

(continued)

Table 8.3: Commonly Abused Drugs (continued)

Category	Representative Drugs	Method of Administration	Intoxication Effects and Health Risks
Hallucinogens	LSD (street names: acid, blotter) *Shown at left*	Ingested	*Effects:* Effective even at very low doses, this drug is known for producing powerful hallucinations. Other effects include nausea, increased heart rate, tremors, and headaches. *Risks:* Shortened attention span, miscarriage and pre-term labor in pregnant women, paranoia, disordered thinking
	PCP (street name: angel dust)	Inhaled, ingested, injected	*Effects:* This synthetic drug can lead to both euphoria and extreme unhappiness, and can also produce hallucinations. *Risks:* Slurred speech, poor coordination, loss of sensitivity to pain, nausea, vomiting, violent behavior, coma, and even death
	Psilocybin (street names: shrooms, magic mushrooms)	Ingested	*Effects:* This group of mushrooms, if ingested, has effects similar to those of LSD. Effects last for up to 6 hours. *Risks:* Paranoia, disordered thinking, nausea, erratic behavior
Club Drugs	MDMA (street names: ecstasy, E, X, XTC)	Ingested	*Effects:* This synthetic drug creates feelings of warmth and friendliness, and also increases heart rate and blood pressure. *Risks:* Hallucinations, brain damage, disordered thinking, disturbed sleep. Extremely dangerous if mixed with alcohol.
	GHB (street name: G)	Ingested	*Effects:* A central nervous system depressant that disrupts memory and can lead to unconsciousness. *Risks:* Temporary amnesia, nausea, vomiting, seizures, memory loss, hallucinations, coma
	Rohypnol (street name: roofies)	Ingested	*Effects:* This drug is a powerful tranquilizer that slows physical and mental responses, and is the best known of the so-called "date rape" drugs. *Risks:* Temporary amnesia, slowed physical and mental reactions, semi-consciousness, unconsciousness
	Ketamine (street names: K, special K) *Shown at left*	Inhaled or injected	*Effects:* Used legally as an anesthetic for animals, this drug produces hallucinations. *Risks:* Sensory distortion, disordered thinking, sensory detachment, impaired attention, delirium
Inhalants	Solvents (e.g., paint thinner), aerosols (e.g., spray paint), gases (e.g., nitrous oxide), nitrites (e.g., leather cleaner)	Inhaled	*Effects:* Found in ordinary household products, these substances can produce a feeling of being "high" or drunk. *Risks:* Dizziness, impaired speech, impaired physical coordination, vomiting, hallucinations, loss of consciousness, death
Depressants	Barbiturates (street names: barbs, downers)	Ingested or injected	*Effects:* This group of drugs slows the functions of the central nervous system and is legally prescribed for anxiety and insomnia. *Risks:* Slowed pulse and breathing, slurred speech, impaired memory, addiction, sleep problems, impaired coordination
	Benzodiazepines (street names: downers, benzos) *Shown at left*	Ingested or injected	*Effects:* This subset of barbiturates functions as tranquilizers, and includes common medications such as Valium. *Risks:* Same as for other barbiturates
Opioids	Heroin (street names: smack, H, brown sugar, junk, horse) *Shown at left*	Injected or inhaled	*Effects:* This depressant produces a feeling of drowsiness, dreaminess, and euphoria, and can also lead to dramatic mood swings. *Risks:* Addiction, cardiovascular damage, respiratory illnesses, internal infections, death
	Prescription opioids (street names: Oxy, Captain Cody)	Ingested	*Effects:* This group of drugs produces feelings of sleepiness, dreaminess, and a reduced sensitivity to pain. *Risks:* Addiction, dangerous interactions with other drugs, nausea, vomiting, lack of physical coordination

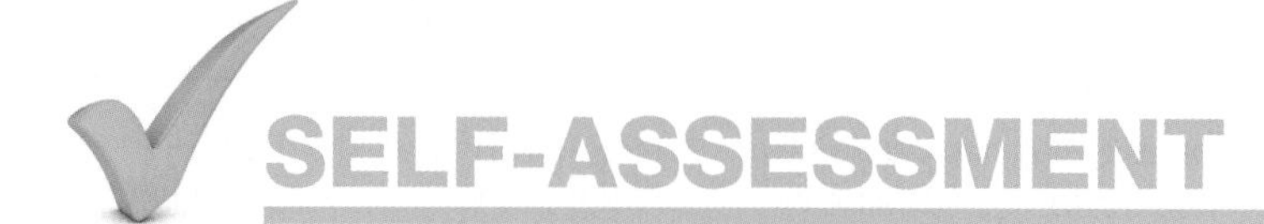
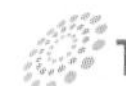 Take this self-assessment online at www.pearsonhighered.com/lynchelmore.

Should You Seek Drug Treatment?

Answer Yes or No to the following 20 questions.

1. Have you used drugs other than those required for medical reasons?
2. Have you abused prescription drugs?
3. Do you abuse more than one drug at a time?
4. Do you use drugs more than once a week?
5. Have you tried to stop using drugs and were not able to do so?
6. Have you had blackouts or flashbacks as a result of drug use?
7. Do you ever feel bad or guilty about your drug use?
8. Does your spouse or parents ever complain about your involvement with drugs?
9. Has drug abuse created problems between you and your spouse or your parents?
10. Have you lost friends because of your use of drugs?
11. Have you neglected your family because of your use of drugs?
12. Have you been in trouble at work because of your use of drugs?
13. Have you lost a job because of drug abuse?
14. Have you gotten into fights when under the influence of drugs?
15. Have you engaged in illegal activities in order to obtain drugs?
16. Have you been arrested for possession of illegal drugs?
17. Have you ever experienced withdrawal symptoms (felt sick) when you stopped taking drugs?
18. Have you had medical problems as a result of your drug use, such as memory loss, hepatitis, convulsions, bleeding, etc.?
19. Have you gone to anyone for help for a drug problem?
20. Have you been involved in a treatment program especially related to drug use?

HOW TO INTERPRET YOUR SCORE

The more "Yes" answers you gave, the more likely it is that you should seek treatment for your drug use.

Value Your Values

What are your values? Health, independence, financial security, achievement, caring relationships, honesty, integrity...? What about your goals? Do you want to be accepted into medical school, get a job in high tech, or land a role on Broadway? Challenging yourself to identify how your choices about drugs reflect and support—or deny and derail—your values and goals can be an enlightening exercise. The next step is identifying what specific steps you need to take to live in closer alignment with your values and to achieve your goals.

Make Some Trade-Offs

If you're tempted to abuse drugs, or to continue to abuse them, you may believe that they'll provide a quick fix for your boredom, emotional pain, concern about your grades, or whatever else might be troubling you. Although it's true that, for a few minutes or hours, you'll escape, what about those short- and long-term consequences? Make a better trade-off. **Endorphins** are your body's own "feel-good" chemicals. When they bind to opiate receptors in the brain, they increase pleasure and decrease pain. There are many healthful ways to prompt your brain to produce this "natural high," including exercise, team sports, meditation, volunteer work, and spending time with people you love. Many people find that challenging themselves to overcome fears—by performing, for instance, or public speaking, or rock climbing—boosts their endorphins.

Another important trade-off you might have to make is in your circle of friends. Tell them in unambiguous language that you're drug free. True friends will not only accept, but respect your decision. Those who ridicule you about it, or try to talk you out of it, may still deserve your care and concern, but not your time. Let them know you have no hard feelings, but won't be able to hang out with them anymore.

Taking this step means you'll also need to change how you spend your free time. Accept invitations only to events and with friends that you know are clean. Recognize your vulnerable times—for instance, Friday and Saturday nights—and schedule some drug-free activities in advance to make sure your calendar is filled. That way, you can honestly say, "Sorry, I'm busy," if someone asks you to a party where drugs will be available.

Build a Healthier Lifestyle

If you're in recovery, the experience will go more smoothly if you take care of yourself. Although withdrawal often disturbs sleep patterns, go to bed at a reasonable hour and try to get 7 to 8 hours of sleep. If your mind races, try repeating a positive affirmation, or sending loving thoughts to any friends who you know are struggling with abuse and addiction, too.

Don't ignore your diet. Depending on the drug you used, you may have lost significant weight. In addition, you may be dehydrated. Yet withdrawal from certain drugs can promote gastrointestinal problems such as diarrhea, vomiting, and nausea, just at a time when you need nutrients, including fluids, to support your recovery. Guidelines from the National Institutes of Health recommend that you:[69]

- Stick to regular mealtimes.
- Eat a diet that is relatively low in fat and has adequate protein and complex carbohydrates (including plenty of vegetables and whole grains).
- Take a multivitamin-mineral supplement.
- Eat nutritious snacks.
- Don't mistake hunger or thirst for a drug craving. If a craving hits, eat a healthy meal or snack, or drink a glass of water, milk, or 100% juice.

Finally, exercise. The endorphins released during vigorous physical activity will help decrease cravings and elevate your mood.

endorphins Hormones that act as neurotransmitters and bind to opiate receptors, stimulating pleasure and relieving pain.

Ask for Help

If you're trying to quit, but a craving hits you in the middle of the night, who is the one person you know you could call on for help? Maybe it's your mom or dad, maybe a close sibling or your best friend

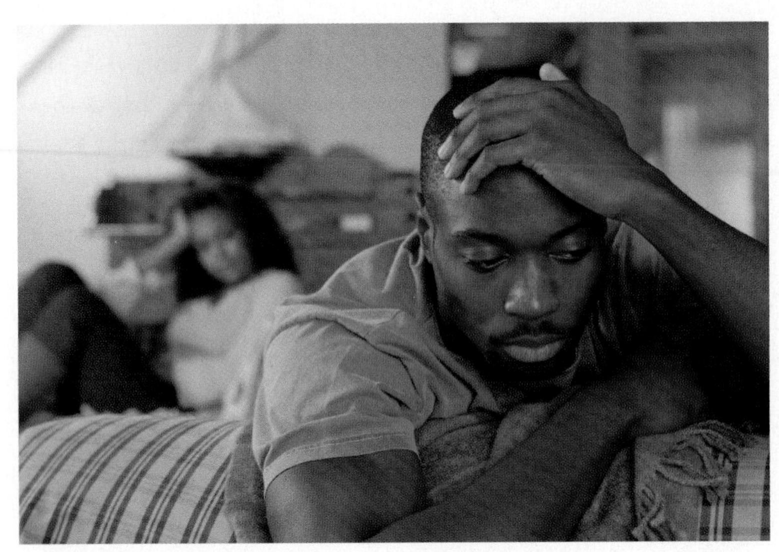

Don't be afraid to **talk to someone** if you're suffering with addiction.

. . . or maybe a member of your 12-step program or support group. Whoever it is, tell that person what you're going through and ask him or her to be "on call" for you. And remember, you don't have to "tough it out"—medications and clinical counseling are a phone call away. The Substance Abuse and Mental Health Services Administration's nationwide treatment referral help line is available 24 hours a day at 1-800-662-HELP.

You can also locate treatment centers in your area by clicking on the map at http://findtreatment.samhsa.gov.

Deal With Relapse

Relapse is a common and unfortunate fact of drug treatment. Experts stress that "falling off the wagon" does not mean treatment does not work or that a user will never be free of the drug. Relapse can, however, be extremely demoralizing. It is better to look at relapse not as a failure, but as practice. As with every challenge in life, you may need to try several times before finally getting something right.

Research points to three factors that can trigger intense renewed drug craving and cause a relapse (see Chapter 1 to review strategies for identifying and overcoming triggers):[70]

- **Priming.** One small exposure to a formerly abused substance can cause an addict to use again, sometimes more heavily than before. For a recovering addict, "just one joint" is rarely that.
- **Environmental cues.** Seeing people, places, or things that were heavily associated with past drug use can sometimes prompt a recovering addict to use again.
- **Stress.** Acute and chronic stress can contribute to the resumption of drug abuse.

It can take years to kick a habit, but through proper treatment and perseverance, people with drug addictions can recover and lead productive lives. Few health-related behaviors are harder to change than those involving addictive drugs. All of us trying to make healthy changes can draw inspiration from those who have successfully overcome a drug habit. A common misperception is that a person has to hit "rock bottom" before he or she can recover from a drug addiction. This is not true; early treatment or intervention is often successful.

intervention A technique used by family and friends of an addict to encourage the addict to seek help for a drug problem.

Helping a Friend

Often, addicts do not realize they have a problem or that it is interfering with their lives. In such cases, friends and family may stage what is called an **intervention,** an organized attempt by an individual, family, or other group to encourage a loved one to get professional help. Interventions usually involve direct, face-to-face demonstrations of love, support, and encouragement to enter treatment. Before you consider an intervention, meet with a substance abuse counselor for guidance and for information about available treatment options.

An excellent resource for helping a loved one with a drug addiction is the Partnership for a Drug-Free America website at www.drugfree.org.

Campus Advocacy

How can you promote a campus environment where drug abuse and addiction are not seen as expected or even hip behaviors, but recognized as serious health problems? Here are some ways to get involved:

- Recognize that, every time you say no to drugs, you're challenging the idea that drug use is normal. Still, it's hard to "just say no," especially if you value fitting in. So be ready with "a line"; for instance: "No thanks, I've got a paper due tomorrow." Or, "I'm working on a health challenge right now, and that would only make it worse." Or try humor: "Sorry, but I need to preserve all the brain cells I have!"
- Spread the word. Although information alone usually isn't enough to stop drug abuse, when combined with other prevention and treatment efforts, it does make a difference, especially when the information comes from peers. For instance, let's say you know that a friend is abusing a prescription drug, but mistakenly thinks that, because it was prescribed for a family member, it's safe and legal. Take the opportunity to ask some questions: *Do you know about the health risks of using this drug? Do you know that what you're doing is illegal?* Let your friend know you're concerned and offer to help.
- Get your message out online. Use your social networking sites to raise awareness, and send short articles about the consequences of student drug abuse to your school's online newspaper.
- Visit the office of your dean of students or your student government association and lobby for chem-free housing and campus-sponsored activities. Join drug-free organizations on campus, and attend their activities. If a club you belong to doesn't have a drug-abuse policy, suggest that the members establish one.
- Volunteer to become a peer mentor. Many colleges have peer mentoring associations (PMAs) whose volunteers help their peers overcome substance abuse and other challenges.

Watch videos of real students discussing drugs and addiction at www.pearsonhighered.com/lynchelmore.

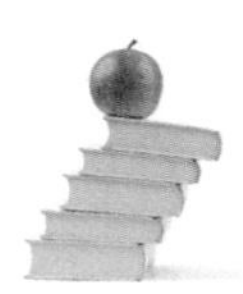

Choosing to Change Worksheet

To complete this worksheet online, visit **www.pearsonhighered.com/lynchelmore**.

Although you may not realize it, you might routinely use one or more psychoactive drugs. If you drink caffeinated beverages like coffee, tea, cola, or energy drinks, or drink alcohol or smoke cigarettes, or take pain relievers, sleeping pills, or allergy medicine, you are using a psychoactive drug. Monitor your drug use for a week.

Part I. Keep a Drug Diary

List the drugs you consumed daily over the course of a week. Did you drink coffee? List the number of cups. How about energy drinks or caffeinated sodas? Tea? Did you smoke cigarettes? How many? Drink alcohol? Did you take prescription medications? Over-the-counter medications? Also make note of your stress level and mood at the time you used the drug.

Example:

Day	Substance	Amount	Drug	What did it do for you?	Stress Level 1 = low stress 2 = moderate stress 3 = high stress	Mood (angry, happy, depressed, bored, frustrated, etc.)
1	Coffee	3 cups	Caffeine	Helped me wake up	3	Frustrated

Your Turn:

Day	Substance	Amount	Drug	What did it do for you?	Stress Level 1 = low stress 2 = moderate stress 3 = high stress	Mood (angry, happy, depressed, bored, frustrated, etc.)
1						
2						
3						
4						
5						
6						
7						

Review and Reflect on Your Drug Diary

1. Were you surprised about anything from your drug diary? ____________ If yes, what surprised you?

____

2. Did you notice any patterns in your use of drugs? ____________ If yes, what patterns were apparent?

____

3. Are you using any drugs as a coping mechanism to deal with your stress levels or moods? ____________
If yes, which drugs?

____

4. Looking at your drug diary, are there any substances you would like to reduce or eliminate?

____

Part II: Reducing or Eliminating Drug Use

Directions: Fill out your stage of change in Step 1 and complete the remaining steps depending on which one applies to your stage of change.

Step 1: Your Stage of Behavior Change. Please check one of the following statements that best describes your readiness when it comes to reducing or eliminating the drug listed in question 4, above.

____________ I do not intend to eliminate or reduce use of this drug in the next 6 months. (Precontemplation)

____________ I might eliminate or reduce the use of this drug in the next 6 months. (Contemplation)

____________ I am prepared to eliminate or reduce the use of this drug in the next month. (Preparation)

____________ I eliminated or reduced use of this drug less than 6 months ago. (Action)

____________ I have eliminated or reduced use of this drug for more than 6 months and want to maintain it. (Maintenance)

Step 2: Precontemplation, Contemplation, and Preparation Stages. Write down a healthier behavior you could replace your drug use with.

____

____

____

Tell someone what you plan to do. Being accountable to others motivates you and also offers you the support and encouragement of others. Who did you tell? ____.

Step 3: Action and Maintenance Stages. Track your progress. For 3 days after you start reducing or eliminating your drug use, keep track of the results. Evaluate your progress and explain whether or not you intend to modify your plan.

____

____

____

If you still have trouble cutting back on your drug use, see a health professional for help. Reread pages 226–228 of the chapter for information on where to find professional help. List the professional resources that will help you achieve your goal:

____

____

Step 4: I don't use drugs but am concerned about someone who does. According to the National Council on Alcoholism and Drug Dependence, Inc., you should ask yourself the following questions.

1. Do you worry about how much your friend or loved one uses alcohol or drugs? Yes No

2. Do you lie or make excuses about their behavior when they drink or use drugs? Yes No

3. Do they get angry with you if you try to discuss their drinking or drug use? Yes No

4. Have you ever been hurt or embarrassed by their behavior when they're drunk, stoned, or strung out? Yes No

5. Do you have concerns about how much time and money they spend on alcohol and/or drugs? Yes No

6. Do you resent having to pick up their responsibilities because they are drunk, high, or hung over? Yes No

7. Do you ever get scared or nervous about their behavior when they're drinking or using drugs? Yes No

8. Do you ever feel like you're losing it—"going crazy"—just really stressed out? Yes No

9. Have you ever considered calling the police because of this person's alcohol or drug use or behavior while under the influence? Yes No

Source: *Concerned about Someone?* by the National Council on Alcoholism and Drug Dependence, Inc., (NCADD). Available at http://www.ncadd.org/index.php/for-youth/concerned-about-someone. Reprinted with permission from NCADD. www.ncadd.org.

If you answered Yes to any of the nine questions, you may want to talk to your friend or loved one right away. Also, reread pages 226–228 of the chapter for information on professional resources that may help and the information on page 230 about how to help a friend with addiction.

Chapter Summary

- *Addiction* is a chronic disease of brain reward, motivation, memory, and related circuitry. One of its most fundamental characteristics is craving.
- Many determinants interact to influence an individual's risk for addiction. In drug addiction, the precise type of drug used and the method of administration also influence the addictive potential.
- Two recognized behavioral addictions are pathological gambling and hypersexual disorder. Some psychologists recognize other behavioral addictions, such as compulsive spending.
- *Drug misuse* is the inappropriate use of a legal drug. *Drug abuse* is the use of any drug that results in harm to your health.
- As a group, college students greatly overestimate how many of their peers are using illicit drugs. Self-reported marijuana use is below 16%.
- Five common ways that people self-administer drugs are ingestion, injection, inhalation, mucosal absorption, and topical administration.
- Chemicals called neurotransmitters—including dopamine, serotonin, and others—facilitate the transport of messages throughout the nervous system. Psychoactive drugs typically trigger a surge of these chemicals, resulting in a sense of euphoria.
- *Psychological dependence* is a mental attachment to a drug. *Physical dependence* occurs when the body requires the regular use of a drug in order to function. Withdrawal from a drug that has created a physical dependence provokes a variety of challenging symptoms, from nausea and vomiting to insomnia and panic attacks.
- Physiological responses to drugs vary widely from individual to individual. Factors may include the individual's physical build, sex, ethnicity, and history of drug use.
- Commonly abused drugs include prescription and over-the-counter medications, marijuana, stimulants (e.g., caffeine, cocaine, amphetamines, and methamphetamine), hallucinogens (e.g., LSD, PCP, and psilocybin), "club drugs" (e.g., MDMA, GHB, Rohypnol, and ketamine), inhalants, and depressants (e.g., opioids, barbiturates, and benzodiazepines).

- The costs of drug abuse include an increased risk for illness, injury, and early death, birth defects and disabilities in children born to women who abused drugs during pregnancy, sexual and other forms of violence, academic problems, broken family relationships, job loss, financial ruin, and homelessness. Substance abuse also costs Americans hundreds of billions of dollars annually.
- Prevention efforts, including public awareness campaigns, can be effective, especially when combined with treatment.
- Most people who need drug treatment do not receive it. Community-based programs such as Narcotics Anonymous, which is free to members, can help. A growing number of colleges are offering on-campus support services and "communities" for students attempting to overcome substance abuse.
- Types of clinical drug treatment include walk-in clinics and on-site residential programs, both of which may offer medications and counseling.
- In attempting behavior change for drug abuse or addiction, you may need to commit to several trade-offs—in the way you attempt to manage your mood, the people you hang out with, and the activities you engage in. It also helps to practice good sleep habits, eat a nourishing diet, and get exercise, as well as to have someone you've prearranged to call should you need help.
- An intervention is an organized attempt by an individual, family, or other group to encourage a loved one to get professional help.

Test Your Knowledge

1. Uncontrollable craving for a drug, despite harmful or potentially harmful consequences, is characteristic of
   a. drug misuse.
   b. drug abuse.
   c. euphoria.
   d. addiction.

2. What are *drugs?*
   a. chemical substances prescribed by a doctor only
   b. only prescription medications and over-the-counter medications
   c. illegal substances only
   d. any chemical taken in order to alter the body physically or mentally for a non-nutritional purpose

3. James is visiting his parents when he suffers from spring allergies. His father offers him some of his prescription allergy medication, and James takes it. This is an example of
   a. drug misuse.
   b. drug abuse.
   c. drug addiction.
   d. tolerance.

4. Using a syringe to direct a drug into the bloodstream is an example of
   a. ingestion.
   b. absorption.
   c. injection.
   d. inhalation.

5. Which of the following can affect an individual's physiological response to a drug?
   a. physical build
   b. gender
   c. past drug history
   d. all of the above

Get Critical

What happened:

In February 2012, pop singer Whitney Houston was scheduled to sing at a pre-Grammy Awards party. Instead, the party was held in her memory. Singer Tony Bennett dedicated his performance to her, then added, "I'd like every person in this room to campaign to legalize drugs."[1] Bennett gave no explanation for why he felt that legalization would have prevented the singer's death.

Voicing an opposing view is a celebrity who got clean. Actor Robert Downey, Jr. struggled for years with drug addiction, cycling in and out of rehab and serving two prison sentences before finally throwing his drugs into the Pacific Ocean. Now, Downey publicly opposes legalization of any drug, including marijuana. Of his stints in prison, he says, "I wouldn't wish that experience on anyone else, but it was very, very educational for me..."[2]

What do you think?

- Do you think Bennett's suggestion to legalize drugs would prevent overdose deaths? Why or why not?
- Downey was introduced to drugs at age 6, when his father gave him a joint. How might this early experimentation with his father have contributed to the severity of his addiction?
- Downey seems to suggest that incarceration for drug use might be an effective form of treatment for some people. What do you think of this claim—and why?

References: **1.** "Tony Bennett Calls for Drug Legalization in Wake of Whitney Houston's Death," by S. A. Schillaci & S. Halperin, February 11, 2012, *The Hollywood Reporter.* Retrieved from http://www.hollywoodreporter.com/news/whitney-houston-death-tony-bennett-drug-legalization-grammys-289618. **2.** "Been Up, Been Down. Now? Super," by D. Carr, April 20, 2008, *The New York Times.* Retrieved from http://www.nytimes.com/2008/04/20/movies/20carr.html?pagewanted=1&8dpc&_r=2.

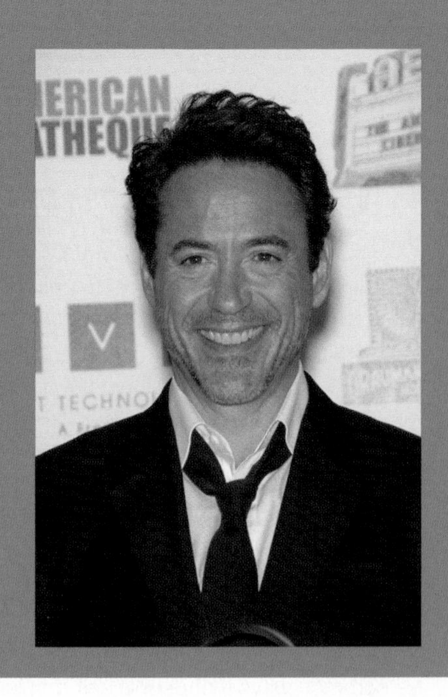

6. What is the most commonly abused illicit drug in the country?
   a. heroin
   b. cocaine
   c. marijuana
   d. prescription drugs for nonmedical use

7. What is the second most commonly abused illicit drug in the country?
   a. heroin
   b. cocaine
   c. marijuana
   d. prescription drugs for nonmedical use

8. Caffeine is an example of a(n)
   a. depressant.
   b. opioid.
   c. hallucinogen.
   d. stimulant.

9. What is psilocybin more commonly known as?
   a. ecstasy
   b. roofies
   c. hashish
   d. magic mushrooms

10. The return to drug abuse after a period of conscious drug abstinence is called
    a. intervention.
    b. remediation.
    c. relapse.
    d. codependency.

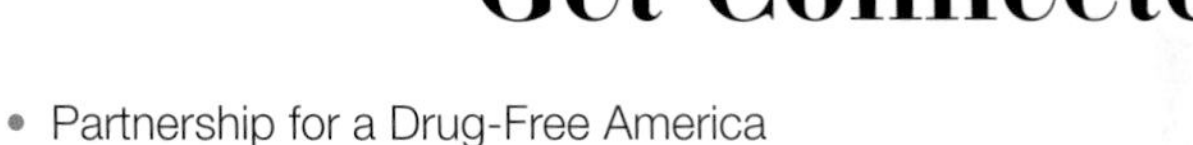

Get Connected

Mobile Tips!

Scan this QR code with your mobile device to access additional tips about avoiding drug misuse or abuse. Or, via your mobile device, go to **http://mobiletips.pearsoncmg.com** and navigate to Chapter 8.

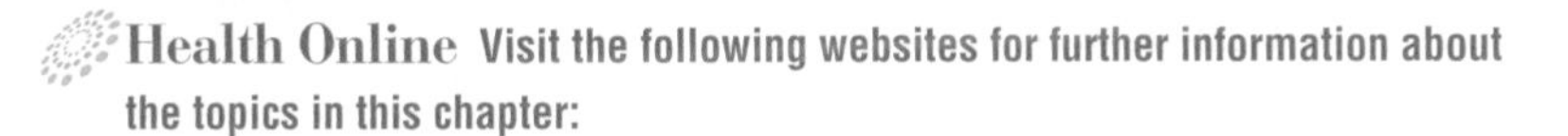

Health Online Visit the following websites for further information about the topics in this chapter:

- The Science of Addiction
  www.drugabuse.gov/publications/science-addiction
- Drugs of Abuse Information
  www.drugabuse.gov/drugs-abuse
- Partnership for a Drug-Free America
  www.drugfree.org
- Narcotics Anonymous
  www.na.org
- National Center on Addiction and Substance Abuse at Columbia University
  www.casacolumbia.org

Website links are subject to change. To access updated web links, please visit ***www.pearsonhighered.com/lynchelmore.***

References

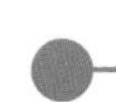

i. National Council on Problem Gambling. (2011, April). FAQs: Problem gamblers. Retrieved from http://www.ncpgambling.org.

ii. Substance Abuse and Mental Health Services Administration, Office of Applied Studies. (2010, September). *Results from the 2009 national survey on drug use and health: Volume I: Summary of national findings.* Retrieved from http://oas.samhsa.gov/nsduh/2k9nsduh/2k9ResultsP.pdf.

iii. American College Health Association. (2012). *American College Health Association national college health assessment (ACHA-NCHA II): Reference group executive summary, fall 2011.* Retrieved from http://www.acha-ncha.org/reports_ACHA-NCHAII.html.

1. Xu, J., Kochanek, K. D., Murphy, S. L., & Tejada-Vera, B. (2010, May 20). Deaths: Final data for 2007. *National Vital Statistics Reports 58* (19). Available at http://www.cdc.gov/NCHS/data/nvsr/nvsr58/nvsr58_19.pdf.

2. Lawyer, S., Resnick, H., Bakanic, V., Burkett, T., & Kilpatrick, D. (2010, March–April). Forcible, drug-facilitated, and incapacitated rape and sexual assault among undergraduate women. *Journal of American College of Health, 58* (5), 453–460.

3. Substance Abuse and Mental Health Services Administration. (2011). *Results from the 2010 national survey on drug use and health: Summary of national findings.* NSDUH Series H-41, HHS Publication No. (SMA) 11-4658. Rockville, MD: Substance Abuse and Mental Health Services Administration. Retrieved from http://www.oas.samhsa.gov/NSDUH/2k10NSDUH/2k10Results.pdf.

4. National Council on Problem Gambling. (2011, April). FAQs: Problem gamblers. Retrieved from http://www.ncpgambling.org.

5. American Society of Addiction Medicine. (2011, April 12). Definition of addiction. *ASAM Public Policy Statement.* Retrieved from http://www.asam.org/DefinitionofAddiction-ShortVersion.html.

6. Leshner, A. I. (2001, April 9). Addiction is a brain disease. *Issues in Science and Technology*. Retrieved from http://www.issues.org/17.3/leshner.htm#.

7. Frances, A. (2010, Fall). DSM-5 suggests opening the door to behavioral addictions. Addiction Medicine Forum. *California Society of Addiction Medicine News*, 14–15.

8. National Institute on Drug Abuse. (2010, August). *Drugs, brains, and behavior: The science of addiction.* NIH Pub. No. 10-5605. Retrieved from http://www.nida.nih.gov/scienceofaddiction/sciofaddiction.pdf.

9. Lynch, W. J. (2006). Sex differences in vulnerability to addiction. *Experimental and Clinical Psychopharmacology*, *14* (1), 34–41.

10. National Institute on Drug Abuse. (2003, October). Risk factors and protective factors. *Preventing Drug Abuse Among Children and Adolescents*. NIH Pub. No. 04-4212(b). Retrieved from http://www.nida.nih.gov/prevention/risk.html.

11. National Center on Addiction and Substance Abuse at Columbia University. (2001). Spirituality and religion reduce risk of substance abuse. Retrieved from http://www.casacolumbia.org/templates/PressReleases.aspx?articleid=115&zoneid=48.

12. Karim. R. (2010, Fall). Out of control behaviors: Should behavioral addictions be classified as real disorders? Addiction Medicine Forum. *California Society of Addiction Medicine News, 3,* 13.

13. Welte, J. W., Barnes, G. M., Tidwell, M. C., & Hoffman, J. H. (2008, December 21). The prevalence of problem gambling among U.S. adolescents and young adults: Results from a national survey. *Journal of Gambling Studies*, *24* (2), 119–133.

14. Task Force on College Gambling Policies. (2009). Executive summary: A call to action: Addressing college gambling: Recommendations for science-based policies and programs. Division on Addictions at the Cambridge Health Alliance and the National Center for Responsible Gaming. Retrieved from http://www.ncrg.org/files/ncrg/uploads/docs/publiceducation_outreach/a_call_to_action_executive_summary_92909.pdf.

15. Slavina, I. (2010, January 13). Don't bet on it: Casinos' contractual duty to stop compulsive gamblers from gambling. *Chicago-Kent Law Review*, *85* (1), 369–400. Retrieved from http://cklawreview.com/wp-content/uploads/vol85no1/Slavina.pdf.

16. Petry, N. M., Ammerman, Y., Bohl, J., Doersch, A., Gay, H., Kadden, R., Molina, C., & Steinberg, K. (2006, June). Cognitive-behavioral therapy for pathological gamblers. *Journal of Consulting and Clinical Psychology*, *74* (3), 555–567.

17. Society for the Advancement of Sexual Health. (2011). *Sexual addiction*. Retrieved from http://www.sash.net.

18. Koran, L. M., Faber, R. J., Aboujaoude, E., Large, M. D., & Serpe, R. T. (2006). Estimated prevalence of compulsive buying behavior in the United States. *American Journal of Psychiatry, 163* (10), 1806–1812.

19. Christenson, G. A., Faber, R. J., De Zwaan, M., Raymond, N. C., Specker, S. M., Ekern, M. D., . . . Eckert, E. D. (1994). Compulsive buying: Descriptive characteristics and psychiatric comorbidity. *Journal of Clinical Psychiatry, 55*, 5–11.

20. Harris Interactive. (2009, December 23). Internet users now spending an average of 13 hours a week online. Retrieved from http://www.harrisinteractive.com/vault/HI-Harris-Poll-Time-Spent-Online-2009-12-23.pdf.

21. Greenfield, D. (2009). Frequently asked questions about Internet addiction. Center for Internet Behavior. Retrieved from http://www.virtual-addiction.com/faq.htm.

22. CTIA Media. (2011). 50 wireless quick-facts. Retrieved from http://www.ctia.org/media/industry_info/index.cfm/AID/10379.

23. Lenhart, A. (2010, September 2). Adults, cell phones, and texting. *Pew Internet and American Life Project.* Retrieved from http://pewresearch.org/pubs/1716/adults-cell-phones-text-messages.

24. The National Center on Addiction and Substance Abuse at Columbia University. (2007). *Wasting the best and the brightest: Substance abuse at America's colleges and universities.* Retrieved from http://www.casacolumbia.org.

25. American College Health Association. (2012). *American College Health Association national college health assessment (ACHA-NCHA II): Reference group executive summary, fall 2011.* Retrieved from http://www.acha-ncha.org/reports_ACHA-NCHAII.html.

26. Levinthal, C. F. (2002). *Drugs, behavior, and modern society* (3rd ed.). Boston, MA: Allyn & Bacon.

27. Gelenberg, A. J., & Bassuk, E. (Eds.). (1997). *The practitioner's guide to psychoactive drugs* (4th ed.). New York, NY: Plenum.

28. Miller, L. (Ed.). (2006). *Chain pharmacy industry profile* (9th ed.). Alexandria, VA: NACDS Foundation.

29. Kaufman, D. W., Kelly, J. P., Rosenberg, L., Anderson, T. E., & Mitchell, A. A. (2002). Recent patterns of medication use in the ambulatory adult population of the United States: The Slone survey. *Journal of the American Medical Association, 287* (3), 337–344.

30. Robert Wood Johnson Foundation. (2004). *California pilot program creates Rx fact sheets, ads to inform consumers.* Retrieved from http://www.rwjf.org/reports/grr/041745.htm.

31. United States Office of National Drug Control Policy. (2011). Epidemic: Responding to America's prescription drug abuse crisis. Drug Enforcement Agency. Retrieved from http://www.whitehousedrugpolicy.gov/publications/pdf/rx_abuse_plan.pdf.

32. McCabe, S. E., Schulenberg, J. E., Johnston, L., O'Malley, P. M., Bachman, J., & Kloska, D. D. (2005). Selection and socialization effects of fraternities and sororities on U.S. college student substance use: A multi-cohort national longitudinal study. *Addiction, 100*, 512–524.

33. Substance Abuse and Mental Health Services Administration, Center for Behavioral Health Statistics and Quality. (2010). Drug abuse warning network, 2008: National estimates of drug-related emergency department visits. Retrieved from http://www.oas.samhsa.gov/DAWN/2K8/ED/DAWN2k8ED.pdf.

34. Substance Abuse and Mental Health Services Administration, Office of Applied Studies. (2009, February 5). *The NSDUH report: Trends in nonmedical use of prescription pain relievers: 2002 to 2007.* Rockville, MD: Substance Abuse and Mental Health Services Administration.

35. U.S. Food and Drug Administration and the Consumer Healthcare Products Association. (2010). *Over-the-counter medicines: What's right for you?* Retrieved from http://www.fda.gov/Drugs/ResourcesForYou/Consumers/BuyingUsingMedicineSafely/UnderstandingOver-the-CounterMedicines/Choosingtherightover-the-countermedicineOTCs/ucm150299.htm.

36. National Institute on Alcohol Abuse and Alcoholism. (1997). Alcohol metabolism. *Alcohol Alert,* No. 35; PH 371.

37. Substance Abuse and Mental Health Services Administration, Office of Applied Studies. (2008, January 10). Misuse of over-the-counter cough and cold medications among persons aged 12 to 25. National Survey on Drug Use and Health. Retrieved from http://www.oas.samhsa.gov/2k8/cough/cough.pdf.

38. National Institute on Drug Abuse. (2010, November). NIDA InfoFacts: Marijuana. Retrieved from http://www.nida.nih.gov/PDF/InfoFacts/Marijuana.pdf.

39. Block, R. I., & Ghoneim, M. M. (1993). Effects of chronic marijuana use on human cognition. *Psychopharmacology, 100* (1–2), 219–228.

40. Daling, J. R., Doody, D. R., Sun, X., et al. (2009, March 15). Association of marijuana use and the incidence of testicular germ cell tumors. *Cancer*, *115* (6), 1215–1223.

41. U.S. Department of Justice. Drug Enforcement Agency. (2011, January). The DEA position on marijuana. Retrieved from http://www.justice.gov/dea/marijuana_position.pdf.

42. Frary, C., Johnson, R., & Wang, M. (2005). Food sources and intakes of caffeine in the diets of persons in the United States. *Journal of the American Dietetic Association, 105* (1), 110–113.

43. Graham, T. E. (2001). Caffeine and exercise: Metabolism, endurance and performance. *Sports Medicine, 31* (11), 785–807.

44. Higdon, J., & Frei, B. (2006). Coffee and health: A review of recent human research. *Critical Reviews in Food Science & Nutrition, 46* (2), 101–123.

45. Weng, X., Odouli, R., & Li, D. (2008). Maternal caffeine consumption during pregnancy and the risk of miscarriage: A prospective cohort study. *American Journal of Obstetrics & Gynecology*, *198* (3), 279e1–279e8.

46. National Institute on Drug Abuse. (2010). NIDA InfoFacts: Methamphetamine. Retrieved from http://www.drugabuse.gov/infofacts/methamphetamine.html.

47. Scott, M. (2002). *Clandestine drug labs* (2nd ed.). Rockville, MD: National Criminal Justice Reference Service.

48. National Institute on Drug Abuse. (2010). NIDA InfoFacts: MDMA (ecstasy). Retrieved from http://www.drugabuse.gov/Infofacts/ecstasy.html.

49. Johnston, L. D., O'Malley, P. M., Bachman, J. G., & Schulenberg, J. E. (2009). *Monitoring the future: National survey results on drug use, 1975–2008, volume I: Secondary school students* (NIH Publication No. 09-7402). Bethesda, MD: National Institute on Drug Abuse. Retrieved from http://monitoringthefuture.org.

50. U.S. Drug Enforcement Administration. (n.d.). Depressants. Retrieved from http://www.justice.gov/dea/concern/depressants.html.

51. National Institute on Drug Abuse. (2005). Heroin. Retrieved from http://www.nida.nih.gov/researchreports/heroin/heroin3.html.

52. Substance Abuse Policy Research Program. (2010, March). Overview of substance abuse and healthcare costs. Retrieved from http://saprp.org/knowledgeassets/knowledge_detail.cfm?KAID=21.

53. National Institute on Drug Abuse. (2011). Health effects of specific drugs. Drug InfoFacts. Retrieved from http://www.nida.nih.gov/infofacts/infofactsindex.html.

54. National Institute on Drug Abuse (2010, December). Drugged driving. Retrieved from http://www.nida.nih.gov/PDF/Infofacts/driving.pdf.

55. Davidson, M., London, M., & Ladewig, P. (2012). *Olds' maternal-newborn nursing and women's health* (9th ed.). Upper Saddle River, NJ: Pearson. 923–924.

56. National Coalition for the Homeless. (2009, July). Substance abuse and homelessness. Retrieved from http://www.nationalhomeless.org/factsheets/addiction.pdf.

57. National Center on Addiction and Substance Abuse. (2009, May). Shoveling up: The impact of substance abuse on federal, state, and local budgets. Retrieved from http://www.casacolumbia.org/templates/PressReleases.aspx?articleid=556&zoneid=85.

58. National Institute on Drug Abuse. (2008, July). Addiction science: From molecules to managed care. Retrieved from http://www.drugabuse.gov/publications/addiction-science.

59. United States Department of Justice. (2011). Substance abuse and crime. Office of Justice Programs. Retrieved from http://www.ojp.usdoj.gov/programs/substance.htm.

60. Partnership for a Drug-Free America. (2011). Preventing teen abuse of prescription drugs. Retrieved from http://www.drugfree.org/wp-content/uploads/2010/10/Preventing-Teen-Abuse-of-Prescription-Drugs-Fact-Sheet-2draft-Cephalon-sponsored.pdf.

61. Office of National Drug Control Policy. (2011). National youth anti-drug media campaign. Retrieved from http://www.mediacampaign.org.

62. Occupational Safety and Health Administration. (2011). Workplace substance abuse. Retrieved from http://www.osha.gov/SLTC/substanceabuse/index.html.

63. Executive Office of the President of the United States. (2010). Executive summary: *2010 national drug control strategy*. Retrieved from http://www.whitehousedrugpolicy.gov/strategy/2010StrategyExecutiveSummary.pdf.

64. Narcotics Anonymous. (2010, May). Information about NA. Retrieved from http://www.na.org/admin/include/spaw2/uploads/pdf/PR/Information_about_NA.pdf.

65. U.S. Department of Education. (2004). Higher education center for alcohol, drug abuse, and violence prevention: Treatment. Retrieved from http://www.higheredcenter.org/environmental-management/intervention/treatment.

66. Augsburg College. (2011). StepUP program: Outcomes. Retrieved from http://www.augsburg.edu/stepup/outcomes.html.

67. National Institute on Drug Abuse. (2009, September). NIDA InfoFacts: Treatment approaches for drug addiction. Retrieved from http://www.drugabuse.gov/infofacts/treatmeth.html.

68. Drug and Alcohol Services Information System. (2005). Polydrug admissions: 2002. *The DASIS Report.* Retrieved from http://www.oas.samhsa.gov/2k5/polydrugTX/polydrugTX.htm.

69. National Institutes of Health. (2010, March). Diet and substance abuse recovery. Retrieved from http://www.nlm.nih.gov/medlineplus/ency/article/002149.htm.

70. Hanson, G. (2002). New insights into relapse. *NIDA Notes, 17* (3). Retrieved from http://www.drugabuse.gov/NIDA_Notes/NNVol17N3/DirRepVol17N3.html.

Alcohol: Choices and Challenges

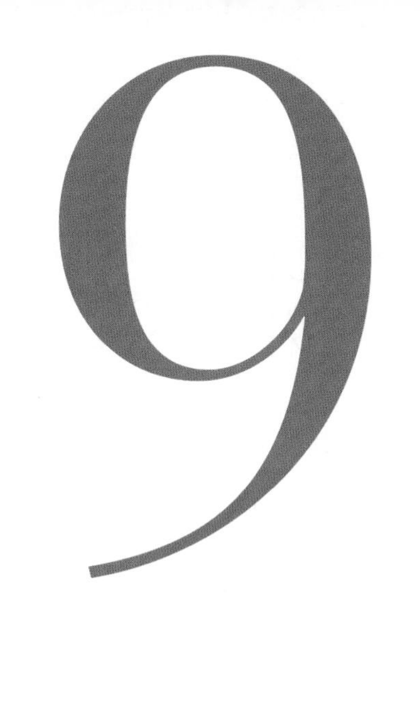

- Alcohol is a factor in about 60% of fatal burns, 50% of severe trauma injuries and sexual assaults, and 40% of deaths in motor vehicle crashes.[i]

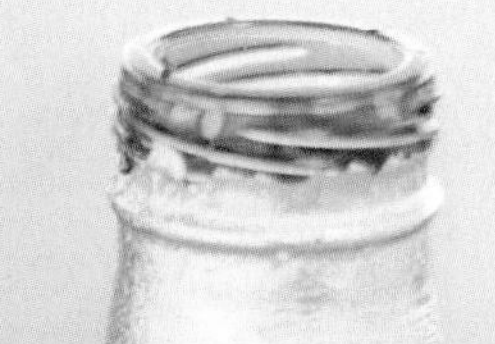

- Around 24% of U.S. college students do not drink at all.[ii]

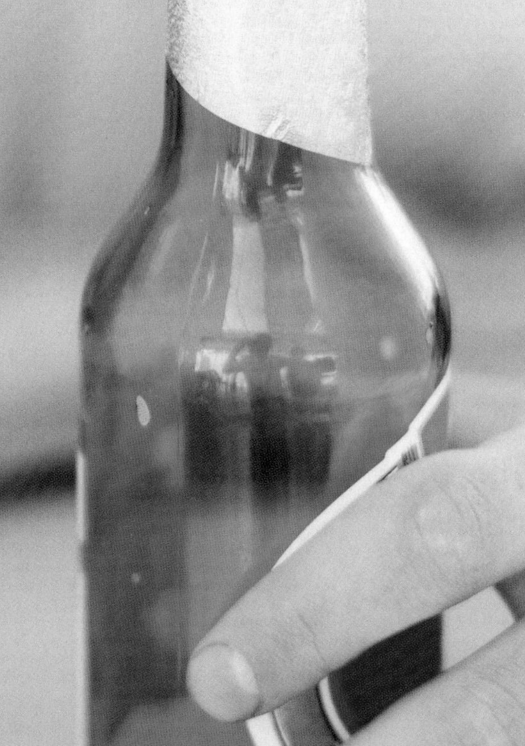

- Each year, about 1 out of every 20 U.S. undergraduates is involved with police or campus security as a result of his or her drinking.[iii]

LEARNING OBJECTIVES

DISTINGUISH between *moderate drinking* and *social drinking*.

IDENTIFY four common types of high-risk drinking on campus.

EXPLAIN how the body absorbs and metabolizes alcohol.

DESCRIBE the short-term and long-term physical effects of high-risk drinking.

DESCRIBE the behavioral effects of high-risk drinking.

DISTINGUISH between alcohol abuse and dependence.

DESCRIBE several options for treatment of alcohol dependence.

IDENTIFY appropriate actions to take to help a friend with a drinking problem.

DISCUSS how you can get involved in reducing high-risk drinking on your campus.

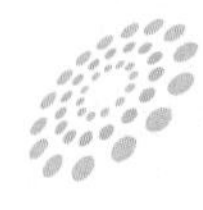

Health Online icons are found throughout the chapter, directing you to web links, videos, podcasts, and other useful online resources.

During the past month, how many times were you offered alcohol?

Although you may be younger than the U.S. legal drinking age of 21, alcohol is probably easily available on your college campus, and many students feel pressured to try it. Although experimenting with alcohol may seem like a harmless rite of passage, it can leave you vulnerable to alcohol poisoning, accidental injury, and assault. What's more, alcohol is highly addictive, and many adults with alcoholism report that their problem began in their college years. Even in the absence of addiction, alcohol abuse can ruin your relationships, your finances, your grades, and your college career.

By abstaining from alcohol altogether, you can eliminate the possibility that it will harm your health or lead to an addiction that could one day control you. You might also find that your peers respect your stance and—in part because it's totally clear—may be less likely to pressure you to change. Total abstinence is not realistic for everyone, however, and just limiting your use of alcohol can also be a valid choice. We begin this chapter with a look at the potential health benefits and risks of moderate alcohol intake.

Moderate Drinking

A 2009 government survey reports that slightly more than half the adults in the United States (51.9%) are "current drinkers"; that is, they have consumed alcohol within the last 30 days. This translates into more than 130 million Americans.[1] Among full-time college students, the rate is 63.9%—considerably higher than the national average. See the **Diversity & Health** box for a detailed snapshot of drinking in the United States.

The *Dietary Guidelines for Americans, 2010* advises adults who drink to do so "in moderation." It defines **moderate drinking** as "the consumption of up to one drink per day for women and up to two drinks per day for men."[2] One **standard drink** contains approximately 14 grams (half an ounce) of absolute alcohol.[3] To see how this translates into beer, wine, and other alcoholic beverages, see **Figure 9.1.**

Moderate drinking is a level of consumption well below what many people think of as "social drinking," which refers to drinking patterns that are accepted by one's peers.[3] On many college campuses, for example, social drinking may cause a variety of health and behavioral problems. In contrast, moderate drinking does not generally cause problems either for the drinker or for society and, in fact, it may confer some health benefits.

Potential Health Benefits of Moderate Drinking

A considerable body of evidence links moderate drinking with an overall reduction in the risk of death from coronary heart disease (CHD).[3] In studies of men and women from a range of ethnic groups, both people who abstain from alcohol and people who report greater than moderate consumption have higher risks of CHD mortality than do moderate drinkers. **Figure 9.2** shows the effect of alcohol consumption on mortality rate. As you can see, the lowest risk of mortality occurs with consumption of a single alcoholic drink per day for both men and women. Notice that the risk of mortality rises sharply thereafter.

moderate drinking The consumption of up to one alcoholic drink per day for women and up to two alcoholic drinks per day for men.

standard drink A drink containing about 14 grams pure alcohol (one 12-oz. can of beer, one 5-oz. glass of wine, or 1.5 oz. of 80-proof liquor).

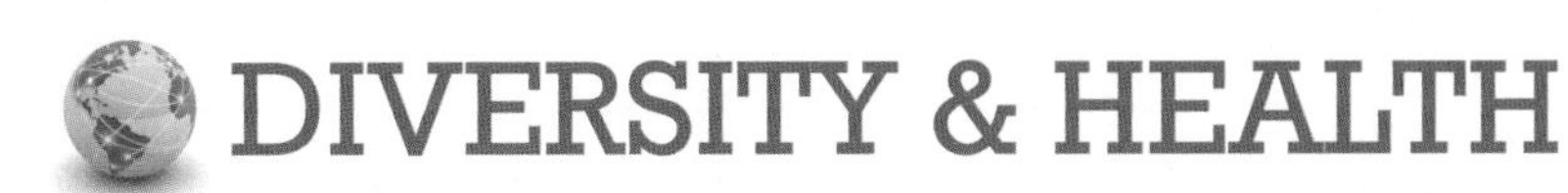

DIVERSITY & HEALTH

Alcohol Use Through the Lenses of Gender and Age, Race/Ethnicity, Education, and Geography

Although alcohol use and abuse cuts across all demographic groups, some groups show heavier patterns of drinking than others. The 2010 National Survey on Drug Use and Health conducted by the Substance Abuse and Mental Health Services Administration revealed the following patterns.

Overall

- Among people aged 12 or older, 51.8% are current drinkers: over 131 million people.
- Nearly one-quarter (23.1%) participated in binge drinking (having five or more drinks on the same occasion) at least once in the 30 days prior to the survey.
- In the same population, 6.7% reported heavy drinking (having five or more drinks on the same occasion on each of 5 or more days in the past 30 days).

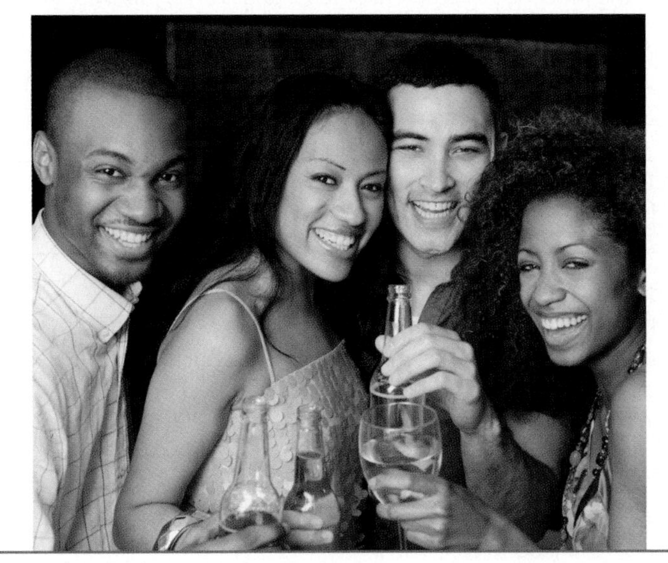

Gender and Age

- Overall, 57.4% of males aged 12 or older are current drinkers, compared to 46.5% of females in the same age group.
- Prevalence of alcohol use reaches its peak among young adults aged 18 to 25. In this group, 65.9% of males are current drinkers, and 57.0% of females.
- Among youths aged 12 to 17, rates are much lower: 13.6% are current drinkers.

Race/Ethnicity

- Among Caucasians, 56.7% report being current drinkers, the highest rate of any racial/ethnic group.
- Among mixed-race individuals, 45.2% report being current drinkers.
- Among African Americans, 42.8% report being current drinkers.
- Among Hispanics, 41.8% report being current drinkers.
- Among Asian Americans, 38.4% report being current drinkers.
- Among Native Americans, 36.6% report being current drinkers.
- Rates of binge drinking are highest among Hispanics (25.1%), followed by Native Americans (24.7%), Caucasians (24.0%), those of mixed race (21.5%), African Americans (19.8%), and Asian Americans (12.4%).

Education

- Among individuals aged 18 and older, the rates of alcohol use increase with increasing levels of education. For example, 36.8% of adults without a high school education are current drinkers, as compared with 69.1% of college graduates.
- Similarly, adults aged 18 to 22 enrolled full time in college are more likely than their part-time or unenrolled peers to engage in heavy drinking and binge drinking.
- However, these trends reverse after graduation: Binge drinking and heavy drinking are a few percentage points lower among college graduates than among those without a college degree.

Geography

- The rates of alcohol use are lower in the South (47.5%) than in the Northeast (57.8%), the Midwest (54.7%), or the West (51.0%).

Source: Substance Abuse and Mental Health Services Administration. (2011). *Results from the 2010 national survey on drug use and health. Summary of national findings.* (HHS Publication No. SMA 11-4658). Retrieved from http://www.oas.samhsa.gov.

In addition to reducing mortality risk, moderate alcohol consumption can temporarily reduce stress. If you've tried alcohol, you probably already know that a single drink can relieve feelings of tension and self-consciousness, and help you to feel more relaxed and sociable.[3]

That said, there are certain groups of adults who should abstain from drinking alcohol, even in moderation. These include:[3]

- Women who are pregnant or trying to conceive
- People who are planning to drive or engage in any other activity requiring attention or skill
- People taking medication, whether prescription or over-the-counter
- People with a medical condition for which alcohol use is contraindicated
- People recovering from alcohol abuse or dependence (defined later in this chapter)
- People under the age of 21

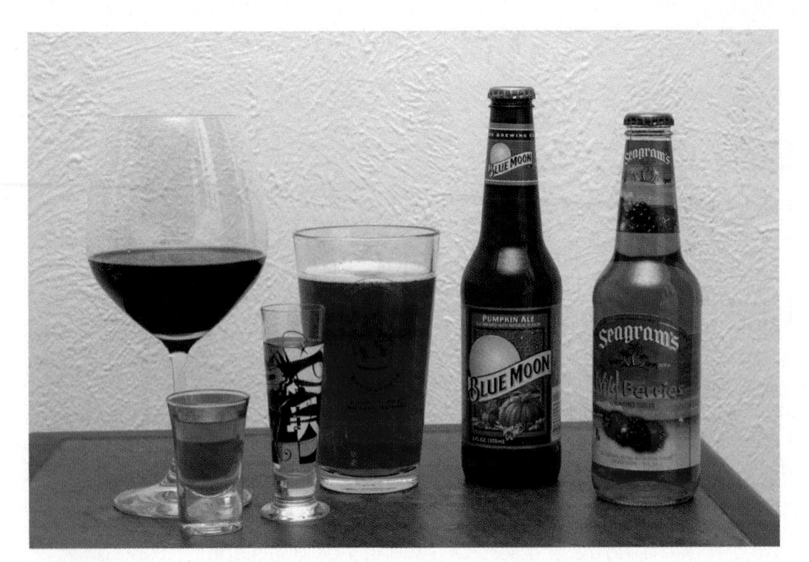

Figure 9.1 **"Standard" serving sizes.** A 5-ounce glass of wine, a 1.5-ounce shot of liquor, and a 12-ounce can of beer are all "standard" servings containing about the same amount of alcohol: 14 grams (1/2 ounce).

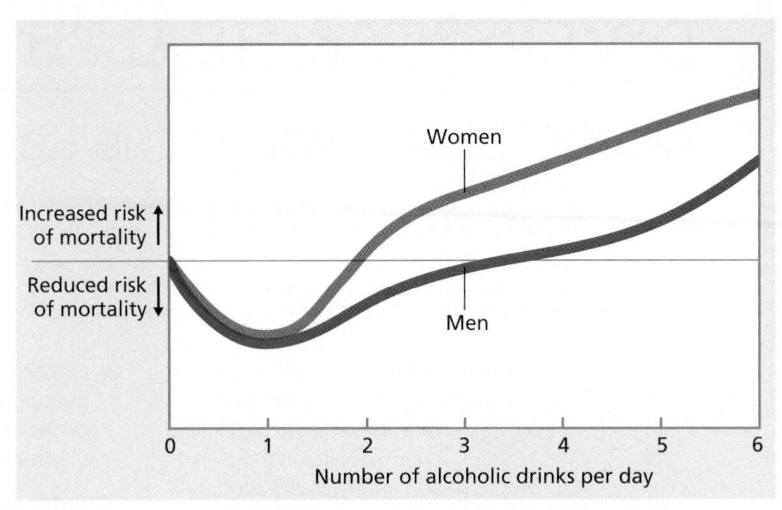

Figure 9.2 **Effect of alcohol consumption on mortality risk.** Drinking one "standard" serving of alcohol per day is associated with the lowest risk of death for both males and females. At intake levels above one drink, the risk of death rises.

Source: The Science of Nutrition, 2nd ed. by Janice Thompson, Melinda Manore, & Linda Vaughan, ©2011. Reprinted and Electronically reproduced by permission of Pearson Education, Inc., Upper Saddle River, New Jersey.

Potential Risks of Moderate Drinking

Although the cardiovascular and social benefits may sound appealing, moderate drinking is not risk free. For instance, moderate drinking may increase your risk for a type of stroke involving bleeding (hemorrhagic stroke). It is also weakly related to an increased risk of breast cancer in women. Moreover, some evidence suggests that even moderate drinking can erode driving skills. Finally, some individuals who drink moderately eventually shift to heavier drinking, incurring the risks of all of the health and behavioral problems associated with this increase. People with family members who have struggled with alcohol abuse or dependence are especially at risk for this shift to heavier drinking.[3]

High-Risk Drinking on Campus

The **Student Stats** feature provides a snapshot of the results of a survey of self-reported alcohol use among 2-year and 4-year college and university students. Although such statistics are helpful, they don't reveal much about the drinking behavior of greatest concern: **high-risk drinking.** This term may be unfamiliar to you, but it is increasingly preferred by many governmental health agencies because it emphasizes the negative consequences of misuse of alcohol.[4] Many specific drinking behaviors come under the broad umbrella of high-risk drinking. Discussed here are underage drinking, pre-drinking, binge drinking, and heavy drinking.

Underage Drinking

What is **underage drinking**? In the United States, it has been defined by the 1984 Federal Uniform Drinking Age Act (FUDAA), which established financial penalties for any state that failed to prohibit the purchase or public possession of any alcoholic beverage by a person under the age of 21. Because all states ultimately complied, the Act effectively raised the national minimum legal drinking age to 21. Although the FUDAA governs purchase and public use of alcohol, many states have laws allowing minors to consume alcohol in private residences. In some of these states, the presence of a parent or legal guardian is required; in others, the only restriction is that consumption occur in a private residence.[5] Still, research shows that the FUDAA has had positive effects on health and safety, primarily in decreasing traffic crashes and fatalities, suicide, and consumption by those under age 21.[6, 7]

To find the laws governing underage drinking in your state, visit this website and click your state on the map: www.alcoholpolicy.niaaa.nih.gov/State_Profiles_of_Underage_Drinking_Laws.html.

How widespread is underage drinking? About 26% of 16 to 17-year-olds drink. Among people aged 18–20, the percentage increases to 49.7, almost half of this age group.[1] Alcohol is the most commonly used and abused drug among youths: the U.S. Centers for Disease Control (CDC) report that people aged 12 to 20 drink 11% of all alcohol consumed in the United States. Moreover, in 2008, there were nearly 200,000 emergency room visits by people under age 21 for injuries and other conditions linked to alcohol.[8]

In addition to an increased risk for injury and illness, underage drinking can result in social problems, legal problems, memory problems and failing grades, disruption of normal growth and sexual development, and unwanted, unplanned, and unprotected sexual activity.[8] These and other effects of high-risk drinking are described in more detail later in this chapter.

high-risk drinking An episode or pattern of alcohol consumption that is likely to result in harm to the drinker and/or to others.

underage drinking The drinking of an alcoholic beverage by a person who is under the age of 21.

pre-drinking Planned heavy drinking, usually at home, that takes place prior to attending a public drinking establishment such as a bar or a club. Also called *pre-gaming.*

Pre-Drinking

Pre-drinking or "pre-gaming" involves planned heavy drinking, usually at home, before going to a

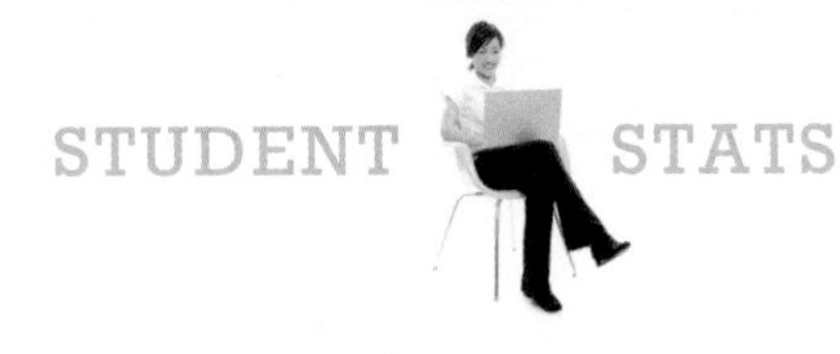

Alcohol Use on Campus

A recent national survey of college students revealed that:

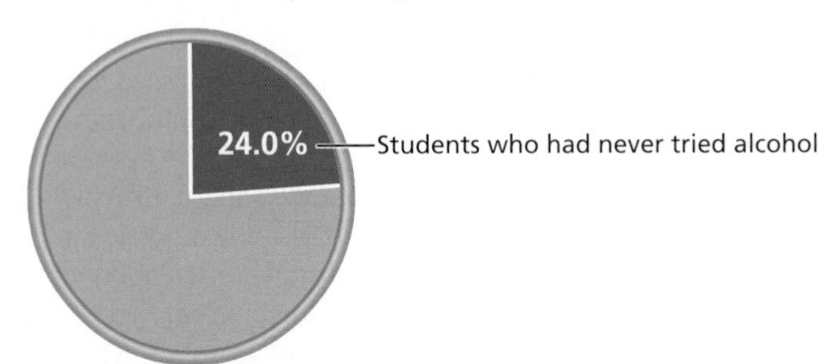

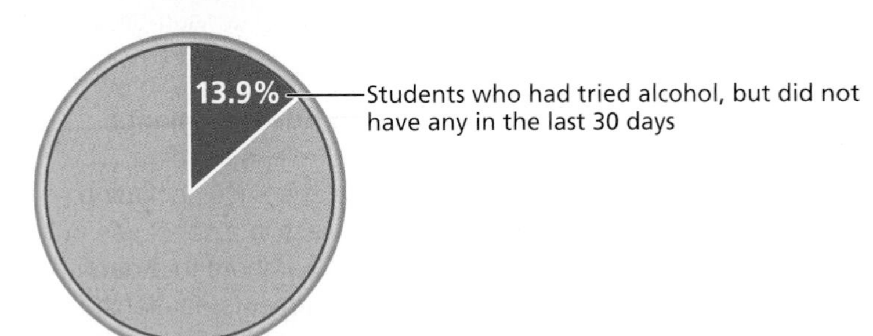

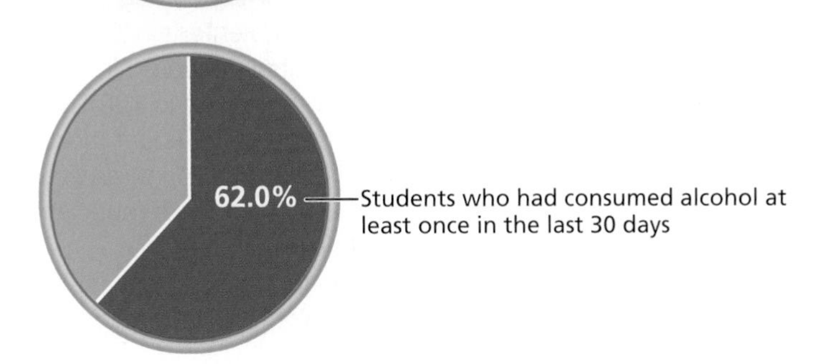

Data from *American College Health Association National College Health Assessment (ACHA-NCHA II) Reference Group Executive Summary, Fall 2011* by the American College Health Association, 2012.

public drinking establishment such as a bar or nightclub. It has become increasingly popular among college students who want to save money on alcoholic beverages purchased at a public establishment. A recent study on pre-drinking found that a primary motive of young people engaging in the behavior was, not surprisingly, to get drunk.[9] Because pre-drinking often involves the rapid consumption of large quantities of alcohol, young people who engage in it are at high risk for blackouts and other severe effects of high-risk drinking.

Binge Drinking

An estimated 40% of college students nationwide report **binge drinking.**[10] Binge drinking, or *heavy episodic drinking*, is defined by the National Institute on Alcohol Abuse and Alcoholism (NIAAA)

> *"Nearly 200,000 emergency-room visits by people under age 21 are for injuries and other conditions linked to alcohol."*

as a pattern of drinking alcohol that results in a blood alcohol concentration (BAC) of 0.08% or above.[11] For a typical adult, this corresponds to consuming five or more drinks (for men), or four or more drinks (for women), in about 2 hours. Note that some organizations define binge drinking even more narrowly as consuming four or more drinks (for men) and three or more drinks (for women) within 2 hours.

Binge drinking is arguably the most significant high-risk behavior among college students today. If you consider the consequences—discussed shortly—and how widespread binge drinking is, it is easy to see why. The incidence of binge drinking is highest among young adults aged 18 to 24, whether they are in college, the military, or the workforce. Studies indicate that 12th graders heading to college are consistently less likely than their non–college-bound counterparts to report binge drinking; however, once at college, these same students report more binge drinking than their peers who entered the workforce.[12] In 2009, 43.5% of full-time college students were binge drinkers. Among those of the same age not enrolled full time in college, the rate was 37.8%.[1]

Although college students of all types may binge drink, the behavior is most common among fraternity and sorority members, athletes, sports fans, and extremely social students.[13] It often occurs in the context of drinking games, in which participants compete to determine who can drink the most or the fastest, or who can better perform tasks involving memory or physical skill—such as playing ping-pong, throwing darts, or flipping quarters—while drinking. One study of campus drinking games concluded that drinkers engaging in games quickly lose track of how much they are consuming: during a game of beer pong lasting just 20 minutes, for example, both males and females developed blood alcohol levels that met the criteria for intoxication.[14]

binge drinking An episode of alcohol consumption that results in a blood alcohol concentration of 0.08% or above.

Listen to a Centers for Disease Control podcast on the dangers of binge drinking at www2c.cdc.gov/podcasts/player.asp?f=11157.

Heavy Drinking

Heavy drinking is the consumption of five or more drinks on the same occasion on each of 5 or more days in the past 30 days.[1] In other words, heavy drinking is frequent binge drinking. College students who "reserve" their binge-drinking episodes for weekends would fall into the category of heavy drinkers. Because each episode of binge drinking is highly toxic to the body, heavy drinkers are at significant risk of experiencing the most severe consequences of excessive alcohol intake, including liver disease and alcohol dependence. Among full-time college students in 2009, 16% were heavy drinkers.[1]

Is your drinking pattern risky? Assess yourself at http://rethinkingdrinking.niaaa.nih.gov/IsYourDrinkingPatternRisky/WhatsYourPattern.asp.

What Makes Students Vulnerable to High-Risk Drinking?

Students themselves cite many different reasons for reaching for a drink: coping (to avoid problems), conformity (to gain peer acceptance), enhancement (to induce a positive mood), and socializing (to make parties and outings more enjoyable).[15] But what factors increase the chances that a student will engage in high-risk drinking?

Peer Pressure and the Campus Environment

Peer pressure is often a major factor. When students are frequently offered alcoholic beverages at parties or goaded into consuming multiple drinks at a time by their friends, they may come to think that heavy drinking is normal behavior and therefore acceptable. Aware of the impact of social norms on students' drinking behaviors, alcohol abuse prevention experts try to counter student perceptions of their peers' drinking behaviors with the fact that the majority of students drink responsibly or don't drink at all. In fact, 56.5% of college students do not engage in binge drinking.[1] In a recent survey from the American College Health Association, 13.9% of U.S. college students who had tried alcohol reported that they had not had a single alcoholic beverage within the past 30 days, and 26.5% reported that they had never tried alcohol at all.[16] Moreover, a 2010 survey at one private New England college found that 91% of students expressed a preference for being around students who drink moderately or not at all.[17]

On some campuses, advertisements for alcoholic beverages are in full view, flyers announcing keg parties and other activities involving alcohol are posted everywhere, and local liquor stores do not always check ID. Such aspects of the social and built environment encourage alcohol consumption and high-risk drinking. Campus-based strategies to reduce high-risk drinking are discussed later in this chapter.

Want to find out the alcohol policy at your college or university? For a state-by-state list of campus policies, click on the interactive map at www.collegedrinkingprevention.gov/policies/default.aspx.

Family Exposure

Parents also influence the drinking patterns of college students. Parental disapproval of drinking in high school seems to have a protective effect against alcohol misuse in college.[18] Moreover, research suggests that college students whose parents allowed alcohol consumption in high school are significantly more at risk for high-risk drinking.[18] However, the precise situation in which the drinking occurs must be taken into account, as studies also show that those who grow up in families that allow them to consume alcohol during family meals are significantly less likely as adults to binge drink or to get drunk.[19]

Mental Health and "Hidden Disabilities"

Research has consistently shown a strong correlation between mental disorders and substance abuse, including high-risk drinking.[20] For example, the U.S. Department of Health and Human Services reports that, among adults aged 18 to 25 who had not used alcohol previously, almost 34% of those who experienced a major depressive episode in the past year began using alcohol. In contrast, just under 25% of young adults who had not experienced a major depressive episode in the past year began drinking.[20] Moreover, a recent national survey reported that more than half of first-year college students with so-called "hidden disabilities," including psychological problems, attention deficit hyperactivity disorder (ADHD), and dyslexia, reported alcohol consumption in their senior year of high school.[21]

heavy drinking The consumption of five or more drinks on the same occasion on each of five or more days in the past 30 days.

ethyl alcohol (ethanol) The intoxicating ingredient in beer, wine, and distilled liquor.

proof value A measurement of alcoholic strength, corresponding to twice the alcohol percentage (13% alcohol equals 26 proof).

The Role of Media and Advertisements

The media play a crucial role in shaping perceptions about substance use, including high-risk drinking. Increases in alcohol use in the 1990s were linked by researchers to a decline in public service announcements cautioning against alcohol use and a corresponding increase in pro-use messages from the entertainment industry. For example, alcohol appeared in 93% of the 200 most popular movie rentals in 1997, and the same year, the alcohol industry spent more than $1 billion on television, radio, print, and outdoor advertising.[22] Other studies have found that frequent exposure to television and video portrayals of alcohol consumption as desirable can overwhelm an adolescent's ability to make logical decisions about drinking.[23]

The Body's Response to Alcohol

Alcohol is a type of drug classified as a central nervous system depressant. In more than moderate amounts, it is toxic to the body. The key ingredient in every can of beer, glass of wine, and shot of tequila is **ethyl alcohol,** or **ethanol.** This intoxicating substance is produced through a process called *fermentation,* in which natural sugars are converted into alcohol and carbon dioxide with the help of yeast. To produce beer and wine, manufacturers add other ingredients, such as water, that dilute the drinks. To create hard liquor, they put the ethyl alcohol through another process, known as *distillation.* Distillation involves boiling the fermented liquid to evaporate its alcohol. This vapor is collected and cooled so that it condenses back into a liquid with a higher alcohol concentration than before.

Stronger beverages are often referred to by their **proof value,** a measure of their ethyl alcohol content. A proof is double the actual alcohol percentage—for example, a bourbon labeled *100 proof* contains 50% alcohol by volume. Many red wines have a proof value of 26, which means they contain 13% alcohol by volume.

Because different alcoholic beverages have different proof values, a standard serving size varies greatly by drink type. As you saw in Figure 9.1, a 5-ounce glass of table wine has the same alcohol content as 1.5 ounces—roughly one shot glass—of 80-proof liquor. Although these amounts may seem intuitive enough, researchers at the University of California at Berkeley found that when people were asked to serve themselves a standard drink at home, they poured considerably more alcohol than they should have.[24] Sometimes the packaging can fool you. For instance, two 12-ounce bottles of different types of *alcopops*—flavored alcoholic beverages such as wine coolers, rum teas, or fruity malt beverages—may each appear to be a single serving. Yet these drinks can vary in proof value from 8 to 25, which means that one bottle may qualify as a single standard drink, whereas the other may constitute two or three.

Absorption and Metabolism

When you consume an alcoholic beverage, the alcohol passes through cells lining your stomach and small intestine into your bloodstream, a process known as **absorption.** The alcohol then travels to your liver, where it is broken down by enzymes in a process known as **metabolism (Figure 9.3).** (A small amount of alcohol is metabolized in the stomach as well, but 80% of alcohol metabolism takes place in the liver.) One enzyme in particular, *alcohol dehydrogenase* (ADH), converts alcohol into a byproduct called *acetaldehyde.* The acetaldehyde is then quickly transformed into acetate by other enzymes and is eventually metabolized to carbon dioxide and water. Some alcohol, however, is not metabolized, and is excreted in urine, sweat, and breath. It can be detected in breath and urine tests such as the Breathalyzer test. The Breathalyzer test is based on the fact that increases in the level of alcohol in the blood correspond to increases in the level of alcohol in breath vapor.

To check your own understanding of what constitutes a "standard drink," visit http://pubs.niaaa.nih.gov/publications/Practitioner/pocketguide/pocket_guide2.htm.

The liver can metabolize only a small amount of alcohol at a time, roughly one standard drink per hour. Alcohol that is not immediately metabolized by the liver continues to circulate in the bloodstream to other parts of the body, including the brain. If a person consumes alcohol at a faster rate than the liver can break it down, the person will become intoxicated.

absorption The process by which alcohol passes from the stomach or small intestine into the bloodstream.

metabolism The breakdown of food and beverages in the body to transform them into energy.

blood alcohol concentration (BAC) The amount of alcohol present in blood, measured in grams of alcohol per deciliter of blood.

Blood Alcohol Concentration (BAC)

The amount of alcohol contained in a person's blood is known as **blood alcohol concentration (BAC).** Also referred to as *blood alcohol level*, BAC is measured in grams of alcohol per deciliter of blood, and is

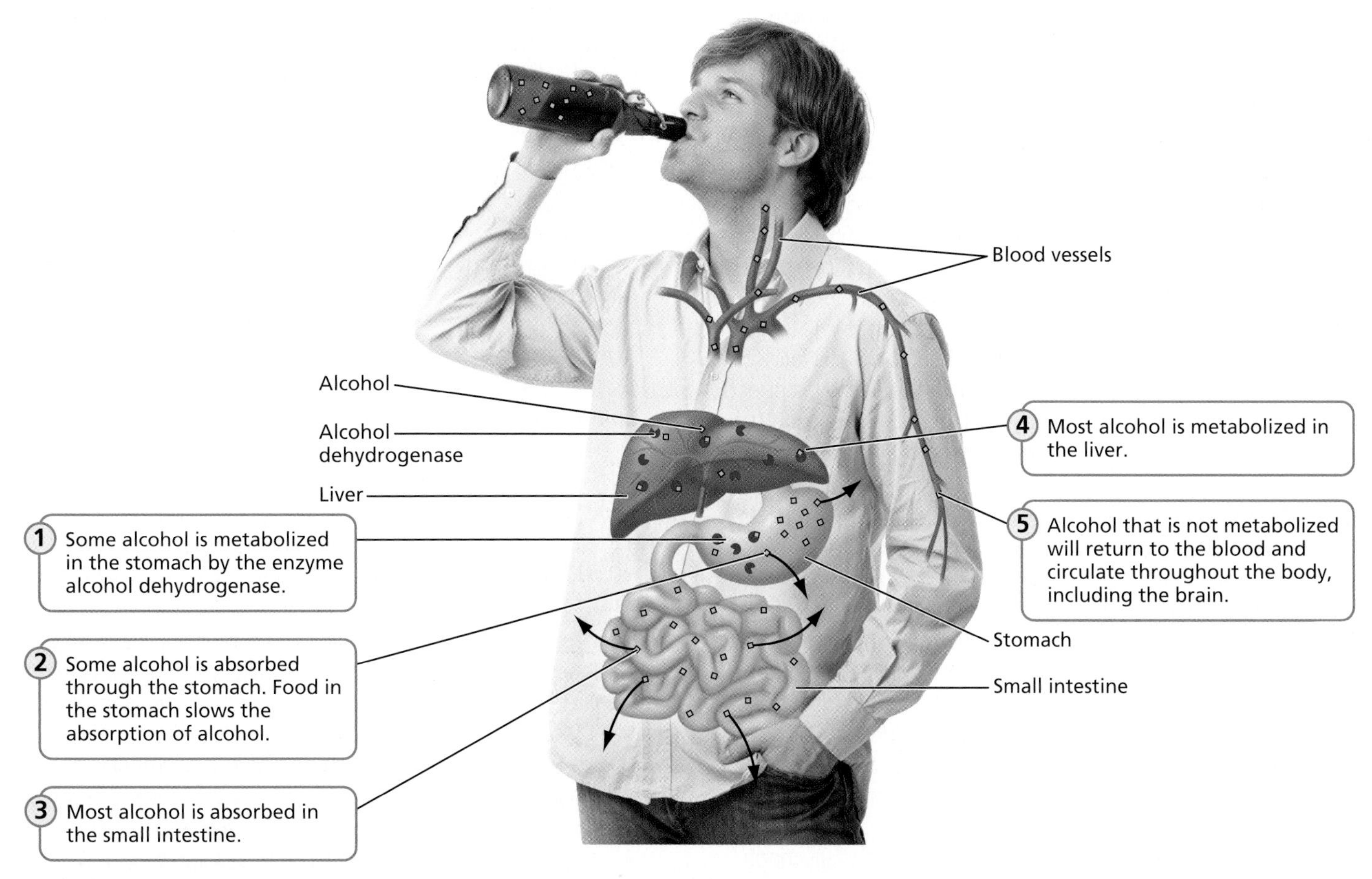

Blood vessels
Alcohol
Alcohol dehydrogenase
Liver
1 Some alcohol is metabolized in the stomach by the enzyme alcohol dehydrogenase.
2 Some alcohol is absorbed through the stomach. Food in the stomach slows the absorption of alcohol.
3 Most alcohol is absorbed in the small intestine.
4 Most alcohol is metabolized in the liver.
5 Alcohol that is not metabolized will return to the blood and circulate throughout the body, including the brain.
Stomach
Small intestine

Figure 9.3 Alcohol absorption and metabolism. Alcohol is absorbed into the bloodstream through the stomach and small intestine. Metabolism takes place in the stomach and in the liver.

Source: Adapted from Blake, Joan Salge, *Nutrition and You, 2nd ed.*, ©2012, Reprinted and Electronically reproduced by permission of Pearson Education, Inc., Upper Saddle River, New Jersey.

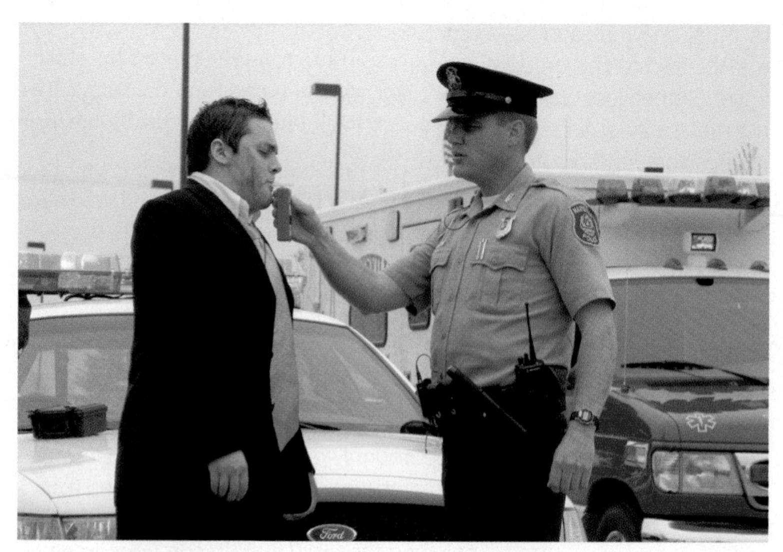

A **Breathalyzer test** can be used to estimate a person's blood alcohol content.

usually expressed in percentage terms. Having a BAC of 0.08% means that a person has 8 parts alcohol per 10,000 parts blood in the body.

Factors Affecting BAC

BAC can be affected by several factors, including:

- **How much and how quickly you drink.** Binge drinking causes a large amount of alcohol to enter your body in a very short period of time. Because your liver cannot process alcohol at a fast pace, this results in a higher BAC.
- **What you drink.** All drinks are not created equal. The water in beer and wine dilutes the alcohol and slows its absorption, so people feel the effects of these beverages a bit less than if they had downed a straight shot of hard liquor. Champagne, on the other hand, contains carbon dioxide, which increases the pressure of the fluid and thereby the rate of absorption of its alcohol content. This causes a more rapid intoxication. Mixers can also make a big difference. Water and fruit juices mixed with alcohol may slow the absorption and intoxication process, whereas soda and other carbonated beverages speed it up. The temperature of the alcohol also affects absorption, with a hot toddy moving into the bloodstream more quickly than a frosty margarita.
- **Your sex.** Women are more vulnerable to alcohol than men and will have a higher BAC after drinking the same amount of alcohol. This occurs for several reasons. First, women typically are smaller, and consequently have less blood volume than men. They also have a higher percentage of body fat. Because alcohol is not easily stored in fat, it will enter the bloodstream more quickly in women. Men have significantly more muscle and consequently have a higher percentage of water in their bodies. The added water helps dilute the alcohol men consume. Women absorb about 30% more alcohol into the bloodstream than men do. This is primarily because women produce less alcohol dehydrogenase, the enzyme responsible for the breakdown of alcohol in the stomach. **Figure 9.4** shows how BAC levels differ between men and women of similar weights.

For Women

Drinks per hour	Body Weight in pounds 100	120	140	160	180	200
1	0.05	0.04	0.03	0.03	0.03	0.02
2	0.09	0.08	0.07	0.06	0.05	0.05
3	0.14	0.11	0.10	0.09	0.08	0.07
4	0.18	0.15	0.13	0.11	0.10	0.09
5	0.23	0.19	0.16	0.14	0.13	0.11
6	0.27	0.23	0.19	0.17	0.15	0.14
7	0.32	0.27	0.23	0.20	0.18	0.16
8	0.36	0.30	0.26	0.23	0.20	0.18
9	0.41	0.34	0.29	0.26	0.23	0.20
10	0.45	0.38	0.32	0.28	0.25	0.23

For Men

Drinks per hour	Body Weight in pounds 100	120	140	160	180	200
1	0.04	0.03	0.03	0.02	0.02	0.02
2	0.08	0.06	0.05	0.05	0.04	0.04
3	0.11	0.09	0.08	0.07	0.06	0.06
4	0.15	0.12	0.11	0.09	0.08	0.08
5	0.19	0.16	0.13	0.12	0.11	0.09
6	0.23	0.19	0.16	0.14	0.13	0.11
7	0.26	0.22	0.19	0.16	0.15	0.13
8	0.30	0.25	0.21	0.19	0.17	0.15
9	0.34	0.28	0.24	0.21	0.19	0.17
10	0.38	0.31	0.27	0.23	0.21	0.19

Figure 9.4 Blood alcohol concentration (BAC) tables. A woman's BAC tends to increase faster than that of a man who has had the same number of drinks, due to differences in weight and body composition. The orange areas indicate legal intoxication.

Source: Adapted by permission of Pennsylvania Liquor Control Board's Bureau of Alcohol Education and The National Clearinghouse for Alcohol and Drug Information, Substance Abuse and Mental Health Services Administration.

- **Your age.** Research indicates that as people age, they become more sensitive to alcohol's effects.[25] The same amount of alcohol can have a greater effect on an older person than on a younger one.
- **Your weight.** The less you weigh, the less blood and water you have in your body to dilute alcohol. As a result, a lighter person will have a higher BAC than a heavier person who drinks the same amount.
- **Your genes.** Research shows that different people carry different versions of the genes that code for production of the enzymes that break down alcohol. Some of these genes code for enzymes that don't work as efficiently as others. This in turn means that some people can't break down alcohol as quickly as others do.[26]
- **Your food intake.** Eating a meal before or along with an alcoholic beverage, especially if the meal is high in protein and fat, helps slow the absorption of alcohol into the bloodstream. Conversely, drinking on an empty stomach speeds absorption, and BAC rises more rapidly.

BAC and Intoxication

In the most basic sense, **alcohol intoxication** is just another term for being drunk. In a legal sense, it means having a BAC of 0.08% or greater. Intoxication levels vary, but generally a person weighing 150 pounds can expect the following symptoms:[27]

alcohol intoxication The state of physical and/or mental impairment brought on by excessive alcohol consumption (in legal terms, a BAC of 0.08% or greater).

- At a BAC of 0.03% (after about one drink), you feel relaxed and slightly exhilarated.
- At a BAC of 0.06% (after two drinks), you feel warm and relaxed, as well as experience decreased fine motor skills.
- At a BAC of 0.09% (after three drinks), you notice a slowed reaction time, poor muscle control, slurred speech, and wobbly legs.
- At a BAC of 0.12% (after four drinks), you have clouded judgment, a loss of self-restraint, and an impaired ability to reason and make logical decisions.
- At a BAC of 0.15% (after five drinks), you have blurred vision, unclear speech, an unsteady gait, and impaired coordination.
- At a BAC of 0.18% (after six drinks), you find it difficult to stay awake.
- At a BAC of 0.30% (after ten to twelve drinks), you are in a stupor or deep sleep.
- At a BAC of 0.50% you are in a deep coma and in danger of death.

Use this calculator to estimate your blood alcohol concentration under a variety of circumstances: http://health.discovery.com/tools/calculators/alcohol/alcohol.html.

Excretion of Alcohol: Sobering Up

We've said that, in a healthy state, the liver can break down alcohol at a rate of approximately one standard drink per hour. When people drink at a faster rate, the extra alcohol stays in their bloodstream until—over time—their liver catches up. Is there any proven way to speed up the process? Websites are full of advice about sobering up fast, but unfortunately, their suggestions are based on myth. It doesn't help to walk around or do other kinds of exercise, because muscles don't metabolize alcohol. Nor does it help to sit in a hot bath, sauna, or steam room. You can't force alcohol out of your body via sweat.

What about drinking coffee or other beverages containing caffeine? Once again, the advice is misguided. Caffeine is a stimulant, but it doesn't cancel out the depressant effects of alcohol: It just makes you drunk and wired. For a closer look at caffeine and other so-called strategies for curing hangovers, see the **Myth or Fact?** box.

Physical Effects of High-Risk Drinking

Excessive alcohol consumption negatively affects the health of the drinker on many different levels **(Figure 9.5).** Not only does it increase the risk of accidental injury and death in the short term, but it also increases the risks of developing serious health problems in the long term.

Short-Term Physical Effects of High-Risk Drinking

Within moments of ingestion, alcohol begins to cause changes in the body. As mentioned in the previous section, as BAC increases, the drinker will experience symptoms such as lightheadedness, relaxation, loss of inhibition, compromised motor coordination, slowed reaction times, slurred speech, dulled senses (i.e., less acute vision, hearing, smelling, and taste), and clouded judgment.

Another short-term effect of alcohol use is dehydration. Alcohol is a diuretic, triggering more frequent urination. This can lead to dehydration—a dangerously low level of fluid in the body's tissues—and an electrolyte imbalance. Symptoms of mild to moderate dehydration include thirst, weakness, dryness of mucous membranes, dizziness, and lightheadedness. Incidentally, caffeine can also increase the need to urinate, so the consumption of both drugs in a short period of time can increase the risk of dehydration.[28]

Short-term effects:
- Lightheadedness
- Relaxation
- Loss of inhibition
- Compromised motor coordination
- Slowed reaction times
- Slurred speech
- Dulled senses (i.e., less acute vision, hearing, smelling, taste)
- Clouded judgment
- Dehydration
- Digestive problems
- Sleep disturbance
- Low blood sugar levels due to alterations in metabolism
- Hangover
- Memory loss
- Alcohol poisoning
- Drug-drug interactions

Long-term effects:
- Increased risk of cancer
- Increased risk of cardiovascular disease
- Increased risk of liver disease (fatty liver disease, hepatitis, cirrhosis)
- Neurological problems
- Tolerance and addiction
- Fetal alcohol syndrome in infants (if alcohol is consumed during pregnancy)

Figure 9.5 **Short- and long-term physical effects of high-risk drinking.**

Alcohol also irritates the stomach and intestines, causing inflammation and indigestion. This is especially true when a person drinks a beverage with an alcohol concentration greater than 15%.[29] Also, while the liver is busy breaking down alcohol, its functioning in other aspects of digestion and metabolism is altered, resulting in low blood glucose levels.

Although alcohol has sedative effects that can make people feel sleepy, once they fall asleep, they are actually likely to experience *disrupted* sleep. The effect tends to occur after most of the alcohol has been metabolized, which is typically in the second half of the sleep period, after four or five hours of sleep.[30] As a result, alcohol-induced sleep is often shorter in duration and poorer in quality. In addition, alcohol relaxes the throat muscles, promoting snoring.

Hangover

The effect many drinkers fear most is a **hangover,** which begins within several hours after drinking has stopped and can last for up to 24 hours. A hangover is the constellation of unpleasant physical and mental symptoms that accompany a bout of heavy drinking. These include fatigue, headache, increased sensitivity to light and sound, redness of the eyes, dry mouth, muscle aches, thirst, vomiting, diarrhea, dizziness, depression, and irritability. In general, the more alcohol people drink, the more likely they are to develop a hangover and the more uncomfortable the hangover is likely to be.

hangover Alcohol withdrawal symptoms, including headache and nausea, caused by an earlier bout of heavy drinking.

That said, some types of drinks are more likely to induce a hangover than others. Researchers believe that key contributors to hangovers are *congeners,* byproducts of fermentation that contribute to the essential characteristics—such as the taste, smell, and appearance—of distinct alcoholic beverages.[31] The body metabolizes congeners very slowly, and they are more toxic than ethanol. Research has shown that beverages containing a large number of congeners, such as whiskey, brandy, and red wine, cause greater hangover effects than beverages composed of more pure ethanol, such as gin and vodka.[32]

Because hangovers are so unpleasant, there are many popular ideas about how to reduce their effects. One of the most common is that coffee will help reduce the pain, tiredness, and headache of a hangover. For a closer look at caffeine and other so-called strategies for curing hangovers, see the **Myth or Fact?** box.

Memory Loss

Alcohol disturbs the functioning of the hippocampus, an area of the brain that plays a key role in our ability to form memories. In research studies, the impairment was detectable after as little as one or two drinks.[33] As the amount of alcohol consumed increases, so does the magnitude of the resulting amnesia: from fragmentary memory loss to complete memory blackouts. Blackouts are periods of memory loss for entire events—conversations, parties, and even sexual encounters—that occurred while a person was drinking.[33]

MYTH OR FACT?

Can Coffee Cure a Hangover?

A hangover is the body's reaction to being poisoned . . . poisoned with too much alcohol. Excessive drinking traumatizes the central nervous system, resulting in headaches, dizziness, nausea, dehydration, and even a weakened immune system.

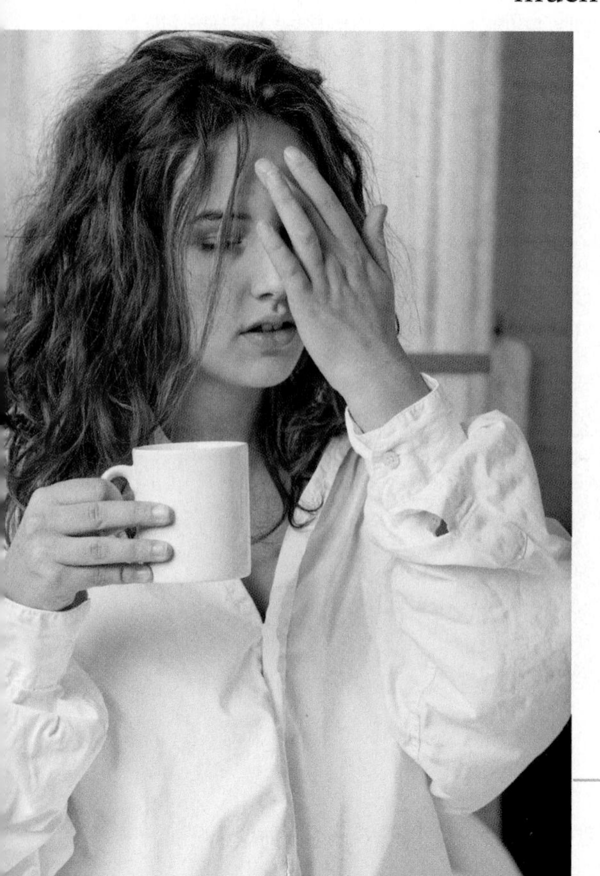

Alcohol is a diuretic and consequently increases urination, which leads to dehydration. Coffee is not an effective hangover cure because the caffeine in it causes even more dehydration. In fact, coffee could actually make your hangover worse! The morning after, you should avoid caffeinated beverages and stick to water for rehydration. Sports drinks might also be a good choice because they will both counter dehydration and replace lost electrolytes.

While we're at it, let's examine a few additional supposed hangover "cures":

- Can a Bloody Mary (vodka and spiced tomato juice) cure a hangover? No. Drinking additional alcohol the morning after may *postpone* the symptoms of a hangover, but cannot prevent them.
- Will eating before you go to bed help alleviate your hangover symptoms the next day? No. In order for food to have any impact, it needs to be in your stomach *while* you are drinking, when it can slow the absorption of alcohol and reduce your level of intoxication. Eating after the fact isn't going to help.
- What about taking over-the-counter painkillers before going to bed? No. These painkillers peak in about four hours, so unfortunately, the effect of a bedtime dose will be gone by morning. Also, note that taking acetaminophen (e.g., Tylenol) immediately after drinking can be downright dangerous. Alcohol disrupts how the liver processes acetaminophen, which can lead to liver inflammation and permanent damage.

The only sure-fire way to avoid the effects of a hangover is to not drink to excess in the first place.

Alcohol Poisoning

Every year in the United States, thousands of college-age adults are transported to local hospitals for treatment of **alcohol poisoning** (also called *alcohol overdose*). A medical emergency, alcohol poisoning occurs as a result of a dangerously high level of alcohol consumption and the toxic byproducts that result when alcohol is metabolized by the body.

When the body absorbs too much alcohol, it can depress the central nervous system, slowing breathing, heart rate, and the gag reflex that is needed to prevent choking. Inebriated students can lose consciousness, choke on their own vomit, and die from asphyxiation. Others may fall asleep and even be heard snoring, but might never wake up. Between 1999 and 2005, an average of 26 college-age adults died each year from alcohol poisoning.[34] In addition, victims can experience *hypothermia* (low body temperature) and *hypoglycemia* (low blood glucose), which can lead to seizures resulting in permanent brain damage. Moreover, when intoxication impairs the gag reflex, vomit can be inhaled into the lungs, leading to aspiration pneumonia and possible respiratory failure.

Signs of alcohol poisoning include mental confusion, vomiting, seizures, slow or irregular breathing, low body temperature, and skin that is pale or bluish in color. If a person who is intoxicated "falls asleep" and cannot be roused—*even if that person is snoring*—he or she needs emergency medical care. It is dangerous to assume the person will be fine if left alone to "sleep it off." A person's blood alcohol concentration can continue to rise even while he or she is passed out.

Alcohol poisoning should be taken as seriously as any other kind of poisoning. Call 911 immediately if a person has been drinking and:

- Is experiencing slow, shallow or irregular breathing (10 seconds or more between breaths).
- Is experiencing seizures.
- Is injured.
- Is unconscious and you can't rouse him or her even by shaking.
- Has consumed other drugs. Simultaneous use of any other drug increases the risk of alcohol poisoning and death. For example, use of marijuana inhibits vomiting, so the body cannot expel the alcohol. Even the simultaneous use of an over-the-counter drug such as an allergy medication can promote serious adverse drug interactions.

Many college students think they can avoid alcohol poisoning by choosing a "caffeinated cocktail"—an alcoholic beverage that also contains caffeine. Read the nearby **Consumer Corner** to find out the truth behind these increasingly popular concoctions.

Drug–Drug Interactions

A number of common over-the-counter and prescription drugs—from simple pain relievers to antidepressants—are labeled with a warning: *Do not take with alcohol.* Why not? One of the liver's hundreds of jobs is to break down toxic substances in the blood, including alcohol and other drugs. Because the liver prioritizes alcohol metabolism over the breakdown of many other types of drugs, the risk of taking these drugs with alcohol is that the medication will persist intact in the bloodstream. This can lead to an intensified effect—in essence, an overdose. Drug–drug interactions can be fatal, and the safest bet is to avoid alcohol if you are taking any medications.

alcohol poisoning A dangerously high blood alcohol level, resulting in depression of the central nervous system, slowed breathing and heart rate, and compromised gag reflex.

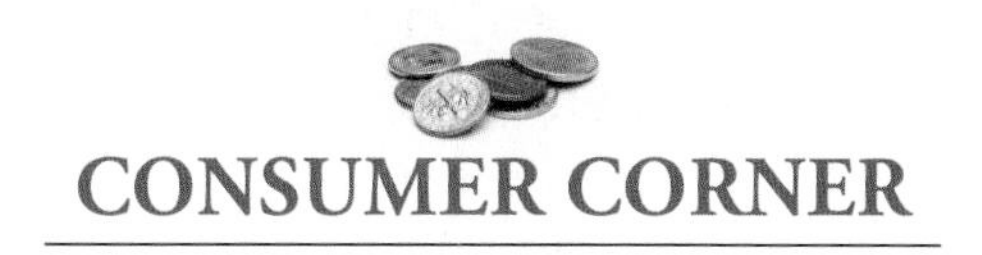

CONSUMER CORNER

Caffeinated Cocktails: A Dangerous Brew?

A few weeks into the fall semester of 2010, nine university students attending an off-campus party in Washington State didn't make it home at the end of the night. Instead they were transported by ambulance to the emergency room of the local hospital, victims of severe alcohol poisoning. Police called to the party found the students unconscious and learned they had been downing cans of a popular fruity, fizzy, alcohol-spiked energy drink.[1]

In response to many such incidents, the U.S. Food and Drug Administration (FDA) conducted a scientific review of alcoholic energy drinks, which concluded in November 2010 that the products presented a public health concern. Manufacturers were asked to reformulate the beverages or face seizure of their products.[2]

End of problem? Unfortunately, not. Long before the introduction of these drinks, students were mixing "home brews" combining beer or hard liquor with commercial energy drinks like Red Bull, Full Throttle, and Spike Shooter, which contain from 80 to 300 mg of caffeine per 8-ounce can. With the withdrawal of the commercial drinks from the market, the practice has made a comeback.

The myth that caffeine (a stimulant) somehow neutralizes alcohol (a depressant) appears to be behind the ongoing popularity of so-called caffeinated cocktails. The fact is that the jolt of caffeine makes the drinker feel wired, reducing the sense of drunkenness and the protective responses, such as sleepiness, that would otherwise help keep a person from drinking to the point of toxicity. The concoctions thereby increase the likelihood that people will drink more, and that their BAC will rise to dangerous levels.

In one study, college students mixing alcohol with energy drinks reported consuming an average of almost 6 drinks per drinking episode, as compared with an average 4.5 drinks for those drinking caffeine-free alcoholic beverages. They also reported drinking more than 8 drinks on at least one occasion within the past 30 days.[3] Health authorities explain that the students keep drinking until they drop. Not surprisingly, students who mix alcohol and caffeine also experience more than twice as many alcohol-related injuries than students who consume the same amount of alcohol without the caffeine.[3]

As successive studies raise more and more questions about the potential dangers of consuming alcohol with caffeine, one thing seems certain: the two don't mix. Whether combined in the same glass, or on the same night, they're a dangerous brew.

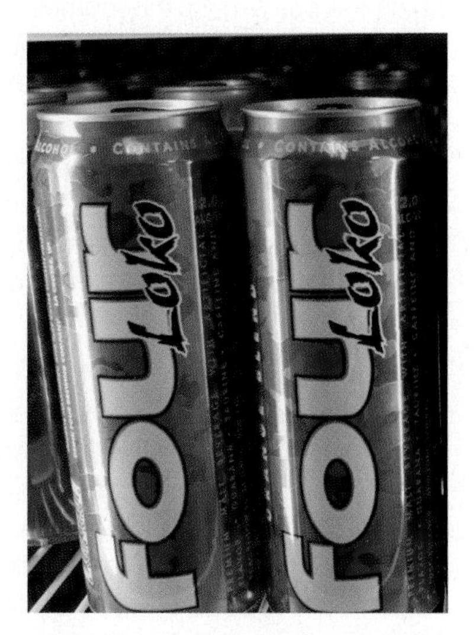

In response to FDA pressure, alcoholic energy drinks such as Four Loko have been removing caffeine from their formulations.

References: **1.** "'Blackout in a Can' Blamed for Student Party Illnesses," by A. Duke, 2010. *CNN*. Retrieved from www.cnn.com/2010/US/10/25/washington.students.overdose/index.html. **2.** U.S. Food and Drug Administration. (2010). "FDA Warning Letters Issued to Four Makers of Caffeinated Alcoholic Beverages." *FDA News Release.* Nov. 17, 2010. Retrieved from www.fda.gov/NewsEvents/Newsroom/PressAnnouncements/ucm234109.htm. **3.** O'Brien, M. C., McCoy, T. P., Rhodes, S. D., Wagoner, A., & Wolfson, M. (2008). "Caffeinated Cocktails: Energy Drink Consumption, High-Risk Drinking, and Alcohol-Related Consequences among College Students." *Acad Emerg Med. 15* (5), 453–460.

Long-Term Effects of High-Risk Drinking

It is difficult to find a part of the body that alcohol does not damage if it is repeatedly exposed to excessive levels. Chronic, heavy use of alcohol has been linked to cancer, heart disease, liver disease, and neurological disorders.

Increased Risk for Cancer

Cancers of the liver, breast, esophagus, mouth, larynx, and throat have all been associated with chronic drinking patterns.[35] Oral cancers are six times more common in alcohol users than in non-drinkers.[33] Drinkers who also smoke are at an even higher risk.[35]

Certain populations may be more at risk for certain alcohol-related cancers. Scientists have observed that approximately 36% of East Asians (Japanese, Chinese, and Koreans) experience a facial flushing response to alcohol.[36] This flush occurs because of an inherited deficiency in an enzyme that helps metabolize alcohol, aldehyde dehydrogenase 2 (ALDH2). There is accumulating evidence that ALDH2-deficient people are at much higher risk of esophageal cancer from alcohol consumption than those with fully active ALDH2.

Effects on Cardiometabolic Health

We said earlier in this chapter that there is some evidence that *moderate* alcohol use may lower the risk of some types of heart disease. In contrast, chronic heavy drinking can raise blood levels of triglycerides, a type of fat. It can also lead to high blood pressure, heart failure, and, in some chronic drinkers, stroke.

Excessive use of alcohol can also have a direct toxic effect on the heart muscle cells, causing *cardiomyopathy,* a serious disease in which the heart muscle becomes inflamed and weakened. As a result, it cannot pump blood efficiently. The lack of blood flow affects all parts of the body, resulting in damage to multiple tissues and organ systems.

Although there is no evidence that alcohol consumption directly contributes to type 2 diabetes, alcohol can cause fluctuations in the blood's glucose level, and heavy drinking can cause it to drop dangerously low.[37] Alcohol can also interfere with the action of diabetes medications.

Weight Gain

Excessive alcohol intake can contribute to overweight and obesity. Alcohol provides 7 calories per gram: This makes it more fattening than carbohydrates or proteins, which provide 4 calories per gram. If you maintain a balanced diet all week, then have five beers per evening on Friday and Saturday nights, you take in an additional 1,500 calories, on average. Over the course of a 14-week semester, that's a weight gain of about 6 pounds!

The calorie counts of alcoholic beverages can also vary quite a bit. Beers average 150 calories for a 12-ounce serving, but the calorie count can vary from as little as 100 to more than 200. In general, the darker the brew, the higher the calorie count. Meanwhile, a 5-ounce glass of wine has about 100 calories, but again, the number can vary—sweet wines, such as Rieslings, can pack 225 calories in a 5-ounce glass. For further comparison, a 1.5-ounce shot of vodka, gin, rum, or another 80-proof liquor provides 100 calories. If the shot is blended with a bar mix, the count can double or triple. For instance, a daiquiri can pack over 300 calories.

Calories in alcoholic beverages can add up. A strawberry daiquiri can contain over 300 calories.

Nutritional Deficits

Chronic heavy drinking can result in nutritional deficits, because alcohol supplies calories but no nutrients. Heavy drinking is particularly associated with losses of body protein as well as many vitamins and minerals. For example, a deficiency of vitamin B_1—thiamine—causes beriberi, a disorder rarely seen in developed nations except in people who are heavy drinkers. The signs of beriberi include damage to the peripheral nerves, especially in the extremities, causing tremors, a staggering gait, and other mobility problems, as well as memory loss and heart disease.

Effects on the Liver

Alcohol can cause two types of reversible liver disease:

- **Fatty liver.** A buildup of fat cells in the liver that can occur after only a few days of heavy drinking. It may cause abdominal discomfort, but often produces no symptoms. The condition is completely reversible with cessation of drinking.
- **Alcoholic hepatitis.** Also called inflammation of the liver. About a third of heavy drinkers will develop alcoholic hepatitis, which causes progressive liver damage and is marked by nausea, vomiting, fever, and jaundice. In some cases, alcoholic hepatitis is fatal. As with fatty liver, if the person stops drinking, the liver can repair itself.

Unfortunately, the most serious form of alcohol-related liver disease is not reversible. Called **alcoholic cirrhosis**, it is a condition in which many years of heavy drinking produce such chronic stress to liver cells that they cease to function and are replaced with scar tissue **(Figure 9.6).** Because the liver is responsible for over 500 body functions, its reduced function causes problems throughout the body, including fatigue, weight loss, significant edema (swelling), jaundice (yellowish discoloration of the skin), tendency to bruise easily, and bleeding into the gastrointestinal tract. Cirrhosis also increases the risk for liver cancer. An estimated 40% of the 26,000 people who die from cirrhosis each year have a history of alcohol abuse, according to the American Liver Foundation.[38]

fatty liver A buildup of fat cells in the liver that can occur after heavy drinking.

alcoholic hepatitis Inflammation of the liver, which results in progressive liver damage and is marked by nausea, vomiting, fever, and jaundice.

alcoholic cirrhosis A condition in which many years of heavy drinking produce such chronic stress to liver cells that they cease to function and are replaced with scar tissue.

Neurological Problems

Alcohol can cause severe and possibly lasting brain damage in people under age 21, according to the American Medical Association. The brain grows and changes during adolescence and into the college years and alcohol can negatively affect brain areas involved in learning and behavior. Moderate drinking impairs learning and memory far more in

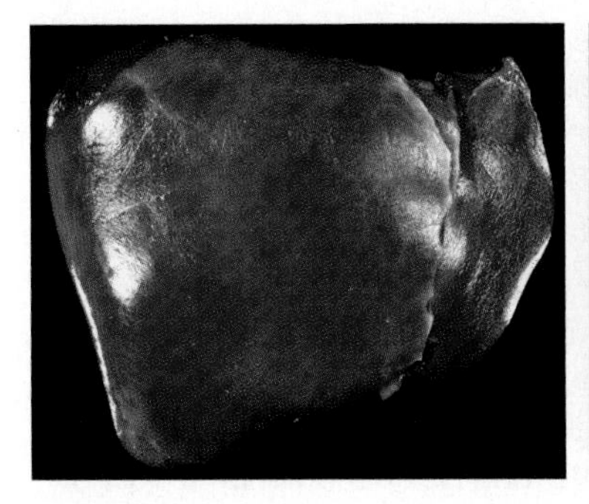

(a) A healthy liver

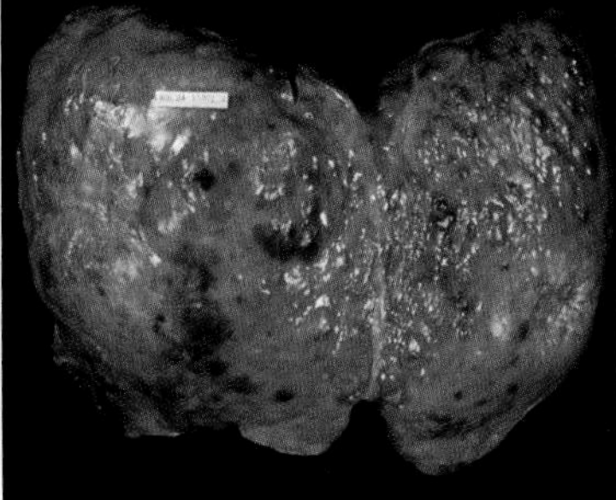

(b) A liver damaged by cirrhosis

Figure 9.6 **In cirrhosis, which is commonly caused by chronic heavy drinking, functioning liver tissue is replaced by scar tissue.** (a) A normal, healthy liver. (b) A liver scarred by cirrhosis.

youth than in adults, researchers have determined, with adolescents only needing to drink half as much to suffer the same negative brain effects.[39]

Other neurological effects include *hepatic encephalopathy*, a term that simply means liver-related brain disease. In hepatic encephalopathy, declining liver function allows a buildup in the blood of substances that are toxic to brain cells. As this load of toxins progressively damages brain cells, the drinker can experience disturbances in sleep patterns, mood, and personality; psychiatric conditions such as anxiety and depression; severe cognitive effects such as shortened attention span; and problems with coordination. In the most serious cases, patients may slip into a coma and die.[40]

Tolerance

With chronic alcohol consumption, the drinker often develops tolerance to at least some of alcohol's effects. **Tolerance** means that, after continued drinking, consumption of a constant amount of alcohol produces a lesser degree of the physical effects of alcohol on the body—or that increasing amounts of alcohol are necessary to produce the same effects.[41] Because of the development of tolerance, chronic heavy drinkers may show few obvious signs of intoxication even at a BAC that in others would be incapacitating or even fatal. Moreover, because the drinker does not experience significant impairment as a result of drinking, tolerance may facilitate the consumption of increasing amounts of alcohol. This can result in physical dependence and liver damage.[41]

A related concern is the development of tolerance for other types of drugs. With chronic heavy drinking, certain liver enzymes are activated that speed up the metabolism and excretion of alcohol. This is referred to as *metabolic tolerance*. At the same time, these enzymes can increase the metabolism of some other drugs, causing a variety of harmful effects on the drinker. For example, rapid breakdown of some prescription medications reduces their effectiveness. Metabolic tolerance to sedatives can increase the risk for their abuse, including the risk for accidental overdose. Moreover, increased breakdown of the common pain reliever acetaminophen (sold as Tylenol and other brand names) produces substances that are toxic to the liver and that can contribute to liver damage.[41]

tolerance A condition in which the body becomes so accustomed to a drug (such as alcohol) that increasing amounts of the drug are required to achieve the same physical effects as when the drug was first taken.

fetal alcohol syndrome (FAS) A pattern of mental and physical birth defects found in some children of mothers who drank excessively during pregnancy.

Alcohol and Pregnancy

A pregnant woman is not only "eating for two," she is also "drinking for two." If that drink contains alcohol, it will reach her developing fetus, in whom it can cause a wide range of mild to severe physical and mental birth defects, collectively referred to as *fetal alcohol spectrum disorders* (*FASDs*).[42] These include mental retardation; learning, emotional, and behavioral problems; and defects involving the heart, face, and other organs. In addition, the ingestion of high levels of alcohol during the first trimester of a pregnancy can cause a miscarriage.

The most severe group of alcohol-related effects is known as **fetal alcohol syndrome (FAS).** The condition was identified more than three decades ago by researchers who noticed a characteristic cluster of health problems in the children of women who had consumed alcohol while pregnant. The telltale signs of the condition include facial abnormalities such as a short nose and flattened upper lip, retarded growth, and permanent intellectual and behavioral problems **(Figure 9.7).**

Today, drinking while pregnant is recognized as the leading cause of birth defects, developmental disabilities, and mental retardation. In the United States, the prevalence of fetal alcohol syndrome is estimated to be between 0.5 and 2 for every 1,000 births, and approximately

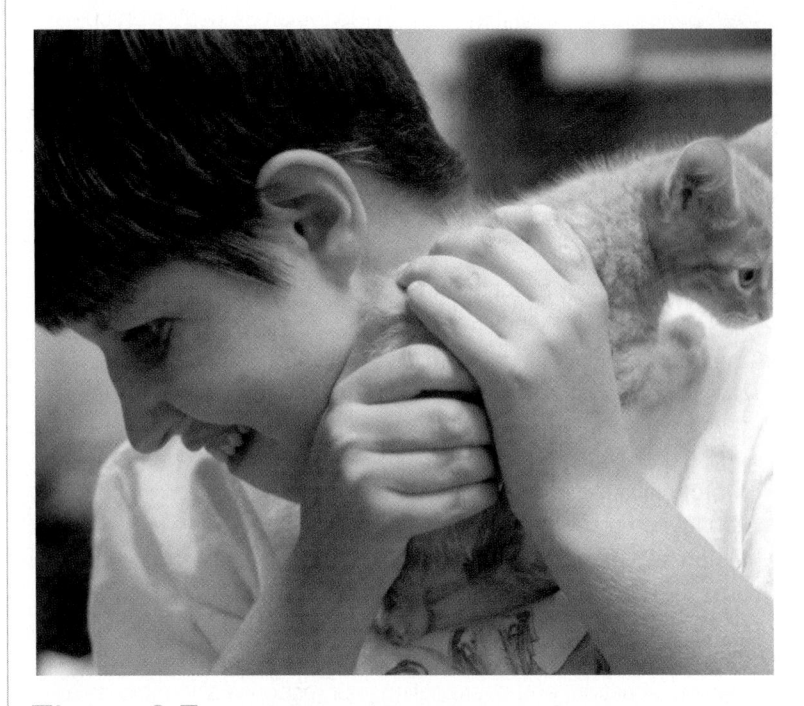

Figure 9.7 **The effects of fetal alcohol syndrome last a lifetime.** Heather is 22 years old and was born with FAS. She is autistic, has cerebral palsy, a seizure disorder, a severe gastrointestinal disorder, and the mental capabilities of a 3 year old. Her adoptive mother has found that once Heather became an adult, most social service help that she needed ceased.

40,000 newborns are affected by an alcohol-related disorder each year.[43] Despite the known risks, an estimated 10.6% of pregnant women reported consuming alcohol while pregnant in a recent national survey.[44]

The highest risk is to babies whose mothers are heavy drinkers, but scientists are unsure whether there is any safe level of alcohol use during pregnancy. In 2005, the U.S. surgeon general issued an advisory to pregnant women urging them to abstain from alcohol altogether. Stating that it is "in the child's best interest for a pregnant woman to simply not drink alcohol," Dr. Richard Carmona said studies also indicate that babies can be affected by alcohol just after conception, before a woman even knows she is pregnant. For that reason, the federal government has begun recommending that women who may possibly be pregnant avoid alcohol.

Behavioral Effects of High-Risk Drinking

Alcohol does not just have physical effects on the body—it is also associated with an increased risk for injury, physical and sexual assault, suicide, impaired decision-making, and failing grades. Among the most serious risks associated with alcohol use are drunk driving and alcohol-related sexual activity.

Motor Vehicle Accidents and Deaths

Every year, more than 160 million incidents of *driving while intoxicated (DWI),* also known as *driving under the influence (DUI),* occur in the United States. Every day, they result in more than 36 deaths on our roadways—jumping to 45 per day during winter vacation and 54 per day over the New Year's holiday.[45]

College students are disproportionately affected by drunk driving. In 2005 alone, more than 1,825 students aged 18 to 24 died from alcohol-related car crashes and unintentional injuries.[46] The same year, more than one-fourth of college students in the United States drove under the influence of alcohol.[46]

How does alcohol affect driving skills? The following are only some of the common impairments:

- **Judgment.** Alcohol reduces reason and caution, so you're more likely to take risks, from speeding to failing to stop at a light that's changing to red. A recent study showed that as few as one or two drinks could seriously impair judgment and driving decisions.[47]
- **Motor skills.** After one or two drinks, drivers have trouble with skid control and other maneuvering tests.[47]
- **Vision and hearing.** Alcohol reduces the acuity of hearing and vision, including depth perception, which helps you relate the position of your vehicle to others on the road.
- **Reaction time.** Impairments in focusing your attention, understanding your situation, and coordinating your response all contribute to significantly slowed reaction time.

Having a BAC of 0.08% or greater will qualify you for a DWI arrest in all 50 states if you are 21 years of age or older. Under *zero-tolerance laws*, it is illegal to have ***any*** alcohol in your system if you are underage and driving a vehicle. In practice, many states have a cut-off of 0.02% to allow for consumption of minute amounts of alcohol—for instance in cough syrups or wine sipped in religious services. Still, teenagers who are caught operating a motor vehicle after having even half a drink could be charged in civil or criminal courts with a DWI or similar charge, and if convicted, could have their license suspended—in some states for one year or until they reach age 21, whichever is longer.

Although penalties vary by state, a first conviction for DWI may result in jail time, a fine ranging from several hundred to several thousand dollars, and/or community service. The offender's driver's license will be suspended for a period of time, and he or she will be required to enroll in an alcohol rehabilitation program. In some states, a DWI conviction—even if a first offense—may remain on the person's criminal record for life.

A second offense may involve mandatory prison time and a much higher fine. In addition, in 22 states, repeat offenders are required to have an *ignition-interlock system* installed in their vehicle.[48] These prevent people from starting their vehicle if they have been drinking. Before starting the vehicle, the driver breathes into the device. If the driver's BAC is over a pre-set limit, the device will not allow the vehicle to start. Studies show that use of ignition-interlock systems reduces subsequent DWI arrest by 50–90%.[48] The National Highway Traffic Safety Administration is advocating for more widespread use of the devices, as intoxicated drivers involved in fatal crashes are eight times more likely to have had a prior conviction for DWI.[48]

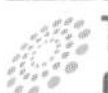
The Mothers Against Drunk Driving (MADD) website includes statistics on drunk driving, victim services, and opportunities to help eliminate drunk driving: www.madd.org.

Other Injuries and Assaults

A common refrain on vintage T-shirts states, "I don't have a drinking problem. I drink, I get drunk, I fall down. No problem!" Health experts, however, are not laughing. More than 500,000 college students are hurt or injured each year because of their drinking.[49] On average, alcohol is a factor in 60% of fatal burn injuries and drownings; 50% of severe trauma injuries; and 40% of fatal falls.[50]

Binge drinkers not only place themselves in harm's way, they also raise risks for those around them. Those who live with or near heavy drinkers are exposed to more property damage, fights, and noise disturbances than those who do not.[51] Of even more concern is the fact that each year, more than 696,000 students between the ages of 18 and 24 are assaulted by another student who has been drinking.[52] Sometimes the assault is fatal: 60% of homicides involve alcohol.[50]

Women face an additional risk. Heavy drinking increases the odds that a woman will become a victim of rape or another form of sexual assault. Conservative estimates indicate that one in four women in the United States has experienced sexual assault, with alcohol being involved in approximately half the cases.[53] Each year, more than 97,000 students between the ages of 18 and 24 are victims of alcohol-related sexual assault or rape.[52]

A Harvard School of Public Health study of rapes occurring among college students found that nearly three-quarters of the victims were raped while they were intoxicated.[54] The study also found several factors in addition to intoxication that increase the risk of rape: These include age younger than 21, residence in a sorority house, illegal drug use, and enrollment in a college that has a high rate of binge drinking. One of the study authors advised that male students become informed about what constitutes consent to sex. "One of the first questions they must ask themselves before initiating sex with a woman is whether she is capable of giving consent. College men must be educated for their own protection that intoxication is a stop sign for sex. College women need to be warned not only about the vulnerability created by heavy drinking, but also about the extra dangers imposed in situations where many other people are drinking heavily."[54] For a list of strategies to protect yourself from risky alcohol-related behavior, see the **Practical Strategies for Health** box.

Increased Risk of Suicide

Alcohol use is closely associated with depression, and can increase the risk that a depressed person will attempt suicide. Alcohol intoxication increases suicide risk up to 90 times, as compared with abstinence.[55] Moreover, intoxication increases the risk that the suicide attempt will succeed. Evidence from completed suicides suggests that intoxication predicts the use of more lethal means (for example, a firearm) in the suicide.[55]

Impaired Decision-Making

High-risk drinking often leads to vandalism, risky sex, and other examples of impaired decision-making. About 11% of college drinkers report that they have damaged property while under the influence of alcohol. And in one study, half of all schools with high drinking levels reported that their campuses had a "moderate" or "major" problem with alcohol-related property damage.[56]

Engaging in sexual intercourse while inebriated is an especially dangerous example of poor decision-making. In one study, 21.3% of college students reported participating in unplanned sexual activities after having too much to drink.[57] More than one in ten said they did not use protection while having sex under the influence, possibly exposing themselves to sexually transmitted infections such as AIDS or hepatitis B, as well as unplanned pregnancy.[57] Moreover, in some studies, male college students—but not females—have reported that their motive in participating in mixed-gender drinking games was to get a woman intoxicated in order to facilitate sex.[58] As we've noted, consent to engage in sexual intercourse is an act of reason and deliberation, requiring that the person giving consent have the capacity to make intelligent decisions. No one who is intoxicated can consent to sex.

Academic Consequences

One of the most common consequences of high-risk drinking among college students is difficulty keeping up with academic responsibilities. In one survey, 25% of college students said they had missed class, fallen behind, flunked exams, or received lower grades as a result of their drinking.[52] **Figure 9.8** on page 252 shows how different levels of alcohol consumption affect average GPA. Moreover, students who engage in high-risk drinking risk being suspended or expelled from their college or university for alcohol-related incidents.

The academic consequences of high-risk drinking aren't limited to the students doing the drinking. Students who share a dorm or apartment with binge or heavy drinkers often experience "bystander effects" that rob them of time and create significant stress. These include, for example, having their studies or sleep interrupted by partying or alcohol-induced aggression, or being called on when a party gets out of hand and a sober driver is needed to transport a student to the local emergency room.

Practical Strategies for Health

How to Protect Yourself from Risky Alcohol-Related Behavior

Accidents or injuries resulting from alcohol-related behavior are all too common on college campuses. The following guidelines can help keep you safe.

- **Don't get drunk.** Alcohol-related risks increase dramatically with intoxication, so if you drink, drink moderately. Eat before you start consuming any alcohol, and keep eating while you drink. During the evening, take breaks between drinks by alternating alcoholic beverages with non-alcoholic ones. Avoid drinking games. They can make you feel pressured to drink alcohol more quickly than your body can handle.
- **Pair up with a friend.** If you are drinking away from home, don't do it alone. Always pair up with a friend and make a pact to stick together.
- **Make arrangements for getting home safely.** If you are heading to a drinking event, arrange for a sober driver or contact a cab company ahead of time. Most colleges have "safe ride" systems that provide safe late-night transportation services from popular nightspots. Program the number into your cell phone.
- **Don't accept drinks from strangers.** While at a party, club, or bar, don't give anyone the opportunity to slip drugs like Rohypnol or GHB into your drink. Never put your drink down. If your drink is out of sight, even for a few minutes, don't finish it. Get yourself a new one. Don't accept an open drink from anyone. If you order a drink in a bar, make sure you watch the bartender open the bottle or mix your drink.

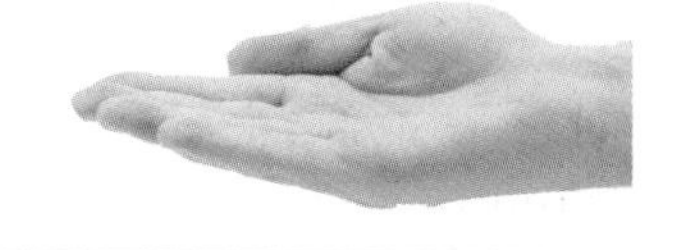

Alcohol Dependence: Causes and Costs

Thus far in this chapter, we've been focusing on high-risk drinking. But what about those people whose behavior doesn't fit the criteria for binge drinking, yet clearly causes problems for them and their loved ones? For instance, what about the commuter student who routinely has a few beers with his friends after classes, then drives home for the night? Or the student who experiences chronic sleep disturbances

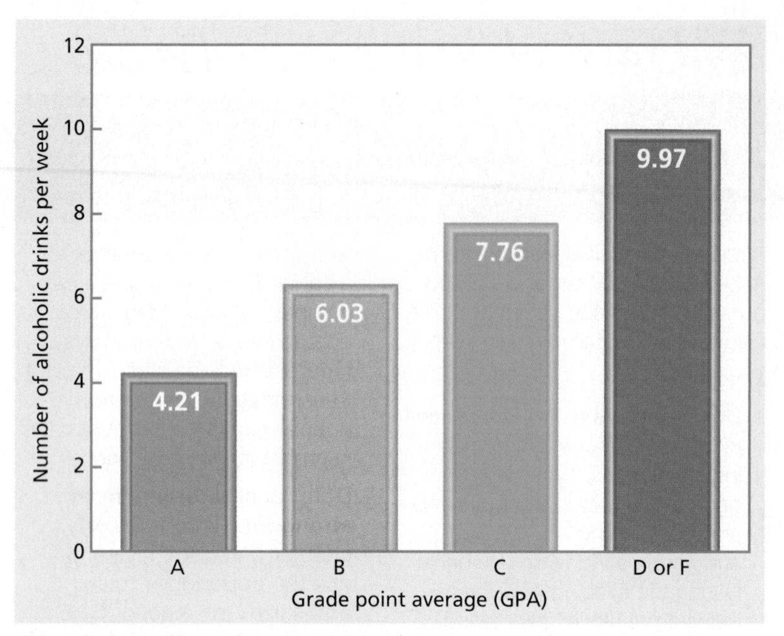

Figure 9.8 Effect of Drinking on GPA. As the average number of drinks consumed per week goes up, the GPA goes down.

Source: Data from *Alcohol and Drugs on American College Campuses: Findings from 1995, 1996, and 1997. A Report to College Presidents*, by C. A. Presley, J. S. Leichliter, & P. W. Meilman, 1999, Carbondale, IL: Southern Illinois University.

because she's in the habit of drinking a couple of glasses of wine before going to bed "to wind down"? These kinds of drinking behavior are referred to as **alcohol abuse;** that is, drinking that gets in the way of work, school, or home life, and causes interpersonal, social, or legal problems. High-risk drinking falls within this broader category of alcohol abuse. **Alcohol dependence,** commonly known as *alcoholism*, is alcohol abuse taken a step further—people who are dependent on alcohol do not just enjoy drinks, they crave them and experience withdrawal symptoms whenever they stop drinking.

alcohol abuse Drinking alcohol to excess, either regularly or on individual occasions, resulting in disruption of work, school, or home life and causing interpersonal, social, or legal problems.

alcohol dependence (alcoholism) A physical dependence on alcohol characterized by intense craving and by withdrawal symptoms when the drinker stops drinking.

In the United States, 17.6 million adults meet the criteria for either alcohol abuse or alcohol dependence.[59] Approximately one-third of college students meet the diagnostic criteria for alcohol abuse, and 1 in 17 meet the criteria for alcohol dependence.[60]

Defining Alcohol Dependence

Alcohol dependence is defined as exhibiting at least three of the following characteristics during a one-year period:

- **Tolerance.** As we noted earlier, tolerance is a physiologic adaptation that results in the drinker needing to consume more and more alcohol to experience the same effects.
- **Withdrawal symptoms.** These include nausea, sweating, shakiness, tremors, seizures, and anxiety experienced after stopping drinking.
- **Loss of control.** Drinking more or longer than intended.
- **Desire to reduce or quit drinking or inability to do so.** Having a persistent desire to cut down on or stop drinking or attempting unsuccessfully to quit.
- **Overwhelming time commitment.** Spending an excessive amount of time buying alcohol, drinking it, and recovering from its effects.
- **Interference with life.** Experiencing a reduction in social, recreational, or work activities due to alcohol use.
- **Continued use.** Drinking despite the knowledge that it is causing physical or psychological problems.

A drinking problem often starts with a few mild signs and symptoms, which the person might not recognize as warnings. Over time, with continued heavy drinking, the number, pattern, and severity of problems can add up to an "alcohol use disorder," a medical condition that physicians can diagnose when a patient's drinking causes distress or harm.[50] Do you have signs or symptoms of an alcohol use disorder? Take the **Self-Assessment** on page 254.

STUDENT STORY

Negative Effects from Drinking

"Hi, I'm Courtney. Out of my friends, most of us drink. There have been a lot of negative effects from drinking. This year alone, one of my sorority sisters fell and broke her hand. Another one has fallen and chipped a tooth. A lot of us spend way too much money when we go out. There's lots of negative effects.

A lot of people drink because it loosens them up to be able to socially interact. But I would tell someone who doesn't want to drink to definitely join organizations on campus. There are a lot of things that you can do to meet other people that have nothing to do with drinking."

1: Courtney lists injuries and financial impacts as negative effects from drinking. What other negative effects can you think of?

2: What factors make Courtney vulnerable to high-risk drinking?

Do you have a story similar to Courtney's? Share your story at www.pearsonhighered.com/lynchelmore.

> *"Approximately one-third of college students meet the criteria for alcohol abuse."*

Risk Factors for Alcohol Dependence

Genetic, psychological, and other factors play a role in determining a person's susceptibility to alcohol dependence. To what extent each factor influences a person's susceptibility depends on the individual.

Genetics and Physiology

Alcohol dependence runs in families and is at least partly inherited.[61] The risk of alcoholism is higher for people who have a parent who abused alcohol, but not all children of alcoholics become alcoholics themselves. The genetic inheritance may be explained to some extent by differences in genes producing enzymes involved in alcohol metabolism; however, research over the past several decades has identified at least a dozen different genes that influence an individual's risk for alcohol dependence.[62]

Once people begin abusing alcohol, the problem often becomes physiological. Heavy drinking can trigger imbalances in the levels of certain chemicals in the body, causing the person to crave or need alcohol to feel good again. Some people keep drinking simply to avoid the uncomfortable withdrawal symptoms.

Ethnicity

Whereas European Americans and African Americans have similar rates of alcohol dependence, about 3.5%, the rates for Native Americans overall and for Mexican Americans are somewhat higher, about 5.5%.[63] However, abuse and dependence vary greatly among different Native American tribes, and non-Mexican Hispanics, including Cuban Americans, Puerto Ricans, and others, have lower rates of dependence than do Mexican Americans.[63]

Asian Americans tend to have very low rates of alcohol dependence, in part because of genetic factors that affect enzymes involved in alcohol metabolism (which can produce a flushing reaction when alcohol is consumed) and in part because of religious and cultural prohibitions against excessive alcohol intake.[63]

When thinking about ethnic factors in alcohol dependence, it's essential to bear in mind the many other health determinants that are related to ethnicity. These include, for example, country of origin, age, level of acculturation, religious affiliation, experience of discrimination or oppression, and level of education, among many others. In short, ethnicity statistics can tell us about percentages of alcohol dependence within a population; they cannot be used to predict alcohol dependence or tell us why an individual becomes dependent on alcohol.

Age at Initiating Drinking

The younger the age at which a person begins drinking, the greater the risk for alcohol dependence. People who begin drinking prior to age 13 are especially vulnerable.[64] Both environmental and genetic factors are thought to play a role: Drinking in early adolescence may create an environment in which the behavior can more easily progress to chronic drinking. At the same time, early alcohol abuse may trigger changes in the brain that in turn may "switch on" genes related to alcohol dependence. Another theory is that the same set of genes increases the likelihood of both early drinking and alcohol dependence.[64] Although 22 is the average age when alcohol dependence begins, it can appear as early as the mid-teens.[65]

Gender

Statistics suggest that men are more likely to become dependent on alcohol than women are.[1] Approximately 24% of men who drink and 15% of women who drink meet the criteria for alcohol dependence. However, females have lower rates of binge drinking in adolescence and young adulthood, and this factor may explain much of the gender difference in rates of dependence.

Psychosocial Factors

Other factors that increase a person's risk for alcohol dependence include low self-esteem, impulsiveness, a need for approval, peer pressure, poverty, and being a victim of physical or sexual abuse. Individuals who are under a great deal of chronic stress are also vulnerable. They may turn to alcohol to cope with their problems and try to make themselves feel better, a potentially destructive behavior that is called **self-medicating.**

self-medicating Using alcohol or drugs to cope with problems and/or emotional distress.

Profiles in Alcohol Dependence

Alcohol dependence knows no demographic boundaries. It can affect men and women of any race, class, age, and social group. That said, researchers have identified five types of alcoholics that are the most prevalent in our society.[66]

- **The young adult subtype.** Usually alcohol-dependent by their 21st birthday, these young adult drinkers typically do not abuse other drugs and are free of mental disorders. They usually lack a family history of alcohol dependence, and rarely seek help for their drinking problem. They may drink less often than members of the other subtypes discussed here, but they tend to binge drink when they do. They account for 31.5% of alcohol-dependent people in the United States.
- **The young antisocial subtype.** These drinkers start at an earlier age than the young adult subtype, and tend to come from families suffering from alcohol dependence. About half could be considered antisocial, and many have major depression, bipolar disorder, or anxiety problems. They are more likely to smoke cigarettes and marijuana, as well as use cocaine. They account for 21% of all alcohol-dependent people.
- **The functional subtype.** Typically middle-aged, well-educated, and smokers, these drinkers have stable jobs, good incomes, and families. About one-third have a family history of alcohol dependence, and about one-fourth have had a major bout of depression. They make up 19.5% of the alcohol-dependent population.

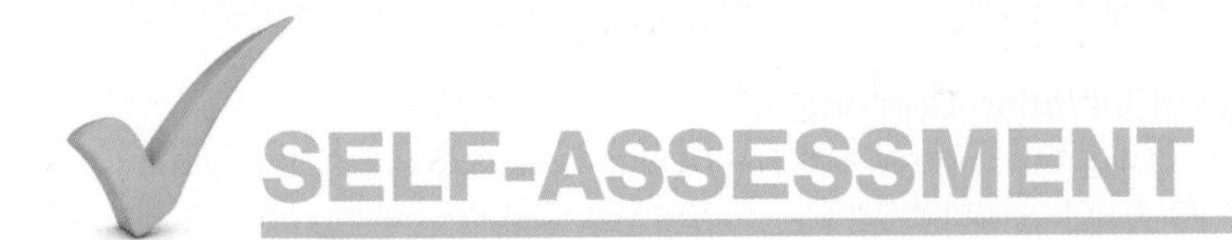

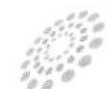

Take this self-assessment online at www.pearsonhighered.com/lynchelmore.

Alcohol Use Disorders Identification Test (AUDIT)

Is the way or amount you drink harming your health? Should you cut down on your drinking? Taking the following self-assessment will help you answer these questions.

Please circle the answer that is correct for you.

1. How often do you have a drink containing alcohol?
   - ☐ Never
   - ☐ Monthly or less
   - ☐ 2 to 4 times a month
   - ☐ 2 to 3 times per week
   - ☐ 4 or more times per week
2. How many drinks containing alcohol do you have on a typical day when you are drinking?
   - ☐ 1 or 2
   - ☐ 3 or 4
   - ☐ 5 or 6
   - ☐ 7 to 9
   - ☐ 10 or more
3. How often do you have six or more drinks on one occasion?
   - ☐ Never
   - ☐ Less than monthly
   - ☐ Monthly
   - ☐ 2 to 3 times per week
   - ☐ 4 or more times a week
4. How often during the last year have you found that you were not able to stop drinking once you had started?
   - ☐ Never
   - ☐ Less than monthly
   - ☐ Monthly
   - ☐ 2 to 3 times per week
   - ☐ 4 or more times a week
5. How often during the last year have you failed to do what was normally expected from you because of drinking?
   - ☐ Never
   - ☐ Less than monthly
   - ☐ Monthly
   - ☐ 2 to 3 times per week
   - ☐ 4 or more times a week
6. How often during the last year have you needed a first drink in the morning to get yourself going after a heavy drinking session?
   - ☐ Never
   - ☐ Less than monthly
   - ☐ Monthly
   - ☐ 2 to 3 times per week
   - ☐ 4 or more times a week
7. How often during the last year have you had a feeling of guilt or remorse after drinking?
   - ☐ Never
   - ☐ Less than monthly
   - ☐ Monthly
   - ☐ 2 to 4 time per s week
   - ☐ 4 or more times a week
8. How often during the last year have you been unable to remember what happened the night before because you had been drinking?
   - ☐ Never
   - ☐ Less than monthly
   - ☐ Monthly
   - ☐ 2 to 3 times per week
   - ☐ 4 or more times a week
9. Have you or someone else been injured as a result of your drinking?
   - ☐ No
   - ☐ Yes, but not in the last year
   - ☐ Yes, during the last year
10. Has a relative or friend, or doctor or other health worker, been concerned about your drinking or suggested you cut down?
    - ☐ No
    - ☐ Yes, but not in the last year
    - ☐ Yes, during the last year

HOW TO INTERPRET YOUR SCORE

The Alcohol Use Disorders Identification Test (AUDIT) can detect alcohol problems experienced in the last year. Questions 1–8 are scored as 0, 1, 2, 3, or 4 points from first to last option. Questions 9 and 10 are scored 0, 2, or 4 only. A score of 8+ on the AUDIT generally indicates harmful or hazardous drinking.

Source: Alcohol Alert (2005). Screening of Alcohol Use and Alcohol-Related Problems. National Institutes of Health, National Institute on Alcohol Abuse and Alcoholism. Available at http://pubs.niaaa.nih.gov/publications/aa65/aa65.htm

- **The intermediate familial subtype.** These middle-aged drinkers tend to have parents who are alcohol-dependent. About half have been depressed. Most smoke cigarettes, and nearly one in five has had problems with cocaine and marijuana use. They account for 19% of the alcohol-dependent population.
- **The chronic severe subtype.** Chronic severe drinkers typically start drinking early in life—and develop alcohol problems at a young age, too. They tend to be middle-aged, antisocial, and prone to psychiatric disorders, including depression. They exhibit high rates of smoking, marijuana use, and cocaine dependence. Although they account for only 9% of alcohol-dependent Americans, about two-thirds of chronic severe drinkers seek help for their drinking problems, making them the most prevalent subtype in treatment.[66]

Costs to Family Members

Al-Anon, a fellowship of relatives and friends of people who are alcohol-dependent, estimates that every alcohol-dependent person affects the lives of at least four others. Here are just a few ways that a person's drinking affects his or her loved ones.[67]

- The loved one is less likely to feel contented, loving, or proud, and more likely to feel disappointed, frustrated, resentful, and angry.
- When the person is actively drinking, the loved one is more likely to be diagnosed with an anxiety disorder; when the person is not actively drinking, the loved one is more likely to be diagnosed with a mood disorder such as depression.
- Fatigue and sleeping problems are common, as is disordered eating.
- The loved one is less likely to feel safe, and is three times more likely to be currently experiencing abuse.

Costs to Society

Excessive alcohol consumption is associated with approximately 75,000 deaths per year in the United States.[68] These are preventable deaths. The direct health-care costs cited in various studies range from 9 billion dollars to over 20 billion dollars, but these costs do not include the costs of care for related problems such as anxiety, depression, health effects on loved ones, and birth defects among children born to alcohol-dependent women.

In addition, we've discussed the role of alcohol in motor vehicle accidents and fatalities, fires, and other dangers to the community, including violent crime. Social costs also include the financial burden of incarceration of criminals. An estimated 80% of all violent crimes committed between 2004 and 2008 involved alcohol. Moreover, 37% of state prisoners serving time for a violent offense in 2004 said they were under the influence of alcohol at the time of the offense.[69]

The Body's Response to Quitting

When a person develops a tolerance to and craving for alcohol, the body's response to quitting can present a tremendous physical and psychological challenge.

Withdrawal Symptoms

As little as five to ten hours after the last drink, a person who is alcohol-dependent can begin to feel the effects of alcohol withdrawal. The physical symptoms may include:[70]

- Pale, clammy skin
- Headache
- Loss of appetite, nausea, and vomiting
- Rapid heart rate
- Delirium tremens—tremors, agitation, confusion, fear, and visual hallucinations
- Fever
- Seizures

In addition, the person may experience psychological symptoms such as anxiety, depression, irritability, and mood swings. The person may be fatigued, yet have difficulty sleeping, and have nightmares when they do fall asleep.[70] Symptoms typically peak in 48 to 72 hours, but may persist at some level for weeks or even months.

Alcohol withdrawal can range from an uncomfortable to a life-threatening experience, and the person experiencing it needs skilled medical care. Although most people recover completely in time, a small percentage of cases result in death.[70]

Benefits of Quitting

The health benefits of quitting drinking begin with a reduced risk for liver disease, heart disease, cancer, and other physical disorders, as well as a reduced risk for psychological disorders, suicide, and traumatic injury. People in recovery may feel more energetic, less prone to headaches, and, after full recovery, may find that they sleep better. Because of alcohol's calorie count, a former drinker may lose weight, especially if he or she exercises as part of the recovery regimen. Relationships with family members, friends, and co-workers will likely improve, and the person may develop a new sense of meaning and purpose in life.

Getting Help for a Drinking Problem

Few people who abuse alcohol acknowledge that they have a drinking problem. Fewer still seek treatment or counseling for it. It can take a major health problem, accident, or hitting "rock bottom" to motivate a problem drinker to change his or her behavior. Even when drinkers decide that they want to quit, they may not know how to do so on their own. An estimated 19 million people in the United States need treatment for an alcohol use problem (about 7.6% of the population aged 12 or older), but only 1.6 million receive treatment at a specialized facility.[1] Among youths between the ages of 12 and 17, an estimated 1.2 million need treatment for an alcohol use problem, but only 77,000 receive treatment.[1]

"An estimated 19 million people in the United States need treatment for an alcohol use problem."

This site provides self-help strategies for cutting back on or quitting drinking: http://rethinkingdrinking.niaaa.nih.gov/Support/ChooseYourApproach.asp.

Looking for an alcohol treatment center? Visit http://findtreatment.samhsa.gov, which allows you to search for a treatment program near you.

Options on Campus

College students struggling to control their drinking need look no further than their campus health center. The health-care options for alcohol intervention may range from psychotherapy to medical care, and may be free of charge to enrolled students. Many campuses participate in intervention programs specifically developed for college students, such as the BASICS program. The acronym BASICS stands for Brief Alcohol Screening and Intervention for College Students. First implemented in 1992, it has been used in over 1,000 sites nationwide, and has reached many thousands of college students. The program is partially funded by the National Institutes of Health, which also has conducted several studies supporting its effectiveness in reducing frequency of high-risk drinking over follow-up periods of 2 to 4 years.[71]

Students entering the BASICS program typically drink heavily and are at risk for—or have already experienced—alcohol-related problems. Over the course of two brief interviews, a trained counselor gathers information about the student's drinking behaviors, beliefs about alcohol, and other factors, and then helps the student to discover the discrepancies between the student's risky drinking behavior and his or her goals and values.[71]

Community-Based Programs

Mutual-help organizations within most communities include the 12-step program Alcoholics Anonymous (AA). AA was founded in 1935 by Bill Wilson and Dr. Bob Smith, both recovering alcoholics, in Akron, Ohio. Now an international mutual-aid movement with more than 2 million members, its mission remains to help members achieve and maintain sobriety.[72] People in AA and similar groups attend general meetings and support each other by sharing advice and their personal experiences with alcohol abuse and recovery.

Clinical Options

Clinical options for treatment of alcohol dependence include outpatient and residential treatment, which in turn typically include some form of psychotherapy as well as medications.

Outpatient and Residential Treatment Programs

People with mild-to-moderate alcohol dependence are often treated in outpatient programs. These may include daily clinic visits for blood tests and other monitoring of withdrawal symptoms, as well as medications, and individual and family therapy.[70]

For patients with more severe dependence, inpatient treatment at a hospital or other facility is important to achieve detoxification while maintaining the patient's safety. In addition to medical care, these 14- to 28-day residential programs typically employ a 12-step approach combined with individual and group therapy and close monitoring for abstinence. They also include longer-term (3 to 4-month) programs and halfway houses that offer life-skill and job training as well as treatment for substance dependence and mental health problems.

Psychotherapy

Several group therapy approaches are about equally effective. Getting support in itself appears to be more important than the particular approach used, as long as it offers empathy, avoids heavy confrontation, strengthens motivation, and provides concrete ways to change drinking behavior. These programs usually focus on abstinence from alcohol. They may offer therapy, provide informational lectures, and include other activities.

Specialized counseling may focus on the individual or family, and may involve months of psychotherapy sessions or just occasional appearances. Short, one-on-one counseling sessions known as "brief interventions" have been increasing in popularity in recent years. Unlike traditional alcoholism treatments that emphasize complete abstinence from alcohol, these interventions may encourage sensible drinking at healthy levels. They require minimal follow-up and can be very effective.[73]

Medications

Medications such as naltrexone, topiramate, and acamprosate can make it easier to quit drinking by offsetting some of the changes in the brain characteristic of alcohol dependence and reducing the craving for alcohol. They don't make you sick if you drink, unlike an older medication (disulfiram). None of these medications is addictive. They can also be combined with support groups or alcohol counseling. Antidepressants may also be prescribed.

Alternative Therapies

Despite the hundreds of offers for supplements and services on Internet websites, there is little research evidence to either confirm or refute the effectiveness of alternative therapies in the treatment of alcohol dependence. The National Center for Complementary and Alternative Medicine is currently investigating two Chinese herbal preparations and a technique called electroacupuncture for effectiveness in treatment of alcohol addiction.[74] Although the studies are ongoing, some preliminary evidence suggests that electroacupuncture (acupuncture combined with electrical stimulation) may be able to counteract addiction by affecting related chemicals (opiates) in the brain.

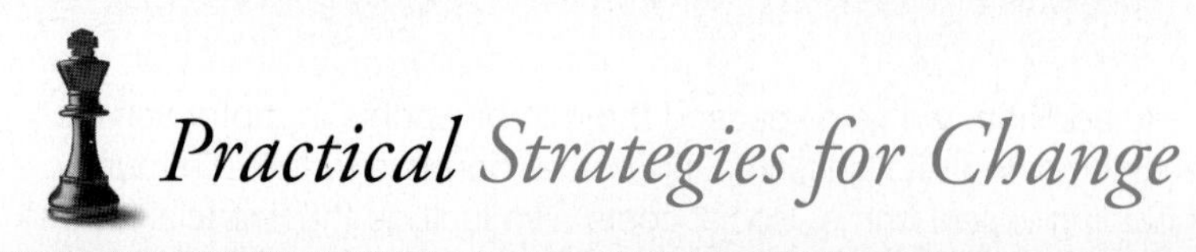

Beating Relapse

If you relapse while trying to quit drinking, don't give up. Follow these tips:

- **Get right back on track.** Stop drinking—the sooner the better.
- **Remember, each day is a new day to start over.** Although it can be unsettling to slip, you don't have to continue drinking. You are responsible for your choices.
- **Understand that setbacks are common when people undertake a major change.** It's your progress in the long run that counts.
- **Don't run yourself down.** It doesn't help. Don't let feelings of discouragement, anger, or guilt stop you from asking for help and getting back on track.
- **Get some help.** Contact your counselor or a sober and supportive friend right away to talk about what happened, or go to an AA or other mutual-help meeting.
- **Think it through.** With a little distance, work on your own or with support to better understand why the episode happened at that particular time and place.
- **Learn from what happened.** Decide what you need to do so that it won't happen again, and write it down. Use the experience to strengthen your commitment.
- **Avoid triggers to drink.** Get rid of any alcohol at home. If possible, avoid revisiting the situation in which you drank.
- **Find alternatives.** Keep busy with goals and activities that are not associated with drinking: academics, fitness, volunteer work, hobbies, or spending time with friends or relatives who don't drink.

Dealing With Relapse

Once an alcoholic has decided to curb or stop drinking altogether, he or she must confront the possibility of relapse—often referred to as "falling off the wagon"—which is experienced by up to 90% of drinkers when they first try to quit.[75] With hard work and commitment, however, it can be overcome. Research from the NIAAA reveals that 20 years after the onset of alcohol dependence, about three-fourths of individuals were fully recovered.[75] Even more surprising, more than half of these individuals were able to drink at low levels without showing symptoms of alcohol dependence.[75] That said, many alcoholics find that abstinence is ultimately the only way to keep alcohol use from disrupting their lives.

Beating any addiction requires both patience and practice. The body has to be weaned off a substance it has been dependent upon, and the mind has to give up a long-held emotional crutch. Recovering alcoholics often have to change their social patterns and entire lifestyle. The box **Practical Strategies for Change: Beating Relapse** provides some tips for recovering from a relapse.

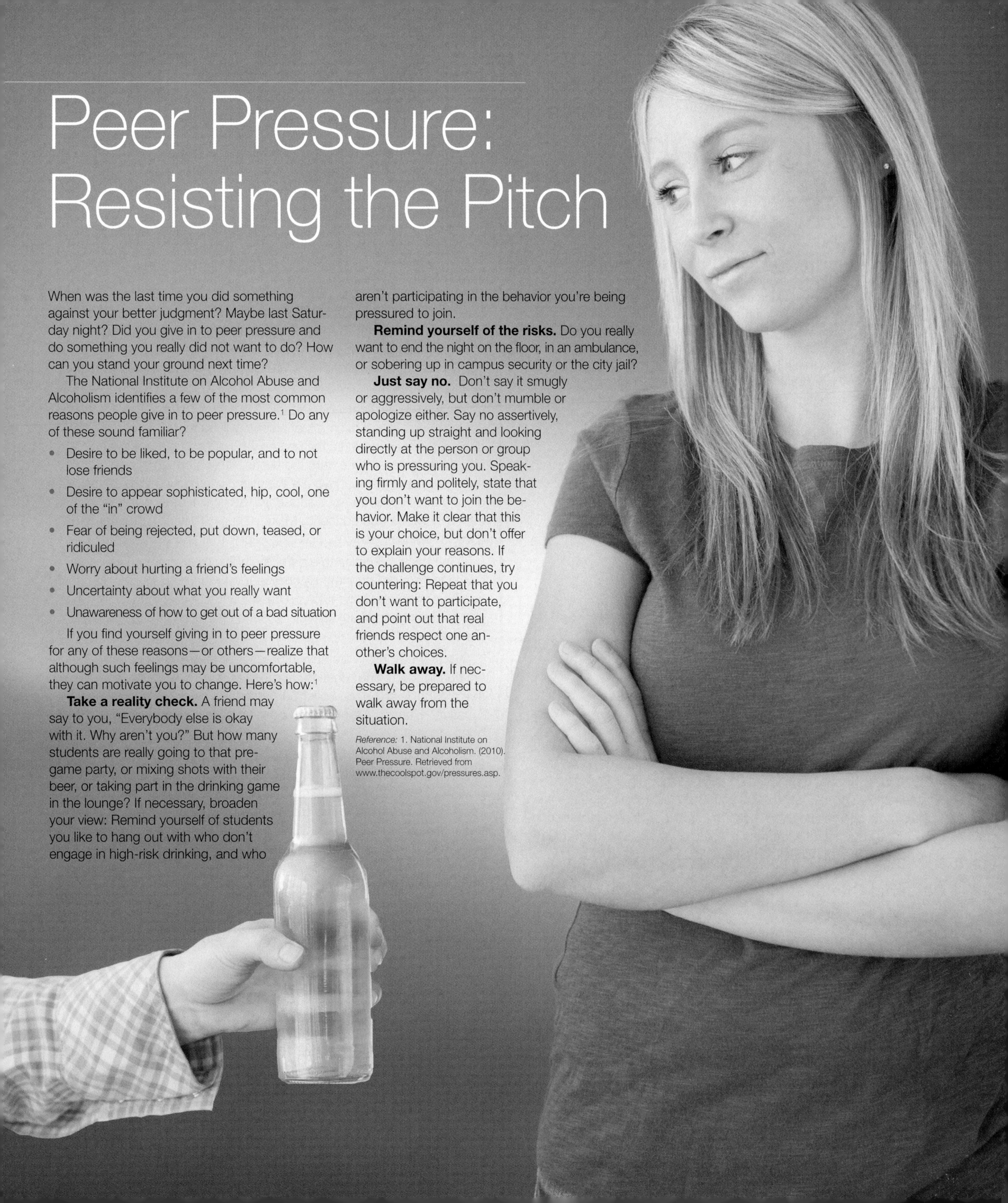

Peer Pressure: Resisting the Pitch

When was the last time you did something against your better judgment? Maybe last Saturday night? Did you give in to peer pressure and do something you really did not want to do? How can you stand your ground next time?

The National Institute on Alcohol Abuse and Alcoholism identifies a few of the most common reasons people give in to peer pressure.[1] Do any of these sound familiar?

- Desire to be liked, to be popular, and to not lose friends
- Desire to appear sophisticated, hip, cool, one of the "in" crowd
- Fear of being rejected, put down, teased, or ridiculed
- Worry about hurting a friend's feelings
- Uncertainty about what you really want
- Unawareness of how to get out of a bad situation

If you find yourself giving in to peer pressure for any of these reasons—or others—realize that although such feelings may be uncomfortable, they can motivate you to change. Here's how:[1]

Take a reality check. A friend may say to you, "Everybody else is okay with it. Why aren't you?" But how many students are really going to that pregame party, or mixing shots with their beer, or taking part in the drinking game in the lounge? If necessary, broaden your view: Remind yourself of students you like to hang out with who don't engage in high-risk drinking, and who aren't participating in the behavior you're being pressured to join.

Remind yourself of the risks. Do you really want to end the night on the floor, in an ambulance, or sobering up in campus security or the city jail?

Just say no. Don't say it smugly or aggressively, but don't mumble or apologize either. Say no assertively, standing up straight and looking directly at the person or group who is pressuring you. Speaking firmly and politely, state that you don't want to join the behavior. Make it clear that this is your choice, but don't offer to explain your reasons. If the challenge continues, try countering: Repeat that you don't want to participate, and point out that real friends respect one another's choices.

Walk away. If necessary, be prepared to walk away from the situation.

Reference: 1. National Institute on Alcohol Abuse and Alcoholism. (2010). Peer Pressure. Retrieved from www.thecoolspot.gov/pressures.asp.

Talking to a Friend about Alcohol

STUDENT STORY

"Hi, I'm Charles. I have a friend that I've actually been really concerned with lately. He's been drinking probably every day, except for like Sunday, a significant amount, and he's kinda been worrying me about his habits. I haven't confronted him about it yet but I do plan on at least saying something in the next week or two if he keeps it up. I'm just going to word it as nicely as I can to not make him feel like he's already an addict, but I'm just going to give him a warning to let him know that he's getting himself into something that he really could regret."

1: How should Charles bring up his friend's drinking? Where and when do you think he should do it? What types of things should he say?

2: What organizations or resources could Charles look to for help with talking to a friend about drinking?

Do you have a story similar to Charles's? Share your story at www.pearsonhighered.com/lynchelmore.

Change Yourself, Change Your World

This chapter has presented statistics on alcohol-related disease, injury, crime, and death that may seem daunting, especially if high-risk drinking seems like normal behavior on your campus. However, there are some simple choices you can make to keep your drinking under control, reduce your risk of becoming a victim of others' drinking, and help your peers make more healthful choices, too.

Personal Choices

If your drinking is getting out of hand, what can you do to take control? Step one: Make sure you haven't given someone else—for instance, your peer group—the power to control your decisions about drinking. Check out page 257 for tips on resisting peer pressure. In addition, here are other personal choices you can make to cut down on your drinking and reduce your risk of alcohol-related consequences.

Respect Your Limits

Remember that your liver can break down the amount of alcohol in just one standard drink per hour, on average. So if you're at a party, try these tips to stay within that limit:[76]

- **Pace and space.** Sip slowly. Add water, juice, or another non-carbonated non-alcoholic beverage to your drink. Make every other drink totally alcohol free.
- **Include food.** Don't drink on an empty stomach. Eat some food before the party, and continue to snack for as long as you are consuming any alcohol. This will help slow the absorption of alcohol into your system.
- **Shuffle things up.** Don't just drink. Get out on the dance floor, join the group watching a movie down the hall, help out with dishes in the kitchen, or invite a friend to sit outside and talk for a while.

Take Precautions

One of the smartest precautions you can take is to host your own party. Seek out friends who don't drink—or who don't expect alcohol at every social event—and invite them to an alcohol-free gathering. Suggest they bring along a bottle or six-pack of their favorite alcohol-free beverage for others to try. Make sure you control your guest list: Don't let strangers crash your party.

What if you're planning to attend a club or off-campus party, and you've heard ahead of time that alcohol will be there? Offer to be the designated driver; that is, the person who doesn't consume alcohol and drives others home from the event. If that's not an option, and there is no designated driver for the event, arrange in advance for a cab or a ride from your campus safe-driver service. If at all possible, attend the party with a trusted friend. Make a pact with each other not to engage in high-risk drinking, and help each other stick to it.

Don't bring valuables to a party, including large amounts of cash. Do bring your cell phone, fully charged, with the number of a cab company programmed in should you need it. If there is any possibility that you could engage in sexual activity during the evening, bring a latex condom.

Another potentially life-saving precaution is to avoid consuming alcohol during swimming, boating, or other water activities. We noted earlier that alcohol is involved in over 60% of fatal drownings. Moreover, the American Boating Association reports that alcohol is involved in 31% of boating fatalities.[77]

Also avoid using other potentially dangerous machinery and equipment if you've been drinking. This includes other types of vehicles, power tools, sharp instruments, and so forth. The truth is, when you're intoxicated, anything from a candle flame to a flight of stairs could become a life-threatening hazard. So the most sensible precaution to take is to avoid getting drunk in the first place.

Helping a Friend

What if you suspect that someone you care about is engaging in high-risk drinking? Although you can't know for sure, you should recognize that your friend could have a problem if his or her typical weekend involves drinking, or if you find yourself having to get your friend home from parties or bars. If your friend calls you the day after a party to find out what he or she said or did the night before, then your friend's drinking is causing blackouts, and it's something you should definitely be concerned about. Trust your feelings. Confronting your friend now might save his or her academic career, health, or life. Here are some guidelines from the University of Texas at Dallas for talking to your friend about getting help for his or her high-risk drinking:[78]

- **Don't talk about it when either of you has been drinking.**
- **Be informed.** Know before your talk where help is available, just in case he or she is ready to seek it.
- **Be objective.** Don't allow your or your friend's emotions to distract you from your goal of getting your friend to recognize the problem and seek help.
- **Use "I" statements.** Say things like, "I'm afraid you'll get kicked out," or "I worry that you'll be charged with a DWI, or even worse—that you'll get killed . . . or kill somebody else." Pointing the finger or using the word "you" too much, as in "You've got to change," will only back your friend into a corner.
- **Don't judge and don't interrupt.** If your friend starts talking about the problem, don't break in. Sometimes just talking can lead to a huge revelation.
- **Don't expect your friend to seek help after just one discussion.** It's difficult to predict how any individual person will react when confronted with his or her drinking problem. But it's still important to begin the process.
- **Stand by your friend.** If your friend is ready to get help, offer to go along to the initial appointment. Don't let the situation change the dynamics of your friendship. Your friend needs some constants. Be supportive and listen when necessary.

Campus Advocacy

As you read this, students nationwide are helping to reduce high-risk drinking on their campuses. If you'd like to get involved, visit your Dean of Students or campus health center. Two national programs that may be active on your campus—and looking for student volunteers—include the following:

- **The BACCHUS Network.** Since 1975, the mission of the BACCHUS Network has been to actively promote student leadership on health and safety issues such as alcohol abuse. One of its goals is to train a network of peer educators who in turn empower other students to voice their opinions and needs to create healthier and safer campus environments. BACCHUS knows that students can play a uniquely effective role in encouraging their peers to consider, talk honestly about, and develop responsible habits and attitudes toward high-risk drinking and other health and safety issues.[79] For instance, a recent campaign urged students to "Be an Everyday Hero" by making safe choices, taking care of friends, securing safe rides, and never riding with a driver who has been drinking. For information on starting a chapter or getting involved on your campus, visit the BACCHUS website at **www.bacchusnetwork.org.**
- **Students Against Destructive Decisions.** Founded 30 years ago in Wayland, Massachusetts in response to the impaired driving deaths of local teens, SADD's original mission was to help young people say "No" to drinking and driving. Today, its broader mission is to provide students with the best prevention tools to deal with issues of underage drinking, other drug use, impaired driving, and other destructive decisions.[80] SADD's approach engages young people in delivering education and prevention messages to their peers. Projects may include peer-led classes and theme-focused forums, workshops, conferences, and rallies, prevention education and leadership training, awareness-raising activities, and legislative work. To get involved, check out **www.sadd.org.**

A recent study from the NIAAA found that student participation is vital to the success of campus programs aimed at reducing high-risk drinking.[81] The study noted that student participation in prevention programs not only improved a school's policy, but also increased campuswide "ownership" of the efforts. In other words, if you're concerned about high-risk drinking on your campus, chances are, your campus is looking for you. Get active, and choose health not only for yourself, but for your friends and your world.

Watch videos of real students discussing their experiences with alcohol at www.pearsonhighered.com/lynchelmore.

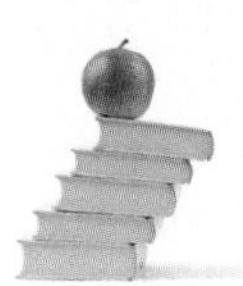

Choosing to Change Worksheet

To complete this worksheet online, visit www.pearsonhighered.com/lynchelmore.

You have acquired extensive information about drinking alcohol by reading this chapter. If you drink, you have had the opportunity to make observations about whether or not your drinking may be harmful or hazardous by completing the **Self-Assessment** on page 254. If you scored 8 or more points, your drinking habits may not be safe or healthy for yourself or others. Limit how much you drink or quit altogether. If you are one of the many college students who do not drink alcohol or drink only moderately and infrequently, then use this **Choosing to Change Worksheet** to interview a friend who struggles with his or her alcohol use.

Directions: Fill in your stage of change in Step 1 and complete Steps 2 or 3, depending on which one applies to your stage of change. Step 4 provides information for finding help with a drinking problem.

Step 1: Your Stage of Behavior Change. Check one of the following statements that best describes your drinking habits if you have more than 2 drinks (men) or more than 1 drink (women) on any single day or are at risk for alcohol related problems based on your self-assessment.

________ I do not intend to quit or cut back on my drinking in the next 6 months (Precontemplation)

________ I might quit or cut back on my drinking in the next 6 months (Contemplation)

________ I am prepared to quit or cut back on my drinking in the next month (Preparation)

________ I do not drink or have cut back on my drinking less than 6 months ago (Action)

________ I do not drink or have cut back on my drinking more than 6 months ago. (Maintenance)

Step 2: Precontemplation and Contemplation Stages. Reread the sections on the physical and behavioral effects of high-risk drinking on pages 245–251 and consider your own costs and benefits for quitting or cutting back on your drinking. Fill in the "Perceived Costs and Benefits" grid as it relates to your excessive drinking.

Perceived Cost of Continuing Excessive Drinking *How is my excessive drinking hurting me?*	Perceived Benefit of Continuing Excessive Drinking *What do I give up if I change?*
1.	1.
2.	2.
3.	3.
4.	4.
5.	5.
6.	6.
7.	7.

Perceived Benefit of Stopping or Modifying Excessive Drinking *How will this help me?*	Perceived Cost of Stopping or Modifying Excessive Drinking *How much will this change "cost" or hurt?*
1.	1.
2.	2.
3.	3.
4.	4.
5.	5.
6.	6.
7.	7.

Now, add up your totals: ______________ reasons to change ______________ reasons to stay the same

What one benefit do you think will motivate you the most? ____

What one "cost" or barrier do you think will present the biggest obstacle for you? ______________________________

Step 3: Preparation, Action, and Maintenance Stages. If you are ready to quit or cut back on your drinking, or have already started, complete the following.

A. Identify emotional or situational "triggers." What are your top five triggers? That is, what situations or emotions make you most want to drink? Common triggers include anxiety, boredom, peer pressure, and socializing with friends, especially to celebrate the end of a stressful week or semester.

____

____

____

____

____

B. Target one of the triggers and substitute an alternate healthier behavior instead of drinking. For example, if you know that you are more likely to drink at the end of a stressful day, instead decide to take a walk or go work out at the gym to reduce the stress from the day.

Target trigger: ____

Alternate healthy behavior response: ____

C. Reduce or remove the trigger in the first place. Temptations to drink can be eliminated by changing your environment to eliminate the trigger. For example: *Instead of going to BJ's Bar before the game, I'll meet everyone at the gate.*

Target trigger: ____

How you can reduce or remove it: ____

D. Other people can help or hinder your willingness to quit or cut back on your drinking. Identify at least one person who can support your efforts, and list one or more thing he or she can do to provide support.

Person: ____

Supportive actions: ____

E. Reward your progress. Permanently quitting or cutting back on your drinking takes patience and consistent reinforcement. List several rewards you could give yourself for meeting your goals:

Select a reward for quitting or cutting back on your drinking for 7 days: ______________________________

Select a reward for quitting or cutting back on your drinking for 1 month: ______________________________

Select a reward for quitting or cutting back on your drinking for 1 semester: ____________________________

Step 4: Finding Help. If you or a friend still have trouble cutting back or quitting drinking, see a health professional for help. A great place to start is on your campus. Most college campuses have a student health center or counseling center staffed with health professionals who can support you or your friend in cutting back or quitting drinking. In addition, you can find an alcohol abuse treatment program with the Substance Abuse Treatment Facility Locator at **http://findtreatment.samhsa.gov.** This searchable directory of drug and alcohol treatment programs shows the location of facilities around the country that treat alcoholism, alcohol abuse and drug abuse problems.

Chapter Summary

- Moderate drinking is the consumption of up to one drink per day for women and up to two drinks per day for men.
- High-risk drinking includes underage drinking, pre-drinking, binge drinking, and heavy drinking.
- Factors that increase the likelihood that a college student will engage in high-risk drinking include peer pressure, the campus environment, family exposure, and media and advertising.
- Alcohol is absorbed into the bloodstream from the stomach and small intestine. It is metabolized by the liver. If a person consumes alcohol at a faster rate than the liver can break it down, intoxication occurs.
- Blood alcohol concentration (BAC) is affected by numerous factors, including how much and how quickly alcohol is consumed, type of alcohol, sex, age, weight, physical condition, food intake, and medications.
- The short-term effects of high-risk drinking use include lightheadedness, loss of inhibition, compromised motor coordination, slowed reaction times, slurred speech, dulled senses, clouded judgment, dehydration, irritation of the stomach and intestines, disrupted sleep, hangover, memory loss, and drug interactions. Alcohol poisoning is a potentially fatal risk of binge drinking.
- Long-term effects of high-risk drinking include increased risk of cancer, cardiometabolic disease, weight gain, nutritional deficiencies, liver disease, and neurological problems. Also, with chronic alcohol consumption, the drinker often develops tolerance to at least some of alcohol's effects.
- Alcohol consumed during pregnancy will reach the developing fetus, in whom it can cause a wide range of mild to severe physical and mental birth defects.
- Behavioral effects of high-risk drinking include increased risk for injury, including motor vehicle fatalities, physical and sexual assault, suicide, impaired decision-making, and failing grades.
- Alcohol dependence is characterized by a tolerance to and craving for alcohol. Breaking the addiction can be challenging, but most people recover completely in time.
- Campus and community-based programs, clinical outpatient and residential treatment, psychotherapy, medications, and even reputable Internet resources can help people quit drinking and avoid relapse.
- To control your own drinking, set limits on your alcohol consumption, and take precautions before events where alcohol will be served, such as volunteering to be the designated driver or making a pact with a trusted friend to stay sober. To help a friend with an alcohol problem, talk to him or her. Confronting your friend now might save his or her academic career, health, or life.

Test Your Knowledge

Get Critical

What happened:

On July 23, 2011, the body of singer Amy Winehouse was found in her apartment. Winner of five Grammy awards, Winehouse had struggled with drug and alcohol abuse for years, but on June 1st had been released from rehab. Several people close to the singer knew that in the days before her death she had begun drinking again, but no one guessed how heavily. On October 26, the results of her autopsy were made public. The cause of death was alcohol poisoning. The level of alcohol in her blood was more than five times the legal limit for driving and much higher than the level known to be lethal.

Dr. Sam Zakhari, a spokesperson for the NIAAA, said what befell Winehouse is not unlike what happens on college campuses on weekends. "You hear it quite frequently here in the U.S. about college students who drink themselves to death."[1]

What do you think?

1. Winehouse's personal security guard, friends, and at least one physician were aware that she had begun drinking again, but did not take action to stop it. Are these witnesses at least partly to blame for her death?
2. If you had a friend recovering from alcohol abuse, and discovered that the friend had begun drinking again, what would you do?

Reference: 1. Kaufman, G. (2011, October 26). Amy Winehouse's Death: Alcohol Expert Weighs In. *MTV.* Retrieved from www.mtv.com/news/articles/1673223/amy-winehouse-death-alcohol.jhtml.

1. Blood alcohol concentration may be somewhat reduced by
   a. engaging in physical activity during drinking.
   b. consuming caffeine with the alcohol.
   c. consuming food with the alcohol.
   d. doing all of the above.

2. A standard drink is
   a. equivalent to 1.5 ounces of 80-proof liquor.
   b. equivalent to 5 ounces of table wine.
   c. equivalent to 12 ounces of beer.
   d. equivalent to any of the above.

3. *Binge drinking* is described as
   a. consuming about five or more drinks within 2 hours for men, or four or more drinks within 2 hours for women.
   b. consuming about five or more drinks a day for men, or four or more drinks a day for women.
   c. consuming seven or more drinks over the course of a week.
   d. drinking more than two shots of hard liquor on any one occasion.

4. Factors associated with an increased risk for alcohol dependence include
   a. female gender.
   b. poverty.
   c. Asian ethnicity.
   d. initiating drinking at age 21 or older.

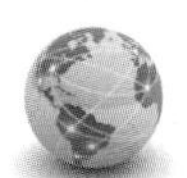

DIVERSITY & HEALTH

Tobacco Use Through the Lenses of Sex, Race/Ethnicity, Age, Education, and Geography

A recent national survey conducted by the Substance Abuse and Mental Health Services Administration revealed the following:

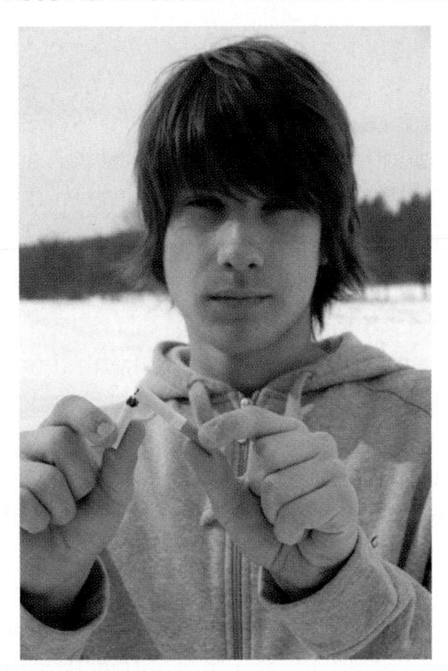

Smoking rates are highest among those aged 18 to 25.

Overall

- An estimated 27.4% of those aged 12 or older (about 69.6 million people) use a tobacco product: cigarettes, cigars, pipes, and/or smokeless tobacco.

Sex

- Men are more likely to use a tobacco product than women. Of males aged 12 or older, 33.7% use a tobacco product, compared with 21.5% of females.
- However, among those aged 12 to 17, there is not much difference in the rate of smoking in males (8.6%) versus females (8.1%).

Race/Ethnicity

- Among Native Americans, 35.8% report current tobacco use, the highest of any racial/ethnic group.
- Among people of mixed race background, 32.0% use tobacco.
- Among Caucasians, 29.5% use tobacco.
- Among African Americans, 27.3% use tobacco.
- Among Hispanics, 21.9% use tobacco.
- Among Asian Americans, 12.5% use tobacco.

Age

- People aged 18 to 25 report a higher rate of current tobacco use (40.8%) than any other age group.

Education

- Adults with college degrees are less likely to use tobacco than those with less education.

Geography

- Rates of smoking are higher in the South (24.1%) and Midwest (24.8%) than in the West (20.0%) and Northeast (22.2%).

Data from *Results from the 2010 National Survey on Drug Use and Health: National Findings*, by the Substance Abuse and Mental Health Services Administration, 2011, retrieved from http://oas.samhsa.gov/NSDUH/2k10NSDUH/2k10Results.htm.

wealth of a country's population; however, the very poorest nations (per capita income averaging $5,000 or less) do tend to have lower smoking rates.[3]

Smoking on Campus

Of all tobacco users, 41.4% are between the ages of 18 and 25.[7] About 30% of college students have tried smoking cigarettes at least once, though only 14.4% report smoking in the previous 30 days, and just 4.6% report smoking daily.[8] If you thought the rates of smoking on your campus were higher, you're not alone: The **Student Stats** box on the next page examines actual versus perceived use of cigarettes among college students.

Why Do Some Students Smoke?

It would be difficult to find a student who has *not* heard that smoking can kill you. Why, then, do some students smoke? There are as many different factors and reasons as there are individuals.

Genetics

Substantial evidence from a number of twin and adoption studies suggests that persistent smoking is significantly influenced by hereditary factors.[9] In addition, molecular studies suggest that genetic variations account for at least some of the susceptibility to become addicted to **nicotine,** the key psychoactive and addictive ingredient in tobacco.[10] Still, no specific genes have been reliably identified, and many researchers emphasize that persistent smoking and addiction to nicotine develop as a result of complex genetic–environmental interactions.[11]

nicotine A compound in the tobacco plant that is responsible for smoking's psychoactive and addictive effects.

Family and Peer Exposure

One environmental factor is family exposure. Research shows that if children have a parent who smokes, they are twice as likely to become smokers themselves by the time they finish high school.[12] Moreover, students whose friends smoke may begin smoking so that they can maintain acceptance from their peer group, or may begin smoking simply because they are more often in environments in which smoking is the norm. In one study, nonsmoking young adults who frequented bars, clubs, and similar establishments where smoking was unrestricted were at significantly higher risk for becoming smokers themselves.[13]

Age at Initiating Smoking

The younger people are when they start smoking, the more likely they are to become adult smokers. Research findings conclude that approximately 90% of adults who are regular smokers began at or before age 19.[14]

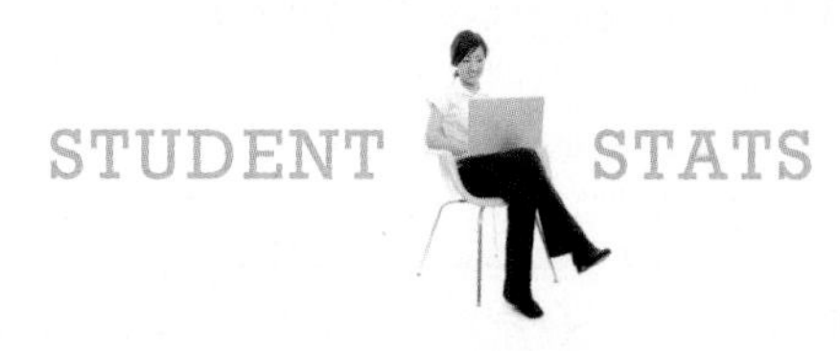

Smoking on Campus

Students often greatly overestimate how many of their peers regularly smoke cigarettes.

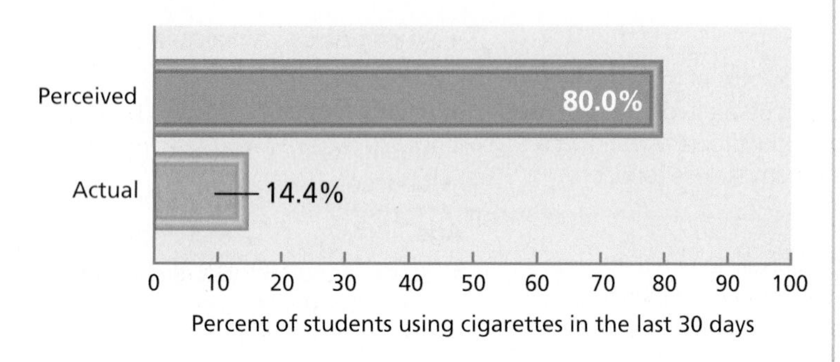

Data from *ACHA-NCHA II: Reference Group Executive Summary, Fall 2011*, by the American College Health Association, 2012.

Psychosocial Factors

Stress is certainly a factor in tobacco use. Schoolwork, family tensions, and complicated social relationships with classmates have all been cited as reasons why students smoke. In one study of adolescent girls, almost half of those who smoked said they started because they had a lot of stress in their lives.[15]

Young people experiencing interpersonal stress may rebel by experimenting with substances that their parents—and other authority figures in their lives—would not approve of. The fact that smoking is "bad" can actually make it more appealing to a teen wishing to challenge authority. In addition, some teens curious to experiment with a variety of recreational drugs may begin with smoking.

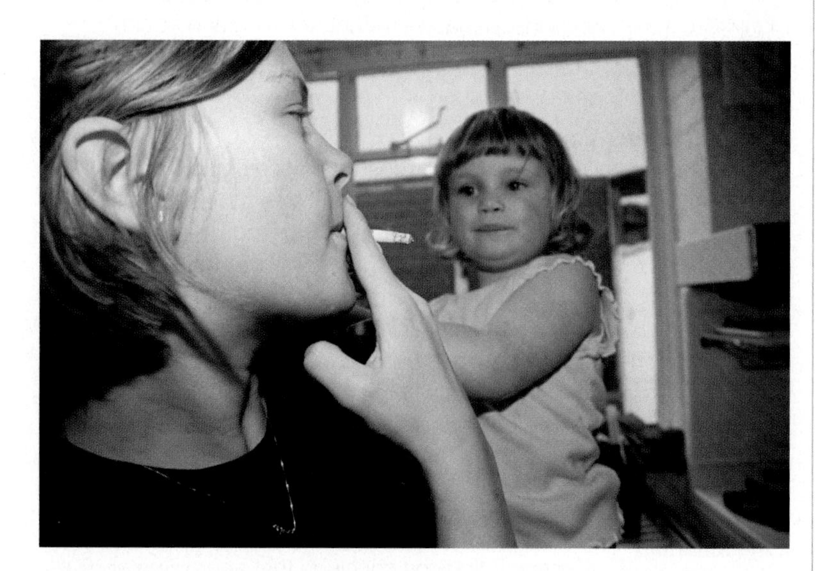

Parents can influence their children to smoke or not smoke.

Behind such experimentation, there's often a failure to appreciate the real risks of tobacco use. Young adults typically have poor decision-making and risk-judging skills, leading them to believe they're invulnerable to harm. In one study, adolescents who had the lowest appreciation for the long-term health risks of smoking were more than three times as likely to start smoking as adolescents with the highest appreciation of the risks.[16] In another study, Florida community college students who smoked rated the health risks of smoking to be less significant than did their nonsmoking peers. Moreover, the smokers viewed their personal risk as lower than the risk to other smokers![17]

Desire to Lose Weight

For decades, public health researchers have speculated that concerns about body weight were important factors in initiation of tobacco use among adolescents, particularly females. A recent study supports this theory. It found that, in general, females who perceived themselves to be overweight in grades 8 and 11 were more likely to be smokers as young adults.[18] Though it is true that nicotine can suppress appetite, taking up smoking to lose weight is one of the worst decisions anyone can make. The damage to health caused by smoking far outweighs any benefits in weight management.

Role of Media and Advertising

The major cigarette manufacturers spend more than $27.2 million every day to promote their products in the U.S., and many of their efforts directly reach young adults.[19] One study found that adolescents who owned a tobacco promotional item such as a T-shirt with a tobacco company logo and could name a brand whose advertisements attracted their attention were more than twice as likely to become established smokers as adolescents who did neither.[20] Overall, the total weight of evidence from multiple types of studies worldwide demonstrates not just an association, but a *causal* relationship, between tobacco promotion and increased tobacco use.[21]

The depiction of smoking is pervasive in films, occurring in three-quarters or more of contemporary box-office hits.[21] Perhaps no form of media is more powerful in influencing smoking initiation: A 2008 report from the National Cancer Institute reached "the government's strongest conclusion to date" that smoking in films encourages smoking in youth.[21]

View video clips about the effects of tobacco advertising and more at www.tobaccofree.org/clips.htm.

What Keeps Most Students from Smoking?

Research on what prevents young people from smoking is limited. However, a recent study in which over 700 students wrote down their reasons for not smoking revealed the following motivators:[22]

- **To avoid health problems.** Overwhelmingly, students chose this as their primary reason for not smoking, even though the majority could identify only the increased risk for cancer. As we'll discuss shortly, smoking also causes heart disease, reduced lung function, and other problems.
- **Aesthetic aversion.** More than 38% of students said they avoid smoking because—essentially—it disgusts them. Students mentioned bad breath, smelly clothes, stained teeth, and similar factors.
- **To avoid wasting money.** More than a fourth of students said they couldn't perceive any benefit to smoking—any reason why it would be worth the health risks, cosmetic effects, and cost.

The Makeup of Tobacco

Tobacco is a plant in the nightshade family, which also includes foods like tomatoes, potatoes, and eggplant, as well as poisonous plants like Jimson weed and belladonna (*deadly nightshade*). It is grown as a cash crop all over the world. After harvesting, the leaves are dried, then rolled, shredded, or otherwise processed into cigarettes, cigars, snuff, and other products.

carcinogenic Cancer causing.

tar A sticky, thick brown residue that forms when tobacco is burned and its chemical particles condense.

carbon monoxide A gas that inhibits the delivery of oxygen to the body's vital organs.

Learn more about the chemicals found in cigarette smoke at www.smokefreeunion.com/shs/documents/WhatsinTobaccoSmoke_000.pdf.

What's in a Cigarette?

Smoking cigarettes is by far the most common form of tobacco use. A typical cigarette in the United States contains 50% shredded tobacco leaf, 30% reconstituted tobacco (made from other parts of the tobacco plant), and 20% expanded tobacco (tobacco that has been "puffed up" like popcorn and functions as "filler."[23] It also contains nearly 600 additives with a wide range of functions. Cocoa, licorice, and vanilla, for example, are among the additives that help hide the harsh taste of tobacco. Meanwhile, ammonia—a chemical commonly used for household cleaning—boosts the delivery of nicotine into the lungs and bloodstream.

When a cigarette is lit and smoked, it releases approximately 7,000 different chemicals, at least 69 of which are **carcinogenic,** meaning they cause cancer. These carcinogens include **tar,** a thick, sticky residue that accumulates in the lungs when tobacco is burned and its chemical particles condense, and **carbon monoxide,** an odorless gas that impairs the delivery of oxygen to the brain, heart, and other organs. Other toxic chemicals in cigarette smoke are identified in **Figure 10.1**.

Until recently, many smokers believed that they would reduce their risk of cancer and other tobacco-related diseases by using a "light" or "mild" brand. They were mistaken. In the summer of 2010, the U.S. Food and Drug Administration (FDA) moved to prohibit the sale of cigarettes with such labels, asserting that they do not reduce smokers' risks for cancer and other diseases, and do not help smokers to quit. To find out more, see the **Consumer Corner** on the next page.

Flavored Cigarettes

Tobacco has a harsh taste, so it makes sense that one of the most popular additives in the history of cigarette manufacturing has been flavorings. Whether fruit, candy, or clove, flavorings make the smoking experience more pleasant, and so are thought to increase smoking prevalence, especially among young people. Yet these cigarettes are at least as dangerous as unflavored brands. For example, clove cigarettes, which have a distinctly sweet, pungent odor and an anesthetic effect in the throat, may deliver more nicotine, carbon monoxide, and tar than

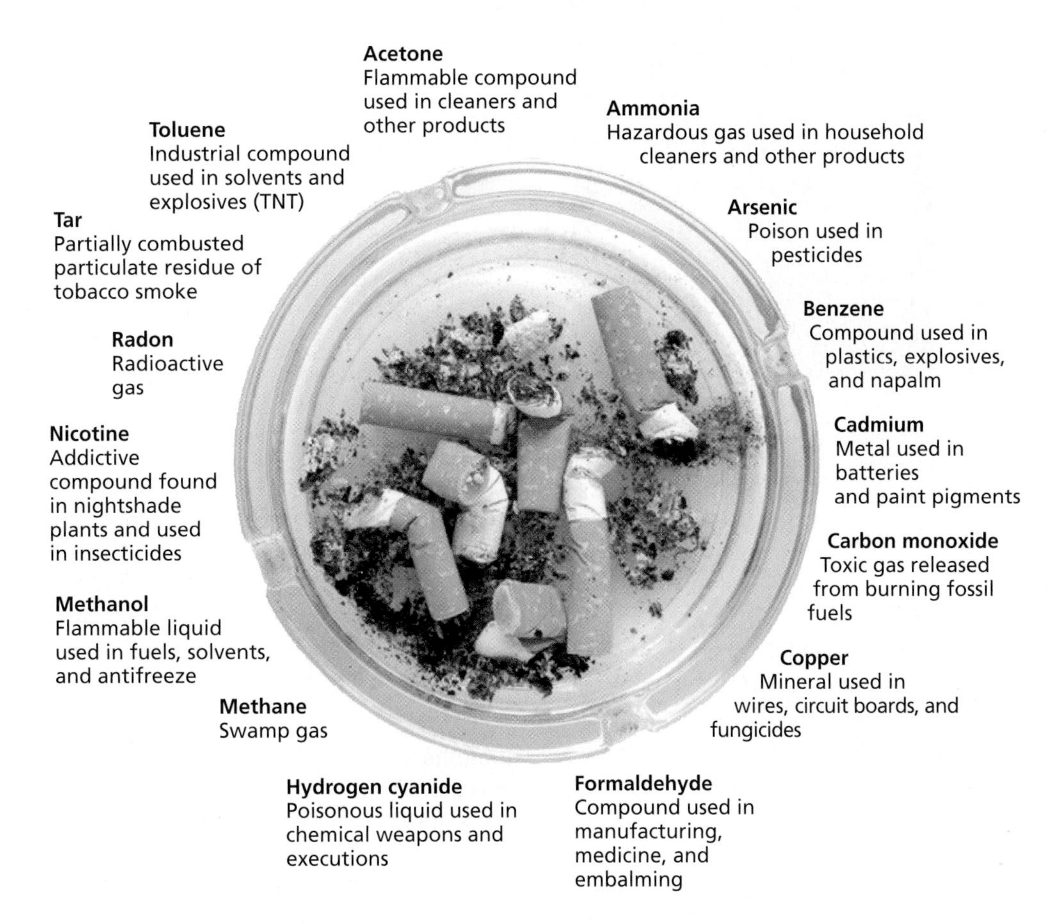

Acetone
Flammable compound used in cleaners and other products
Ammonia
Hazardous gas used in household cleaners and other products
Toluene
Industrial compound used in solvents and explosives (TNT)
Arsenic
Poison used in pesticides
Tar
Partially combusted particulate residue of tobacco smoke
Benzene
Compound used in plastics, explosives, and napalm
Radon
Radioactive gas
Cadmium
Metal used in batteries and paint pigments
Nicotine
Addictive compound found in nightshade plants and used in insecticides
Carbon monoxide
Toxic gas released from burning fossil fuels
Methanol
Flammable liquid used in fuels, solvents, and antifreeze
Copper
Mineral used in wires, circuit boards, and fungicides
Methane
Swamp gas
Hydrogen cyanide
Poisonous liquid used in chemical weapons and executions
Formaldehyde
Compound used in manufacturing, medicine, and embalming

Figure 10.1 **Care for some rat poison?** Arsenic is just one of the 4,000 toxic chemicals in cigarette smoke. Above are some others.

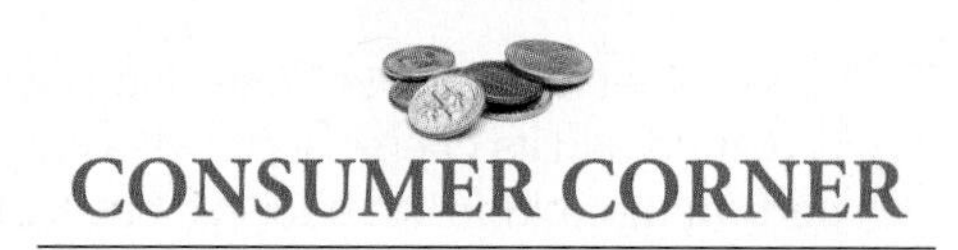

CONSUMER CORNER

"Light" Cigarettes Are No Safer to Use

You have probably seen advertisements for cigarettes that are "low-tar," "mild," "light," or "lite." Some even purport to be "ultra-light." Such messages imply that these cigarettes are less dangerous than regular brands, but this is simply not true.

Although it's true that some of these cigarettes deliver less tar or nicotine than regular cigarettes in machine-based tests, the U.S. Food and Drug Administration (FDA) states that there is no convincing evidence that they are less harmful to a person's health.[1] On the contrary, studies have shown that when smokers switch to low-tar cigarettes, they change the way they smoke, smoking more cigarettes, taking bigger puffs, and holding smoke in their lungs longer.[2]

- The U.S. Surgeon General has concluded that "smoking cigarettes with lower machine-measured yields of tar and nicotine provides no clear benefit to health."[3]
- The National Cancer Institute has determined that people who switch to light cigarettes are likely to inhale the same amount of hazardous chemicals as those smoking regular or "full-flavored" cigarettes. They also remain at high risk for developing smoking-related cancers and other diseases.[4]
- There is no evidence that switching to light cigarettes actually helps smokers kick their habit.

The bottom line: "Light" cigarettes are harmful to health. There is no such thing as a safe cigarette.

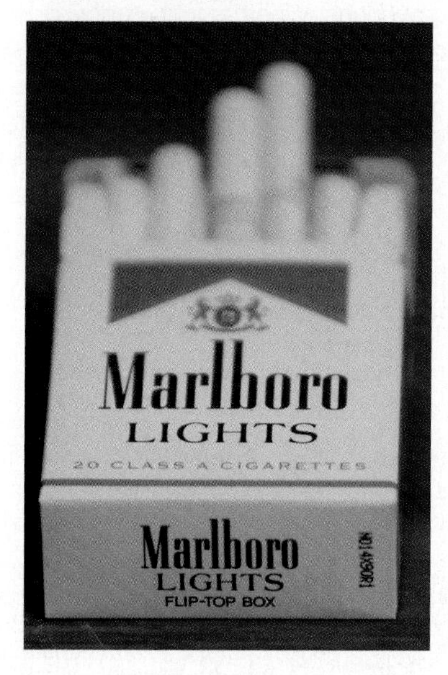

References: **1.** "Putting Out the Myth on Light, Low, and Mild Cigarettes," by the U.S. Food and Drug Administration (FDA), July 22, 2010, retrieved from www.fda.gov/TobaccoProducts/Labeling/MisleadingDescriptors/default.htm. **2.** "The Health Consequences of Smoking: The Changing Cigarette, a Report of the Surgeon General," by the U.S. Department of Health and Human Services, 1981. **3.** "The Health Consequences of Smoking: A Report of the Surgeon General," by the U.S. Department of Health and Human Services, 2004. **4.** "Risks Associated with Smoking Cigarettes with Low Machine-Measured Yields of Tar and Nicotine (Monograph 13)," by the National Cancer Institute, October 2001, retrieved from http://cancercontrol.cancer.gov/tcrb/monographs.

traditional cigarettes.[24] Clove cigarette smokers have higher rates of asthma and up to 20 times the risk for reduced lung function compared with nonsmokers.[25] For these reasons, in 2009, the FDA banned the addition of most types of flavorings from cigarettes produced in the United States.[26] It is not illegal to smoke flavored cigarettes, but it is illegal to sell them.

One flavoring that has escaped the ban—at least temporarily—is menthol. In 2010, the FDA announced that it would begin an investigation aimed at developing new regulations for menthol cigarettes, which account for almost a third of the total $70 billion cigarette market. Menthol, a minty flavoring, cools the sharpness of the tobacco taste and many smokers mistakenly believe it makes the cigarettes safer to smoke. Menthol has no effect—positive or negative—on the toxicity of cigarettes, but because it mellows the smoking experience, like other flavorings, it is thought to contribute to smoking initiation and persistence.[27]

Other Tobacco Products

Cigars, bidis, the loose tobacco used in pipes and hookahs, and smokeless "spit" tobacco are other commonly used tobacco products. Like cigarettes, they are associated with serious health problems.

Cigars

Cigars are rolled tobacco leaves, up to 7 inches in length, and can take up to 2 hours to smoke. Whereas cigarettes ("little cigars") contain less than 1 gram of tobacco, a premium cigar can contain up to 20 grams—as much tobacco as an entire pack of cigarettes.[28] Cigars contain many of the same addictive, toxic, cancer-causing substances that cigarettes do. The smoke from cigars also contains many of the toxins found in cigarette smoke, but in much higher concentrations.

The risk of cancers of the mouth and esophagus is similar in people who smoke cigars and those who smoke cigarettes. Because most cigar smokers do not inhale, their risk of developing lung cancer is lower than it is for cigarette smokers. However, cigar smokers still have higher rates of lung cancer, heart disease, and pulmonary disease than nonsmokers do.[29] In addition, a single cigar can provide as much nicotine as an entire pack of cigarettes, and addiction is common.[29]

Bidis

Whereas cigars are longer and thicker than traditional cigarettes, bidis (pronounced bee-deez) are shorter and thinner. Imported from India and other Southeast Asian countries, bidis are hand-rolled leaves from local trees packed with tobacco flakes and dust, sometimes tied at the ends by a colorful string. They are typically strongly flavored to mask the poor quality of the tobacco, with licorice, cinnamon, clove, chocolate, and fruit flavorings.

Contrary to a popular misconception, bidis are *not* safer than cigarettes. Bidi smoke contains three to five times more nicotine than is found in a regular cigarette.[25] Bidi smokers are at increased risk for several types of cancer, including oral, lung, stomach, and esophageal cancer, as well as heart disease and reduced lung function.[25]

Pipes

Pipes have a small bowl that the smoker fills with loose tobacco, tamps down, then lights. Typically, the smoke is drawn into the mouth and held for several seconds before the smoker exhales. Because pipe smokers don't typically inhale smoke into their lungs, their risk for lung cancer is lower than that of cigarette smokers. However, a 2004 study found pipe smokers' risk of lung cancer and other tobacco-related disease and death similar to or greater than that of people who smoke cigars.[30]

Hookahs

Hookahs originated in ancient Persia and India but are now popular around the globe. They are often referred to as "water pipes" because the device causes the tobacco smoke to pass through a bowl of water, thereby cooling it before it is drawn through a hose and mouthpiece to the user. Many hookah smokers mistakenly believe that this process purifies the smoke of harmful chemicals, but researchers say this is a myth: A typical hour-long session of hookah smoking involves inhaling

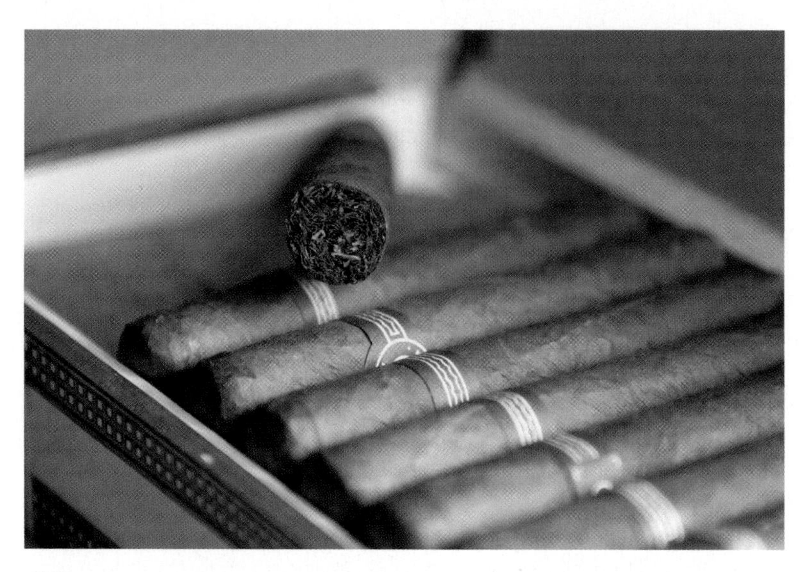

Cigars, clove cigarettes, bidis, and smokeless tobacco all increase the risk of cancer and cardiovascular disease.

100–200 times the volume of smoke inhaled from a single cigarette, but the device filters out only 5% of the nicotine. Smokers may also absorb higher concentrations of the tar, heavy metals, and other toxic chemicals found in cigarette smoke.[31] Thus, hookah smokers are at risk for the same kinds of diseases caused by cigarette smoking, including a variety of cancers, heart disease, and reduced lung function.[31]

In addition, hookah smoking confers two unique risks: First, the devices are typically used by many smokers in a single session, and passing the mouthpiece from one person to another promotes the transmission of communicable infectious diseases, including herpes and tuberculosis. Second, the tobacco is heated with charcoal, a practice that dangerously increases the level of carbon monoxide in the air. This risk is significant even for those not smoking themselves. A 2010 study found that the amount of carbon monoxide in the smoke released during one hookah session was comparable to the amount released from smoking 30 cigarettes.[32] In a 2011 study, people exiting a hookah "café" had more than three times the level of carbon monoxide in their blood as people exiting traditional bars.[33] Carbon monoxide is a known carcinogen, and is also associated with heart disease, headaches, confusion, memory loss, and cognitive problems. It is also extremely toxic to a developing fetus.

"In a 2011 study, people exiting a hookah "café" had more than three times the level of carbon monoxide in their blood as people exiting traditional bars."

Smokeless ("Spit") Tobacco

Baseball fans are used to seeing their heroes use smokeless tobacco, also known as "spit" or "chew." Indeed, one in three major league baseball players uses smokeless tobacco.[34] Viewers watching one game of the 2004 World Series were exposed to a full 9 minutes and 11 seconds of players' perceptible use of smokeless tobacco.[35] No wonder, then, that many young fans have adopted the habit of their role models, using smokeless tobacco at alarming rates. About 1 in every 10 male college students is a current user of smokeless tobacco, compared with just 1 in every 250 female college students.[36] Use is especially common among intercollegiate athletes, and among students enrolled in colleges in rural areas or small towns.[36]

Smokeless tobacco comes in two forms. *Snuff* is a fine-grained tobacco that is often sold in teabag-like pouches that users "pinch" or "dip" between their lower lip and gum. *Chewing tobacco* comes in wads of shredded or "bricked" tobacco leaves that people put between their cheek and gum. No matter the type, smokeless tobacco is meant to stew in the mouth for several minutes to an hour at a time. Users suck on the tobacco juices and then spit to get rid of the saliva that builds up, hence the nickname "spit."

Both chewing tobacco and snuff are typically laden with sweeteners and flavorings to make them taste more pleasant. Although they don't emit harmful plumes of smoke, both forms are loaded with nicotine. It is absorbed into the bloodstream through the mucous membranes that line the mouth, and users can quickly become addicted. The average dose of smokeless tobacco, in fact, contains up to four times the amount of nicotine found in the average cigarette. One can of snuff is

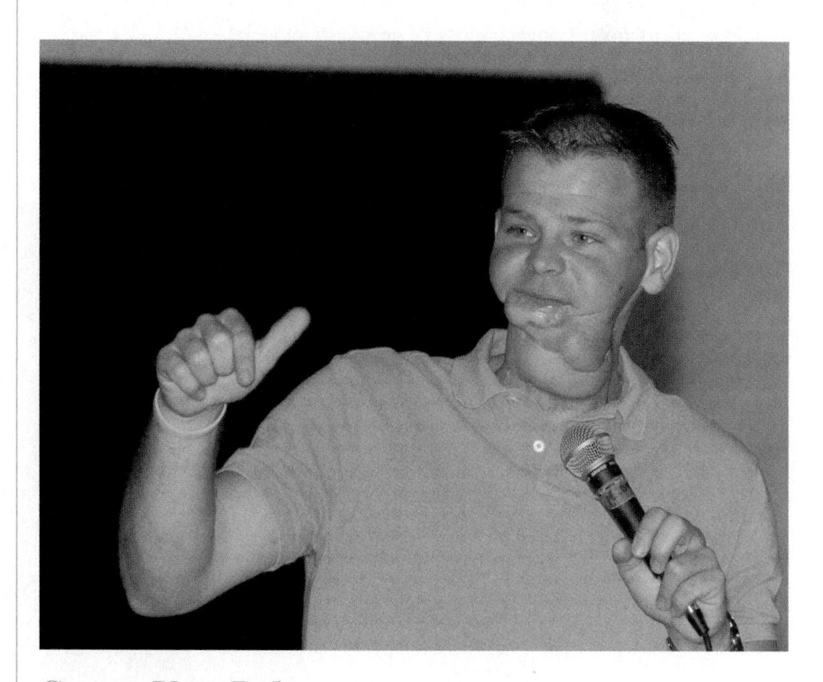

Gruen Von Behrens was hooked on chewing tobacco at age 14, and diagnosed with oral cancer at age 17. He has lost his jaw, lower teeth, and part of his tongue in his fight to beat the disease.

equivalent, nicotine-wise, to about four packs of cigarettes.

The health effects of using smokeless tobacco are varied. Regular use increases a person's risk for cancers of the lip, tongue, cheeks, gums, and mouth. The products stain and wear down the teeth, cause gums to recede, and can cause a condition called **leukoplakia,** characterized by whitish lesions in the mouth. These lesions may become cancerous, and are frequently found in snuff and chew users in their 20s.

leukoplakia White spots on the mucous membranes in the mouth that may become cancerous.

dopamine A neurotransmitter that stimulates feelings of pleasure.

Check out this article on the history of baseball and chewing tobacco from *Slate* magazine: www.slate.com/id/2234341.

Effects of Smoking on the Smoker

One-half of all long-term smokers, particularly those who began smoking in adolescence, will eventually die from their use of tobacco. Furthermore, one-half of the deaths caused by smoking will occur in middle age (35 through 69 years), resulting in the loss of 20 to 25 years of normal life expectancy.[37] That's because smoking irritates and inflames body tissues, damages nearly every organ of the body, including blood vessels, and weakens the immune system.

Short-Term Effects of Smoking

From the moment a person takes the first puff of a cigarette, physiological changes take place in the body. Within 8 seconds of entering the body, nicotine is absorbed by the lungs and quickly moved into the bloodstream, which circulates it throughout the brain. There, it triggers the release of **dopamine,** a neurotransmitter that stimulates feelings of pleasure. The effect is short-lived, however, and smokers quickly crave more nicotine. We'll explore nicotine addiction later in this chapter.

Other short-term health effects of smoking include:

- **Increased heart rate and blood pressure.** Nicotine causes the heart to beat faster. It also raises blood pressure.
- **Shortness of breath and reduction in stamina.** The carbon monoxide in cigarette smoke binds to a protein in red blood cells, disrupting these cells' ability to effectively deliver oxygen to the rest of the body.
- **Coughing.** Cigarette smoke irritates the respiratory passageways, prompting inflammation and increasing the production of mucus. It also damages the microscopic hair cells—called *cilia*—that normally sweep mucus upward. This means that mucus is more likely to pool in the lungs, triggering the need to cough and increasing the risk for infection.
- **Heightened alertness.** Smoking induces the release of the hormone adrenaline, which increases heart rate, pulse, and feelings of alertness.
- **Decreased skin temperature.** Nicotine constricts blood vessels, resulting in less blood flow to the skin (reducing its temperature) and to the legs and feet. Recall that, because of carbon monoxide, the circulating blood cells are also carrying less oxygen.
- **Increased blood glucose.** Smoking triggers the liver to convert stored glycogen to glucose. This results in an increase in the level of glucose circulating in the blood. In one study, smokers had an average 20% higher blood glucose level than nonsmokers.[38]
- **Dulled sense of smell and taste.** Studies over many years have shown that smoking reduces a smoker's ability to smell and taste. A recent study comparing young smokers and nonsmokers not only confirmed that smoking decreases taste sensitivity, but suggested a mechanism: fewer and flatter taste buds were found in 79% of the smokers.[39]

Smoking also results in a number of short-term cosmetic problems, from bad breath to smelly hair, clothes, furniture, car, and other belongings.

Figure 10.2 summarizes the short- and long-term effects of smoking.

Short-term effects:
- Increased heart rate
- Increased blood pressure
- Shortness of breath
- Reduction in stamina
- Coughing
- Heightened alertness
- Decreased skin temperature
- Increased blood glucose
- Dulled sense of smell and taste
- Bad breath
- Smelling like smoke
- Health risks to developing fetus

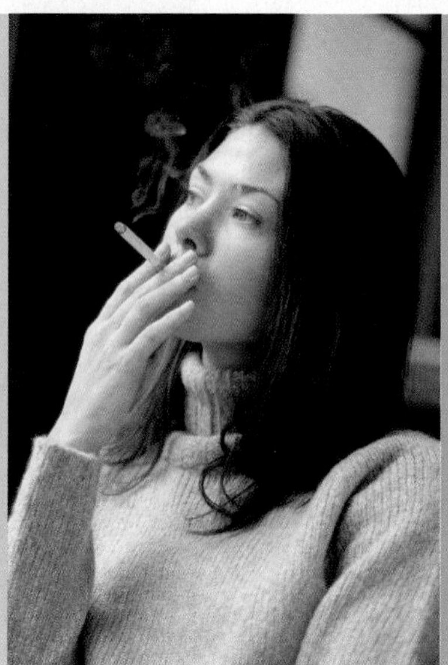

Long-term effects:
- Greatly increased risk of cancer
- Greatly increased risk of cardiovascular disease
- Reduced lung function
- Periodontal disease
- Increased risk of gastroesophageal reflux
- Increased risk of peptic ulcers
- Reduced liver function
- Increased risk of Crohn's disease
- Increased risk of type 2 diabetes
- Erectile dysfunction
- Decreased fertility
- Loss of bone density
- Vision impairment
- Premature aging and wrinkling of skin
- Stained teeth
- Nicotine addiction

Figure 10.2 **Short- and long-term health effects of smoking.**

Long-Term Effects of Smoking

The U.S. Centers for Disease Control and Prevention (CDC) calls tobacco use "the nation's leading killer."[40] Let's look at the reasons.

Cancer

Although you've probably heard claims that the link between smoking and lung cancer is a myth, smoking has long been established as the primary cause of lung cancer throughout the world.[41] In 2012, there were estimated to be over 226,000 new cases of lung cancer in the United States, and over 160,000 lung cancer deaths.[42] That high mortality rate is typical: Lung cancer is the leading cause of cancer death **(Figure 10.3).** Despite this fact, some smokers try to justify their habit by pointing to an elderly acquaintance who, they say, "has smoked a pack a day his whole life!" But statistics tell another story: Male smokers are more than 23 times more likely than male nonsmokers to develop lung cancer, and women who smoke are 13 times more likely to develop the disease.[43] Moreover, smoking is responsible for 85% of all lung cancer deaths.[37]

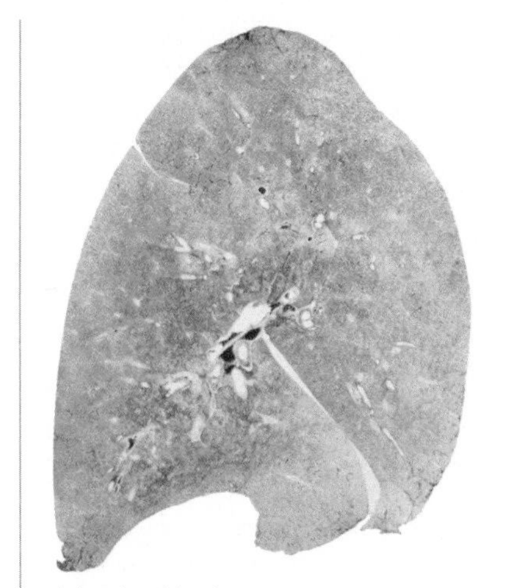

(a) A healthy lung

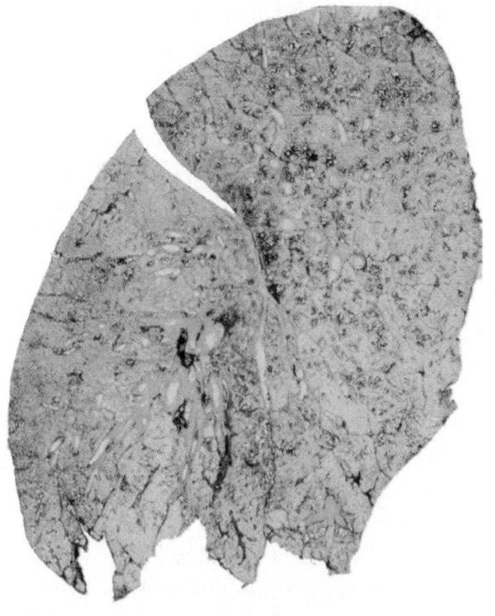

(b) A smoker's lung permeated with deposits of tar

Figure 10.3 Effects of smoking on the lungs. (a) The lungs of a 50-year-old nonsmoker. (b) The lungs of a 50-year-old smoker with lung cancer.

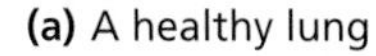

MYTH OR FACT?

Is Social Smoking Really All That Bad?

Although precise statistics are hard to come by, experts guess that about one out of every five smokers doesn't smoke every day.

If you're one of these so-called "social smokers," you probably believe that your behavior is unlikely to cause any harm. Are you right? Here's what the research says about social smoking.

- **Social smokers smoke more than they think.** Although gathering precise data is challenging, researchers find that most self-described social smokers actually smoke a few cigarettes per day. One nicotine addiction specialist notes that people who smoke just one or two cigarettes a week—true social smokers—are very rare indeed.[1]
- **Social smoking leads to addiction.** Tobacco researchers point out that the majority of social smokers are on the road to addiction. Initially they may only bum a cigarette from friends occasionally, but soon they find themselves bumming cigarettes more often. It's only a matter of time before they find themselves buying a pack a week, then two or three packs a week. Although they believe that they can quit whenever they want, on average, social smokers end up addicted, and smoking for years.[1] One-third of people who have ever tried smoking become daily smokers.[2]
- **Social smoking increases risk of cardiovascular disease.** Studies have shown an increased risk of cardiovascular disease at all levels of smoking. Moreover, smoking begins to exert this effect—causing fatal heart attacks and strokes—as early as age 35. The risk is especially acute for women who also use a hormonal method of birth control (pills, patch, etc.). One mechanism by which smoking, even at low levels, promotes heart disease is by causing inflammation and dysfunction of the lining of blood vessels.[2] In one study, young, healthy people who smoked less than one pack per week were found to have a 35% reduction in blood vessel functioning compared with nonsmokers.[3]
- **Social smoking increases cancer risk.** Tobacco smoke itself is a carcinogen, as are at least 69 of its component chemicals. Because inherited genetic variations influence cancer rates, as do other determinants such as diet, stress, etc., the influence of social smoking on cancer promotion is difficult to determine. However, any level of smoking increases the frequency of DNA mutations known to be associated with cancer. And the risk of cancer is more closely tied to the number of years you've smoked—at any level—than to the number of cigarettes smoked per day. As one expert put it, you wouldn't go out to your car four times a week and inhale exhaust fumes. But that's the health equivalent of smoking cigarettes four times a week.[1]

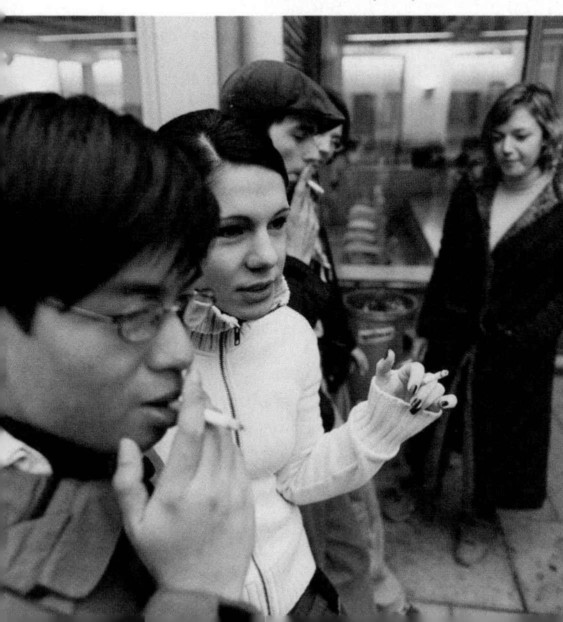

The bottom line? There is no safe level of exposure to cigarette smoke.[2] If you smoke at all, you are at increased risk of nicotine addiction, cardiovascular disease, cancer, and other illnesses. Get help, and quit.

References: **1.** "Can You Get Away With Social Smoking?" by D. DeNoon, 2003, *WebMD*, retrieved from http://www.webmd.com/smoking-cessation/features/can-you-get-away-with-social-smoking. **2.** "How Tobacco Smoke Causes Disease: The Biology and Behavioral Basis for Smoking-Attributable Disease: A Report of the Surgeon General," by the U.S. Department of Health and Human Services, 2010, retrieved from www.surgeongeneral.gov/library/tobaccosmoke/report/index.html. **3.** "Occasional Cigarette Smoking Chronically Affects Arterial Function," by L. Stoner, M. J. Sabatier, C. D. Black, & K. K. McCully, December 2008, *Ultrasound Med Biol, 34*, pp. 1885–1892.

But lung cancer is not the only form of cancer associated with smoking. Smoking is also associated with cancers of the mouth, throat, larynx, esophagus, stomach, pancreas, colon, kidney, bladder, cervix, and blood. A smoker's risk of developing these cancers increases with the number of cigarettes and the number of years of smoking. The risk, however, does begin to drop over time in those who are able to quit for good.

Cardiovascular Disease

Many people can readily identify cancer as a major health risk of smoking, but have little awareness that smoking is also a key risk factor for three types of cardiovascular disease:

- **Coronary heart disease.** The leading cause of death in the United States, coronary heart disease often stems from the development of *atherosclerosis*, a condition in which deposits form on the lining of the arteries supplying blood to the heart (the coronary arteries). Smoking also narrows arteries and damages their lining in a way that accelerates the accumulation of these deposits. Moreover, smoking increases the likelihood that a *thrombus*—a blood clot—will form. This can block an already narrowed coronary artery. At the same time, the carbon monoxide in tobacco smoke reduces the delivery of oxygen to the heart muscle. All of these factors greatly increase a smoker's risk for a heart attack and sudden death.[37]
- **Stroke.** A stroke occurs when a blood vessel carrying oxygen and nutrients to the brain either bursts or is blocked by a clot. When that happens, part of the brain cannot get the blood and oxygen it needs and starts to die. This can cause speech problems, vision problems, memory loss, and paralysis on one side of the body. It can also be fatal. Cigarette smoking doubles a person's odds of having a stroke. The risk, however, steadily decreases after quitting smoking, with former smokers having roughly the same stroke risk as nonsmokers about four years after quitting.[37]
- **Abdominal aortic aneurysm.** The aorta is the largest artery in the body. It exits directly from the heart and travels into the abdomen before it begins to branch into the many smaller arteries that bring blood to the rest of the body. An abdominal aortic aneurysm is a dangerously weakened and bulging area in the aorta. If the area ruptures, it can cause life-threatening internal bleeding. Smoking is clearly associated with the condition. Several studies show that the risk of death from abdominal aortic aneurysm is significantly higher in smokers.[37]

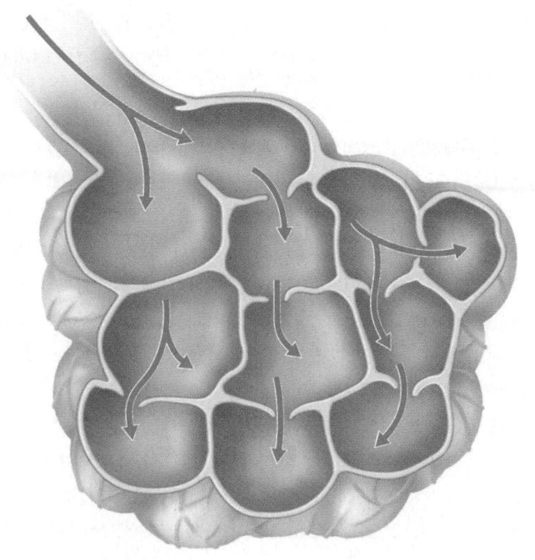

(a) Healthy alveoli

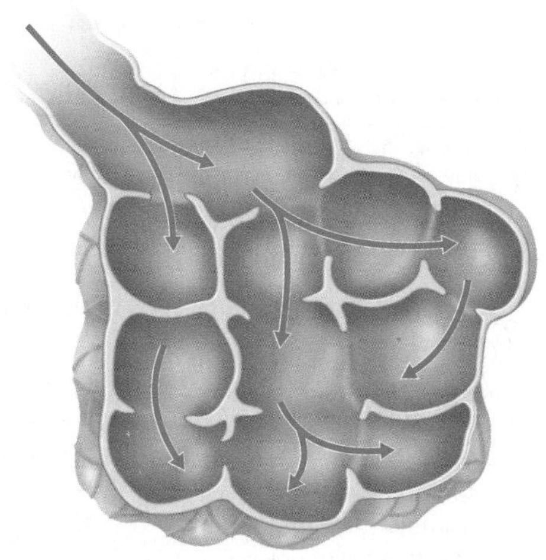

(b) Damaged alveoli due to emphysema

Figure 10.4 **Emphysema.** (a) Normal alveoli are small, so it is easy for air to contact the alveoli walls, and for gas exchange to occur. (b) In emphysema, destruction of alveoli walls creates larger air spaces with less potential for gas exchange.

Reduced Lung Function

We noted earlier that smoking damages the upper respiratory passageways, leading to a characteristic "smoker's cough." Over time, smoking also destroys the microscopic air sacs—called *alveoli*—of the lungs, resulting in reduced lung function. In many smokers, lung function deteriorates to the point of **chronic obstructive pulmonary disease (COPD),** a term that includes emphysema, chronic bronchitis, and chronic asthmatic bronchitis.

When you inhale, air from the environment enters the alveoli in your lung tissues. There, tiny blood vessels in the alveoli walls absorb oxygen from the air, and unload carbon dioxide—a normal waste product—which you then breathe out. Smoking causes an inflammatory reaction in the alveoli that causes their walls to dissolve. In *emphysema*, the walls of many alveoli are destroyed. As a result, adjacent alveoli merge to form larger sacs that do not have the capacity to take in as much oxygen or unload as much carbon dioxide **(Figure 10.4)**. As the condition progresses, it becomes more and more difficult for the lungs to exchange oxygen for carbon dioxide. As a result, oxygen-depleted air stagnates in the lungs, and the patient feels "short of breath." Emphysema sufferers often have trouble performing simple physical activities such as shopping or climbing stairs. As the disease progresses, many emphysema patients must rely on an oxygen tank to help them breathe. The final weeks of life can be agonizing. Some have described the experience as feeling like drowning, only worse, because it takes so long to die.[44]

chronic obstructive pulmonary disease (COPD) A group of diseases characterized by a reduced flow of air into and out of the lungs. COPD includes emphysema, chronic bronchitis, and chronic asthmatic bronchitis.

Recall that smoking also irritates the respiratory passageways (the *bronchi*), causing inflammation and increasing the production of mucus. When this condition persists for at least three months, the patient is said to have *chronic bronchitis*. Symptoms include a chronic cough that produces mucus, shortness of breath, and frequent respiratory infections. Some patients with chronic bronchitis experience episodes of wheezing referred to as *chronic asthmatic bronchitis*. Because essentially all patients with chronic bronchitis or chronic asthmatic bronchitis also have emphysema, the preferred term for all three conditions is now chronic obstructive pulmonary disease.

In 2012, COPD was the third leading cause of death in the United States.[45] Smoking is considered the "primary causative factor" in 80% of COPD deaths.[1] Moreover, the reduced lung function caused by smoking means that respiratory infections, such as colds, influenza, and pneumonia, are more likely to be serious, even fatal, in smokers.

Oral and Gastrointestinal Problems

Smoking and other forms of tobacco use are harmful to the health of your mouth and your gastrointestinal (GI) tract. We've already noted the link between tobacco use and cancers of the mouth, throat, esophagus, stomach, pancreas, and colon. But that's only the beginning.

Many studies suggest that tobacco use may be one of the most significant factors in **periodontal disease.**[46] The word *periodontal* means "around the tooth," and periodontal disease can degrade both the gums and the bone of the lower jaw supporting the teeth **(Figure 10.5)**. It begins when the bacteria in *plaque*, the sticky film that forms on teeth, produce toxins that cause the gum tissue to become inflamed and pull away from teeth. Eventually, gum and bone tissue breaks down, deep pockets—filled with bacteria—form around the teeth, and the teeth loosen. Smokers are much more likely than nonsmokers to have excessive plaque formation, deep pockets between the teeth and gums, and tooth loss. In fact, whereas only 20% of nonsmokers over age 65 have lost teeth, over 40% of smokers over age 65 are toothless.[46]

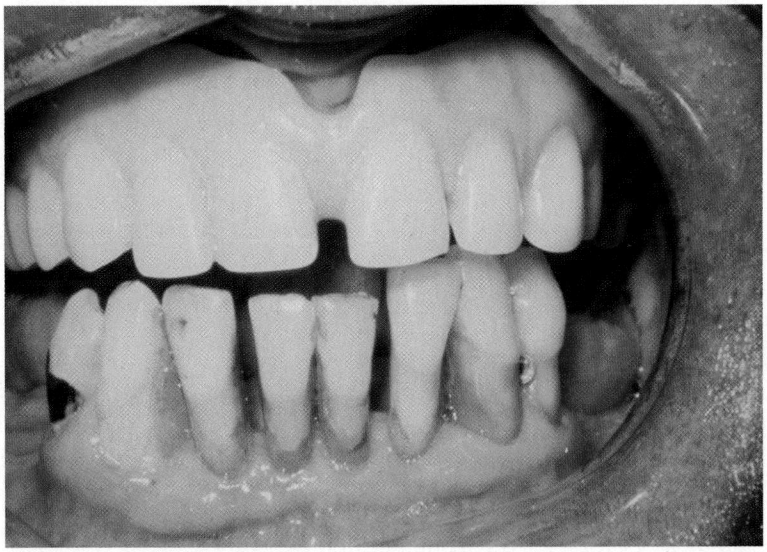

Figure 10.5 Periodontal disease. In advanced periodontal disease, both gums and supporting bone erode, and tooth loss is likely.

periodontal disease Excessive plaque deposition, infection, and inflammation involving the gums and supporting bone, leading to degradation of gum and bone tissue and potentially tooth loss.

gastroesophageal reflux (GER) Condition in which stomach acid leaks back into the lower portion of the esophagus, causing irritation and burning.

peptic ulcer Deep, solitary erosion in the lining of the stomach or the first part of the small intestine.

Crohn's disease Painful intestinal disorder characterized by inflammation and ulceration of one or more regions of the intestinal wall.

Smokers have an increased risk for **gastroesophageal reflux (GER),** commonly known as *heartburn*.[47] Normally a muscular sphincter between the end of the esophagus and the beginning of the stomach (*gastro-* refers to the stomach) keeps the two organs entirely separate except when food is moving from the esophagus into the stomach. The sensation of heartburn occurs when this gastroesophageal sphincter weakens, allowing stomach acid to seep back up into the lower esophagus. When it does, this acidic reflux burns the sensitive esophageal tissues. Over time, the irritation and inflammation of GER can lead to esophageal cancer. The nicotine in tobacco weakens smooth muscle, including that of the gastroesophageal sphincter, and tobacco use is an established risk factor for GER.[47]

Research has also shown that smoking increases the risk of developing a **peptic ulcer,** an erosion in the lining of the stomach or the first portion of the small intestine. Ulcers can cause aggressive abdominal pain. How does smoking promote the formation of ulcers? Some studies suggest that smoking increases the risk of infection with the bacterium responsible for most ulcers. Other studies propose that smoking causes the stomach to produce too much acid, or that smoking reduces the pancreas's production of bicarbonate, a base that neutralizes stomach acid. Whatever the mechanism, smokers are more likely to develop an ulcer, and even with treatment, if they continue smoking, their ulcer is less likely to heal.[47]

The liver is responsible for hundreds of body functions, from packaging nutrients to manufacturing bile for the breakdown of fats to clearing the body of toxins. Smoking deposits into the bloodstream many toxic chemicals that directly damage liver cells, reducing the organ's ability to process alcohol, medications, and other toxic substances.[47] It also contributes to iron overload, which further stresses the liver. Throughout the body, smoking impairs immune functioning. This increases the liver's vulnerability to infection as well as cancer, because certain immune cells are responsible for surveying and destroying tumor cells.

Crohn's disease is characterized by inflammation of the lining of the GI tract, usually the small intestine. It causes pain and diarrhea. Both current and former smokers have an increased risk for Crohn's disease and are more likely to experience relapses. The reason behind this link is not clear, but researchers propose that smoking might decrease blood flow to the intestines, lower intestinal defenses, or prompt an immune system response that results in inflammation.[47]

Type 2 Diabetes

For many years, observational studies have suggested an association between smoking and an increased prevalence of type 2 diabetes, a disorder of glucose regulation. As noted earlier, smoking increases blood glucose. It also decreases the body's ability to use insulin, a hormone essential for glucose control. In 2007, a systematic review of more than 40 years of research concluded that smoking is significantly associated with an increased risk of type 2 diabetes.[48] (For more information about diabetes, see Chapter 11.)

smoking

THE ULTIMATE IN SEX APPEAL?

Tobacco companies, the media, or even your friends might tell you that smoking is sexy, but look at the evidence and decide for yourself. Smoking leads to premature aging, bad breath, hacking coughs, and erectile dysfunction. Is that attractive to you?

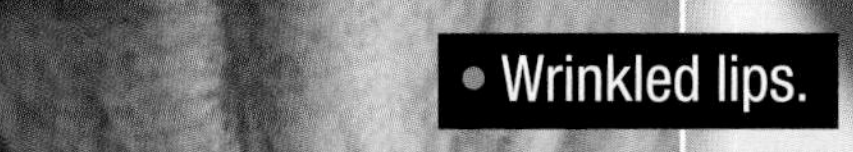

• Wrinkled lips.

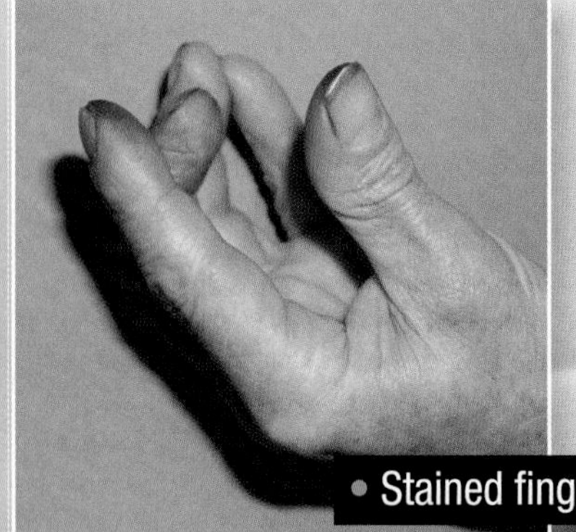

• Stained fingers.

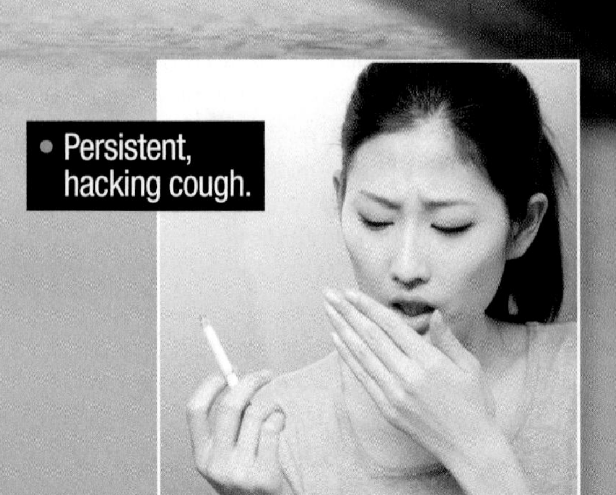

• Persistent, hacking cough.

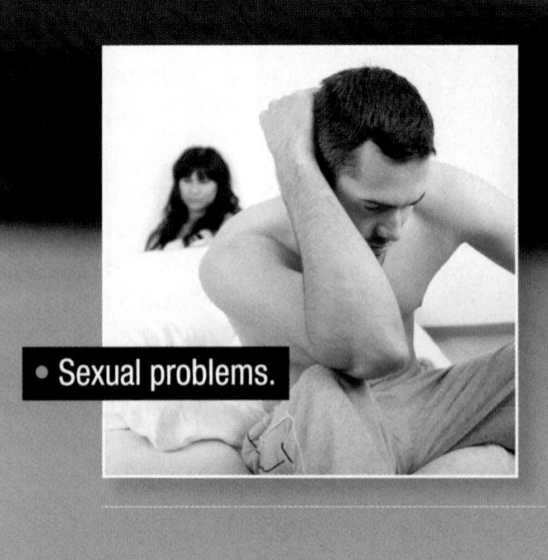

• Sexual problems.

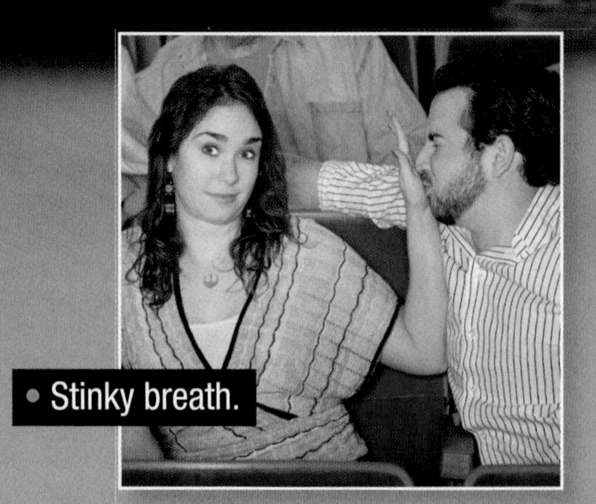

• Stinky breath.

Reproductive Health Effects

Smoking can affect your love life and your ability to become a parent.

Erectile dysfunction in men. A growing body of research literature supports an association between smoking and erectile dysfunction (ED) in men.[49, 50] Although the reasons are not entirely clear, both current and past smokers have been shown to experience higher rates of ED than men who have never smoked. Moreover, the greater the number of cigarettes smoked per day, the greater the likelihood of experiencing ED.[50]

Decreased fertility in both men and women. Smoking has a negative impact both on the ability to become pregnant and the ability to carry a pregnancy to term. Men show a lower sperm count, reduced sperm motility, and increased abnormalities in sperm shape and function. In women, smoking appears to damage the ovaries, accelerate the loss of eggs, reduce reproductive functioning, and accelerate menopause by several years. Toxins in cigarette smoke also increase the likelihood that a woman's eggs will have a genetic abnormality, and that the woman will experience a miscarriage.[51]

Other Health Effects

Many studies have demonstrated a loss of bone density in older men and women who smoke. The longer a person smokes and the more cigarettes smoked per day, the greater the risk of fracture in old age.[52]

Smoking also appears to increase the risk of vision impairment as we age. Two age-related vision disorders—macular degeneration (a loss of central vision) and cataracts (cloudy vision)—are increased among smokers.[53, 54]

Moreover, smoking causes premature aging and wrinkling of the skin, stained teeth, and other cosmetic effects. Still, films, music videos, and other media often portray smoking as sexy. Not sure whether you might agree? Check out page 276.

Effects of Smoking on Others: Health Risks and Costs

Whether or not you smoke, you suffer health and financial consequences from other people's smoking.

Health Risks of Secondhand Smoke

Secondhand smoke is a mixture of **sidestream smoke**—the smoke emanating from the burning end of a cigarette or pipe—and **mainstream smoke,** which is exhaled from the lungs of smokers. Also called *environmental tobacco smoke (ETS),* it contains more than 250 chemicals known to be toxic or capable of causing cancer, including arsenic, ammonia, formaldehyde, and benzene.[55] These chemicals can linger in the air for hours after a cigarette has been extinguished.

Notice that sidestream smoke is not filtered through a cigarette filter or a smoker's lungs. As a result, it actually has higher concentrations of some harmful chemicals than the smoke inhaled by the smoker! For instance, sidestream smoke has at least twice the amount of nicotine and tar as mainstream smoke. It also has five times the amount of carbon monoxide, and higher levels of ammonia and cadmium.

secondhand smoke (environmental tobacco smoke) The smoke nonsmokers are exposed to when someone has been smoking nearby; a combination of sidestream smoke and mainstream smoke.

sidestream smoke Smoke emanating from the burning end of a cigarette or pipe.

mainstream smoke Smoke exhaled from the lungs of smokers.

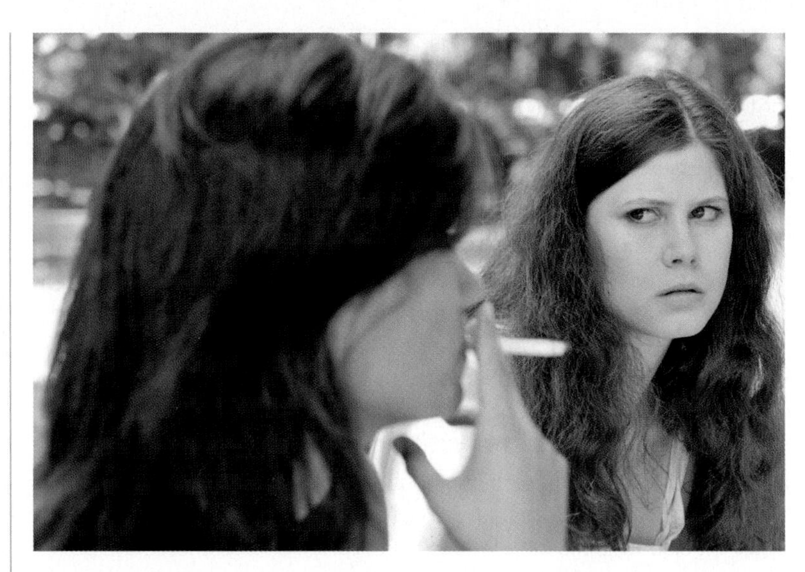

Besides being annoying, secondhand smoke is **dangerous.**

Millions of people in the United States are essentially *passive smokers:* people who breathe in secondhand smoke from their environment. In national surveys, 43% of passive smokers have been found to have detectable levels of *cotinine*—the major breakdown product of nicotine—in their blood.[55]

A 2006 *Report of the Surgeon General* spanning more than 700 pages concluded, "The health effects of secondhand smoke exposure are more pervasive than we previously thought. The scientific evidence is now indisputable: secondhand smoke is not a mere annoyance. It is a serious health hazard that can lead to disease and premature death in children and nonsmoking adults."[55] Let's take a closer look at a few of the most severe health effects of exposure to secondhand smoke.

Health Risks to a Developing Fetus

Smoking while pregnant is like gambling—with the baby's life and health. When a pregnant woman smokes, the nicotine, carbon monoxide, benzene, and other toxic chemicals that enter her bloodstream are passed on to her fetus. This may increase the baby's risk for birth defects such as cleft lip and cleft palate, as well as lifelong health problems such as cerebral palsy, developmental delay, and learning disorders.[56] The Surgeon General also found evidence that was "suggestive but not sufficient" that prenatal smoking increases the risk for childhood cancers.[55]

Nicotine also reduces the amount of oxygen that reaches the fetus, impairing its growth. Babies born to women who smoke are more likely to be born too early or to have a low birth weight, conditions that increases their risk for illness or death.[57] In addition, babies of smokers have 30% higher odds of being born prematurely. Premature newborns are at increased risk for respiratory distress, jaundice, and other complications. Smoking during pregnancy has also been linked in some studies to miscarriages and stillbirths.[58]

Smoking also endangers the mother and fetus because of changes it induces in the placenta, the organ through which nutrient and gas exchange occurs between mother and fetus. Among pregnant smokers, the placenta is more likely to peel away from the uterine wall prior to birth, or to grow in such a way that it covers part or all of the opening of the birth canal. Vaginal bleeding is also more common in pregnant women who smoke.[56]

Health Risks to Infants and Children

Because their bodies are growing and developing, infants and children are particularly vulnerable to the effects of secondhand smoke. Babies born to women who smoked during pregnancy are two to three times more likely to die of *sudden infant death syndrome* (SIDS) than babies born to women who did not smoke.[57] Moreover, infants of women who currently smoke have been shown to have an impaired ability to be aroused from sleep that may increase their risk for SIDS.[59]

Secondhand smoke also contributes to disease in children. Parental smoking causes more than 750,000 ear infections in children each year.[60] It also reduces lung function in children, and promotes the development of persistent wheezing. Evidence suggests that exposure to parental smoking increases the risk of asthma in children. It also increases the child's risk for experiencing a lower respiratory infection such as bronchitis or pneumonia.[55]

Health Risks to Adults

On a basic level, secondhand smoke can irritate the eyes, nose, throat, and lungs. It can also cause chest pain, coughing, and production of excessive phlegm. More significantly, the U.S. Surgeon General concluded that secondhand smoke causes premature death and disease in adults who do not smoke. Here's what we know:

- **Lung cancer.** Exposure to secondhand smoke causes 3,400 lung cancer deaths in lifetime nonsmokers in the United States each year. Moreover, adults living with a smoker have a 20–30% increased risk of lung cancer.[55]
- **Other cancers.** Evidence suggests that secondhand smoke exposure may increase a nonsmoker's risk for cancer of the sinuses, nose, throat, and breast. However, a causal relationship has not been established.
- **Cardiovascular disease.** A nonsmoker's risk of heart disease increases by 25% to 30% with exposure to secondhand smoke. Heart disease claims almost 600,000 lives each year in the United States.[61] As many as one in ten of these deaths are caused by exposure to secondhand smoke.[55]
- **Respiratory distress.** Evidence suggests—but is not conclusive—that secondhand smoke exposure may cause wheezing, cough, chest tightness, and difficulty breathing in nonsmokers.

What's more, smoking is the number-one cause of deaths in residential fires, including fires in dorms and private homes.[62] Each year, about 1,000 Americans are killed in fires caused by smoking. Of these victims, 34% are children.[62]

Check out this article on the dangers of secondhand smoke from *Time* magazine: www.time.com/time/health/article/0,8599,1638535,00.html.

STUDENT STORY

Secondhand Smoke

"Hi, I'm Erica. I don't smoke but my boyfriend does. I tell him it's dangerous but he says he doesn't smoke enough to really hurt him and that he's going to quit when we graduate anyway. If he smokes in the car, I open the window all the way, and I make him go outside to smoke if we're hanging out together. The worst, though, is if I'm hanging out with him and his friends who all smoke. Even though I try to avoid it, I can smell the smoke on my clothes and hair even the next day. It's really gross."

1: How does Erica's exposure to secondhand and thirdhand smoke put her health at risk?

2: Do you think there's a level of smoking that's light enough that it won't really hurt Erica's boyfriend? Do you think his plan to quit smoking when he graduates is a good one?

Do you have a story similar to Erica's? Share your story at www.pearsonhighered.com/lynchelmore.

What Is Thirdhand Smoke?

You may have noticed the acrid smell that clings to a smoker's hair and clothing. But have you ever considered that the same chemicals producing that smell are polluting the environment? **Thirdhand smoke** is a concoction of toxic chemicals released during smoking that linger on environmental surfaces for hours and even days. These deposits build up over time, in a smoker's car, on clothing, in carpets, bedding, and drapes, and are thought to be a health hazard, especially for infants and children. For example, although research into thirdhand smoke is only beginning, researchers are investigating whether exposure to thirdhand smoke could impair normal brain development or increase the risk for childhood respiratory illnesses.

thirdhand smoke Deposits of toxic chemicals generated from smoking that build up on environmental surfaces.

Financial Burden of Tobacco Use

The average cost of a pack of cigarettes in the United States ranges from about $4.50 to $5.00, not including federal and state excise taxes.[63] This means that, before taxes, smoking a pack a day costs a minimum of $1,642 each year—and that doesn't include the cost for lighters or matches, breath mints, dry cleaning, or the higher insurance premiums you're charged, not to mention the costs of health-care visits and medications to treat your more frequent respiratory infections and other illnesses each year. According to one estimate, if you were to quit smoking at age 20 and invest the savings, you'd have almost $250,000 by your 50th birthday.

If you don't smoke, maybe you're thinking that you escape the costs. Not so: The economic burden of tobacco use on Americans is enormous. We spend more than $96 billion per year in smoking-related health-care costs to cover increased physician visits, medications, medical devices such as portable oxygen tanks, surgeries, and time spent in critical care units on mechanical respiration. We lose another $97 billion per year in disability payments and other economic aspects of lost productivity.

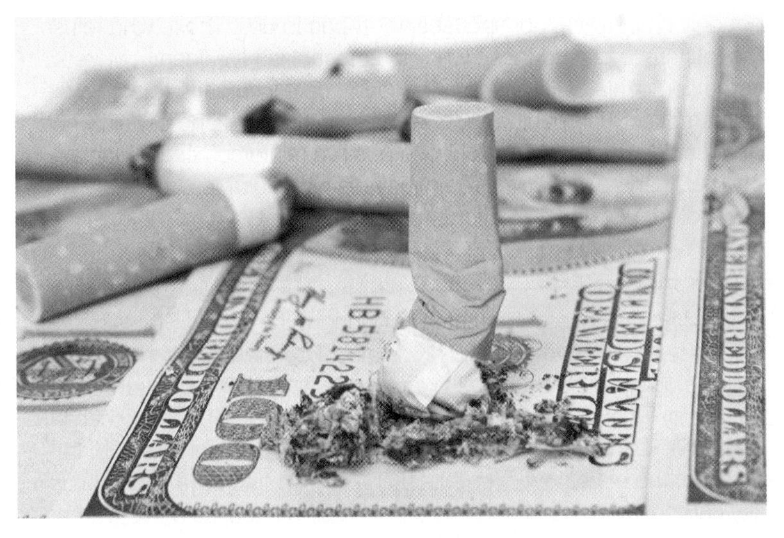

Tobacco is hugely **expensive,** not only to smokers, but to society as a whole.

Together, that's $629 for every man, woman, and child in America. In addition, every household in America pays over $600 a year in federal and state taxes due to smoking.[63]

Reducing Tobacco Use

Given the staggering burden of disease and death, and the economic costs of smoking to society, it's no wonder that the United States Congress, numerous federal agencies, state governments, public health organizations, and even private businesses have been working for decades to reduce tobacco use. These efforts have not been in vain: Research has documented the effectiveness of media campaigns, laws, and policies to reduce tobacco use and protect the public from exposure to secondhand smoke.[40] Here are a few of these efforts.

Campaigns to Discourage Tobacco Use

Evidence from both controlled experiments and population studies shows that mass media campaigns designed to discourage tobacco use can change people's attitudes about smoking, keep people from taking up the habit, and encourage smokers to quit. Many studies document reductions in smoking prevalence when mass media campaigns are combined with other strategies, including school- and community-based programs.[21]

ASSIST

One example of such a "combination" program was the American Stop Smoking Intervention Study (ASSIST) funded by the National Cancer Institute (NCI). Between1991 and 1999, the NCI provided over $128 million to 17 states to change the factors that promote smoking.[64] ASSIST funded public service announcements, promoted smoke-free environments, restricted access to tobacco products among young people, and raised excise taxes on tobacco products. These measures significantly reduced smoking rates: If ASSIST had been implemented in all 50 states, it is estimated that a million fewer Americans would currently smoke.[64] Unfortunately, ASSIST was opposed by the tobacco industry, which during the same eight-year period spent $47 billion—more than 350 times as much money—to market its products.[64]

MPOWER

The U.S. Centers for Disease Control and Prevention (CDC) is the leading federal agency for tobacco control.[40] It supports implementation of a series of interventions similar to those in ASSIST, including media campaigns to warn about the dangers of tobacco. The six interventions—collectively known as MPOWER—include the following:[40]

Monitor tobacco use and prevention policies.

Protect people from tobacco smoke.

Offer help to quit.

Warn about the dangers of tobacco.

Enforce bans on tobacco advertising.

Raise taxes on tobacco.

The CDC implements MPOWER by supporting state efforts, including in schools, by funding tobacco research, and by sponsoring public information campaigns using printed materials, public service announcements, videos, Internet sites, and other media.

College Students' Response to Antismoking Campaigns

Despite the success of antismoking media campaigns among Americans in general, their effectiveness among college students is not clear. For example, a 2006 study suggests that antismoking messages may trigger "boomerang" effects—such as anger and defiance—among college students.[65] In contrast, a 2010 study found that messages identifying health consequences of smoking are highly effective among college students, and that messages unmasking tobacco-industry manipulation of smokers are moderately effective.[66]

Federal Regulations

In the summer of 2009, the U.S. Congress passed the Family Smoking Prevention and Tobacco Control Act. The purpose of the act was to protect public health by providing the U.S. Food and Drug Administration (FDA) with authority to regulate the content, marketing, and sale of tobacco products.[67] Earlier, we described some FDA regulations that have stemmed from this act, including the removal of "light" and "flavored" cigarettes from the market. Other provisions of the act affected tobacco advertising and packaging.

Regulations on Tobacco Advertising

Congress prohibited the advertising of cigarettes on television and radio in 1971. Although tobacco companies are free to advertise in print magazines with a readership over the age of 21, the ads must include warnings from the Surgeon General about the dangers of tobacco use. By 2008, two major cigarette manufacturers had voluntarily removed their ads from most print magazines.

The 2009 act provided for further restrictions on tobacco advertising. For example, ads for tobacco products within 1,000 feet of schools and playgrounds were prohibited, and in 2010, the FDA prohibited the sale or free distribution of hats, T-shirts, and other gear with tobacco slogans or logos. Tobacco brand-name sponsorship of sports activities, theatrical performances, and other events was also banned.

Regulations on Tobacco Packaging

Product packaging was also affected by the 2009 act: New warning labels must cover 50% of the front and back of every package of cigarettes. As a result, the FDA is currently developing a policy requiring that all cigarette packages and promotional materials carry color, graphic images depicting the negative health consequences of cigarette

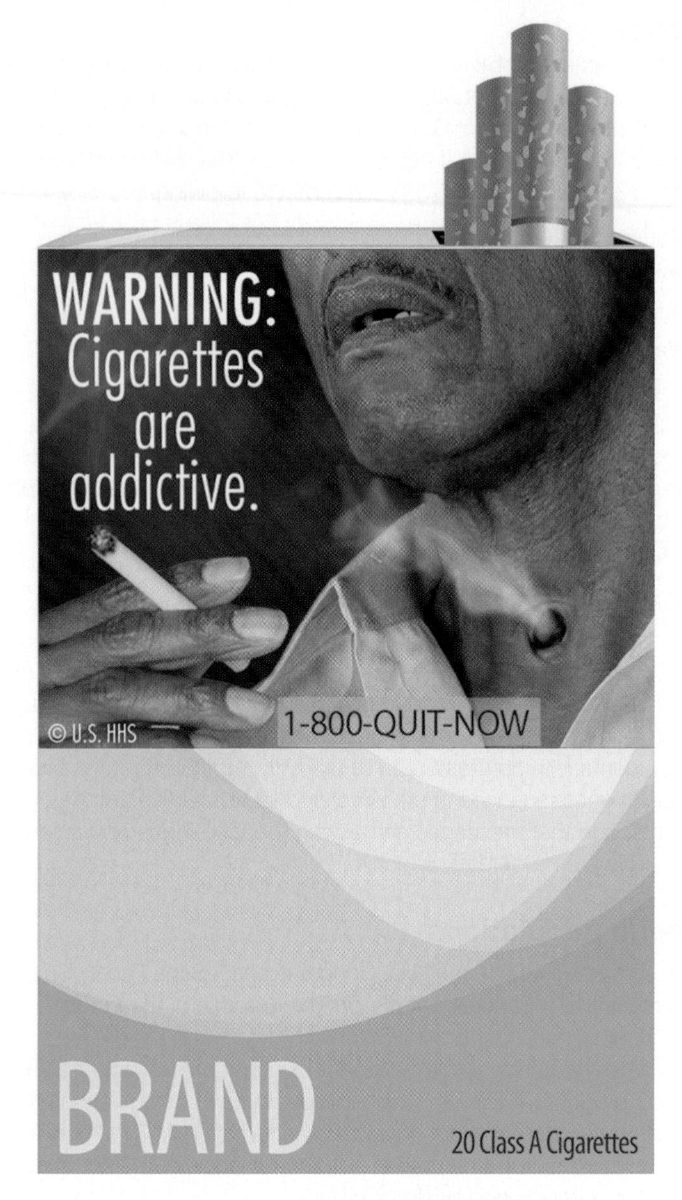

Figure 10.6 Look before you light. U.S. cigarette manufacturers are now required to display graphic health warnings on all packs of cigarettes.

Source: "Proposed Cigarette Product Warning Labels," by the U.S. Food and Drug Administration, retrieved from www.fda.gov/TobaccoProducts/Labeling/CigaretteProductWarningLabels/default.htm.

smoking **(Figure 10.6)**.[68] As of late 2012, U.S. manufacturers are no longer allowed to sell cigarettes that do not display the new graphic health warnings.

Access to Tobacco-Related Health Care

Another recent law related to tobacco use is the Patient Protection and Affordable Care Act of 2010. One provision of this act is to give Americans in private and public health-care insurance plans access to smoking cessation programs at no additional cost.[68]

Corporate Regulations

Antismoking regulations are also becoming common in private business. For example, some large employers—such as the Massachusetts Hospital Association, Alaska Airlines, and Union Pacific Railroad—no longer hire smokers.[63, 69] One employer in Michigan has begun testing not only employees, but spouses, for tobacco use. Those who refuse the test are fired, and those who don't test clean are fined.[63] Moreover, some companies charge more for health-care insurance to employees who smoke. Such punitive policies are controversial and certainly not common: Many employers choose positive reinforcements, such as offering financial incentives to employees who complete a company-sponsored smoking cessation program.

Bans and Taxes

Many cities, counties, and states throughout the United States ban indoor smoking. As of April 2012, a total of 35 states and more than 3,400 municipalities had laws in effect requiring 100% smoke-free non-hospitality workplaces, and/or restaurants, and/or bars.[70] Another 11 states had bans on smoking in workplaces or in restaurants only. In addition, there are now over 700 100% smoke-free college and university campuses in the United States.[71] These campuses don't just ban smoking indoors. Students and staff who want a cigarette have to walk off campus property before they light up.

Want to find out if your campus is 100% smoke free? The list is at www.no-smoke.org/pdf/smokefreecollegesuniversities.pdf.

Recall that both the ASSIST and the MPOWER programs support the use of excise taxes to increase the cost of cigarettes and provide funds for antismoking education and media campaigns. Federal and state excise taxes are shown to discourage smoking, especially among teens and young adults.[72] In 2011, the federal tax on cigarettes was $1.01. State taxes vary widely: In 2011, they ranged from a low of $0.17 in Missouri to a whopping $4.35 in New York, where the total retail price of a pack of cigarettes now ranges from $12 to $15. Many states use cigarette taxes to fund their tobacco control programs.

Getting Help to Quit Smoking

If you smoke, the odds are that you've thought about quitting. Perhaps you've already tried to quit. An estimated 38–50% of smokers under the age of 65 try to break their addiction each year.[73] If they try to quit on their own, more than 85% of them return to smoking, most within a week.[74]

Why Is Nicotine Addiction So Hard to Break?

Most smokers continue to use tobacco for one simple reason: because they are addicted to nicotine.[74] Why is nicotine addiction considered one of the hardest addictions to break? Here are some reasons:[74]

- Nicotine activates "reward pathways" in the brain; that is, brain centers that regulate feelings of pleasure. It does this, in part, by increasing the brain's level of dopamine, a key neurotransmitter involved in the desire to consume drugs. The effect is similar to that seen with other drugs of abuse, including heroin and cocaine.
- Continued nicotine exposure results in long-term changes in the brain, such as an increase in nicotine receptors—"docking stations" on the surfaces of brain cells that provide nicotine access to the cells. Such changes promote addiction.
- Smoking produces a rapid distribution of nicotine to the brain, with drug levels peaking within 10 seconds of inhalation. However, the pleasurable effects dissipate quickly, so the smoker must continue smoking in order to maintain the pleasure and avoid the discomfort of withdrawal.

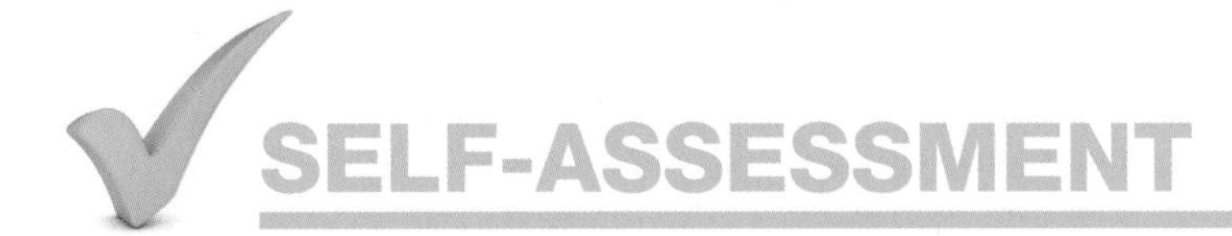

Take this self-assessment online at www.pearsonhighered.com/lynchelmore.

Are You Addicted to Nicotine?

This is a modified version of the well-known Fagerstrom Tolerance Questionnaire (mFTQ). Most smokers continue to use tobacco because they are addicted to nicotine. Take a minute to answer the following seven questions to see if you are addicted to nicotine. For each statement, circle the answer that best describes you.

1. How many cigarettes a day do you smoke?
   a. Over 26 cigarettes a day (2 points)
   b. About 16–25 cigarettes a day (1 point)
   c. About 1–15 cigarettes a day (0 points)
   d. Less than 1 a day (0 points)
2. Do you inhale?
   a. Always (2 points)
   b. Quite often (1 point)
   c. Seldom (1 point)
   d. Never (0 points)
3. How soon after you wake up do you smoke your first cigarette?
   a. Within the first 30 minutes (1 point)
   b. More than 30 minutes after waking but before noon (0 points)
   c. In the afternoon (0 points)
   d. In the evening (0 points)
4. Which cigarette would you hate to give up?
   a. First cigarette in the morning (1 point)
   b. Any other cigarette before noon (0 points)
   c. Any other cigarette in the afternoon (0 points)
   d. Any other cigarette in the evening (0 points)
5. Do you find it difficult to refrain from smoking in places where it is forbidden (church, library, movies, etc.)?
   a. Yes, very difficult (1 point)
   b. Yes, somewhat difficult (1 point)
   c. No, not usually difficult (0 points)
   d. No, not at all difficult (0 points)
6. Do you smoke if you are so ill that you are in bed most of the day?
   a. Yes, always (1 point)
   b. Yes, quite often (1 point)
   c. No, not usually (0 points)
   d. No, never (0 points)
7. Do you smoke more during the first 2 hours than during the rest of the day?
   a. Yes (1 point)
   b. No (0 points)

Total Points____________

HOW TO INTERPRET YOUR SCORE

A total score is obtained by summing the points for questions 1 to 7. What is your level of dependence based on the following three classifications?

0–2 = no dependence
3–5 = moderate dependence
6–9 = substantial dependence

Source: "Measuring Nicotine Dependence among High-Risk Adolescent Smokers," by A. V. Prokhorov, U. E. Pallonen, J. L. Fava, L. Ding, & R. Niaura, 1996, *Addictive Behaviors, 21*, pp. 117–127. Available online at the National Cancer Institute http://cancercontrol.cancer.gov/TCRB/mftq.html.

- Withdrawal symptoms are disturbing enough to quickly drive most people back to tobacco use. They include irritability, craving, depression, anxiety, having trouble thinking clearly and staying focused, disturbed sleep, and increased appetite. These symptoms may begin within hours after the last cigarette.
- Studies have shown that acetaldehyde, another chemical found in tobacco smoke, dramatically increases the effects of nicotine and may also contribute to addiction.

To gauge your level of addition to nicotine, complete the **Self-Assessment** above.

Recent research demonstrates that for up to 6 weeks after people stop smoking, nicotine receptors still exist.[73] This may help explain why the first months of smoking cessation are very difficult for many people. Moreover, many people trying to quit experience unexpected behavioral cravings, such as the desire to light and hold a cigarette, or to keep something in their mouth.[74] These neurologic and behavioral cravings, in addition to the withdrawal symptoms identified above, can overwhelm an individual's desire to quit.

Still, there is some good news: After 6–12 weeks of abstinence, a former smoker's nicotine receptor levels match those of a nonsmoker and relapse is less likely.[73] In addition, former smokers begin to experience the health benefits of quitting almost immediately (**Figure 10.7** on the next page). These health benefits may be rewarding enough in themselves to keep a smoker from relapsing.

Quitting—and remaining tobacco free—is possible, a fact demonstrated by the 47 million Americans who have succeeded.[75] Indeed, the number of smokers able to quit has so outpaced the rate of young adults taking up smoking that today there are more former smokers than current ones.[75] So how do successful quitters go about it?

Options on Campus

A 2001 survey of directors of college health centers revealed that about 56% of college and university student health centers offer smoking cessation programs. However, these programs are often underutilized.[76] A more recent study suggests that smoking cessation programs developed for college students offer students the following five targeted interventions:[77]

- A two-credit smoking cessation course
- Training about the effects of smoking and strategies to quit
- Therapy in problem-solving and stress reduction
- Peer counseling
- Mentors

The study authors propose that offering credits would give students incentive to enroll in the program, the training and therapy components would help students succeed, and the peer counselors and mentors would provide social support to maintain motivation and prevent relapse.

Community-Based Options

A variety of smoking cessation support groups may be available within a smoker's community. For example, Nicotine Anonymous is a 12-step program similar to Alcoholics Anonymous in which members help one another lead tobacco-free lives. It holds meetings in over 600 locations

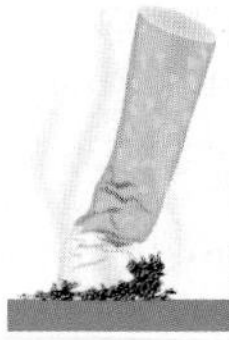

QUIT SMOKING

First 48 hours:

20 minutes
- Blood pressure drops to normal.
- Pulse rate drops to normal.
- Body temperature of hands and feet increases to normal.

8 hours
- Carbon monoxide level in blood drops to normal.
- Oxygen level in blood increases to normal.

24 hours
- Chance of heart attack decreases.

48 hours
- Nerve endings start regrowing.
- Ability to smell and taste is enhanced.

First year:

2 weeks to 3 months
- Circulation improves.
- Walking becomes easier.
- Lung function increases up to 30%.

1 to 9 months
- Coughing, sinus congestion, fatigue, and shortness of breath decrease.
- Cilia regrow in lungs, increasing ability to handle mucus, clean the lungs, and reduce infection.
- Overall energy level increases.

1 year
- Excess risk of heart disease is half that of a smoker.

Future years:

5 years
- Lung cancer death rate for average former smoker (one pack a day) decreases by almost half.

10 years
- Lung cancer death rate similar to that of nonsmokers.
- Precancerous cells are replaced.
- Risk of cancer of the mouth, throat, esophagus, bladder, kidney, and pancreas decreases.

15 years
- Risk of cardiovascular disease is that of a nonsmoker.

Figure 10.7 **Benefits of quitting smoking.** The health benefits of quitting smoking begin the moment you stop.

throughout the United States.[78] In addition, many Internet social networking sites are dedicated to helping smokers quit. There are also commercial programs, such as the Cooper Clayton method developed by faculty at the University of Kentucky.

Free counseling is also available nationwide through "quitlines." These are staffed with trained counselors who can help the caller reach a decision to quit or avoid relapse. For example, the National Cancer Institute's smoking quitline is 1-877-44U-QUIT.

Clinical Options

Using a *nicotine replacement therapy* (*NRT*) at least doubles the chances that a smoker will succeed in quitting.[79] All NRT products supply a controlled amount of nicotine, which helps smokers gradually reduce their dependence and decreases the severity of nicotine withdrawal symptoms. Over-the-counter options include nicotine gum, lozenges, and patches that are applied to the skin like an adhesive bandage. These can be purchased by anyone age 18 and older. Prescription NRT options include inhalers and nasal sprays, both under the brand name Nicotrol.

Two prescription drugs, bupropion (Zyban) and varenicline (Chantix), do not contain nicotine at all. Instead, they reduce the smoker's craving for tobacco and ease withdrawal symptoms by binding with nicotine receptors in the brain in a way that produces effects similar to those of nicotine. However, serious safety concerns have recently arisen about both of these drugs. These include an increased risk for depressed mood, hostility, and suicidal thoughts or actions.[80]

If you plan to quit smoking, tell your health-care provider, who should approve of any smoking cessation products you decide to use. This is especially important if you have allergies, asthma, or other health problems, are taking any other medications, or are pregnant or planning to become pregnant. In addition, you should not continue smoking while taking a smoking cessation product. You should also avoid taking more than one smoking cessation product at the same time, as improper use can result in nicotine overdose.

In addition to nicotine replacement therapies, clinical smoking cessation programs are effective for approximately 20–40% of smokers.[55] There are several types, including residential programs and individual or group therapy.

Alternative Therapies

The National Center for Complementary and Alternative Medicine is currently conducting a clinical trial to determine the effectiveness of yoga—a therapy involving physical and breathing exercises and meditation—in helping people quit smoking. Some studies suggest that other forms of exercise—including walking, jogging, and cycling—may help smokers quit by producing effects in the brain that reduce the craving for nicotine.[81] In addition, many herbal remedies, including teas, pills, and aromatic oils, are marketed as antismoking aids, but these are currently unproven.

A new nicotine product often advertised as a smoking cessation aid is the so-called *electronic cigarette* (or *e-cigarette*), a battery-powered device that delivers a dose of nicotine in vapor form. Invented in China in 2003, it quickly became popular in the United States. In 2010, the FDA classified the electronic cigarette as both a drug and a "drug-delivery device" subject to FDA approval. It also announced that it had taken action against five manufacturers of electronic cigarettes because of health risks, poor manufacturing practices, and unsubstantiated claims of benefits.[82]

Change Yourself, Change Your World

Earlier in this chapter we said that, each year, about half a million Americans die because of their own or someone else's smoking. Whether you're a smoker and want to quit, or you'd like to support a friend trying to quit, or you just want to reduce the threat of secondhand smoke, there are powerful choices you can make to reach your goal.

Personal Choices

If your goal is to quit smoking and avoid relapse, you'll want to follow a plan that works. The plan here, adapted from the National Cancer Institute (NCI), is one you can trust.[83]

Prepare to Quit

Quitting is more likely to succeed if you're prepared. Start by thinking about why you want to quit. Write down your reasons, and keep them with you—in your pocket or backpack, on your refrigerator, programmed into your phone. Or make your list your screen saver, so you see your reasons for quitting every time you use your computer. Wherever you put them, make sure the reasons you list are meaningful to you and your life. For instance:

- I'll have more stamina on the basketball court.
- The sores inside my mouth will heal.
- I won't have to be embarrassed about bad breath and smelly clothes.
- I'll save all the money I'd have spent on cigarettes, and take my kid brother on a skiing trip.
- I'll know that I'm the one in control of my life.

Next, it helps to know your enemy, so take a good, hard look at how strong your addiction to nicotine really is. For instance, do you smoke only socially, when out with friends? Or do you smoke throughout the day? If the latter, how soon after you wake up in the morning do you crave your first cigarette? How many cigarettes do you typically smoke in a day? Your honest answers may help you to decide whether or not you need professional support in your efforts to quit. For example, going "cold turkey" usually works for only a very small percentage of smokers who have a low level of nicotine dependency.[83] Others need support.

Next, identify your triggers—the activities, feelings, and other factors that make you want to smoke. According to the NCI, many smokers say that drinking coffee—or even just smelling freshly brewed coffee—makes them want to smoke. Or they might reach for a cigarette whenever they're with other smokers. Some are triggered by driving or studying or watching TV. Some crave a cigarette when they're feeling bored, depressed, anxious, angry, or impatient. Anything sound familiar? List your own triggers, then beside each, list a strategy for avoiding the trigger entirely, or for substituting a behavior other than smoking when the trigger arises. For example, if you're triggered when you're around other smokers, start hanging out with your nonsmoking friends! If you typically smoke when you drive, replace cigarettes and lighters in your car with a stash of lollipops, pretzels, or chewing gum. If a craving still comes on strong, take a long, deep breath and remind yourself that it will go away, usually in just a few minutes.

Finally, learn your options. Earlier in this chapter, we discussed campus and community-based support, as well as medications and clinical smoking cessation programs. Stay open to the option of combining two or more of these methods.

Start

Now that you've prepared yourself, how do you actually get a plan in gear? START is a five-step strategy for quitting smoking from the NCI. **Practical Strategies for Change: Quitting Smoking** summarizes the steps of the START method. Notice that these are *actions*, like telling your friends about your plan to quit, so they may take some time to implement. Once you're sure you've completed all five steps, the only thing left is to take the plunge.

Take the Plunge

Today's the big day: the day you begin to take back your smoke-free life. Today of all days, it's essential that you stay busy and physically active. In light of those studies suggesting that exercise reduces nicotine cravings, you might want to start your day off with a brisk walk or jog, or bike to campus instead of driving. Throughout the day, find nonsmoking places to spend your time, eat at a nonsmoking restaurant or cafeteria, and when you've finished eating, "fool your mouth" with a toothpick, straw, lollipop, or chewing gum. Brush your teeth often, and follow up with mouthwash. This is a perfect time for a craft or hobby that keeps your hands busy, from wood carving to knitting to playing the recorder. Whenever you find it hard to stay mentally focused, go for a quick walk or bike ride, or if time allows, take a yoga class or stroll through a museum with a friend.

When a craving hits, wait it out. Take slow, deep breaths, drink water, repeat an affirmation, or sing a song. Go to a different room, or leave the building you're in and run around the block. If you're at home, clean something, organize your computer desktop, vacuum out your

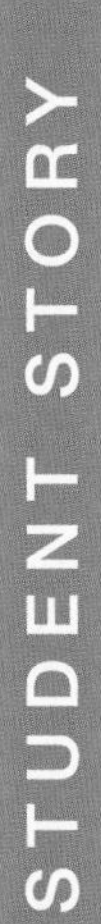

Quitting Cold Turkey

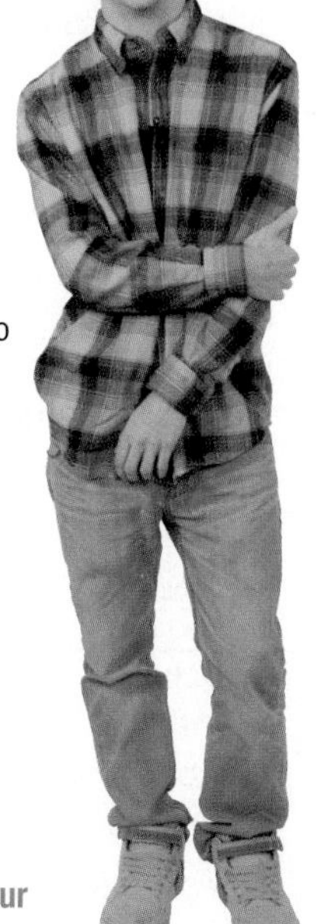

"Hi, I'm Addison. When I first started smoking I was 16 years old. I've tried to quit numerous times—always cold turkey. I'd last maybe a week if I was lucky. Recently I tried to quit again. This time I went cold turkey *and* I started working out too. I tried to replace a bad habit with a healthier habit. I go to the gym every day, I haven't smoked in two weeks, and I hope to keep it that way."

1: What stage of behavior change is Addison in? (Review Chapter 1 if you can't remember the stages of behavior change.)

2: What do you think of Addison's plan to "replace" smoking with working out?

3: How can Addison improve his chances of quitting smoking for good?

Do you have a story similar to Addison's? Share your story at www.pearsonhighered.com/lynchelmore.

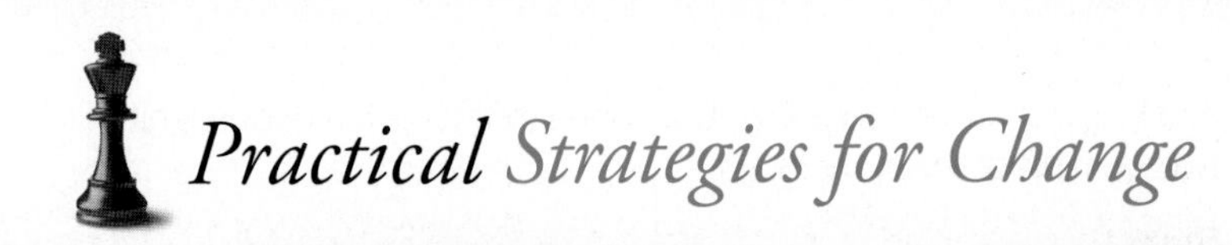

Practical Strategies for Change

Quitting Smoking

The National Cancer Institute promotes the START method as an effective smoking cessation strategy.

S = Set a quit date.

Choose a date within the next two weeks as your official quit date. Smoking cessation experts suggest that you pick a special date as your quit date. Consider your birthday, a special anniversary, New Year's Day, the Fourth of July, "World No-Tobacco Day" (May 31), or the "Great American Smokeout" (the third Thursday of November).

T = Tell family, friends, and coworkers that you plan to quit.

If you are going to be successful in your attempt to quit, you will need the help and support of others. So inform the important people in your life and let them know exactly how they can help you in your efforts.

A = Anticipate and plan for the challenges you'll face while quitting.

Studies show that most people who return to smoking do so within the first three months. Make plans ahead of time for dealing with cravings and withdrawal symptoms when they hit. Have a peer, mentor, or counselor you can call on when challenges hit, or call 1-877-44U-QUIT to talk to a smoking cessation counselor from the National Cancer Institute. For help within your own state, call 1-800-QUITNOW or visit www.smokefree.gov.

R = Remove cigarettes and other tobacco products from your home, car, and work.

Get rid of everything you can that reminds you of smoking. Throw away all cigarettes and smoking paraphernalia such as lighters, matches, and ashtrays. Change your routine, so that certain events and places don't prompt a cigarette craving. Clean your car, your carpets, your curtains, your clothes.

T = Talk to your doctor about getting help to quit.

Your health-care provider can prescribe medication that can help you quit. Many over-the-counter products are also helpful in dealing with nicotine withdrawal.

car, or call a friend. No matter what, don't give in. Know that the craving will go away.

At the end of your first smoke-free day, give yourself a reward! Then plan for bigger rewards when you make it to a week, a month, and your first smoke-free anniversary. With all the money you're saving by not smoking, you'll be able to afford new apps for your iPod, theater tickets, camping trips . . . it's up to you.

Ready to quit smoking today? Visit the National Cancer Institute's www.smokefree.gov. The American Cancer Society also offers helpful tips for quitting smoking at www.cancer.org/Healthy/StayAwayfromTobacco/index.

Deal with Relapse

Smokers commonly experience withdrawal symptoms when they first quit smoking, including difficulty concentrating, a negative mood, and the urge to smoke. These symptoms usually peak within one or two weeks. Not surprisingly, you're most likely to relapse early in the quitting process, although sometimes relapse can occur months or even years after quitting. Any smoking—even taking a single puff—increases the likelihood of a full relapse.

Beating nicotine addiction requires patience and strategy. Your brain has to be weaned off a substance it has become dependent on, and your mind has to stop using tobacco as a means of stress relief or a boost to self-confidence. You need to change your thoughts, behaviors, social patterns, and perhaps your entire lifestyle. So it's not unusual for people to slip up. In fact, most people make several unsuccessful attempts before they finally quit smoking for good.[83] If you do relapse, here are some tips for recovering:[83]

- Do not allow the incident to discourage you! If you smoked one or two cigarettes, remind yourself that that's better than having smoked an entire pack. Admit that you've had a setback, but slam the door shut on any thought that says, "Now I'm a smoker again." You're not. You've made a mistake, and you can learn from it.
- Figure out what happened. What triggered your relapse? How can you avoid that trigger in the future, or what can you substitute for a cigarette if you can't avoid it?
- Return to your support system. Talk to your peer or mentor, phone a quitline, or visit your health-care provider again.
- Resume your healthy life. Work out, stick to your healthy diet, avoid alcohol, get plenty of sleep. If you think you could benefit from counseling, get it.

Helping a Friend

If you've successfully quit smoking, you're in an ideal position to support peers who are trying to quit. You've been there. You know the challenges, and you know how they can be overcome. But even if you're one of the majority of college students who has never smoked a single cigarette, you can still help a friend who is trying to quit. Here are some tips from the American Cancer Society:[84]

- Respect that the quitter is in charge. This is their lifestyle change and their challenge, not yours.
- Find out whether your friend wants you to ask regularly how he or she is doing. Let the person know that it's okay to talk to you whenever he or she needs to hear encouraging words.
- Spend time doing things with the quitter to keep his or her mind off smoking—go to the movies, or take a walk or a bike ride together.
- If your friend seems to be having a tough time, try to see it from his or her point of view—a smoker's habit may feel like an old friend who has always been there when times were tough. It's hard to give that up.

- Finds ways to celebrate along the way. Let your friend know that *you* know that quitting smoking is a big deal!
- Don't doubt the smoker's ability to quit. Your faith in them reminds them they can do it.
- If your friend gets grumpy, don't take it personally. Nicotine withdrawal symptoms usually pass in about two weeks.
- Don't judge, nag, preach, tease, or scold. This is only likely to make the smoker feel worse.
- Finally, don't offer advice. Just ask how you can help.

Campus Advocacy

If you've never smoked or have quit smoking, you'd probably prefer to attend school without being exposed to other people's tobacco smoke. In fact, smokers themselves sometimes say that they support smoke-free zones because they don't like to breathe in secondhand smoke, plus when they're in a smoke-free zone, they're forced to reduce the number of times they light up. Many national public health organizations, from the U.S. Centers for Disease Control to the American College Health Association, support not only indoor smoking bans on college and university campuses, but outdoor bans as well. This is in part because indoor smoking bans may encourage smokers to cluster just outside of buildings, saturating these areas with tobacco smoke, which can then drift back into the building through doors, air intakes, and walkways.[85]

Watch videos of real students discussing their experiences with tobacco at www.pearsonhighered.com/lynchelmore.

If you'd like to advocate for a smoke-free campus, the American Cancer Society recommends you address the issue on multiple fronts. Specifically, it advises that you lobby for a policy that includes the following provisions:[86]

- Prohibit smoking within all buildings, including residence halls and fraternities and sororities, and at all indoor and outdoor campus events.
- Prohibit the sale and the free distribution of tobacco products on campus.
- Prohibit tobacco advertisements in college-run publications.
- Provide free, accessible tobacco treatment on campus, and advertise it.
- Prohibit campus organizations from accepting money from tobacco companies.
- Prohibit the university from holding stock in or accepting donations from the tobacco industry.

You can take action to clear your campus of secondhand smoke! For more information, visit the American Cancer Society's website at www.cancer.org and download the publication: *Advocating for a Tobacco-Free Campus: A Manual for College and University Students*. Or visit your student health center, share your concerns, and ask how you can get involved.

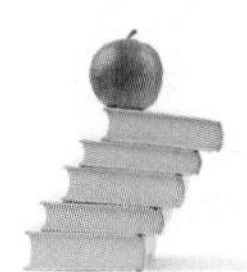

Choosing to Change Worksheet

To complete this worksheet online, visit www.pearsonhighered.com/lynchelmore.

Directions: If you currently smoke, complete Part I. If you don't smoke, complete Part II.

Part I. Smokers

Step 1: Your Stage of Behavior Change. Select the statement that best describes your intention about quitting smoking.

________ I do not intend to quit smoking in the next 6 months. (Precontemplation)

________ I might quit smoking in the next 6 months. (Contemplation)

________ I am prepared to quit smoking in the next month. (Preparation)

________ I quit smoking less than 6 months ago. (Action)

________ I quit smoking more than 6 months ago. (Maintenance)

Next fill out the Step that applies to the stage of change that you are in.

Step 2: Precontemplation or Contemplation Stages. If you are in the early stages of change, it is recommended that you reread the sections on the effects of smoking on pages 272–278 and consider your own costs and benefits for quitting smoking. Fill in the "Perceived Cost and Perceived Benefit" grid as it relates to your smoking.

Perceived Cost of Continuing Smoking *How is my smoking hurting me?*	Perceived Benefit of Continuing Smoking *What do I give up if I change?*
1.	1.
2.	2.
3.	3.
4.	4.
5.	5.

Perceived Benefit of Quitting Smoking *How will this help me?*	Perceived Cost of Quitting Smoking *How much will this change "cost" or hurt?*
1.	1.
2.	2.
3.	3.
4.	4.
5.	5.

Now add up your totals: ____________ reasons to change ____________ reasons to stay the same

What one benefit do you think will motivate you the most? ____

What one "cost" or barrier do you think will present the biggest obstacle for you? ____________________________

LEARNING OBJECTIVES

EXPLAIN the differences between type 1 and type 2 diabetes.

DISCUSS some of the long-term effects of uncontrolled diabetes.

IDENTIFY the major risk factors for type 2 diabetes.

DISCUSS the structure and function of the heart and blood vessels.

COMPARE AND CONTRAST the four major types of cardiovascular disease.

DISCUSS the clinical management of cardiovascular disease.

LIST the nine factors associated with cardiometabolic risk.

IDENTIFY choices you can make to improve your cardiometabolic scorecard.

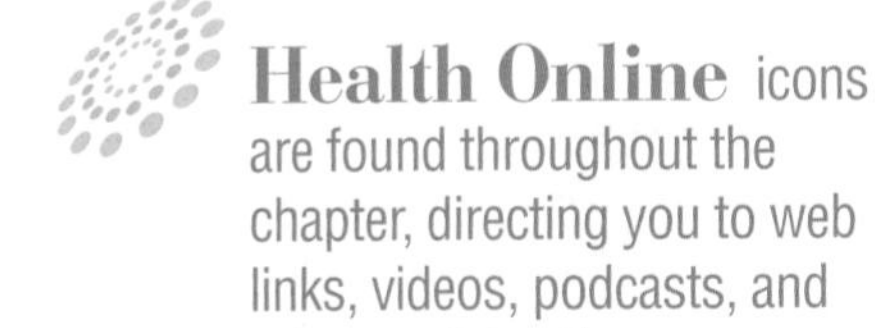

Health Online icons are found throughout the chapter, directing you to web links, videos, podcasts, and other useful online resources.

College is all about preparing for your future.

Where will your major take you? Will you go to graduate school? What will your career be like? How will the friendships and relationships you make on campus shape your life in your postcollege years?

To that list of questions, we'd like to add one more: Will the behaviors you practice today help maintain your health or increase your risk for disease?

It's an important question because, when we consider your risk of developing two specific diseases—diabetes and cardiovascular disease—the odds are against you. If 100 students were enrolled in your health course, and you and your classmates were to follow current U.S. health trends, here is where national statistics suggest your class would wind up:

- About 27 of your group would develop diabetes.[1] As a result, some would die of kidney failure, some would go blind, and some would have to undergo toe, foot, or leg amputations.
- About 36 class members would develop cardiovascular disease. About 29 would eventually die of a heart attack, stroke, or other disease of the heart or blood vessels.[2]

These facts are sobering. But they do not necessarily predict your fate. Just as you can use your time in college to shape your career, you can also use these years to start reducing your *cardiometabolic risk*; that is, your risk of developing diabetes and cardiovascular disease, two chronic diseases that often occur together, especially in people who are overweight. We'll define cardiometabolic risk more precisely later in this chapter. First, to help you appreciate why it's important, let's explore each of the disorders associated with a high cardiometabolic risk: diabetes and cardiovascular disease.

Diabetes

Do you know someone with diabetes? Do you have it yourself? Your answer is far more likely to be "Yes" than was your parents' reply at your age.

Once a condition found mainly in adults over age 65, diabetes, an inability of the body to regulate the level of glucose in the blood, is now one of the most common serious illnesses among American adults of all ages. The number of cases continues to grow rapidly: Between 1980 and 2009, the number of people in the United States with diabetes more than tripled **(Figure 11.1)**. Currently, more than 11% of American adults aged 20 or older has some form of diabetes, and another 35% is on its way to developing it.[1] At this rate of growth, public health experts anticipate that one out of every three U.S. children born in the year 2000 will develop diabetes.[3]

This growing epidemic of diabetes is of concern not only because of the devastating effects of the disease—including blindness, loss of limbs, and early death—but also because of the staggering costs to American society. Medical expenses for a patient with diabetes are more than two times higher than for a patient without diabetes, and overall, direct medical costs of diabetes were $116 billion in 2007. In addition, another $58 billion was lost to the American economy in 2007 from indirect costs such as disability, work loss, and premature death.[1]

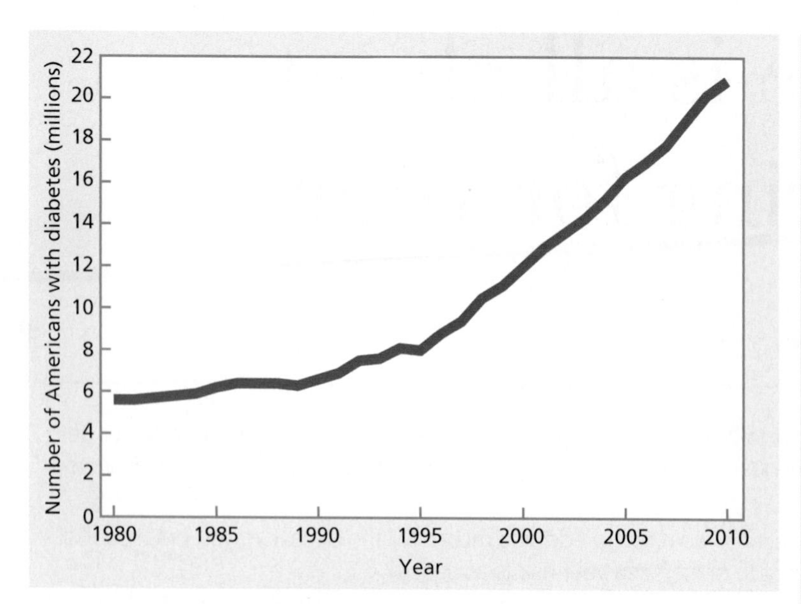

Figure 11.1 Diabetes is on the rise. From 1980 to 2010, the number of people in the United States with diabetes almost quadrupled, from 5.6 million to 20.9 million.

Source: Number (in Millions) of Civilian/Noninstitutionalized Persons with Diagnosed Diabetes, United States, 1980–2010, by the Centers for Disease Control and Prevention, retrieved from http://www.cdc.gov/diabetes/statistics/prev/national/figpersons.htm.

Forms of Diabetes

Diabetes, known formally as **diabetes mellitus,** is a broad term that covers a group of diseases characterized by high levels of the simple sugar *glucose* in the blood. In fact, the word *mellitus* is derived from the Latin word for honey. These high levels of blood glucose arise from problems with the body's production or use of **insulin,** a hormone secreted by the **pancreas** that is necessary for transportation of glucose into the body's cells.

When you eat carbohydrate, your body metabolizes it into glucose, which is absorbed across the lining of the small intestine into the bloodstream **(Figure 11.2)**. In response to this surge of glucose, your pancreas secretes insulin into your bloodstream. Glucose molecules are too large to pass unassisted into most body cells. Insulin helps them cross into cells by encouraging proteins called *glucose transporters* to move to the cell membrane. There, the glucose transporters enable cells to take up the glucose, which they then use for energy to accomplish their functions. You can imagine what might happen in people whose pancreas doesn't make any insulin, or doesn't make enough to adequately clear their bloodstream of glucose. Or in people whose pancreas produces enough insulin, but whose body cells don't respond to the insulin properly. In such cases, glucose builds up within the blood vessels, causing a variety of problems, while the body's cells—unable to take the glucose in—suffer from lack of nourishment.

Type 1 Diabetes

Type 1 diabetes arises when the body's own immune system destroys the beta cells in the pancreas that manufacture insulin. As a result, when the type 1 diabetic eats carbohydrate, the glucose from the meal remains in the bloodstream (see Figure 11.2). This excessive glucose "pulls" water out of the interior of body cells and into the blood vessels. This leaves the person feeling perpetually thirsty, despite increased fluid intake. Also, because body cells are deprived of glucose, the person may become tired, irritated, and intensely hungry, even after eating. Brain cells cannot survive without glucose, so to provide it, the body turns to alternate metabolic pathways that, unfortunately, release acids. High blood acidity can cause the person to slip into a diabetic coma.

Type 1 diabetes usually appears in childhood or adolescence, and researchers are investigating the role of specific genes in its development, as well as the possible role of external factors such as viruses. People with type 1 diabetes must monitor their blood sugar level throughout each day, and take insulin through injections or a pump implanted in their bodies. For this reason, type 1 diabetes is also known as *insulin-dependent diabetes*. Insulin can't be taken as a pill because it is a protein, and would be digested in the gastrointestinal tract.

Type 1 diabetes accounts for the majority of diabetes in children and up to 5% of diabetes cases overall.[1] There is no cure, but the condition is the focus of intense research, including studies into the use of stem cell therapy to replace the pancreas's insulin-making beta cells.

Type 2 Diabetes

Type 2 diabetes is more common than type 1, accounting for close to 95% of all adult diabetes cases.[4] Once known as *adult-onset diabetes,* it is still most common after age 60; however, the incidence of type 2 diabetes has surged among all age groups, including teenagers. One study of prescription medication use found that preteen and teenage use of type 2 diabetes drugs more than doubled between 2002 and 2005.[5] And new cases of type 2 diabetes now exceed or match the number of new type 1 diagnoses in youth aged 10 to 19 of Hispanic, African American, or Native American ancestry.[1]

Whereas in type 1 diabetes, the cells of the pancreas stop making insulin, most cases of type 2 diabetes begin as *insulin resistance* (see Figure 11.2). The pancreas makes normal amounts of insulin, but the body's cells don't respond to it properly—they resist its effects. One factor in this resistance is interference due to an overabundance of fatty acids concentrated in fat cells. This explains why type 2 diabetes is linked not only to age but also to obesity. If the body's cells can't respond to insulin, they can't take up glucose, and it remains in the bloodstream. The resulting **hyperglycemia** (persistent high blood glucose) signals the pancreas to produce more insulin to get more glucose into the cells. As the demand for insulin continues to rise, the beta cells of the pancreas begin to fatigue. Over time, they can completely lose their ability to produce insulin, just as in type 1 diabetes. And as blood glucose levels remain elevated, the same thirst, fatigue, and other effects seen with type 1 diabetes occur.

Other Forms of Diabetes

Less common varieties of diabetes resemble type 2, but also have differences that set them apart:

- *Gestational diabetes* develops in a woman during pregnancy, and affects up to 5% of pregnant women. The condition usually disappears after childbirth, but researchers have learned that

diabetes mellitus A group of diseases in which the body does not make or use insulin properly, resulting in elevated blood glucose.

insulin A hormone necessary for glucose transport into cells.

pancreas An abdominal organ that produces insulin as well as certain compounds helpful in digestion.

type 1 diabetes A form of diabetes that usually begins early in life and arises when the pancreas produces insufficient insulin.

type 2 diabetes A form of diabetes that usually begins later in life and arises when cells resist the effects of insulin.

hyperglycemia A persistent state of elevated levels of blood glucose.

Healthy person

Person with diabetes

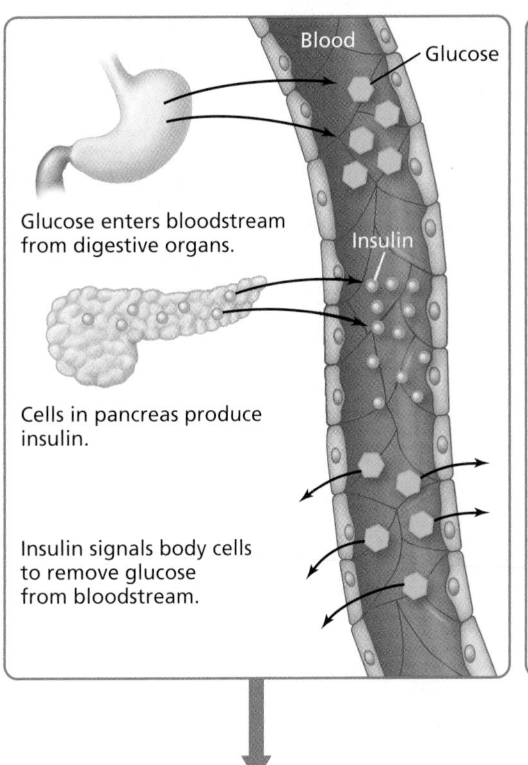

Type 1 diabetes

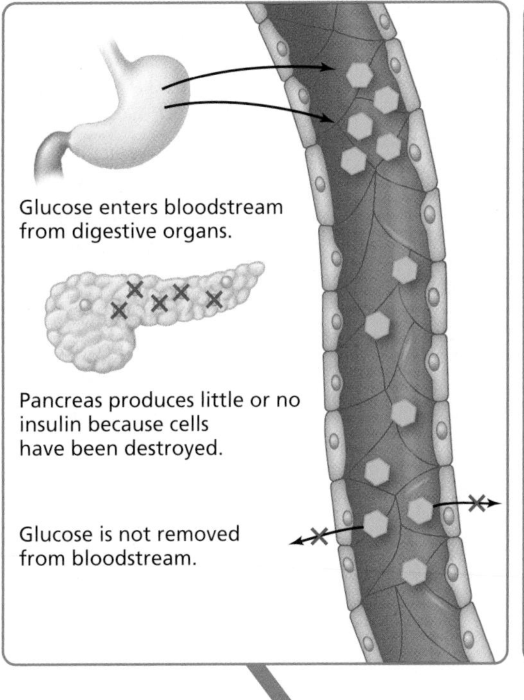

Type 2 diabetes

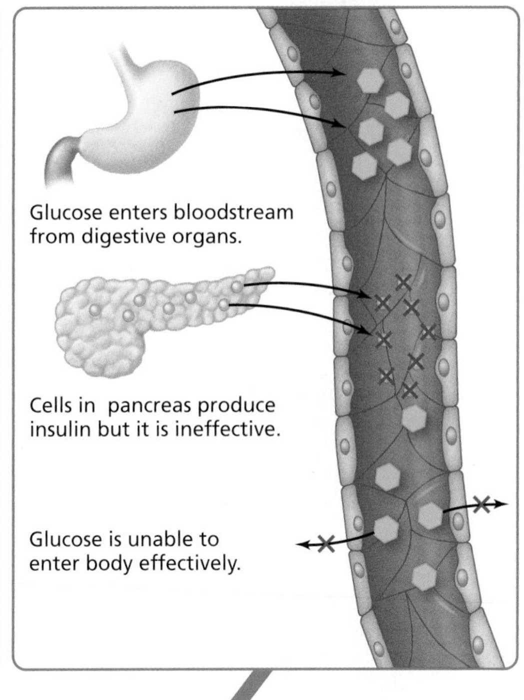

Glucose enters bloodstream from digestive organs.
Pancreas produces little or no insulin because cells have been destroyed.
Glucose is not removed from bloodstream.
Cells in pancreas produce insulin but it is ineffective.
Glucose is unable to enter body effectively.

- Blood glucose level is regulated.
- Body cells take in and utilize energy from glucose.

- Glucose accumulates in blood and causes high glucose levels.
- Body cells lack energy.
- Nerves and blood vessels are damaged.

Figure 11.2 **Two types of diabetes.** In type 1 diabetes, the beta cells of the pancreas stop producing insulin entirely, or produce an amount insufficient for normal body functioning. In type 2 diabetes, the body is unable to use insulin properly. In advanced cases, the pancreas becomes exhausted and, as with type 1 diabetes, stops producing insulin. In either case, the body's cells are unable to take in glucose from the bloodstream.

women who develop gestational diabetes are at greater risk for type 2 diabetes later in life.[6]

- *Type 1.5* is a general term for several varieties of diabetes that blend aspects of type 1 and type 2. For instance, a physician may suspect type 1.5 in a newly diagnosed adult diabetic who is not overweight. Also called *latent autoimmune diabetes of adults* (LADA), type 1.5 is often revealed when blood tests show some immune-system destruction of pancreatic beta cells—but healthy, insulin-producing beta cells as well. Researchers estimate that perhaps 10% of all diagnoses of type 2 diabetes are actually due to type 1.5, and the number of cases may be growing.[7]

Watch a video showing how diabetes affects blood sugar at www.mayoclinic.com/health/blood-sugar/MM00641.

Signs and Symptoms of Diabetes

The classic physical signs and symptoms of diabetes include:

- Frequent urination
- Excessive hunger and thirst
- Tendency to tire easily
- Numbness or tingling in the hands and feet
- Frequent infections, including in women a tendency to develop vaginal yeast infections

These symptoms, while common across all types of diabetes, can develop differently from person to person. Moreover, early stages of diabetes may not be accompanied by any symptoms at all.

Long-Term Effects of Diabetes

Persistent hyperglycemia causes damage throughout the body, especially to blood vessels **(Figure 11.3)**. This damage in turn can lead to a variety of complications:[1]

- Damage to the blood vessels that supply the heart and brain raises the risk of heart attack and stroke two to four times above the risk for people without diabetes. High blood pressure occurs in 67% of people with diabetes.
- The kidneys have microscopic blood vessels that filter excessive glucose from the blood into urine. Hyperglycemia stresses this delicate filtration system, leading to kidney disease, a serious

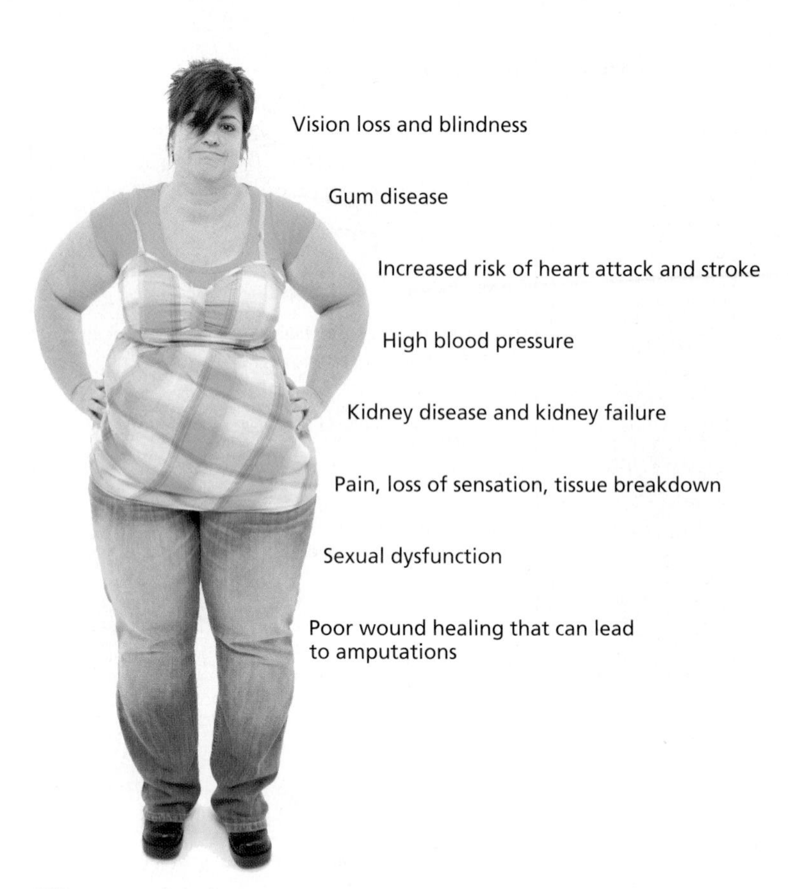

Figure 11.3 Long-term complications associated with diabetes.

complication of diabetes. Diabetes is the most common cause of kidney failure, and end-stage kidney disease is a common cause of death among diabetics.

- Hyperglycemia also damages blood vessels that serve nerves, causing pain, loss of sensation, and tissue breakdown, as well as an increased risk for non-healing wounds. Such wounds are especially likely in the feet, ankles, and lower legs, and surgical amputation of toes, then foot, then the entire leg below the knee, is not uncommon among even middle-aged adults with diabetes. On average, more than 60% of nontraumatic lower-limb amputations occur in people with diabetes.
- Damage to the nerves and blood vessels that serve the genitals can cause both men and women with diabetes to experience sexual dysfunction. Many men will be unable to maintain an erection, and women may experience a failure of vaginal lubrication or a decreased or absent sexual response.
- When hyperglycemia damages the tiny blood vessels serving the retina of the eye, vision deteriorates. In the early stages, the person may notice only blurred vision, but without appropriate management, this can progress to blindness. In fact, diabetes is the leading cause of new cases of blindness among U.S. adults.
- Gum disease is also more common in people with diabetes, about one-third of whom experience loss of attachment of the gums to the teeth.

Overall, diabetes is now the seventh most common cause of death in the United States, and shaves 10 to 15 years off a person's life.[3]

Risk Factors for Type 2 Diabetes

After age 50, body cells become increasingly less responsive to the effects of insulin. This explains in part the gradual increase in blood glucose levels that occurs as we age. But aging doesn't by any means consign us to diabetes. Other risk factors may be much more important. These include the following:

- **Overweight.** Being overweight or obese increases your risk, and the more overweight you are, the more that risk goes up at a young age. In one national study that gauged lifetime diabetes risk according to body mass index (BMI), 18-year-old men who were very obese had a 70% risk of developing diabetes, while the risk for very obese women of the same age was 74%.[8]
- **Disproportionately large waist.** People who carry more of their excess weight around their abdominal area are at greater risk for diabetes. Greater amounts of abdominal fat have been linked to insulin resistance.
- **Diet.** We've said that overweight increases your risk, but a few types of foods also play a role—independently of the number of calories. For instance, foods high in fiber slow the release of glucose into the bloodstream, so a high-fiber diet is thought to reduce your risk for diabetes. Foods high in saturated fats are also likely to be high in cholesterol, which further increases the vulnerability of your blood vessels to disease. These foods are also higher in calories, so contribute to being overweight. Beyond that, eating a nutritious diet with plenty of whole grains, vegetables, and lean protein foods is recommended. What about sweets? Does eating a lot of sugar cause diabetes? Check out the **Myth or Fact?** box for the answer!
- **Lack of exercise.** When you had some free time over the weekend, did you opt for an activity like going for a bike ride, or crash on the couch to play a video game? Exercise helps control weight, burns glucose, and makes your body cells more receptive to insulin. Physi-

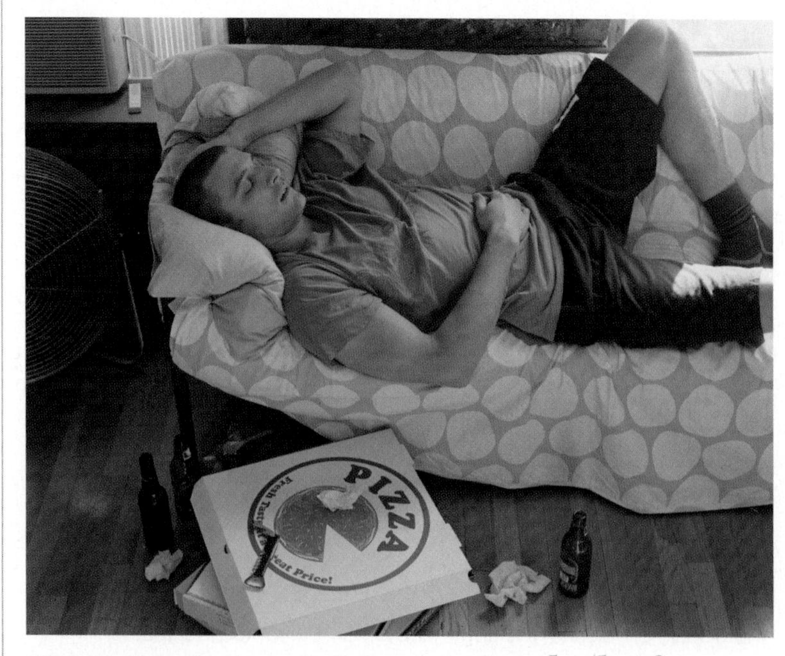

Risk factors for type 2 diabetes include **lack of physical activity** and being overweight.

cal activity also builds up muscle mass, and muscle cells absorb most of the glucose in your blood. In contrast, a sedentary lifestyle increases your risk for type 2 diabetes.

- **Genetic factors.** Do members of your family have type 2 diabetes? If so, you are at higher risk. Several common genetic variants can increase a person's risk of type 2 diabetes. This inherited risk is seen both within families and within ethnic groups. In addition, African Americans, Hispanics, and Native Americans develop diabetes at higher rates than other U.S. population groups.[9] For more information on racial/ethnic differences in diabetes rates, see the **Diversity & Health** box.

You can also determine your risk for diabetes by taking the **Self-Assessment** on page 299.

Clinical Management of Diabetes

Symptoms of type 1 diabetes often appear suddenly and are severe; for instance, a teen may begin losing weight, then pass out one day at school. In type 2 diabetes, symptoms come on more gradually. But in either case, blood tests are necessary to make the diagnosis. In addition, most physicians perform a routine blood glucose screening in all of their patients over age 45.[10]

Detecting Diabetes

Two simple laboratory tests can reveal whether or not you have—or are developing—diabetes. One of the most common is the *fasting blood glucose test* (*FBG*), which requires you to fast (consuming nothing other than plain water) overnight. A technician then draws a blood sample, and the level of glucose in your blood is measured. Here is what the measurement values mean:

- A blood glucose level below 100 mg/dL is normal.
- A blood glucose level between 100 and 125 mg/dL means that you have **prediabetes.** That is, your FBG is higher than normal but not high enough to warrant a diagnosis of diabetes. Prediabetes indicates that your body is struggling to regulate your blood glucose, and you are at significant risk for developing diabetes.
- A blood glucose level of 126 mg/dL or higher indicates true diabetes.

A second test, known as the *glycated hemoglobin test*, or *A1C test*, measures how much glucose is attached to the hemoglobin—the oxygen-carrying compound—in your red blood

prediabetes A persistent state of blood glucose levels higher than normal, but not yet high enough to qualify as diabetes.

MYTH OR FACT?

Does Eating Too Much Sugar Cause Diabetes?

Doughnuts for breakfast. Grape soda at lunch. A bag of licorice stashed in your backpack . . . No doubt about it. You've got a sweet tooth. But does that mean you're going to develop diabetes?

Not necessarily. The American Diabetes Association explains that type 1 diabetes is caused by genetics and unknown factors.[1] The development of type 2 diabetes is influenced by genetics and a variety of lifestyle factors—but these don't include a high-sugar diet specifically. Still, there is an *indirect* link between consumption of lots of sweets and type 2 diabetes: Being overweight sharply increases your risk, and a diet high in calories, whether from sugar or from fat, can contribute to weight gain.[1] The *Dietary Guidelines for Americans* calls calories from sweets *empty calories*, and encourages you to limit them in order to avoid weight gain. Especially if you have a history of diabetes in your family, you should build a healthy plate at every meal, cut back on foods high in solid fats and added sugars, eat the right number of calories for you, and exercise regularly to manage your weight.[2]

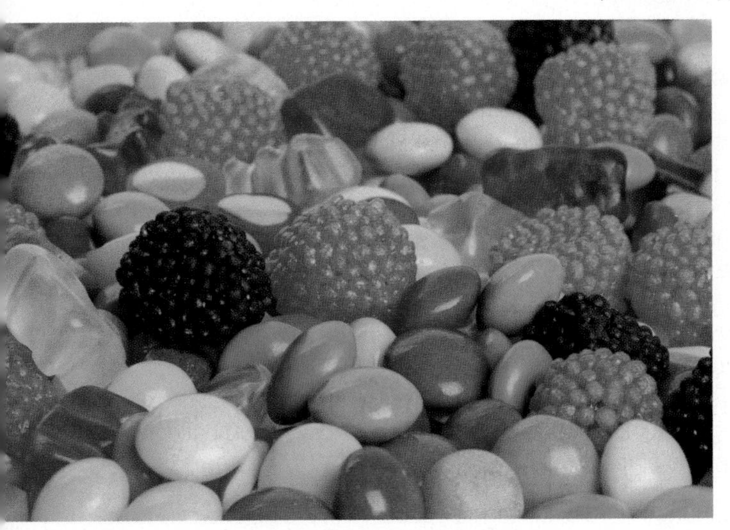

Eating sugar won't cause diabetes directly.

If eating sweets doesn't directly cause diabetes, how come people with diabetes have to eat sugar-free versions of candies, cookies, and other treats? The answer is: They don't. Diabetic and "dietetic" foods offer no special advantage over standard foods. Most of them still raise blood glucose levels, and are usually more expensive. On the other hand, if eaten in moderation as part of a healthy meal plan, standard sweets and desserts can be enjoyed by people with diabetes. They are no more "off limits" to them than to people without diabetes.[1]

References: **1.** "Diabetes Myths," by the American Diabetes Association, 2011, retrieved from www.diabetes.org/diabetes-basics/diabetes-myths. **2.** "Let's Eat for the Health of It," by the U.S. Department of Health and Human Services & U.S. Department of Agriculture, June 2011, Washington, DC: U.S. Government Printing Office, retrieved from http://www.choosemyplate.gov/downloads/MyPlate/DG2010Brochure.pdf.

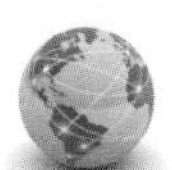

DIVERSITY & HEALTH

Racial Disparities in Incidences of Diabetes

Even as broad public health efforts focus on reducing the risks of chronic diseases such as diabetes, significant racial and ethnic disparities remain. Consider the following:

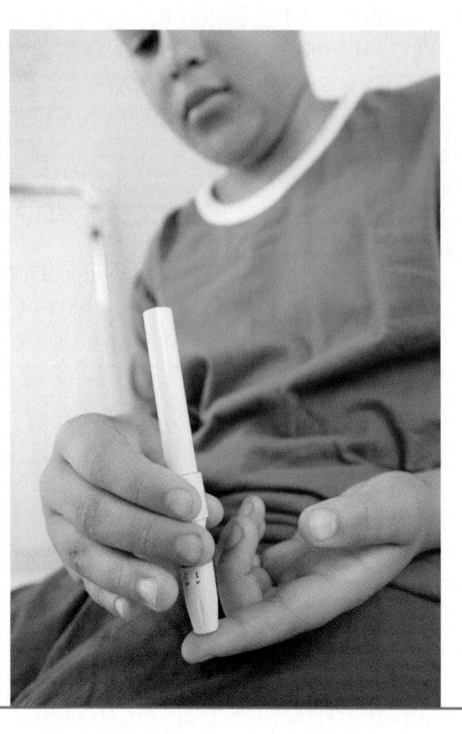

- Among American adults, non-Hispanic whites have the lowest rate of diabetes: 7.1%. The rate within certain Hispanic subgroups, including Cuban Americans and Central and South Americans, is only slightly higher: 7.6%. The rate for Asian Americans is 8.4%.[1]
- In general, Hispanics have disproportionately higher rates of diabetes than non-Hispanic whites. Overall, their rate is 11.8%, but it climbs to more than 13% among Mexican Americans and Puerto Ricans.[1]
- African Americans also have a higher rate of diabetes than whites—12.6% for non-Hispanic blacks—and are more likely to die of diabetes than members of other racial and ethnic groups.[1, 2, 3] Socioeconomic factors such as inequities in income, education, standard of living, and access to health care are believed to play a role in this higher mortality rate, more so than any biological differences associated with race.
- Native Americans have the highest rates of diabetes in the world. Overall, more than 16% of Native American adults have diagnosed diabetes. The rate is highest among American Indian adults in southern Arizona, 33.5% of whom have diabetes.[1]

If your race/ethnicity puts you at higher risk for type 2 diabetes, talk to your health-care provider to find out what you can do to reduce your risk. Remember that maintaining a healthy weight, exercising, eating a nutritious diet, not smoking, and limiting your alcohol intake can go a long way toward keeping you healthy—regardless of your race.

References: **1**. "National Diabetes Fact Sheet, 2011," by the Centers for Disease Control and Prevention, 2011, retrieved from http://www.cdc.gov/diabetes/pubs/pdf/ndfs_2011.pdf. **2**. "Health, United States, 2009: With Special Feature on Medical Technology," by the National Center for Health Statistics, 2009, retrieved from http://www.cdc.gov/nchs/data/hus/hus09.pdf#032. **3**. "Diabetes Death Rate by Race/Ethnicity," by the Kaiser Family Foundation, 2010, retrieved from http://www.statehealthfacts.org/comparemaptable.jsp?cat=2&ind=76.

cells. An A1C level of 6.5% or higher on two separate occasions indicates that you have diabetes.[10]

If type 1 diabetes is suspected, the physician will order a further test to see whether or not there is evidence of an immune system response against the beta cells of the pancreas. The urine may also be tested to look for waste chemicals suggesting that the body cells—given their inability to use glucose for energy—are breaking down fats or proteins for energy.

Treating Diabetes

If you are diagnosed with diabetes or prediabetes, your doctor will work with you toward one central goal—stabilizing your body's use of glucose. The approach prescribed will depend on the type and severity of diabetes you have.

Glucose monitoring. To stay healthy, people with diabetes must maintain a continual awareness of their blood glucose levels. That means measuring and recording blood glucose levels as often as three times a day. In the past, blood glucose monitoring required pricking the finger. Now, devices are available that can read glucose levels through the skin, or from a small needle implanted in the body.

Insulin therapy. All people with type 1 diabetes, and many with type 2, need insulin daily to survive. Many diabetics inject their insulin using a fine needle and syringe, or an insulin pen—a device that looks like an ink pen, except the cartridge is filled with insulin. Others use an insulin pump worn on the outside of the body. A tube connects the reservoir of insulin to a catheter that's inserted under the skin of your abdomen. The person programs the pump to dispense specific amounts of insulin **(Figure 11.4)**.[10] Most of the new devices are about the size and weight of an MP3 player, and some are even free of tubing, delivering insulin via skin absorption from a "pod" attached to the skin with a gentle adhesive.

Weight loss. For people with prediabetes or with type 2 diabetes who are overweight—whether or not they are using insulin—weight loss is important. The good news is that losing just 5% to 10% of your body weight can significantly improve your cells' ability to respond to insulin.[10] In obese patients with diabetes, especially those with a BMI of 35 or higher who are at high risk for severe complications, bariatric (weight-loss) surgery may be an option. Bariatric surgery reduces the size of the stomach and may also bypass the first section of the small intestine, so weight loss can be dramatic. However, patients will gradually begin to gain weight again if they do not follow a healthful diet and engage in regular exercise. Moreover, bariatric surgery in obese patients carries a high risk of adverse consequences, and 1 in 200 patients dies within 3 months of the surgery.[11]

Exercise. Along with a balanced, reduced-calorie diet, exercise is essential. During exercise, glucose is transported into body cells for use as energy. Moreover, exercise increases the sensitivity of body cells to

SELF-ASSESSMENT

Are You at Risk for Type 2 Diabetes?

Fill in the points that correspond to your answer on each line.

1. Are you age 45 or older? ____________
   Yes (1 point) No (0 points)
2. What is your weight status? (See the BMI chart in Figure 7.1 on p. 176.)?
   ____
   BMI is less than 25 (0 points)
   BMI is 25–29.9 (1 point)
   BMI is 30–39.9 (2 points)
   BMI is 40 or above (3 points)
3. Do you have a parent, brother, or sister with diabetes? ____________
   Yes (1 point) No (0 points)
4. Is your family background African American, Alaska Native, American Indian, Asian American, Hispanic/Latino, or Pacific Islander American? ____________
   Yes (1 point) No (0 points)
5. Have you had gestational diabetes? ____________
   Yes (1 point) No (0 points)
6. Have you given birth to at least one baby weighing more than 9 pounds?
   ____
   Yes (1 point) No (0 points)
7. Is your blood pressure 140/90 or higher, or have you been told that you have high blood pressure? ____________
   Yes (1 point) No (0 points) Don't know (1 point)
8. Are your cholesterol levels higher than normal? Is your HDL, or good, cholesterol, below 35, or is your triglyceride level above 250? ____________
   Yes (1 point) No (0 points) Don't know (1 point)
9. Are you fairly inactive? ____________
   Yes (1 point) No (0 points)
10. Do you have a history of cardiovascular disease? ____________
    Yes (1 point) No (0 points)
    Add up your score: ____________

HOW TO INTERPRET YOUR SCORE

The higher your score, the higher your risk for type 2 diabetes. If you scored 3 or higher, it is recommended that you take immediate action to reduce your risk for type 2 diabetes. If you answered "Don't know" to any questions, visit your health care provider to get checked.

Source: Adapted from *Am I at Risk for Type 2 Diabetes?*, by the National Diabetes Information Clearinghouse, U. S. Department of Health and Human Services, available at http://diabetes.niddk.nih.gov/dm/pubs/riskfortype2/index.aspx, and Diabetes Risk Test, by the American Diabetes Association, available at http://www.diabetes.org/diabetes-basics/prevention/diabetes-risk-test/risk-test-flyer-2012.pdf.

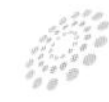

Take this self-assessment online at www.pearsonhighered.com/lynchelmore.

insulin, so less insulin is needed to clear glucose from the bloodstream. For these reasons, a personalized program of aerobic exercise is typically prescribed.

Oral medications. If someone with type 2 diabetes is not successful in losing weight, or weight loss doesn't reduce blood glucose significantly enough, the physician may prescribe an oral medication. Diabetes medications work in a variety of ways. Some, for instance, prompt the pancreas to manufacture and release more insulin, whereas others help increase the cells' response to insulin. If A1C tests continue to show, however, that medication isn't reducing blood glucose levels effectively, then the physician is likely to recommend a type 1 approach to treatment involving insulin therapy.

As you've seen, controlling diabetes requires consistent attention to diet, exercise, body weight, blood glucose levels, and all prescription therapies. But the rewards, including a longer life and a reduced risk of serious diabetes-related complications, are worth it.

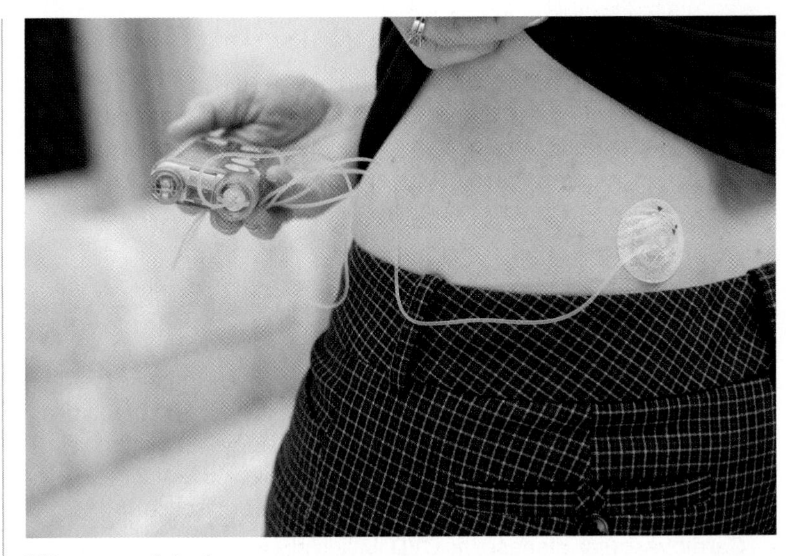

Figure 11.4 Controlling diabetes. Insulin pumps allow many people to control their blood glucose levels throughout the day without painful injections.

STUDENT STORY

A Family History of Diabetes

"Hi, I'm Michael. Chronic disease runs in my family, particularly diabetes on both my mom's and dad's sides. Just recently, my mom, my sister, and my dad were all diagnosed with type 2. It has affected me because I have to watch them take all their pills and recover from injuries and sicknesses and see the pain that they're going through, particularly with the circulation in their legs.

I am doing things to stop the risk of getting diabetes. I'm eating better. I'm exercising. I'm studying diabetes and other chronic diseases just to make sure that I protect myself to the fullest. I'm also teaching my mom and my dad as well about it.

I would tell other students to eat right, eat your fruits and vegetables, and exercise a minimum of 30 minutes a day every day, to help you fight against chronic diseases such as diabetes."

1: Why is it that Michael's family members are having problems with pain and circulation in their legs? What are other short- and long-term effects of diabetes?

2: Michael is paying attention to his diet and staying physically active. What else could he do to lower his risk for developing diabetes?

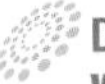

Do you have a story similar to Michael's? Share your story at www.pearsonhighered.com/lynchelmore.

Cardiovascular Disease

Every so often, a sad piece of news arrives. A favorite teacher from high school has died of a heart attack. A friend's grandmother has had a stroke. You take note of these losses, but you may not see any direct connection to your own health. After all, these people were a lot older than you, right? Their health issues are altogether different—aren't they?

The answer to that last question is a resounding "No." Although both heart attacks and strokes typically occur later in life, the conditions that lead to these events often begin to develop far earlier. As the rates of obesity and type 2 diabetes rise in children and adolescents, researchers are becoming increasingly concerned about an accompanying rise in cardiovascular disease. For instance, a 2006 study involving more than 2,000 youth with diabetes, aged 3 to 19, revealed that 21% already had at least two risk factors for cardiovascular disease.[12]

Cardiovascular disease, or **CVD,** is actually a group of disorders that includes hypertension (high blood pressure), coronary heart disease (including heart attacks), congestive heart failure, and stroke. It is present in nearly 15% of college-age males and nearly 9% of college-age females, and as we age, the prevalence skyrockets. Moreover, CVD is the leading cause of adult mortality in the United States, responsible for more than 3 in 10 deaths.[2]

Research shows that many college students don't realize their risks of joining this epidemic. One survey of undergraduates found that most rated their own risk as lower than that of their peers, an indication of thinking that CVD is "someone else's problem."[13] Two further studies found that female students tended to overestimate their risk of breast cancer but underestimate their risk of CVD.[14, 15] Rethinking your real risks may seem depressing, but it can actually be empowering. As with diabetes, cardiovascular disease is closely linked to lifestyle. By choosing to live healthfully now, you can reduce your risk for many forms of CVD.

A meaningful understanding of CVD requires that you become familiar with the structures and activities of your cardiovascular system.

The Healthy Cardiovascular System

The cardiovascular system is made up of blood vessels and the heart, which together form the blood-delivery network that keeps the body functioning. Blood, circulating through blood vessels, ferries oxygen, nutrients, and wastes to and from cells through **arteries,** which carry blood away from the heart, and **veins,** which carry blood back to the heart **(Figure 11.5a)**.

At the center of this system is the heart, which is only about the size of a fist, but is surprisingly strong. That's because it's almost entirely made up of a thick layer of muscle called the **myocardium.** The contractions of the myocardium keep blood moving, ensuring that it transports oxygen and nutrients to, and eliminates wastes from, every region of the body.

Although the heart is a single organ, it's surprisingly complex, consisting of four hollow, muscular chambers **(Figure 11.5b)**. The two upper chambers are the **atria.** Each atrium is connected by a valve to a corresponding lower chamber. These are the two **ventricles.** A thick wall of tissue divides the right-hand pair of chambers from the pair on the left, creating two side-by-side pumps. This division lets each side of the heart focus on a different task—either sending oxygen-poor blood to the lungs for replenishment or pumping that reoxygenated blood back out to the rest of the body.

Here's how the blood circulates (see Figure 11.5b). The right atrium receives oxygen-depleted blood from the superior and inferior vena cava, the largest veins in the body, and then pushes it to the right ventricle, which sends it into the pulmonary arteries, which take it to the lungs. There, blood cells collect freshly inhaled oxygen and dispense with carbon dioxide (a metabolic waste), which we exhale. Now the pulmonary veins bring the oxygen-rich blood to the left atrium and ventricle. They receive this blood and pump it out into the body via the aorta, a large artery that branches off into smaller arteries. These include the coronary arteries, which sustain the heart muscle itself.

The body's blood vessels divide into a network of smaller and smaller branches, eventually fanning out into **capillaries,** tiny blood vessels that deliver oxygen and nutrients to individual cells and collect their wastes. Once blood in the capillaries has exchanged oxygen and nutrients for wastes, it is returned to the heart via the veins. As with any system of pipes or tubes, the arteries, capillaries, and veins work best when they are free of blockage or damage, allowing blood to flow smoothly.

This entire process is complex—yet remarkably quick. The average person has about five to six quarts of blood, all of which is pumped by the heart throughout the body in a single minute. In adults at

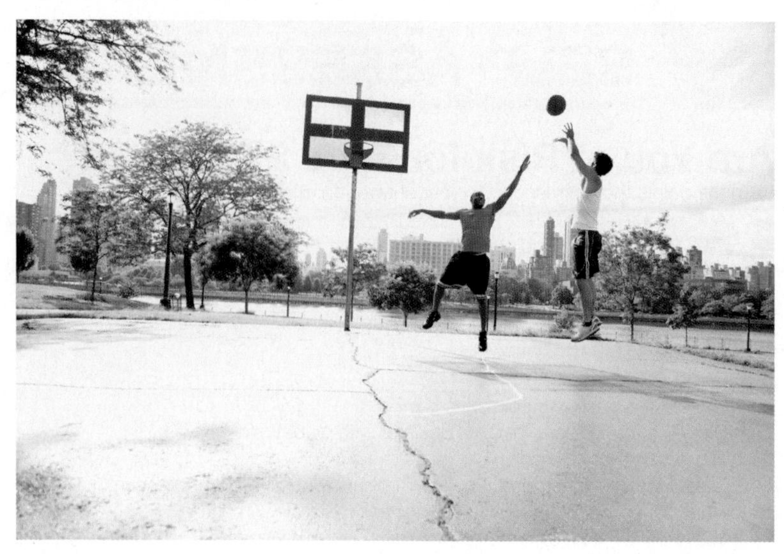

Aerobic exercise can help keep your cardiovascular system healthy.

cardiovascular disease (CVD) Diseases of the heart or blood vessels.

arteries Vessels that transport blood away from the heart, delivering oxygen-rich blood to the body periphery and oxygen-poor blood to the lungs.

veins Vessels that transport blood toward the heart, delivering oxygen-poor blood from the body periphery or oxygen-rich blood from the lungs.

myocardium The heart's muscle tissue.

atria The two upper chambers of the heart, which receive blood from the body periphery and lungs.

ventricles The two lower chambers of the heart, which pump blood to the body and lungs.

capillaries The smallest blood vessels, delivering blood and nutrients to individual cells and picking up wastes.

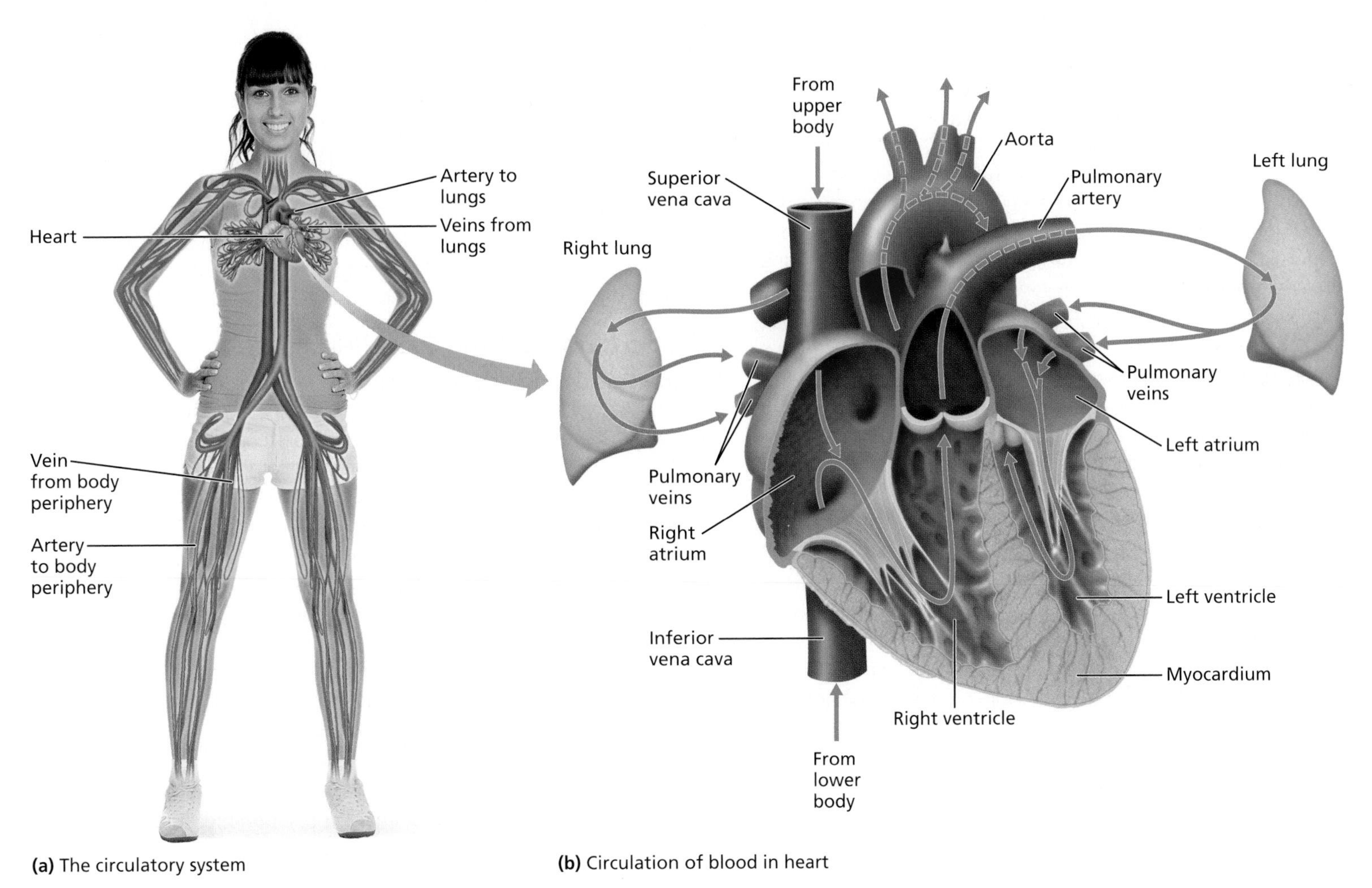

(a) The circulatory system

(b) Circulation of blood in heart

Figure 11.5 **The cardiovascular system.**

rest, the heart typically beats 60–120 times per minute, pumping a few ounces of blood with each beat until all the blood has been circulated. To keep up this rapid rhythm, the heart relies on electricity. A bundle of specialized cells in the heart's sinus node, located in the right atrium, generate electrical impulses and transmit them throughout the myocardium at a steady, even rate, setting the heart to beat about 100,000 times a day.

If your cardiovascular system is healthy, this delivery network generally runs smoothly. Your heart pumps strongly, and your blood vessels deliver blood efficiently. Your heartbeat thumps at the steady, even pace required for healthy blood flow through all parts of your body. But if damage occurs to even one part of this interconnected system, the entire network will begin to struggle to perform its functions. Next, we'll look at the physiologic mechanism that most commonly damages the cardiovascular system: atherosclerosis.

Atherosclerosis

Atherosclerosis is an arterial condition characterized by inflammation, scarring, and the buildup of mealy deposits along artery walls. In fact, the word's root, *athere,* is Greek for porridge! Together, these factors cause a narrowing of arteries, which restricts blood flow to cells and tissues "downstream" of the narrowed area. Cells starved of oxygen and nutrients cannot function; thus, when atherosclerosis affects the coronary arteries, the person can suffer a heart attack. When it affects arteries in the brain (cerebral arteries), the person can suffer a stroke.

Let's take a closer look at how atherosclerosis develops. The condition begins when the delicate inner lining of an artery becomes damaged. Although the cause of this damage is not always known, in some cases it is thought to result when **blood pressure**—the force of blood pulsating against the artery walls—is excessive. In others, it reflects the lining's encounter with irritants, and as you now know, a high level of blood glucose is a major irritant of blood vessels. Excessive lipids in the bloodstream, including triglycerides and cholesterol, can also irritate the vessel lining. In addition, the toxins in tobacco smoke and even certain types of infection can promote this initial damage.

The body responds to injury with inflammation, and at injured arterial sites, the resulting inflammation spreads into the artery wall. This leaves it

Watch a video showing how the heart and blood vessels work at www.mayoclinic.com/health/circulatory-system/MM00636.

atherosclerosis Condition characterized by narrowing of the arteries because of inflammation, scarring, and the buildup of fatty deposits.

blood pressure The force of the blood moving against the arterial walls.

weakened, scarred, and stiff (sclerotic). As a result, two types of lipids circulating in the bloodstream—triglycerides and cholesterol—can seep between the damaged lining cells and become trapped within the artery wall. Soon they are joined by white blood cells, calcium, and other substances. Eventually, this buildup, called *plaque,* narrows arteries significantly enough to impair blood flow **(Figure 11.6).** When this occurs in a coronary artery, the person may experience chest pain (called *angina*), weakness, shortness of breath, and other symptoms.

hypertension (high blood pressure) A persistent state of elevated blood pressure.

Plaque may build up to the point where it significantly blocks or even stops the flow of blood through an artery. This causes death of the tissues that are normally served by that vessel. Sometimes plaque can become hardened and rupture, causing microscopic tears in the artery wall that allow blood to leak into the tissue on the other side. When this happens, blood platelets rush to the site to clot the blood. This clot can obstruct the artery and—if it occurs in a coronary or cerebral artery—cause a sudden heart attack or stroke. Alternatively, softer plaque can break off and travel through the bloodstream until it blocks a more distant, smaller artery.

As noted earlier, cholesterol, a lipid made by the body and found in the food you eat, is a major component of plaque. We all need cholesterol for our bodies to function, but excessive amounts can be a key contributor to atherosclerosis. We'll look more closely at types of cholesterol, and what levels are considered healthful, when we talk about CVD detection and prevention later in this chapter.

Atherosclerosis is difficult to detect without specific medical tests, and most people who are developing the condition are unaware it is occurring. But researchers have found that the condition can start early in life, especially in people with known risk factors. For example, in one study of young adults (most were in their early 30s) who were overweight and had high blood glucose levels but otherwise appeared healthy, participants showed significant development of atherosclerosis in their cerebral arteries.[16]

If your physician suspects that you are developing atherosclerosis, you will likely be advised to improve the quality of your diet and increase your level of exercise. If your cholesterol levels are high and don't respond to lifestyle changes, cholesterol-lowering medications, most commonly *statins*, may help. Millions of people in the United States use statins to control cholesterol levels, but their use must be monitored for rare but serious side effects.

Atherosclerosis is dangerous because it directly contributes to each of the forms of CVD discussed next: hypertension (high blood pressure), coronary heart disease, congestive heart failure, and stroke. As you read about these disorders, bear in mind that they rarely develop in isolation; rather, one condition typically contributes to or occurs simultaneously with another. In addition, as noted earlier, the damage to the body's blood vessels caused by diabetes also contributes to CVD.

Hypertension (High Blood Pressure)

Hypertension, more commonly known as *high blood pressure,* is a chronic condition characterized by consistent blood pressure readings above normal. (We'll define normal and hypertensive readings shortly.) Hypertension in and of itself is considered a form of CVD. In addition, it's also a risk factor for other forms of CVD, including coronary heart disease, congestive heart failure, and stroke.

The level of your blood pressure is typically measured in an artery in your upper arm, but it's determined, in part, by the pumping actions of your heart. When your heart contracts, an action called *systole,* the pressure of the blood in your arteries momentarily increases. When it relaxes, an action called *diastole,* your blood pressure drops. But the force of your heart isn't the only actor. Blood pressure is also affected by the *compliance*—the ability to stretch and recoil—of your arteries.

We noted earlier that atherosclerosis can lead to both narrowing and stiffening of the arteries. When it does, blood pressure rises. To appreciate why, imagine the difference between trying to pump a pulsing stream of water into a network of wide, soft rubber tubes versus narrow, stiff metal pipes. The wide rubber tubing would stretch and bounce back with each pulsation, absorbing some of the pressure and allowing the turbulence to quickly settle down and the water to flow. In contrast, the narrow metal pipes would not accommodate the pulsating flow. This means the pump would have to work harder to propel the water against their resistance. Now imagine that atherosclerosis has stiffened your arteries and narrowed them with plaque! The more stiff and narrow your arteries become, the more they impede blood flow and drive your blood pressure up.

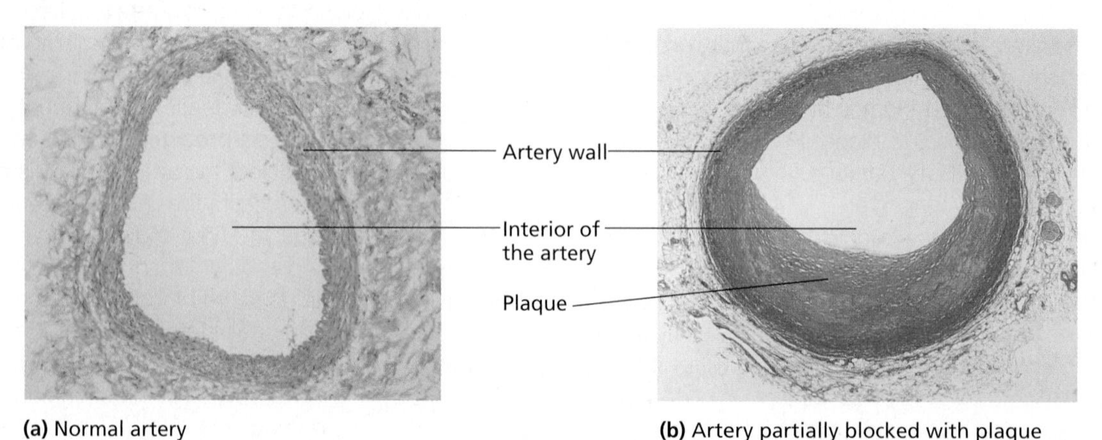

Figure 11.6 Atherosclerosis. These light micrographs show a cross section of (a) a normal artery allowing adequate blood flow and (b) an artery that is partially blocked with plaque, which can lead to a heart attack or stroke.

Signs and Symptoms of Hypertension

Most people with hypertension experience no symptoms. This fact, together with its contribution to heart attacks and strokes, explains the reputation of hypertension as a "silent killer." A very few people with dangerously advanced hypertension may experience headaches and dizziness.

Long-Term Effects of Hypertension

Left untreated, hypertension can lead to the other forms of CVD discussed in this section. It can also cause vision loss and kidney disease, and can reduce your ability to think clearly, remember, and learn.[17]

Risk Factors for Hypertension

Although atherosclerosis contributes to hypertension in many people, usually the causes aren't entirely clear. But your age, weight, ethnic background, and diet all play a role, with a high-sodium diet putting you at especially significant risk. In the United States, the prevalence of hypertension is rising, especially among women. One study found that almost 30% of the U.S. adult population, or about 73 million people, have hypertension, with increased body weight emerging as a key factor in this trend.[18] Though risk for everyone rises with age, more and more young people are also developing the condition. One study of hypertension in young people found that as many as 1.5 million children and teenagers in the United States may have the condition, and many of them don't know it.[19]

Clinical Management of Hypertension

How do physicians diagnose hypertension? Blood pressure is measured using a stethoscope and a device called a *sphygmomanometer.* Readings are recorded in millimeters of mercury (mm Hg). The systolic pressure—the pressure in your arteries as your heart contracts—is given first, and the diastolic pressure—the pressure when the heart is momentarily relaxed—is given second. So "125 over 70" means your systolic pressure is 125 and your diastolic is 70. Incidentally, this reading would qualify as prehypertension, even though, as you can see in **Table 11.1,** a diastolic reading of 70 is normal. In other words, if either number is elevated, the reading is considered abnormal.

Most physicians recommend that patients with hypertension follow a balanced, low-sodium diet. Sodium is an essential mineral, but if consumed in excess, it draws water out of cells and into the bloodstream. This increases the total volume of your blood, and therefore the pressure that your blood exerts against the walls of your arteries. Sodium is bound to chloride in table salt, but is also a prominent ingredient in most processed foods, from tomato soup to macaroni-and-cheese dinners. The DASH diet from the National Institutes of Health is a low-sodium diet that has been shown in numerous studies to reduce blood pressure. DASH stands for "Dietary Approaches to Stop Hypertension," and its menus provide no more than 2,300 mg of sodium per day.[20] The 2010 *Dietary Guidelines for Americans* suggests that people with hypertension, as well as African Americans and all Americans over age 50, consume no more than 1,500 mg per day. Over 95% of American adults consume more than their recommended amount of sodium (1,500 or 2,300 mg) per day.[21]

Download a colorful guide to the DASH eating plan at www.nhlbi.nih.gov/health/public/heart/hbp/dash/new_dash.pdf.

In addition to a diet low in sodium, people with hypertension should follow a diet with an appropriate number of calories to help them achieve and maintain a healthy weight. Regular moderate exercise can also help reduce blood pressure and body weight. Smoking damages blood vessels, and anyone with hypertension who smokes should seek professional help to quit. Alcohol consumption should not exceed one drink per day for women and two drinks for men. Drinking in excess of this level raises blood pressure.[22]

Many patients with hypertension take prescription medications. Some of the most common are diuretics (commonly called "water pills"), which help the body to eliminate sodium and water. This in turn reduces the total volume of blood flowing within the arteries. Other medications work by helping to relax and dilate blood vessels, and still others slow the heartbeat. These prescription medications can help control hypertension, but many doctors recommend a remedy straight off the drugstore shelf: low-dose aspirin. Although better known as a pain reliever, aspirin also works as a mild blood thinner.

coronary heart disease (coronary artery disease) Atherosclerosis of the arteries that feed the heart.

angina pectoris Chest pain due to coronary heart disease.

Table 11.1: Blood Pressure Classification

Classification	Systolic Reading (mm Hg)		Diastolic Reading (mm Hg)
Normal	< 120	and	< 80
Prehypertension	120–139	or	80–89
Hypertension			
Stage 1	140–159	or	90–99
Stage 2	≥ 160	or	≥ 100

Source: Data from *The Seventh Report of the Joint National Committee on Prevention, Detection, Evaluation, and Treatment of High Blood Pressure* (NIH Publication No. 03-5233), by the National Heart, Lung, and Blood Institute, 2005 (Bethesda, MD: National Institutes of Health).

Coronary Heart Disease

Of all types of CVD, **coronary heart disease (CHD)** causes the most deaths **(Figure 11.7).** In fact, CHD is the single leading cause of death in the United States. The American Heart Association estimates that the condition causes about 1 out of every 6 deaths and kills more than 405,000 people each year.[23]

Also called *coronary artery disease,* CHD arises when plaque in the coronary arteries builds up to the point that it impairs the heart's ability to function. Partial coronary artery blockages can cause *angina,* or chest pain that occurs when the heart muscle doesn't get enough blood. Larger or even total blockages can trigger a *myocardial infarction* (heart attack) or a disruption in heart rhythm known as *sudden cardiac arrest.* We'll look at these conditions next.

Angina

If your coronary arteries have been narrowed or obstructed, they can still deliver some blood to your heart—but not necessarily as much as this powerful muscle needs. If your heart's need for nutrients and oxygen exceeds what your coronary arteries can provide, you may feel chest pain, or **angina pectoris.** Angina can feel like pressure or like a

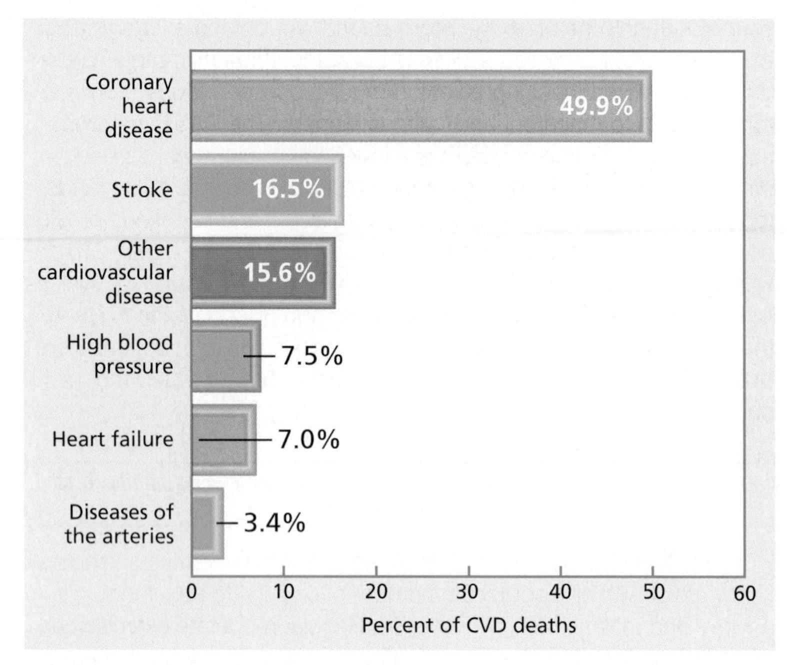

Figure 11.7 Deaths from cardiovascular disease in the U.S. The majority of deaths resulted from coronary heart disease.

Source: Data from: *Heart Disease and Stroke Statistics: 2012 Update,* by the American Heart Association, 2012. Used with permission.

squeezing pain in the chest. These sensations can also radiate out to your shoulders, arms, neck, jaw, or back, or even resemble indigestion.

myocardial infarction (MI) (heart attack) A cardiac crisis in which a region of heart muscle is damaged or destroyed by reduced blood flow.

Nearly 7 million people in the United States suffer from angina. Once considered more of a health concern for men, recent research has found that angina is equally common in women.[24]

Angina itself may not be life-threatening, but it signals that a person is at greater risk of a life-threatening cardiac event. If angina isn't correctly recognized or treated, the arterial narrowing behind it may progress to a full blockage, leading to the next condition we'll discuss—heart attack.

Myocardial Infarction (Heart Attack)

When blockage of a coronary artery deprives a region of the myocardium of its blood supply, that region can stop working effectively. Its cells can even die if they go too long without blood and the oxygen and nutrients it carries. During a heart attack, or **myocardial infarction (MI),** the more time that passes without treatment to restore blood flow, the greater the damage. Warning signs of a heart attack include angina, discomfort in the chest or other parts of the upper body, shortness of breath, and sweating, nausea, or dizziness. Chest pain, which is a hallmark symptom in men, doesn't occur as often in women, who are somewhat more likely to experience less specific forms of pain and discomfort **(Figure 11.8).** Because of this, women are more likely to be

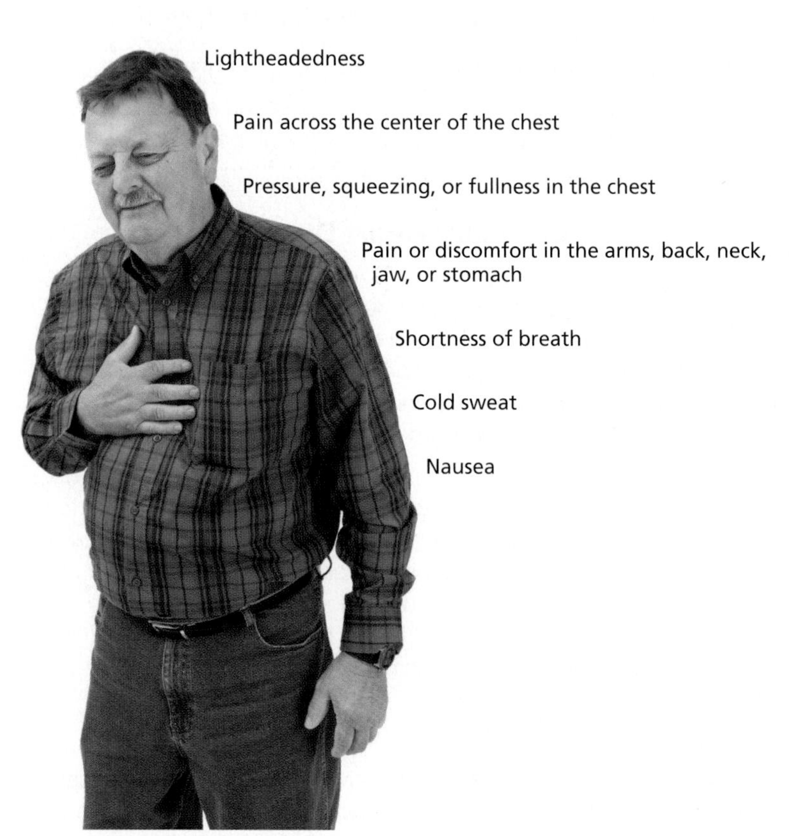

(a) Warning signs in men

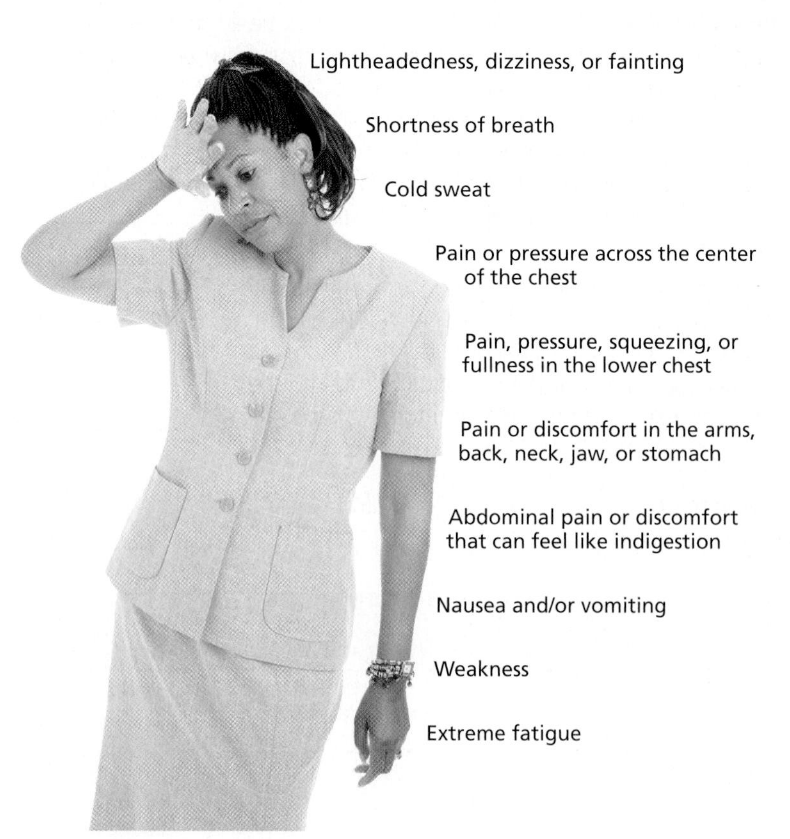

(b) Warning signs in women

Figure 11.8 Warning signs of a heart attack differ somewhat in men and women. These warning signs can occur individually, or several can occur simultaneously.

misdiagnosed and released from emergency rooms with unrecognized acute myocardial infarctions.

When a heart attack strikes, it may seem sudden. But as you are learning in this chapter, a heart attack is actually the end result of a steady, silent buildup of CVD, often over many years or even decades. According to the American Heart Association, more than 1.2 million people in the United States have a heart attack each year, and many die as a result.[23] Those who survive often continue to face significant health risks and functional impairment as they try to recover. The good news is that the U.S. death rate from heart attack has dropped in recent years. We'll discuss the prevention and control of CVD shortly.

Arrhythmia and Sudden Cardiac Arrest

If the heart is starved of blood, its muscle wall isn't the only aspect of its structure that is at risk. The nerve cells that set the pace of the heart's pumping can also be affected, resulting in an irregular heartbeat called an **arrhythmia.** As you learned earlier, your heartbeat is regulated by your sinus node, which sets a series of electrical currents flowing through your heart in a steady, even pattern. If this electrical conduction is disrupted, your heart can beat too slowly, too quickly, or unevenly. Arrhythmias come in many forms that affect different aspects of the heart's function, and some are more serious than others. More than 2 million people in the United States live with some form of arrhythmia.[25]

A slow heart rate of less than 60 beats per minute is called **bradycardia.** A fast heart rate—more than 100 beats per minute—is called **tachycardia.** An especially dangerous type of tachycardia is *fibrillation*. In fibrillation, an improper electrical signal causes either the atria or the ventricles to contract so quickly and unevenly that they quiver rather than pump, unable to move blood effectively. Many people live with atrial fibrillation and have no symptoms at all, or symptoms that are troubling but not life-threatening, such as palpitations or fainting spells. In contrast, ventricular fibrillation completely stops heart functioning and is a medical emergency. It is the most common type of arrhythmia seen in cases of **sudden cardiac arrest.** The person's heart must be restarted within 6 minutes via electrical shock to prevent death. Even if the heart is restarted within 6 minutes, the patient may sustain irreversible brain damage from lack of oxygen to the brain.

Many factors increase the risk for arrhythmias. These include stress, smoking, genetic factors, heavy alcohol use, strenuous exercise, certain medications, and even air pollution. But atherosclerosis and coronary heart disease, which affect how well your heart is nourished, are especially important factors.

Clinical Management of CHD

The diagnosis and treatment of CHD depends on the precise form it takes: angina, MI, or sudden cardiac arrest. So let's look at each separately.

Management of angina. Because chest pain can be due to a respiratory infection or other cause unrelated to CHD, a physician will conduct one or more tests before making the diagnosis of angina. An **electrocardiogram,** also called an *ECG* (or *EKG*), measures the heart's electrical activity. This test can detect not only arrhythmias, but other problems such as restricted blood flow. You can take an ECG while sitting quietly, which will give you a baseline measurement, or have the test done while you are exercising. This more vigorous form, called a *stress test*, shows how your heart performs under increased physical demands. An *echocardiogram* may be done during the stress test, to produce images of the heart using sound waves. You may also have a chest X-ray to rule out other conditions and to check the size of your heart, which can be enlarged in some types of CVD.

Whether angina is mild or severe, lifestyle changes can help. These include weight loss, eating a healthy diet, engaging in a prescribed gentle, safe exercise plan, avoiding smoking, and managing blood glucose levels. The first medication a physician might try is aspirin, which helps prevent blood clots and improves blood flow. You may also have heard of people with angina placing nitroglycerin tablets under their tongue or using a nitroglycerin spray: These work by dilating blood vessels. Statins, which we mentioned in the treatment of atherosclerosis, may be prescribed to reduce blood cholesterol, and beta blockers may be needed to help slow the heartbeat. Other prescription drugs can be tried to relax the muscles of the blood vessel walls.

Management of an MI. When a person arrives in a hospital emergency department complaining of chest pains, the ER team typically hooks the person up to a heart monitor, administers oxygen so that the heart doesn't have to work as hard, and provides medication—typically by IV—to relieve the pain. A variety of tests may then be performed. A special blood test can determine if there is damage to the heart muscle indicative of an MI, and a test of the blood vessels, called *coronary angiography* (*angio-* refers to a vessel), may be done to see how and where the blood is being blocked from flowing through the heart.[26]

In patients whose arteries are dangerously obstructed, procedures are available to open them. One common artery procedure, called a **balloon angioplasty,** involves threading a catheter through the artery and inflating a small balloon at the obstructed spot, flattening plaque against the arterial walls and opening the vessel **(Figure 11.9).** To keep the vessel open, the physician may place a *stent,* a small metal tube that keeps the plaque flat, in the vessel. Some stents contain slow-release medication to further reduce the risk of blockage.

If a blockage is extremely dangerous, especially if it involves coronary arteries, **bypass surgery** may be recommended. This procedure circumvents the blocked vessel rather than opening it. Using a healthy blood vessel from another part of your body, the surgeon builds an alternative route for blood to flow around the arterial obstruction. If more than one artery is blocked, multiple bypasses can be performed.

Once the immediate crisis has been resolved, a special program of *cardiac rehabilitation* may be advised. In "cardiac rehab," patients learn to make lifestyle changes to improve their cardiovascular health. A physical activity program is usually designed, and is tailored to the patient's abilities and needs. The activity is initially performed in a clinical setting to ensure that heart rate and blood pressure remain in healthful ranges. Over time, the patient progresses to more strenuous activity. Counseling and support

arrhythmia Any irregularity in the heart's rhythm.

bradycardia A slow arrhythmia.

tachycardia A fast arrhythmia.

sudden cardiac arrest A life-threatening cardiac crisis marked by loss of heartbeat and unconsciousness.

electrocardiogram (ECG) A test that measures the heart's electrical activity.

balloon angioplasty An arterial treatment that uses a small balloon to flatten plaque deposits against the arterial wall.

bypass surgery A procedure to build new pathways for blood to flow around areas of arterial blockage.

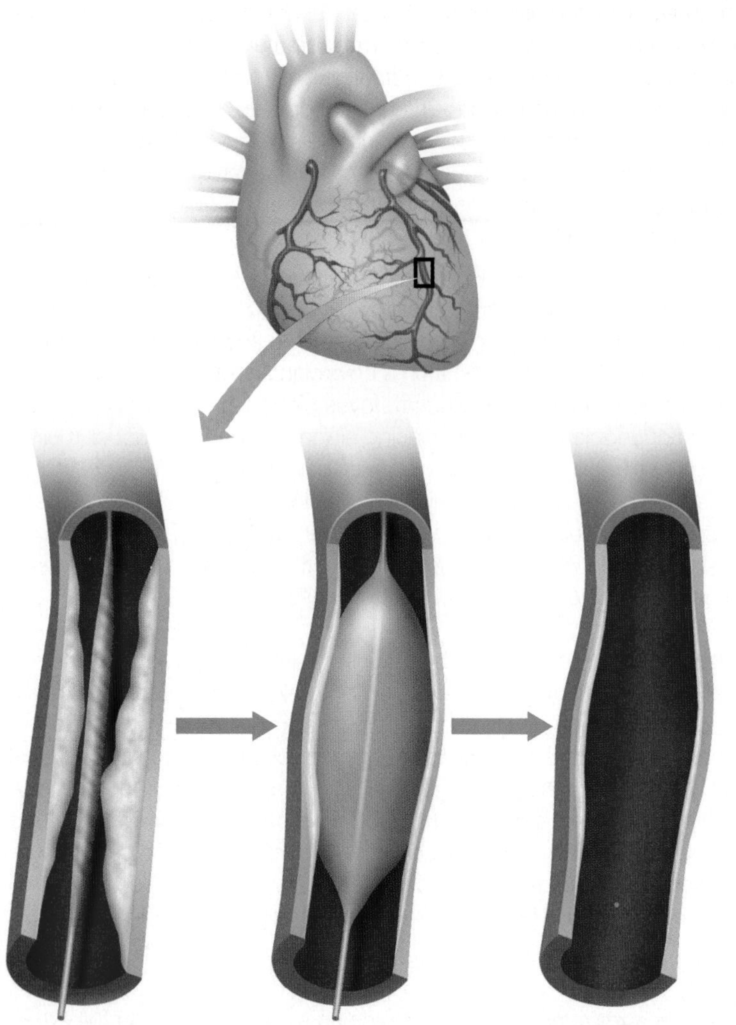

Balloon-tipped catheter inserted into artery narrowed by plaque

Balloon is inflated, pushing plaque against artery lining

Balloon is deflated and removed, leaving artery open

Figure 11.9 **Balloon angioplasty.**

are also offered. Low-dose daily aspirin or other medications may also be prescribed.

Management of sudden cardiac arrest. In cases of sudden cardiac arrest, there is rarely time for transport to a hospital emergency department. The person's heart must be restarted within minutes with a device called an *automated external defibrillator* (*AED*), or the person will die. This device sends an electric shock to the heart and can restore a normal heartbeat, allowing time for transport to a medical center. Public places, including college campuses, usually have AEDs, but for obvious reasons, their location must be generally known and immediately accessible. Police, firefighters, and emergency medical technicians usually are trained and equipped to use a defibrillator.

If a person suddenly loses consciousness, failing to respond when asked if okay, tilt his or her head upright. If the person does not take a normal breath within 5 seconds, he or she may be experiencing a sudden cardiac arrest. If an AED is not available, the American Heart Association recommends that you call 9-1-1 and then begin "hands-only" CPR. The technique is simple, involving only pushing hard and fast in the center of the victim's chest until help arrives.

If you have 2 minutes to spare, you can learn "hands-only" CPR. Watch this video from the American Heart Association at http://handsonlycpr.org.

If a person survives a sudden cardiac arrest, hospital staff will attempt to determine the cause. If the cause is found to be an MI, then treatment will be similar to that described above. The patient may also have surgery to place an *implantable cardioverter defibrillator* (*ICD*), which is similar to a pacemaker, but transmits stronger electric pulses to help prevent further dangerous arrhythmias. For information on helping someone "on the scene" in a CVD emergency, see page 308.

Congestive Heart Failure

All of the conditions we've just discussed can be serious on their own. But they can also contribute to a gradual loss of heart function. In **congestive heart failure,** the heart can no longer pump enough blood to meet the body's needs. As a result, blood may pool—or become congested—in other areas of the body, such as the lungs, the abdomen, or the arms and legs. This pooled blood quickly becomes depleted of oxygen and nutrients, so the affected regions become damaged and unable to function properly. More than 6 million adults in the United States live with congestive heart failure.[23]

congestive heart failure A gradual loss of heart function.

We noted earlier that the forms of CVD are interrelated, and indeed a common cause of congestive heart failure is CHD, which damages heart muscle, reducing its ability to beat strongly. Persistent tachycardia may also cause the heart to work too hard, slowly wearing it out. However, a landmark heart health study found that hypertension, which forces the heart to work harder than it should to pump blood against resistance, is the most common risk factor for congestive heart failure. Less than one-third of adults found to have hypertension-related heart failure are still alive 5 years after their diagnosis.[27] Other factors, including having diabetes or an infection that triggers inflammation of your heart muscle, can also cause heart failure.

Regardless of the cause, a failing heart results in a failing body. When congestion occurs in the arms and legs, they swell with fluid. Fluid pooling in the lungs makes it difficult to breathe. The abdomen may swell, and the person may gain "water weight." Heart failure also typically causes weakness and exhaustion, loss of appetite, and an inability to concentrate or stay alert. Thus, the individual may find it difficult to perform everyday tasks.

A low-sodium diet, smoking cessation, and maintenance of a healthful weight are all essential in slowing the progress of congestive heart failure. The physician may prescribe diuretics to rid the body of excessive sodium and water, and beta blockers and other prescription medications to slow the heartbeat, dilate blood vessels, and reduce the total workload on the heart. If congestive heart failure cannot be managed with lifestyle changes and medication, heart surgery may be necessary, either to open blocked coronary arteries or to insert a pacemaker or ICD.[28]

Stroke

As you've learned in this chapter, a blockage in an artery that feeds the heart can cause angina, a heart attack, or even sudden cardiac arrest. What would

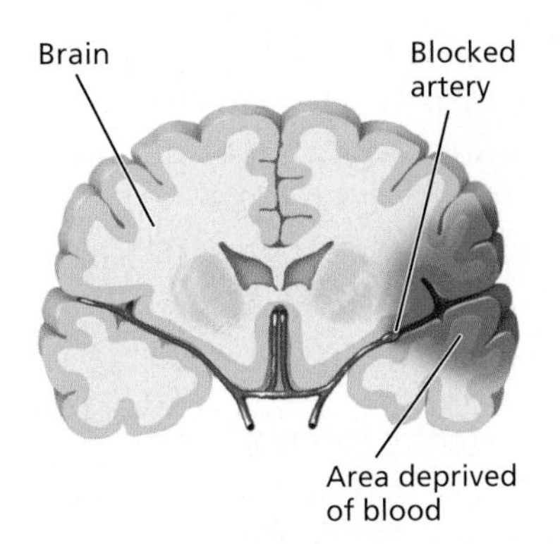

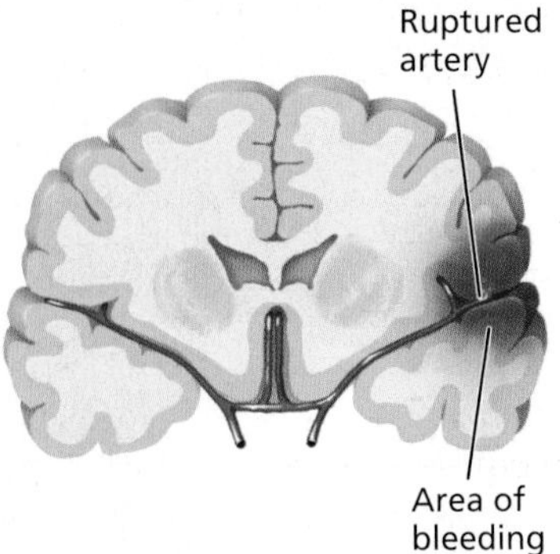

Figure 11.10 Two types of stroke. (a) In an ischemic stroke, a blocked artery damages brain tissue by depriving it of blood. (b) In a hemorrhagic stroke, a ruptured artery damages brain tissue by flooding it with too much blood.

happen if a similar obstruction or other serious damage hit an artery serving the brain? The answer is a **stroke,** a medical emergency in which the blood supply to a part of the brain ceases.

Types of Stroke

Strokes can take either of two forms **(Figure 11.10).**

Ischemic stroke. In **ischemic stroke,** either a cerebral artery or one of the carotid arteries that run through the neck into the brain becomes blocked. The blockage may be due to either of two materials:

- A *thrombus* is a clot that originates in the affected artery, usually as a result of atherosclerosis.
- An *embolus* is a plug of foreign matter such as a detached blood clot or other debris that originates in a larger vessel and is swept into a narrowed cerebral artery, entirely obstructing it.

In either case, all brain tissues normally served by the blocked artery become starved of oxygen and nutrients. Ischemic strokes represent about 80% of the more than 700,000 strokes that occur each year in the United States.[29]

Hemorrhagic stroke. The term *hemorrhage* means uncontrolled bleeding. In **hemorrhagic stroke,** a cerebral artery ruptures, spilling blood into brain tissue and depriving of oxygen and nutrients regions that would normally have been served by the broken vessel. In some cases, the bleeding occurs in an area of surface brain tissue and seeps into the space immediately beneath the skull. The two most common causes of hemorrhagic stroke are uncontrolled hypertension and the presence of an *aneurysm,* a weak spot in an artery wall that may rupture.

stroke A medical emergency in which blood flow to or in the brain is impaired. Also called a *cerebral vascular accident (CVA)*.

ischemic stroke A stroke caused by a blocked blood vessel.

hemorrhagic stroke A stroke caused by a ruptured blood vessel.

transient ischemic attack (TIA) A temporary episode of strokelike symptoms, indicative of high stroke risk.

Signs and Symptoms of an Impending Stroke

Brain cells deprived of blood quickly die. The outward signs of stroke often portray this damage as it unfolds. A person having a stroke may suddenly feel weak, numb, or paralyzed in the arm, leg, or face, especially on one side of the body. He or she may stumble and have other difficulty walking. Vision may become blurry, or the person may start seeing double. Slurred speech is a common sign, as is an inability to find the right words or to repeat a simple sentence. A sudden and severe headache is also common, and may be accompanied by dizziness or vomiting. Consciousness may be altered, and the person may suddenly seem confused or experience delusions.

Some people at risk for stroke may experience a fleeting episode of a milder version of these symptoms days, weeks, or months before having a full stroke. Such a mini-stroke, known as a **transient ischemic attack,** or TIA, isn't always easy to recognize, but it is a clear warning sign of an impending stroke.

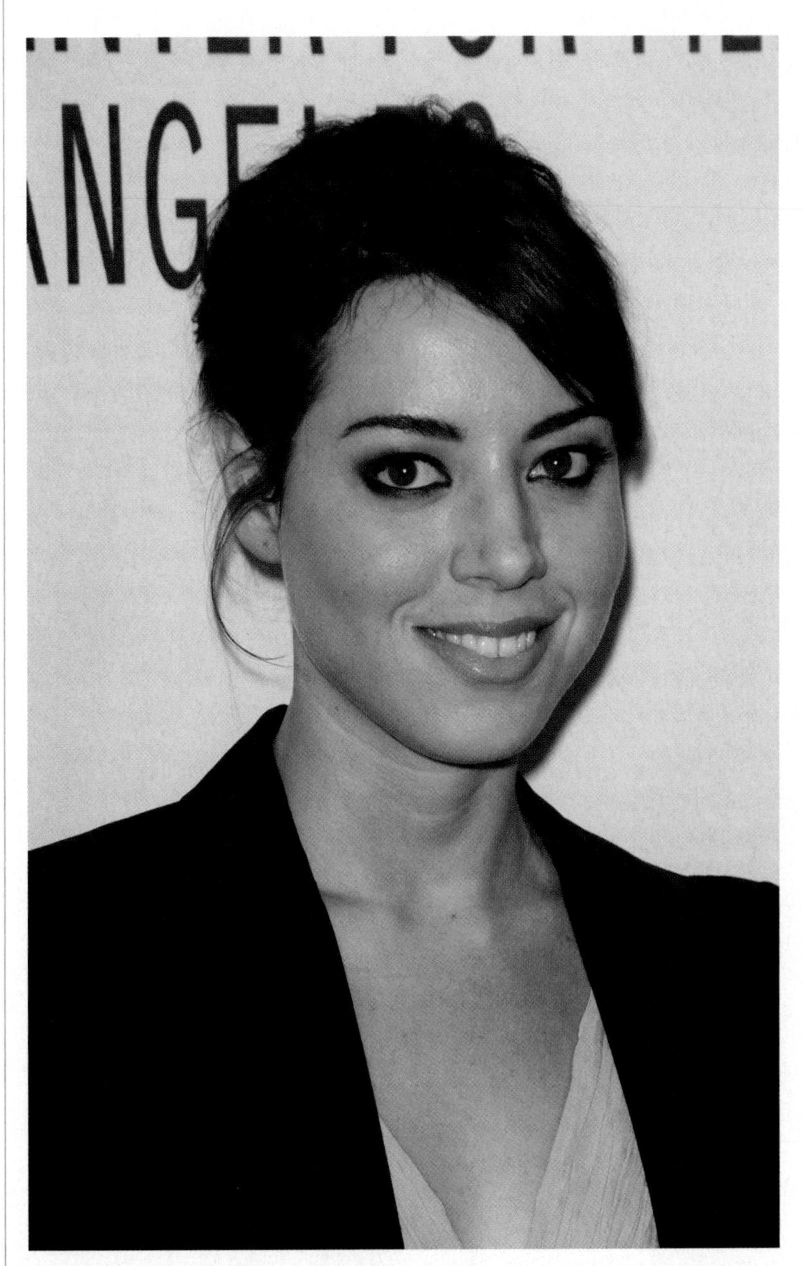

Being young doesn't mean you're immune from cardiovascular disease. Aubrey Plaza, one of the stars of TV's Parks and Recreation, suffered a **stroke** when she was only 20 years old.

Helping Someone in a CVD Emergency

We all know that someone showing signs of a heart attack, cardiac arrest, or stroke needs to head for the nearest hospital. But before the person is under medical care, you can take steps to help.

- If you see someone showing the signs of a heart attack, cardiac arrest, or stroke, the first thing you should do is call 9-1-1. If possible, make this call from a land line, not a cell phone. Land line calls to 9-1-1 are usually routed straight to local emergency dispatch centers, whereas calls from cell phones are often routed to local highway safety agencies, who must then reroute the call to the correct dispatch center, sometimes costing valuable time.
- Once you call 9-1-1, wait with the person until emergency medical services arrive rather than driving to the hospital yourself. Paramedic and ambulance units have lifesaving equipment and skills that they can deploy immediately and sustain during the trip to the hospital. If you drive the person to the hospital, he or she can't benefit from this faster access to medical help.

In addition, here are ways you can help in specific types of emergencies:

Heart Attack

- Although the symptoms of a heart attack aren't always clear cut, don't hesitate to call 9-1-1 if you suspect one is occurring. Trying a "wait and see" approach could cost the person important time and even raise his or her risk of cardiac arrest.
- Have the person chew an aspirin, unless he or she is allergic to aspirin or is under medical orders to avoid it. Aspirin has blood-thinning properties that can help in a heart attack. The drug used must be aspirin, not another type of pain reliever.
- Have the person take nitroglycerin, but only if already prescribed. This drug is often used in people with CVD.
- If the person falls unconscious, begin "hands-only" CPR. If you don't know how, ask the dispatcher to instruct you on the proper technique until help arrives.

Sudden Cardiac Arrest

- If you suspect cardiac arrest, call 9-1-1 immediately. People in cardiac arrest need their heart restarted within 6 minutes or they will die.
- Check the unconscious person for a pulse *after* you call 9-1-1. The side of the neck is a more reliable place to feel for a pulse than the wrist.
- If you don't find a pulse, begin "hands-only" CPR. If you need help, the 9-1-1 dispatcher will instruct you on the proper technique until help arrives.
- If you are in a public place such as a campus or office building, an airport, or a shopping mall, ask someone nearby to look for a device called an *automated external defibrillator*, or AED. AEDs are electrical heart-starting machines, and they are designed for anyone to use. Just open the box and follow the instructions. Don't worry about shocking someone unnecessarily—AEDs are designed to scan for a heartbeat and not deliver a shock if a heartbeat is detected.

Stroke

- The signs of stroke aren't always obvious, but if you suspect a stroke, call 9-1-1 immediately. The faster medical help arrives, the more likely it is that permanent brain damage can be avoided.
- Make note of the time you first noticed the symptoms. This information is vital for paramedics and doctors trying to provide treatment as fast as possible.
- While you wait for help, don't administer cardiac aid such as "hands-only" CPR unless the person goes into cardiac arrest. A person having a stroke may be disoriented or have trouble moving, but CPR should be reserved for people who are unconscious and have no pulse. Otherwise, it could be harmful.

References: **1.** "Cardiopulmonary Resuscitation (CPR): First Aid," by the Mayo Clinic, 2010, retrieved from http://www.mayoclinic.com/health/first-aid-cpr/FA00061. **2.** "Heart Attack First Aid," by Medline Plus, 2010, retrieved from http://www.nlm.nih.gov/medlineplus/ency/article/000063.htm. **3.** "How to Use an Automated External Defibrillator," by the National Heart, Lung, and Blood Institute, (n.d.), retrieved from http://www.nhlbi.nih.gov/health/dci/Diseases/aed/aed_use.html. **4.** "Stroke: Preventing and Treating 'Brain Attack'," by Harvard Health Publications, (n.d.), retrieved from http://www.harvardhealthcontent.com/70,BA0908?Page=Section1. **5.** "Learn to Recognize a Stroke," by the American Stroke Association, 2010, retrieved from http://www.strokeassociation.org/presenter.jhtml?identifier=1020.

Long-Term Effects of a Stroke

Prompt treatment can greatly reduce the long-term effects of a stroke. Depending on the severity of the stroke, how long the brain was deprived of oxygen, and the quality of follow-up health care, the person may experience a range of effects, including:

- Temporary or resistant paralysis, especially on one side of the body
- Impaired speaking, swallowing, and chewing, due to difficulty controlling the muscles of the mouth and throat
- *Aphasia*, a difficulty in understanding and expressing ideas in spoken or written words
- Loss of memory and the ability to reason and make decisions
- Pain, cold, and other uncomfortable sensations, especially on the side of the body affected by the stroke
- Personality changes, including dependency and impulsivity

Rehabilitation efforts, including speech therapy and physical and occupational therapy, can help reduce some of these effects, but many people who survive a stroke must learn to live with some level of disability and discomfort.

Clinical Management of a Stroke

Anyone showing signs of a TIA or stroke requires immediate medical attention to prevent or reduce brain damage. In addition to a physical examination, blood tests will be conducted to check the patient's clotting response and to rule out other problems such as infection. The physician may order one or more types of scans. For example, in a *computerized tomography angiography* (*CTA*), a dye is injected into the patient's circulation prior to scanning to help reveal narrowed or ruptured cerebral arteries. In *magnetic resonance imaging* (*MRI*), a scan using radio waves may detect areas of damaged brain tissue.

In an ischemic stroke, the goal of emergency treatment is to open the blocked cerebral artery and restore blood flow to that area of the brain. Believe it or not, aspirin is the best-proven immediate treatment for ischemic stroke. If the patient is treated within 4.5 hours, the physician may also administer an injection of a clot-busting drug that can help the patient recover more fully. In some cases, the physician may be able to thread a device into the brain that can grab and remove the clot.[30]

In a hemorrhagic stroke, aspirin is never given, as it promotes bleeding. Instead, drugs are used to reduce the force of blood moving into the damaged area, to help control the bleeding, and to prevent seizures. Surgery can sometimes repair the ruptured vessel, or the surgeon may be able to clip the aneurysm, isolating it from the rest of the circulation and preventing further bleeding.[30]

Once a stroke patient is stabilized, rehabilitation can begin. This often requires admission to a special rehabilitation unit or facility, where the patient works with a neurologist and a variety of therapists to improve speech, movement, etc.

Other Forms of Cardiovascular Disease

Less common types of CVD in the United States include the following:

- **Congenital heart disease.** About 9 in every 1,000 babies are born with some type of heart defect.[31] Some of the more frequent forms these defects take include holes in the walls that divide the chambers of the heart, abnormal narrowing of the coronary arteries, and malformations of the arteries that connect the heart and lungs. Most congenital heart defects can now be accurately diagnosed and treated with drugs or surgery.
- **Heart valve disorders.** Blood flows through your heart in only one direction, from atrium to ventricle, because the chambers of your heart are gated with valves. These flaps of connective tissue swing open and shut like one-way doors, allowing blood to pass from atrium to ventricle but preventing it from pooling or streaming backward. Congenital defects, infections, or heart disease can damage these. In some cases, a valve may let too little blood pass. In others, a valve may leak. Medications can ease some valve problems, whereas more serious malfunctions may require surgical repair or replacement.
- **Hypertrophic cardiomyopathy.** Up to half a million Americans have hypertrophic cardiomyopathy (HCM), a genetic disorder in which the heart muscle cells grow excessively, resulting in a thick, stiffened muscle wall that cannot pump enough blood during vigorous activity, especially exercise. Children with HCM are not allowed to play competitive sports but in some cases may be allowed to participate in moderate physical activity. This restriction is critical, because HCM can cause sudden death in an athlete. Although there is no cure, medications can help manage the symptoms.[32]
- **Rheumatic heart disease.** Although it is rare in the United States, around the globe rheumatic heart disease is the leading cause of cardiovascular death among people younger than age 50.[33] It begins when a bacterial infection—caused by the same *Streptococcus* bacterium that causes strep throat—flares into rheumatic fever. Along with an elevated temperature, the illness causes inflammation of connective tissues throughout the body. Sometimes that damage includes the heart valves. Rheumatic heart disease is easily prevented by taking antibiotics in the early stages of a strep infection, stopping it before it can progress to rheumatic fever.
- **Peripheral artery disease.** Along with the heart and brain, blood vessels throughout the body can suffer from damage due to atherosclerosis, hypertension, and high blood glucose. Peripheral artery disease (PAD) is a narrowing and stiffening of the arteries that serve the legs and feet. This causes pain, aching, burning, and tingling sensations that are sometimes severe, and in advanced cases can occur even when the person is at rest. Poorly managed diabetes is a significant risk factor in PAD, as is smoking. As we discussed earlier, damage to peripheral blood vessels increases the risk for nonhealing wounds, tissue death, and surgical amputation of the toes, foot, or leg.

Risk Factors for Cardiovascular Disease

This section identifies the risk factors for CVD—including those you can't change and those you can. We've encountered many of them already, in our discussion of type 2 diabetes. And as we'll see shortly, several of them are defining factors in cardiometabolic risk.

- **Your age.** Most cases of heart attack, sudden cardiac arrest, and stroke occur in people older than 65. You can't stop yourself from aging, but you can work to make sure every year of life is as healthy as possible.
- **Your sex.** Men face greater heart attack risks than women, and they tend to have heart attacks earlier in life. However, CVD is still the top killer of women in the United States over the course of their lifetime, and women need to pay attention to CVD risks as well. The

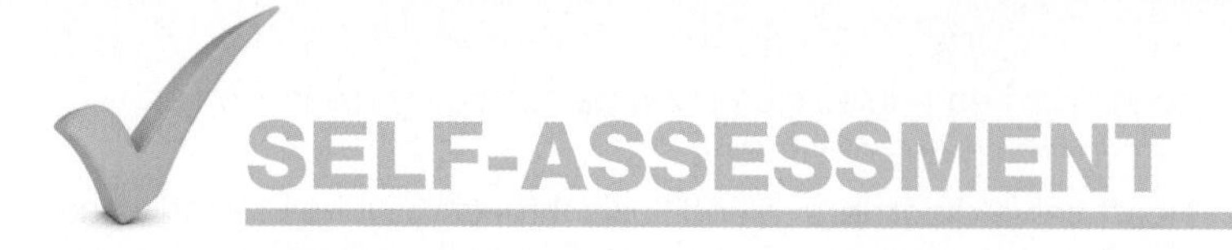

What's Your Risk for a Heart Attack?

Circle your answers.

1.	Do you smoke?	Yes	No	
2.	Is your blood pressure 140/90 mmHg or higher, OR have you been told by your doctor that your blood pressure is too high?	Yes	No	Don't Know
3.	Has your doctor told you that your LDL ("bad") cholesterol is too high, OR that your total cholesterol level is 200 mg/dL or higher, OR that your HDL ("good") cholesterol is less than 40 mg/dL?	Yes	No	Don't Know
4.	Has your father or brother had a heart attack before age 55, OR has your mother or sister had one before age 65?	Yes	No	Don't Know
5.	Are you over 55 years old?	Yes	No	
6.	Do you have a BMI score of 25 or more? (See Figure 7.1 on page 176)	Yes	No	Don't Know
7.	Do you get less than a total of 30 minutes of moderate-intensity physical activity on most days?	Yes	No	Not Sure
8.	Has a doctor told you that you have angina (chest pains), OR have you had a heart attack?	Yes	No	Don't Know

HOW TO INTERPRET YOUR SCORE

If you circled any of the "Yes" answers, you're at an increased risk of having a heart attack. If you circled "Don't Know" for any questions, ask your doctor for help in answering them.

Source: Adapted from *The Healthy Heart Handbook for Women*, NIH Publication No. 07-2720, by the U.S. Department of Health and Human Services, National Heart, Lung, and Blood Institute (NHLBI), National Institutes of Health (NIH), 2007, available at http://www.nhlbi.nih.gov/educational/hearttruth/materials/online-toolkit.htm.

Take this self-assessment online at www.pearsonhighered.com/lynchelmore.

Diversity & Health box explores some of the factors behind gender differences in CVD rates.

- **Your genetic inheritance.** Children of parents with hypertension, stroke, and heart disease are more likely to develop these conditions themselves. Some ethnic groups, especially African Americans, are also at increased risk for these conditions.[34] You can't change your genetics. But when it comes to CVD, your DNA isn't destiny. By reducing the CVD risks you can control, you can help make sure that your genes don't equal your fate.
- **Your blood pressure.** At a doctor's visit or health fair, have your blood pressure measured. Hypertension increases your risk for CHD, congestive heart failure, and stroke. As noted earlier, hypertension in adults is defined as blood pressure equal to or greater than 140 over 90. For more detailed guidelines, see Table 11.1 on page 303.
- **Your blood lipids.** If you have abnormal levels of various lipids circulating in your bloodstream, a condition known as **dyslipidemia,** the health of your heart and blood vessels is at risk. A simple blood test can give you a variety of data about your blood lipid levels (**Table 11.2**). These include your total cholesterol score, the level of triglycerides circulating in your bloodstream, and your readings for two cholesterol-carrying protein compounds:
    - LDL, short for **low-density lipoprotein,** is a molecule that packs a lot of cholesterol (about 50%) with very little protein. It's often dubbed "bad" cholesterol because excess LDLs degrade over time, releasing their cholesterol load into your bloodstream. This circulating cholesterol can then become trapped in injured blood vessels. A high LDL score means there's a lot of cholesterol "**l**ittering" your bloodstream, so it increases your risk for CVD.
    - HDL, an abbreviation of **high-density lipoprotein,** is half protein with very little cholesterol. It's often called "good" cholesterol because it picks up free cholesterol in the bloodstream and transports it to your liver for recycling. You can think of HDL as your arteries' "**h**ousekeeper." A high HDL score therefore decreases your risk for CVD.
- **Your blood glucose.** A blood glucose level of 110 mg/dL or higher increases your risk for CVD. Given that 110 is considered prediabetes, you don't have to have full-blown diabetes before your blood glucose level begins to increase your CVD risk.
- **Inflammatory markers.** As noted earlier, inflammation plays a key role in atherosclerosis. Physicians can detect inflammation in the body by measuring your blood level of a protein—called *C-reactive protein (CRP)*—produced by the liver during an inflammatory re-

dyslipidemia Disorder characterized by abnormal levels of blood lipids, such as high LDL cholesterol or low HDL cholesterol.

low-density lipoprotein (LDL) A cholesterol-containing compound that, as it degrades, releases its cholesterol load into the bloodstream; often referred to as "bad cholesterol."

high-density lipoprotein (HDL) A cholesterol-containing compound that removes excess cholesterol from the bloodstream; often referred to as "good cholesterol."

Table 11.2: Classification of Blood Lipid Levels for Adults

LDL Cholesterol	
< 100	Optimal
100–129	Near optimal/above optimal
130–159	Borderline high
160–189	High
≥ 190	Very high
HDL Cholesterol	
< 40	Low
≥ 60	Optimal
Total Cholesterol	
< 200	Desirable
200–239	Borderline high
≥ 240	High
Triglycerides	
< 150	Normal
150–199	Borderline high
200–499	High
≥ 500	Very high

Source: Data from the *Third Report of the Expert Panel on Detection, Evaluation, and Treatment of High Blood Cholesterol in Adults* (NIH Publication No. 05-3290), by the National Heart, Lung, and Blood Institute, 2005, retrieved from www.nhlbi.nih.gov/health/public/heart/chol/wyntk.htm.

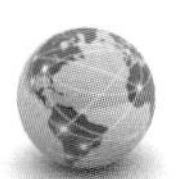

DIVERSITY & HEALTH

Why Do Men Have Greater CVD Risk?

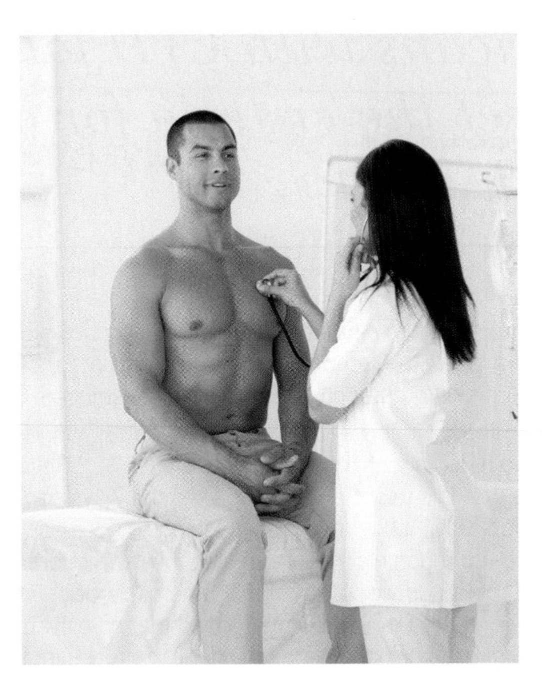

Although cardiovascular disease is the leading killer of both men and women in the United States, men typically develop heart disease and suffer cardiac crises about 10 to 20 years earlier than women.[1]

When this disparity first became apparent, some researchers theorized that the differences were due to lifestyle factors. Men, they assumed, experienced more stress, drank more, smoked more, and ate more heavily than women. But eventually, they came to recognize that many women share these lifestyle factors. So something else had to be going on. Further research revealed that "something else" to be hormones.

Estradiol, a form of the female reproductive hormone estrogen, is produced in significant amounts by a woman's ovaries from the time she begins to menstruate until she experiences menopause. While it's circulating in the bloodstream, estradiol appears to exert a protective effect against heart disease. For example, it is associated with decreased LDL and increased HDL cholesterol, and it is thought to help blood vessels guard against atherosclerosis.[2] This theory fits with general patterns of heart disease in men and women. Whereas men are at greater risk earlier in life, women's risks increase greatly after menopause, when estradiol production drops.

This doesn't mean, however, that young women should be any less vigilant about lowering their CVD risks. More than 80,000 American women under age 50 experience heart attacks annually, and these are twice as likely to be fatal as heart attacks in men.[3] The bottom line? Both men and women can benefit from adopting heart-healthy behaviors as early in life as possible.

References: **1.** "Prediction of Coronary Heart Disease Using Risk Factor Categories," by P. Wilson, R. D'Agostino, D. Levy, A. Belanger, H. Silbershatz, & W. Kannel, 1996, *Circulation, 97* (18), pp. 1837–1847. **2.** "Estrogen Protection, Oxidized LDL, Endothelial Dysfunction and Vasorelaxation in Cardiovascular Disease: New Insights into a Complex Issue," by C. Packer, 2007, *Cardiovascular Research, 73* (1), pp. 6–7. **3.** "Women and Heart Disease Facts," by the Women's Heart Foundation, 2007, retrieved from http://www.womensheart.org/content/HeartDisease/heart_disease_facts.asp.

sponse. A high level of CRP (above 3.0 mg/L) indicates that inflammation is going on somewhere in the body, but not necessarily in the blood vessels. So it's not likely that a physician would order a CRP test unless you had other significant risk factors, such as hypertension and dyslipidemia.

- **Homocysteine.** The amino acid homocysteine can only be metabolized by the body when we consume adequate amounts of the B vitamins folate, B_6, and B_{12}. Low levels of homocysteine in the blood are associated with a reduced risk of MI and stroke.[35] High levels suggest an increased risk. Although the reasons for this are not known, researchers speculate that homocysteine may injure blood vessels, stimulate atherosclerosis, and increase blood clotting.
- **Your weight.** Of all Americans with CVD, 27% are overweight and another 44% are obese.[23]

  Obesity is an independent risk factor for CVD, and worsens other risk factors.[36] A variety of mechanisms contribute to this increased risk:[23]
  - Obesity increases the total volume of blood circulating in the body as well as the total metabolic demand of body cells. Therefore, at any given level of activity, the cardiac workload is greater for people who are obese.
  - The left ventricle of the heart grows excessively large in obese people, a condition called *left ventricular hypertrophy*, and this increases the risk for ventricular dysfunction.
  - In obese people, fat cells can actually infiltrate and replace heart muscle, disturbing regions such as the sinus node where the heart's electrical impulses are generated.
  - Fat cells—especially those stored in abdominal fat—manufacture and release into the bloodstream a variety of inflammatory chemicals, including CRP, as well as chemicals that interfere with the body's response to insulin.
- **Your diet.** In a study from the American Heart Association, 100% of Americans with CVD failed to meet the criteria for a healthy diet score.[23] What is a heart-healthy diet? A large-scale analysis of published studies on diet and heart disease identified fish, nuts, fresh fruits and vegetables, plant oils, and whole grains as protective against CVD. In contrast, foods containing saturated fat, cholesterol, or *trans* fatty acids and foods with a high glycemic index increase your CVD risk.[37] What about chocolate? Is it off limits, or does it protect against heart disease? Visit the **Consumer Corner** for answers!
- **Your level of physical activity.** Exercise reduces blood sugar, increases HDL cholesterol, combats atherosclerosis, strengthens the heart muscle, and expends calories, helping you to maintain a healthful body weight. Among Americans with CVD, 45% report participating in no regular physical activity.[36]
- **Smoking.** Nicotine constricts the blood vessels, and carbon monoxide damages their walls, increasing their susceptibility to atherosclerosis. Smoking also increases blood pressure, increases the

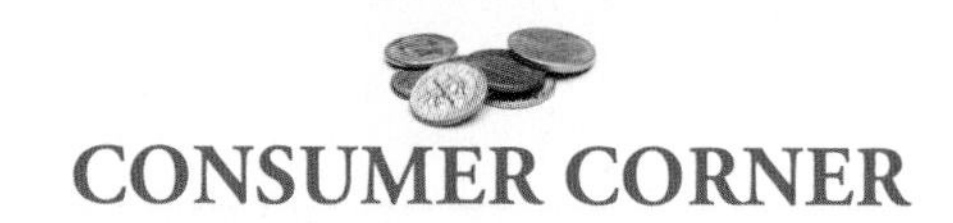

CONSUMER CORNER

Dark Chocolate: A Heart-Healthy Indulgence

If you're a "chocoholic," your years of guilt have come to an end. Researchers now believe that chocolate—especially dark chocolate—is good for your blood vessels and heart. Over the past two decades, many studies have associated regular consumption of a modest amount of dark chocolate with improved cardiovascular functioning and a reduced risk for heart disease. Here are a few examples:

- In one study of healthy adults, participants who ate one small dark chocolate bar every day for two weeks showed improved blood vessel functioning and blood flow over the placebo group.[1]
- A similar placebo-controlled study in overweight adults found that consumption of both solid dark chocolate and liquid cocoa improved blood vessel functioning and lowered blood pressure.[2]
- A study of middle-aged and elderly women found a reduced incidence of heart-failure hospitalizations and deaths in women who reported eating chocolate.[3]
- Another study asked nearly 1,200 patients who had experienced a heart attack about their chocolate consumption, then followed them for 8 years. During the course of the study, those who had reported that they eat chocolate were less likely to die of heart disease than those who said they never eat chocolate, and the more often chocolate was consumed—up to two or more times a week—the lower the incidence of cardiac death.[4]

The ingredients thought to be responsible for chocolate's beneficial effects are members of the flavonoid group of antioxidant phytochemicals, especially a flavonoid called epicatechin. Flavonoids reduce the buildup of cholesterol in blood vessels, blood vessel inflammation, and the platelet action that results in blood clots. They also improve blood pressure and blood lipid profiles, and reduce insulin resistance.[5] Dark chocolate has higher levels of flavonoids than does milk chocolate, and some chocolate manufacturers are producing less-processed "extra-dark" chocolates that preserve even more flavonoids.

Still, most research studies support only modest consumption of dark chocolate—such as one small, slender (1.5-ounce) bar, 3 tablespoons of dark chocolate chips, or 4 individual pieces of dark chocolate daily. Even these modest amounts pack about 180 empty calories, which is about two-thirds of the empty calorie allowance for someone consuming 2,000 calories a day. So if you love chocolate and want to indulge, go ahead—but go easy.

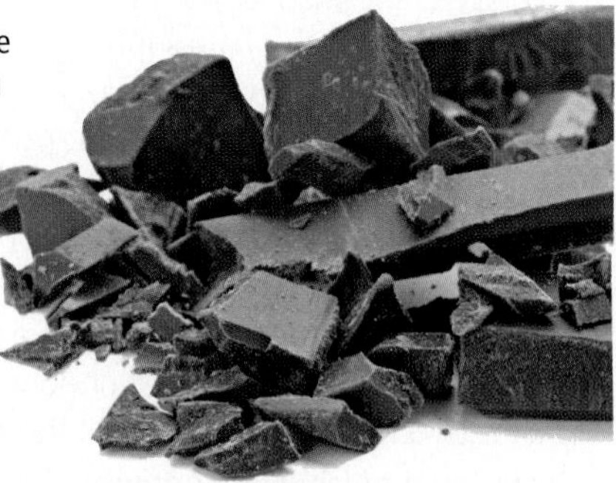

References: **1.** "Flavonoid-Rich Dark Chocolate Improves Endothelial Function and Increases Plasma Epicatechin Concentrations in Healthy Adults," by M. B. Engler, M. M. Engler, C. Y. Chen, M. J. Malloy, A. Browne, E. Y. Chiu, . . . M. L. Mietus-Snyder, June 2004, *Journal of the American College of Nutrition, 23* (3), 197–204. **2.** "Acute Dark Chocolate and Cocoa Ingestion and Endothelial Function: A Randomized Controlled Crossover Trial," by Z. Faridi, V. Yanchou Njike, S. Dutta, A. Ali, & D. L. Katz, July 2008, *American Journal of Clinical Nutrition, 88* (1), pp. 58–63. **3.** "Chocolate Intake and Incidence of Heart Failure: A Population-Based Prospective Study of Middle-Aged and Elderly Women," by E. Mostofsky, E. B. Levitan, A. Wolk, & M. A. Mittleman, 2010, *Circulation, 3*, pp. 612–616. **4.** "Chocolate Consumption and Mortality Following a First Acute Myocardial Infarction: The Stockholm Heart Epidemiology Program," by I. Janszky, K. J. Mukamal, R. Ljung, S. Ahnve, A. Ahlbom, & J. Hallqvist, September 2009, *Journal of Internal Medicine, 266* (3), pp. 248–257. **5.** "Cocoa and Cardiovascular Health," by R. Corti, A. J. Flammer, N. K. Hollenberg, & T. F. Luscher, 2009, *Circulation, 119*, pp. 1433–1441.

> *"In a study from the American Heart Association, 100% of Americans with CVD failed to meet the criteria for a healthy diet score."*

tendency for blood to clot, and decreases HDL cholesterol. Smokers also have a greatly reduced tolerance for exercise. Smokers have a two to four times greater risk of CHD than nonsmokers.[34]

- **Your emotions.** Negative emotions like depression and anxiety, as well as too much stress, can raise your CVD risk.[38] Researchers speculate that this might be due in part to the ways some people find to cope with these emotions—such as by overeating, smoking, or drinking too much alcohol. Moreover, these emotions may change body metabolism in ways that trigger atherosclerosis. For instance, one study of more than 1,800 men found that an elevated level of cortisol, a stress hormone, was an independent risk factor for atherosclerosis.[39]
- **Your sleep.** Short sleep increases your CVD risk. For instance, getting fewer than 5 hours of sleep a night doubles your risk for hypertension.[38] Obesity can be a factor in sleep problems, so weight loss can help.
- **Your income.** Research shows that lower income adults have an increased rate of CVD, and children born into lower income families are more likely to develop CVD as adults. This may be because low-income adults are less likely to eat a heart-healthy diet and be physically active; it can be difficult to find healthful foods in poor neighborhoods, and to find a safe, affordable place to be physically active. Lower income Americans are also more likely to smoke.[38]

What's your risk for a heart attack or stroke? Find out at www.heart.org/gglRisk/locale/en_US/index.html?gtype=health.

Cardiometabolic Risk

Now that you've learned about diabetes and CVD, you're ready to tackle a concept that has recently emerged as a critical public health concern: cardiometabolic risk. For decades, researchers have noted that obesity and insulin resistance together promote a variety of serious metabolic abnormalities. They used the term **metabolic syndrome** to refer to this cluster of abnormalities, which includes, for example, high fasting blood glucose and low HDL cholesterol. More recently, researchers have come

> **metabolic syndrome** A set of unhealthy physical and metabolic conditions together linked to an increased risk for type 2 diabetes and cardiovascular disease.

Father's Heart Attack

STUDENT STORY

"Hi, I'm Mark. When I was in the 5th grade, my dad had a heart attack. It was really frightening because I was 11 years old and I was faced with the prospect of maybe one of my parents dying. That was definitely a point when I realized that not only was it something that I needed to think about as far as my parents' health, but that there's a chance that I too could someday have a heart attack because those things tend to run in the family.

After my dad's heart attack, he met with the cardiologist and they talked about some of the changes he could make to improve his health. He started to take a lot of medicine. He also decreased the amount of tobacco he used. He still is sadly using dipping and chewing tobacco. However, he doesn't use as much and also he has gone from drinking perhaps two to three cans of beer a day to one, if that. Decreasing his tobacco and alcohol usage has made a huge difference in his health because I think in the past 11 years he's only had one minor recurrence of heart issues and that's pretty good."

1: If cardiovascular disease runs in Mark's family, is that a risk factor he can control? What risk factors for CVD can he control and what risk factors are not controllable?

2: Even though Mark's father cut down his use of tobacco, do you think it is still a contributing risk factor for CVD for him? Why do you think he continues to use tobacco even after a heart attack?

Do you have a story similar to Mark's? Share your story at www.pearsonhighered.com/lynchelmore.

to recognize that these abnormalities increase a person's risk not only for type 2 diabetes, but also for CVD. As a result, many public health groups have expanded the concept of metabolic syndrome to include the risk factors traditionally associated with CVD, such as smoking. Their name for this expanded concept is cardiometabolic risk.[40]

In 2009, the Agency for Healthcare Research and Quality (part of the Department of Health and Human Services) published lengthy guidelines defining **cardiometabolic risk (CMR)** as a cluster of modifiable factors that identify individuals at increased risk for type 2 diabetes mellitus and cardiovascular disease. CMR includes all five of the factors that make up the definition of metabolic syndrome, plus four other factors **(Figure 11.11):**[41]

1. Abdominal obesity (a waist circumference ≥ 40 inches for males and ≥ 35 inches for females)
2. Elevated blood pressure (≥ 130/85 mm Hg)
3. Elevated fasting blood glucose (≥ 110 mg/dL)
4. Elevated blood triglycerides (> 150)
5. Low HDL cholesterol (< 40)
6. High LDL cholesterol (≥ 130)
7. Smoking
8. Inflammatory markers (notably CRP)
9. Insulin resistance

Although the first factor—abdominal obesity—is particularly dangerous, obesity in general has become a "gold standard" for identifying people at high cardiometabolic risk. Men and women whose BMI is 30 or higher are at significantly increased risk of cardiometabolic disease and early death.[42]

The AHRQ (Agency for Healthcare Research and Quality) recommends that all males have an initial CMR screening at age 35, and females at age 45. If you're obese, or if you have already been diagnosed with type 2 diabetes, hypertension, or dyslipidemia, you should have a CMR screening immediately, and annually. In addition, because depression is the most frequently cited psychological disorder associated with diabetes, you can anticipate that, if your physician finds any of the factors associated with CMR, he or she is likely to also screen you for depression.[41]

cardiometabolic risk (CMR) A cluster of nine modifiable factors that identify individuals at risk for type 2 diabetes and cardiovascular disease.

When college students are screened for CMR, studies show that several CMR factors are already present. For example, one study conducted over 7 years at a large university found that 60% had body fat percentages associated with elevated triglycerides and LDL, along with decreased HDL.[43] Another study using data from university health centers found that 43% of students had at least one CMR factor, and more than 14% had two or more factors.[44]

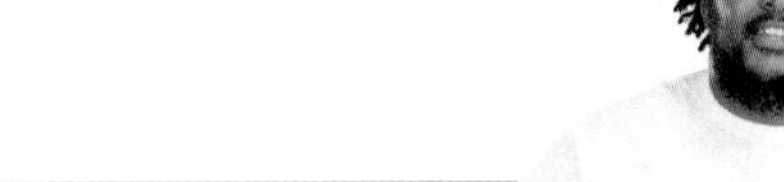

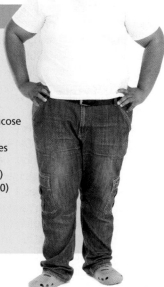

Figure 11.11 Cardiometabolic risk. These nine factors dramatically increase your risk of developing type 2 diabetes and cardiovascular disease.

Individuals found to be at cardiometabolic risk are treated with a variety of therapies. Lifestyle measures—discussed shortly—are essential. If these measures didn't significantly reduce CMR, or if the patient were unable to practice them, then the same kinds of prescription medications discussed earlier in this chapter would likely be prescribed.

Change Yourself, Change Your World

Notice that the definition of CMR classifies all nine risk factors as modifiable—meaning they are within your power to change! And the sooner you start, the better for your body. So get a physical exam, and find out your CMR. If you discover that you don't have any of the risk factors now, the advice ahead can help keep you from developing them. If you do have one or more of the risk factors, following the guidelines here could quite literally save your life.

Personal Choices

Several large-scale research initiatives, both nationally and internationally, have identified proven steps you can take to reduce your CMR. Two recent studies have shown that people who practice most of the following healthy lifestyle behaviors have a 65–70% reduced CMR.[45,46] Believing in your ability to make healthy choices and lower your risk is an important first step. One study of college students found that higher self-efficacy, or a belief in your own ability to control events in your life, indicated a better likelihood of making healthy choices.[47]

Below are the top behaviors you can start practicing today. If they sound familiar—they should! Although researchers link these behaviors specifically to CMR reduction, they're the same choices we've been advocating throughout this text to benefit every aspect of your life.

Don't Smoke

If you smoke, get the help you need to quit. Start with a visit to your campus health center. Do it *today*. As you've just learned, smoking drives up your cardiometabolic risk. Researchers have established that the ingredients in tobacco smoke constrict and irritate artery walls, trigger inflammation, promote atherosclerosis, and increase blood pressure.[48] Moreover, smoking causes many types of cancer and is directly responsible for 80% to 90% of all lung cancer deaths. Overall, smoking causes 1 out of every 5 deaths that occurs in the United States each year.[49] (For more information on smoking cessation, see Chapter 10.)

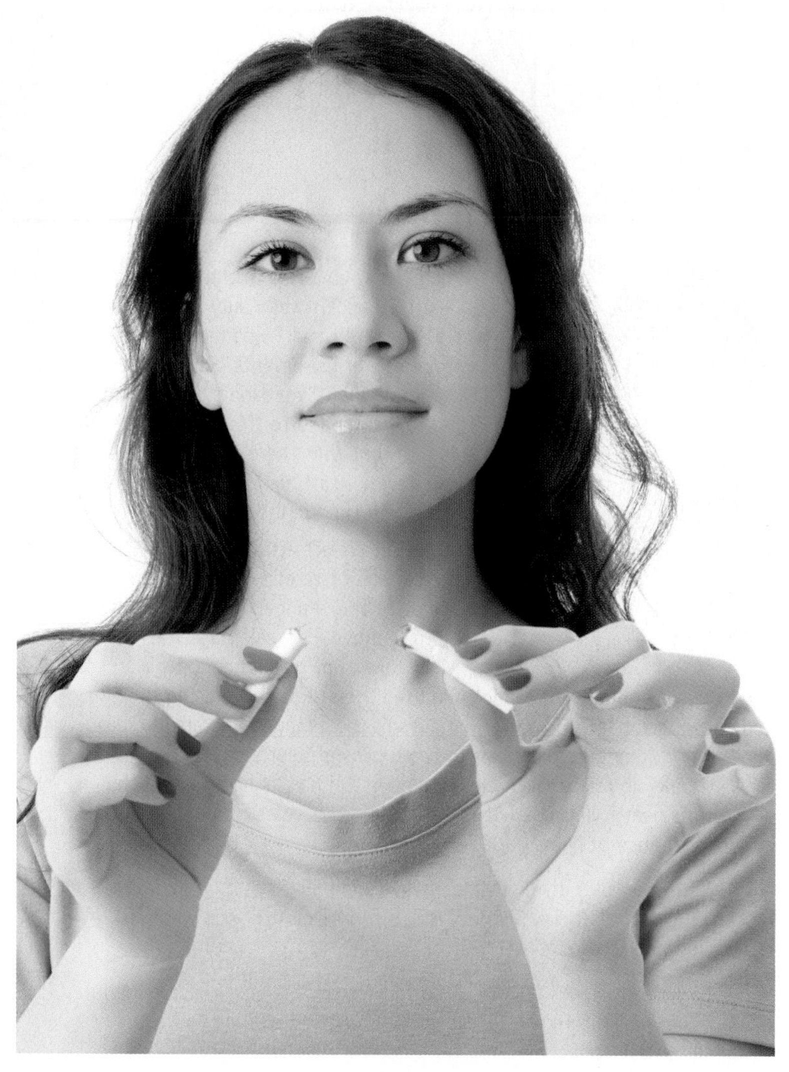

Quit. Not smoking is one of the best things you can do to reduce your cardiometabolic risk.

Shed Any Extra Pounds

If you're overweight or obese, shedding even a few pounds can reduce your CMR. But remember to watch more than the number on the scale. Aim for a waist measurement of less than 40 inches if you are a man or less than 35 inches if you are a woman. And keep your BMI within the range for normal weight (18.5 to 24.9). (See Chapter 7 for a refresher on BMI and waist circumference.) We can't all hit an ideal weight or body shape and freeze ourselves there. But we can all work to stay within a weight range that is healthy and right for our body type.

Eat Right

Not sure how to begin reducing your CMR? Try starting with what you eat for lunch. Choose foods that include complex carbohydrates, lots of fiber, and low levels of sodium and saturated fat. In one study of more than 80,000 women, researchers found that following a diet low in red meat and processed meats, high in produce and whole grains, and moderate in plant-based fats and alcohol reduced diabetes risk by 36%.[50] Some cardiologists recommend adopting a plant-based diet, one of the most popular of which is the Mediterranean diet. The foods that are basic to this plan include legumes and other vegetables, fruits, whole grains, nuts, olives, and olive oil, along with some cheese, yogurt, fish, poultry, eggs, and wine. A 2011 analysis of 50 studies linked the Mediterranean diet to a lower risk of metabolic syndrome.[51]

Download a poster identifying the main elements and benefits of the Mediterranean diet at http://meddietexperience.weebly.com/mediterranean-diet-poster.html.

Nutrition information can also help people improve their cardiometabolic scores. Among college students taking a nutrition course, 10% significantly reduced their BMI, and at least 14% improved their blood lipids levels and blood pressure, and reduced their fasting blood glucose.[52] (For a detailed discussion of nutrition, see Chapter 5.) The nearby **Practical Strategies for Change** has specific suggestions on changing your diet to reduce your CMR.

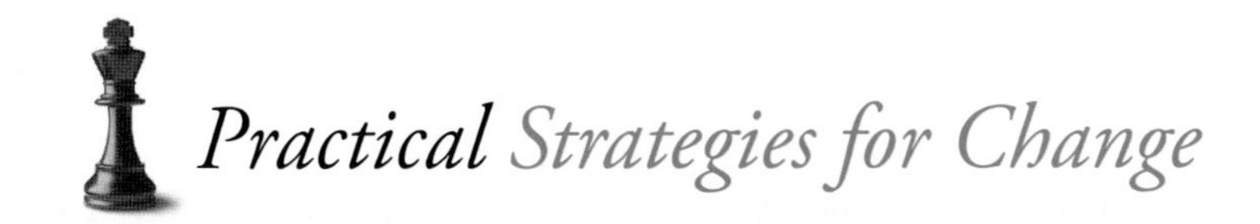

Practical Strategies for Change

Heart-Healthy Food Choices

Making heart-healthy diet choices can substantially reduce your cardiometabolic risk. Here are a few suggestions:

- **Reduce your intake of saturated fat and cholesterol.** Eat less red meat, and avoid processed meats like pepperoni and sausage. Several times a week, replace meat with plant-based protein choices such as beans, lentils, tofu, and tempeh. Choose nonfat or low-fat versions of milk, yogurt, cheese, and other dairy products. Replace butter with *trans* fat–free margarine, nut butters, and plant oils. Snack on fruits and nuts instead of potato chips.
- **Boost your consumption of omega-3 fatty acids.** Fatty fish such as salmon provides EPA and DHA, two omega-3 fatty acids known to reduce triglyceride levels, inflammation, and arterial plaque formation. The 2010 *Dietary Guidelines for Americans* suggests that you eat fish at least twice a week.
- **Increase your fiber intake.** Fiber not only helps you feel full and eat less, but can help slow the release of glucose into your bloodstream as well as reduce arterial inflammation, blood pressure, and blood levels of LDL cholesterol. Whole grain breads and cereals and fresh fruits and vegetables are good sources.
- **Decrease your sodium intake.** Cut back on processed foods, which tend to contain a great deal of sodium. One serving of regular canned soup, for example, can contain almost half of a day's recommended allowance of sodium. Opt for fresh foods when possible, or choose low-sodium versions of prepared foods.
- **Put some color in your diet.** Brightly colored fruits and vegetables, such as blueberries, raspberries, red grapes, tomatoes, black beans, and parsley, contain phytochemicals called *flavonoids,* which have been associated with reduced CVD risk. You don't need to carry around a detailed list of foods to find those higher in flavonoids—just focus on choosing colorful fruits and vegetables, and aim for a mix of colors.
- **Eat yogurt.** Yogurt and other fermented dairy products contain *probiotics*, strains of bacteria beneficial to human health. By reducing blood vessel inflammation, for example, they reduce the formation of atherosclerotic plaque in arteries. Probiotics also create acids that disrupt the liver's production of cholesterol, and actually break down and consume cholesterol for food. Blend with fresh fruit for an even more nutritious treat.
- **What about alcohol?** A moderate alcohol intake—no more than two drinks per day for males and one drink per day for females—increases levels of HDL cholesterol while decreasing LDL cholesterol; it also reduces the risk of abnormal clot formation in the blood vessels. However, alcohol packs 7 calories per gram, more than either protein or carbohydrate, and calories from alcohol tend to be stored in the abdomen. If you consider that a bottle of beer provides about 150 calories, if you drink just two per day and don't adjust your intake of foods and other beverages to compensate, you'll gain a pound about every 12 days. And that weight gain will more than offset any potential cardiovascular benefit.

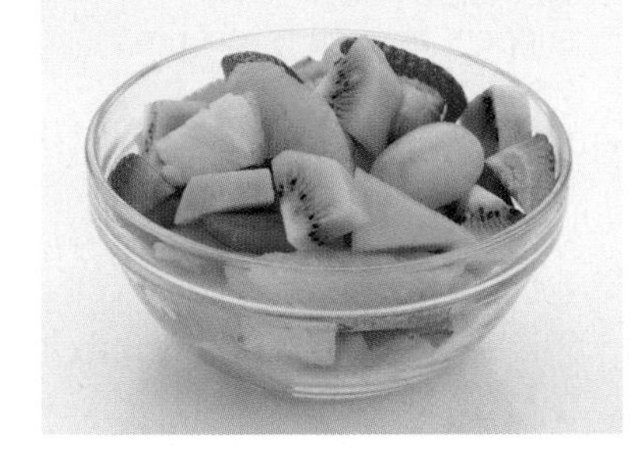

Get Moving

Physical activity helps control blood sugar, burn calories, control weight, and strengthen your heart. This fact holds true throughout your life:

- A study of elementary school children found that those with low levels of physical activity already showed more risk factors for cardiovascular disease.[53]
- A study in adolescents found that higher levels of physical activity consistently corresponded to a reduced CMR.[54]
- In a study of college students, those classified as fit, even if their body fat percentages were higher than desirable, had lower triglycerides, higher HDL, and lower blood glucose levels.[43]
- A study of obese adults found that those who followed a weight-loss diet and engaged in a program of physical activity lost more weight on average (24 pounds) than those who only followed the diet (18 pounds).[55]

If you aren't exercising right now, aim for at least 30 minutes of physical activity a few days a week. If you already meet that level, start exercising every day, and work on slowly increasing the intensity and duration of your workouts. Remember to balance cardiorespiratory fitness, or activities that build heart and lung capacity, with strength training. (For more information on physical activity, see Chapter 6.)

Limit Your Alcohol Intake

Excessive drinking is bad for your health overall and your heart specifically. This holds true even at a young age. One study of college students found that those on their way to developing hypertension were also far more likely to drink heavily.[56] Another study associated heavy drinking in young adulthood with a significantly increased CMR later in life—even among those who had stopped drinking entirely by middle adulthood.[57]

Get Enough Sleep

Chronic short sleep is linked to insulin resistance, high blood pressure, poor blood lipids, and other cardiometabolic risk factors. One study of teenagers between the ages of 13 and 16 found that those sleeping less than 6.5 hours a night were 2.5 times more likely to have elevated blood pressure.[58] Another study of adult women associated short sleep with high total triglycerides and low HDL cholesterol.[59] Aim for 8 hours of sleep a night.

Maintain Good Oral Hygiene

The health of your mouth and your cardiovascular system may not seem connected, but scientists have found clear links between dental problems and CVD.[60] Periodontal disease, or disorders of the gums and bones that surround your teeth, are a prime concern. Researchers are still trying to nail down why, but suspect that the pathogens involved in gum disease trigger an inflammatory reaction that can cascade throughout the body and contribute to atherosclerosis. In addition, as mentioned earlier, gum disease is a common complication of uncontrolled diabetes. So brush and floss daily, and visit the dentist regularly.

Manage Your Emotions

People who carry stress, anger easily, or are prone to hostility, anxiety, or depression are at increased cardiometabolic risk. Just as physical factors such as cholesterol or excess weight strain the body's coping mechanisms, so do negative emotions. If you need some help, get it. (See Chapter 2 for information on psychological resources.)

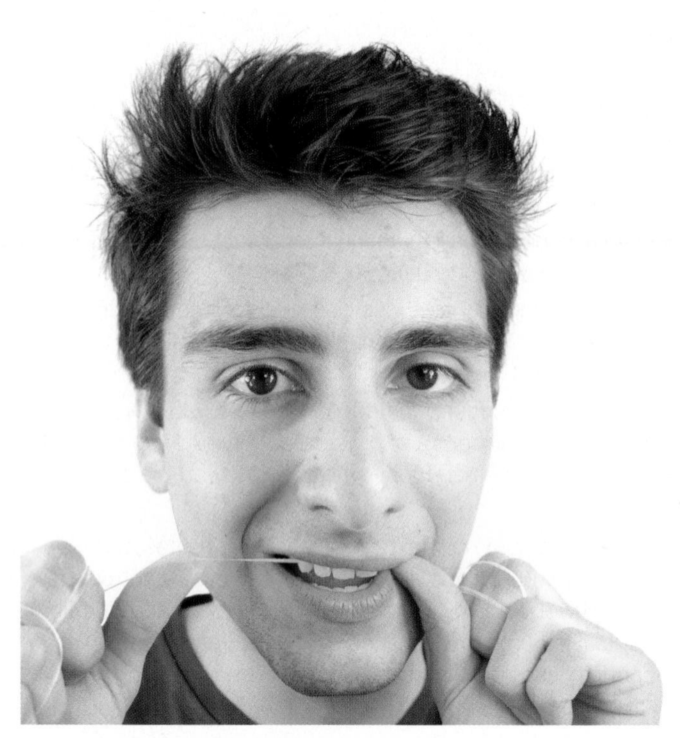

Good **dental hygiene** can help keep your heart healthy.

Offset Your Non-Modifiable Risk Factors
Be aware of the risks in your background. Do you know your family's history of diabetes? If not, ask. Awareness of your family history is especially important if your ethnicity puts you at increased risk. Becoming aware of inherited risks is important because it allows you to discuss them with your health-care provider and to take steps, such as improving your diet and exercise habits, to reduce those risks.[61]

Get Screened
Take advantage of annual physicals and health fairs to have your blood pressure and blood lipids monitored. Because your body's functioning changes as you age, don't assume that the numbers you show now will last a lifetime. Have your blood pressure checked at least once every 2 years, and talk to your physician about how often you should have your blood tested for glucose, lipid levels, and other cardiometabolic indicators.

If you already know you have diabetes, hypertension, or dyslipidemia, take steps to keep your condition under control. Stick to a regular schedule of health-care check-ups, and follow your health-care provider's advice.

Supporting a Friend with Diabetes or CVD

If you're fit, slender, and have none of the metabolic factors associated with CVD, it can be tough to empathize with people you care about who may be struggling with overweight or obesity, especially if they've recently been diagnosed with prediabetes, prehypertension, or full-blown diabetes or CVD. Though you may be tempted to tell them to just "shape up," such advice may only cause them to avoid you—when what they really need right now is a caring, supportive friend. So what *can* you do? The American Diabetes Association offers these tips:[62]

- **Learn more.** Ask your friend to tell you more about his or her condition—how it affects life day to day, what treatments seem helpful, and what the frustrations might be. You could also offer to attend a patient education class or workshop with your friend. Discover what your friend would find most helpful by asking these simple questions:
  1. What is the hardest thing about living with this condition?
  2. What do I and your other friends do that makes things a little easier? What do we do that makes things harder?
  3. What can I do to help that I'm not doing now?
- **Provide the help your friend asks for.** Whether it's keeping junk food out of sight or offering to go for a walk, do your best to follow through.
- **Share your own feelings.** How does your friend's situation affect you? Do you feel as if you can't indulge in a pastry whenever your friend is around, or that you can't share your elation over completing a strenuous hike, road race, or other athletic challenge? Opening up about such feelings can help clear the air and allow you and your friend to support each other.
- **Know when to get help.** If your friend is clearly not sticking to the treatment plan—for instance, if he or she is refusing to take prescribed medication, smoking, abusing alcohol, or binge-eating—consider the behavior a cry for help, and encourage your friend to get it. For example, offer to go with your friend to your campus health services center.

Campus Advocacy

Throughout this text, we've identified ways to promote a healthier campus environment—everything from advocating for more healthful food choices in dining halls and neighborhood restaurants to lobbying for a tobacco-free campus. Here, we discuss a few more ways you can specifically address the problems of diabetes and CVD:

- Find out the location of the AEDs on your campus, including in campus housing and in classrooms, labs, and other buildings you regularly use. If anyone were to suffer a sudden cardiac arrest on campus, that information could very well enable you to save the person's life.
- In addition, next time it's offered on your campus, register for training in CPR. Both the American Red Cross and the American Heart Association commonly offer certification classes, which usually are just a few hours long, and held on an evening or a Saturday at very low cost.
- Consider getting a group of students together to sponsor a "heart walk" to raise money for the American Heart Association. For more information, visit www.heartwalk.org.
- If you have type 1 diabetes, contact your campus chapter of the College Diabetes Network. This group can provide information, peer support, and many other resources to help make managing your diabetes a little easier.
- Finally, most campus health services sponsor special health-screening events offering free or very low-cost blood pressure checks, and blood tests for lipids and glucose levels. Volunteering to help at such events is a great way to learn more about cardiometabolic risk, and to meet other students. At the very least, take advantage of such screenings whenever they're offered.

LEARNING OBJECTIVES

DEFINE cancer and identify the factors involved in its initiation and spread.

ASSESS your personal risk factors for developing cancer.

DISCUSS the clinical detection, classification, and treatment of cancer.

IDENTIFY and **DESCRIBE** the most common cancers, including signs and symptoms, risk factors, and diagnosis and treatment.

DISCUSS some of the challenges of living with cancer.

DEVELOP a plan for reducing your risk for cancer.

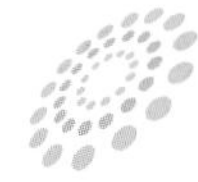

Health Online icons are found throughout the chapter, directing you to web links, videos, podcasts, and other useful online resources.

Who's afraid of cancer? Just about everyone.

And with good reason: In the course of your lifetime, you have about a 1 in 3 chance of developing cancer, and a 1 in 4 chance of dying from it.[1, 2] But as you saw in the opening statistics, there are also reasons for optimism: Every year, researchers are learning more about what causes and contributes to cancer, and how you can reduce your risk. And as new technologies provide new treatments, more and more Americans are surviving this frightening disease.

An Overview of Cancer

Cancer is a group of diseases characterized by uncontrolled reproduction of abnormal cells and, in some cases, the spread of these cells to other sites in the body. If the reproduction and spread of cancer cells is not checked, the person is likely to die. But how many people develop cancer, and how many of these survive? Let's look at some cancer facts and figures.

> cancer A group of diseases marked by the uncontrolled multiplication of abnormal cells.

Cancer by the Numbers

Worldwide, cancer causes about 13% of all deaths.[3] In the United States, it is second only to coronary heart disease as a leading cause of death. In a given year, more than 1.6 million new cases of cancer will be diagnosed in the United States, and more than 500,000 people will die from the disease.[1] Some types of cancer occur more frequently or have higher death rates than others. Statistics on cancer cases and deaths by body site are identified in **Table 12.1.**

Despite these disturbing figures, more people are surviving cancer than ever before. The 5-year survival rate for cancer is now 67%, up from 49% in 1975. This progress reflects advances in screening and detection, meaning that we are now able to diagnose certain cancers in earlier stages, and improved methods of treatment.[1]

However, cancer survival rates reflect significant health disparities. Americans living in poverty have enjoyed little or no decrease in cancer death rates, and the decreased death rates seen in minority groups has been slower than that for Caucasians. Level of education also makes a difference. For instance, in 2007, the cancer death rate was nearly three times higher for the least educated Americans than for the most educated. Eliminating such disparities is a key focus of national cancer prevention efforts.[1] For more information on cancer health disparities, see the **Diversity & Health** box on page 327.

In addition to causing pain, anguish, and death, cancer places an enormous financial burden on American society. Cancer costs the U.S. economy over $200 billion annually. This amount includes over $100 billion in direct medical expenditures, along with the costs of lost productivity due to illness and premature death.[1]

If those 1 in 3 odds seem frightening, bear in mind that they don't apply to everyone equally. That's because the vast majority of cancer cases don't result from inherited genetic defects but from damage to genes that occurs during our lifetime—often as a result of our own behaviors. Let's take a look at how such damage occurs, and what factors are responsible.

How Does Cancer Develop?

Cancer begins when, for any of a variety of reasons, entirely normal cells undergo changes in their operating instructions that turn them into rogue agents of abnormal growth. Understanding how this happens starts with a look at DNA.

Table 12.1: Leading Sites of New Cancer Cases and Deaths, 2012 Estimates

Estimated New Cases		Estimated Deaths	
Site	Incidence (% of all cases)	Site	Mortality (% of all cases)
Male			
Prostate	241,740 (29%)	Lung and bronchus	87,750 (29%)
Lung and bronchus	116,470 (14%)	Prostate	28,170 (9%)
Colon and rectum	73,420 (9%)	Colon and rectum	26,470 (9%)
Urinary bladder	55,600 (7%)	Pancreas	18,850 (6%)
Melanoma of the skin	44,250 (5%)	Liver and intrahepatic bile duct	13,980 (5%)
Kidney and renal pelvis	40,250 (5%)	Leukemia	13,500 (4%)
Non-Hodgkin lymphoma	38,160 (4%)	Esophagus	12,040 (4%)
Oral cavity and pharynx	28,540 (3%)	Urinary bladder	10,510 (3%)
Leukemia	26,830 (3%)	Non-Hodgkin lymphoma	10,320 (3%)
Pancreas	22,090 (3%)	Kidney and renal pelvis	8,650 (3%)
All sites	848,170 (100%)	All sites	301,820 (100%)
Female			
Breast	226,870 (29%)	Lung and bronchus	72,590 (26%)
Lung and bronchus	109,690 (14%)	Breast	39,510 (14%)
Colon and rectum	70,040 (9%)	Colon and rectum	25,220 (9%)
Uterine corpus	47,130 (6%)	Pancreas	18,540 (7%)
Thyroid	43,210 (5%)	Ovary	15,500 (6%)
Melanoma of the skin	32,000 (4%)	Leukemia	10,040 (4%)
Non-Hodgkin lymphoma	31,970 (4%)	Non-Hodgkin lymphoma	8,620 (3%)
Kidney and renal pelvis	24,520 (3%)	Uterine corpus	8,010 (3%)
Ovary	22,280 (3%)	Liver and intrahepatic bile duct	6,570 (2%)
Pancreas	21,830 (3%)	Brain and other nervous system	5,980 (2%)
All sites	790,740 (100%)	All sites	275,370 (100%)

Data from *Cancer Facts & Figures, 2012,* by the American Cancer Society, 2012, p. 10, available at http://www.cancer.org/acs/groups/content/@epidemiologysurveilance/documents/document/acspc-031941.pdf.

The structures and functions of just about every cell in the body are controlled by DNA, a compound packed into the cell nucleus—the "command center" of every active cell. DNA controls cells in two ways:

- Regions of DNA called *genes* carry the instructions—the "recipes"—for assembling all of the proteins the body requires. Proteins in turn are the substance of all of our cells, tissues, and organs, as well as thousands of compounds that enable the body to function.
- DNA instructs cells to divide and multiply, ensuring that the body's tissues are as fresh and vital as possible. For instance, the cells lining your digestive tract are replaced every few days, and your skin cells are continually being shed and replaced. If you're injured, the replacement process speeds up to help you heal. Genes control cell reproduction by coding for the proteins involved in the process. You can think of them as operating a bit like the accelerator and brakes on a car. If you need lots of new cells quickly, growth-promoting proteins become more active. Once enough new cells are in place, growth-opposing proteins slow the process back down to normal.

If something damages DNA, and the damage is not repaired, the cell will begin to produce defective—malfunctioning—proteins. This is precisely what happens in the first stage in the development of cancer, known as *initiation*.

Initiation

DNA can be damaged by a variety of external hazards. These include the toxins in tobacco and tobacco smoke, alcohol, many chemicals used in industry, radiation from sunlight, sunlamps, or tanning beds, and even certain viruses.[4] When we come into contact with such agents—whether by absorbing them via our skin, or breathing or ingesting them—they can cause dangerous *mutations,* or DNA changes, that can lead to cancer **(Figure 12.1).** These cancer-generating agents

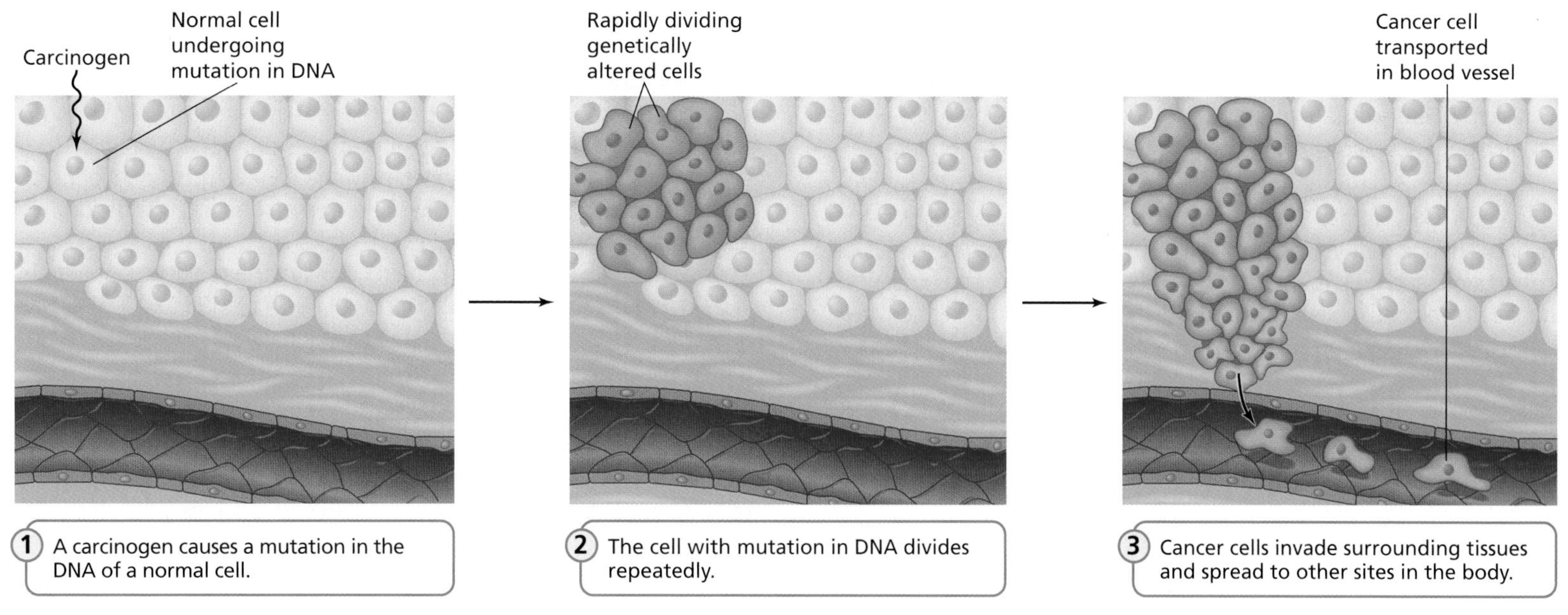
Carcinogen
Normal cell undergoing mutation in DNA
Rapidly dividing genetically altered cells
Cancer cell transported in blood vessel
1 A carcinogen causes a mutation in the DNA of a normal cell.
2 The cell with mutation in DNA divides repeatedly.
3 Cancer cells invade surrounding tissues and spread to other sites in the body.

Figure 12.1 Progression of cancer.

Source: From Thompson, Janice; Manore, Melinda; and Vaughan, Linda. *The Science of Nutrition*, 2nd edition, p. 605, Fig. 15.11. © 2011. Reprinted by permission of Pearson Education, Inc., Upper Saddle River, NJ.

are known as **carcinogens** (from *carcino-* meaning "cancer" and *-gen* as in generator, so a "cancer-maker").

Fortunately, many mutations are quickly repaired. And our body's immune system has specialized cells—for instance, the aptly named *natural killer cells*—that seek out body cells with mutated DNA and cause them to self-destruct. We all have natural killer cells roaming our tissues; that is, they're part of our inborn defenses. But when mutations are more severe than the body can fix, or the number of natural killer cells is reduced by stressors, or our encounters with a carcinogen such as tobacco are too frequent, the body's defenses become overwhelmed. And that's when cells with defective DNA can take hold, multiply, and form cancerous tumors.

Tumor Formation

Defective growth-control genes cause the production of proteins that either stimulate or fail to stop excessive cell reproduction. As cells begin reproducing out of control, they form clusters of immature cells that serve no purpose. Their only function is to keep multiplying. Such clusters of cells eventually form clumps of abnormal tissue called **tumors.** The defective genes that promote tumor formation are called **oncogenes** (*onco-* is a Latin prefix meaning "tumor").

Not all tumors are cancerous. Many are **benign tumors**—that is, they grow only very slowly, do not invade surrounding tissues, and do not spread to other parts of the body. Still, even benign tumors can be harmful if they are growing in a location—such as the brain—where their presence causes pressure and pain and disrupts normal functioning. In contrast, **malignant tumors** are by definition cancerous (see Figure 12.1). They invade surrounding tissue, and can shed tumor cells into blood and lymph (fluid that seeps out of body tissues and is eventually returned to the bloodstream).

For a one-minute explanation of the role of the immune system in halting the initiation of cancer, check out www.youtube.com/watch?v=ESJd4lAsekA&feature=related.

carcinogen A substance known to trigger DNA mutations that can lead to cancer.

tumor An abnormal growth of tissue with no physiological function.

oncogene A mutated gene that encourages the uncontrolled cell division that results in cancer.

benign tumor A tumor that grows slowly, does not spread, and is not cancerous.

malignant tumor A tumor that grows aggressively, invades surrounding tissue, and can spread to other parts of the body; all cancers are malignant.

metastasis The process by which a malignant tumor spreads to other body sites.

relative risk A measure of the strength of the relationship between known risk factors and a particular disorder.

Metastasis

Once malignant cells have broken away from the tumor and entered the blood or lymph, they can travel to distant body regions and find new places to take root. This aggressive spreading process, called **metastasis,** makes malignant tumors very dangerous: Metastasis causes 90% of all cancer deaths.[5] When malignant cells have metastasized to multiple body sites, the cancer is far more challenging to treat.

It's important to note that, whereas cancer can spread throughout the body, it cannot be spread from person to person. Though certain cancer-associated viruses, such as HIV or hepatitis, are contagious, cancer itself is not.

What Factors Increase Your Risk for Cancer?

Anyone can develop cancer. In the United States, men have slightly less than a 1 in 2 lifetime risk; for women, the lifetime risk is a little more than 1 in 3. Lifetime risk is meaningful when considering populations, but for individuals, it can be misleading. For a more helpful picture of your own cancer risk, you need to consider your **relative risk,** which is a measure of the strength of the relationship between known risk factors and a particular disorder. For example, if you're a female with a mother or sister diagnosed with breast cancer, you have twice the relative risk of developing breast cancer as women without this family history. And if you're a male and you smoke, you have a 23 times higher risk of developing lung cancer than male nonsmokers.[1]

In some instances, of course, relative risk is related to prevention. Someone with a family history of a cancer linked to a genetic defect cannot change that factor, but a smoker can stop smoking. In fact, all cancers caused by smoking can be entirely prevented, as can cancers caused by alcohol abuse, obesity, and excessive exposure to UV radiation. Moreover, regular screening can be preventive when it allows health-care providers to detect and remove precancerous growths. Screening is known to reduce mortality for cancers of the breast, colon, rectum, and cervix. The American Cancer Society estimates that at least half of all new cancer cases could have been prevented or detected earlier by screening.[1]

Non-Modifiable Risk Factors

Many risk factors for cancer are, unfortunately, beyond your control. These include age, genetics, ethnicity, and certain biological factors.

Age

The risk of being diagnosed with cancer increases with age. This increased risk is thought to be due to two factors. First, our cells are exposed to more and more carcinogens with each passing year. Second, our cellular repair mechanisms are thought to become less effective as we age.[3] About 77% of all cancers are diagnosed in people age 55 or older.[1]

Genetics and Family History

About 5% of cancers are strongly hereditary.[1] Foremost among these are cancers of the breast and ovaries, colon and rectum, and prostate.[6] Hereditary cancers occur when defective versions of genes are passed through the family bloodline. For instance, most people have normal versions of the genes researchers identify as BRCA1 and BRCA2. These genes are involved in cell growth, cell division, and repair of damaged DNA. When the genes are defective, they cannot function appropriately, so the affected person is more prone to developing cancer when he or she encounters carcinogens. Women who inherit an altered BRCA1 or BRCA2 gene are at increased risk for breast and ovarian cancer, and men who inherit the altered gene are at increased risk for prostate cancer.[7] Similarly, people who inherit altered forms of the MLH1 or MSH2 gene—which normally work to fix "copying errors" in DNA—are at increased risk for colorectal cancer.[8]

Ethnicity

The incidence of cancer in the United States is highest among African Americans, as are deaths from cancer. Researchers acknowledge that, in addition to ethnicity itself, a variety of complex factors are likely to contribute to this disparity.[9] The most obvious include a lower level of health insurance coverage and, thus, access to health care. When health care is obtained, discrimination may influence options for diagnosis and treatment. Inequalities in work and housing environments, such as a higher level of air pollution and toxic wastes in water and soil from nearby industries, as well as overall standard of living, may contribute. Culturally based practices and beliefs also may contribute by keeping some people from seeking screenings and early diagnosis. For more information on disparities in cancer rates, see the **Diversity & Health** box.

Biological Factors

Cancer can also be related to biological factors, such as the body's hormones. Researchers theorize, for instance, that excessive stress hormones disrupt normal cell mechanisms—such as DNA repair and regulation of cell reproduction—that help cells protect against cancer.[10] Also, reproductive hormones play a role in women's cancer risk. Hormones influence the age at which a woman has her first period and enters menopause, both of which factor into breast cancer risk. Similarly, use of hormonal birth control or hormone replacement therapy (HRT) increases a woman's risk for breast cancer, and in 2009, the National Cancer Institute confirmed an increased risk of ovarian cancer in women who had used HRT as well.[11]

What About Gender?

Cancer death rates are higher in men; however, the reason for this difference may be less biology and more lifestyle. For instance, men are 24% less likely than women to have visited a doctor within the past year.[12] Also, more men (23.5%) than women (17.9%) smoke[13] and more men than women are heavy drinkers and become alcohol dependent.[14]

Modifiable Risk Factors

When you think about the vegetables you eat, do you picture a colorful salad or a bag of fries? How often do you exercise? Are your BMI and waist size within a healthful range? Do you smoke, or spend time with someone who does? Do you drink alcohol, and if so, how much? These are all modifiable risk factors that can play a major role in the development of cancer.

Diet

It seems as if every day you hear about some new food that supposedly either causes or protects against cancer. When you encounter such claims, keep in mind that no single research study is conclusive: Our understanding of the role of specific foods in health is still evolving. Here's what we can say with some confidence:

- **Antioxidants.** Certain essential chemical reactions in the body release chemicals called *free radicals* that can damage body cells. (For more detail, see Chapter 5.) Substantial research evidence suggests that a diet rich in antioxidants—consumed in foods, not supplements—reduces your risk for cancer. Antioxidants oppose the cell damage caused by free radicals, enhance the immune system's ability to remove from the body cells with DNA mutations, and inhibit the growth of cancer cells and tumors.[15] A wide variety of plant foods, from blueberries to bell peppers, are rich in antioxidant phytochemicals; thus, a plant-based diet is recommended.
- **Fiber.** For decades, researchers have debated whether or not a high-fiber diet protects against colon cancer, and possibly cancers at other sites. The jury is still out. Many experts now suggest that, if fiber-rich foods play a role, it's not because of their fiber![16] Foods high in fiber also tend to be high in antioxidant phytochemicals, as well as vitamins and minerals, so teasing out any specific contribution from fiber is challenging. Moreover, high-fiber foods help you feel full with fewer calories, so they help you maintain a healthful weight. And as we discuss shortly, that's one of the most important things you can do to reduce your risk for cancer. The bottom line is that a diet rich in fruits, legumes and other vegetables, and whole grains is associated with a reduced risk for some common cancers, including mouth, throat, larynx, esophageal, stomach, and colorectal.[16]

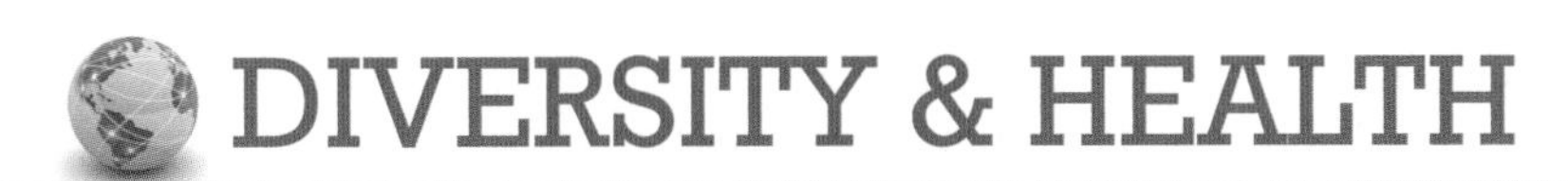

DIVERSITY & HEALTH

Cancer Disparities by Race and Socioeconomic Status

In 2009, 1 in 4 African Americans and 1 in 4 Hispanic Americans lived below the poverty line, compared with 1 in 11 Caucasian Americans. Poverty is an obstacle to receiving quality health care. Poor Americans are more likely to lack health insurance, as well as to engage in behaviors that increase cancer risk, such as smoking, physical inactivity, and poor diet. As a result, the American Cancer Society estimates that, in 2007, if all segments of the population had experienced the same cancer death rate as that of wealthy Americans, 37% of cancer deaths could have been avoided.

Among all populations, deaths due to cancer and heart disease have fallen, however, deaths due to heart disease have fallen more rapidly. Among Hispanics, Asian-Americans, and Pacific Islanders, cancer has recently overtaken heart disease as the leading cause of death.[1]

The table at right from the National Cancer Institute compares overall cancer cases and deaths by race/ethnicity. In addition, certain minority groups have higher rates of cancers at specific sites. For example:[2]

- African Americans have the highest rates of lung, colorectal, and prostate cancer in the United States and are much more likely than Caucasian Americans to die of these diseases.
- Native Americans have the highest rate of kidney cancer, as well as the poorest survival rate for this cancer.
- Asian Americans have the highest rates of stomach and liver cancer of all groups, and are more than twice as likely to die of these cancers as Caucasian Americans.
- Caucasian American women have the highest incidence rate for breast cancer, although African American women are most likely to die from the disease.
- Hispanic American women have the highest rate of cervical cancer in the United States, but the death rate for this cancer is highest among African American women. Hispanic Americans also have higher incidence and death rates for cancers of the stomach, liver, and gallbladder.[1]

Overall Cancer Incidence and Death Rates*

	All Sites	
Racial/Ethnic Group	**Incidence**	**Death**
All	470.1	192.7
African American/Black	504.1	238.8
Asian/Pacific Islander	314.9	115.5
Hispanic/Latino	356.0	129.1
American Indian/ Alaska Native	297.6	160.4
White	477.5	190.7

*Statistics are for 2000–2004, and represent the number of new cases of invasive cancer and deaths per year per 100,000 men and women.

References: **1.** Siegel, R., Naishadham, D., and Jemal, A. (2012, September 17). Cancer statistics for Hispanics/Latinos. *CA: A Cancer Journal for Clinicians.* Vol. 62, Issue 5. DOI: 10.3322/caac.21153. **2.** "Cancer Health Disparities," by the National Cancer Institute, March 11, 2008, retrieved from http://www.cancer.gov/cancertopics/factsheet/disparities/cancer-health-disparities.

- **Dietary fats.** Some studies suggest an increased cancer risk from consuming a diet high in saturated fats. On the other hand, consuming a diet rich in omega-3 fatty acids, which are particularly abundant in fatty fish, including salmon and canned tuna, is associated with a reduced cancer risk.[15] The *Dietary Guidelines for Americans* recommend consuming fish twice a week.
- **Meats cooked at high heat.** Heterocyclic amines (HCAs) and polycyclic aromatic hydrocarbons (PAHs) are chemicals formed when muscle meat, including beef, pork, fish, or poultry, is cooked using high-temperature methods, such as frying, barbecuing, or grilling over an open flame. These chemicals are carcinogenic.[17] Although not all studies agree, some have found that high consumption of well-done, fried, or barbecued meats is associated with increased rates of colorectal, pancreatic, and prostate cancer.[18]
- **Nitrates.** Nitrogen-containing compounds called nitrates are associated with an increased cancer risk. These chemicals are present in agricultural products such as fertilizers and can make their way into groundwater. People living in agricultural areas may consume nitrates if they drink tap or well water. Nitrates and a related chemical, nitrites, are also found in some cured meats such as deli meats, hot dogs, bacon, and ham.

Physical Activity

The American Cancer Society recommends regular physical activity of at least 30 minutes 5 days a week to reduce your risk for cancers of the breast, colon, uterus, and prostate.[19] Exercise may also improve outcomes in people who are recovering from cancer. Two recent studies involving a total of more than 1,000 patients who had been treated for colorectal cancer found a 40–50% reduction in risk of recurrence

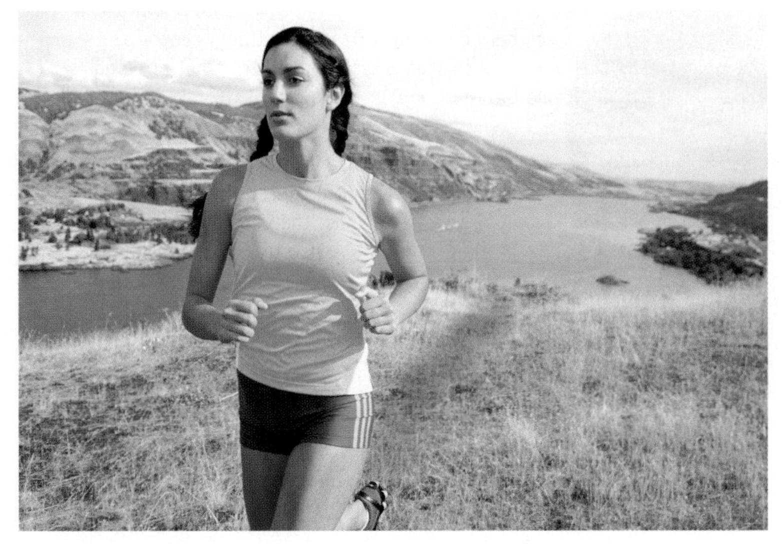

Exercising is one of the best things you can do to reduce your risk of cancer.

and mortality in patients who participated in significant physical activity, such as one hour of walking six times a week.[20]

Need some help getting your body in motion? Meet the American Cancer Society's "virtual trainer" at www.cancer.org/Healthy/eathealthygetactive/getactive/app/meet-our-virtual-trainer.aspx.

Body Weight

The American Cancer Society estimates that about one-third of all cancer deaths are related to overweight or obesity, inactivity, and a poor diet, and are thus preventable. Moreover, overweight and obesity are clearly linked with an increased risk for the following types of cancer:[1]

- Breast cancer in postmenopausal women
- Uterine cancer
- Colorectal cancer
- Cancer of the esophagus
- Pancreatic cancer
- Kidney cancer

Moreover, obesity is thought to increase the risk for cervical and ovarian cancers, for cancers of the liver and gallbladder, and for cancers affecting certain immune cells. The good news is that some studies have shown a link between losing weight and reducing your cancer risk.[1]

Tobacco Use

Tobacco use is the leading cause of preventable illness and death in the United States. It is capable of causing cancer almost anywhere in the body and accounts for at least 30% of all cancer deaths.[1] Smoking is linked to at least 15 cancers, including those of the lungs, esophagus, larynx, mouth, throat, kidney, bladder, pancreas, stomach, and cervix.[21] A 2010 report of the U.S. Surgeon General explains that tobacco causes disease by damaging cells and prompting inflammation. According to the report, inhaling even the smallest amount of tobacco smoke can damage your DNA.[22] One in three cancer deaths in the United States is tobacco related.[22]

Alcohol Use

Alcohol consumption has long been linked to an increased risk for various types of cancer. A statistical analysis of more than 200 studies of alcohol and cancer spanning more than 30 years found that alcohol most strongly increases the risks for cancers of the oral cavity, pharynx, esophagus, and larynx. It also found significant increases in risk for cancers of the stomach, colon, rectum, liver, female breast, and ovaries.[23]

Consumption of more than one drink per day for women and more than two drinks per day for men is associated with an increased mortality rate. But we don't know the precise "threshold level" of alcohol consumption at which cancer risk increases. We also don't know exactly how alcohol acts to promote cancer. Researchers theorize that it irritates or directly damages body cells, especially those of the mouth, throat, and liver, causing an accumulation of "copying mistakes" in their DNA as they try to repair the damage. We also know that, in the colon and rectum, bacteria convert alcohol into acetaldehyde, a chemical that is carcinogenic. Alcohol may also act in combination with other harmful chemicals present in the body—for instance, by reducing the body's ability to break them down and excrete them. It may also reduce the body's ability to absorb folate (one of the B vitamins) from food. Low folate levels are associated with an increased risk for certain cancers. Tobacco use, which is common among drinkers, enhances alcohol's damaging effects.[24]

Sun Exposure

Sunbathing may feel glorious, but is the pleasure worth the harm? Ultraviolet (UV) rays, a form of radiation generated by sunlight, sun lamps, and tanning beds, can penetrate and damage your skin cells. Two types of UV rays are of concern:

- UVA rays penetrate into deeper layers of the skin. Studies suggest that excessive exposure to UVA rays increases your risk for skin cancer. It also contributes to wrinkling and other signs of aging.
- UVB rays don't penetrate as deeply as UVA, but are responsible for sunburns.

The National Cancer Institute states that it is not known whether protecting your skin from UV radiation decreases your risk for skin cancer; however, it suggests avoiding intense sunlight, wearing protective clothing, and applying a sunscreen that reduces your exposure to UVA and UVB radiation.[25] But before you go down to the drugstore and grab the first tube of sunscreen you see, you may want to visit the nearby **Consumer Corner.**

Want to know your risk of UV exposure wherever you are, any day of the year? Go to www.epa.gov/sunwise/uvindex.html and enter your location. You'll immediately learn the UV index and precautions you should take to stay "sunwise."

Environmental Exposure to Carcinogens

Do you have a job that involves working with chemicals or radiation, or live in an area with high levels of air pollution? If so, you may be exposing your body—and your DNA—to carcinogens on a regular basis.

STUDENT STORY

Reducing Cancer Risk

"**Hi, I'm Tara.** My grandfather passed away a week before school started from throat cancer because he smoked a lot of cigarettes. That affected me big time.

I don't smoke at all, but I still try to stay away from secondhand smoke 'cause it really does run in my family. Cervical cancer also runs in my family. I got the vaccine, the Gardisil vaccine, to protect from that. I also try to watch what I eat."

1: Avoiding tobacco smoke reduces Tara's risk for which cancers? How much do you think she's reducing her risk for lung cancer?

2: What non-modifiable risk factors does Tara have for cancer?

3: What else could Tara do to reduce her risk for cancer?

Do you have a story similar to Tara's? Share your story at www.pearsonhighered.com/lynchelmore.

Many jobs involve working with chemicals or radiation, or produce airborne particles, such as wood dust from sanding, that are known carcinogens. Be sure you are aware of all safety procedures used at your workplace and follow them. If you aren't sure about these safety procedures, talk to your boss or human resources department. State and federal laws lay out clear occupational safety requirements that companies must follow. If you devise your own summer job that requires you to work with chemicals—for instance, house painting, house cleaning, or landscaping—research the appropriate safety measures, such as wearing gloves and mask, and follow them!

How safe is the environment at your summer job? Visit www.osha.gov/SLTC/youth/summerjobs.

If you live in an area known for air pollution, you can start reducing your risks by being aware of the ebbs and flows in pollution levels. For example, pay attention to public service announcements identifying days when pollution levels are especially high, and avoid outdoor exercise during those times. If pollutants from nearby industry or a landfill or other waste site are a concern, or the safety of your public water supply is uncertain, consider getting involved in public pollution-reduction efforts. Many communities have environmental and health advocacy groups dedicated to reducing pollution and the diseases connected to it.

Don't forget that secondhand smoke is air pollution! Every year in the United States, about 3,400 nonsmoking adults die of lung cancer caused by breathing secondhand smoke.[26] If your roommate, office mate, or dinner date lights up, tell him or her to take it outside.

Pesticides are chemicals used to protect crops from weeds, animals, insects, or microorganisms. Some pesticides are classified as carcinogens, and studies of people with high exposures to pesticides have found high rates of many cancers, including cancers of the stomach, lung, brain, and others. Pesticide residues remain on conventionally grown produce, and the National Cancer Institute recommends washing fresh fruits and vegetables thoroughly to reduce your exposure.[27] Organic produce is typically grown without the use of synthetic pesticides, and consuming more organic foods can further reduce your risk.

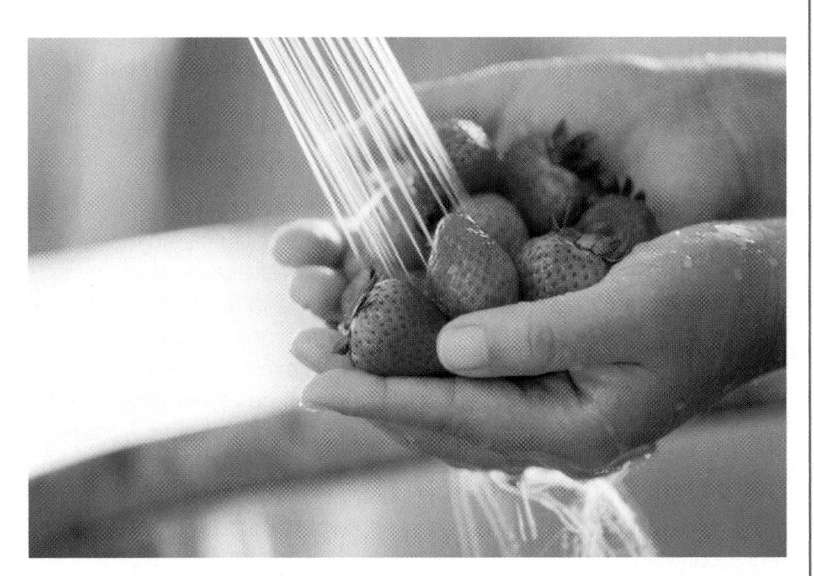

Washing **pesticides** off of produce can reduce your exposure to potential carcinogens.

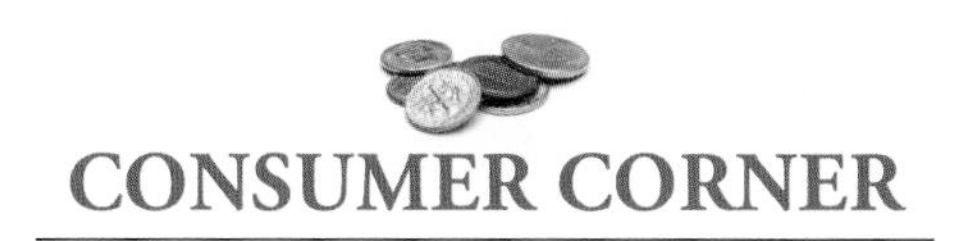

CONSUMER CORNER

Selecting a Sunscreen

In 2011, the U.S. Food and Drug Administration (FDA) released new regulations for the labeling of sunscreens.[1]

- No sunscreen is allowed to boast of a sun protection factor (SPF) higher than "50+" because there's no scientific evidence that protection higher than that level exists. (SPF ratings indicate the length of time the product should protect you from sunburn. For instance, if you would burn within 20 minutes of sun exposure without any sunscreen, application of an SPF 15 sunscreen should theoretically protect you for 5 hours.)
- No sunscreen can claim to be waterproof. Only "water resistant" is now allowed.
- Sunscreens are allowed to be labeled "Broad Spectrum" only if they offer protection against UVB rays, which cause burning, and UVA rays, which penetrate deeply into the skin and can damage DNA.
- Sunscreen products are required to state that those labeled "Broad Spectrum" and "SPF 15" (or higher) not only protect against sunburn, but, if used as directed with other sun-protection measures, have been shown to reduce the risk of skin cancer. By contrast, any sunscreen not labeled as "Broad Spectrum" or that has an SPF value between 2 and 14 has only been shown to help prevent sunburn.

Some consumer groups applauded the new regulations, but others said they didn't go far enough to warn Americans of the dangers of relying on sunscreens for protection against UV radiation. One claim is that the level of UVA protection that can earn a sunscreen a "Broad Spectrum" endorsement is ineffective. Yet consumers wearing a "Broad Spectrum" product may be tempted to stay out in the sun longer, thereby actually increasing their cancer risk. The International Agency for Research on Cancer (IARC) cautions that, whereas sunscreen use reduces rates of squamous cell carcinoma, some studies suggest that it may increase the risk for malignant melanoma, the most dangerous form of skin cancer. The IARC advises that consumers use sunscreen, but only as one step in a five-step program of sun avoidance:[2]

1. Avoid summer sun exposure between 10:00 a.m. and 4:00 p.m.
2. Stay in the shade to the greatest extent possible.
3. Wear a sun-protective T-shirt, a wide hat, and sunglasses while outdoors.
4. Apply sunscreen (SPF 30 minimum, with UVA protection) frequently and generously while in the sun.
5. Do not use sunscreen for tanning or as a means of staying longer in the sun.

Another concern is the potential toxicity of the active ingredients in most sunscreens. In 2011, the Environmental Working Group (EWG) released its annual report on sunscreens, in which it discussed research indicating that a form of vitamin A called retinyl palmitate used in 30% of sunscreen formulations promotes the development of cancer tumors in skin exposed to sunlight.[3] Moreover, the EWG cites studies critical of a chemical called oxybenzone, which is used in a majority of sunscreens sold in the United States. A study published by the U.S. Centers for Disease Control found blood levels of this chemical—which has been linked to cell damage—in 96% of Americans.[4]

The EWG suggests using a mineral sunscreen lotion (not a spray!) containing zinc oxide or titanium dioxide. These products block UV radiation without penetrating the skin.[3]

References. **1.** "FDA Sheds Light on Sunscreens," by the U.S. Food and Drug Administration, September 9, 2011, retrieved from http://www.fda.gov/ForConsumers/ConsumerUpdates/ucm258416.htm. **2.** "Reminder on Solar UV Radiation and Artificial UV Light," Press Release No. 178, by the International Agency for Research on Cancer June 1, 2007, retrieved from http://www.iarc.fr/en/media-centre/pr/2007/pr178.html. **3.** "Sunscreens Exposed: 9 Surprising Truths," by the Environmental Working Group, June 23, 2011, retrieved from http://breakingnews.ewg.org/2011sunscreen/sunscreens-exposed/sunscreens-exposed-9-surprising-truths. **4.** "Concentrations of the Sunscreen Agent Benzophenone-3 in Residents of the United States: National Health and Nutrition Examination Survey 2003–2004," by A. M. Calafat, L.-Y. Wong, X. Ye, J. A. Reidy, & L. L. Needham, 2008, *Environmental Health Perspectives 116*, doi:10.1289/ehp.11269.

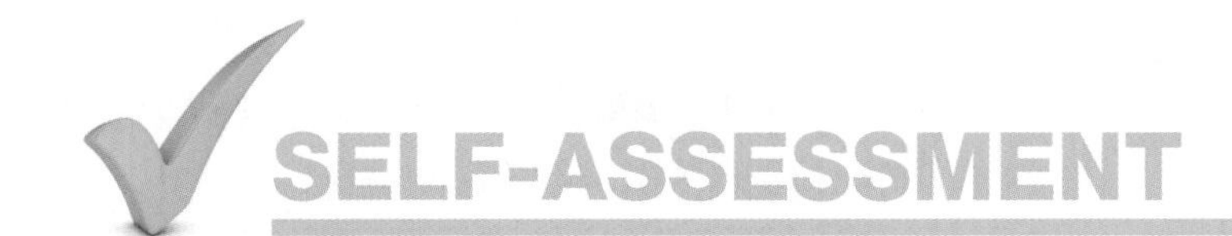

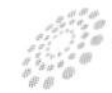
Take this self-assessment online at www.pearsonhighered.com/lynchelmore.

Am I at Risk for Cancer?

Next to each statement, check the answer that applies to you.

1. I eat a variety of vegetables and fruits every day.
   ☐ Always ☐ Sometimes ☐ Never
2. I choose whole-grain foods (breads, pastas, and cereals), rather than foods made from refined grains. I also choose brown rice instead of white rice.
   ☐ Always ☐ Sometimes ☐ Never
3. I avoid excess dietary fat.
   ☐ Always ☐ Sometimes ☐ Never
4. I choose foods rich in omega-3 fatty acids, such as salmon, canned tuna, and other fatty fish.
   ☐ Always ☐ Sometimes ☐ Never
5. If I eat red meat, I choose lean cuts and eat smaller portions.
   ☐ Always ☐ Sometimes ☐ Never
6. I prepare meat, poultry, and fish by baking, broiling, or poaching rather than by frying, barbecuing, or grilling over a flame.
   ☐ Always ☐ Sometimes ☐ Never
7. I limit my intake of processed meats containing nitrates, such as bacon, ham, deli meats, and hot dogs.
   ☐ Always ☐ Sometimes ☐ Never
8. I get at least 150 minutes of moderate intensity or 75 minutes of vigorous intensity activity each week (or a combination of these), preferably spread throughout the week.
   ☐ Always ☐ Sometimes ☐ Never
9. I limit sedentary behavior such as sitting, watching TV, and other screen-based entertainment.
   ☐ Always ☐ Sometimes ☐ Never
10. I have maintained a healthy weight at all ages.
    ☐ Always ☐ Sometimes ☐ Never
11. I avoid tobacco in all its forms.
    ☐ Always ☐ Sometimes ☐ Never
12. I drink no more than one drink a day if I'm a woman or two drinks a day if I'm a man.
    ☐ Always ☐ Sometimes ☐ Never
13. I avoid intense sunlight, or when in the sun, I wear protective clothing and a UVA and UVB sunscreen.
    ☐ Always ☐ Sometimes ☐ Never
14. I am not exposed to environmental carcinogens (chemicals, radiation, airborne particles, air pollution, secondhand smoke, or pesticides) through work or at home.
    ☐ Always ☐ Sometimes ☐ Never
15. I have access to quality health care and receive regular examinations by a health-care provider.
    ☐ Always ☐ Sometimes ☐ Never
16. If I am a woman, I have been vaccinated against HPV.
    ☐ Yes ☐ No
17. I have never been sexually active or I have always practiced safer sex to avoid exposure to STIs that can promote cancer.
    ☐ Yes ☐ No

Totals: _____Always _____Sometimes _____Never _____Yes _____No

HOW TO INTERPRET YOUR SCORE

For questions 1–15, the more "Always" the better. For questions 16–17, each "No" answer increases your risk. Focus on improving the behaviors for which you selected "No," "Never," or "Sometimes." Those answers indicate that these are factors that can contribute to your risk of cancer. The Choosing to Change Worksheet at the end of the chapter will assist you in improving these areas.

Exposure to Infectious Agents

Certain infectious microorganisms are known to be linked to some forms of cancer, and researchers are looking for others. They theorize that these disease-causing agents trigger cancer by causing persistent inflammation, suppressing a person's immune system, or stimulating cells into extended periods of growth. In the United States, some of the more common cancer-causing infectious agents include the following viruses:

- **Hepatitis B and C.** These forms of the hepatitis virus can lead to liver cancer. In people from certain countries in Asia, such as China, where hepatitis B is common, virus-related liver cancer is a top health concern.[28] Vaccination against hepatitis B can prevent infection and significantly reduce the rate of liver cancer in populations.[29]
- **HIV.** This virus, in suppressing the immune system, can lead to certain types of cancer that are otherwise rare. These are called *opportunistic* cancers because they occur when reduced immune defenses allow them the opportunity to develop.[1]
- **HPV.** The human papilloma virus, or HPV, is usually transmitted through sexual contact. Nearly all women with cervical cancer have evidence of HPV, although not all cervical HPV infections turn into cancer. Young women are now also able to receive a vaccine against certain dangerous strains of HPV, and a vaccination has recently been developed for young men. You'll find more information on cervical cancer later in this chapter. HPV is also linked to a rise in cases of mouth and throat cancer, most likely due to transmission during oral sex.[1, 30]

Access to Health Care

Earlier, we talked about the role of health disparities in cancer risk. One of these is reduced access to health care. Regular examinations by a health-care provider can result in the detection and removal of growths that may otherwise develop into cancer. For example, a Pap test performed during a woman's routine gynecologic exam can detect cervical dysplasia—abnormalities in the cells on the surface of the cervix. If left untreated, cervical dysplasia can progress to cervical cancer. Access to quality health care can also allow for the diagnosis and treatment of cancer at an earlier stage, when it is less invasive and has not metastasized. Early diagnosis of mouth cancers, for example, is more likely with regular dental care.

To determine your risk for developing cancer, complete the **Self-Assessment** above.

The Clinical Picture

Clinical diagnosis and treatment of cancer usually begins with the primary health-care provider. If lab tests or other evidence suggest cancer, the patient is likely to be referred to an **oncologist,** a physician specializing in cancer treatment. From an oncologist, the patient is likely to learn more about the precise type of cancer, how advanced it is, and what plan of treatment is recommended.

oncologist A physician who specializes in cancer treatment.

biopsy A test for cancer in which a small sample of the abnormal growth is removed and studied.

Detecting Cancer

Because cancer can occur in sites as varied as lungs, bones, and blood, no single test can detect all cancers. But the increasing variety of detection methods is allowing more cancers to be caught earlier, when they are easier to treat.

Cancer Screening

Cancer may develop silently for years before producing any noticeable signs and symptoms. That's where screening tests come in. These tests "screen" large numbers of people to check for the presence of a disease or conditions associated with a disease. Often, a screening test will detect a "precancerous" mass and allow for its removal long before it has caused any symptoms. For instance, a *colonoscopy* is a screening test in which the clinician uses a tiny camera to examine the walls of the colon (large intestine). It allows the clinician to find and remove benign, precancerous, and cancerous growths called *polyps*, which typically cause no symptoms. Another example of a screening test is the Pap test mentioned earlier for cervical cancer. The American Cancer Society guidelines for cancer screening are identified in **Table 12.2.**

Typical Signs and Symptoms

Researchers have developed screening tests for only a very few cancers. So it's important that you be aware of 10 general symptoms that can tip you off that cancer might be developing in your body. Most often, these symptoms *are not due to cancer*. However, if you notice any of them, and don't see an apparent reason for them, make an appointment with your doctor:[31]

- A thickening or lump in the breast or any other part of the body
- A new mole or a change in an existing mole
- A sore that does not heal
- Hoarseness or a cough that does not go away
- Persistent changes in bowel or bladder habits
- Discomfort after eating
- Difficulty swallowing
- Weight gain or loss with no known reason
- Unusual bleeding or discharge
- Feeling weak or very tired

"Cancer may develop silently for years before producing any noticeable signs and symptoms. That's where screening tests come in."

Diagnostic Tests

When signs and symptoms suggest the possibility of cancer, the physician may perform one or more of a variety of diagnostic tests:

- **Lab tests.** Lab tests of blood, urine, or other body fluids can check for the presence of substances called *tumor markers* that suggest cancer. Alternatively, they can check for organ function, which may be compromised by tumors. And newer lab tests can analyze body fluids for signs of cancer-related DNA. A test being developed for oral cancer, for example, analyzes a saliva sample for the cancer's DNA "signature." If proven effective, this test will allow for earlier detection and treatment.[32]
- **Scans.** Other detection methods rely on imaging technologies. These include ultrasound (US), magnetic resonance imaging (MRI), computed tomography (CT), and positron emission tomography (PET), each of which has advantages and disadvantages for different locations and types of tissues. For example, PET scans involve injecting the patient with a small amount of a radioactive substance, then scanning the body with a machine that records with various colors areas of high chemical activity in the body **(Figure 12.2).** It can detect masses of cancer cells, which have a high rate of metabolic activity that supports their rapid reproduction. Scans also differ in their risk to patients. For example, no known risks are associated with US, whereas CT exposes the body to levels of radiation many times higher than that of conventional X rays.
- **Biopsy.** In a **biopsy,** a physician or surgeon removes a small sample of the abnormal growth so that it can be sent to a lab and studied for

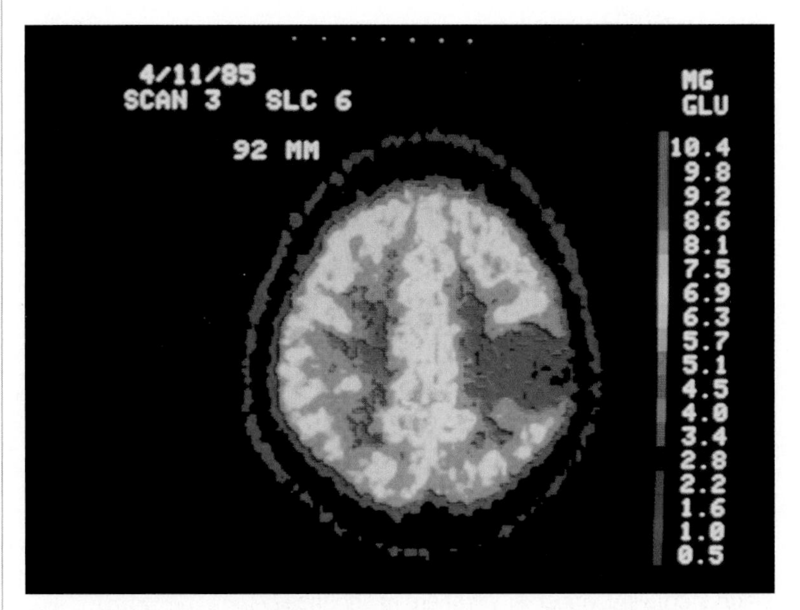

Figure 12.2 **A PET scan of a cancerous growth in the brain.** The cancer appears as the blue spot on the right.

Table 12.2: Screening Guidelines for the Early Detection of Cancer in Average-Risk Asymptomatic People

Cancer Site	Population	Test or Procedure	Frequency
Breast	Women, age 20+	Breast self-examination (BSE)	It is acceptable for women to choose not to do BSE or to do BSE regularly (monthly) or irregularly. Beginning in their early 20s, women should be told about the benefits and limitations of breast self-examination (BSE). Whether a woman ever performs BSE, the importance of prompt reporting of any new breast symptoms to a health professional should be emphasized. Women who choose to do BSE should receive instruction and have their technique reviewed on the occasion of a periodic health examination.
		Clinical breast examination (CBE)	For women in their 20s and 30s, it is recommended that clinical breast examination (CBE) be part of a periodic health examination, preferably at least every 3 years. Asymptomatic women age 40 and older should continue to receive a clinical breast examination as part of a periodic health examination, preferably annually.
		Mammography	Begin annual mammography at age 40.*
Cervix	Women, age 21+	Pap test, HPV test	Cervical cancer screening should begin at 21 years of age. Screening should be done every 3 years with a Pap test. From age 30 through age 65, women should have a Pap test and an HPV test every 5 years. After age 65, women who have had normal test results need no further screening. Women who have been diagnosed with cervical dysplasia should continue screening as for younger women.
Colorectal	Men and women, age 50+	Fecal occult blood test (FOBT) with at least 50% test sensitivity for cancer, or fecal immunochemical test (FIT) with at least 50% test sensitivity for cancer, **or**	Annual, starting at age 50. Testing at home with adherence to manufacturer's recommendation for collection techniques and number of samples is recommended. FOBT with the single stool sample collected on the clinician's fingertip during a digital rectal examination in the health-care setting is not recommended. Guaiac-based toilet bowl FOBT tests also are not recommended. In comparison with guaiac-based tests for the detection of occult blood, immunochemical tests are more patient friendly, and are likely to be equal or better in sensitivity and specificity. There is no justification for repeating FOBT in response to an initial positive finding.
		Stool DNA test, **or**	Interval uncertain, starting at age 50
		Flexible sigmoidoscopy (FSIG), **or**	Every 5 years, starting at age 50. FSIG can be performed alone, or consideration can be given to combining FSIG performed every 5 years with a highly sensitive gFOBT or FIT performed annually.
		Double contrast barium enema (DCBE), **or**	Every 5 years, starting at age 50
		Colonoscopy	Every 10 years, starting at age 50
		CT colonography	Every 5 years, starting at age 50
Endometrial	Women, at menopause	At the time of menopause, women at average risk should be informed about risks and symptoms of endometrial cancer and strongly encouraged to report any unexpected bleeding or spotting to their physicians.	
Prostate	Men, age 50+	Digital rectal examination (DRE) and prostate-specific antigen test (PSA)	Men who have at least a 10-year life expectancy should have an opportunity to make an informed decision with their health-care provider about whether to be screened for prostate cancer, after receiving information about the potential benefits, risks, and uncertainties associated with prostate cancer screening. Prostate cancer screening should not occur without an informed decision-making process.
Cancer-Related Checkup	Men and women, age 20+	On the occasion of a periodic health examination, the cancer-related checkup should include examination for cancers of the thyroid, testicles, ovaries, lymph nodes, oral cavity, and skin, as well as health counseling about tobacco, sun exposure, diet and nutrition, risk factors, sexual practices, and environmental and occupational exposures.	

*Beginning at age 40, annual clinical breast examination should be performed prior to mammography.

Note: The American Cancer Society is currently developing screening recommendations for lung cancer in heavy smokers; please refer to cancer.org for the most current information.

Source: Cancer Facts & Figures, 2012, by the American Cancer Society, 2012, p. 64, available at http://www.cancer.org/acs/groups/content/@epidemiologysurveilance/documents/document/acspc-031941.pdf and American Cancer Society. (2012, March 14). *New screening guidelines for cervical cancer.* Retrieved from http://www.cancer.org/Cancer/news/new-screening-guidelines-for-cervical-cancer.

signs of cancer. In some cases, the physician will do a needle biopsy, using a needle to withdraw fluid from, for example, a breast mass. Some biopsies are done with an endoscope, a thin, flexible tube with which a physician can inspect and remove a sample of tissue from, for example, the stomach. In a surgical biopsy, the surgeon may remove the suspicious mass entirely, or just a portion.[33]

Describing Cancer

The first question likely to enter the mind of a patient diagnosed with cancer is: What are my chances? This question is addressed by evaluating the tumor grade and the cancer stage.

pathologist A physician who specializes in identifying the nature of a disease by examining cells and tissues.

Grading, Staging, and Prognosis

Tumor cells can be classified—or *graded*—according to how abnormal they appear **(Figure 12.3).** A **pathologist,** a physician who specializes in identifying the nature of a disease by examining cells and tissues, examines a specimen under the microscope and assigns a grade of 1 to 4:[34]

- Grade 1 indicates that the cells making up the tumor are well differentiated; that is, they are specialized, somewhat like normal body cells of the same tissue type. Grade 1 cells tend to grow and multiply slowly, so grade 1 tumors are considered less aggressive.

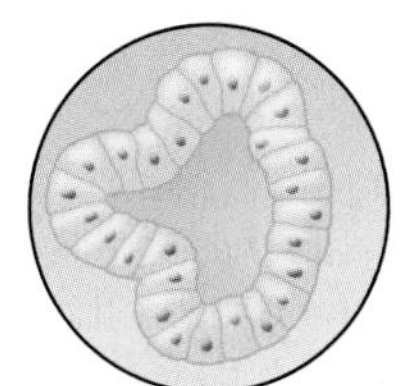
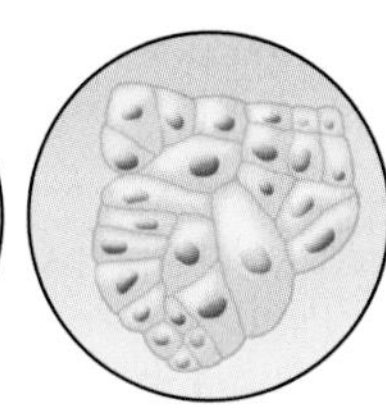
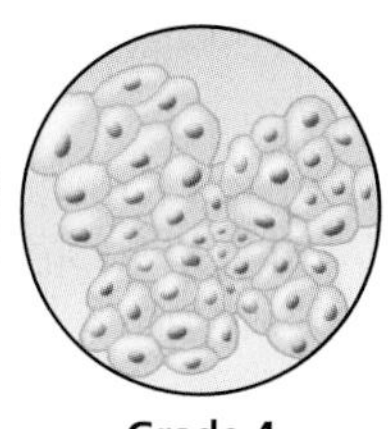

(a) Tumor grading

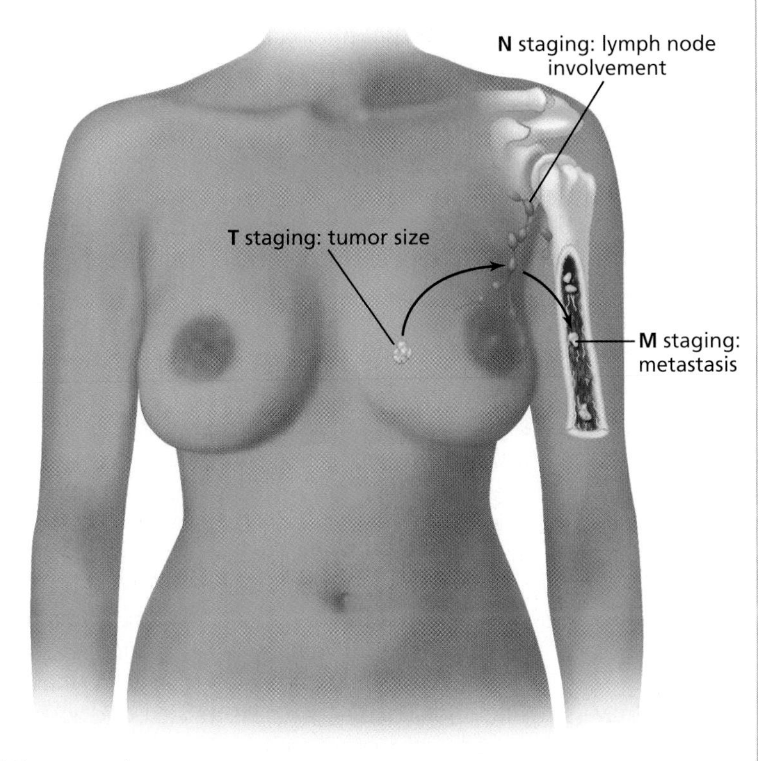

(b) Cancer staging

Figure 12.3 Grading and staging of cancer. Grading classifies tumors by the type of cell; staging classifies tumors according to: tumor size (T), extent of lymph node involvement (N), and whether or not the cancer has metastasized (M).

Source: Adapted from McConnell, T. H. *The Nature of Disease,* 1st edition, page 104. © 2007. Lippincott Williams and Wilkins.

- Grade 2 tumors are made up of cells that are moderately differentiated. They may still have some characteristics of the normal, functional cells in that tissue.
- Grade 3 tumors are made up of poorly differentiated cells. These tumors tend to grow rapidly.
- Grade 4 tumors consist of undifferentiated cells. These cells have no function other than to multiply, and they do so rapidly. Thus, a grade 4 tumor will spread much faster than a tumor with a lower grade.

Tumor grading is important, but it must be combined with cancer staging to provide a complete "picture" of the cancer. Staging describes the extent or severity of the cancer according to the tumor's size and behavior. Accurate staging is essential in determining the choice of treatment plan and estimating the patient's **prognosis;** that is, the clinical estimation of the course and outcome of the cancer. Prognosis (a word that means "knowing in advance") includes an estimation of the likelihood that treatment will be successful and that the patient will survive. Although many staging systems are in use, most facilities use the TNM system:[35]

- **Tumor.** The extent of the primary tumor is either described as *in situ*, meaning that abnormal cells are present but are precancerous, or assigned a number from T1 to T4, with higher numbers indicating a larger tumor size.
- **Nodes.** *Lymph nodes* are small organs containing defensive cells. They are distributed along *lymphatic vessels*, the tiny tubes that carry lymph back to the bloodstream, where they act to filter and cleanse the lymph of harmful agents. Cancer that has spread to lymph nodes is more difficult to treat. N0 indicates no lymph node involvement, whereas N1 to N3 indicate involvement of regional to distant nodes.
- **Metastasis.** M0 means no distant metastasis, whereas M1 means that distant metastasis is present.

For example, breast cancer classified as T3 N1 M0 is a large tumor that has spread to nearby lymph nodes but has not metastasized to distant body sites.

TNM classifications are used in different ways for staging different types of cancer. For example, colon cancer that is T3 N0 M0 is stage II, but bladder cancer with the same TNM classification is stage III. In general, the higher the stage, the more advanced the cancer: Stage IV typically means that the cancer has spread to another organ.

We noted that cancer stage suggests prognosis. For example, in early stages, lung cancer has a 52% survival rate, but this plummets to 4% for lung cancer patients in stage IV. And localized breast cancer has a 99% survival rate, but just 23% of patients with metastatic breast cancer survive.[1] Thus, the wisdom of early detection and treatment cannot be overemphasized.

Classification of Cancer

Cancers can be grouped into five broad categories according to the type of tissue in which the cancer arises:

- **Carcinomas** begin in the body's epithelial tissues, which include the skin and the tissues that line or cover internal organs. These are the most common sites for cancer. *Adenocarcinomas* are a common subtype: these arise in glands that secrete mucus or other types of fluids.
- **Sarcomas** start in the muscles, bones, fat, blood vessels, or other connective or supporting tissue.
- **Central nervous system cancers** begin in the tissues of the brain and spinal cord. These do damage both by directly altering nerve function and by growing large enough to interfere with the function of surrounding tissue.
- **Leukemias** start in the tissues that make your blood. They do not cause solid tumors, instead filling the blood with abnormal blood cells.
- **Lymphomas** begin in the cells of the immune system. These cancers tend to appear first in the lymph nodes, and take the form of solid tumors.

prognosis The clinical estimation of the course and outcome of a disease.

carcinoma Cancer of tissues that line or cover the body.

sarcoma Cancer of muscle or connective tissues.

central nervous system cancer Cancer of the brain or spinal cord.

leukemia Cancer of blood-forming tissue.

lymphoma Cancer of the lymph system.

Cancer Treatment

The type of cancer treatment a patient receives varies according to the type of cancer, the stage, the patient's age, and his or her overall state of health. Unfortunately, where you are treated matters, too: The nation's top cancer centers are likely to have oncologists, surgeons, and other staff far more experienced in treating the less common or more advanced cancers using the latest therapies. This, in turn, affects 5-year survival rates, which tend to be higher at the nation's top cancer centers than at community hospitals. For instance, 5-year survival for patients with prostate cancer treated at top facilities is 72%, but just 62% for those treated in community hospitals. For patients with stage IV cancers, the differences in survival rates are even greater.[36]

Surgery

Surgery is often the first step in cancer treatment. The surgeon typically removes the tumor itself as well as some healthy tissue around it, as nearby tissue may have been infiltrated by cancer cells.[37] The surgeon may also remove some nearby lymph nodes. In some cases, surgery alone may cure the cancer. For instance, a grade 1 or 2 tumor that has not spread to the lymph nodes nor metastasized may be removed and the patient simply followed closely for a period of years to monitor for recurrence.

When the tumor is present on a body surface or the lining of an accessible cavity, laser therapy can be used instead of surgery. Lasers are narrow, high-intensity beams of light that can be aimed precisely to cut away tiny amounts of tissue. Skin cancers, for instance, are typically removed with laser therapy, as are small tumors in the esophagus, stomach, and colon.

palliative care Treatment aimed at improving quality of life rather than curing the disease.

The side effects of surgery depend mainly on the size and location of the tumor, and the type of operation. Of course there is pain at the surgical site, and the anesthesia may leave the patient feeling nauseated, confused, sleepy, or dizzy. The patient may feel tired or weak for months after the surgical wound has healed. With laser therapy, anesthesia may not be used at all, or may be local, and the tissues sustain less damage; therefore, the side effects are minimal.

Radiation Therapy

In radiation therapy, high-energy electromagnetic rays are aimed at the affected site to kill cancer cells and destroy or shrink a tumor. A physician specializing in radiation therapy—called an *interventional radiologist*—may use several types:[37]

- *External radiation* is generated from a large machine outside the body. Most people are treated in a clinic setting for several days a week for a few weeks.
- *Internal radiation* comes from radioactive material covered in protective seeds, needles, or thin plastic tubes that are inserted in or near the tissue. The implants generally remain in place for several days.

In addition, a few types of cancer can be treated with *systemic radiation*, a therapy in which the patient is injected with or swallows a substance containing radioactive material. The material then travels throughout the body—for instance, to the bone marrow.

Radiation may be tightly targeted, but still can kill normal cells. The side effects, which depend mainly on the dose and type of radiation and the site that is treated, may include fatigue, nausea, vomiting, and diarrhea. The skin in the treated area may become tender, or even develop a radiation burn wound. Hair loss in the treated area is common.

A new technique performed by interventional radiologists is *radiofrequency ablation*, in which the radiologist guides a needle through the patient's skin and into the tumor. Through the tip of the needle, the radiologist administers heat that "microwaves" and kills the tumor cells. An opposite technique, called *cryoablation*, uses an extremely cold gas (*cryo-* means "cold") to freeze the tumor.[38]

Chemotherapy

Chemotherapy is the use of drugs that kill cancer cells. Most patients receive chemotherapy in an outpatient clinic, with doses for one or more days, followed by a recovery period of several days or weeks before the next session. The drugs are usually administered by injection or through a vein, but are now sometimes given orally. Once they enter the bloodstream, they can travel to and destroy cancer cells all over the body. Unfortunately, they also destroy other rapidly dividing cells, including blood cells, cells in hair follicles, and cells that line the intestinal tract. This explains the chemotherapy patient's fatigue and vulnerability to infection, hair loss, and nausea, vomiting, diarrhea, and weight loss.[31]

Chemotherapy may follow surgery, with the goal of destroying any cancer cells that may have broken away from the tumor. If a tumor is inoperable—for instance, if it is located next to or has grown into vital structures such as the brain, the heart, or primary blood vessels, or if it is large and has already metastasized—chemotherapy may be the first choice of treatment, or the patient may receive a combination of radiation and chemotherapy. Even for patients with terminal illness, chemotherapy may still be included as part of a broader program of **palliative care;** that is, treatment aimed at improving quality of life rather than curing the disease. Palliative care monitors and relieves a patient's pain, and addresses physical, psychological, and spiritual suffering.

Hormone Therapy

Some cancers cells have receptor sites—docking stations—for certain normal body hormones. When these hormones attach, the cancer cells

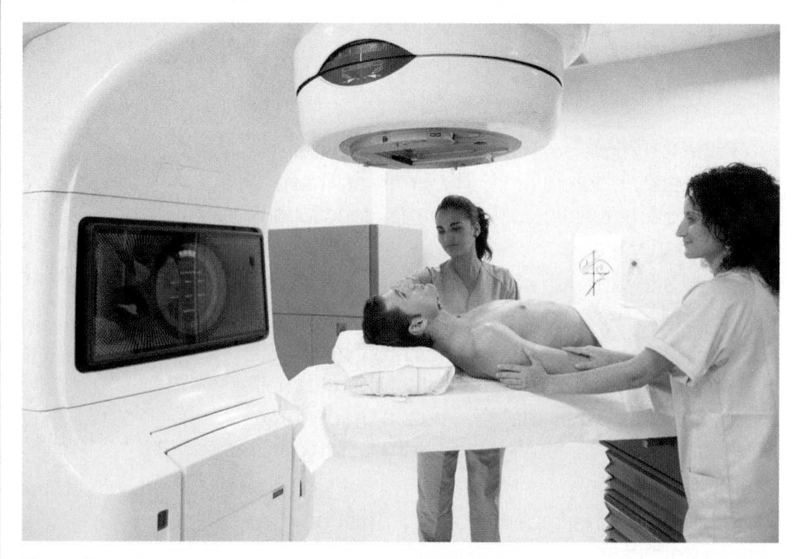

Radiation can treat cancer but can also, unfortunately, kill healthy cells.

use them to boost their ability to multiply. For example, the female reproductive hormones estrogen and progesterone help some types of breast cancer cells to multiply.[39] In hormone therapy, the patient takes medication that stops the production of these hormones, or impairs the hormones' functioning. Alternatively, the patient may undergo surgery in which the body glands producing the hormone—such as the ovaries—are removed.

Biological Therapy

Biological therapy increases the effectiveness of the body's natural defenses against cancer. In biological therapy, substances administered by injection or through a vein travel through the bloodstream to stimulate the immune system to destroy cancer cells. The substances work in a variety of ways, for instance by making cancer cells more recognizable to the immune system, by blocking processes that change precancerous cells to cancer cells, by increasing the destructive power of natural killer cells and other immune cells, and by preventing cancer cells from metastasizing.[40]

Treatments That Target Blood Vessels

Tumors require blood vessels to bring them the oxygen and nutrients they need. As they enlarge and invade other tissues, they need to develop ever more extensive networks of blood vessels. *Angiogenesis* is the process by which the body forms new blood vessels (*angio-* refers to blood vessels). It is controlled by a variety of body chemicals, and occurs normally, for example, in wound healing and during pregnancy. New drugs called *angiogenesis inhibitors* can derail this process, and thus slow or halt the growth of tumors. They are usually administered intravenously about every two weeks.

In addition, interventional radiologists use a targeted technique to directly cut off the blood supply to a tumor. In *chemoembolization*, the radiologist delivers through a flexible tube a dose of chemotherapy that embolizes, or blocks, the arteries feeding the tumor.

Stem Cell Transplantation

Every day, about 200 billion new red blood cells are produced in your bone marrow, the spongy tissue in the core of the larger bones of your body. Recall that high doses of chemotherapy destroy rapidly dividing cells—including these newly forming blood cells. Transplantation of blood-forming *stem cells* enables patients who have received high doses of chemotherapy to "catch up" on red blood cell production. In the technique, the patient receives healthy, blood-forming stem cells through a tube placed in a large vein. New blood cells develop from the transplanted stem cells. Ideally, the stem cells used in the therapy are taken from the patient beforehand. This prevents immune system rejection of the transplanted cells, which can occur when they come from another person.[41]

Gene Therapy: Still Experimental

Gene therapy is any of a variety of techniques used for correcting defective genes responsible for the development of diseases. In gene therapy, the defective gene could be replaced or repaired, or its function could be altered. Gene therapy is still in an experimental stage, and the FDA has not currently approved any human gene therapy product; however, research is ongoing, and does hold some promise. For example, in 2006, researchers at the National Cancer Institute used gene therapy to alter human immune cells so that they would target and destroy cancer cells in patients with melanoma, the most serious form of skin cancer. In 2009, British researchers announced their development of a treatment that delivered genes wrapped in nanoparticles to cancer cells in rats. Once taken up by the cancer cells, the genes produced a protein that destroyed the cells.[42]

Complementary and Alternative Therapies

Ads all over TV and the Internet endorse dietary supplements, "all-natural" beauty products, air-purification devices, and hundreds of other items claiming to reduce cancer risk or even to cure cancer. As you probably suspect, such claims are rarely legitimate. The actor is in most cases simply being paid to read a script. Even when he or she really uses the product or service and genuinely believes it to be beneficial, it still may not be effective or even safe. The National Council Against Health Fraud estimates that Americans spend 3 to 4 billion dollars annually on fraudulent products and services to prevent and treat cancer.[43]

Fortunately, in 1998, the National Cancer Institute founded the Office of Cancer Complementary and Alternative Medicine (OCCAM) to sponsor research into complementary and alternative therapies for cancer treatment and to improve the quality of care for cancer patients. The OCCAM provides the most current facts about complementary and alternative therapies used in cancer, from herbs to meditation, thereby helping patients to avoid wasting their money, or even being harmed by fraudulent treatments.

For information on the safety and effectiveness of available complementary and alternative cancer therapies in alphabetical order, go to www.cancer.gov/cam/health_camaz.html.

Common Cancers Affecting Both Men and Women

Although cancer can arise in hundreds of different sites in your body, some sites are far more prone to cancer than others. We'll start with a look at cancers that affect both men and women, and follow with a separate overview of common sex-specific cancers.

Skin Cancer

More than 3 million Americans are estimated to develop skin cancer each year, yet skin cancer is responsible for only about 12,000 deaths.[1] To see why, let's look at the three forms of skin cancer.

Types of Skin Cancer

The vast majority of skin cancers are carcinomas that develop in the epidermis, the top layer of skin. The two most common types involve either the squamous (flat, scaly) cells on the surface or the somewhat deeper basal cells. When you evaluate statistics on cancer rates, bear in mind that neither squamous cell carcinoma nor basal cell carcinoma is included. That's in part because both tend to grow very slowly and remain localized, and they are highly treatable; however, because some forms can become invasive, they should be removed promptly. Typically, a dermatologist will excise the mass with a scalpel or laser, or use cryosurgery (destruction of tissue via freezing) during an office visit.

In contrast, about 5% of skin cancer cases are **malignant melanomas,** which arise in the melanocytes, the skin cells that produce the pigment

gene therapy Any of a variety of techniques used for correcting defective genes responsible for the development of diseases.

malignant melanoma An especially aggressive form of skin cancer.

melanin that gives us our varied skin tones. UVA radiation can reach the melanocytes and cause changes in their DNA that can then promote uncontrolled growth. Malignant melanoma is much more likely than squamous or basal cell carcinoma to invade other tissues and to metastasize. If caught early and removed, it is unlikely to cause anything more serious than a small scar, but if left untreated, it can be fatal. In 2012, more than 9,000 Americans were expected to die of malignant melanoma.[1]

Risk Factors

Risk factors for all types of skin cancer include:

- Fair skin and light hair or eyes
- Skin that sunburns easily
- Personal or family history of skin cancer
- Frequent excessive sun exposure, including sunburns
- Use of tanning beds

An additional risk factor specific to malignant melanoma is the presence of unusual or numerous moles (more than 50).

Signs and Symptoms

What should you watch for? Squamous and basal cell carcinomas look like round bumps, colored spots, or scaly patches on the skin. These may bleed or ooze, but don't change color. Basal cell carcinomas may even resemble acne. In contrast, melanoma may arise as a new growth on the skin that progresses over a month or more. It also commonly appears as a gradual change to an existing mole. When examining any skin growth, use the ABCDE acronym to remember to look for these signs of malignant melanoma **(Figure 12.4):**

- **A**symmetry, where one side does not match the other
- **B**order irregularity, where edges are uneven or scalloped
- **C**olor changes, where pigmentation is not uniform
- **D**iameter, where the size is more than 6 millimeters (about the size of a pea)
- **E**volving, where the mole looks different from others nearby or changes in size, shape, or color over time

If you notice any of these signs, see your doctor as soon as possible.

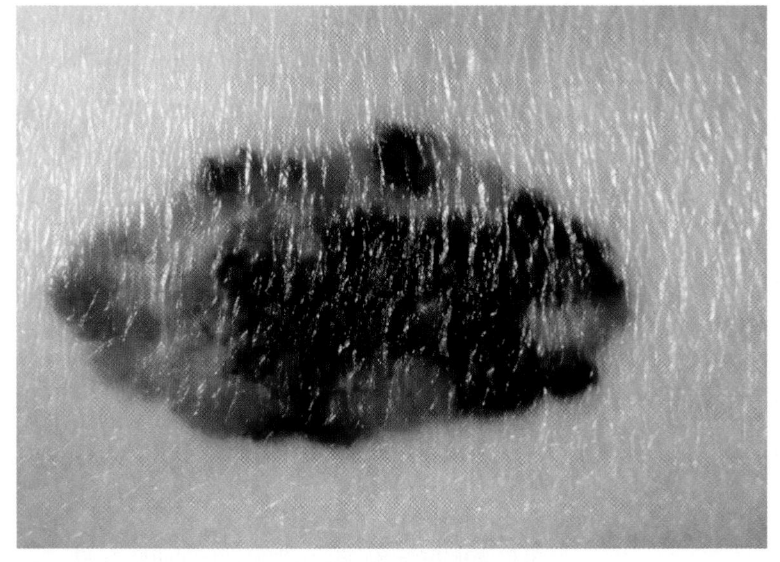

Figure 12.4 Skin cancer.

Diagnosis and Treatment

If you notice an unusual growth on your skin, see a dermatologist, who will likely remove it and send it to a lab for evaluation. If the dermatologist suspects melanoma, he or she may remove a "margin" of surrounding healthy tissue and sometimes a nearby lymph node. Large, invasive melanomas are treated with surgery and often radiation and/or chemotherapy. Again, early treatment is critical: The 5-year survival rate for localized melanoma is 98%, but only 15% of melanoma patients with distant metastasis survive.[1]

Reducing Your Risk

If you don't have a history of skin cancer in your family, doctors don't recommend regular screenings for melanoma. But everyone's risk begins to increase at age 20, so it's a good idea to check your skin periodically for signs of change. If you do have a family or personal history of skin cancer, many doctors recommend augmenting your own checks with a yearly skin exam from a dermatologist.

In a recent survey, only 5% of college students reported using sunscreen, and just 3% said they avoid sun exposure during midday.[44] That's unfortunate, as a lot of unprotected sun exposure increases your skin cancer risk. Allow yourself about 20 minutes in the sun—an amount of sun exposure that experts consider safe and that allows your skin to synthesize vitamin D.[45] For longer sun exposure, put on a hat and other protective clothing, or apply a broad-spectrum, high-SPF sunscreen. Especially avoid sun exposure at midday, when the sun is high in the sky. Don't believe that being in water provides any protection: It doesn't! And even if your sunscreen says it is "water resistant," reapply it after coming out of the waves.

Avoid all forms of tanning. The skin cancer risks of sustained, repeated exposure to UVA rays have been widely documented by medical researchers. Especially in fair-skinned people, tanning is linked to an increased risk of melanoma and other forms of skin cancer. Indoor tanning beds emit doses of UV radiation far more powerful than those that come from the sun, and the American Cancer Society considers them definitively carcinogenic.[1] And though some people like to tan because they think it makes them look better now, they overlook the fact that sun exposure actually prematurely ages your skin and makes it look worse later on.

Lung Cancer

With more than 225,000 new cases expected in 2012, and more than 160,000 deaths, lung cancer is the most common malignancy affecting both males and females in the United States—and the most deadly. Even localized lung cancer has only a 52% 5-year survival rate, and just 4% of lung cancer patients with distant metastasis survive.

Types of Lung Cancer

There are two main types of lung cancer:[46]

- *Small cell cancers* typically develop in the more central areas of the lungs, and spread aggressively. This type of cancer develops almost exclusively in smokers.
- *Non–small cell cancers* may arise in cells lining the respiratory tract, in the tiny air sacs where gas exchange occurs, or in any of several other locations. Adenocarcinoma, the most common type, usually develops on the outermost surface—the periphery—of the lungs, and can spread to blood and lymph.

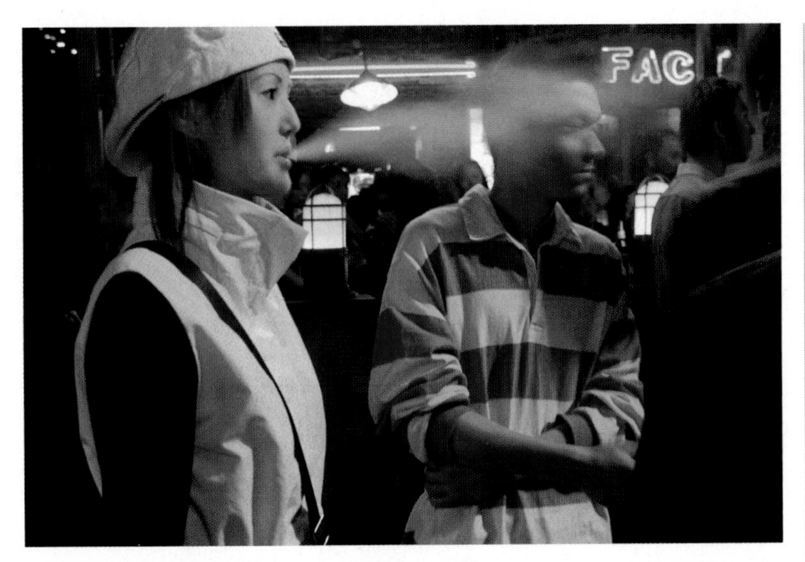

Lung cancer is **the most deadly** cancer in the United States, and smoking is its **largest** risk factor. Consider that before you light up.

Risk Factors

Risk factors for lung cancer include:

- A history of smoking or being exposed to secondhand smoke. The longer you've smoked or been exposed to tobacco smoke, the higher your risk.
- Genetic factors
- Exposure to radon. In some areas, this naturally occurring radioactive gas exists in high concentrations in the soil and, over time, seeps into people's homes or water supplies.
- Exposure to other cancer-causing substances, such as asbestos or arsenic.

Signs and Symptoms

What should you watch for? By the time any of the following symptoms have appeared, a case of lung cancer is usually fairly advanced:

- Spitting up blood-streaked mucus
- Chest pain
- A persistent cough
- Recurrent attacks of pneumonia or bronchitis

Diagnosis and Treatment

So far, this cancer has proven very difficult to detect early, and there are no established general screening guidelines. CT scans have been found effective at catching the disease early in people at higher risk, such as those with a history of heavy smoking, but it is not yet clear if this helps patients live longer.[47] Moreover, the potential risk of cumulative radiation exposure from multiple CT scans has not been adequately evaluated. A new screening technique in which a patient's cheek is swabbed and the cells analyzed under diffuse light is showing promise. It relies on the "field effect"—the ability of cancer to cause changes in distant, healthy tissue, in this case, the surface (epithelial) cells of the cheek. Research into this screening test is currently under way.[48]

The typical treatment protocol for lung cancer varies greatly according to the type and stage at the time of diagnosis. Early-stage non–small cell cancer is usually treated with surgery, which may be followed by radiation and/or chemotherapy. Stages III and IV are usually deemed inoperable, as are all forms of small-cell cancer except in rare cases when found very early. For these patients, chemotherapy and sometimes radiation are options.

> *"Don't make the mistake of waiting: Lung cancer can and does strike people in their 20s. Visit your campus health services today."*

Reducing Your Risk

Lung cancer accounts for 28% of all cancer deaths—more than any other cancer—and smoking accounts for the vast majority of these deaths.[1] If you smoke, get started on a plan to quit and, in the meantime, keep your smoke away from others. Don't make the mistake of waiting: Lung cancer can and does strike people in their 20s. Visit your campus health services today.

If you don't smoke, take steps to reduce your exposure to secondhand smoke. The delicate lining of the lungs becomes inflamed as soon as it is exposed to the toxic chemicals in cigarette smoke. The U.S. Surgeon General reports that even occasional exposure to secondhand smoke causes damage that can lead to cancer.[22] (See Chapter 10 for information on promoting a smoke-free campus.)

In addition, check your home for radon. According to the U.S. Environmental Protection Agency, nearly 1 in 15 U.S. homes has elevated radon levels.[49] You can purchase an inexpensive test kit to check the air in your home. You can also talk to campus officials about radon testing in campus buildings, and ask your employer for test results from your workplace.

Colon and Rectal Cancers

Colon cancer occurs in the large intestine, the last main portion of the gastrointestinal tract. Rectal cancer affects the final few inches of the colon. Together, colon and rectal cancers are referred to as *colorectal cancer*. Most cases begin with a particularly dangerous type of polyp in the gland cells of the colon lining. Although these precancerous polyps grow slowly, they will result in invasive cancer if not removed. Approximately 103,000 cases of colon cancer and over 40,000 cases of rectal cancer are diagnosed each year in the United States, making colorectal cancer the second most common cancer affecting both men and women. Colorectal cancer results in the deaths of more than 50,000 Americans annually.[1]

Risk Factors

Risk factors for colorectal cancer include:

- A family history of colorectal cancer
- A family history of polyps in the colon or rectum

- Being over the age of 50
- African American race. African Americans have the highest rate of colorectal cancer of any ethnic group.
- Presence of an inflammatory bowel disorder, such as colitis or Crohn's disease
- A poor diet. Some studies have found that frequent consumption of red meat may increase the risk for colorectal cancer, whereas other studies have found that diets rich in fruits, legumes and other vegetables, and whole grains reduces the risk.[16] Research also suggests that a high-fat diet increases the risk for colorectal cancer. The culprit is thought to be bile, which the body releases into the digestive tract to break apart the fats that we eat.[50] Bile is therefore important to human health; however, lining cells overexposed to it have been shown to develop cancer.
- Smoking. Long-term smokers have a 30–50% increased risk for colorectal cancer.[51]

Signs and Symptoms

What should you watch for? In its early stages, when it is easiest to treat, colorectal cancer often has no outward symptoms. As the cancer progresses, warning signs include the following:

- Changes in bowel habits, including constipation or diarrhea, or a feeling that the bowel is not emptying fully
- Bleeding from the rectum or blood in the stool
- Abdominal pain or discomfort, including gas or cramps
- Fatigue and weakness
- Unexplained weight loss

Diagnosis and Treatment

Screening is recommended for everyone once they reach the age of 50, using methods that include:

- A yearly test that detects blood in the stool
- Every 5 to 10 years, an internal imaging test that looks for polyps, such as a colonoscopy **(Figure 12.5)**
- For people at higher risk, such as those with a family history of colorectal cancer, doctors usually recommend a more frequent screening schedule

Colon cancer that is localized within a polyp and doesn't invade the colon wall can be removed during a colonoscopy. For larger cancers, the affected segment of the colon is surgically removed. If the surgeon is unable to reconnect the two healthy sections of the colon, the patient may have to eliminate stool via an opening (called an *ostomy*) in the abdominal wall. Radiation and chemotherapy are also common, especially for cancer in advanced stages.

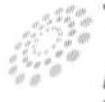

To learn more about colon cancer screening, check out this video from the American Cancer Society: www.cancer.org/Healthy/ToolsandCalculators/Videos/get-tested-for-colon-cancer-english.

Reducing Your Risk

The following measures may help to prevent colorectal cancer:

- Engaging in regular exercise
- Consuming a plant-based diet
- Maintaining a healthy weight
- Limiting alcohol consumption

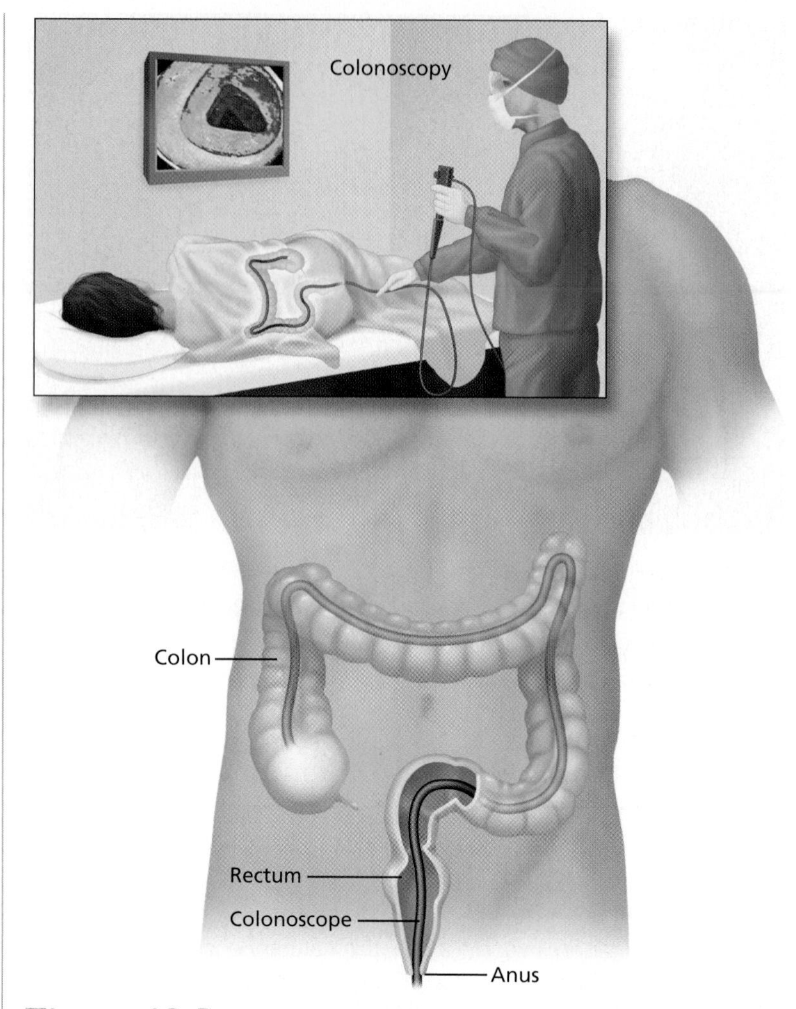

Figure 12.5 **Colonoscopy.** In a colonoscopy, a flexible, thin, lighted tube called a colonoscope is inserted through the anus and rectum into the colon, allowing the examiner to look for tissue abnormalities such as polyps.

- Avoiding smoking
- Following recommended screening guidelines, as precancerous and even some malignant polyps can be removed during a colonoscopy

Oral Cancer

Oral cancer is any malignancy of the lips, tongue, mouth, throat, or other oral tissue. More than 40,000 cases are diagnosed each year, resulting in nearly 8,000 deaths. Since 2008, incidence has been increasing for a type of oral cancer caused by HPV infection transmitted through sexual contact.[1]

In addition to HPV infection, risk factors include:

- Smoking. This includes not only cigarettes, but pipes, cigars, hookahs, and other forms of smoking.
- Use of "smokeless" or chewing tobacco
- Excessive drinking. A mix of heavy drinking and smoking is linked to a 30-fold increase in risk.
- Excessive sun exposure. This is associated with an increased risk of cancer of the lips.

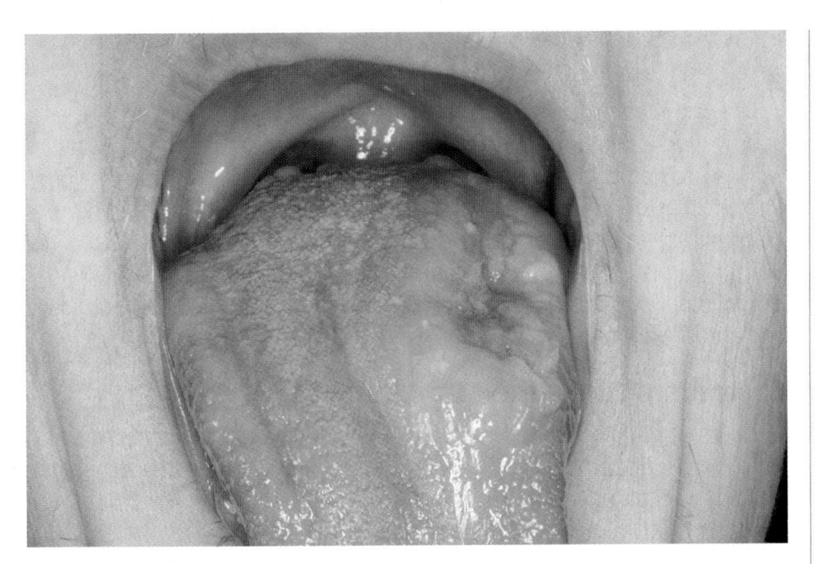

Figure 12.6 **Oral cancer.**

What should you watch for? Symptoms include a sore, discolored, swollen, or numb patch in the mouth or throat that doesn't heal or go away **(Figure 12.6).** Unexplained bleeding and coughing up blood are other signs. A persistent sore throat or even ear pain may be present, and the person may have difficulty chewing or swallowing.

Although there are no general screening guidelines, doctors and dentists usually make checking for oral cancer a routine part of any regular exam. As you learned earlier in this chapter, scientists are also trying to develop a screening test that would detect oral cancer's DNA signatures in a person's saliva.

Treatment of oral cancer includes surgery, which may be disfiguring. Radiation and chemotherapy may be necessary.

The best strategies for reducing your risk are to use a condom or dental dam if you engage in oral sex, avoid all types of tobacco products and, if you drink alcohol, to do so in moderation. When out in the sun, wear a sun-protective lip balm. And have regular dental exams.

Stomach Cancer

Over 21,000 cases of stomach cancer are diagnosed in the United States each year, causing more than 10,000 deaths. Even when stomach cancer is localized, the 5-year survival rate is only 62%. But stomach cancer usually metastasizes quickly, and with metastasis, survival drops to just 4%.[1]

The great majority of cases are adenocarcinomas. These arise in the glands that secrete the mucus that protects the stomach wall from being burned by stomach acid. The primary risk factors are dietary: People who eat a lot of salty and smoked foods and those who eat few fruits and vegetables are at increased risk. Infection with *Helicobacter pylori*, the bacterium that causes ulcers, also increases the risk, as does smoking.

Gastrointestinal distress—such as heartburn, stomach pain, nausea, vomiting, and feeling bloated—is a primary symptom, as are weight loss and fatigue. An endoscopy or scan may be done to view the stomach lining. In early stages, tumors can be removed during endoscopy. Later-stage tumors require surgical removal of the affected portion of the stomach. In some cases, the entire stomach may have to be removed, and the esophagus connected directly to the small intestine. Radiation and chemotherapy are other options.

Pancreatic Cancer

The *pancreas* is an abdominal organ that has two main tasks: During digestion, it releases juices into the small intestine that help break down foods, and after absorption, it releases insulin into the bloodstream to help body cells take up glucose. As you can imagine, any damage to this critical organ is life-threatening. Pancreatic cancer has the lowest overall survival rate of any cancer: just 6% of diagnosed patients survive 5 years. Approximately 44,000 cases are diagnosed each year, with almost 38,000 deaths. This poor survival rate also reflects the fact that pancreatic cancer typically goes undetected until it is quite advanced: More than half of cases are diagnosed in an advanced stage.[1]

Risk Factors

Risk factors for pancreatic cancer include:

- Smoking or the use of smokeless tobacco
- Obesity
- Diabetes
- Physical inactivity
- African American race. African Americans have the highest rate of pancreatic cancer in the world.[52]
- Genetic factors

Signs and Symptoms

Signs of pancreatic cancer rarely appear until the disease is advanced. Many patients report having no significant health concerns until they notice their skin looking yellowed (jaundiced). This prompts a physician visit and eventual diagnosis. Other common signs and symptoms include upper abdominal pain, loss of appetite, and unexplained weight loss.

Diagnosis and Treatment

Currently, no standard screening guidelines exist for pancreatic cancer. Researchers are looking for ways to detect this cancer early and determine who would benefit most from screening.

Treatment is usually palliative because the cancer is typically advanced before it is diagnosed. Fewer than 20% of patients are candidates for surgery.[1] Radiation and chemotherapy can extend survival time for many patients.

Reducing Your Risk

Reduce your risk of pancreatic cancer by following basic health guidelines, which include:

- Not smoking
- Eating a healthy diet high in fruits, vegetables, and whole grains and low in sugar, processed foods, and saturated fats
- Maintaining a healthy weight
- Exercising regularly—at least 30 minutes a day on most days

Liver Cancer

The *liver* is the metabolic workhorse of the human body. Its functions include breakdown of alcohol and other toxins, packaging of nutrients, production of bile, and literally hundreds of others. In 2012, there were more than 28,000 cases of liver cancer and over 20,000 deaths. Most

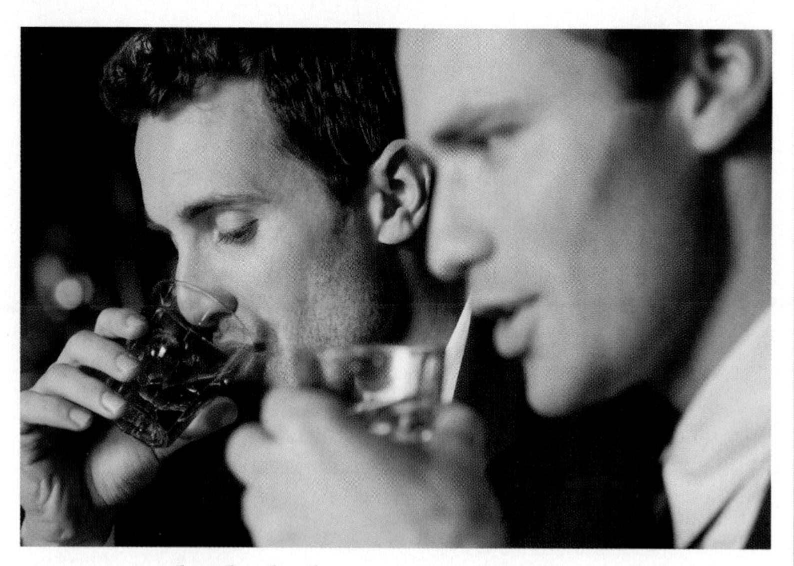

Long-term **alcohol abuse** can lead to liver cancer.

cases arise following damage from long-term alcohol abuse. However, HBV, HCV, and parasitic infections, as well as consumption of foods contaminated with aflatoxin, a toxin produced by molds during food storage, are other risk factors. Liver cancer is more than twice as common in men as in women, and rates are highest among Asian Americans and Hispanic Americans.[1]

Signs and symptoms of liver cancer include enlargement of the liver, jaundice, weight loss, abdominal pain or swelling, and weakness. In patients without alcohol-induced liver damage, surgery may be an option. When tumors cannot be surgically removed, interventional radiologists may try radiofrequency ablation or chemoembolization.

Urinary System Cancers

Cancers of the urinary system may involve the kidneys, bladder, or the system of tubes that transport urine (the ureters and urethra). Together, there are about 141,000 cases of urinary system cancers each year, causing about 29,000 deaths.[1] Smoking and obesity are the most significant risk factors. In addition, exposure to industrial chemicals may be implicated in bladder cancer.

Early stages don't usually cause symptoms. Depending on the precise location of the cancer, advanced cases may prompt pain or swelling in the lower back, swelling of the legs and ankles, fatigue, weight loss, and blood in the urine. Surgery is the primary treatment. If surgery is not an option, either radiofrequency ablation or cryoablation may be used. Angiogenesis inhibitors may also be administered to block the tumor's blood supply. Kidney cancer does not respond well to chemotherapy or radiation, but these are options for bladder cancer, as are certain biological therapies.

Brain Tumors

A *brain tumor* is any abnormal growth—benign or malignant—in the tissues of the brain. Benign tumors have a distinct border, grow slowly, and are not invasive. They can, however, press on sensitive tissues and cause pain and functional problems. Usually, they can be removed surgically. In contrast, malignant tumors grow aggressively, invading surrounding tissues and often metastasizing to other parts of the brain and the spinal cord. There are no known risk factors for either type. An estimated 23,000 cases of brain and other nervous system cancers were diagnosed in 2012, with more than 13,000 deaths.[1]

The most common symptom of a brain tumor is headaches that are usually worse in the morning. There may be nausea and vomiting, as well as problems with vision, hearing, speech, or walking, memory loss, and difficulty concentrating. Diagnosis may involve medical imaging or a spinal tap—analysis of the fluid surrounding the brain and spinal cord. Surgery is the usual first treatment. Typically, radiation therapy follows. Sometimes, patients are treated with chemotherapy, including surgically implanted wafers that release the drug slowly into the brain tissue.[53]

Cancers of the Blood and Lymph

Cancers of the blood and lymph include various forms of leukemias and lymphomas. Together, there are more than 126,000 cases each year in the United States, and more than 43,000 deaths.[1]

Leukemias

Over 47,000 cases of leukemia—cancer of the blood—are diagnosed in the United States each year, and about 23,500 people die from it.[1] Although commonly thought of as a childhood cancer, most cases actually occur in older adults. The disease arises in one of two primary forms: acute and chronic. Research into the genetics of cancer has revealed that these broader categories actually contain dozens of subtypes, each with unique DNA features.

Risk factors for leukemia include:

- Being male
- Having an inborn genetic disorder, such as Down syndrome
- Exposure to carcinogens such as tobacco smoke, certain chemicals, or radiation

The signs and symptoms of leukemia resemble those of many other, less serious illnesses, making leukemia difficult to diagnose early. They include fatigue, nosebleeds, pallor, repeated infections, unexplained fever, bruising, and weight loss.

There are currently no general recommendations for leukemia screening. Doctors are most likely to spot the disease early when they order a routine blood test to check for a variety of risk factors and notice abnormal levels of white blood cells or other signs of leukemia.

Much remains to be learned about the causes of leukemia, so specific preventions are not yet clear. However, recommendations include avoiding carcinogens known to increase leukemia risk, such as tobacco smoke.

Lymphomas

More than 90% of cases of lymphomas are non-Hodgkin lymphomas. These types arise in either of two groups of immune cells: B lymphocytes or T lymphocytes. (These are discussed in more detail in Chapter 13.) Non-Hodgkin lymphomas can develop at any age, and usually the first signs are enlarged lymph nodes, fever, sweating, and weight loss. Some types spread only slowly, whereas others are highly aggressive. Radiation, chemotherapy, and certain biological therapies are treatment options.

Hodgkin lymphoma, also called Hodgkin's disease, is one of the most curable forms of cancer. It typically occurs in people age 15 to 35, or in people over age 50. Hodgkin lymphoma arises in the lymph nodes and can spread to other sites. The earliest sign is usually enlarged lymph nodes, accompanied by sweating, chills, itching, loss of appetite, and weight loss. A lymph node biopsy is used for diagnosis, and treatment is typically radiation, chemotherapy, or both.

Common Cancers in Men

Cancers affecting the male reproductive system include prostate cancer and testicular cancer. Although both are common, prostate cancer tends to occur in older men, whereas testicular cancer more commonly develops in younger men.

Prostate Cancer

The *prostate* is a gland in the male reproductive system that secretes a fluid that assists in the movement of sperm. It is located below the bladder **(Figure 12.7).** Prostate cancer is the most commonly diagnosed malignancy among men in the United States: About 240,000 cases are diagnosed each year.[1]

More than 90% of prostate cancers are discovered in localized or regional stages, and for these, the 5-year survival rate is essentially 100%. Still, over 28,000 deaths each year are caused by prostate cancer; with distant metastasis, survival is just 29%.[1]

Risk Factors

Risk factors include:

- Age. Most cases—97%—occur in men age 50 or older.
- Genetic inheritance. Family history strongly affects the risk.
- African American race. American and Jamaican men of African descent have the highest rates of prostate cancer in the world.
- Diet. A high-fat diet translates into higher risk.
- Being overweight
- A sedentary lifestyle. A low level of physical activity increases risk.

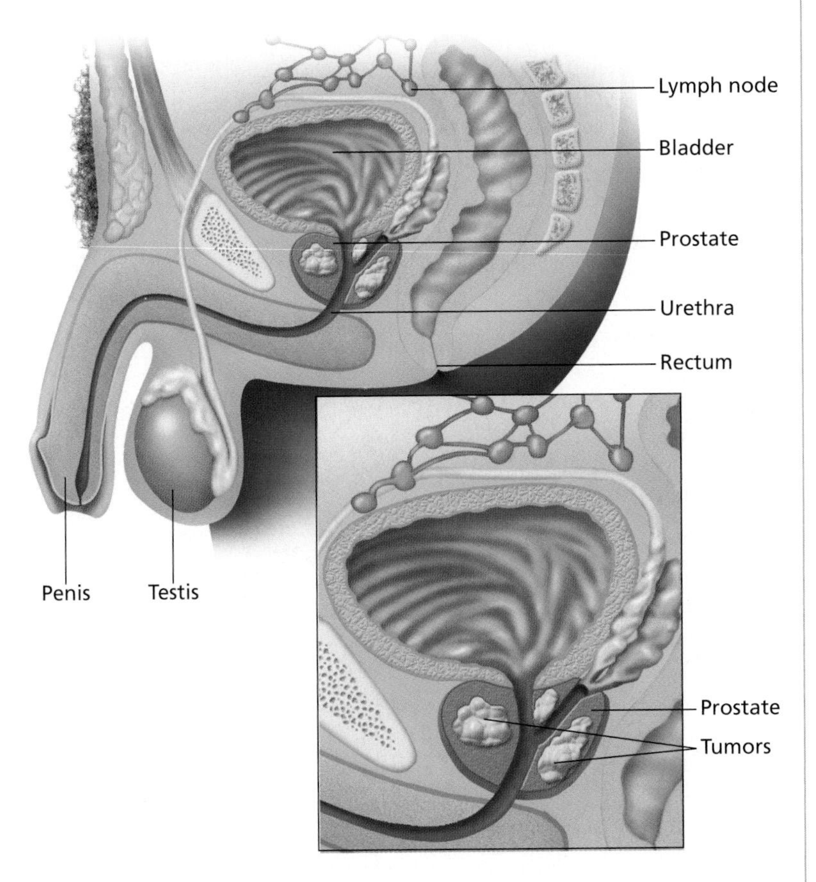

Figure 12.7 **Prostate cancer.**

Signs and Symptoms

Prostate cancer in its early stages is typically silent. Symptoms tend to appear only as the disease becomes more advanced, and may include:

- Difficulty urinating
- The urge to urinate frequently
- Pain or burning with urination
- Blood in the urine
- Pain in the low back, thighs, or pelvis

Diagnosis and Treatment

It is difficult to detect early-stage prostate cancer. A screening test called the PSA test exists, but the American Cancer Society states that, at this time, there is insufficient data to recommend for or against screening. In 2012, the U.S. Preventive Services Task Force recommended against routine PSA screening for American men regardless of age. The Task Force stated that current methods of PSA screening and treatment of screen-detected cancer are not effective in preventing deaths from prostate cancer.[54]

The recommended treatment for less aggressive prostate cancers, especially in older men, is simply "active surveillance"; that is, observing the progress of the condition over time. This is because some types of prostate cancer grow so slowly that the patient is likely to die of other causes before the cancer becomes life-threatening. Hormonal therapy is commonly used to treat more aggressive cases. In 2010, the U.S. Food and Drug Administration approved a new "vaccine" that uses a patient's own immune system to fight advanced prostate cancer that is no longer responding to hormonal therapy. The drug improves survival time, but does not cure the disease.[55] Surgery may be used, but it may produce urinary and erectile difficulties.[1]

Reducing Your Risk

To lower your risk, head for the produce aisle. Fruits and vegetables high in the phytochemical lycopene, a pigment found in tomatoes and other red produce, may lower risk. You can also keep yourself healthier by following a diet low in saturated fats and by maintaining a healthful weight.

Testicular Cancer

Brought to public attention by cycling champion Lance Armstrong, testicular cancer is one of the most common malignancies in young men. It involves the *testes*, the organs within the scrotum that produce male reproductive hormones and sperm. More than 8,500 men are diagnosed with it each year, and about 360 die from it.[1]

The risk factors for testicular cancer include:

- Being a male between the ages of 20 and 39
- Having a family history of cancer
- Caucasian race. Testicular cancer is more common among Caucasian Americans than minorities.
- A history of an undescended testicle; that is, a testicle that did not descend from the abdomen into the scrotum before birth. The risk of cancer is increased for both testicles, and remains whether or not the individual has had surgery to move the testicle into place.

The signs and symptoms of testicular cancer include a lump in either testicle, a feeling of heaviness in the scrotum, pain in the testicle or scrotum, abdominal discomfort, and fatigue.

SPOTLIGHT

Testicular Self-Exam

Some men are at increased risk for testicular cancer. These include men with an undescended testicle, previous testicular cancer, or a family member who has had this cancer. If you have such a risk, discuss it with your health-care provider and ask whether or not you should be performing regular testicular self-exam (TSE). Medical experts do not recommend doing regular TSE if you are not in a high-risk group.

Here are instructions on how to perform TSE if you and your health care provider decide that this is right for you:

If you choose to do TSE, timing is important. Perform the exam during or after a shower, when the skin of the scrotum is warm and relaxed. While standing:

- Feel your scrotal sac until you find one testicle.
- Hold the testicle with one hand while firmly but gently rolling the fingers of the other hand over the testicle as shown in the figure. Examine its entire surface.
- Repeat the procedure on the other testicle.

The epididymis of a normal testis feels like a small "bump" on the side of the testis. Normal testicles also contain blood vessels and other structures. It's easy to confuse these with cancer. If you have any doubts, see a doctor.

Source: Adapted from *Testicular self-examination* by the National Library of Medicine's MedlinePlus. (2011, September 26). Retrieved from www.nlm.nih.gov/medlineplus/ency/article/003909.htm

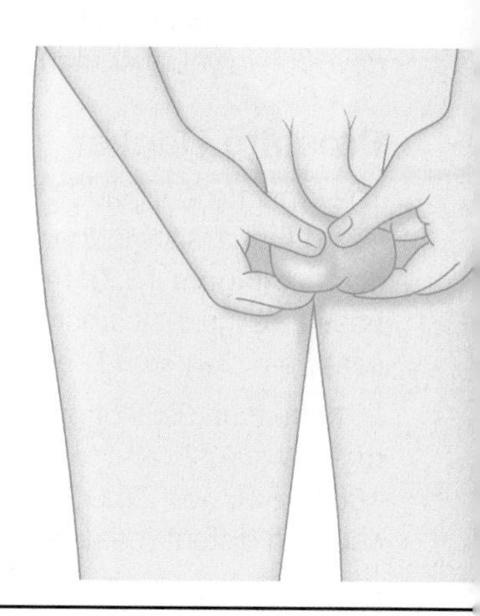

An ultrasound of the testicles can reveal whether the lump is solid or filled with fluid, and exactly where in the scrotum it is located. A blood test may reveal the presence of certain tumor markers. Treatment almost always involves surgery to remove the testicle. In advanced cases, radiation or chemotherapy may follow surgery. The 5-year survival rate for testicular cancer is 95% overall, and even with metastasis, the survival rate is 73%.[1]

Because researchers still haven't uncovered the cause of testicular cancer, the most effective preventions aren't yet clear. Testicular self-exams can aid in detection (see the **Spotlight** box above), but there is no definitive evidence that they lead to a reduction in deaths from testicular cancer, and the U.S. Preventive Services Task Force recommends against routine clinical screening and self-exam. If you are concerned about testicular cancer or have a family history of it, consult your doctor for advice on what preventive measures you can take.

Common Cancers in Women

Cancers affecting the female reproductive system include breast cancer, ovarian cancer, and cervical and uterine cancers.

Breast Cancer

With nearly 230,000 new cases and almost 40,000 deaths each year, invasive breast cancer is the most common cancer among women in the United States and the second leading cause of cancer death in women. Though 99% of women survive localized breast cancer, and 84% breast cancer with lymph node involvement, the survival rate drops to only 23% with metastasis; thus, early detection and treatment remain a top health concern.[1]

Types

Whether or not a woman has ever breast-fed a baby, her breasts are made up of fatty tissue in which are embedded milk-producing glands **(Figure 12.8).** There are 15 to 20 regions of glandular tissue, called lobes, in each breast. These are connected to ducts that transport breast milk to the nipple. Most invasive breast cancers are carcinomas arising in these ducts. Only about 10% involve the lobes. Both types typically begin with a preinvasive *in situ* stage. In 2011, there were more than 57,000 total cases of *in situ* breast cancer, of which 85% were ductal carcinoma *in situ*. If not removed, such cancers can develop into true invasive adenocarcinomas. These can grow into the

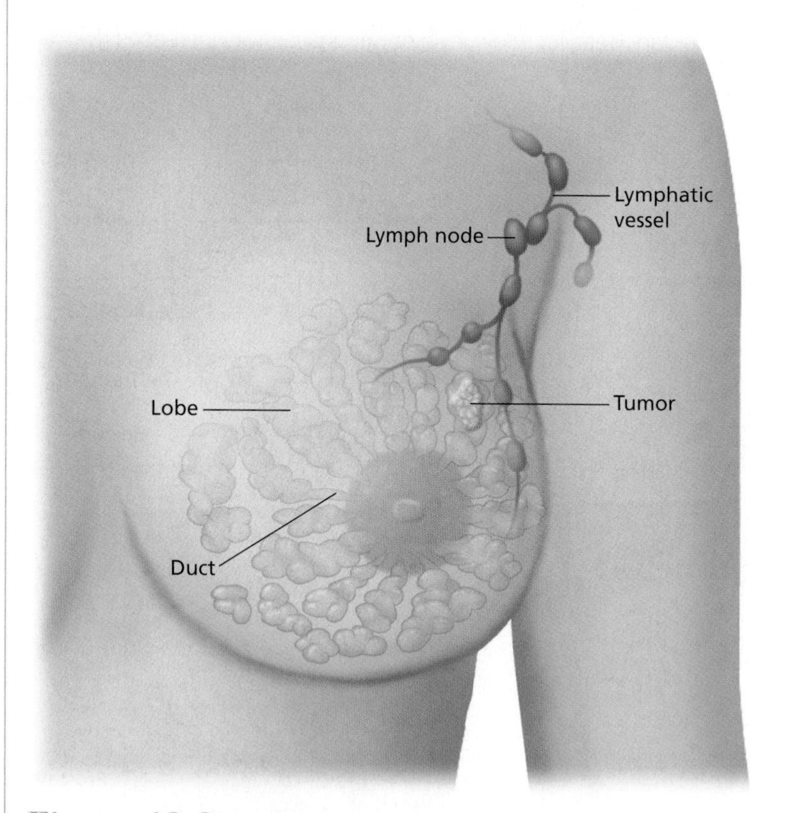

Figure 12.8 **Female breast.** A woman's breast contains 15 to 20 milk-producing regions called lobes, connected to ducts through which breast milk is transported to the nipple during breast-feeding. Each breast is drained by an extensive system of lymphatic vessels through which cancer cells can metastasize to distant body regions.

LEARNING OBJECTIVES

RELATE the concept of self and non-self to the role of your immune system.

IDENTIFY the six links in the chain of infection.

DISCUSS several types of nonspecific body defenses.

DESCRIBE how the body's specific immune response fights infectious disease.

EXPLAIN how immunization prevents infectious disease, both in individuals and in communities.

DISCUSS the most common infectious diseases and their treatment.

DISTINGUISH between immune hypersensitivities and autoimmune disorders, and give examples of each.

EXPLAIN how to reduce your risk for infection and limit the spread of infection on campus.

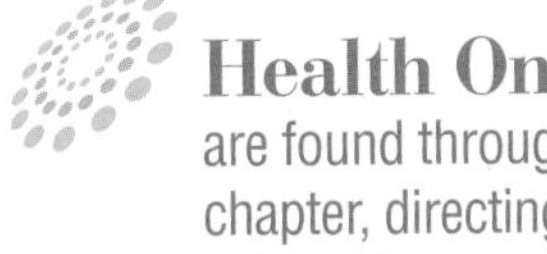

Health Online icons are found throughout the chapter, directing you to web links, videos, podcasts, and other useful online resources.

Ever feel as if it's you against the world?

To the cells of your **immune system,** that's a given. Their entire reason for existing is to protect you from threats originating in your environment. Key to their success is the ability to distinguish between *self* and *non-self*—between the proteins that constitute *you* and those of every other living thing. With the exception of identical twins, every human being is a unique package of proteins, and your immune cells are constantly moving through your bloodstream, surveying your inner landscape for non-self proteins to mark and destroy. Plant pollens, cat dander, the proteins on the surfaces of microbes, and even proteins in blood transfused from another person—all are non-self. What's more, when your own body cells become infected or damaged, they produce alien proteins that make them vulnerable to attack by your immune system.

Most times, your immune system works exceptionally well, killing harmful agents before they've had a chance to reproduce. But sometimes, of course, it gets overwhelmed, and an infectious illness takes hold. And in some people, the immune system goes berserk, overreacting to proteins that wouldn't otherwise provoke any harm, or even attacking the body's own tissues. We'll discuss these immune disorders later in this chapter. First, let's take a look at the immune system's primary role—defending against infection.

How Are Infections Spread?

Despite our best intentions to stay free of illness, it is impossible to make it to adulthood without ever having battled an infection. An **infection** is an invasion of body tissues by *microorganisms*—microscopic living things—that use the body's environment to multiply. In the process, these organisms damage body cells and tissues and make us sick. **Epidemiologists**—scientists who study the patterns of disease in populations—use the term *outbreak* to describe a situation in which infectious disease occurs in an abnormal number of people within the same area at the same time. If four people in your dorm develop a head cold the same week, that's not an outbreak, but if four people experience food poisoning the same day after eating in the dining hall, that is. An outbreak that occurs throughout a geographical region is classified as an *epidemic*.

For infections to spread in a population, six conditions have to be met. These are collectively referred to as the **chain of infection (Figure 13.1).** Disruption of any of the links in this chain reduces the likelihood that an infectious disease will develop into an outbreak. Are you taking steps to reduce your chances of spreading infections? Take the **Self-Assessment** on page 358 to find out.

Pathogens

A **pathogen** is any agent capable of causing disease. The spread of infectious disease begins with a pathogenic microorganism—a harmful strain of viruses, bacteria, fungi, protozoa, or parasitic worms (helminths). Bear in mind that microorganisms live all over the Earth, in environments as diverse as hot springs and cold caves. They also populate every square inch of your skin, and vastly outnumber the human cells in your body. Whereas many of these are neither harmful nor particularly helpful, some—the so-called *normal*

immune system The body's cellular and chemical defenses against pathogens.

infection The invasion of body tissues by microorganisms that use the body's environment to multiply and cause disease.

epidemiologist A scientist who studies the patterns of disease in populations.

chain of infection Group of factors necessary for the spread of infection.

pathogen An agent that causes disease.

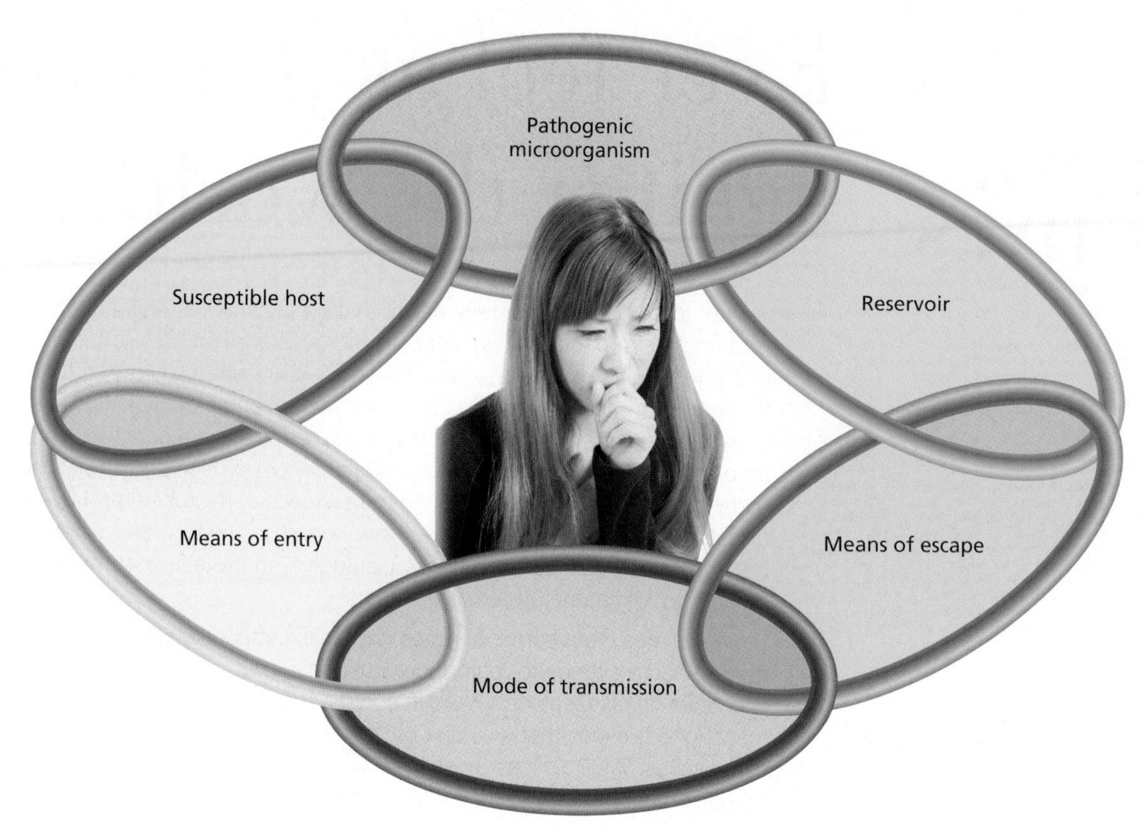

Figure 13.1 Chain of infection. To cause infection, a pathogen such as a cold virus has to have a reservoir, such as a college student's body, in which to multiply and a means of escape, such as a cough. This enables the virus to be transmitted—for instance, by air to another student's eyes (the means of entry). If the student is susceptible—that is, if he has no immunity to the particular virus—he will experience infection.

intestinal flora—are downright healthful, helping your body synthesize nutrients and digest your food. In short, only a tiny fraction of the Earth's microorganisms are pathogenic. **Table 13.1** identifies the five main groups of microorganisms and their most common pathogenic strains.

Reservoir

Any hospitable environment for a particular pathogen, where it can multiply in large numbers, is called a **reservoir.** Soil, water, and foods are potential nonliving reservoirs for microbes, as you've noticed if you've ever stored a half-empty jar of tomato sauce in your refrigerator for more than a couple of weeks. Insects and rodents and other animals are living reservoirs of infection. That's why pest control is an important public health measure for breaking the chain of infection. And as you know from your own experience, human beings are significant reservoirs of infection, especially when they're in close proximity on college campuses. The reason you've probably been advised to stay home from class if you're experiencing a fever is to break the chain of infection by keeping you, the reservoir, from transmitting the pathogen to others.

Mode of Transmission

For pathogens to produce new cases of infection, they have to keep moving from their reservoir to new **hosts**—people, animals, or plants in or on which they can survive and reproduce. They can escape their reservoir in a variety of ways, including via insect, animal, or human bodily secretions such as saliva, mucus, urine, feces, semen, or blood. The **mode of transmission,** or the way pathogens move from reservoir to host, varies according to the pathogen. Infections can be transmitted directly or indirectly.

Direct Transmission

Among the routes of direct transmission, the most common for college students is contact with other people who are infected. Contact with infected animals and vectors are other direct routes.

- **Contact with infected people.** Close person-to-person contact with someone who has an infection is a common mode of disease transmission. Even if a person does not have any symptoms, he or she can still be a **carrier;** that is, a person who is either incubating a pathogen and hasn't yet become sick, or a person who has recovered from an illness but remains a source of infection. Many infections are transmitted sexually, also, via oral, genital, or anal routes. Kissing is not as innocent as you might think: Open-mouth kissing allows exchanges of bodily fluids like saliva, which may be contaminated with pathogenic microbes.[1] Some pathogens can be transmitted through casual hugging, or even through simple touch. Transfer of pathogens from a pregnant woman to

reservoir An environment in which a pathogen is able to multiply in large numbers.

host A person, plant, or animal in or on which pathogens can survive and reproduce.

mode of transmission The route by which a pathogen moves from a reservoir to a host.

carrier A person infected with a pathogen who does not show symptoms, but who can transmit the pathogen to others.

Immunization typically involves exposing a person to a pathogen through a vaccine, often but not always administered by injection. The first vaccines used scrapings from cowpox lesions, which were found to protect against the much more serious disease smallpox. The Latin word for cow is *vacca*, which explains how vaccines got their name. The administration of a vaccine enables the body to develop immunity to a pathogen without actually experiencing the illness. This is called *artificially acquired immunity*.

A few types of vaccines are available:

- **Attenuated vaccines.** To *attenuate* is to weaken in size or strength, and attenuated vaccines are composed of live pathogens that scientists have cultured in a way that weakens them. They are also called modified live vaccines. When they are introduced into the body, these living but weakened microbes pose little threat, yet provoke a full immune response. The immune system produces antibodies as well as memory cells that can stave off that particular type of infectious disease for years to come, perhaps for a lifetime. The risk with attenuated vaccines is that they can produce mild symptoms of the infectious disease, and cannot be used by people with weak immune systems.
- **Killed vaccines.** Some vaccines are made from pathogens that have been killed, but still retain their ability to provoke a specific immune response. Killed vaccines are more stable, and so can be more easily stored than attenuated vaccines. They are also much less likely to provoke symptoms of infection.
- **Subunit vaccines.** New biotechnology techniques have led to the development of subunit vaccines, which use only parts of an organism. These are produced by genetic engineering techniques that manipulate genetic material from the pathogen to cause it to produce the antigenic protein. The hepatitis B vaccine is an example. Subunit vaccines cannot cause the disease and don't provoke symptoms of the disease. They can therefore be widely used.

Vaccination produces *active immunity* because it induces an active immune response. In contrast, injections of ready-made antibodies can provide temporary *passive immunity*. Physicians use passive immunity when protection is needed immediately, for example, in the case of exposure to the virus that causes rabies, or when an unvaccinated person has a wound infected with the tetanus bacterium—either of which can be fatal. The injected antibodies immediately target the pathogen for destruction. Passive immunity lasts only as long as the injected antibodies survive, a few months at most.

The Centers for Disease Control has developed recommended immunization schedules for children, teens, and adults **(Table 13.2)** and all states require certain immunizations before children can enter school. Exemptions to immunization laws can be given if a child has certain medical conditions, as well as for religious reasons. In addition, some people are not immunized because they don't know or understand the recommendations, don't have access to health care, or cannot afford the shots. Sometimes, people avoid vaccines because they believe that they are unsafe. Whereas in the past, a vaccine very infrequently produced the very disease it was administered to protect against, modern vaccines are considered very safe. In the United States, years of testing are required before a vaccine can be licensed, and the CDC monitors vaccines after administration for adverse reactions.[4] Still, challenges to claims of vaccine safety persist. For example, many people believe that vaccines are responsible for autism. Is it true? Check out the **Myth or Fact?** box on the next page and decide for yourself.

Low immunization rates within a community can compromise **herd immunity.** Herd immunity occurs when greater than 90% of people in a community or region are fully vaccinated against a disease, leaving that disease with few potential reservoirs and thus little opportunity to spread through the population. It therefore offers some protection against the disease for individuals who cannot

Table 13.2: Vaccines Recommended for College Students[a]

Vaccine	Number of Doses
Tetanus, diphtheria, pertussis (Tdap, Td)[a]	Single dose of Tdap, then boost with Td every 10 years
Measles, mumps, rubella (MMR)[a]	2 doses recommended for college students
Polio (IPV)[a]	4 doses if given in childhood; 3 doses if given in adulthood
Varicella (Var) (chickenpox)[a]	2 doses
Human papillomavirus (HPV)[a, b]	3 doses
Hepatitis B (Hep B)[a]	3 doses
Meningococcal disease[c]	1 dose
Pneumococcal polysaccharide (PPV)[d]	1 dose with revaccination after 5 years for those with elevated risk factors
Hepatitis A (Hep A)[d]	2 doses
Annual influenza (and H1N1)[d]	1 dose annually

[a]Recommended for those who lack documentation of past vaccination with all recommended doses and have no evidence of prior infection.
[b]Recommended for those ages 26 and under.
[c]Recommended for previously unvaccinated college freshmen living in dormitories.
[d]Recommended if some other risk factor is present.

Source: Vaccines Needed by Teens and College Students, by the U.S. Department of Health and Human Services, Centers for Disease Control and Prevention, 2010, retrieved from http://www.cdc.gov/vaccines/recs/schedules/teen-schedule.htm.

immunization Creating immunity to a pathogen through vaccination or through the injection of antibodies.

herd immunity The condition in which greater than 90% of a community is vaccinated against a disease, giving the disease little ability to spread through the community, providing some protection against the disease to members of the community who are not vaccinated.

> *"In the United States, the cost of infectious disease exceeds $120 billion per year."*

be vaccinated (due to medical conditions) or who haven't been vaccinated yet (such as newborns). This protection is critical because infections remain the world's leading killer of children and young adults. Moreover, the financial burden of infectious disease is immense: even in the United States, the cost of infectious disease exceeds $120 billion per year.[5] Unfortunately, as indicated in the nearby **Student Stats** box, it's unlikely that herd immunity exists on your campus for many common infectious diseases.

virus A microscopic organism that cannot multiply without invading body cells.

parasite Any organism that lives on or in another organism, upon which it depends for its survival.

incubation period Period of time between the initial infection and the onset of signs and symptoms, and during which the person may be contagious.

Common Viral Diseases

Viruses are so small they escape detection by light waves from traditional microscopes, and were unknown until the invention of the electron microscope in 1931. They are also so simple that some microbiologists challenge their status as living organisms. Consisting of a strand of genetic material (DNA or RNA) surrounded by a protein coat, they cannot perform one of the basic functions of life—reproduction—unless they invade cells. In human cells, they hijack the DNA and other cellular "machinery" and use it to force the cell to crank out duplicate viruses at the expense of the cell's normal functions—and at the expense of your health. Eventually, these new viruses burst out of the cell into the blood or other tissues, killing the host cell **(Figure 13.3).** In other words, viruses are **parasites,** organisms that live on or in another organism, upon which they depend for their own survival.

Viruses cannot survive for long outside of a host, but once inside a cell they can multiply very quickly. For example, a cell infected with the common flu virus begins to release new flu viruses only six hours after the virus has entered the cell. Within just a few hours more, it produces enough new viruses to infect 20 to 30 more cells. The infected cell dies about 11 hours after the virus entered.[6]

During the period of time between the initial infection and the appearance of symptoms, the virus is actively reproducing—and the person who is infected may be able to pass the germ along to you. For colds and flu, this **incubation period** may last from just 1 to 5 days. For some viral infections, however, incubation can take much longer. For instance, the incubation period for infectious mononucleosis (mono) is 4 to 6 weeks.[7]

Colds

A cold is a viral infection involving the nose and throat. More than 200 different viruses cause cold symptoms. Common culprits are groups of

MYTH OR FACT?

Do Vaccines Cause Autism?

In 1998, an article appeared in the British medical journal *The Lancet* that claimed that autism—a developmental brain disorder that causes problems in communication, social interaction, and behavior—was caused by the childhood vaccine for measles, mumps, and rubella (MMR).[1] In response, some parents' groups began a movement against vaccinations, and more and more parents stopped vaccinating their children.

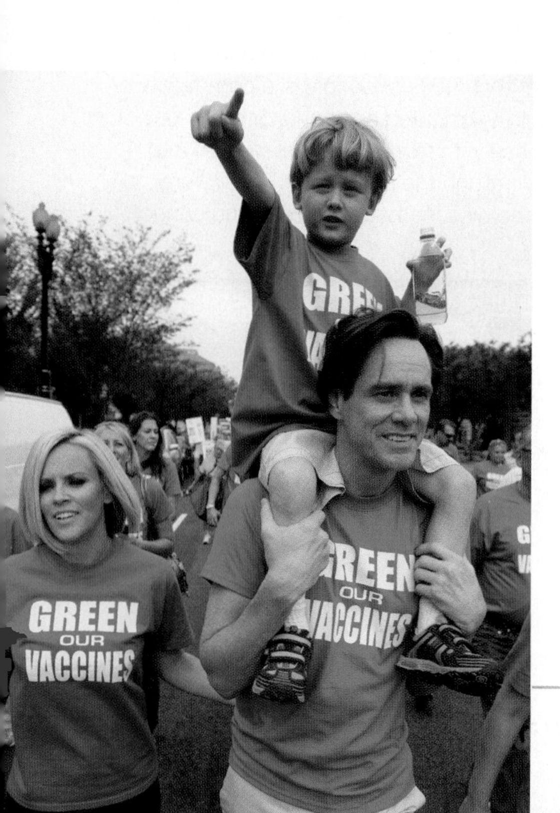

Anti-vaccine groups claim autism is linked to the recommended number and schedule of childhood vaccinations and the use of thimerosal, a preservative that contains mercury, in some vaccines. As evidence of the damage of vaccinations, parents of autistic children publicized "before" and "after" home videos of their children displaying autistic characteristics only after the date of vaccination. Celebrities such as Jenny McCarthy and Holly Robinson Peete advocated for vaccination reform.

However, after much research, there is no evidence of a link between autism and vaccines.[2] Thimerosal, which was never present in the MMR vaccines most blamed for autism, was removed from most common childhood vaccines by 2001 and autism rates did not decline.[3, 4] And in February 2010 *The Lancet* retracted the original paper linking autism to the MMR vaccine, citing a recent British medical panel ruling that the lead author had been deceptive and violated basic research ethics in his study.

The causes of autism remain unknown. However, one thing is clear: It is dangerous to experience an infectious disease that could have been prevented by a vaccine.

References: **1.** "Ileal-Lymphoid-Nodular Hyperplasia, Non-Specific Colitis, and Pervasive Developmental Disorder in Children," by A. J. Wakefield, S. H. Murch, A. Anthony, J. Linnell, D. M. Casson, M. Malik, . . . J. A. Walker-Smith, 1998, *The Lancet, 351*, pp. 637–641. **2.** "Vaccine Studies: Examine the Evidence," by the American Academy of Pediatrics, Updated November 2010, retrieved from http://www.aap.org/immunization/families/faq/VaccineStudies.pdf. **3.** "Thimerosal Content of Vaccines Routinely Recommended for Children 6 Years of Age and Younger," Table 1 in "Thimerosal in Vaccines," in *Vaccines, Blood & Biologics*, by the U.S. Food and Drug Administration, 2010, retrieved from http://www.fda.gov/BiologicsBloodVaccines/SafetyAvailability/VaccineSafety/ucm096228.htm#t1. **4.** "Prevalence of Autism Spectrum Disorders—Autism and Developmental Disabilities Monitoring Network, United States, 2006," by Catherine Rice for the Centers for Disease Control and Prevention, December 18, 2009, *Morbidity and Mortality Weekly Report Surveillance Summaries, 58*, pp. 1–20, retrieved from http://www.cdc.gov/mmwr/preview/mmwrhtml/ss5810a1.htm.

Frontline: The Vaccine War **explores both sides of the vaccine debate: www.pbs.org/wgbh/pages/frontline/vaccines/view.**

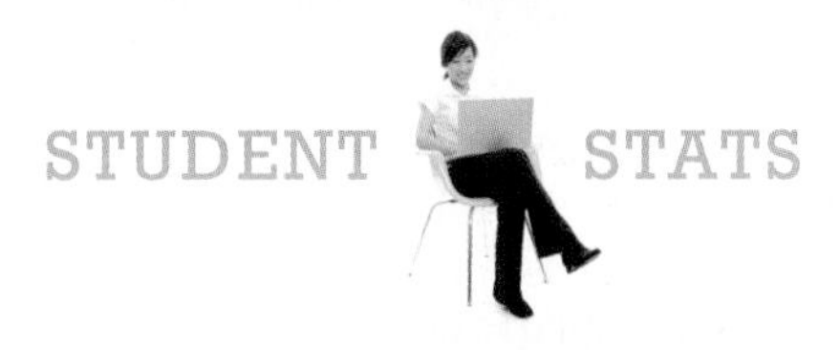

Immunization Status of College Students

A recent national survey of college students found the following rates of vaccination against common infectious diseases:

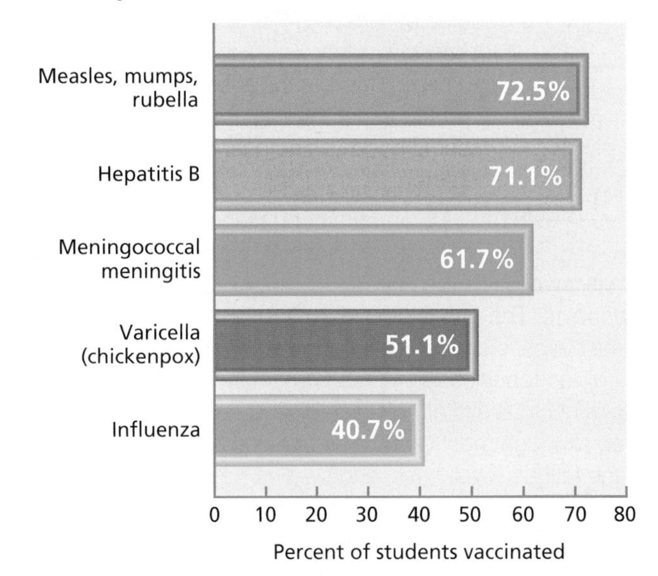

Source: Data from *American College Health Association National College Health Assessment (ACHA-NCHA II) Reference Group Executive Summary, Fall 2011* by the American College Health Association. 2012, retrieved from http://www.acha-ncha.org/reports_ACHA-NCHAII.html.

rhinoviruses and coronaviruses. They are typically spread by touching contaminated objects, through personal contact, or by breathing airborne pathogens. If it seems as if you are often battling a cold, you may not be imagining it. Adults get about one to three colds a year, usually during the fall and winter, and children average twice as many.[8]

Cold symptoms appear about 2 or 3 days after infection. They include a runny or congested nose, sneezing, cough, sore throat, headache, and mild fever. These symptoms generally taper off in about a week.

There is no known cure for the common cold. Over-the-counter medications may provide some relief from some symptoms, but typically have side effects. Acetaminophen may relieve headache or sore throat pain, and cough syrup can help you sleep through the night, but decongestant nasal sprays should not be used for more than a few days because long-term use can damage the delicate membranes of the nose and prompt a rebound inflammation. Surprisingly effective is chicken soup! Researchers say it inhibits the movement of neutrophils, thereby limiting inflammation, and relieves nasal congestion.[9] A saltwater gargle can soothe a sore throat, as can using a humidifier to relieve overly dry room air. Taking vitamin C and/or zinc lozenges at the onset of a cold may help reduce its duration.[9] Beyond that, physicians advise getting plenty of rest and keeping your fluids up.

Colds cannot be treated with antibiotics, because antibiotics are designed to fight bacteria, not viruses. However, sometimes viral infections leave the body susceptible to secondary bacterial infections of the sinuses, ears, or respiratory tract, in which case antibiotics would be prescribed.

To prevent colds, wash your hands frequently, keep your hands away from your face, especially your eyes, and stay away from people who have colds. And if you have a cold, try not to transmit it to others: Always cough or sneeze into a tissue, not into the air. Throw away the tissue immediately. If you don't have a tissue, cough or sneeze into the crook of your elbow. Frequently and thoroughly wash your hands, objects, and surfaces you touch. And stay home when your symptoms are at their peak.

Viral Conjunctivitis

Conjunctivitis is inflammation of the conjunctiva, the thin membrane that lines the inner eyelid and covers the eye. Because it causes a pinkish discoloration of the white of the eye, it is commonly called "pink eye." Other signs and symptoms include itching, a feeling that there is something in the eye, watering, or discharge. Conjunctivitis commonly accompanies a cold, although it can also be caused by bacteria, allergies, or irritation from chemicals such as tobacco smoke or eye makeup. It typically begins in one eye, and can easily spread to the other, especially if you blow your nose and then touch your eyes. It is highly contagious, so if you have conjunctivitis, you should stay home. Treatment is not usually necessary, as the condition typically resolves on its own in a few days.[10] Applying a warm or cool wet compress to the affected eye for a few minutes several times throughout the day can help relieve discomfort. Avoid wearing contact lenses until the conjunctivitis heals.

conjunctivitis Inflammation of the conjunctiva of the eye.

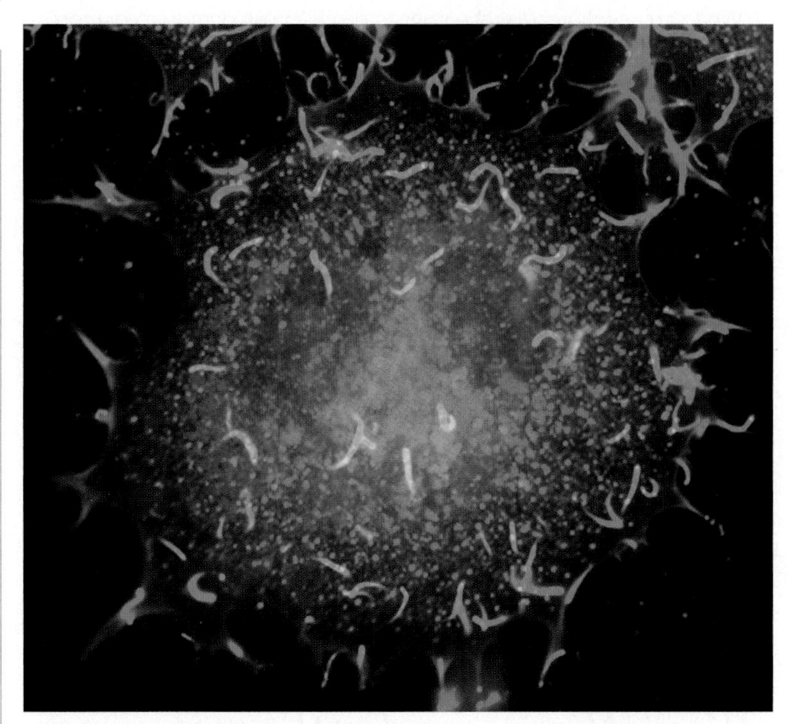

Figure 13.3 **Viral reproduction.** Viruses co-opt the more sophisticated genetic and metabolic "machinery" of cells to enable their own reproduction. Here, dozens of new viruses are bursting out of a human cell.

Influenza

The flu is a contagious respiratory condition caused by a number of **influenza** viruses. Between 5% and 20% of the U.S. population get the flu in any given year. Although it often is a moderate illness, causing a fever, body aches, fatigue, and a dry cough, the flu can be life-threatening in some infants, frail elderly, or people with weakened immune systems. It can also lead to bacterial pneumonia, dehydration, sinus infections, and ear infections and tends to exacerbate underlying medical conditions such as asthma and diabetes. Every year, more than 200,000 people in the United States are hospitalized with flu complications, and at least 36,000 die from an influenza infection.[11]

influenza A group of viruses that cause the flu, a contagious respiratory condition.

pandemic A worldwide epidemic of a disease.

mononucleosis A viral disease that causes fatigue, weakness, sore throat, fever, headaches, swollen lymph nodes and tonsils, and loss of appetite.

This CDC video explains how to "Take 3" to avoid catching or spreading influenza: www.cdc.gov/CDCTV/IR_Take3/index.html.

As with colds, influenza viruses are spread through personal contact, airborne pathogens, or touching inanimate objects covered with a virus. There is no known cure—although antiviral medications may be prescribed to reduce symptoms—and so prevention remains the best medicine. In addition to proper hand washing and coughing and sneezing into a tissue or the crook of your elbow, federal health officials recommend that children, pregnant women, health workers, people over age 65, and people of all ages with chronic medical conditions such as asthma and diabetes get an influenza vaccine annually. Notice that, because the strain of flu virus changes each year, the "flu shot" you got last year will not protect you from this year's strain. Influenza vaccines are available at many campus health centers, doctors' offices, pharmacies, and even grocery stores every fall. You can receive an influenza vaccine as an injection into the arm or as a nasal spray.

When an infectious disease passes quickly from person to person unchecked and eventually spreads worldwide, it is called a **pandemic.** In 1918–1919, an influenza pandemic killed between 20 million and 40 million people, more than died from the infamous bubonic plague of the 14th century. It was unusual in its deadliness as well as in the fact that its victims were more likely to be young adults than children or elderly. Flu pandemics can occur when a new influenza virus emerges to which humans have not been exposed before. This lack of exposure leaves people with no acquired immunity to help defend against the virus, and it can become highly contagious. Often, animals are the reservoir for flu viruses that mutate into new strains that cause pandemics. The most recent pandemic, the 2009 H1N1 flu pandemic, was caused by a virus that started in pigs. It was not nearly as virulent as the strain involved in the 1918 pandemic, and it caused fewer than 19,000 deaths worldwide.[12]

"In 1918–1919, an influenza pandemic killed between 20 million and 40 million people."

Mononucleosis

Infectious **mononucleosis,** or *"mono,"* is often called "the kissing disease" and is caused by the Epstein-Barr virus. It is transmitted through contact with an infected person's saliva. Sharing drinking glasses, straws, eating utensils, or toothbrushes can expose you to the Epstein-Barr virus, as of course can kissing. Recall that the incubation period for mono is a few weeks long; moreover, the virus can persist for months after infection. This means that kissing or sharing utensils with someone who seems healthy is no guarantee that you won't be infected.

Common among teens and young adults, mono causes fatigue, weakness, sore throat, fever, headaches, swollen lymph nodes and tonsils, a swollen spleen, and loss of appetite. The condition usually is not serious, although some people may experience complications involving the liver or spleen. Also, a history of mononucleosis increases your risk for developing multiple sclerosis, a nervous system disease discussed later in this chapter.[13] Moreover, although most symptoms of mono dissipate within 2 or 3 weeks, the fatigue, weakness, and swollen lymph nodes can persist for months. When they do, a student's life can be affected profoundly. A recent study in the UK found substantial illness among some university students with mono, affecting their academic studies, physical exercise, and social activities. Women were more likely to be seriously affected than men; for example, 16% of female students discontinued their studies following mono infection, whereas none of the males in the study did so.[14]

A blood test indicating the presence of antibodies to the Epstein-Barr virus can be used to support a suspected diagnosis of mononucleosis. Primary treatments are as basic as drinking plenty of fluids and getting lots of rest. Gargling with salt water can help relieve a sore throat, and acetaminophen can reduce headache pain and fever. If

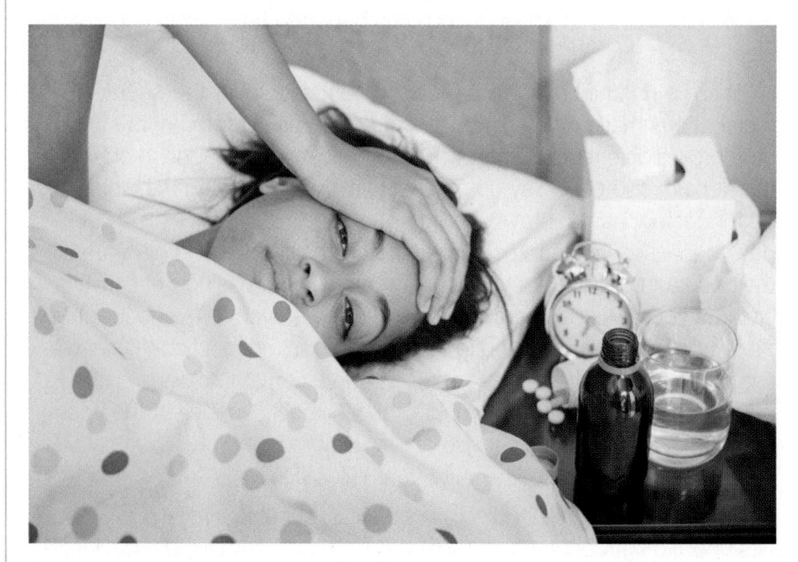

Many infections cause **fatigue**.

swelling of the lymph nodes or tonsils is severe, a physician may prescribe a short course of an anti-inflammatory drug such as prednisone. A ruptured spleen is a potential complication of infectious mononucleosis, so it's essential to avoid heavy lifting, contact sports, or other vigorous activity for at least a month post-infection.[15]

hepatitis Inflammation of the liver that affects liver function.

jaundice A yellowing of the skin, mucous membranes, and sometimes the whites of the eyes, often caused by liver malfunction.

Viral Hepatitis

Hepatitis is an inflammation of the liver. One of its most dramatic signs is **jaundice,** a yellow discoloration of the skin and the whites of the eyes. Jaundice develops because the inflammation reduces the liver's ability to clear from the blood a waste product of dead blood cells called bilirubin, which has a brownish yellow pigment. Other signs and symptoms of hepatitis include fatigue, fever, nausea, abdominal pain, and muscle and joint pain. In some cases it can be deadly. Viral infections are the primary cause of hepatitis, though alcohol, drugs, and some underlying medical conditions can also cause inflammation of the liver.

There are several types of viral hepatitis. Hepatitis A, B, and C are the most common forms in the United States, but there are also rarer hepatitis viruses, known as D and E.

Hepatitis A is the most widespread form of hepatitis. It is contracted through consuming microscopic amounts of feces that can lurk on contaminated fruits, vegetables, and ice cubes. The virus can also be spread during oral-anal sexual contact, or by changing dirty diapers, failing to thoroughly wash your hands afterward, and then putting your hands in your mouth. Symptoms can last for weeks or months, although some people never feel ill. Although the virus can cause liver failure and death in a small portion of the population, most people make a full recovery, sustaining no permanent liver damage. Rates of hepatitis A have decreased in recent years, in part because a vaccine for hepatitis A was introduced in 1995. Physicians recommend that children and teens, travelers to certain countries, and other at-risk individuals get the vaccine.

Hepatitis B is transmitted mostly through sexual contact or needle sharing. It can also cross the placenta from an infected pregnant women to her fetus. A sometimes severe disease, hepatitis B is capable of causing lifelong infection, liver scarring, liver failure, and death. A vaccine is available. (For more information, see Chapter 16.)

Hepatitis C is the primary reason for liver transplants in the United States. More than three-fourths of those who are infected with this highly destructive virus go on to develop chronic infections that can last a lifetime, scarring the liver or triggering liver cancer. Unfortunately, early symptoms of this form of hepatitis are mild or nonexistent, and many people do not realize they have it until liver damage has occurred. Hepatitis C kills between 8,000 and 10,000 people in the United States every year, and typically is spread through sharing syringes and other drug-related paraphernalia.[16] It can also be passed on by unsterilized tattoo needles and piercing equipment, or sexual contact. Before screening tests were developed and made available in the United States, it was also spread through blood transfusions and organ transplants. It is still possible to pick up the infection from needles or other medical instruments in other parts of the world where sterilization practices may not be as rigorous.

People with any hepatitis infection may not be aware that they have the disease, because their symptoms can be so mild; however, they can still transmit it to others. Blood tests can determine whether you have hepatitis. Treatment is usually nothing more than rest, fluids, and proper nutrition for acute cases of hepatitis, but chronic cases sometimes benefit from medications. If you have chronic hepatitis, your doctor should regularly screen you for liver disease. You should avoid alcohol, and check with your doctor before using any drugs, including OTC and prescription medications.

Oral Herpes

Oral herpes, clinically known as *herpes labialis*, is infection of the lips, mouth, or gums by the herpes simplex virus, usually a strain referred to as type 1 (or HSV-1). More than half of all people in the United States are infected with this virus by age 20; however, not all develop clinical signs of infection.[17] The type 2 herpes simplex virus (HSV-2), which typically causes genital herpes, is sometimes involved in oral herpes. On the other hand, HSV-1 often causes genital herpes: A recent study found that, among university students, it was responsible for more cases of genital herpes than HSV-2 was.[18]

The primary feature of oral herpes is a cluster of painful blisters, often called *cold sores*, on the lips or other infected areas **(Figure 13.4).** These can be accompanied by sore throat, fever, or swollen glands. After 2 to 3 weeks, the initial outbreak subsides and the virus goes dormant, producing no symptoms but remaining in the nerves of the face. A variety of situations, from intense sun exposure to stress, can reactivate the virus, causing a new, though less severe, outbreak.

Treatment with an antiviral medication such as acyclovir reduces the severity of recurrences. Prevention of recurrences includes the use of zinc oxide sunblock on the lips when outdoors, stress management techniques, and general health maintenance strategies such as adequate sleep.

All herpes viruses are very contagious. Avoid kissing anyone with lip or mouth blisters, and do not share towels, cups, or other objects. Also be aware that both HSV-1 and HSV-2 can be transmitted during oral-genital contact.[17]

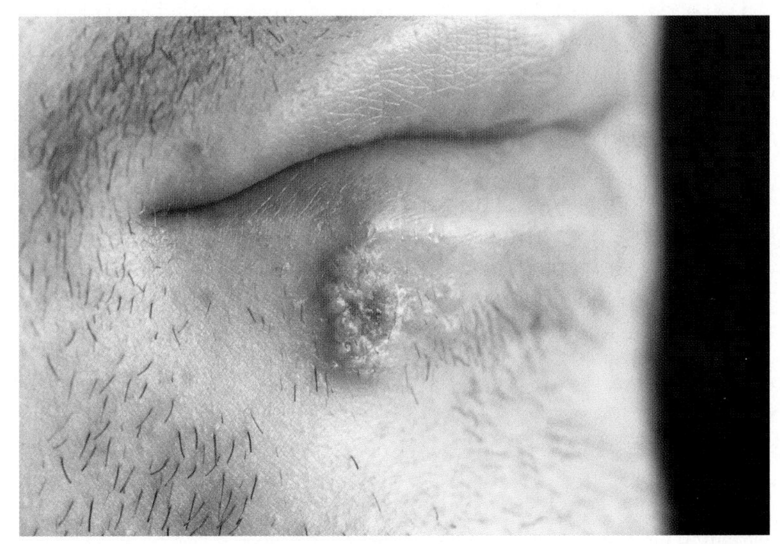

Figure 13.4 The characteristic blisters of oral herpes.

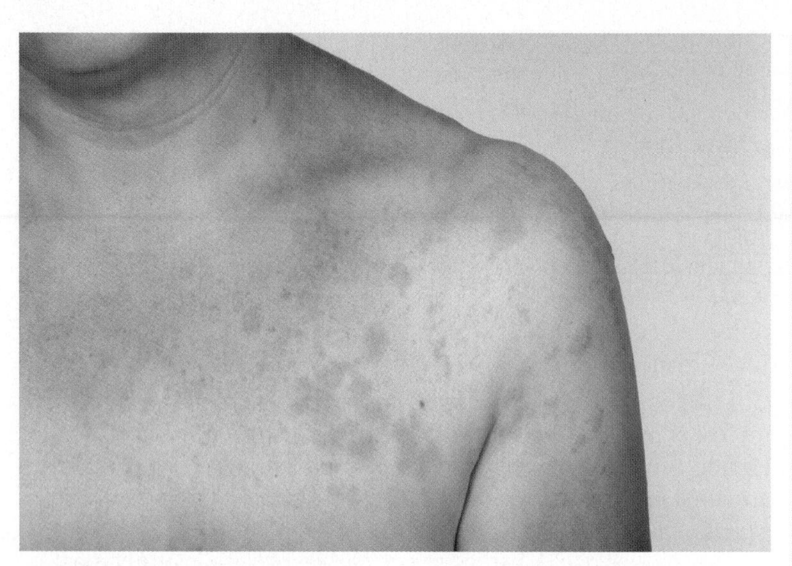

Figure 13.5 Shingles. The painful blisters associated with shingles follow the tracks of nerves branching from the spinal cord, but may appear almost anywhere on the torso or face.

Varicella (Chickenpox and Shingles)

The varicella-zoster virus—another type of herpes virus—is responsible for *varicella*, commonly known as chickenpox. Children normally receive two vaccinations, one before age 2 and a second before age 6, to protect against varicella. Vaccination is important because varicella caused more than 100 deaths on average each year prior to introduction of the vaccine in 1995. Moreover, infection in teens and young adults can be more severe than childhood infection. The main signs and symptoms are itchy blisters on the torso, face, and scalp that last for 5 to 10 days, headache, and fever. An infected person is contagious for 24 to 48 hours before the blisters appear, and until all of the blisters have formed scabs. Usually no treatment is necessary, though oatmeal baths are recommended to soothe the itching.[19]

Like other members of the herpes virus family, varicella remains in the body permanently. It becomes reactivated in about 1 million older adults each year as *shingles*, an outbreak of burning or itching sores on the torso or face **(Figure 13.5).**[20] The blisters may last 3 to 4 weeks. Taking an antiviral medication such as acyclovir right away can help reduce the severity and duration of the attack. Treatment is important because shingles involving the face can spread to the eyes, causing blindness. Another complication is post-herpetic neuralgia, nerve pain that can last for months or even years after the blisters have resolved. Fortunately, a shingles vaccine is now available, and is recommended for adults over age 60.[20]

Common Bacterial Diseases

Whereas viruses are acellular, **bacteria** are single-celled microorganisms that can exist either independently or as parasites, drawing their nourishment from other forms of life. Also unlike viruses, bacteria are able to reproduce on their own without the help of a host cell, by dividing in two.

Less than 1% of the many types of bacteria that exist all over our planet are harmful.[21] Pathogenic bacteria cause harm by producing and releasing toxins into our tissues, or by directly damaging cells or their functions. Our primary weapons in combating bacterial infections are a variety of **antibiotics,** prescription medications that either kill bacteria directly or block key steps in their reproduction. However, bacteria can develop **resistance** to these important drugs. This occurs when a random mutation, or change in a bacterium's genetic code, enables the bacterium to overcome the effects of the antibiotic. Perhaps only 1 bacterium in 10 million gains this advantage, but since it can grow and divide in the presence of the antibiotic, it can quickly take over. Indiscriminate use of antibiotics, whether in farm animals or in humans, promotes resistance. Everyone can help limit the development of resistance by taking antibiotics only when they have been prescribed by a physician, and by taking them for the full course prescribed.

Many bacteria live in and are beneficial to humans. Called *probiotics*, a term meaning "life promoting," they help us digest food, synthesize vitamins, and fight off disease. Manufacturers of yogurt, kefir, and other fermented milk products culture especially vigorous strains of these bacteria in their products because of their healthful properties. Probiotics are also important in keeping competing—and potentially harmful—microbes in check. For instance, helpful bacteria in the female reproductive tract compete for resources with pathogenic fungal species. When a woman takes an antibiotic to combat a bacterial infection, these helpful bacteria may also be killed off, allowing the fungal pathogens to reproduce unopposed. The result is a yeast infection. A similar reaction can occur in the intestinal tract and elsewhere in the body.

Meningitis

Meningitis is an infection of the meninges, the thin membranes that surround the spinal cord and the brain. The infection can be caused by a number of viral and bacterial strains, and is characterized by high fever, stiff neck, headaches, and even confusion or seizures. When caused by a virus, meningitis tends to be much less severe and dissipates on its own. Bacterial meningitis, however, can be life-threatening, and may cause hearing loss, brain damage, and other disabilities. The bacteria that most commonly cause meningitis are *Streptococcus pneumoniae* and *Neisseria meningitidis*; most often, meningitis occurs when these bacteria have infected another part of the body and then enter the bloodstream and migrate to the meninges. Even when treated promptly with the proper antibiotics, bacterial meningitis kills between 5% and 10% of patients worldwide, usually within a day or two of the onset of symptoms.[22]

Adolescents and young adults account for nearly one-third of all cases of bacterial meningitis in the United States, and college students—especially those living in dormitories—are at moderately increased risk.[23] To reduce their risk, the Centers for Disease Control and Prevention recommends that all youths between the ages of 11 and 18 receive the meningococcal vaccine, an inoculation that protects against some but not all of the bacterial strains that cause meningitis. As of 2009, 15 U.S. states had mandated vaccination for college freshmen.[23]

bacteria (singular: *bacterium*) Single-celled microorganisms that can be beneficial, harmless, or harmful, invading and damaging body cells and sometimes releasing toxins.

antibiotic A drug used to fight bacterial infection.

resistance The ability of a bacterium to overcome the effects of an antibiotic through a random mutation, or change in the bacterium's genetic code.

meningitis Infection and inflammation of the meninges covering the spinal cord and brain.

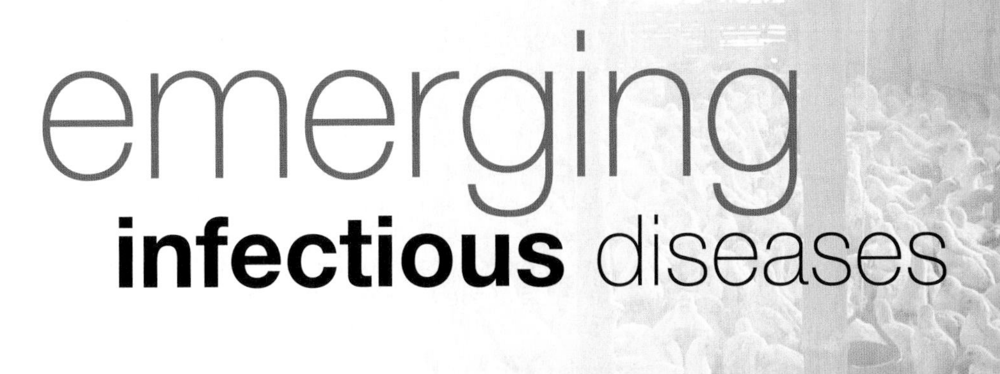

emerging infectious diseases

Although some diseases have plagued humankind for as long as records have been kept, others have only become a human health threat in recent years or have reemerged as worldwide travel has spread them. Some of the more troubling emerging infections are described here.

H1N1 ("Swine flu"). H1N1 is a new influenza virus first detected in the United States in April 2009. The virus contains genes not only from pigs, but also from birds and humans. H1N1 spreads from person to person similarly to the seasonal flu and in June 2009 the World Health Organization declared it a worldwide pandemic. The virus causes cough, sore throat, congestion, body aches, headaches, chills, and fatigue. Most people recover on their own without treatment, but in some cases the illness can cause severe respiratory problems and even death.

H5N1 (Avian influenza or "bird flu"). H5N1 has been diagnosed in hundreds of people in more than a dozen countries since November 2003. Most of them contracted the serious infection after coming into direct contact with infected poultry. It causes conjunctivitis (pink eye), pneumonia, and for more than half its victims, death. The virus has, in a few rare instances, spread from person to person, and it would only take a slight mutation for it to spread very easily. If that were to occur, H5N1 would have the potential of becoming the next influenza pandemic.

SARS (severe acute respiratory syndrome). SARS is caused by a type of coronavirus. It emerged in southeastern China in 2003, and within a matter of months spread to more than two dozen countries throughout the world, including the United States. The virus, which causes pneumonia in most of those who are infected with it, is believed to have made the jump to humans through animals that were sold in Asian food markets. The respiratory illness killed hundreds and sickened thousands worldwide during the outbreak of 2003. It is spread through close person-to-person contact.

West Nile Virus. This infectious disease is spread through the bite of an infected mosquito. Although it appeared in other parts of the world earlier, it was not discovered in the United States until 1999. Since then it has spread rapidly, infecting tens of thousands of people across the country, and killing more than 1,000.[1] Rates of West Nile virus are growing in the U.S., and 2012 experienced the highest U.S. infections on record. Although 80% of infected people experience no effects, about 1 in every 150 people infected goes on to experience severe symptoms ranging from muscle weakness and disorientation to vision loss, paralysis, coma, and death. The only way to avoid getting the virus is to avoid mosquito bites.

Hantavirus. Hantavirus is a disease transmitted by rodents. The respiratory illness causes fatigue, fever, muscle aches, coughing, shortness of breath, and a buildup of fluid in the lungs. Symptoms appear after exposure to the urine, droppings, or saliva of infected rodents.

Reference: **1.** "Statistics, Surveillance, and Control Archive" in *West Nile Virus,* by the Centers for Disease Control and Prevention, June 5, 2012, retrieved from http://www.cdc.gov/ncidod/dvbid/westnile/surv&control.htm#maps.

Close contact with poultry or other animals can pass new diseases to humans.

Staphylococcal Infections

There are more than two dozen types of *Staphylococcus* bacteria, but one—*Staphylococcus aureus*—is responsible for the bulk of all "staph" infections. It causes boils and other minor skin ailments, especially in people with eczema (a chronic, itchy skin rash) or burned skin. Sometimes staph can cause more serious infections of the blood, lungs, heart, or urinary tract, most often in those whose immune system is weakened because of illness or other conditions.

toxic shock syndrome A rare, serious illness caused by staph bacteria that begins with severe flu symptoms but can quickly progress to a medical emergency.

methicillin-resistant *Staphylococcus aureus* (MRSA) A strain of staph that is resistant to many broad-spectrum antibiotics commonly used to treat staph infections.

Staphylococcus aureus also releases toxins that can trigger food poisoning. For instance, if you have *Staphylococcus* on your hands—as most of us do—and fail to wash before preparing food, it can begin to reproduce and secrete its toxins into the food. If you then leave the food out at room temperature for longer than two hours, it may become saturated with toxins. Although cooking the food after this occurs will kill the bacteria, it will not neutralize the toxin, so if you eat it, you'll probably experience food poisoning.

Staphylococcus toxins are also responsible for **toxic shock syndrome,** a rare disease that initially resembles a bad cold or flu but can progress within hours to a medical emergency. Fever, chills, nausea, and diarrhea give way to seizures, low blood pressure, and organ failure and, in about 5% of cases, death.[24] In 1980, more than 800 menstruating women developed the condition, and 38 died from it. Federal investigators linked the cases to use of a new, highly absorbent tampon that was subsequently taken off the market. Menstruating women can avoid toxic shock syndrome by changing their tampons every 4 to 8 hours, using the lowest absorbency tampon possible, and alternating between tampons and pads. About half of TSS cases are not associated with menstruation. They can occur in males or females, typically when burns or surgical wounds become infected.[25]

Some staph bacteria are resistant to the antibiotics that traditionally had been effective against them. Known as **methicillin-resistant *Staphylococcus aureus*** or **MRSA,** these bacteria cause skin and wound infections and are responsible for many cases of pneumonia. See the **Spotlight** on MRSA below.

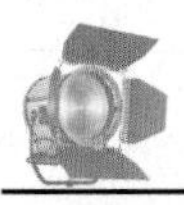

SPOTLIGHT

MRSA

MRSA, or methicillin-resistant *Staphylococcus aureus*, is a strain of staph that is resistant to many broad-spectrum antibiotics commonly used to treat staph infections. MRSA is responsible for serious skin infections, which first appear as painful, red, pus-filled lesions, but it can also cause other infections, including pneumonia. Because it is not treatable with many antibiotics, it poses a threat to anyone who is infected. The Centers for Disease Control and Prevention estimates that nearly 100,000 people in the United States develop a serious MRSA infection in any given year and that about one-fifth of them die from it. These statistics reflect a drastic rise in MRSA: In 1974, 2% of all staph infections were MRSA, in 1995, 22%, and in 2004, MRSA accounted for 64% of all staph infections.[1] It is thought that the development of bacteria like MRSA, which are resistant to multiple antibiotics, is in part due to the misuse of antibiotics.

The infection can be spread by direct skin-to-skin contact or by touching something that has been touched by an infected person. Most people with MRSA become infected when in the hospital or in other health-care settings such as dialysis centers and nursing homes. However, MRSA is becoming more common in schools and on college campuses. School athletes are especially susceptible, due to frequent skin-to-skin contact with others, the higher possibility of cuts or abrasions on the skin, and the use of facilities like locker rooms that may harbor MRSA.

Frequent hand washing, especially when in a clinical setting, is critical to limiting the spread of this serious infection. The following steps will also help you avoid catching or spreading MRSA.

- In addition to hand washing, keep open wounds covered with dry, sterile bandages.
- Shower immediately after exercise or participating in a close-contact sport.
- Do not share personal items such as towels or razors with others.
- If you have a skin infection that does not appear to be getting better after a day or so, see a doctor and request that you be tested for MRSA.

Early detection is important, especially because some MRSA strains, at least for now, respond to the antibiotic vancomycin, and small skin infections can be treated by draining and cleaning the lesion.

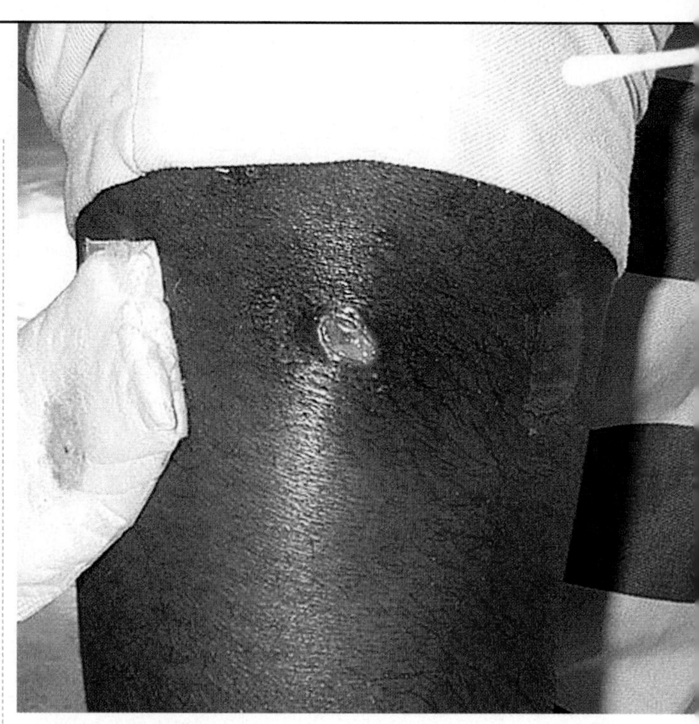

A sore due to MRSA.

Reference: 1. "Overview of Healthcare-Associated MRSA," in *Healthcare-Associated Methicillin-Resistant Staphylococcus aureus (HA-MRSA)*, by the Centers for Disease Control and Prevention, 2010, retrieved from http://www.cdc.gov/ncidod/dhqp/ar_mrsa.html.

Streptococcal Infections

Chances are you or someone you know has been infected with the bacteria *Streptococcus*, perhaps more than once. Group A *Streptococcus* (GAS) causes an itchy, blistery skin condition called *impetigo*, which is more common in children but also occurs in adults, especially in the later stages of a cold. GAS is also behind all bouts of strep throat, a relatively mild illness that causes throat pain, swollen tonsils, fever, headache, and stomachache. Particularly common in children and teens, strep throat is highly contagious through airborne droplets or touching contaminated objects. Strep throat usually requires a course of antibiotics to treat. If left untreated, it can lead within weeks to rheumatic fever, an inflammatory disease that can damage the heart valves and joints.

If you've ever seen a news report about "flesh-eating bacteria," the culprit was almost certainly GAS. Clinically referred to as *necrotizing fasciitis*, the disease occurs when GAS invades body tissues and destroys muscle, fat, and skin. About 25% of patients who develop necrotizing fasciitis do not survive.[26]

Lyme Disease

When hiking in the northern United States, you may have seen warning signs about Lyme disease. The infection is caused by the bacterium *Borrelia burgdorferi* and is transmitted to people through the bite of infected black-legged ticks, commonly called deer ticks. Adult ticks are about the size of a sesame seed, but immature ticks, called *nymphs*, typically spread the disease, and are half the size. Thus, they are difficult to spot, even on fair skin, and can attach to any part of the body, including the scalp.[27] Incidentally, Lyme disease gets its name from Lyme, Connecticut, where 51 cases of an unusual form of arthritis were reported in 1975. Investigators at Yale University eventually discovered the mode of transmission and the pathogen responsible.

Early symptoms of Lyme disease are headache, fatigue, fever, and muscle or joint pain. Within 4 weeks of infection, 70–80% of victims also experience a bull's-eye-shaped skin rash that radiates out from the area of the bite, starting small and growing larger **(Figure 13.6).** If the infection goes untreated, it can lead to swelling and pain in the joints, rapid heartbeat or other heart problems, partial facial paralysis, and neurological problems such as memory loss, which can last for years.

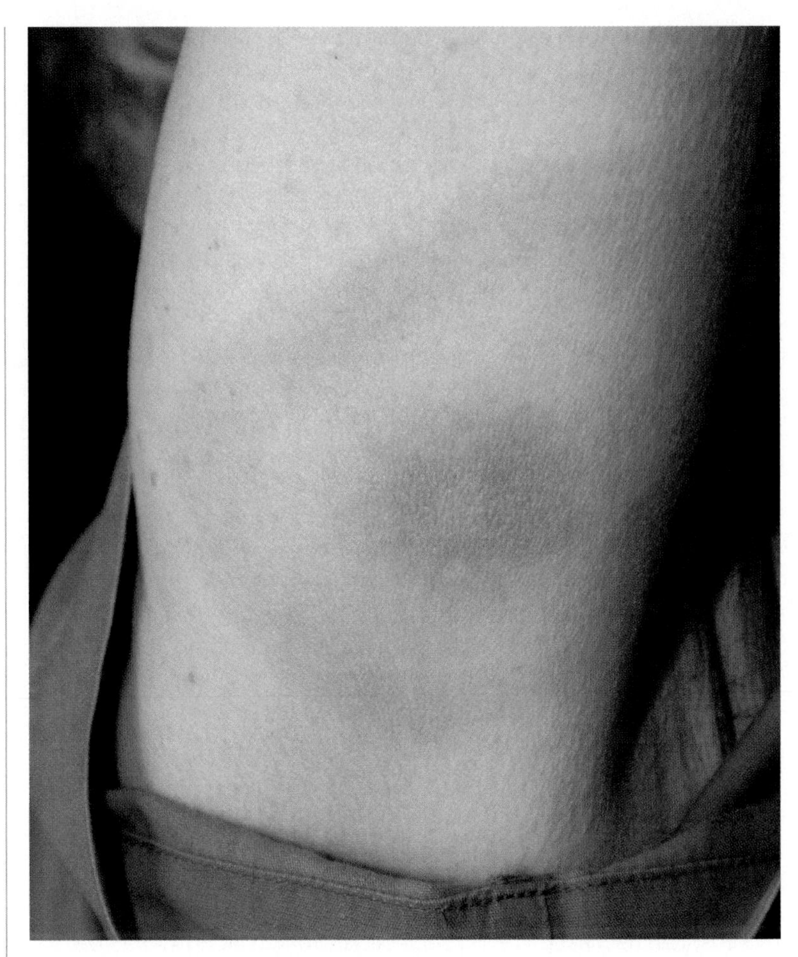

Figure 13.6 **Lyme disease.** This "bull's-eye" rash develops in a majority of people infected with Lyme disease.

If administered in the early stages of infection, antibiotics are usually successful in curing Lyme disease, but some people will have recurring symptoms of the disease for years. Prevention remains the best medicine:

- At home, clear long grasses, rake leaves, and remove trash where ticks can hide.
- If you have a pet that goes outdoors, talk with your vet about using a tick medication, and check your pet for ticks at least once daily from spring through autumn.
- When hiking, stay on the center of trails, avoiding forays into wooded areas or overgrown grass and brush. Wear long sleeves, long pants, and long socks to help keep ticks off your skin. Take a shower and check your body for ticks within an hour or two after your hike. Machine wash your clothes and dry them on high heat.

If you find a tick on yourself or your pet, use a pair of tweezers or small pliers to grasp it firmly as close to the skin as possible. Pull it straight out, as twisting can cause part of the head to remain in the wound. Clean the wound and apply an antiseptic. And don't panic: Ticks normally don't transmit the bacterium until after they have been on the skin for 36 to 48 hours or more.[27]

Bacterial Pneumonia

Pneumonia is an inflammation of the lungs that can be caused by infection with bacteria, viruses, fungi, or parasites. The symptoms vary greatly with the pathogen involved. Mild cases, called *atypical pneumonia* (or "walking pneumonia" because it isn't severe enough to require bed rest), are most commonly due to one of three bacterial species, most commonly *Mycoplasma pneumoniae*, and usually cause no more than chills, cough, a low-grade fever, and shortness of breath on exertion. Other pathogens can cause severe illness, and overall, pneumonia ranks as the ninth leading cause of death in the United States, and the number-one cause of death for children worldwide.[28, 29] The most common and serious of these is the *Streptococcus pneumoniae* bacterium. Infection causes high fever, chest pain, shortness of breath, chills, and a cough with green, yellow, or bloody mucus.

Pneumonia often develops as a complication of a cold or flu, and can be mistaken for these lesser infections. You should see a doctor immediately if you suddenly experience symptoms of pneumonia, as it can lead to ear infections, meningitis, and other complications.

Antibiotics are used to treat bacterial pneumonia infections, but as antibiotic-resistant bacterial strains

pneumonia Inflammation of the lungs.

have become more common, these drugs are becoming ever less effective. Prevention remains the best measure. Health-care experts recommend that people get an annual flu shot, which reduces the risk of developing pneumonia. In addition, infants and children are routinely vaccinated against *Streptococcus pneumoniae*. High-risk adults are encouraged to get the pneumococcal polysaccharide vaccine (PPSV). This includes all people over age 65, as well as people with asthma and other chronic respiratory problems, impaired immunity, or a history of exposure to certain chemicals and environmental pollutants.

Tuberculosis

Tuberculosis, or TB, is a serious disease caused by *Mycobacterium tuberculosis*, which enters the air when an infected person talks, coughs, or sneezes. The bacterium has a waxy wall that can allow it to survive in aerosol droplets for months. Once inhaled by a new host, it typically attacks the microscopic air sacs of the lungs. Macrophages rush to the site and ingest the bacterium, but because of its waxy coat, cannot actually digest it. In most people, however, this stops the progression of the infection, even though the characteristic tubercles (nodules) that give the disease its name remain in the lung tissue. In about 5–10% of people, TB becomes reactivated years later, spreading throughout the lungs, or disseminating widely throughout the body, to settle in the brain, spine, bone marrow, or kidneys.[30] Without proper treatment, disseminated TB can prove fatal.

Symptoms of active TB include weight loss, fatigue, fever, night sweats, and a persistent cough that does not go away after 3 weeks. The latent form does not cause any symptoms, is not infectious, and as noted may never progress to active TB. Medication, taken for many months, can help keep latent TB infections from evolving into active TB disease. However, drug-resistant strains of TB are now common, and some strains are capable of resisting multiple drug regimens.

Once the leading cause of death in the United States, TB cases have been declining in recent years and reached an all-time low in 2011. Infection rates continue to be highest among immigrants and racial and ethnic minorities, with Asian Americans having the highest rates. The poor, the homeless, and those infected with HIV are also at increased risk. Although there were only 10,521 new cases reported in 2011, millions of people in the United States are estimated to be living with a TB infection. Worldwide, about 2 billion people are infected.[31]

Tetanus

Tetanus is a nervous system disease caused by infection with the *Clostridium tetani* bacterium, which releases spores that can survive in soil and dust. The spores are transmitted to humans through breaks in the skin. Once in the body, they germinate and multiply rapidly, producing a potent nerve toxin that causes persistent muscle contraction. The familiar name of this disease, *lockjaw*, describes one of its characteristic signs: an inability to open the mouth because of persistent contraction of the jaw muscles. The patient also develops muscle stiffness and, if the disease is untreated, severe seizurelike contractions that are powerful enough to fracture bones. Death occurs in about 10–20% of cases.[32]

Treatment involves the immediate administration of anti-tetanus antibodies—a form of artificially acquired passive immunity. The antibodies bind to the tetanus toxins before they can bind to nerve cells. Antibiotics and a tetanus vaccine are also given. Infants are routinely vaccinated against tetanus. Adults need booster shots at least every 10 years to maintain immunity.

Urinary Tract Infections

A urinary tract infection (UTI) can involve any part of the urinary tract, including the kidneys, which filter and dilute wastes from the blood to produce urine, and the ureters, which transport urine to the bladder. However, the great majority of cases involve the bladder, which stores urine, and a UTI is often simply referred to as a bladder infection. Symptoms include a frequent urge to urinate, pain or burning on urination, fever, nausea, and sometimes blood in the urine.

In most cases, bacteria enter the urethra (the tube that transports urine from the bladder to the body exterior) after a bowel movement, during sexual intercourse, or through a catheter, a medical device used to drain urine in patients who can't urinate independently. Women are at increased risk because their urethra is much shorter than that of males. Women who use a diaphragm or spermicides for contraception are at even greater risk. Another risk factor is delaying urination: Small numbers of bacteria are typically flushed out of the body during urination, and ignoring the urge allows bacteria time to multiply in the bladder.

UTIs are treated with antibiotics, which unfortunately can wipe out helpful bacteria and prompt a yeast infection. To prevent UTIs, drink at least 6 to 8 glasses of water a day. Drink a glass of water before sex and urinate shortly afterward to flush out any bacteria. Both vitamin C and cranberry juice have also been shown to protect against infections by increasing the acidity of your urine, and cranberry juice also makes the walls of your bladder slippery, so bacteria can't adhere to it.[33]

Other Infectious Diseases

Although viruses and bacteria are the more common culprits in infectious disease, certain strains of fungi and other microbes can also cause infection.

Fungal Infections

Fungi are organisms that, like plants and animals, have cells in which a true nucleus surrounds and holds their DNA. They obtain their food from organic matter, in some cases human tissue. They are found in soil, on plants, in water, and even in the air we breathe. Common examples are multicellular, threadlike molds and single-celled, globular yeasts. Not all fungi are microorganisms, however: Mushrooms are large species. Some fungi reproduce via microscopic spores, which can become airborne and come into contact with skin or surfaces. Mold spores are just about everywhere. In fact, if you've ever wondered how a closed container of leftovers in your fridge developed that fuzzy coating of mold, it probably started with spores that drifted into the container just before you sealed it.

Some of the thousands of fungi that exist are quite beneficial. Penicillin, the powerful antibiotic used to treat a number of bacterial infections, is derived from a mold. Yeasts are used to make bread,

tuberculosis Disease caused by infection with *Mycobacterium tuberculosis* in which the immune response produces characteristic walled-off tubercles (nodules) in the lungs.

tetanus A disorder caused by infection with *Clostridium tetani* and characterized by persistent muscle contraction.

fungi Multicellular or single-celled organisms that obtain their food from organic matter, in some cases human tissue.

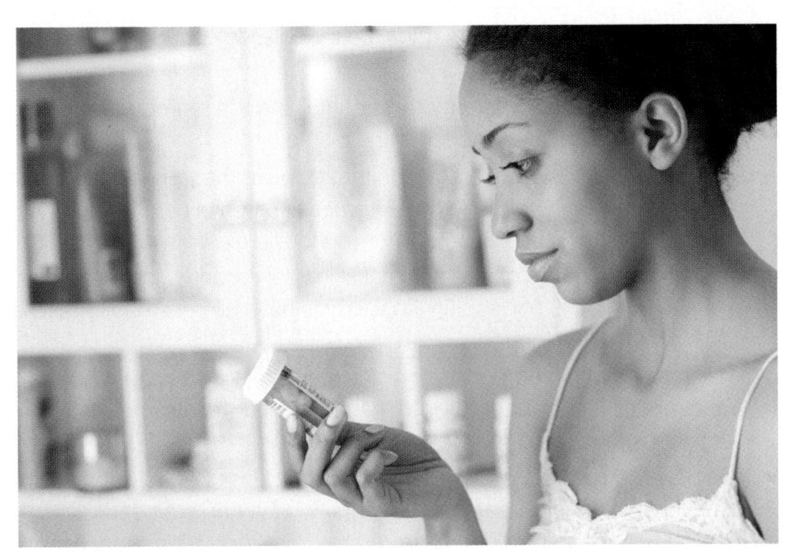

Yeast infections are often caused by taking **antibiotics**.

cheese, and many other food products. But fungi are also behind many minor infections of the skin, scalp, and nail beds, from athlete's foot to a certain type of dandruff! And in the immunocompromised, especially people with AIDS, some fungal pathogens that are easy for healthy people to vanquish can cause unusual infections, such as a rare fungal pneumonia that can be life-threatening.

Yeast infections are some of the most common types of fungal infections. Small amounts of a yeast called *Candida albicans* are always present in a person's body, but if imbalances occur—after taking antibiotics, for example, or, for women, during the normal hormonal changes that come with menstrual periods—this fungus may be able to multiply out of control. It can cause infections in various parts of the body, including the intestinal tract and vagina. Fungal overgrowth in the large intestine can result in bloating, cramps, and diarrhea. Vaginal yeast infections are marked by itching in the vagina and around the genitals, and are often accompanied by an abnormal vaginal discharge that can resemble cottage cheese. Sexual intercourse should be avoided not only because it is likely to be painful but also out of consideration for your partner; although yeast infections are not sexually transmitted, some men do develop an itchy rash after having sex with an infected woman.[34] Over-the-counter treatment, usually a vaginal antifungal cream or suppository, is usually effective, or the patient may be advised to take a single dose of an oral antifungal medication. Other *Candida* infections include thrush (an overgrowth in the mouth), diaper rash, and infections of the nail beds.

Protozoan Infections

Protozoa are single-celled organisms that, like fungi, obtain nutrients from feeding on organic matter. While some are free-living, and even helpful—consuming harmful bacteria or serving as food for fish and other animals—protozoan parasites rely on other living things, such as humans, for food and shelter. These protozoa are capable of causing serious diseases in humans, especially in people living in developing countries. In the United States, where sanitation and food-handling standards have reduced our exposure to them, protozoan infections are less common.

One of the protozoan diseases of global concern is **malaria,** which kills nearly one million people every year, primarily infants, children, and pregnant women.[35] The infection is caused by the protozoa *Plasmodium,* and is typically transmitted to humans through the bites of infected mosquitoes. Malaria is a serious threat throughout much of sub-Saharan Africa and parts of Latin America, Asia, and the Middle East, and fully 50% of the world's population is at risk of contracting it.[19] Although it was controlled in the United States more than five decades ago, occasional outbreaks still occur here. As global temperatures rise, malaria rates might increase if malaria-carrying mosquitoes move into areas that historically have not been affected by the disease.

Initial symptoms include fever, chills, vomiting, and headache. If not treated with antimalarial drugs promptly, the infection can be fatal. Some strains of malaria have become resistant to drugs, making treatment much more difficult. Malaria can be prevented by warding off mosquito bites through the use of insecticides, wearing long pants and long-sleeved shirts, and sleeping beneath mosquito netting imbued with insecticides. Antimalarial drugs can also be taken during trips to malaria-endemic areas.

Giardiasis is a diarrheal disease caused by infection with *Giardia intestinalis*. It typically enters soil and water via animal feces and is transmitted to humans exposed to contaminated soils or water. Unfortunately, treating water with chlorine is not effective, as this microbe has a tough outer shell that helps it tolerate chlorine. Infection may not produce any symptoms at all, or it may cause diarrhea, intestinal cramps, gas, nausea, vomiting, and even itchy skin and hives. Treatment requires a prescription medication such as metronidazole. Prevention includes thorough hand washing after handling animal feces or gardening, and avoiding swallowing water while swimming.

Parasitic Worm Infections

Parasitic worms (helminths) are creatures that compete with a host body for nutrients. Some tiny worms burrow through the skin, while others are contracted from eating microscopic eggs in undercooked foods. Once inside the body, some can grow up to 10–15 feet in length. Others can live for up to 15 years. They are most frequently found in tropical regions and are a problem in areas with poor sanitation. Infections are most common in travelers, refugees, migrant workers, children, and the homeless. Two of the more common parasitic worms in the United States are tapeworms and pinworms.

The tapeworm, the largest of the parasitic worms, is usually spread through poorly cooked beef, pork, or fish. The pork tapeworm is the most dangerous, because its eggs can invade tissues and even the central nervous system, resulting in seizures. The dwarf tapeworm, which only grows to about 2 inches, is the variety most commonly found in the United States, and has been linked to food contaminated with mouse droppings. Oral medications can usually treat tapeworm infections.

Pinworm infections are the most common worm infections in the United States They are generally not serious and are often transmitted in day care

protozoa Single-celled parasites that rely on other living things for food and shelter.

malaria A serious disease that causes fever and chills that appear in cycles. In some cases malaria can be life-threatening.

parasitic worms (helminths) Multicellular creatures that compete with a host body for nutrients.

centers, schools, and summer camps. Infection occurs when the eggs of pinworms are inadvertently swallowed, often by placing dirty fingers in or near the mouth. The eggs then travel to the intestines, where they hatch. Female worms, which have pin-shaped tails, travel at night through the anus and deposit their eggs on the skin. Infections can be treated with oral medications, and topical ointments are often used to relieve anal itching.

Prion Infection

A **prion** is a proteinaceous infectious particle. It lacks genetic material and is not considered a living organism—yet it can reproduce itself by causing normal cell proteins to misfold into prions, typically in the tissue of the central nervous system. This is the hallmark of Creutzfeldt-Jakob disease (CJD), a fatal neurological disorder that affects about 1 in 1 million Americans. CJD is not an infectious disease, because the protein misfolding seems to happen spontaneously, or because of genetic mutations. However, a variant form of CJD, referred to as vCJD, *is* due to infection.

First identified in 1996, vCJD is the "human equivalent" of bovine spongiform encephalitis, commonly known as *mad cow disease*. The term "spongiform" refers to the appearance of affected nerve tissue, which is riddled with holes like a sponge. The resulting neurological impairment is severe, and vCJD typically progresses to death within 13 or 14 months. The pathogen is transmitted from infected animals to humans when humans consume meat—usually beef derived from a sick cow. Prions are not destroyed by cooking. Consumption of contaminated beef is thought to be responsible for the 171 deaths from vCJD that occurred in the United Kingdom from 1994 through 2010, an incidence that has prompted worldwide changes in beef production. Three deaths have been attributed to vCJD in the United States in the same time period.[36]

Immune Disorders

We've seen that, in immunocompromised individuals, the immune response is weak, leaving the person unusually vulnerable to pathogens. But the opposite can also occur. The immune system can go into overdrive and, instead of protecting against disease, actually provoke it. The two main categories of such immune disorders are hypersensitivities and autoimmune diseases.

Immune Hypersensitivities

Immune hypersensitivities are characterized by an exaggerated response to something that is not an irritant to most people. For instance, a peanut butter sandwich is a healthful snack to most of us. When a person can't ingest a peanut fragment without going into shock, an immune hypersensitivity is at work.

Allergies

More than 50 million people in the United States have **allergies,** hypersensitivity reactions to proteins that are otherwise harmless. Allergies are widespread on college campuses, with almost 20% of students in one survey stating that they had been treated for allergies in the last year.[37]

prion An infectious protein particle that lacks genetic material but can reproduce itself by causing normal cell proteins to misfold, typically resulting in destruction of central nervous system tissue.

allergies Abnormal immune system reactions to substances that are otherwise harmless.

mast cell A type of cell in the skin and mucous membranes that releases histamine and other chemicals into the bloodstream during an allergic reaction.

anaphylactic shock A result of anaphylaxis in which the release of histamine and other chemicals into the body leads to a drop in blood pressure, tightening of airways, and possible unconsciousness and even death.

Antigens associated with allergies are called *allergens*. Some of the most common are:

- Plant pollens, the powdery material containing the reproductive grains of cone-bearing and flowering plants.
- Dust mites, microscopic arachnids that thrive in the temperature range and humidity found in most homes. Dust mites are thought to be the most common cause of year-round allergies.[38]
- Pet dander (particles of shed animal skin), saliva, urine, or feathers. From 15% to 30% of people with allergies have allergic reactions to dogs or cats.[39]
- Insect venom injected by stinging bees, wasps, or ants. As many as 3% of adults are thought to be vulnerable to life-threatening reactions to insect stings.[40]
- Food allergens, most commonly proteins from milk, eggs, fish, crustacean shellfish, tree nuts, peanuts, wheat, and soybeans.[41] Food allergies can produce an immediate, life-threatening reaction called anaphylaxis, discussed shortly, or a delayed reaction such as a cough or rash. Many people blame food allergies for vague symptoms such as mild headaches, a runny nose, or loose stools, but researchers believe fewer than 5% of U.S. adults actually have allergic reactions to any foods.[42]

If you have allergies, you may suffer from itching, sneezing, coughing, watery eyes, difficulty breathing, and congestion. When allergic people come into contact with substances they are sensitive to, their immune systems begin to produce antibodies called immunoglobulin E, or IgE. IgE antibodies bind simultaneously to the allergen and to a **mast cell,** a type of cell found in the body's connective tissues, including the skin and mucous membranes (which, among other things, line the nose, throat, and lower airways). As a result of these interactions, the mast cell releases powerful inflammatory chemicals such as histamine into the bloodstream. It is these chemicals—and not the allergens themselves—that make allergy sufferers miserable.

In some instances, allergens provoke a rare, serious allergic reaction known as *anaphylaxis*. In this case, the wave of histamine and chemicals released by mast cells occurs throughout the body, and can cause **anaphylactic shock,** in which blood pressure drops and airways swell. If not treated immediately with an injection of epinephrine (the hormone and neurotransmitter commonly called adrenaline), a person can lapse into unconsciousness and even death. People who know they are at risk for anaphylaxis from bee stings, ingesting peanuts, etc., often carry an "EpiPen"—epinephrine in a form the person can self-inject.

Fortunately, there are strategies for coping with allergies. First and foremost, allergists recommend avoidance: Steer clear of the things you are allergic to whenever possible, staying indoors on high-pollen days and keeping your room clear of dust and dander. Your doctor may recommend prescription or over-the-counter medications that can help alleviate symptoms. Immunotherapy, in which patients are given a series of injections containing increasing amounts of the allergen to desensitize them, is also an option.

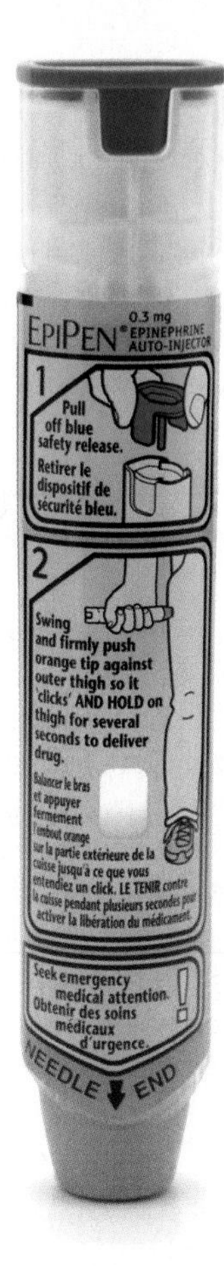

An **Epi-Pen** can save a life if needed to counteract a severe allergic reaction.

The incidence of allergies has increased steadily in recent years. Ironically, this increase may be the unintended result of our antiseptic, health-conscious lifestyle. A possible explanation, the *hygiene hypothesis*, contends that early childhood exposure to microbes, especially parasites, can prevent the development of allergies, and conversely, reduced exposure to microbes can increase the chances of developing allergies. Many factors in developed countries today reduce exposure to microbes: smaller family size (fewer siblings means fewer family members bringing microbes into the home); less exposure to animals, specifically farm animals; use of vaccines, antibiotics, and antimicrobial soaps and cleaning products; and less exposure to general dirt and microorganisms.

The hygiene hypothesis may also explain the increasing rates of asthma, an immune hypersensitivity that we'll look at next.

This video explores the hygiene hypothesis of developing allergies: www.pbs.org/wgbh/evolution/library/10/4/l_104_07.html.

Asthma

Asthma is a chronic, inflammatory disease of the bronchi, the branching tubes that transport air to and from the lungs. An acute episode of asthma, commonly called an "asthma attack," results from three main physiological changes affecting the bronchi:

- Constriction of the bronchial muscles, known as *bronchospasm,* which squeezes the walls of the tubes
- Inflammation of the lining of the bronchi, which decreases their interior space
- Overproduction of mucus by an excessive number of goblet cells within the tubes, which further clogs the narrowed space.

As a result, it becomes increasingly difficult for the person to inhale fresh air or to exhale stale air, an effort sometimes described as trying to breathe through a straw. The person develops a deficit of oxygen and an excess of carbon dioxide waste in the blood, which produces a sensation of suffocation. Just over 8% of the U.S. population currently has asthma, and in 2009, it caused more than 3,300 deaths.[43]

There are two general types of asthma. *Allergic asthma* is caused by exposure to allergens in the air (e.g., pollen), in the blood (e.g., bee venom), or in food (e.g., peanuts). *Intrinsic asthma*, on the other hand, can be induced by exercise, cold temperatures, or respiratory infection, and is not associated with an allergy. It isn't clear why some people have asthma and others do not, but it is likely a combination of genetics (if one of your parents has asthma, you are more likely to have it) and the environment in which you live.

Prevention of asthma episodes includes avoiding known triggers. Many children and adults with chronic asthma take inhaled steroids or other anti-inflammatory medications daily to reduce the immune hypersensitivity. Once an attack has begun, fast-acting inhaled bronchodilators can help open the airways and ease breathing.

About 1 in 10 school-aged children in the United States suffers from asthma, reflecting a doubling of asthma rates over the last 30 years.[44] Also notable is the racial disparity in asthma rates. Whereas 8% of Caucasian children have asthma, 13% of African American children have the disease. This is thought to reflect socioeconomic conditions, with poorer children more likely to be exposed to mold, dust mites, the dried wastes of rodents and roaches, diesel soot, and other types of air pollution.

Autoimmune Diseases

Auto- means "self." When the immune system fails to recognize normal body cells as self, and attacks them as if they were invaders, **autoimmune disease** occurs. In autoimmune disease, the body makes autoantibodies that target self cells. At the same time, regulatory T cells fail to keep the immune response in check.[45] The result is a harmful and sometimes even deadly attack by the body against the body.

Celiac Disease

Celiac disease is an autoimmune disease that damages the lining of the small intestine and interferes with absorption of nutrients from food. In the United States, about 1 in 133 people is affected.[46] The disease is even more common within families—among those with another family member affected, 1 in 22 will develop celiac disease—and specific gene markers have now been linked to the disorder.

People with celiac disease have a total intolerance for a food protein called *gluten*, which is found mainly in wheat, rye, and barley. When they consume gluten, their immune system goes on

asthma Chronic inflammatory disease characterized by bronchospasm, inflammation of the bronchial lining, and overproduction of mucus within the narrowed bronchi.

autoimmune disease General term for any of a number of disorders characterized by inflammation and other immune responses against the body's own tissues.

the offensive, setting off an inflammatory response that erodes the tiny absorptive cells lining the small intestine. In people who are not aware they have the disease, and continue to consume gluten, the body's ability to absorb nutrients becomes so impaired that the person can experience dramatic weight loss, diarrhea (or sometimes, constipation), low bone density from poor calcium absorption, seizures from electrolyte imbalances, and a variety of other signs and symptoms, including a painful rash called *dermatitis herpetiformis*. Celiac disease is also a risk factor for cancer of the small intestine, which otherwise is extremely rare.

Celiac disease is thought to be frequently misdiagnosed, typically as *irritable bowel syndrome* (*IBS*), a disorder in which patients experience bowel cramping and pain shortly after eating, and often either diarrhea or constipation. Celiac disease is also sometimes misdiagnosed as an inflammatory bowel disorder, discussed next. Given the potential for misdiagnosis, the National Institutes of Health is promoting greater awareness of celiac disease among U.S. health-care providers.[47] Although a variety of blood tests can detect the presence of antibodies to gluten or the genetic markers of the disease, definitive diagnosis requires a biopsy of the small intestine that shows the erosion of the lining.

There is no cure for celiac disease, but patients who maintain a strict gluten-free diet—and avoid personal care products such as lip balms and lotions made with gluten—should see their symptoms begin to abate within several weeks.

Inflammatory Bowel Disorders

Inflammatory bowel disease (*IBD*) is a general term covering two related disorders:

- *Crohn's disease* can affect any portion of the gastrointestinal tract, but is most often seen in the small intestine, where one segment will be inflamed and thickened, and another segment will be entirely healthy.
- *Ulcerative colitis* is superficial inflammation and the development of ulcers in the lining of the colon and rectum. The condition extends through a large portion of the colon, rather than "skipping" segments.

Both conditions can produce severe pain, diarrhea, bleeding, and a variety of symptoms beyond the gastrointestinal tract. Both are also associated with an increased risk for cancer.

Mainstays of drug treatment are antibiotics, steroids and other anti-inflammatory agents, and immunosuppressive drugs. Surgical removal of severely diseased regions may be required.[48]

Other Autoimmune Disorders

Many other autoimmune diseases exist. Here we can mention only a few of the most common:[45]

- *Type 1 diabetes*, in which the immune system attacks the cells of the pancreas that produce insulin. (See Chapter 11.)
- *Multiple sclerosis*, in which the immune system damages the protective sheath (called myelin) around nerves. This slows the transmission of nerve impulses, and can lead to tremors, weakness, trouble with coordinated movements such as walking and speaking, and even paralysis.
- *Rheumatoid arthritis*, in which inflammation affects the lining of the joints, causing joint stiffness, pain, and swelling, as well as reduced joint functioning.
- *Sjögren's syndrome* (pronounced SHOW-grins syndrome), in which the immune system targets moisture-producing glands in the body, causing dry eyes, dry mouth, joint swelling, fatigue, and other symptoms.
- *Systemic lupus erythematosus* (pronounced e-rih-thee-ma-TOE-sus), in which immune destruction can occur all over the body, affecting the skin, heart, lungs, kidneys, and other organs. The person may experience hair loss, weight loss, a red facial rash, chest pain, fatigue, and many other symptoms.

Change Yourself, Change Your World

This chapter may be leaving you feeling even more powerfully that it's you against the world. But it's not true. Although we identify ahead some of the most important personal choices you can make to defend against infection, it's not all up to you. Public health experts are continually developing methods to protect everyone against the spread of infection, and to keep us informed of outbreaks of infectious disease and our options for prevention and treatment. And look around campus: Those posters reminding you to wash your hands or get the flu vaccine are just one illustration of the truth that, when it comes to breaking the chain of infection, we work best when we work together.

Personal Choices

Chances are, as you read this, a variety of infectious microbes are roaming your campus. So what can you do to reduce the chance that they'll find you a susceptible host?

Keep Your Immune System Strong

Start with your personal habits. The following are key:

- Don't smoke. If you do, you're setting out the welcome mat to pathogenic microbes. Smoking destroys some of your nonspecific respiratory defenses against pathogens—like the cilia that should sweep microbes out of your lungs—and reduces your immune function overall. So people who smoke are more likely to catch colds and flu.
- Limit your alcohol. Both binge drinking and heavy drinking suppress the immune system, interfering with the functioning of neutrophils, macrophages, and B and T cells, as well as the cytokines that assist their functions.[49] Heavy drinking is also associated with malnutrition, which itself impairs immunity.
- Eat right. Malnutrition is proven to increase susceptibility to infection; in fact, the most common way that malnutrition kills infants and children is by making them more vulnerable to infectious disease.[50] For well-nourished populations, certain substances in foods may help boost immune health. These include probiotics, the plant pigment beta-carotene, vitamin B_6, vitamin C, zinc, and many other components of a healthful, balanced diet.
- Don't shortchange your sleep. Short sleep reduces the number of functioning T cells and thereby can make you more vulnerable to infection.[51]
- Exercise. Researchers have found that regular physical activity can help you fend off infectious diseases by boosting your immune system.[52]

Reduce Your Risk for Common Infections

Keeping your immune system strong helps you avoid becoming the next microbial host. Another way to break the chain of infection is to avoid direct and indirect transmission, whether from someone else to you, or from you to others. The **Practical Strategies for Health** shows how.

See Your Doctor

Have you had a tetanus booster in the last 10 years? If you don't know, phone your health-care provider and find out. While you're at it, make sure all your other immunizations are up to date (see Table 13.2). And don't forget your annual flu shot! The CDC recommends it for all college students.

Join the CDC's "The flu ends with U" vaccination campaign. Submit your pledge at www.cdc.gov/flu/nivw/pledge.

If you feel yourself coming down with a cold or flu, chances are you don't need medical care. Rest, fluids, and the other self-care measures identified in this chapter—along with time—should get you back on your feet. But if you continue to feel exhausted weeks after other signs of infection have passed, or develop a cough that won't quit, a rash, or other alarming signs and symptoms, visit your campus health services center or see your doctor. You might be hosting a bug that's gaining the upper hand, and medication may be important to preserve your health.

Campus Advocacy

Want to help break the chain of infection on your campus? Consider volunteering for an infection control internship! Available on many large campuses, these internships allow students to collect data, staff flu clinics, and increase student awareness of infectious diseases and prevention measures, from vaccination to simple hand washing. In one such program, interns staffed a table at their campus health fair and handed out flyers with vaccination information.

If an internship doesn't fit into your schedule, there are plenty of smaller ways you can help:

- Stay home if you're feverish, have conjunctivitis, or can't control your coughing, sneezing, or runny nose.
- Post a reminder about hand washing in the kitchen and bathroom of your apartment or residence hall.
- Carry a small container of hand sanitizer in your backpack, and share it!
- Encourage your friends to check their immunization status and to get the annual flu vaccine.
- Interview friends who've experienced the flu, mono, hepatitis, or another infection common on campus. Publish their stories on your campus website to increase awareness of the importance of infection control.
- Visit your campus health services center and ask about other ways you might help reduce the spread of infection on campus.

Download a free hand-washing poster at the CDC's website: www.cdc.gov/h1n1flu/pdf/handwashing.pdf.

Watch videos of real students discussing infectious disease at www.pearsonhighered.com/lynchelmore.

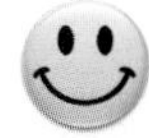 *Practical Strategies for Health*

Protecting Yourself Against Infectious Diseases

To avoid contracting an infection:

- Wash your hands often, or use hand sanitizer with at least 60% alcohol.
- Keep your hands away from your eyes, nose, and mouth. Touching your face is a common way to transmit pathogens from your hands into your body.
- Avoid close contact with people who are sick.
- Routinely clean and disinfect surfaces, including keyboards, phones, and kitchen counters.
- Keep up to date on your vaccinations and get an annual flu shot.
- Make sure your pets are up to date on their vaccinations as well. And talk to your vet about flea and tick preparations.
- Avoid contact with wild animals. Rodents, bats, raccoons, skunks, and foxes can all spread harmful bacteria or viruses.
- Avoid mosquito bites. In mosquito-dense areas, wear insect repellent when you are outdoors, particularly at dusk and dawn; eliminate standing water in flower pots, bird baths, or other containers left outdoors; make sure you have intact window screens; and wear long-sleeved shirts and pants to avoid bites.
- Avoid walking barefoot in locker rooms or on dirt.
- Eat well. Proper nutrition supports your immune system.

If you do contract an infection, take steps to prevent infecting others:

- Stay home, especially if you're feverish.

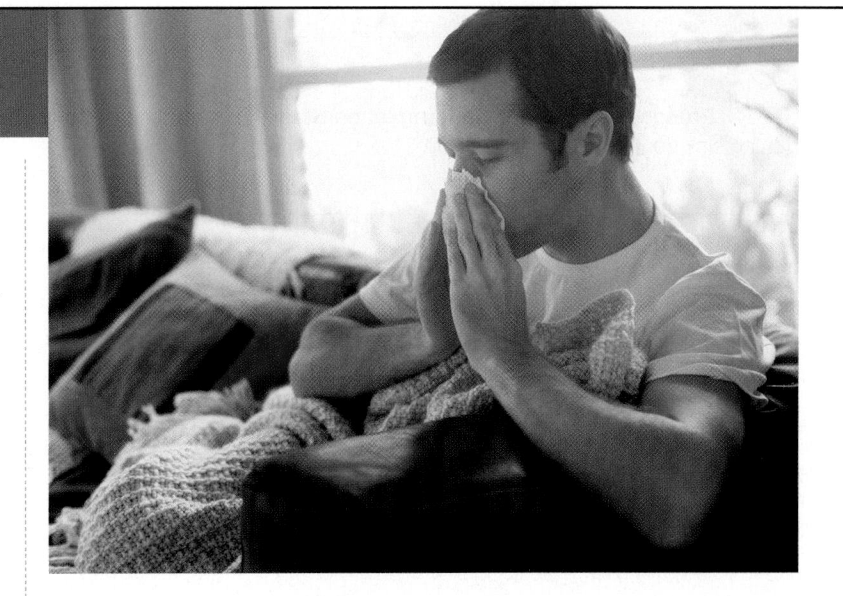

- Keep a distance of about 3 feet from others.
- Cover your mouth or nose with a tissue when you cough or sneeze, or cough or sneeze into the bend of your elbow, and wash your hands afterwards.
- Throw away used tissues immediately.
- Don't share cups, cell phones, or other objects with anyone else unless you've cleaned them first.

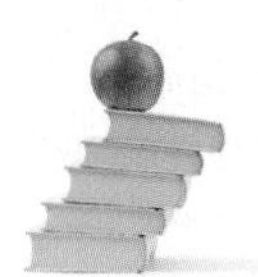

Choosing to Change Worksheet

To complete this worksheet online, visit www.pearsonhighered.com/lynchelmore.

In this chapter you learned about the importance of preventing infectious diseases. To reduce your risk of infection, follow the steps below.

Directions: Fill in your stage of change in Step 1 and complete Step 2 with your stage of change in mind. Then complete Steps 3, 4, or 5, depending on which ones apply to your stage of change.

Step 1: Your Stage of Behavior Change. Please check one of the following statements that best describes your readiness to reduce your infectious disease risk.

_____________ I do not intend to reduce my infectious disease risk in the next 6 months. (Precontemplation)

_____________ I might reduce my infectious disease risk in the next 6 months. (Contemplation)

_____________ I am prepared to reduce my infectious disease risk in the next month. (Preparation)

_____________ I have been reducing my infectious disease risk for less than 6 months. (Action)

_____________ I have been reducing my infectious disease risk for more than 6 months. (Maintenance)

Step 2: Recognizing Infectious Disease Risk. Complete the preventing infectious diseases **Self-Assessment** on page 358 to see if you are at an increased risk of contracting an infection. After completing your self-assessment, did you answer "Sometimes" or "Never" to any of the ways to prevent the spread of infectious diseases? List them:

____

____

Step 3: Precontemplation or Contemplation Stages. How often do you get sick with an infection? How does getting sick negatively impact your life?

____

____

What is holding you back from taking action to reduce your risk of contracting an infectious disease?

____

____

How can you overcome these obstacles to reducing your risk of contracting an infectious disease?

____

____

Step 4: Preparation and Action Stages. The recommendations for reducing your risk of contracting an infectious disease appear in the **Practical Strategies for Health** box on page 377. Select one strategy that you wish you felt more confident in employing. Indicate one action you can take (or already have taken) to strengthen your confidence in your ability to employ that strategy. Be specific. Set a **goal,** including a timeline, for reducing your infectious disease risk.

Strategy to employ and how you will strengthen your confidence: ______________________________

____

Goal: ______________________________

Step 5: Maintenance Stage. Your goal is to stay focused and renew your commitment to reducing your chances of contracting an infectious disease. What benefits of practicing infectious disease prevention are most important to you and why?

____

____

____

How easy has it been to practice infectious disease prevention? Is it truly a habit or do you need to expend some effort to do it?

____

____

____

Chapter Summary

- For infections to spread in a population, six conditions have to be met. Collectively referred to as the chain of infection, these include a pathogen, reservoir, means of escape, mode of transmission, means of entry, and a new susceptible host.
- Pathogens are agents that cause disease. Microbial pathogens include viruses, bacteria, fungi, protozoa, and parasitic worms.
- Infectious diseases can be directly transmitted via contact with an infected person, animal, or vector, or indirectly transmitted via contact with contaminated objects, air, water, or food.
- Your body's first line of nonspecific defense against infection includes your skin, mucous membranes, cilia, bodily fluids, and coughing, sneezing, and other functional defenses. These prevent pathogens from entering the body or trap and expel them if they do.
- Your immune system, a powerful network of cellular and chemical defenses, fights pathogens that enter the body. Neutrophils, macrophages, dendritic cells, and natural killer cells are key nonspecific defenders. B cells and T cells work with precision and focus to produce antibodies and kill specific pathogens. Memory B cells and T cells can provide long-term immunity to an infection, which makes getting the same infection again unlikely.
- Specific immunity can be artificially acquired by immunization or by administration of preformed antibodies.
- Viruses are not cells. Rather, they must invade plant, animal, and microbial cells and use those cells' genetic and metabolic machinery to survive and reproduce. Viruses cause illnesses ranging in severity from the common cold to a potentially fatal hepatitis.
- Bacteria are cellular microorganisms capable of reproducing independently. They cause illnesses ranging from mild to life-threatening pneumonias and from simple skin infections to a quickly fatal form of meningitis.
- Fungi are more similar to plant and animal cells in that their DNA is encapsulated in a true nucleus. They are the most common cause of simple skin, scalp, and nail infections, and of vaginal infections. Some rare fungal infections are opportunistic, taking advantage of a host's immunocompromised state to reproduce and cause severe illness.
- Protozoa, parasitic worms (helminths), and prions also cause infectious disease.
- In hypersensitivity reactions, the immune system mistakes common substances, such as nuts, pet dander, or pollen, for harmful agents, triggering allergies. Allergies can cause asthma.
- Autoimmune diseases such as celiac disease and inflammatory bowel disorders occur when the immune system generates an inflammatory response against its own tissues.
- You can take action to help break the chain of infection, such as by properly washing your hands, staying home when you have a cold or flu, and keeping up to date on your immunizations.

Test Your Knowledge

1. Pathogens
   a. cannot be stopped by your body's nonspecific defenses.
   b. are agents that cause disease.
   c. infect animals but not humans.
   d. include bacteria and other cellular microbes, but not viruses or prions.

2. A person who has no signs or symptoms of infectious disease but can transmit infectious microbes to others is called a
   a. reservoir.
   b. carrier.
   c. contaminator.
   d. vector.

3. Your first line of defense against infection is
   a. natural killer cells.
   b. antibiotics.
   c. cytotoxic T cells.
   d. your skin.

4. Subunit vaccines
   a. provide passive immunity.
   b. typically produce mild symptoms of the disease.
   c. provide artificially acquired immunity.
   d. use killed microorganisms.

5. What type of organism takes over the body's cells, forcing them to make replicas of it?
   a. viruses
   b. fungi
   c. bacteria
   d. protozoa

6. Which of the following is an example of a contagious disease?
   a. malaria
   b. vCJD
   c. mononucleosis
   d. multiple sclerosis

7. Antibiotics are appropriate treatments against
   a. bacteria.
   b. viruses.
   c. fungi.
   d. none of the above.

8. Lyme disease is spread by
   a. fleas.
   b. ticks.
   c. mosquitoes.
   d. mice.

Get Critical

What happened:

In January 2011, while on a trip to Sudan to support a peaceful voting process on the question of independence for South Sudan, actor and activist George Clooney contracted malaria. After an acute 10-day illness, he joined friend and *New York Times* columnist Nicholas Kristof to advocate for malaria prevention and treatment. While expressing gratitude that his own recovery from the illness had been quick, Clooney pointed out that the average Sudanese lacks access to effective medications. "I had drugs to take before, during, and after . . . Life-saving drugs for diseases that kill millions needlessly belong to mankind, not to companies to profit from." Kristof added that, "The average Sudanese in rural areas might not receive any treatment for malaria at all . . . Children and pregnant women are particularly vulnerable to dying from it . . ." Kristof also explained why prevention efforts such as insecticide-treated bed nets can cause malaria rates to plummet: Mosquitoes merely carry malaria from one human to another, so the smaller the pool of infected people, the less likely that mosquitoes will be carrying it.

What do you think?

- Do you agree with Clooney that pharmaceutical companies should donate the medications they make to impoverished populations when lives are at stake? Why or why not?
- Malaria is a preventable disease, and prevention efforts, including the use of insecticide-treated bed nets, have helped reduce malaria rates as much as 90% in some regions. Deaths from malaria have dropped by 25% since 2000. Yet the organization Malaria No More reports that malaria still kills one child every minute worldwide. What actions could college students in the United States take to provide bed nets for poor families in malaria-ridden areas? Go to www.malarianomore.org and find out.

Source: "George Clooney Answers Your Questions about Malaria," by N. Kristof, February 8, 2011, *The New York Times*. Retrieved from http://kristof.blogs.nytimes.com/2011/02/08/george-clooney-answers-your-questions-about-malaria.

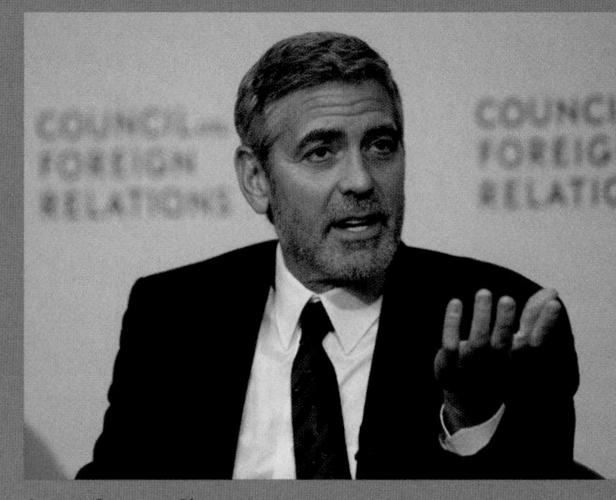

Actor George Clooney

9. A release of histamine throughout the body
   a. is known as anaphylaxis.
   b. produces a hot, itchy skin welt.
   c. produces a dangerous rise in blood pressure.
   d. is characteristic of shingles.

10. A disease characterized by the presence of autoantibodies and the failure of regulatory T cells is known as
    a. an infectious disease.
    b. a pandemic.
    c. a hypersensitivity disorder.
    d. an autoimmune disease.

- **Take responsibility.** Own what is yours and admit when you've made mistakes. But don't negate an apology by following it with blame, as in, "I'm sorry I blew up, but you shouldn't have touched my laptop!" Instead, try following an apology with a promise: "I'm sorry I blew up. I totally overreacted, and in the future, I'll do my best to handle things more calmly. In return, I'd really appreciate your promising to ask me before you use my computer."
- **Use "I" messages.** Begin the discussion with an "I feel" statement, explaining how the other person's behavior has affected you, and why you think you've reacted this way. For example, "I felt sad when you asked me why I was back so late from rehearsal, because this concert is really important to me." Making the discussion about yourself may help the other person focus on your feelings. In contrast, "You" messages—such as, "You don't trust me!"—can make the other person feel attacked and are likely to trigger defensiveness.
- **Be solution focused.** Try to look for a win-win compromise. Effective communication requires that you find a resolution that enables both parties to feel satisfied.
- **Step away if necessary.** Sometimes the timing isn't right for resolving a relationship conflict. If tempers flare and the conversation is headed toward an unproductive argument, take a break. But don't storm out. Assure the person you're not giving up, but explain that you need some distance. Then walk away calmly. Return to the issue when it can be approached with a more constructive attitude.
- **Resist antagonizing the other person.** For example, resist correcting grammatical errors or bringing up details that do not matter to the real issue at hand.
- **Seek help if you need it.** If you or your partner continues to have difficulty communicating about relationship issues in a constructive way, it may be time to seek help from a counselor or other professional who can help. Your campus health services center should be able to recommend someone you can work with, or you can locate a therapist in your area by visiting the American Association of Marriage and Family Therapy's website at **www.aamft.org.**

Nonverbal Communication

Sometimes you can get a message across without saying a single word. Imagine a teenager who has been out way past her curfew. When she arrives home, she unlocks the front door and tiptoes inside, hoping to make it to her bedroom unnoticed. But in the living room, she sees her father, still awake in his easy chair, tapping his feet, arms crossed, face scowling. Message received.

Savvy communicators know that it isn't just what you say but *how* you say it that matters. Nonverbal cues such as posture, gestures, eye contact, and even touch help us broadcast our thoughts, whether we realize it or not. This is known as **nonverbal communication,** sometimes called *body language*. If a friend has a glazed-over look in her eyes or is checking her phone while you are talking, that body language can communicate that she is bored. A person with upright posture and good eye contact conveys confidence, whereas someone who is hunched over and whose eyes dart back and forth communicates nervousness and discomfort. Crossed arms can convey defensiveness—or simply that someone is cold. The ability to ensure that your body language is in tune with what you intend to say is a key characteristic of an effective communicator.

nonverbal communication Communication that is conveyed by body language.

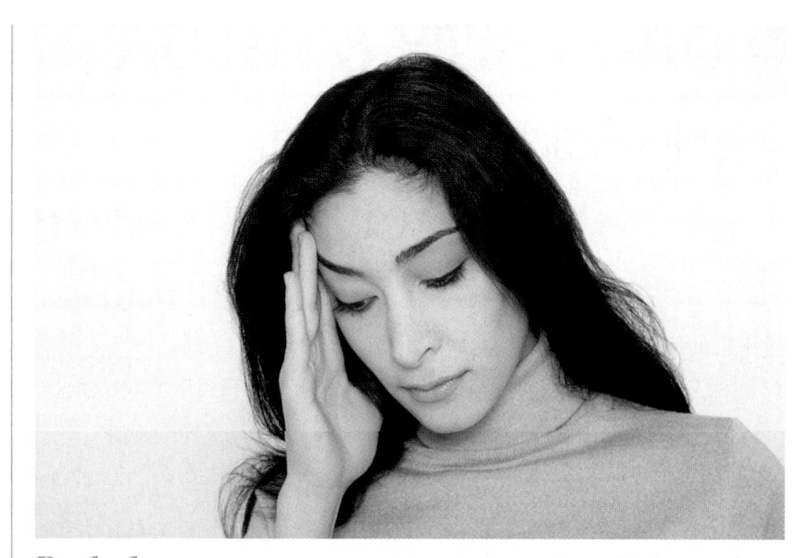

Body language can communicate a lot of information. Do you think this person is relaxed, or anxious?

Being a Good Listener

Listening is an integral part of successful communication because it enables you to understand your partner. Though it might seem like a simple skill, good listening is more than just hearing the other person's words. It involves picking up nonverbal cues like facial expression and hand gestures that can help you to understand how the person feels about what's being said. And that, in turn, requires concentration and attentiveness. Some strategies for effective listening include the following:

- **Be silent while another person is sharing his or her feelings or concerns.** Speak up only when you have a question or want to summarize what you have heard.
- **Overcome the urge to interrupt.** You may be tempted to finish the other person's sentences to show that you understand, but it's best to let others complete their thoughts before you speak.
- **Empathize with what the other person is saying.** If you put yourself in the other person's shoes, you will gain a better perspective of his or her viewpoint.
- **Avoid jumping to conclusions or making quick judgments.** Let the other person complete his or her thought before judging. If you have a question about what another person means, ask for a clarification.
- **Try to set aside any anger or resentment you may be feeling.** These emotions can interfere with your ability to truly listen.
- **Make other people feel comfortable speaking to you.** This can be done by maintaining eye contact, keeping a relaxed posture, and nodding and smiling so that others know you are listening. Avoid smirking, frowning, or crossing your arms.
- **Give the speaker your undivided attention.** Get rid of any distractions. Close the door and turn off your cell phone.

Resolving Conflicts

Sporadic interactions with others may be consistently pleasant, but all enduring relationships involve

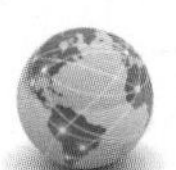

DIVERSITY & HEALTH

He Said, She Said: Gender and Communication

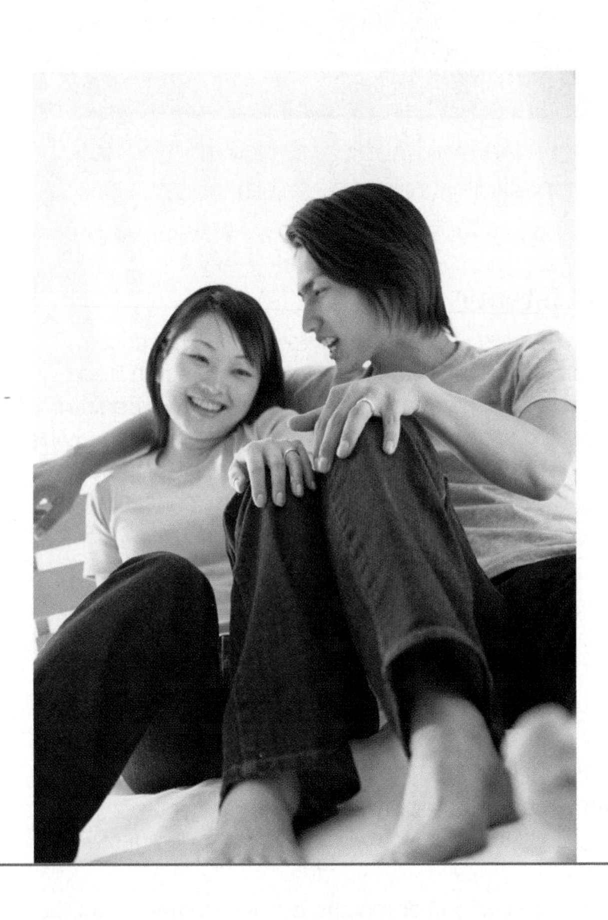

Although both men and women share a common need to communicate information, thoughts, and feelings, research suggests that there are differences in how they go about it. One of the most fundamental differences appears to be the motivation, or driving force, behind a man's or woman's communication.[1] Men often communicate in order to achieve social status and to avoid failure, whereas women are more likely to communicate to build personal connections and avoid social isolation. So a man wants to *report* and a woman wants *rapport*. Though individuals may vary, in general:

- Women seek to connect to others in conversation, whereas men want to be independent information givers.
- Women want to build consensus before making a decision, whereas men want to make decisions quickly on their own.
- Women avoid competitive conversation and attempt to minimize differences, whereas men are more comfortable giving orders and pointing out areas of superiority.[1]

There are also gender differences in overall communication style. In general, these include the following:

- Men tend to speak significantly fewer words each day than women, probably because men like to get to the main point and women like to notice and share details.
- Women are more likely to process their problems out loud. They will use conversation to think through a problem and work toward a solution. In contrast, men tend to think through a problem silently, and then verbalize their solution.
- Men are more likely to speak bluntly and state requests directly. Women are more likely to be tactful, use indirect speech, listen, and to offer feedback or make requests. Similarly, women are more likely to give feedback with sensitivity to another person's feelings. Men give feedback more directly, making the assumption that the other person won't take it personally.
- Women are more likely to use "circular" speech and change the topic in the middle of a conversation, returning to it later. Men are more likely to be linear communicators and thinkers; they want to finish one topic before going on to another.[2]

Neither communication style is better or worse, just different. And understanding the differences can improve male–female communication and relationships.

References: **1.** *You Just Don't Understand: Women and Men in Conversation,* by D. Tannen, 1991, New York: Ballantine Books. **2.** *Men Are from Mars, Women Are from Venus,* by J. Gray, 1992, New York: HarperCollins.

conflict, an experience prompted by a difference of opinion, principles, needs, or desires in which the partners involved perceive a threat to their self-interest. Although it can certainly be stressful, conflict is a normal aspect of relationships, arising naturally from differences between the partners' experiences and values. What's more, conflict negotiation is healthy, contributing to the personal growth of the individuals as well as to the growth of their relationship. That's because each successful resolution of a conflict proves to the partners that they can withstand challenges and grow. Over time, they gain confidence that, no matter what life throws at them, they'll be able to cope.

Methods of Approaching Conflict

Because an ability to resolve conflict is a critical interpersonal skill, it's unfortunate that so many people practice **conflict avoidance.** That is, they consciously or subconsciously avoid discussing their concerns or annoyances, believing it is better to keep the peace than start what could become an ongoing feud. Conflict avoidance is rarely a healthy strategy because, if you refuse to acknowledge the existence of a problem, then nothing can be done about it. In the end, everyone loses out on an opportunity for growth.[3]

Another potentially unsuccessful approach to conflict is **accommodation,** in which you acknowledge the conflict, but let the other person have his or her way. When the issue is not highly significant, accommodation can be a loving gesture. For instance, let's say that you're not a football fan, but when you visit your parents on break, you agree to

conflict An experience prompted by a difference of opinion, principles, needs, or desires in which the partners involved perceive a threat to their self-interest.

conflict avoidance The active avoidance of discussing concerns, annoyances, needs, or other potential sources of conflict with another person.

accommodation A practice of giving in to the other person's needs or wishes and denying one's own.

watch the Sunday afternoon game with your dad. As long as you know that your act is freely chosen, and can bring to mind instances when your dad, in turn, has accommodated you, there's give and take. But consistent accommodation to satisfy the other person's needs or desires can quickly become a one-sided effort: You're giving up, not only on yourself, but on the possibility of a better relationship. And it builds resentment.

Competition is another potentially unhealthy strategy, in which each of the people involved strive for an all-out "win" rather than to find a mutually agreeable solution.[3] It's a stance that says only one of us can benefit from the situation, so it virtually guarantees arguing, hurt feelings, even harm.

The most effective approaches to conflicts are compromise and collaboration. In **compromise,** everyone involved gives in a little so that everyone can also gain. For instance, in planning an evening out, you choose the restaurant and your partner chooses the movie. In **collaboration,** everyone works together to find an agreeable solution to the problem. Not only does collaboration enhance feelings of bonding, it also has the potential to produce innovative solutions that the individuals hadn't previously considered. Thus, collaboration is considered the best method of resolving conflict.[3]

Strategies for Resolving Conflict

Compromise and collaboration require that the people involved voice their concerns maturely and constructively, and listen attentively. These are acquired skills. To keep the conflict from escalating, the opposing parties must agree to fight fair, be respectful, and avoid personal attacks, name-calling, finger-pointing, and other put-downs.

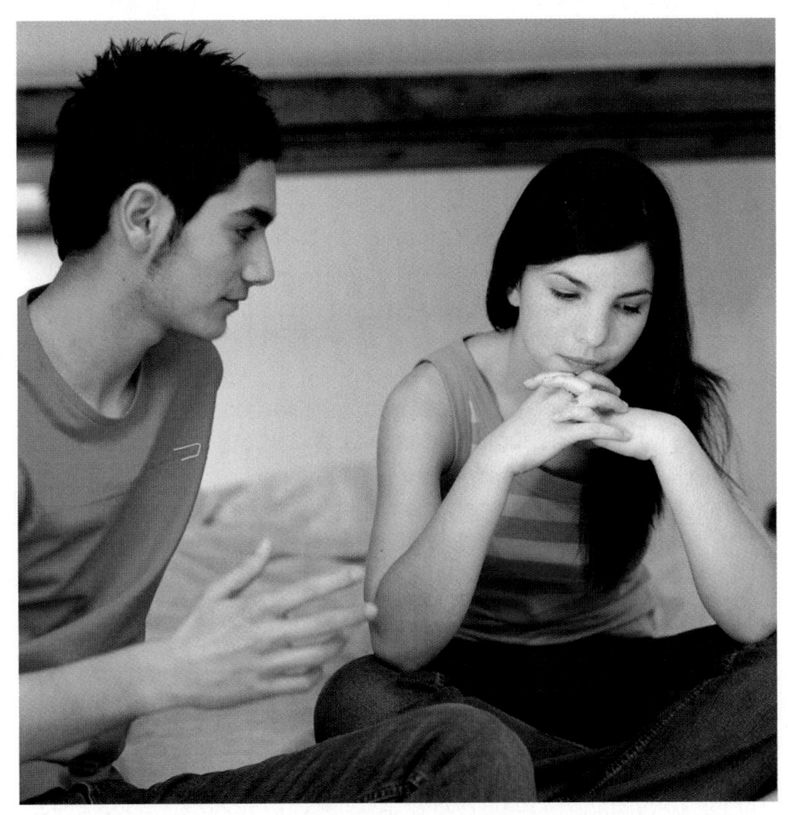

To keep conflict from **escalating,** fight fair, be respectful, and avoid personal attacks.

Strategies for effective **conflict resolution** include the following:

- Strive to resolve conflict, rather than to "win."
- Voice your frustrations as soon as possible, rather than allowing them to build up.
- Approach the conflict as you would any other problem that needs to be solved: Together, define the problem, express the facts (and your feelings) regarding the problem, and listen to possible solutions. Evaluate each possible solution, agree upon one, and make specific plans on how and when to implement it. After a solution is adopted, evaluate it. Is everyone satisfied with the outcome, or would another solution work better?
- Communicate your concerns and opinions clearly, honestly, and directly, instead of expecting the other person to read your mind.
- Listen to the other person's feedback and summarize what you think he or she has said.
- Do not ridicule the other person's feelings.
- Stay on the subject, arguing only one point at a time.
- Make sure you are arguing about what is truly bothering you.
- Do not fight while drunk or drinking.
- Postpone a discussion to an agreed-upon time if one person is tired or not ready to work on the problem.
- Admit when you are wrong.
- Find a way to collaborate when at all possible.
- Forgive, forget, and start over.[4]

competition An approach to conflict in which the parties involved strive to fulfill their own needs or desires at the expense of the needs and desires of the others involved.

compromise An approach to conflict in which each party agrees to accept less than what they had fully wanted so that a resolution can be reached.

collaboration An approach to conflict in which all parties work together to achieve a mutually acceptable resolution.

conflict resolution Process in which a solution to a conflict is reached in a manner that both people can accept and that minimizes future occurrences of the conflict.

Finding Forgiveness

That final bullet point above advises you to forgive. But what does that really mean? Buddhist physician Alex Lickerman writes that forgiveness is, at its core, an acknowledgment that the other person is a complex human being who isn't defined solely by his or her negative behavior toward you. In other words, forgiveness acknowledges that the person still has the capacity for good. It also prompts you to let go of your anger and resentment, and so keeps you from becoming, in turn, someone who harms. If you're finding it hard to forgive, recognize that forgiving someone is not the same as saying that what they did is okay! You're not condoning the person's action, but rather refusing to allow it to influence your life. In other words, forgiveness sets you free.[5]

Factors Influencing Relationships

Most of us are social creatures from the time we are born, craving closeness and connections to others. And whether we are at home, school, or work, we spend much of our time in the presence of other people. Several personal factors influence how we develop relationships with others, including our self-perception, our early relationships, gender roles, and aspects of our social environment.

Self-Perception

How we relate to others depends, in part, on how good we feel about ourselves. Self-esteem is a sense of positive self-regard that results in elevated levels of self-respect, self-worth, self-confidence, and self-satisfaction. People with low self-esteem are more likely to feel lonely and socially isolated. They tend to be preoccupied with the thought of rejection and often behave agreeably toward others because they want to be liked.[6] One psychology professor found that college students with low self-esteem often blame themselves for a boyfriend's or girlfriend's unhappiness, even when other factors are clearly responsible.[6] The study stated that overly insecure people may "read nonexistent meaning into their partners' ambiguous cues," and wind up sabotaging their relationships, "thus leading their relationships to the outcome they wish to avoid." The finding is true not only of young lovers but of couples in long-term relationships. Researchers have found that even after a decade of marriage, people with low self-esteem misread subtle cues and believe their partners love them far less than they actually do.[7]

Early Relationships

The first relationship we ever experience is the family relationship. Early experiences with our families are important because they help form the template for all subsequent relationships we experience in our lives. Some experts theorize that our relationships with others are patterned after the attachment we had with parents and other caregivers when we were children, a concept known as **attachment theory.**[8] These early interactions may shape our expectations of adult relationships and be responsible for the individual differences in relationship behaviors and needs.[9]

Exactly what constitutes a "family" changes over time, but it is generally defined as a domestic group of people with some degree of kinship, be it through marriage, blood, or adoption. Families today take many different forms, including households headed by single parents, blended families with stepparents and stepsiblings, extended-family households with relatives or family friends all living under the same roof, foster families, and gay and lesbian partnerships, to name just a few. There is no perfect or "right" kind of family, but in a healthful family environment, children are respected and nurtured, and learn how to have strong relationships of their own.

Gender Roles

Gender roles are the behaviors and tasks considered appropriate by society based upon whether we are a man or a woman. Just as many girls are trained at an early age to play with dolls and stuffed animals, boys are encouraged to appreciate cars and trains and to emulate seemingly all-powerful "super-heroes." As children grow up, girls tend to place greater value on interpersonal connections than boys do. Some experts think that this tendency can make adolescent girls more vulnerable to depression and low self-esteem.[10]

attachment theory The theory that the patterns of attachment in our earliest relationships with others form the template for attachment in later relationships.

gender roles Behaviors and tasks considered appropriate by society based on whether someone is a man or a woman

Gender roles often extend into adulthood. A generation ago, men were traditionally expected to work and support the family while women were encouraged to stay home to raise the children. Today, many women opt to juggle both family and career, while some men make the decision to be stay-at-home fathers. Yet attitudes and stereotypes about gender roles remain. For instance, couples in which the man earns less than the woman—only about 4% of all couples in 1970, but 22% of all couples in 2007—may experience more stress than couples for whom the reverse is true.[11] In addition, some research has shown that traditional gender roles become more pronounced in married couples after the birth of a child.[12]

Social Factors

Relationships don't arise solely from the interactions of the people involved. They are social bonds that are influenced by level of education, economics, and many other aspects of the social environment in which they occur. For example, since at least the year 2000, women have represented about 57% of all college students.[13] This means that, for college students seeking a committed romantic relationship, the number of potential male partners is smaller than the number of female partners. Still, most college graduates are finding spouses: A 2010 survey found that both incidence of and satisfaction with marriage is much higher among college-educated Americans than among those with lower levels of education, who also experience more nonmarital childbearing and more divorce.[14] And in part because a higher level of education correlates with a higher earning potential, Americans with the highest incomes are also the most likely to be married.[10]

Spirituality and religious behavior also influence the quality and duration of relationships. A substantial body of research shows that relationship quality tends to be higher among more-religious people and among couples who share religious beliefs and practices.[15]

Friendships

Do you have a best friend? If so, you benefit in more ways than one. Besides offering someone to hang out with and confide in, friendships are important for your health. Consider the following research:

- A study tracking thousands of residents in a Northern California county for nine years found that people who lacked social and community ties were two to three times more likely to die during that time than those with a solid social network.[16]
- Another study found that people who are isolated are at increased risk of dying from a number of causes, and that social support is especially related to survival after a heart attack.[17]
- A study of college freshmen found that those who had a small social circle and considered themselves lonely had a weaker immune response to a flu vaccine than nonlonely students.[18]
- Epidemiologic studies associate loneliness with stress, depression, and poor life satisfaction.[19]

Unfortunately, friendships are less numerous today than they have been in the past. A recent study found that between 1985 and 2004, the number of Americans who feel they have someone to discuss important matters with dropped by almost a third. The study also found that the percentage of people who spoke about important matters only with family members jumped from 57% to 80%.[20]

Building New Friendships

If you're like most students, your first few weeks on campus were filled with one introduction after another. Don't feel embarrassed if you know you've already met someone but need to ask their name again. They've probably forgotten your name, too! If you're shy, build new friendships by taking small steps that feel safe. For instance, while waiting in line at the cafeteria, comment to the person ahead of you in line about the food choices, or compliment something they're wearing. If that goes well, ask some simple questions—people love to talk about themselves! Here are a few more ideas:[21]

- Keep your door open when you're in your dorm room and don't mind being disturbed—it's a subtle invitation to your hallmates to stop by.
- Make an effort to get to know people outside of your dorm, too. Stay back after class and talk to your classmates. If it's lunchtime, invite them to join you in the cafeteria. The campus fitness center is another good place to meet new people. Or join a student organization that reflects your interests, and get involved!
- Introduce people you've met to other people and ask to meet your friends' friends. The more people you meet, the greater your chances of finding the few who will become close friends.
- Get to know the following "connectors": your resident advisor or building superintendent; your academic advisor, instructors, coaches; department secretaries and other administrative personnel; anyone else who could help you plug in to the network you're hoping to connect to.

Finally, try not to predict whether or not the people you meet today will become lasting friends. Just find people who share your interests and values, and with whom you have fun. The rest will come.[21]

Listen to this National Public Radio story on college friendships: www.npr.org/templates/story/story.php?storyId=112330125.

STUDENT STORY

Good Friends

"Hi, I'm Brittany and this is my friend Sandy. We're both freshmen and we've been friends for about a semester now, ever since we became neighbors in our dorm. We started eating dinner together occasionally and then began hanging out more and more often. We like the same music, we study together, go to the gym, and just hang out and have fun. Recently both of my parents were laid off, and Sandy has been really great in helping me deal with it; she listens to me talk and I feel like she's really there for me. In a few weeks, a group of us are going to Florida for spring break, and next year, we're even going to get an apartment together. I thought it was going to be difficult making friends in college but I'm so glad I've found such a good one already!"

1: What are the benefits of Brittany and Sandy's friendship? What personal and environmental factors helped make them friends?

2: Why do you think Brittany confided in Sandy about her parents being laid off? How did Sandy help?

3: What can Brittany and Sandy do to make sure that they have a good living situation when they move in together next year?

Do you have a story similar to Brittany and Sandy's? Share your story at www.pearsonhighered.com/lynchelmore.

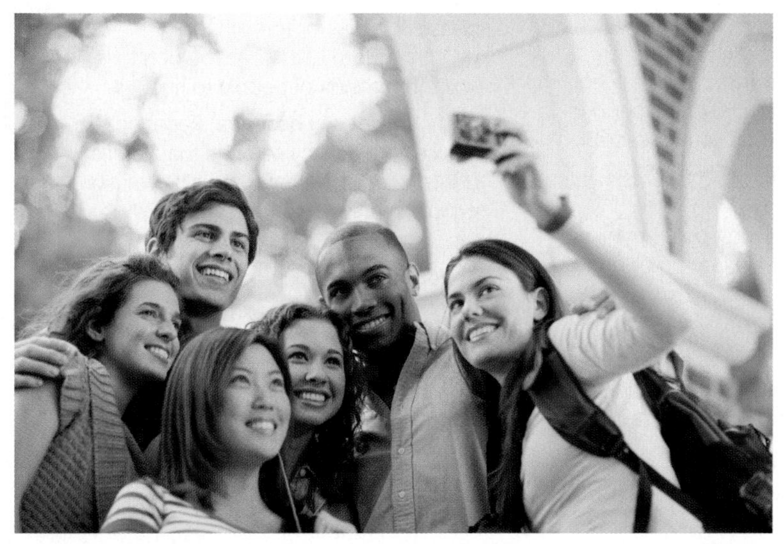

Friendships with others can boost emotional and physical health.

Maintaining Old Friendships

Friendships can be some of the longest, most-fulfilling relationships in your life, outlasting even marriages. But the demands of being a student can make it hard to keep them up. If you're struggling to maintain your tried-and-true friendships now that you're in college, follow these tips:

- **Understand that you and your friends are changing.** Don't be afraid to show how you're changing, and don't expect your friends to stay the same, either.
- **Don't overwhelm old friends with information about your college life.** It's exciting to exchange stories, but avoid dominating the conversation with too much talk about your new friends or activities.
- **Keep in touch.** Phone, email, voice over Internet services like Skype, instant messaging, and social networking applications like Facebook and Twitter are all great ways to update your friends about what you're doing and hear from them. However, be warned: The strongest friendships can't survive on your Facebook status updates alone. If you really want to maintain a friendship with someone, take the time to send him or her a personal message or pick up the phone.
- **Don't be afraid to reconnect.** If you've lost touch with an old friend, research indicates that you can still rekindle the friendship even after years without contact.[22]

the Facebook REVOLUTION

On February 4, 2004, Harvard computer science student Mark Zuckerberg launched "Thefacebook" and forever changed the world of social connections and friendships.[1]

Originally used only by Harvard students, the network quickly spread to colleges across the U.S. and Canada. In 2005, Facebook launched a high school version and by late 2006, anyone with a valid email address could join. Facebook is the leading social networking site with more than 400 million active members throughout the world.[2] Half of its members visit the site every day.[2]

Despite the popularity of Facebook, it is not without its critics. Privacy proponents worry that members' information is too easily accessed by those with both personal and business motives. Facebook has also received criticism for hosting controversial group pages, including ones that support anorexia and holocaust denial. Other critics point out that Facebook has been used to facilitate cyberbullying and stalking. University professors complain that students are wasting a tremendous amount of time on Facebook that could be spent studying and that students are distracted in class because they are using Facebook. Professors at some U.S. colleges have even banned laptops from classrooms because of Facebook.[3]

Critics also contend that Facebook and other social network sites are redefining the very meaning of "relationship" or "friend," and not for the better. They worry that people may be losing the ability to build intimate relationships through meaningful communication because they increasingly rely on online communication that is absent of body language and vocal intonation—important signifiers in communication.[4] In contrast, some researchers have found a strong association between Facebook use and the building and maintaining of social bonds, especially an increased ability to bridge to new networks of relationships.[5] These researchers also suggest that Facebook use improves the psychological well-being of users experiencing low self-esteem and low life satisfaction.

Who's right? The jury is still out, and more research into the consequences of social networking is clearly needed. In the meantime, sites like Facebook continue to attract new fans. If you're one of them, learn to use them safely and effectively by following a few tips:

- **Limit your number of friends.** Do you really care about all of those thousands of Facebook "friends" you've been collecting since high school? Limit your friends list to those you really care about and don't let it become a way of keeping score of your popularity or a substitute for social interaction with your real friends.
- **Don't accept friend requests from people you don't know.**
- **Don't tag friends in unflattering photos.**
- **Manage your profile settings.** You may not want your boss or professor seeing your photos from last weekend. So, if you have both personal and professional "friends," make sure you know how to edit your profile information.
- **Think before you post.** Don't post anything you wouldn't say out loud in person or don't want the entire Internet to read.
- **Use personal messaging instead of wall posts.** Be careful about posting something on your or a friend's wall that might get one or both of you in trouble. Instead, use Facebook's personal message feature to say anything you don't want thousands of people to read about.
- **Don't list personal info.** Never post your address, phone number, class schedule, or any other personal information that you don't want thousands of people to know.
- **Activate privacy settings.** Facebook has several privacy settings that you can use to control the amount of information other people see.[6]
- **Limit the amount of time you spend on Facebook.** Because information (even if it is trivial information) is updated constantly on Facebook, it can become addicting and lead to social isolation. Why not ignore your virtual friends for a while and spend some face-to-face time with your real live friends?[7]

References: **1.** "Hundreds Register for New Facebook Website," by Alan Tabak, February 9, 2004, *Harvard Crimson*, retrieved from http://www.thecrimson.com/article.aspx?ref=357292.

2. *Statistics*, Facebook Press Room, retrieved November 23, 2011, from http://www.facebook.com/press/info.php?statistics.

3. "Facing the Facebook," by M. Bugeja, January 3, 2006, *The Chronicle of Higher Education*, retrieved from http://chronicle.com/jobs/news/2006/01/2006012301c/careers.html.

4. "Archbishop Vincent Nichols Voices Fears over Social Networking Sites," August 2, 2009, *The Guardian*, retrieved from http://www.guardian.co.uk/media/2009/aug/02/vincent-nichols-social-networking-bebo.

5. "The Benefits of Facebook 'Friends': Social Capital and College Students' Use of Online Social Network Sites," by N. Bl Ellison, C. Steinfield, & C. Lampe, 2007, *Journal of Computer-Mediated Communication, 12*(4), article 1, retrieved from http://jcmc.indiana.edu/vol12/issue4/ellison.html.

6. "10 Privacy Settings Every Facebook User Should Know," by N. O'Neill, February 2, 2009, *All Facebook*, retrieved from http://www.allfacebook.com/2009/02/facebook-privacy.

7. "Are Social Networks Messing with Your Head?" by D. DiSalvo, Jan/Feb 2010, *Scientific American Mind*, pp. 48–55.

The Role of Social Networking

College students are using social networking websites such as Facebook, MySpace, and Twitter like never before. Of people aged 18 to 34, 74% have either Facebook or MySpace accounts, and people who are attending or have attended college are more likely than average to use these sites.[23] Social networking sites allow you to keep loose tabs on a wide number of friends through a constant stream of status updates. These online friendships can range from close ties with good friends to weak affiliations with people you've never met. One of the benefits of this wide range, according to one researcher, is that social networking expands your resources beyond just close friends who are similar to you.[24] Friendships with some of your online friends may be weak, but they allow you to access new ideas, information, or support from people who come from different backgrounds, which enables you to learn about new things that you may not otherwise be exposed to. See the special feature for more on how Facebook is changing the way we relate to each other.

These videos explore the effects of social networking: www.pbs.org/wgbh/pages/frontline/digitalnation/relationships/socializing.

> *"Of people aged 18 to 34, 74% have either Facebook or MySpace accounts, and people who are attending or have attended college are more likely than average to use these sites."*

Intimate Relationships

Intimacy is the emotionally open and caring way of relating to another person. An intimate relationship is usually one that is deep and has evolved over time, in which two people feel safe and comfortable sharing their innermost thoughts and secrets.

Sternberg's Triangular Theory of Love

Psychologist Robert Sternberg theorized that there are three primary components of healthy, loving relationships:

- **Intimacy.** The emotional component. Intimacy is the feeling of closeness and connectedness experienced in loving relationships.
- **Passion.** The motivational component. Passion is the intensity that fuels romance, physical attraction, and sex.

intimacy A sense of closeness with another person formed by being emotionally open and caring.

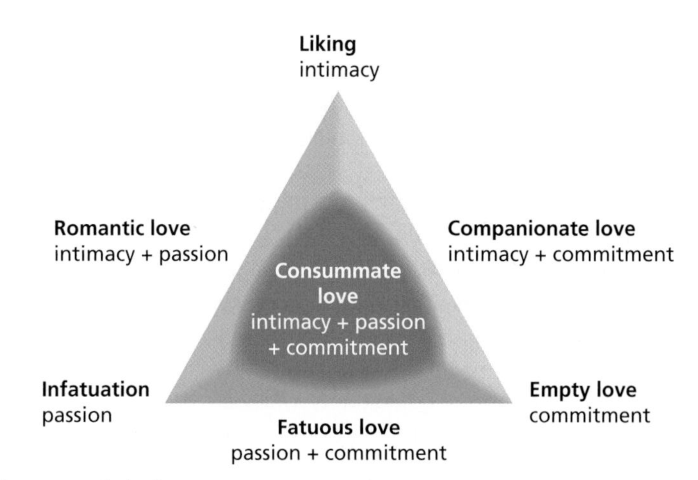

Figure 14.1 Sternberg's triangular theory of love.

Source: "A Triangular Theory of Love," by R. J. Sternberg, 1986, *Psychological Review, 93*, pp. 119–135. © 1986.

- **Commitment.** The cognitive component. Commitment is the short-term decision to love another person and the long-term decision to stay committed to maintaining that love.[25]

Sternberg used the shape of a triangle to illustrate his theory, which he called the triangular theory of love **(Figure 14.1).** Sternberg postulates that the type and intensity of love a couple experiences depends upon the strength of each of the three components in their relationship. The factors can be combined to characterize seven different types of love:

- **Liking.** Liking is intimacy alone. A closeness to another person, without passionate feelings or a long-term commitment.
- **Infatuation.** Infatuation is passion alone. Also known as "love at first sight."
- **Empty love.** Empty love is commitment alone. The passion is not there and neither is the intimacy. This can be found in some stagnant relationships or just before a couple breaks up.
- **Romantic love.** Romantic love is passion and intimacy without commitment. Physical attraction with an emotional bond.
- **Companionate love.** Companionate love is commitment and intimacy without passion. It is essentially a committed friendship in which the passion has died down, as sometimes occurs in people who have been married a long time.
- **Fatuous love.** Fatuous love is commitment and passion without intimacy—such as a whirlwind romance that does not last very long.
- **Consummate love.** Consummate love is the whole package: intimacy, passion, and commitment. This is the kind of love many of us strive for.[25]

Sternberg also identified an eighth category—nonlove—which is the absence of intimacy, passion, and commitment. This type of casual interaction makes up the majority of our relationships with other people.

What Causes Attraction?

You have probably heard the saying "opposites attract," but that's a myth. Studying the factors that bring two people together for a romantic relationship reveals that we tend to pick partners who are a lot like us—who are of similar economic class, educational level, religion, and racial or ethnic group and who share the same interests or values. Emerging research indicates that we even seek out partners who have similar body shapes to our own.[26] This tendency to be attracted to people who share some of our characteristics is known as **assortative mating.** Some studies have also found that we look for people who have a similar level of physical attractiveness to us, with more attractive people being more particular about the physical attractiveness of their potential partners.[27]

assortative mating The tendency to be attracted to people who are similar to us.

dating Spending time with another person one on one to determine whether there is an attraction or a desire to see more of each other.

hooking up Casual, noncommittal, physical encounters that typically range from kissing to oral sex but may involve intercourse.

Beauty, of course, is more than skin deep. Who we are and how we behave also influence whether others are attracted to us. One study found that men and women who were honest or helpful were perceived as better looking. Those who were rude or unfair or displayed other negative traits were generally considered less attractive.[28]

Although similarities in physique may bring us together, it is similarity in personality that appears to be most indicative of whether the relationship will be a happy one.[29] Why? "Once individuals are in a committed relationship, it is difficult to ignore personality differences," the study concluded. And personality differences, the researchers noted, "may result in more friction and conflict in daily life."[29] In the couples they studied, there were very few signs that opposites attract—or endure as a couple.

How To Be a Healthy Couple

STUDENT STORY

"Hi, we're Jonathan and Yeani, and we've been a couple for six months. There are a lot of obstacles that we face in our relationship, especially when it comes to juggling our schoolwork in addition to all the other aspects of our lives. At times, things seem hard. We each get stressed out by school and we can get on each other's nerves, but it's nice to have someone to lean on, and to know that you don't have to go through all your problems alone. For us, communication and trust have really helped make our relationship successful. Our best advice to new couples trying to make things work in college is to be open with one another, and don't be afraid to express your concerns, doubts, fears, or any other emotions with your partner."

1: Do you think juggling a relationship with school is a common source of stress for college couples? What can you do to help balance school and relationship time?

2: Why do you think Jonathan and Yeani chose to be in a relationship rather than just hooking up?

3: Do you agree with their advice for new couples in college? What else do you think college couples should do to keep their relationship healthy?

Do you have a story similar to Jonathan and Yeani's? Share your story at www.pearsonhighered.com/lynchelmore.

Dating

Dating—that is, spending time with another person one on one to determine whether there is an attraction or a desire to see more of each other—has evolved over the years.

Formal Dating

Until a few decades ago, most young Americans followed an expected sequence of steps in a culturally accepted dating ritual:

1. You were introduced to or met someone new. Frequently, a family member or close friend arranged the introduction.
2. One of you—usually the male—asked the other to go out for coffee, a meal, a walk, or a movie.
3. Presuming the first formal date went well, you'd go out again. Soon, you'd introduce each other to a wider circle of friends and family members.
4. Eventually, you might make some sort of declaration that you were "going steady," such as exchanging a class ring.
5. Steady dating would be considered a "courtship" intended to lead to marriage.

This ritual is rarely practiced today. In a study by Rutgers University's National Marriage Project, people reported meeting through groups of friends and spending time together more casually. A formal date is "the old way," said one man. "I'll meet them and we'll just hang out," added another.[30]

Hooking Up

One relationship behavior among college students that has been the subject of considerable controversy is **hooking up**—casual, noncommittal, physical encounters that typically range from kissing to sexual intercourse. Although media accounts of hook-ups involving sexual intercourse between strangers are common, a recent study of over 14,000 college students found that only about one-third of hook-ups involve sexual intercourse, and that hook-ups between total strangers are uncommon.[31] The same study found that hook-ups have not replaced committed relationships: By their senior year, 69% of heterosexual college students had been in a relationship for at least six months.[31]

Some of the negative effects from hook-ups involving sexual intercourse include an increased likelihood of STIs and unplanned pregnancy.[32, 33] This is more likely when hooking up is fueled by alcohol or other drugs, impairing the participants' judgment during the encounter. Some studies also suggest that hook-ups involving sex can have a negative impact on psychological well-being.[31, 32]

Still, for at least part of their college years, many men and women find hook-ups easier to deal with than committed relationships, which they view as too time-consuming and stressful. Some students report that committed relationships have threatened their academic success, interfered with friendships, or even involved jealousy or abuse.[30]

What's clear is that, since the demise of the old courtship rituals, no common standards for relationship behavior on campus have emerged. According to National Marriage Project research, this

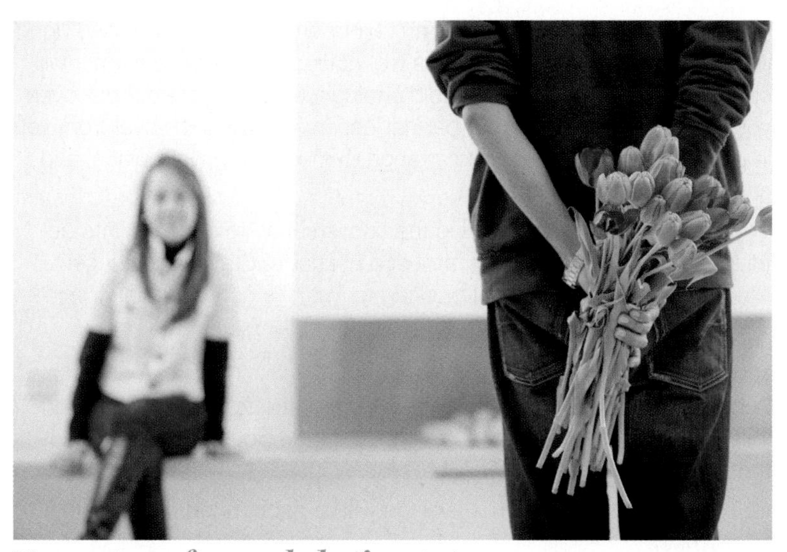

These days, **formal dating** is less common among young people than hanging out or hooking up.

absence of rules and rituals has left some singles "mystified, frustrated, and confused."[30] Some experts are concerned that today's singles are not learning the skills to build intimacy, and to test out whether someone would be a good marriage partner. Others counter that, freed from rules imposed by the culture, students do eventually learn to build intimate relationships—on their own terms.

Online Dating

Although a greater percentage of people in relationships (32%) still report that they met their partner through a friend, the Internet has become the second most common way to get acquainted. A 2010 survey of more than 3,000 adults who had begun a romantic relationship within the two years prior to the survey found that 23% of heterosexual and 61% of gay and lesbian couples met online.[34]

Popular sites such as eHarmony, Match.com, and OKCupid report millions of users each month. These services assist members in finding suitable partners by providing a place where they can both advertise themselves online with a personal profile and view the profiles of others looking for partners. Members search profiles using criteria such as sex, age, location, and interests. Online dating easily and effectively increases the pool of potential partners, a real selling point for the busy, technologically savvy 21st-century dater. Also, because face-to-face meetings are not immediate, potential partners have the opportunity to build their relationships via phone calls, texting, email, or Skype without the sexual tension of an in-the-flesh encounter.

If you use an online dating service, remember that the people you meet are basically strangers. So in order to stay safe, follow these precautions:

- Never give out your full name, address, or other personal information until you have met the person and are sure he or she is trustworthy.
- Meet your date in a public place, like a restaurant or café. Avoid going to isolated places with a new date. Always tell a friend beforehand what you are doing and where you are going.
- Do not have a new date pick you up at your home. Wait to reveal where you live until you trust the person.
- If something doesn't feel right when you meet the person, don't be afraid to cut your date short.

Same-Sex Relationships

homosexual A person sexually attracted to someone of the same sex.

heterosexual A person sexually attracted to someone of the opposite sex.

homophobia Fear and hatred of homosexuality.

Around 8.8 million people in the United States identify as lesbian, gay, or bisexual (LGB).[35] In many ways committed **homosexual** couples are similar to committed **heterosexual,** or straight, couples; for example, studies conclude that long-term same-sex couples are just as satisfied in their relationships as are heterosexual married couples.[36, 37] In at least one study, same-sex couples reported more positive feelings toward their partners and less conflict than married straight couples.[37] Indeed, same-sex couples often have more equality in relationships because they do not subscribe to traditional gender roles. This is especially true of lesbian couples—whom scientists have found are "especially effective at working together harmoniously."[36]

Yet one striking difference for LGB couples is the disapproval and discrimination they often face from society or even from family members. Most states do not allow homosexual couples to marry, and many do not allow them to adopt children. Some religions frown upon homosexuality. This can make homosexual couples feel stigmatized, isolated, and powerless. **Homophobia,** the fear and hatred of homosexuality, can also discourage intimacy between same-sex friends if it makes them fear being labeled as gay or lesbian.[38]

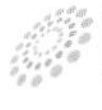

Online support for students struggling with their sexual identities can be found at www.hrc.org/resources/category/coming-out and www.thegyc.com.

Maintaining a Healthy Relationship

Successful relationships are built on trust, respect, and communication. They enable each individual to retain his or her own identity and foster personal growth rather than smothering it.

> *"Some people have an idealized view of healthy relationships, believing that they are free of conflict and require little effort to maintain. However, no deep, intimate relationship is without challenges."*

Some people have an idealized view of healthy relationships, believing that they are free of conflict and require little effort to maintain. However, no deep, intimate relationship is without challenges. Well-adjusted couples learn how to steer clear of avoidable problems and to be respectful, supportive, and sensitive to each others' feelings when they encounter challenges they must overcome. With compromise, collaboration, and a commitment to work together, couples can help each other through some of the most trying times of life—the loss of a job, the death of a parent or child, the diagnosis of a debilitating disease. **Practical Strategies for Health** provides tips for maintaining a strong and healthy relationship.

How do you know if your intimate relationship is a healthy one? Are there aspects of your relationship that concern you or that could be improved? Are you at a point in your relationship where the negatives are outweighing the positives? Taking a step back and assessing the strength of your relationship can be illuminating. The **Self-Assessment** on the next page is one place to start.

When an Intimate Relationship Ends

Many healthy relationships eventually end. Even though they may still care about each other, the partners might simply recognize that they have grown apart. Or perhaps infidelity, jealousy, competitiveness, addiction, or other problems have overwhelmed the couple's ability to cope. Raising children can also put a strain on a relationship.

How to Break Up

Breaking up is hard to do. Some people remain in a relationship long after it has died simply because they can't face "a scene." But there are ways to break up compassionately.

First, make it face to face. Don't text or email that it's over. And don't just change your Facebook status to single and hope your partner will catch on. Even worse, don't avoid ending it until your partner discovers you with someone new. Your partner deserves to hear it's over from you in person, and in advance. So arrange to meet in a private place, and say what you need to say.

When you do, avoid allowing the conversation to descend into details. Don't bring up the past, and don't criticize. Stay on message: "I'm breaking this off. It's not working for me. It's not your fault or mine. We're just not suited to each other."

How to Recover

Especially if you were not the initiator, recovering from a failed relationship can take a surprisingly long time and conscious effort. Strategies that can facilitate the recovery process include:

- **Talk about it.** Share your feelings with a good friend or family member.
- **Focus on what is good about you.** Resist the urge to blame yourself and exaggerate your faults while mending a broken heart.
- **Take care of yourself.** Exercise, eat well, and get plenty of sleep.
- **Let your emotions out.** Do not be afraid to cry.
- **Do things you normally enjoy.** Have some fun.
- **Keep yourself busy.** Get your mind off your pain for a while.
- **Give yourself time to recover.** Recognize that your hurt will not go away overnight.[39]

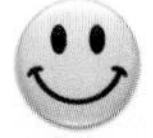 *Practical Strategies for Health*

Tips for Maintaining a Strong Relationship

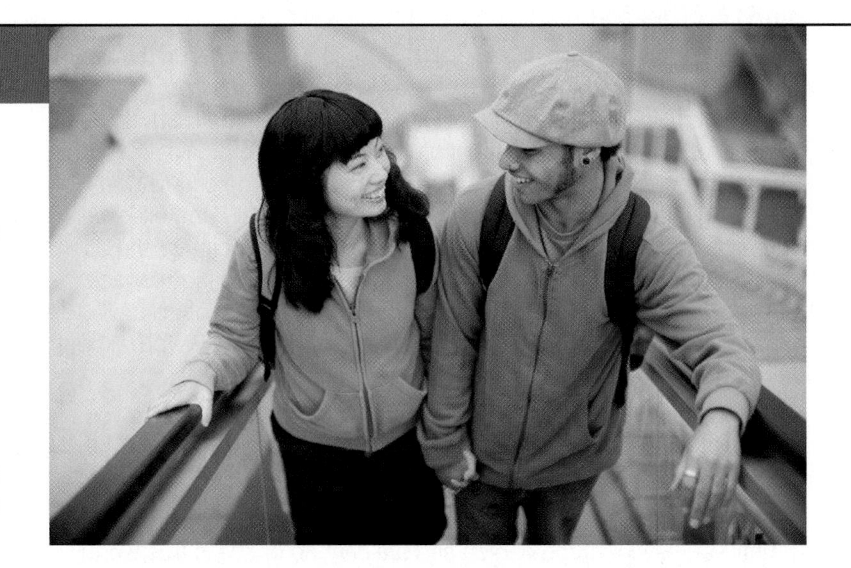

Although there is no simple recipe for success, the following strategies can help you maintain a strong, healthy relationship with your partner:

- **Be honest with the other person.** Strive to maintain a warm, comfortable relationship in which you can confide in each other about virtually anything.
- **Trust each other.**
- **Respect each other.** Be able to disagree without using put-downs or threats. Try to understand the other person's feelings, even if you don't share his or her ideas.
- **Communicate effectively.** Ask how your loved one thinks and feels, rather than expecting him or her to be a mind reader. Offer empathy when needed. Take the time to make sure you understand what the other person is attempting to say.
- **Give your loved one freedom and encouragement.** Recognize that each person has the right to his or her own opinions, feelings, friends, and dreams. Encourage each other's enjoyment and success in life.
- **Encourage common interests and shared activities.** Engage in activities and hobbies you both like. Be able to enjoy each other's company.
- **Be kind to one another.** Help each other out and show care through consistent respect rather than abuse followed by apologies.
- **Have mutual affection for one another.** Be appreciative and remind yourself of all the good things that you like about your loved one.
- **Share decision making.** Make decisions together, instead of telling each other what to do.[1]

Reference: 1. Adapted from "Characteristics of a Healthy and Enjoyable Friendship or Dating Relationship," *Employee Assistance*, retrieved November 8, 2008, from http://www.eap.partners.org/WorkLife/Relationships/Healthy_Relationships/Characteristics_of_a_Healthy_and_Enjoyable_Friendship_or_Dating_Relationship.asp.

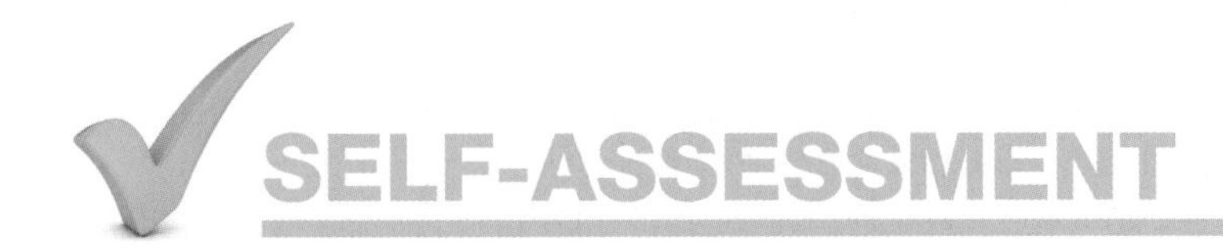

SELF-ASSESSMENT

Is My Relationship Healthy?

Circle "yes" or "no" in response to each of the following questions.

1.	I am very satisfied with how we talk to each other.	yes	no
2.	We are creative in how we handle our differences.	yes	no
3.	We feel very close to each other.	yes	no
4.	My partner is seldom too controlling.	yes	no
5.	When discussing problems, my partner understands my opinions and ideas.	yes	no
6.	I am completely satisfied with the amount of affection from my partner.	yes	no
7.	We have a good balance of leisure time spent together and separately.	yes	no
8.	My partner's friends or family rarely interfere with our relationship.	yes	no
9.	We agree on how to spend money.	yes	no
10.	I am satisfied with how we express spiritual values and beliefs.	yes	no

HOW TO INTERPRET YOUR SCORE

The more you replied "yes" to these statements, the more likely you are to be involved in a healthy relationship.

Source: Empowering Couples: Building on Your Strengths, by D. H. Olson & A. K. Olson, 2000, Minneapolis, MN: Life Innovations, Inc., retrieved from www.prepareenrich.com/pe_main_site_content/pdf/research/national_survey.pdf.

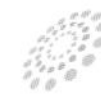

Take this self-assessment online at www.pearsonhighered.com/lynchelmore.

Dysfunctional Relationships

Whereas some relationships are uplifting, others are toxic, becoming more of a burden than a joy. Dysfunctional relationships can come in many forms, with one or both partners being manipulative, controlling, mean, disrespectful, or even verbally or physically abusive.

This kind of negative behavior is often learned early. Children observe how their parents relate to each other, and often think the hostile or unhealthy ways they interact are normal. Research has shown that adolescents who witnessed their parents' marital violence were more likely to be physically aggressive toward romantic partners themselves.[40] Similarly, adolescents exposed to marital discord tended to have conflict in their own marriages many years later.[41]

Characteristics of Dysfunctional Relationships

You might be in a dysfunctional relationship, yet not recognize it as such. That's because the signs that a relationship is dysfunctional are often subtle:[42]

- You focus on the other person at the expense of yourself.
- You feel pressured to change to meet your partner's ideals.
- Your partner expects you to justify what you do and whom you see, or you expect your partner to.
- You don't have any personal space.
- One of you makes all the decisions without listening to the other's input.
- You are afraid to disagree with your partner, and your ideas are criticized.
- You lie to each other.
- You feel stifled and trapped, unable to escape the pressures of the relationship.
- You or your partner is addicted to drugs or alcohol and it affects your relationship.

If you have noticed any of these signs in your relationship, it may be dysfunctional. Don't wait until more obvious problems surface. Consider a trip to your campus health center for some counseling, and be willing to go alone if your partner won't accompany you.

Problems That Threaten Relationships

In addition to the subtle signs just identified, the following attitudes and behaviors can damage or destroy relationships.

Inflexibility

Many people in relationships assume that there is a universal standard of behavior by which they are entitled to hold their partner accountable. The reality is that most relationship breakdowns arise when partners have conflicting values, priorities, and beliefs for which there is no generally accepted standard, yet insist that their partner adhere to their standards.[43] For example, consider the following sampling of issues about which couples commonly become inflexible:

- To what extent is it appropriate to socialize with members of the opposite sex?
- How much time should be devoted to academic pursuits, family responsibilities, friendships, job, and hobbies versus the relationship?
- How much should we keep each other informed about where we've been and whom we've been with?
- What kind of intimate behavior is acceptable (or expected)?
- How much and what kind of arguing is acceptable?
- How much of our time together should be planned versus "making it up as we go"?[43]

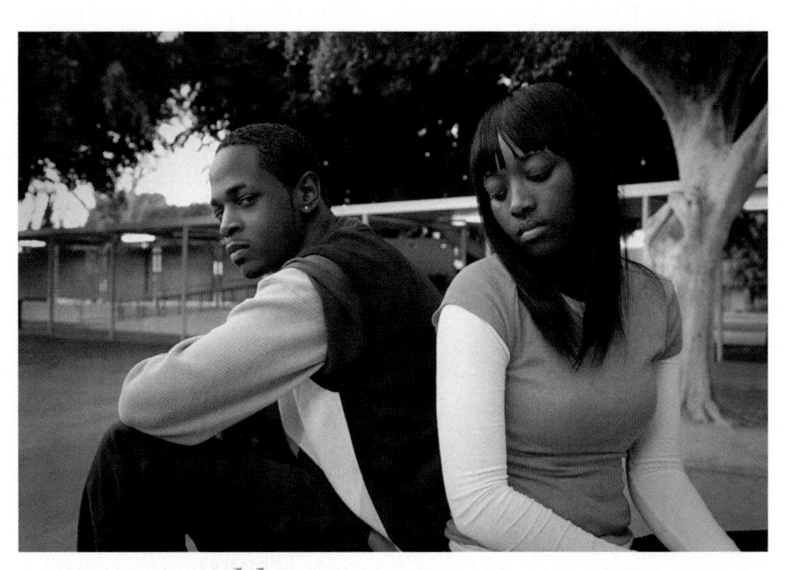

Addressing **problems** in relationships can help you fix them.

People who are happy together may have very different answers to these questions, but they have one thing in common: They avoid labeling their partner's answers as wrong, and instead accept that there are many legitimate ways to live.[42] "My way or the highway" is the slogan of dysfunctional relationships.

Power Plays

Does it drive you crazy when your partner leaves dirty dishes in the sink, drives with the windows down on a frigid day, or wears ear plugs when studying and therefore can't hear his or her cell phone when you're trying to get in touch? All of these minor issues can have a perfectly legitimate explanation . . . or they may be signs of a **power play**—that is, an attempt to control a person or situation by manipulating power. In hockey games, power plays occur when one team has a numerical advantage—more players on the ice than the other team. In relationships, power plays are typically much more subtle. For instance: "I'll show you that I'm the one in control by 'failing to hear' your phone calls—and when you complain, I'll point out how unreasonable you're being by explaining that I had my ear plugs in because I was studying." Sometimes, even the individual performing the power play is unaware of the dysfunctional game he or she is playing.

Infidelity

According to the 2010 General Social Survey, about 10% of married Americans are unfaithful to their spouses in any given year. The rate of **infidelity** over a lifetime is, of course, higher: 28% of males and 15% of females admit to having had at least one extramarital affair.[44] Infidelity is often a symptom of a relationship that has become dysfunctional for other reasons. In such cases, it can act as "the last straw," shattering the relationship beyond repair. One study implicated infidelity in more than 21% of divorces, making it the most cited reason for seeking divorce.[45]

But sexual infidelity is not the only type that threatens relationships; recently, sociologists have begun studying *financial infidelity*—that is, deception with a partner about money. This can involve hiding a bill or purchase from a partner; failing to divulge to a partner the existence or extent of credit-card debt; deceiving a partner about one's salary; or hiding cash or the existence of a savings account from a partner. In a 2011 survey, 31% of people who had combined finances with a significant other admitted such deceptions.[46] Television sitcoms often portray spouses hiding purchases or debts from each other, but statistics suggest it's no laughing matter: The 2011 survey found that, among those who had been affected by a partner's financial infidelity, 16% said it had resulted in divorce.[46]

power play An attempt to control a person or situation by manipulating power.

infidelity Unfaithfulness, especially participation of a married person in a sexual act with someone other than one's spouse.

jealousy The response to a threat to a relationship from an actual or imagined rival for a partner's attention.

cohabitation The state of living together in the same household; usually refers to unmarried couples.

Jealousy

Sociologists define **jealousy** as the response to a threat to a relationship from an actual or imagined rival for a partner's attention.[47] Although it is natural to feel jealous once in a while, jealousy becomes serious when it is a precursor to domestic violence or interferes with the relationship in other ways. Jealousy is associated with low self-esteem, irrational thinking, depression, divorce, and physical violence. It is not a marker of true love, but rather of insecurity, immaturity, and a need to be in control. An underlying cause of extreme jealously is a fear of abandonment. Ironically, the behavior of extremely jealous partners often makes these fears come true. Not only can it destroy a relationship, it can be destructive to everyone in it.

Experts suggest that couples deal with jealousy directly and attempt to talk about the feelings underlying it. Often, talking about what sparks the jealousy may be enough to reduce it. If you are suffering from jealousy yourself, work on building your self-esteem, since low self-esteem is one of the sources of jealousy. If your partner is jealous, be available and respond to his or her concerns, offer reassurance, and keep in mind that changes do not happen immediately. Sometimes counseling may be needed to help you and your partner move forward.[48]

Physical Abuse

There is one situation that demands that you immediately leave a relationship: physical abuse. If a partner is threatening you physically or being physically abusive to you—or to your children if you have any—remove yourself and your children from the relationship as soon as possible. If you need immediate help, dial 9-1-1, or call the National Domestic Violence Hotline at 1-800-799-SAFE. Chapter 20 discusses physical abuse and domestic violence in more detail.

Committed Relationships

Most adults value having a committed relationship with another person. Nationwide surveys reveal that about two-thirds of unmarried adults say a long-term committed relationship is integral to having a fulfilling life.[49]

Types of Committed Relationships

Committed relationships come in various forms, including cohabitation, marriage, and domestic partnerships.

Cohabitation

One of the greatest transformations in family life in the United States during the last century has been the significant increase in **cohabitation**—unmarried couples living together under the same roof. Whereas traditional courtship progressed from dating to engagement to marriage, many couples today opt to live together before getting engaged or married. Some continue in long-term, committed relationships without ever tying the knot. Cohabitation is now so common and accepted in our society that an estimated 50–60% of couples in the United States now live together before getting married.[50]

For some, cohabitation represents a chance to get to know each other better before taking marriage vows. Others choose to cohabitate to benefit from the companionship, intimacy, and shared living costs cohabitation allows.

There is a downside to cohabitation. Most cohabitating couples are denied the legal and financial benefits afforded to married couples. These include family leave, Social Security benefits after the death of a partner, and access to a lover's pension, health insurance coverage, and untaxed retirement savings.[51] In addition, cohabitating couples in the United States report the lowest levels of wealth among household types. Research indicates that nearly half the couples that live together remain unmarried five years later, and that most of them are no longer in a relationship with each other.[52] Those who do get married are

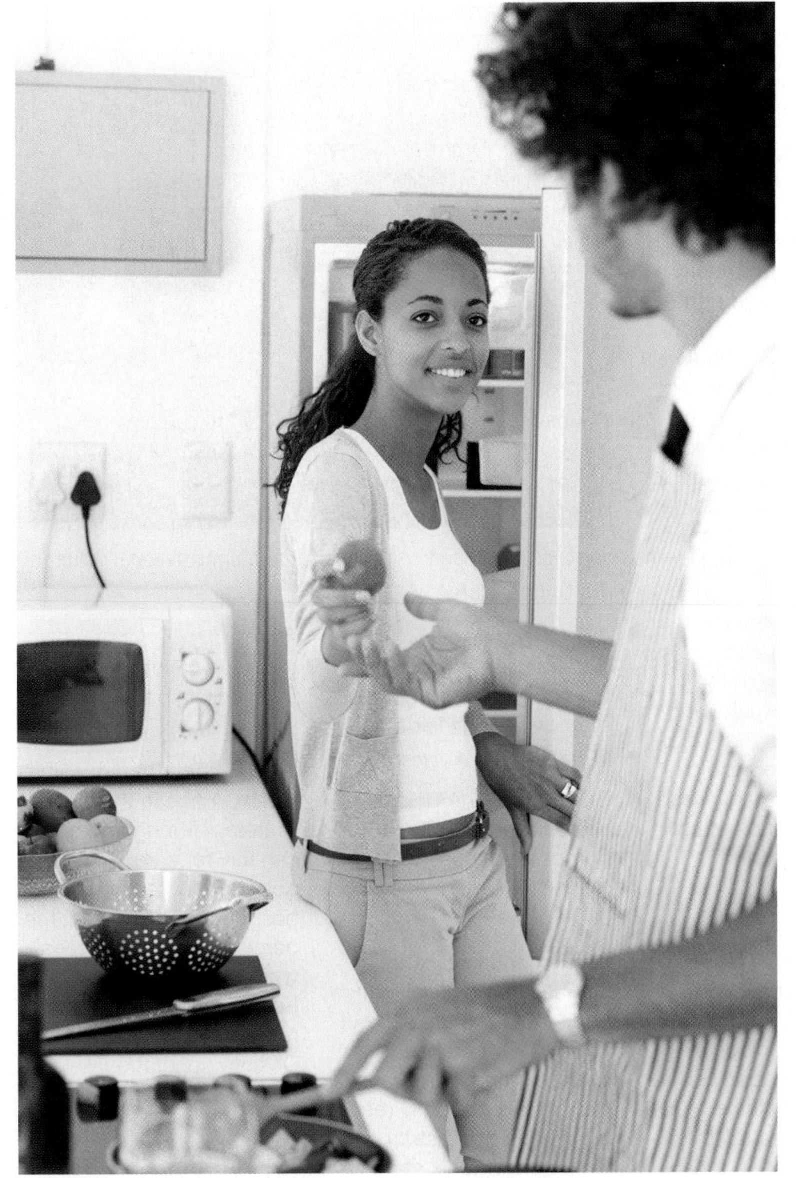

Cohabitation can have benefits, but it also has drawbacks.

actually more likely to get divorced than couples who did not cohabitate. Moreover, couples who cohabitate or who cohabitated before marriage report higher rates of depression and marital conflict, lower marital satisfaction, higher relational dependency, more infidelity, less life satisfaction, lower self-esteem, and lower levels of marital interaction compared with couples who did not live together before marriage. One theory for these differences is that marriage fosters certain behavior changes by the couple and those around them that cohabitation just doesn't encourage.[53]

More recent research suggests that these trends may be changing as cohabitation becomes more common and accepted in society. It also shows that cohabitating couples who are engaged before they move in together may be more successful than couples who live together but have no plans to marry.[54]

Marriage

Between 85% and 90% of Americans will marry during their lifetime.[55] An overwhelming majority of high school seniors say that having a happy marriage is "extremely important" to them.[56] Meanwhile, same-sex couples have been waging an intense legal and political battle around the country to have their unions recognized as legal marriages. Find out what's at stake for same-sex couples in the accompanying **Spotlight.**

Benefits of Marriage. What makes marriage so appealing? Aside from its romantic associations, marriage has practical benefits. It is a legally binding contract, giving a sense of legitimacy to the relationship in the eyes of society and the law.[57] It signals to others that each spouse has entered into a long-term commitment that carries with it expectations of fidelity, mutual support, and lifetime partnership.

Study after study has shown that marriages in general—and good marriages in particular—provide a wealth of physical, psychological, and financial benefits. The longer a person stays married, in fact, the more the benefits accrue.[57] The benefits include:

- **Better mental health.** Married people tend to be happier and more satisfied with their lives, on average, than unmarried people, according to an analysis of 22 studies.[58]
- **Better physical health and longer life expectancies.** Being married is linked to fewer sick days, less use of hospital facilities, and less likelihood of having chronic health conditions.[59] Married men can expect to live, on average, at least seven years longer than never-married men, while married women tend to live at least three years longer than their never-married counterparts.[60]
- **Better financial health.** Married couples tend to have higher household incomes than unmarried people.[56]

Are married people healthier because they are married? Or is it that healthier people are somehow more likely to get married? Although researchers suspect that both could be at play, there is evidence that marriage fosters healthful and helpful behaviors. For example, married couples generally drink less, exercise more, get more sleep, and visit the doctor more often than people who are not married.[61]

Issues That Married Couples Argue About. Most marriage experts agree that the top issues behind marital spats are money, sex, in-laws, housework, and career. But all of these issues can act as "smokescreens," obscuring for the couple the more fundamental issues that need attention, such as inflexibility and power plays (discussed earlier). For instance, couples often argue about how much money is acceptable to spend and how much they should save. These values in turn are typically influenced by each individual's experiences, both in their childhood homes and in interactions with mentors, colleagues, and peers. Because no single approach to the household budget is objectively right, the key is respect for the other partner's standards and collaboration to find a mutually acceptable solution.

On the other hand, experts say that the occasional blow-up keeps marriages—and marriage partners—healthy, whereas conflict avoidance can be toxic. For example, one study found that early death is more than twice as likely among spouses who suppress their anger than among spouses who express their anger and resolve the conflict.[62]

The American Psychological Association has created a list of nine psychological tasks for a good marriage. You can find it here: www.apa.org/helpcenter/marriage.aspx.

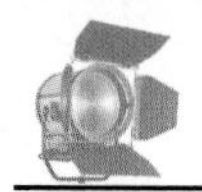

SPOTLIGHT

Same-Sex Marriage: The State of Our Current Debate

When Barbara Bush, daughter of former President George W. Bush, publicly endorsed same-sex marriage early in 2011, she joined a growing cohort of adult children of conservative politicians who have openly split with their parents on the issue. Bush's declaration of support for same-sex marriage was particularly stunning, since her father, as President, pushed for a constitutional amendment banning such unions. Journalists and activists are now pointing to a growing "generation gap" on the issue. And statistics suggest it exists: In 2010, a nationwide poll found that 53% of young Americans (those born in 1990 or later) support same-sex marriage, whereas only 29% of older Americans (those born before 1945) support it.[1] The same poll also found a significant political gap on the issue: 53% of registered Democrats favor legalizing same-sex marriage, whereas just 24% of Republicans do. Regional differences are also striking: nearly all of the states that recognize same-sex marriage are in the Northeast.

There's no question that the issue of same-sex marriage is polarizing. Perhaps that's because it exposes differences in our interpretation of certain doctrines we hold "sacred"—from constitutional law to the American ethic of fairness to religious and cultural teachings. For instance, some proponents of same-sex marriage argue that the guarantees of equal protection and due process in the United States Constitution require that same-sex couples be treated no differently from heterosexual couples. At the same time, opponents argue that marriage is an institution founded to promote and protect the need to procreate, and therefore can only occur between a male and a female. To answer this argument, those in favor of same-sex marriage point out that no states require couples applying for a marriage license to swear that they will attempt to have children, and that men and women who are infertile and women past child-bearing age are allowed to marry. They also point out that both adoption and advances in fertility technology provide many paths to parenthood for same-sex couples.[2]

What's at stake? Although the debate is certainly fueled by a clash of values surrounding the marriage rite itself, far more significant are the rights and protections that marriage guarantees—and denies to couples lacking a marriage license. In 2004, a report of the U.S. General Accounting Office identified a total of 1,138 federal statutory provisions classified to the United States Code in which marital status is a factor in determining or receiving benefits, rights, and privileges.[3] A couple's status can affect whether they are entitled to certain tax advantages, health-care benefits, community property rights, and rights to surviving children. Moreover, homosexual couples have been denied the right to become foster parents and adoptive parents, to petition for their partners to immigrate, and to become residents in the same nursing home. Until recently, same-sex partners could even be denied the right to visit each other in the hospital: A ruling of the Department of Health and Human Services requiring hospitals to recognize gay and lesbian partners' visitation rights just took effect in 2011.

Currently, federal law does not recognize same-sex marriages. The Defense of Marriage Act (DOMA), passed in 1993, prohibits federal recognition of same-sex marriages and allows individual states to refuse to recognize such marriages performed in other states.[4] Section 3 of DOMA requires that federal benefit programs define marriage as the union of one man and one woman. Recently, state courts have begun to address DOMA's constitutionality. For instance, in May 2012, a U.S. Court of Appeals in Boston ruled that section 3 of DOMA discriminates against married same-sex couples. Legal experts anticipate that the constitutionality of DOMA will be challenged in the U.S. Supreme Court in 2013. And state courts in five states have held that denying gay and lesbian couples the right to marry violates their state constitution.[4]

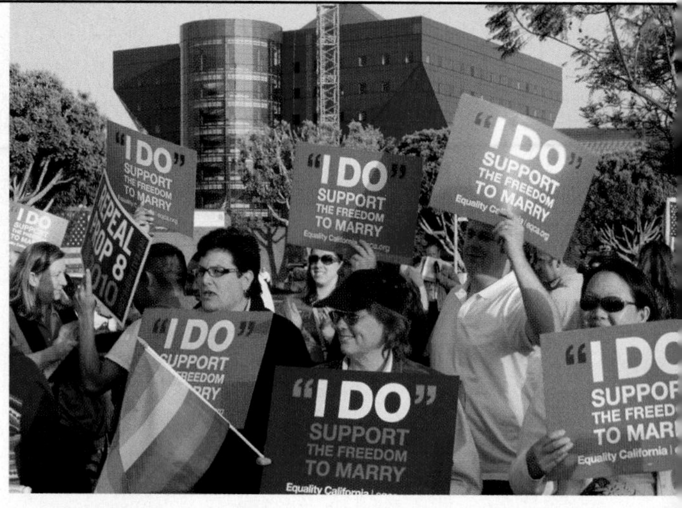

Same-sex marriage continues to be a controversial issue in the United States.

So where in the United States is it possible for homosexual partners to marry?

The answer to this question is continually changing, as state judicial rulings and state laws are subject to appeal and repeal. As of this writing, same-sex marriage is currently recognized in the District of Columbia and six states: Connecticut, Iowa, Massachusetts, New Hampshire, New York, and Vermont.[5] This list is provisional. For example, in February 2012, a California court of appeals overturned a state ban on gay marriage as unconstitutional; however, that ruling is expected to be appealed. In addition, New Jersey has an "all but marriage" ruling that grants homosexual partners in domestic partnerships and civil unions the same benefits as marriage partners. In addition, several more states have same-sex marriage initiatives on the ballots for voters.

What is the future of same-sex marriage in the United States? Although no one can say for sure, dozens of polls conducted over the past decade show that the percentage of Americans who favor legal marriage between homosexual partners is inching upward. Despite generational, political, and regional differences, America's overall support for same-sex marriage is growing.

References: **1.** "Fewer Than Half of Americans Oppose Gay Marriage, Poll Finds," CNN, October 6, 2010, retrieved from http://articles.cnn.com/2010-10-06/us/poll.gay.marriage_1_gay-marriage-americans-favor-new-poll?_s=PM:US. **2.** "Same-Sex Couples and the Law," FindLaw Family Law Center, 2011, *Thomson Reuters*, retrieved from http://family.findlaw.com/same-sex-couples/defense-of-marriage-act.html. **3.** *Defense of Marriage Act: Update to Prior Report,* U.S. General Accounting Office, January 23, 2004, GAO-04-353R, Washington, D.C. **4.** "Same-Sex Marriage: Legal Issues," by A. M. Smith, August 18, 2010, *Congressional Research Service,* 7-5700; RL31994, retrieved from http://assets.opencrs.com/rpts/RL31994_20100818.pdf. **5.** "New York Allows Same-Sex Marriage, Becoming Largest State to Pass Law," by N. Confessore and M. Barbara, June 24, 2011, *The New York Times*, retrieved from http://www.nytimes.com/2011/06/25/nyregion/gay-marriage-approved-by-new-york-senate.html?pagewanted=all.

One of the greatest hurdles single mothers face is economic hardship. An estimated 30% of women who have a child born out of wedlock live in poverty, compared with just 8% of women who were married at the time of their child's birth.[92] Single mothers, on average, also have lower levels of education than other women, which can hurt their job prospects and lower their earnings potential.

Just how children fare growing up in a single-parent household varies, and has been the source of some controversy. Experts recognize that a family's structure is not as important as how it functions. Yet children from single-parent families have a risk of negative life outcomes that is two to three times higher than children from married, two-parent families.[68] Children born out of wedlock are more likely to experience a wide range of behavioral and emotional problems, reaching adulthood with less education and earning less income. They are more likely to be "idle"—out of school and out of work—in their late teens and early 20s. They experience more symptoms of depression, and have more troubled marriages and higher rates of divorce. They are also more likely to have a child out of wedlock themselves.[93]

But do these gloomy predictions hold for children born to women who deliberately choose single motherhood? A growing number of sociologists are saying no. Women who are financially independent and well-educated—whether lesbian or heterosexual—are increasingly choosing to have children without men. Sociologist Suzanne Bianchi of the University of Maryland explains that these women make sacrifices in their personal lives and careers to make single parenting work, putting their children first. Wellesley College sociologist Rosanna Hertz agrees: "The child really becomes the focal point of their lives."[94] A 2004 study involving 1,500 U.S. multiethnic 12- and 13-year-olds supports these observations: Cornell professor Henry Riciutti found that, when income and level of education are factored in, there's "little or no difference" between the intellectual development, academic achievement, and behavior of children in single-parent and two-parent families. The study also suggests that any risks of single parenting can be greatly reduced with increased access to economic, social, educational, and parenting support.[95]

Characteristics of Happy Families

Researchers have devoted a great deal of time to looking at strong families, measuring their affection and communication, trying to decipher their secrets for success. What they found is that a happy family is not one without trouble. Most have experienced a variety of setbacks. But strong families learn how to adapt and endure, taking a constructive approach to dealing with crises.[96]

Members of strong families share and value these traits:

- **Commitment.** They are dedicated to the family and promoting each other's happiness. They are honest, faithful, and dependable.
- **Appreciation and affection.** They care for each other and are not afraid to express it. They give compliments and show their affection freely.
- **Positive communication.** They are good talkers and good listeners. They do argue, but avoid blaming each other and are able to compromise and collaborate.
- **Time together.** They spend quality time together as often as they can, and arrange their schedules to ensure that this happens.
- **Spiritual well-being.** They have hope, faith, and compassion, as well as shared ethical values.
- **The ability to manage stress and crises.** They see crises as both challenges and opportunities for growth. They pull together during tough times and give support to each other.[97]

Change Yourself, Change Your World

Healthy relationships have many challenges, from misunderstandings and hurt feelings to episodes of significant emotional pain. Still, failing to build healthy relationships simply is not an option! In the words of civil rights leader Martin Luther King, Jr., "We must learn to live together as brothers, or perish together as fools."[98] The rewards of healthy relationships are abundant.

Personal Choices

If you want to build and maintain healthy relationships, a smart first step is to practice the skills—including effective communication and conflict-resolution skills—described earlier. In addition, it's important to adopt the following behaviors:

- **Stay true to who you are.** Everyone wants to experiment with different beliefs, values, and behaviors. That's a natural aspect of human development that continues, in healthy people, right through old age. But when you adopt attitudes and behavior patterns that don't feel authentic, just because you think doing so will help you fit in or keep a relationship going, you're doomed to dishonest, superficial relationships. Give yourself and the people you interact with a real chance to bond: Be yourself, right from the start.
- **Respect others for who they are.** Have you ever found yourself thinking about breaking off a relationship because you're just "too different"? If so, it might be time to think again. If you can learn to value your differences—in beliefs, standards, experiences, skills, behaviors, style—you might find that you're able to forge a highly energetic relationship in which you and your partner become more productive and creative than you'd be if you stuck with people in your own crowd. Sociologist Mark Granovetter refers to this phenomenon as "the strength of weak ties," and it's a key reason to value diversity in your relationships.[99]

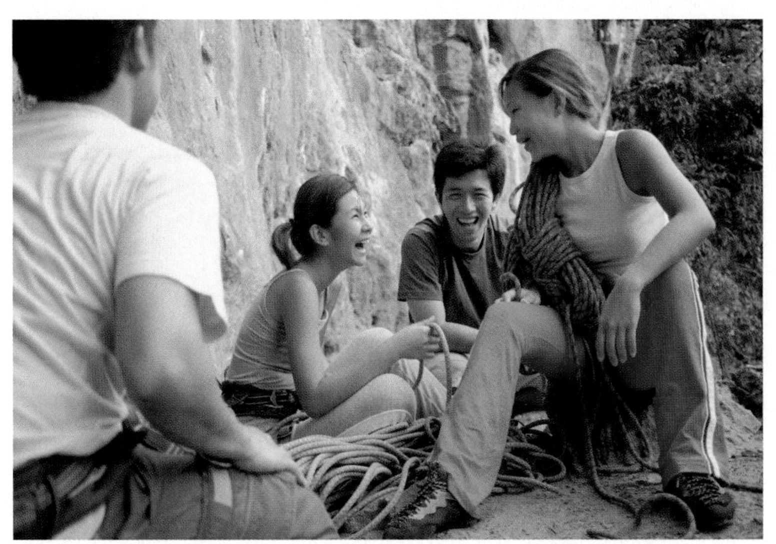

Taking the time to appreciate your friends and partners for who they are can **strengthen your relationships.**

- **Affirm.** What about the more subtle qualities your friend or partner brings to your relationship? Take a moment alone to jot down the unique attributes you enjoy about the other person. If you get stuck at "beauty" or "sense of humor," dig a little deeper. Perhaps your friend's wisdom helped you figure out a solution to a challenge, or maybe his or her compassion during a time of self-doubt gave you a deep sense of being understood. After you've made your list, let the person know how much you appreciate these qualities.
- **Learn to give and receive.** This doesn't mean the two of you have to be rich! The most meaningful gifts in lasting relationships are gifts of time, attention, listening, honest feedback, and emotional support. Give of these gifts unselfishly, and accept them from your partner with gratitude.
- **Lighten up.** Finally, make room in your relationship for fun! Take a break from studying and take a bike ride, or keep a Saturday free for a trip to the beach. Keep humor a part of your daily interactions, too.

Campus Advocacy

College students come together from regions all over the world not only to acquire knowledge, but to learn to respect and negotiate differences. These include differences in culture, religion, language, ability, sexual orientation, and much more. What can you do to build bridges to others on your campus? Here are some simple ideas.

Keep the Lines of Communication Open

One international student described her two years of study at an American university as "a challenging experience."[100] She noted that students on her campus tended to associate only with those like themselves, and often avoided even speaking to students from other countries. She offered this advice for keeping the lines of communication open:[100]

- Initiate a conversation. If the person has difficulty speaking English, give them some time to think through a translation, or to take out their electronic dictionaries and find the right words.
- Words are not the most important part of human communication. Observe the person's facial expression and gestures; take a look!
- During a conversation, empathize. Try to see the world through the other person's perspective.

Join a Campus Organization That Promotes Tolerance

Many different organizations provide training and tools to combat *bias*—unfair preferences—and promote an atmosphere of tolerance on campus. For example:

- The National Educational Association of Disabled Students (NEADS) has a network of 40 campus-based groups to support students with disabilities. Membership is open to all students, regardless of level of ability. For information about forming a group or becoming a member, go to **www.neads.ca/en/norc/campusnet/leadership_starting.php.**
- Campus Pride is a national nonprofit group working to create a safer college environment for LGBT (lesbian, gay, bisexual, or transgender) students across the United States. Find out more at **www.campuspride.org.**
- The Association for Non-Traditional Students in Higher Education (ANTSHE) is a partnership of academic professionals and students that supports adult learners. Find it on Facebook, or at **www.antshe.org.**

These are just a few examples, so find out what's happening on your campus and get involved. An added benefit is that you are likely to form strong bonds with others in the organization as you work together to achieve your goals.

Explore New Options

You don't have to join an organization to build diverse relationships on campus. Try attending a few services of a campus religious organization that you're not familiar with. Drop in on a meeting of a political group on the other side of the spectrum. Or volunteer to help plan a social or cultural event sponsored by an international students' organization. You might argue that you're only one person, but in reality, you're part of a vast network of relationships. By reaching out in simple ways like these, you challenge the belief that differences can keep us from building strong, meaningful relationships.

Watch videos of real students discussing communication and relationships at www.pearsonhighered.com/lynchelmore.

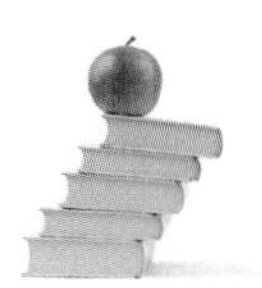

Choosing to Change Worksheet

To complete this worksheet online, visit **www.pearsonhighered.com/lynchelmore**.

Successful healthy relationships are built on trust, respect, and communication. They enable each individual to retain his or her own identity and foster personal growth rather than smothering it. With this in mind, think about one relationship that is important to you and needs improvement. Write down this relationship in Step 1.

Directions: Fill in your stage of change in Step 1 and complete the remaining steps with your stage of change in mind.

Step 1: Your Stage of Behavior Change. My relationship with ______________________ is important to me and needs improvement. Please check one of the following statements that best describes your readiness to improve this relationship.

________ I do not intend to participate in building a healthy relationship in the next 6 months. (Precontemplation)

________ I might participate in building a healthy relationship in the next 6 months. (Contemplation)

________ I am prepared to participate in building a healthy relationship in the next month. (Preparation)

________ I have been building a healthy relationship for less than 6 months but need to do more. (Action)

________ I have built a healthy relationship for more than 6 months, and want to maintain it. (Maintenance)

Step 2: Communication Skills. It is important to know how to communicate effectively with others. Think about the communication skills listed on pages 384–385. List the skills that you feel you have mastered in your own life. Then, list one area in particular that you would like to improve.

Mastered: ____

____

Needs improvement: ____

____

Step 3: Reflecting on Past Communication. Reflect on a recent conversation with the person listed in Step 1 that would have benefited from changes to the communication skill you want to improve. Now that you are more informed about successful communication, what could you have done differently?

____

____

____

Step 4: Listening. Listening is a major component of communication. Consider the good listening skills that were discussed on page 385. Which techniques can you try to become a better listener? Provide examples of how you will apply these skills within your chosen relationship.

Techniques: ____

____

Examples: ____

____

Step 5: Putting Yourself in Someone Else's Shoes. Another way to improve a relationship is to try to see things through the other person's eyes. Take a moment to think about your chosen relationship and write down key factors in that person's life and situation. Answer the following questions: Who are the important people in his or her life and why? What other people is he or she having problems with and why? What are his or her current stressors? What is he or she looking forward to or worried about?

____

____

____

Step 6: Writing a Note. Imagine that you are writing a note to the person with whom you want to improve relations. What would you say? Write it down.

____

____

____

____

Step 7: Your Next Step. Given your current stage of behavior change, what will be your next step in building the relationship you want to improve?

____

____

____

____

Chapter Summary

- Good communication includes being able to articulate your honest thoughts and feelings, being aware of how body language can affect how others interpret what you are saying, and being a good listener.
- Methods of approaching conflict include avoidance, accommodation, and competition, which are typically unhealthful, and compromise and collaboration, which can help strengthen relationships and produce innovative solutions. Effective conflict resolution requires that both parties voice their concerns maturely and engage in constructive criticism, rather than resorting to personal attacks and put-downs.
- Self-perception, early relationships, gender roles, and a variety of social factors affect how we develop relationships throughout life.
- Strong friendships and social ties contribute to greater overall health.
- Sternberg's triangular theory of love identifies intimacy, passion, and commitment as the three primary components of healthy, loving relationships.
- Formal dating rituals have become much less common on campus than hooking up, engaging in casual, noncommittal, physical encounters. Still, a majority of college students do form committed relationships.
- Most people in relationships met their partner through a friend; however, online dating has become the second most common way partners meet.
- Overall, same-sex couples are just as satisfied in their relationships as heterosexual couples.
- Healthy relationships are based on trust, respect, and communication. Dysfunctional relationships are characterized by manipulation, disrespect, cruelty, or abuse. Problems that commonly threaten relationships include inflexibility, power plays, infidelity, and jealousy. Any relationship in which physical abuse occurs should be ended immediately.
- Cohabitation, marriage, and domestic partnerships are examples of different kinds of committed relationships.
- About half of all marriages eventually end in divorce.
- Raising children can be rewarding as well as stressful. Couples should ask themselves how having a baby would change their lives, and whether they are truly ready for those changes.
- The influence of four classic parenting styles—neglectful, authoritarian, indulgent, and authoritative—on children's development is controversial. New research suggests that parenting style may not have as great an influence as children's innate characteristics and their interactions with peers.
- Strong families are characterized by commitment, appreciation, affection, positive communication, time together, spiritual well-being, and the ability to adapt to changes.

- To build healthy relationships, stay true to yourself, respect differences, affirm your partners and friends, learn to give and receive, and make room in your relationship for fun.
- On campus, you can learn to build relationships of mutual respect and tolerance by keeping the lines of communication open, getting involved in campus organizations that support diversity, and exploring new options when attending social, cultural, and other events.

Test Your Knowledge

1. All of the following are examples of nonverbal communication except
a. eye contact.
b. email.
c. arm movements.
d. facial expressions.

2. The best method for resolving conflict is
a. avoidance.
b. accommodation.
c. collaboration.
d. compromise.

3. In Sternberg's triangular theory of love, the primary components of healthy relationships include all of the following except
a. passion.
b. contentment.
c. commitment.
d. intimacy.

4. Assortative mating refers to the tendency of people to
a. be attracted to people who have opposite interests to their own.
b. fall in love at first sight.
c. "hook up" instead of date.
d. select romantic partners who are similar to themselves.

5. Healthy relationships are characterized by all of the following except
a. honesty.
b. respect.
c. good communication.
d. constant contact.

6. How many people in the United States identify themselves as homosexuals?
a. 880,000
b. 8.8 million
c. 18.8 million
d. 80 million

7. What is the best way to deal with jealousy in an intimate relationship?
a. Ignore it.
b. Limit what you do until your partner is no longer jealous.
c. Talk openly about it.
d. Reduce the jealous person's self-esteem.

8. In general, married people
a. enjoy better mental and physical health than unmarried people.
b. live longer than unmarried people.
c. are financially better off than unmarried people.
d. experience all of the above.

9. What is the divorce rate in the United States?
a. around 30%
b. around 40%
c. around 50%
d. around 60%

10. What proportion of people in the United States are part of a stepfamily?
a. one in three
b. one in four
c. one in five
d. one in ten

Get Critical

What happened:

Is there such a thing as love at first sight? Researchers at Ohio State University decided to find out, recruiting 164 first-year students and pairing them off on the first day of class.[1] Students were instructed to introduce themselves and spend just a few minutes talking. They were then given a questionnaire and asked to predict how close they would become to each other over the course of the next few months. Nine weeks later, were they on target? Researchers found that most students did indeed guess correctly during that first brief meeting the kind of relationship that would develop.

In a separate study, Florida State University psychologists found that it takes just half a second to decide whether someone is attractive and a potential mate.[2] They also noticed that people gazed at attractive faces for a little bit longer than the faces that were not appealing to them.

What do you think?

- **Do you find these studies compelling proof that "love at first sight" exists?**
- **How do you define "love"? Do you agree with Sternberg's triangular theory of love? Why or why not?**

References: **1.** "At First Sight: Persistent Relational Effects of Get-Acquainted Conversations," by M. Sunnafrank & A. Ramirez, 2004, *Journal of Social and Personal Relationships, 21*, pp. 361–379. **2.** "Can't Take My Eyes Off You: Attentional Adhesion to Mates and Rivals," by J. K. Maner, M. T. Gailliot, D. A. Rouby, & S. L. Miller, 2007, *Journal of Personality and Social Psychology, 93*, pp. 389–401.

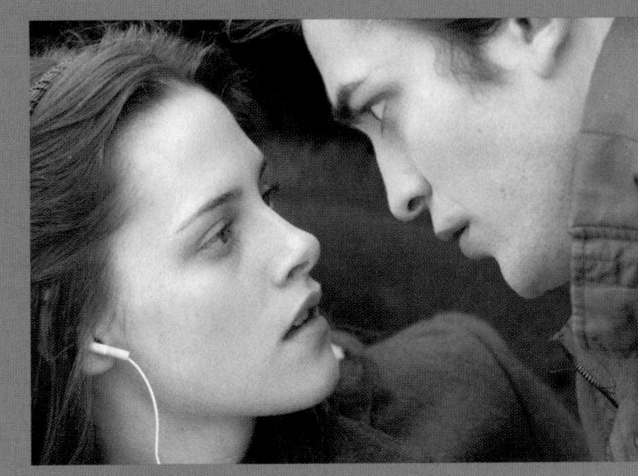

In the movie *Twilight,* Edward and Bella experienced love at first sight.

Get Connected

Mobile Tips!

Scan this QR code with your mobile device to access additional tips about relationships and communication. Or, via your mobile device, go to **http://mobiletips.pearsoncmg.com** and navigate to Chapter 14.

Health Online Visit the following websites for more information about the topics in this chapter:

- Conflict Resolution Information Source
  www.crinfo.org
- American Psychological Association
  www.apa.org
- Human Rights Campaign
  www.hrc.org
- National Teen Dating Abuse Helpline
  www.loveisrespect.org
- The National Marriage Project
  http://nationalmarriageproject.org
- American Association for Marriage and Family Therapy
  www.aamft.org

Website links are subject to change. To access updated web links, please visit ***www.pearsonhighered.com/lynchelmore***.

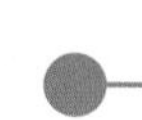

References

i. Facebook Press Room. (2010). Statistics. Retrieved March 15, 2010, from http://www.facebook.com/press/info.php?statistics.

ii. Stanley, S. M., Rhoades, G. K., & Markman, H. J. (2006). Sliding versus deciding: Inertia and the premarital cohabitation effect. *Family Relations, 55,* 499–509.

iii. Karasu, S. R. (2007). The institution of marriage: Terminable or interminable? *American Journal of Psychotherapy, 61* (1), 1–16.

1. Jourard, S. M. (1971). *The transparent self.* New York: D. Van Nostrand Company.

2. Baugh, E. J., & Humphries, D. (2010, January). Can we talk? Improving couples' communication. University of Florida Department of Family, Youth, and Community Services. Document FCS2178. Retrieved from http://edis.ifas.ufl.edu/pdffiles/fy/fy04400.pdf.

3. Thomas, K. (1976). Conflict and conflict management. In *Handbook of industrial and organizational psychology*. Chicago: Rand McNally.

4. University of Pennsylvania Faculty/Staff Assistance Program. (n.d.). *Conflict resolution: How to fight fair so that everyone wins.* Retrieved October 5, 2008, from http://www.upenn.edu/fsap/conflict.htm.

5. Lickerman, A. (2010, February 1). How to forgive others. *Psychology Today*. Retrieved from http://www.psychologytoday.com/blog/happiness-in-world/201002/how-forgive-others.

6. Schuetz, A. (1998). Autobiographical narratives of good and bad deeds: Defensive and favorable self-description moderated by trait self-esteem. *Journal of Social and Clinical Psychology, 17,* 466–475.

7. Bellavia, G., & Murray, S. (2003). Did I do that? Self-esteem–related differences in reactions to romantic partners' moods. *Personal Relationships, 10* (1), 77–95.

8. Bowlby, J. (1982). *Attachment and loss: Vol. 1., Attachment* (2nd ed.). New York: Basic Books.

9. Kilmann, P. R., Urbaniak, G. C., & Parnell, M. M. (2006). Effects of attachment–focused versus relationship skills–focused group interventions for college students with insecure attachment patterns. *Attachment & Human Development, 8* (1), 47–62.

10. Gurian, A. (n.d.). *Depression in adolescence: Does gender matter?* NYC Child Study Center. Retrieved from http://www.aboutourkids.org/articles/depression_in_adolescence_does_gender_matter.

11. Cohn, D., & Fry, R. (2010, January 19). Women, men, and the new economics of marriage. Pew Research Center. Retrieved from http://pewsocialtrends.org/2010/01/19/women-men-and-the-new-economics-of-marriage.

12. Katz-Wise, S. L., Priess, H. A., & Hyde, J. S. (2010). Gender-role attitudes and behavior across the transition to parenthood. *Developmental Psychology, 46* (1), 18–28.

13. American Council on Education. (2010). *Gender equity in higher education: 2010.* Available at http://www.acenet.edu/genderequity2010.

14. National Marriage Project. (2010). *The state of our unions: Marriage in America 2010.* Retrieved from http://www.virginia.edu/marriageproject/pdfs/Union_11_12_10.pdf.

15. Ellison, C. G., Burdette, A. M., & Wilcox, W. B. (2010, August). The couple that prays together: Race and ethnicity, religion, and relationship quality among working-age adults. *Journal of Marriage and Family, 72* (4), 963–965.

16. Berkman, L. F., & Syme, S. L. (1979). Social networks, host resistance, and mortality: A nine-year follow-up study of Alameda County residents. *American Journal of Epidemiology, 109* (2), 186–204.

17. Berkman, L. F. (1995). The role of social relations in health promotion. *Psychosomatic Medicine, 57* (3), 245–254.

18. McPherson, M., Smith-Lovin, L., & Brashears, M. E. (2006). Social isolation in America: Changes in core discussion networks over two decades. *American Sociological Review, 71* (3), 353–375.

19. Pressman, S. D., Cohen, S., Miller, G. E., Barkin, A., Rabin, B. S., & Treanor, J. J. (2005). Loneliness, social network size, and immune response to influenza vaccination in college freshmen. *Health Psychology, 24* (3), 297–306.

20. Swami, V., Chamorro-Premuzic, T., Sinniah, D., Maniam, T., Kannan, K., & Stanistreet, D. (2007). General health mediates the relationship between loneliness, life satisfaction and depression. *Social Psychiatry and Psychiatric Epidemiology, 42,* 161–166.

21. Students Helping Students. (2005). *Navigating your freshman year: How to make the leap to college life—and land on your feet.* New York: Penguin Group.

22. Ledbetter, A. M., Griffin, E. M., & Sparks, G. G. (2007). Forecasting "friends forever": A longitudinal investigation of sustained closeness between best friends. *Personal Relationships, 14* (2), 343–350.

23. Harris Interactive. (2009, April 16). *Just under half of Americans have a Facebook or MySpace account.* Retrieved from http://www.harrisinteractive.com/vault/Harris-Interactive-Poll-Research-Social-Network-Sites-2009-04.pdf.

24. University of Kansas. (2009, March 30). In the age of Facebook, researcher plumbs shifting online relationships. *ScienceDaily.* Retrieved from http://www.sciencedaily.com/releases/2009/03/090330091555.htm.

25. Sternberg, R. J. (1986). A triangular theory of love. *Psychological Review, 93,* 119–135.

26. Rowett Research Institute (2007, August 13). Love at first sight of your body fat. *ScienceDaily*. Retrieved from http://www.sciencedaily.com /releases/2007/08/070812095324.htm.

27. Association for Psychological Science. (2008, February 14). Beauty bias: Can people love the one they are compatible with? *ScienceDaily*. Retrieved from http://www.sciencedaily.com/releases/2008/02/080211094943.htm.

28. Blackwell Publishing, Ltd. (2007, November 30). Personality traits influence perceived attractiveness. *ScienceDaily*. Retrieved from http://www.sciencedaily.com/releases/2007/11/071129145852.htm.

29. Luo, S., & Klohnen, E. C. (2005). Assortative mating and marital quality in newlyweds: A couple-centered approach. *Journal of Personality and Social Psychology, 88* (2), 304–326.

30. Whitehead, B. D., & Popenoe, D. (2002). *The state of our unions: The social health of marriage in America.* Piscataway, NJ: National Marriage Project, Rutgers University. Retrieved from http://www.virginia.edu/marriageproject/pdfs/SOOU2002.pdf.

31. Armstrong, E. A., Hamilton, L., & England, P. (2010, summer). Is hooking up bad for young women? *Contexts: A Publication of the American Sociological Association*. Retrieved from http://contexts.org/articles/summer-2010/is-hooking-up-bad-for-young-women.

32. Daniel, C., & Fogarty, K. (2007). *"Hooking up" and hanging out: Casual sexual behavior among adolescents and young adults today* (Publication FCS2279). Department of Family, Youth, and Community Sciences, Florida Cooperative Extension Service, Institute of Food and Agricultural Sciences, University of Florida. Retrieved from http://edis.ifas.ufl.edu/fy1002.

33. Kruse, A. (2009, December 2). Liquid courage: The dangers of drinking and hooking up. *California University Cal Times*. Retrieved from http://sai.cup.edu/caltimes/index.php/2009/12/02/liquid-courage-the-dangers-of-drinking-and-hooking-up.

34. American Sociological Association. (2010, August 16). Internet access at home increases the likelihood that adults will be in relationships. Press Release. Retrieved from http://www.asanet.org/press/Internet_Access_and_Relationships.cfm.

35. Romero, A. P., Baumle, A. K., Lee Badgett, M. V., & Gates, G. J. (2007, December). *Census snapshot: The United States.* The Williams Institute, UCLA School of Law. Retrieved from http://www.law.ucla.edu/williamsinstitute/publications/USCensusSnapshot.pdf.

36. Roisman, G. I., Clausell, E., Holland, A., Fortuna, K., & Elieff, C. (2008). Adult romantic relationships as contexts of human

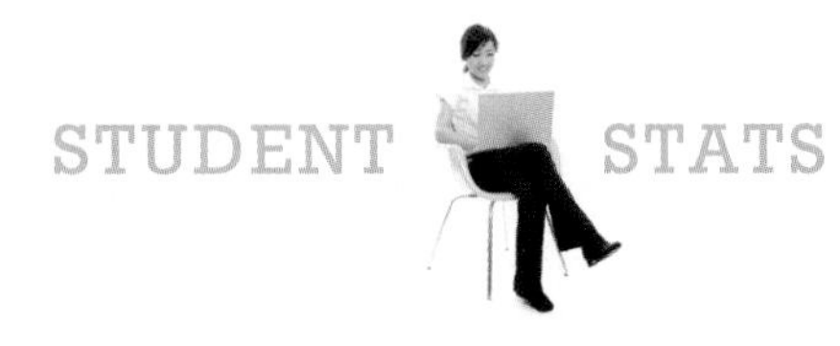

Sex and the College Student

Number of sexual partners college students reported having over the past year

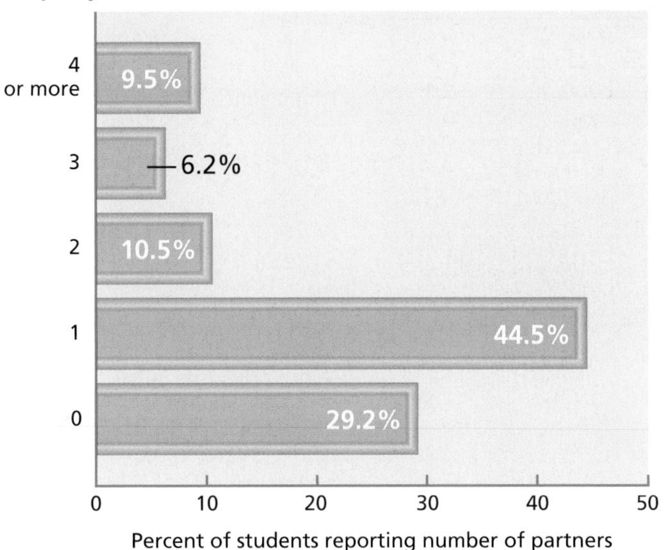

Data from *American College Health Association-National College Health Assessment (ACHA-NCHA II) Reference Group Executive Summary, Spring 2011* by the American College Health Association, 2011, retrieved from http://www.achancha.org/docs/ACHA-NCHA-II_ReferenceGroup_ExecutiveSummary_Spring2011.pdf.

- **Emotional reasons.** Love, commitment, communication, and desire to express feelings of closeness and gratitude were frequent motivators.
- **Insecurity.** Many students reported feeling pressure to be sexually active—either from a partner, or from the peer group in general. Others wanted to feel more attractive, mature, or powerful, or to prevent a breakup.
- **Goal achievement.** Some students engaged in sex to achieve a goal: pregnancy, increased social status, or even revenge—for instance, engaging in sex with a new partner to punish an established partner for openly flirting with a rival at a party.

Sexual Anatomy and Health

Whether we engage in sexual activity or not, and regardless of our reasons for doing it, our sexual anatomy evolved for one reason: reproduction. To ensure the survival of our species, a female's ovaries release an egg each month, while a male's testes are constantly manufacturing new sperm. Given these biological realities, the sexual decisions we make in a split second can alter the course of our lives dramatically, by leading to an unintended pregnancy or a sexually transmitted infection that permanently affects fertility.

"One in five women said they regretted the sexual activity they had engaged in while intoxicated."

vulva All of the female external organs, collectively. Also called *genitals*.

mons pubis The fatty, rounded areas of tissue in front of the pubic bone.

labia Two pairs (majora and minora) of fleshy lips surrounding and protecting the clitoris and the vaginal and urethral openings.

clitoris An organ composed of spongy tissue and nerve endings which is very sensitive to sexual stimulation.

vagina The tube that connects a woman's external sex organs with her uterus.

uterus (womb) The pear-shaped organ where a growing fetus is nurtured.

cervix The neck, or narrowed lower entrance, of the uterus that serves as a passageway to and from the vagina.

Female Sexual Anatomy

A woman's sexual anatomy includes both external and internal sex organs **(Figure 15.1).** The term **vulva** refers to all of the female external organs collectively—also known as *genitals*. These include the following structures:

- **Mons pubis.** The fatty, rounded area of tissue in front of the pubic bone; covered in pubic hair in teens and adults.
- **Labia majora.** The fleshy, larger outer lips (*labia* means lips) surrounding the labia minora.
- **Labia minora.** The thin, inner folds of skin, which rest protectively over the *clitoris,* the *vaginal opening,* and the *urethral opening*, through which urine is released from the body.
- **Clitoris.** An organ composed of erectile tissue with an abundance of nerve endings that make it very sensitive to sexual stimulation. During sexual arousal, the clitoris fills with blood and plays a key role in producing the female orgasm. In fact, the clitoris is the only organ in either sex with the sole purpose of sexual arousal and pleasure.

The internal organs include the following:

- **Vagina.** The tube that connects a woman's external sex organs with her *uterus*. It serves as the passageway through which menstrual flow leaves the body, as well as the passageway through which sperm enters the body during heterosexual intercourse. During childbirth, it functions as the birth canal.
- **Uterus.** Also known as the *womb.* The uterus is a pear-shaped organ, normally about the size of a fist. It is here that a growing fetus is nurtured. The lining of the uterus is called the *endometrium*. It is shed monthly in nonpregnant women of childbearing age.
- **Cervix.** The narrowed neck of the uterus that projects into the top of the vagina. Sperm deposited into the vagina swim through the opening of the cervix into the body of the uterus.

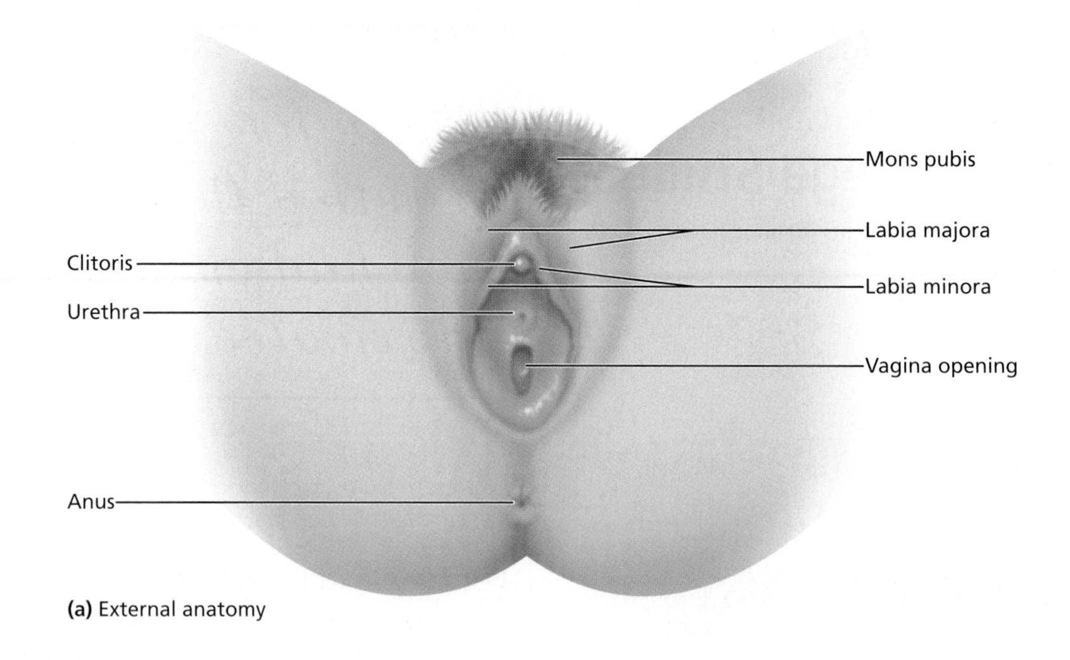

(a) External anatomy

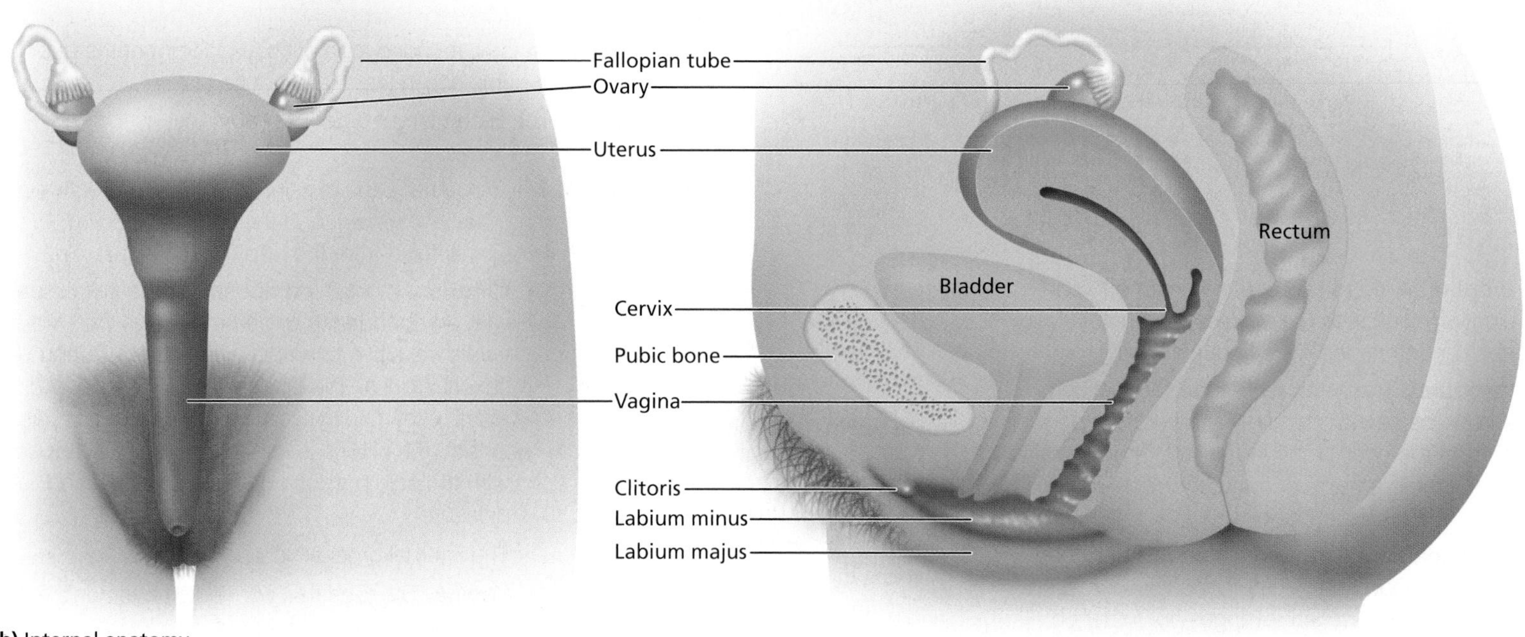

(b) Internal anatomy

Figure 15.1 Female sexual anatomy.

- **Ovaries.** The two organs, one on either side of the pelvic cavity, where a woman's eggs, or *ova,* are stored. Every month, at approximately midway through her **menstrual cycle,** a woman *ovulates*; that is, one of her ovaries releases an egg. The ovaries produce the hormone *estrogen*.
- **Fallopian tubes.** The tubes—one on either side of the uterus—that extend from the uterus to the ovaries. These tubes end in fringelike extensions called *fimbriae* that are lined with hair cells (cilia). After a woman ovulates, these structures sweep the egg into the interior of the fallopian tube, which is lined with muscle tissue that contracts, propelling the egg toward the uterus. If it encounters sperm within the tube, the egg may become fertilized. Whether fertilized or not, the egg will eventually reach the uterus.

ovaries The two female reproductive organs where ova (eggs) reside.

menstrual cycle A monthly physiological cycle marked by *menstruation.*

fallopian tubes A pair of tubes that connect the ovaries to the uterus.

puberty A 2- to 3-year period of transition from childhood to adolescence, during which reproduction becomes possible.

Sexual Development in Girls

Although the organs of reproduction are of course in place at birth, reproductive functioning is delayed until **puberty,** a 2- to 3-year period of transition during which reproduction becomes possible. Under the influence of female reproductive hormones such as estrogen, girls develop secondary sex characteristics, such as underarm and pubic

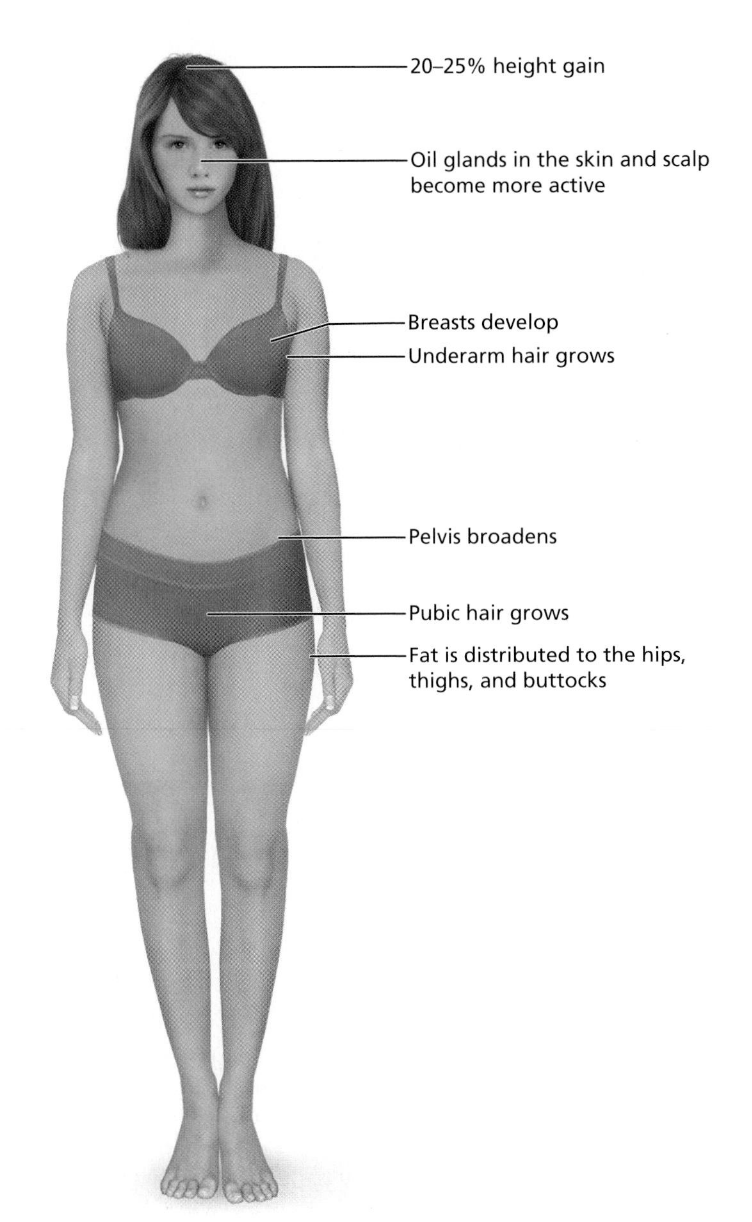
20–25% height gain
Oil glands in the skin and scalp become more active
Breasts develop
Underarm hair grows
Pelvis broadens
Pubic hair grows
Fat is distributed to the hips, thighs, and buttocks

Figure 15.2 Changes of puberty: girls.

hair, breasts, and changes in fat distribution **(Figure 15.2).** Girls may begin to develop so-called *breast buds* as early as age 8 to 10, but full breast development may not be complete until age 12 to 18. Underarm and pubic hair may first appear earlier or later than breast buds. The unmistakable sign of puberty is **menarche** (pronounced *me-NAR-kee*), the onset of a girl's first menstrual period. It typically begins about two years after the first signs of breast buds and pubic hair appear.

Puberty is accompanied by a growth spurt, especially between ages 12 to 14. Girls may experience a 20–25% gain of height by the time they reach their full adult height around age 18. At the same time, a girl develops more pronounced curves as the pelvis broadens and fat is distributed to the hips and buttocks. Many girls become concerned for the first time about their weight, and may try fad diets or other types of disordered eating. Estrogen causes the oil glands in the skin and scalp to become more active, so adolescent girls may also become fixated on acne and oily hair.

As adolescents begin to separate from their parents, their relationships with peers become all-important. In early puberty, girls typically prefer to hang out with other girls in nonromantic friendships. By about age 14 to 16, the peer group expands and may include dating and romantic relationships.[6]

menarche The first onset of menstruation.

penis The male sexual and reproductive organ.

erection The process of the penis filling up with blood as a result of sexual stimulation.

circumcision The surgical removal of the foreskin.

scrotum The skin sac at the base of the penis that contains the testes.

Common Sexual Health Problems in Females

Good sexual health includes good preventive care. Guidelines vary among different public health agencies, but in general, women should have their first pelvic exam and Pap test by age 21. After that, sexually active women should follow their health-care provider's advice about screenings for cervical cancer and sexually transmitted infections. Unfortunately, about half of all college-age women do not get screened regularly.[2] Not only does this reduce the odds that any medical problems will be detected early, it also deprives women of the opportunity to discuss important sexual health issues and reproductive concerns with a trusted expert.

Sexually transmitted infections are a major health concern for sexually active women of all ages, not only for the harm they cause directly, but also because of their association with other serious disorders. For example, infection with the human papillomavirus (HPV), which is sexually transmitted, is known to be the most important risk factor for cervical cancer.[7] And sexually transmitted bacterial infections can result in *pelvic inflammatory disease*, a common cause of infertility.

A fungal infection affecting females is *vulvovaginal candidiasis* (VVC), an inflammation of the vagina that can produce itching, pain, and discharge. Although it is not sexually transmitted, the condition is common and is often referred to as a "yeast infection." It is typically caused by an overgrowth of *Candida albicans,* a species of yeast (a type of fungus) that is normally present in the vagina in controlled amounts. VVC most commonly occurs when a woman takes a broad-spectrum antibiotic that kills off the normal vaginal bacteria that usually compete with *Candida* for nutrients.

Male Sexual Anatomy

A man's reproductive anatomy also includes both internal and external organs **(Figure 15.3).** The external organs are the following:

- **Penis.** The male sexual and reproductive organ consists of the shaft (body) and a slitted tip called the glans (head). Made up of soft, spongy tissue, the penis fills with blood during sexual arousal and becomes firm and enlarged, a state known as an **erection.** Boys are born with a hood of skin, known as the *foreskin,* covering the head of the penis. In more than half of boys born in the United States, parents opt to have the skin surgically removed through a procedure called **circumcision** (see **Myth or Fact? Should Boys Be Circumcised for Health Reasons?**).
- **Scrotum.** The skin sac at the base of the penis contains the *testes* (testicles). The scrotum is responsible for regulating the temperature of the testes, which need to be kept cooler than the core body temperature to enable production of *sperm*, the male reproductive cells.

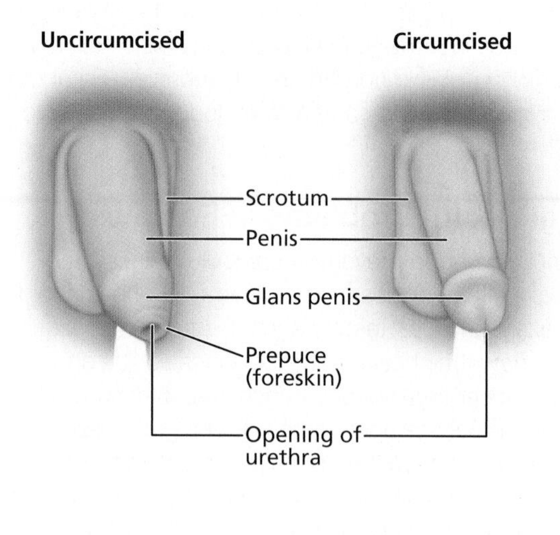

(a) External anatomy

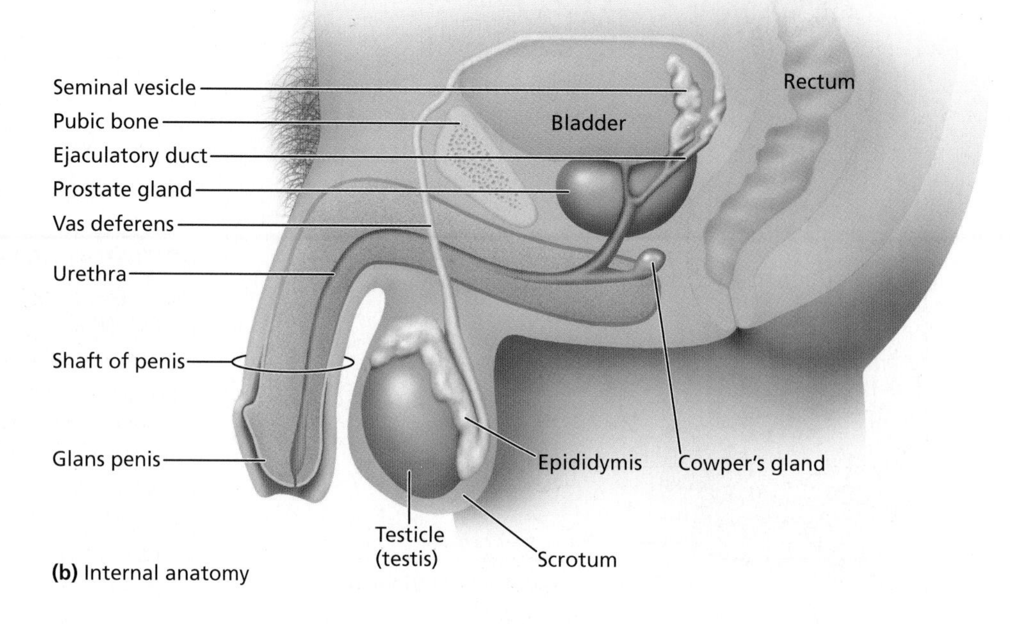

(b) Internal anatomy

Figure 15.3 Male sexual anatomy.

MYTH OR FACT?

Should Boys Be Circumcised for Health Reasons?

Infant boys are born with a hood of skin, known as the *foreskin,* covering the head of the penis. In more than half of boys born in the United States, parents opt to have the foreskin surgically removed through a procedure called *circumcision.*

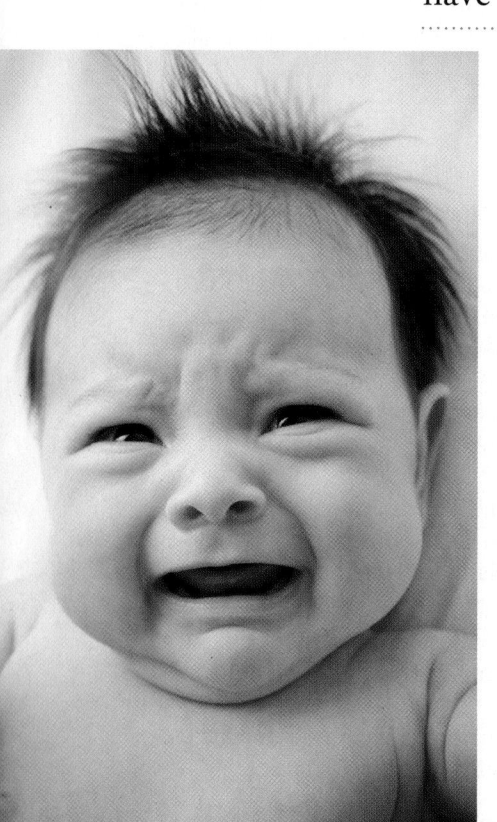

Circumcision rates vary greatly across the country and throughout the world, with the surgery being much more popular in the Midwest and Northeast than in the West, where slightly less than one-third of boys were circumcised in 2005.[1] Circumcision is also widely performed in the Middle East and Canada, but in Europe, Latin America, China, and India it is uncommon.

In some families, the decision to circumcise is primarily a religious one. In both the Jewish and Muslim faiths, circumcision is a common rite of passage. In others, it is more of a cultural determination—boys are circumcised because their fathers were. What remains most controversial is circumcising for health-related reasons.

Most medical experts agree on certain potential health benefits of circumcision. They point out that circumcision boosts personal hygiene, making it somewhat easier to clean the penis. It also reduces the risk of urinary tract infections in infancy. Men who have been circumcised have lower rates of penile cancer, and several types of research studies have documented a reduced risk of both acquiring and transmitting some sexually transmitted infections, including HIV.[2] Safe-sex practices, however, are much more important at stopping the spread of those diseases than circumcision.

Opponents of circumcision point out that the procedure can be painful. It also comes with risks, including the potential for infection and excessive bleeding. Rarely, the penis may not heal properly or a second surgery may be needed. Some opponents argue that circumcision reduces penile sensation and sexual function; however, well-designed studies of these issues are few and inconclusive.[2]

The American Academy of Pediatrics has declared that "existing scientific evidence demonstrates potential medical benefits of newborn male circumcision; however, these data are not sufficient to recommend routine neonatal circumcision."[3] Whether to circumcise their son is a decision that parents should make after weighing both the benefits and the risks, the organization determined. When parents do go forward with a circumcision, the Academy advises that pain medication be given to the newborn.

References: **1.** Raw data from the National Center for Health Statistics, 2007, retrieved from http://nchspressroom.files.wordpress.com/2007/07/circumcision-1979-2005.pdf. **2.** "Male Circumcision and Risk for HIV Transmission and Other Health Conditions: Implications for the United States" by the Centers for Disease Control, 2008, retrieved from http://www.cdc.gov/hiv/resources/factsheets/circumcision.htm. **3.** "Circumcision Policy Statement" by the American Academy of Pediatrics, 1999, *Pediatrics, 103* (3), pp. 686–693.

testes (testicles) The two reproductive glands that manufacture sperm.

epididymis A coiled tube on top of each testicle where sperm are held until they mature.

vas deferens A tube ascending from the epididymis that transports sperm.

accessory glands Glands (seminal vesicles, prostate gland, and Cowper's gland) that lubricate the reproductive system and nourish sperm.

semen The male ejaculate consisting of sperm and other fluids from the accessory glands.

urethra A duct that travels from the bladder through the shaft of the penis, carrying fluids to the outside of the body.

The internal male organs are the following:

- **Testes (testicles).** Paired glands that secrete the reproductive hormone *testosterone*, which prompts production of sperm.
- **Epididymis.** The coiled tube—one above each testicle—where sperm are held until they mature.
- **Vas deferens.** The tube that ascends from the epididymis—one on each side of the scrotum—and transports sperm into the *ejaculatory duct*.
- **Accessory glands.** A set of glands that lubricate the reproductive system and nourish the sperm. They include the *seminal vesicles,* small sacs that store *seminal fluid,* which provides sugars and other nutrients that feed and activate sperm. The seminal vesicles secrete seminal fluid into the ejaculatory duct, which also receives sperm from the vas deferens. This mixture of sperm and seminal fluid is called **semen.** Another accessory gland that contributes to semen is the *prostate gland,* a walnut-shaped structure below the bladder. It secretes into semen an alkaline fluid that helps protect sperm from the acidic environment of the vagina. Below the prostate are the *Cowper's glands,* pea-shaped glands on each side of the urethra that discharge a lubricating secretion into the urethra just before ejaculation.
- **Urethra.** Within the prostate, the ejaculatory duct joins the urethra, a much longer duct that travels from the bladder through the shaft of the penis, and carries fluids to the outside of the body. Both urine from the bladder and semen from the ejaculatory duct pass through the urethra, although not at the same time.

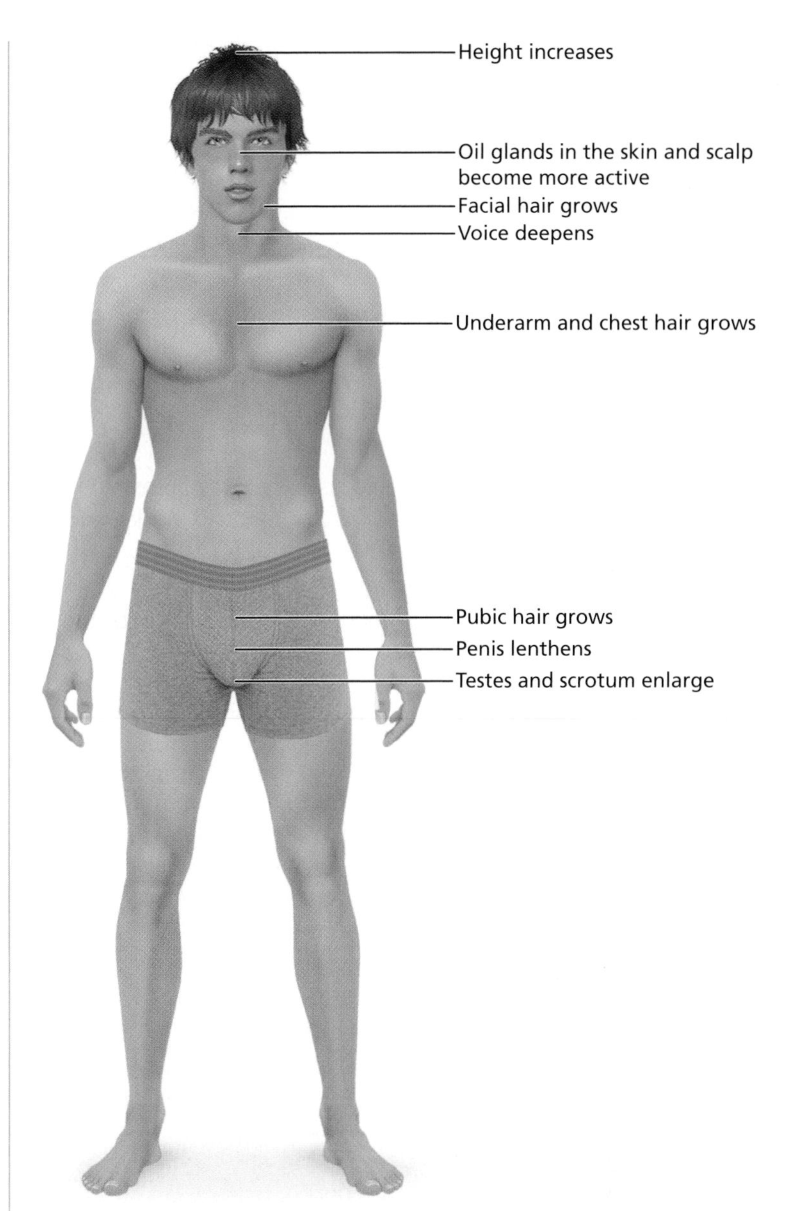
Height increases
Oil glands in the skin and scalp become more active
Facial hair grows
Voice deepens
Underarm and chest hair grows
Pubic hair grows
Penis lenthens
Testes and scrotum enlarge

Figure 15.4 **Changes of puberty: boys.**

Sexual Development in Boys

Boys may begin to notice enlargement of the testes and scrotum as early as 9 years of age, followed closely by lengthening of the penis. Adult size and shape is usually reached by about age 16 or 17.[6] Secondary sex characteristics such as deepening of the boy's voice typically begin simultaneously with these changes **(Figure 15.4).** Growth of facial, underarm, chest, and pubic hair begins around age 12 and continues until about age 15 or 16. Like girls, boys experience a growth spurt, reaching their full adult height around age 21. At the peak of the growth spurt, usually around age 14 to 15, the boy begins to experience nocturnal emissions (commonly called wet dreams) in which he involuntarily ejaculates semen during sleep.

Acne is a common concern for boys as well as girls, as both testosterone and estrogen increase the activity of the oil glands responsible for the condition. Acne in boys is often severe, affecting not only the face, but also the shoulders and upper chest and back.

Early adolescent boys typically prefer to hang out with other boys in nonromantic friendships. Romance becomes more likely as boys mature, around age 14 to 16, but may not occur until boys develop a stronger sense of their sexual identity, around age 16 to 18.[6]

Brain centers involved with logical reasoning and decision-making do not fully mature until the third decade of life; therefore, adolescents—girls as well as boys—are unable to fully think through the consequences of their actions. Believing they are "indestructible" and that bad things only happen to others, they are more likely than adults to take risks, such as having unprotected sex.

Common Sexual Health Problems in Males

Like women, men should take their sexual health seriously and get regular medical checkups. Sexually active men should regularly examine their genitals for blisters or other sores. These may be signs of a sexually transmitted infection. If you notice these—or any other changes to your genitals—be sure to discuss them promptly with your health-care provider. A hard lump in a testicle may be a sign of testicular cancer, which is most often diagnosed in men in their 20s and 30s.

A common disorder in males is *cryptorchidism*, usually referred to as an undescended testicle; that is, a testicle that has failed to move down into the scrotum before birth. It is routinely discovered during infancy, and usually descends before the boy's first birthday. If it has not descended by toddlerhood, surgery can be done to bring the testicle into the scrotum. Surgical correction is necessary because an undescended testicle cannot produce viable sperm and is at increased risk for testicular cancer.

In addition, several common sexual health problems in men involve the prostate:

- **Prostatitis.** An infection or inflammation of the **prostate gland.** Symptoms range from the frequent need to urinate to pain in the pelvic region and lower back.
- **Prostate gland enlargement.** An excessive growth of prostate tissue that presses on the urethra, impairing or blocking the flow of urine. This usually develops in men over age 60.
- **Prostate cancer.** A typically slow growth of cancerous tissue from which cancer cells can spread to other parts of the body. Prostate cancer most commonly affects men over age 65.[8]

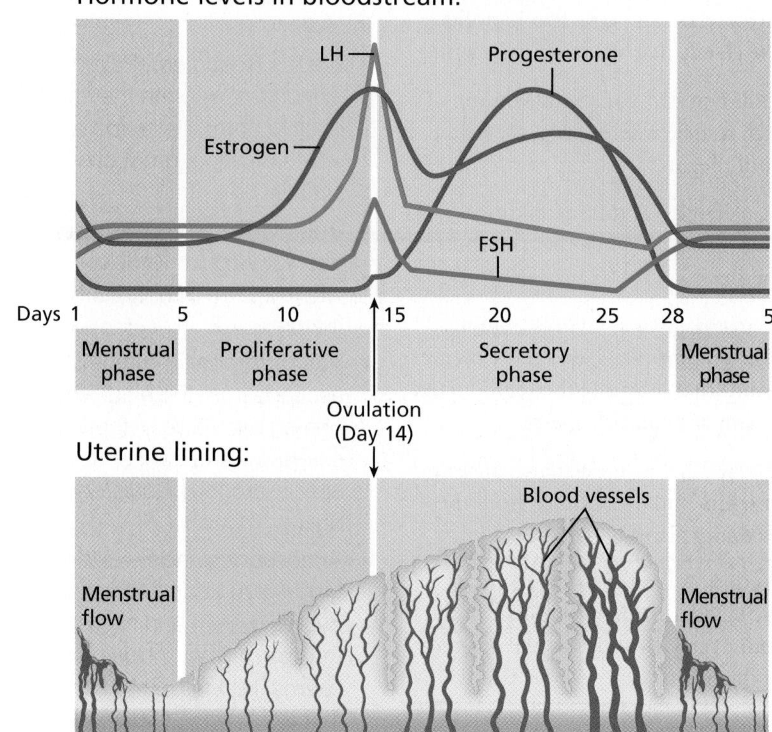

Figure 15.5 Phases of the menstrual cycle. The menstrual cycle consists of a menstrual phase, a proliferative phase, and a secretory phase.

The Menstrual Cycle

Menstruation is the discharge of blood and endometrial tissue from the vagina. Also called a *period* or *menstrual period,* menstruation usually lasts from three to seven days. In the United States, the average age at menarche is 12, although it is considered normal to start as early as 8 or as late as 15.[9] **Menopause,** the time at which women stop menstruating, usually occurs in a woman's early 50s.

Menstruation is just one of several physiologic events in a woman's *menstrual cycle* **(Figure 15.5).** Because it is controlled by hormones, the menstrual cycle can be interrupted by anything that affects hormone production. This includes illness, excessive dieting with or without excessive exercise, and breastfeeding. The menstrual cycle also ceases during pregnancy. Otherwise, in women of childbearing age, it repeats approximately every month, spanning from 21 to 35 days (the average is 28 days) each time.[9]

View an animation of the menstrual cycle at www.womenshealth.gov/publications/our-publications/fact-sheet/menstruation.cfm#b. (Click Start on the diagram.)

Phases of the Menstrual Cycle

The menstrual cycle is characterized by a series of events involving both the uterus and the ovaries. As indicated in Figure 15.5, fluctuations in the levels of four female reproductive hormones control these events, which are typically grouped into three phases: the **menstrual phase,** the **proliferative phase,** and the **secretory phase.**

Menstrual Phase

The first day of a woman's menstrual flow is arbitrarily designated as day 1 of the menstrual cycle. Menstruation results from the breakdown of the endometrium after the body "recognizes" that a pregnancy has not occurred. During this phase, a hormone called *FSH—follicle-stimulating hormone—* is released from the pituitary gland in the brain. A woman's ovary contains hundreds of thousands of cavities called *follicles,* each of which contains an immature egg cell. FSH stimulates the maturation of the immature egg within a few of these follicles. As they develop, the follicles begin releasing an ovarian hormone, *estrogen,* into the bloodstream. As estrogen reaches the uterus, it causes menstruation to end (around day 6).

Proliferative Phase

Estrogen is also responsible for causing the lining of the uterus to thicken (proliferate) in preparation for the entry into the uterus of a fertilized egg. Also during this phase, a woman may notice a copious, slippery discharge of mucus from her vagina. This characteristic *cervical mucus* helps facilitate the mobility of sperm and protect them from the otherwise acidic environment of the vagina. Its presence also indicates that a woman is about to **ovulate,** that is, release an egg. In fact, the proliferative phase ends when, around day 14 of a 28-day cycle, the pituitary gland releases another hormone, *LH,* or *luteinizing hormone,* which triggers just one of the several maturing follicles to release a mature egg (an *ovum*).

prostate gland A walnut-sized gland that produces part of the semen.

menstruation The cyclical discharge of blood and tissue from the vagina.

menopause The time when a woman stops having menstrual cycles.

menstrual phase Phase of the menstrual cycle characterized by menstrual flow, the release of FSH from the pituitary gland to the brain, and the release of estrogen.

proliferative phase Phase of the menstrual cycle characterized by a thickening of the lining of the uterus and discharge of cervical mucus. This phase ends when luteinizing hormone triggers the release of a mature egg.

secretory phase Phase of the menstrual cycle characterized by the degeneration of the follicle sac, rising levels of progesterone in the bloodstream, and further increase of the endometrial lining.

ovulate To release an egg from the ovary.

In some women, ovulation is accompanied by a sharp pain on one side of the lower abdomen. This pain is caused by irritation from the stretching of the ovary wall and the release of fluid into the lower abdominal cavity. Although it may last for several minutes to several hours, this "mid-cycle pain" is entirely normal and can help a woman pinpoint more precisely the time when she is fertile.

Secretory Phase

Once the ovum has been ejected, the remaining follicle sac degenerates into a *corpus luteum,* a tiny gland that begins releasing a fourth reproductive hormone, progesterone. Rising levels of progesterone enter the bloodstream and travel to the uterus, further thickening the endometrial lining in preparation for the arrival of a fertilized egg.

As noted earlier, the released ovum is swept into the nearby fallopian tube and begins to travel toward the uterus. If sperm are present in sufficient numbers in the fallopian tube, fertilization is likely to occur. The fertilized egg will then produce the hormone *human chorionic gonadotropin* (hCG), which is needed to sustain a pregnancy. In fact, over-the-counter pregnancy test kits work by detecting the presence or absence of hCG in a woman's urine. Within 3 to 4 days, the fertilized ovum reaches the uterus.

A woman's ovum is viable only for about 12 to 24 hours. If fertilization does not occur within this time period, it will quickly deteriorate, and the levels of all four reproductive hormones will begin to dramatically decrease. Thus, around day 25, the endometrium will start to degenerate. Within approximately 3–4 days, menstruation will begin and the cycle repeats itself again.

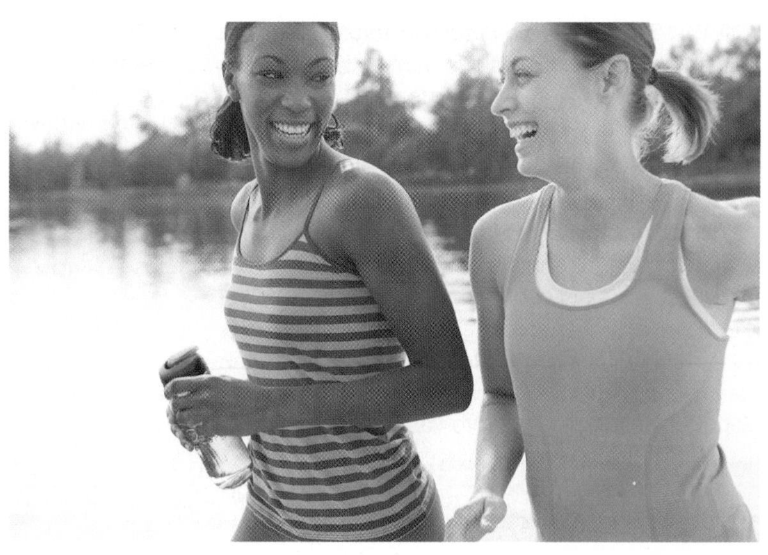

Exercise can help relieve the symptoms of **premenstrual syndrome**.

Disorders Associated with the Menstrual Cycle

Although normal menstruation is a sign of health and maturity, in some women it's accompanied by pain, excessive bleeding, or other problems that interfere with their ability to carry out their daily activities. We discuss the most common of these disorders here.

premenstrual syndrome (PMS) A collection of emotional and physical symptoms that occur just prior to menstruation.

premenstrual dysphoric disorder (PMDD) Severe and debilitating psychological symptoms experienced just prior to menstruation.

Premenstrual Syndrome

As many as 85% of women experience mildly disturbing emotional and physical symptoms just prior to menstruation.[10] These symptoms can include breast tenderness, fluid retention, headaches, backaches, uterine cramping, irritability, mood swings, appetite changes, depression, and anxiety. Approximately 15% of women experience a constellation of the symptoms at a "sufficient severity to interfere with some aspect of life" and consequently are considered to have **premenstrual syndrome,** or **PMS.**[11] The symptoms of PMS typically appear in the week or two before the period begins, and dissipate after menstrual bleeding starts.

Exactly what causes PMS isn't entirely clear. Some women may simply be more sensitive to the changes in female reproductive hormones that occur during the menstrual cycle. Chemical changes in the brain may also play a role. Stress and psychological problems do not cause the syndrome, although there is evidence that they can intensify it.[12]

Some lifestyle changes can reduce the symptoms of PMS. These include avoidance of smoking, alcohol, caffeine, salt, and sugary foods. A balanced diet rich in whole grains, fruits, and vegetables is important, along with regular exercise and adequate, restful sleep. In addition, some women find that a multivitamin and mineral supplement providing adequate levels of B vitamins, magnesium, and vitamin E is helpful, and women aged 19–50 should consume 1,000 milligrams of calcium daily. Over-the-counter remedies such as aspirin and ibuprofen can also relieve symptoms. In more severe cases of PMS in women who do not want to become pregnant, a woman's physician may prescribe birth control pills, which stop ovulation and reduce menstruation.[12]

Premenstrual Dysphoric Disorder (PMDD)

Some women experience the psychological symptoms of PMS in a more severe and debilitating way. This condition, known as **premenstrual dysphoric disorder (PMDD),** can interfere with daily functioning and social relationships. (*Dysphoria* refers to a generalized feeling of sadness, anxiety, or discontent.) About 3–8% of women suffer from true PMDD.[12] A diagnosis of PMDD means that a woman experiences at least five of its symptoms, which include:

- Anxiety
- Panic attacks
- Mood swings
- Feelings of despair
- Persistent irritability or anger
- Sleep disturbances
- Food cravings
- Low energy
- Difficulty focusing
- Loss of interest in daily activities and relationships

The lifestyle changes and medications prescribed for PMDD are the same as for PMS. In addition, the woman's physician may prescribe an antidepressant.

Dysmenorrhea

More than half of all menstruating women experience some pain for 1–2 days each month.[13] In most of these women, the pain is mild; however, sometimes the pain is severe enough to interfere with normal activities. This is called **dysmenorrhea,** or painful menstruation, and can include severe abdominal cramps, back or thigh pain, diarrhea, or even headaches in the days immediately preceding and during menstruation.[14] Dysmenorrhea is the leading cause of absenteeism from school in adolescent girls.[14]

The cramping pain of dysmenorrhea is due to *prostaglandins,* chemicals that regulate many body functions, including contraction of smooth muscle—like the muscle in a woman's uterus. Prostaglandins cause uterine muscle cells to contract, expelling the uterine lining. This is why over-the-counter prostaglandin inhibitors like ibuprofen and naproxen are usually effective in treating dysmenorrhea. The discomfort also usually wanes spontaneously with age and often disappears after pregnancy.

dysmenorrhea Pain during menstruation that is severe enough to limit normal activities or require medication.

endometriosis A condition in which endometrial tissue grows in areas outside of the uterus.

amenorrhea Cessation of menstrual periods.

toxic shock syndrome (TSS) A rare bacterial infection linked to tampon use.

Endometriosis

Endometriosis is a condition in which endometrial tissue grows in areas outside of the uterus such as the fallopian tubes, ovaries, and other structures in the pelvic region.[15] This tissue responds to the same hormonal signals that affect the uterus, and so breaks down and bleeds monthly into the abdominopelvic cavity. The condition can cause severe pain in the pelvic region that may be associated with the menstrual cycle, as well as scarring that can result in infertility. Endometriosis occurs most commonly in women in their 30s and 40s, but can occur at any time during the reproductive years. Although a physician can evaluate a woman for endometriosis during a physical examination, it is confirmed by laparoscopic surgery, in which a thin, lighted tube is inserted into the abdominopelvic cavity. If endometrial tissue is found, it can often be removed during the same procedure.[15]

Amenorrhea

As much as some young women would love to stop menstruating, a lack of periods can be a sign that the body is in distress. Missed periods, also known as **amenorrhea,** can usually be traced to severe weight loss with or without excessive exercise, a hormonal imbalance, or significant stress. Some medications, including certain birth control pills, can also suppress menstruation.

Amenorrhea is clinically defined as having no periods for at least three consecutive months.[16] It occurs normally in women who are pregnant, and usually throughout the first few months of breast-feeding. However, it can also signal a serious underlying disorder of the reproductive organs. Amenorrhea is also a common consequence of disordered eating. For example, it is somewhat common among athletes—especially gymnasts and long-distance runners—who train vigorously while restricting their calorie intake to maintain a competitive weight.

Amenorrhea is not without long-term consequences. Symptoms can include headaches and vaginal dryness, but doctors are most concerned about its effect on bone health. Recall that the female reproductive hormone estrogen is produced by the ovaries during the normal menstrual cycle. Estrogen plays a key role in building new bone tissue, so amenorrhea puts women at significant risk for low bone density. This means that women who experience long-term amenorrhea can suffer from osteoporosis and bone fractures at a relatively early age. In fact, stress fractures in female athletes are often an outward sign of the *female athlete triad*, in which failure to consume enough calories to maintain a healthy body weight prompts amenorrhea, which in turn leads to osteoporosis.

Toxic Shock Syndrome

In 1980, scientists had an alarming announcement for women who used one brand of super-absorbent tampons: They could kill you. The feminine hygiene products were linked to **toxic shock syndrome,** a rare disease characterized by a sudden high fever, vomiting, diarrhea, chills, muscle aches, a rash, and low blood pressure leading to dizziness or fainting. The bacterium *Staphylococcus aureus* is the primary culprit, and researchers determined that super-absorbent tampons, especially when left in place for longer than 8 hours, could encourage the growth of the bacteria, which release a virulent toxin. Before the tampons were removed from store shelves, they sickened hundreds and killed dozens of women.[17]

Today, toxic shock syndrome is extremely rare, but can still occur in women—usually aged 15 to 24—who use tampons. To reduce the risk of developing the syndrome, experts recommend that women use the lowest absorbency tampons needed, and alternate between tampons and pads. Tampons should also be changed at least every 4 to 8 hours.

The Physiology of Sex

In 1986, it was Mark Harmon. Twenty-five years later, Bradley Cooper won the title. Not best actor, not best dressed, but *People* magazine's "Sexiest Man Alive." Why? What makes us find one person sexier than another—and what happens when the person we find sexy just happens to think we're sexy, too?

Sexual Attraction

Sex researchers believe that, even today, sexual attraction is powerfully influenced by the evolutionary drive to reproduce. Thousands of years ago, our female ancestors were likely to be attracted to males who exhibited characteristics suggesting they could provide for and protect their future children, as well as participate in parenting activities. In turn, males were drawn to females who appeared suitable for bearing and raising numerous children. Although most men and women today aren't consciously driven by such considerations, they may unconsciously be influenced by them. For example, studies have shown that, when women are ovulating—that is, when they are most fertile—they produce a scent that attracts men and causes their testosterone levels to rise. The men in turn secrete a chemical with an odor that repels women who are not ovulating.[18] Another study has found that women are unconsciously attracted to men who exude a scent indicating that a vital component of their immune system is different; such differences in immunity promote the survival of any future children. Moreover, couples whose immune systems are similar in this component have higher rates of infertility.[18]

Scents are not the only ploys nature uses to ensure species survival: Men find women's voices more attractive when they are slightly higher in pitch—a change that occurs under the influence of estrogen when women are ovulating.[19] And guess what? Those same ovulating women are more attracted to "masculine" faces with a strong jaw, wide cheekbones, and a heavy brow.[20] Bradley Cooper, perhaps?

Another factor related to evolution is income: When women are asked to look at faces of male strangers and rate their attractiveness,

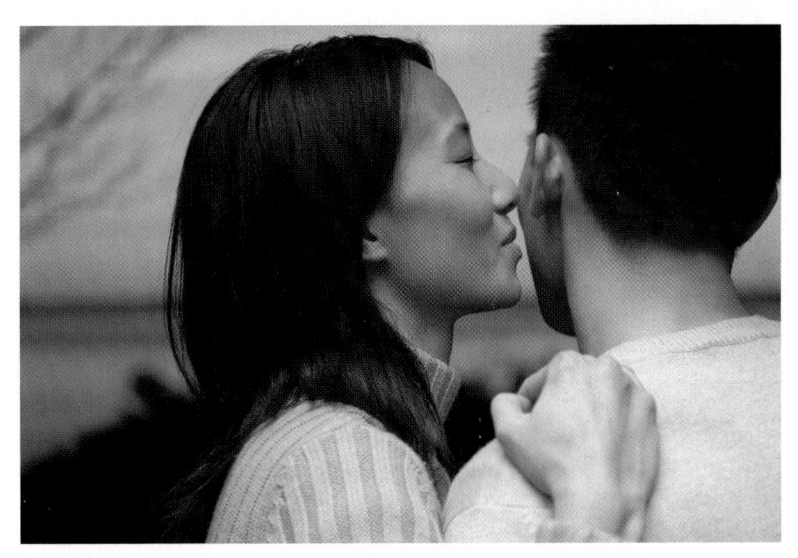

Touch can be one of the most powerful means of sexual arousal.

they rate them differently when the same face is shown with a corresponding income. Faces assigned a low income are rated as less attractive than faces assigned a high income.[18] Because women's earnings in the United States have grown 44% since 1970, and 22% of women now earn more than their spouses, this factor may become less influential—at least among Americans—over time.[21]

Sexual Arousal

We take in information about our environment with our five senses, and appropriate stimulation of any of these—a glimpse of bare skin, a musky odor—can get us "in the mood." But our sense of touch is perhaps most key to our arousal. **Erogenous zones** are areas of our body that are likely to arouse us sexually when they're touched. For nearly everyone, these include the genitals. Beyond that, our erogenous zones are unique to each of us. Different people find that the sensation of touch on one or more other parts of the body—the neck, nipples, buttocks, or even the arms, fingers, legs, or toes—can make them feel aroused.[22] What's more, the reaction isn't automatic! The person touching us and the way they touch both influence whether or not we become aroused.

Kissing between sexual partners appears in more than 90% of human cultures, and even in some nonhuman species.[23] A kiss produces a complex and rich exchange of tactile and chemical cues, and a recent study of over 1,000 college students found that a majority of both males and females reported experiences in which they were turned off to someone they had previously been attracted to because of a "bad" kiss.[23] On the other hand, a "good" kiss promotes sexual arousal and receptivity. The same study found that both men and women value kissing before sex—though women were far more likely than men to say they would not proceed to sex without first kissing.

> *"Kissing between sexual partners appears in more than 90% of human cultures, and even in some nonhuman species."*

erogenous zones Areas of the body likely to cause sexual arousal when touched.

human sexual response cycle Model of sexual response proposed by Masters and Johnson in which distinct phases occur in an essentially linear fashion from excitement to the calm after orgasm.

excitement The first phase of the sexual response cycle, marked by erection in men and by lubrication and clitoral swelling in women.

Arousal is also influenced by psychological factors, including developmental experiences within our families, our mood, stress level, and even memories of shared experiences with our partner. Feelings of closeness, acceptance, and gratitude can kindle the flame, whereas unacknowledged resentment, anger, or guilt can put it out.

The Sexual Response Cycle

Famed sex researchers William H. Masters and Virginia E. Johnson were the first to scientifically study the body's physiological reactions to sexual stimulation and subsequent release through orgasm. In their groundbreaking 1966 book, *Human Sexual Response*, they described a **human sexual response cycle** which, despite their use of the word "cycle," actually describes an essentially linear progression of four distinct phases extending from the first moment of sexual desire until the calm after sexual fulfillment **(Figure 15.6):**[24]

- **Excitement.** The first phase occurs as the result of any erotic mental or physical stimulation that leads to arousal. In both sexes it is

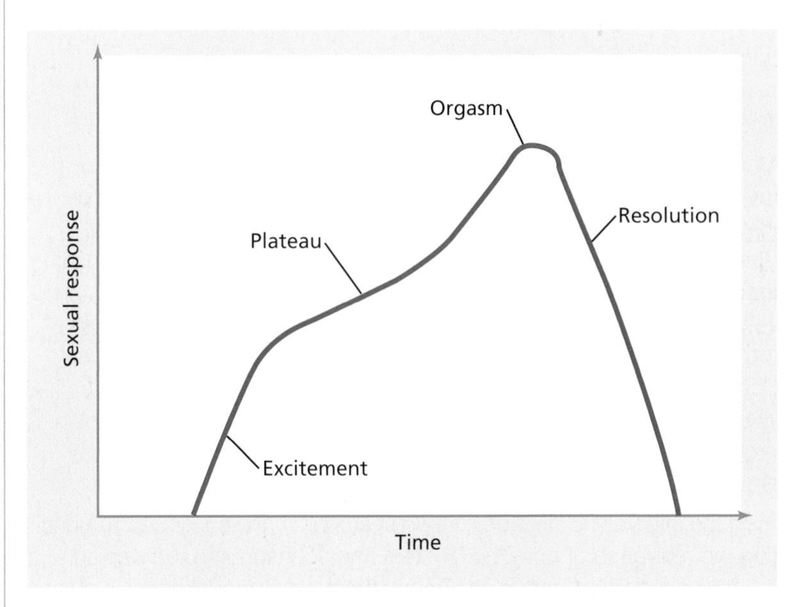

Figure 15.6 Human sexual response. The Masters and Johnson model proposes an essentially linear progression of four distinct phases.

characterized by increased heart and respiration rate and also increased blood pressure. Nipple erection, especially as the result of direct stimulation, occurs in almost all females and in approximately 60% of males. Both may also experience a "sex flush," which is the reddening of the skin due to vasocongestion (blood vessel engorgement). In males, the penis becomes mostly erect and the testicles draw upward. In females, the labia increase in size and the clitoris swells. Lubrication occurs as the result of vasocongestion of the vaginal walls.

- **Plateau.** This more intense excitement takes partners to the edge of orgasm, leaving hearts beating rapidly and genitals sensitive to touch. In males, the urethral sphincter, a valve at the base of the penis that prevents urination during ejaculation, closes. Muscles at the penis base also begin to contract rhythmically. Males also secrete a pre-ejaculatory fluid (that may contain small amounts of sperm) and the testicles rise closer to the body. In females, the outer third of the vagina swells and the pelvic muscle tightens, creating what Masters and Johnson refer to as the *orgasmic platform.*
- **Orgasm.** This event concludes the plateau phase and is the peak or climax of sexual response. It is accompanied by rhythmic muscle contractions of the genitals and surrounding areas. Most describe it as an intensely pleasurable feeling of release of sexual tension. In men, orgasm is accompanied by ejaculation.
- **Resolution.** In this phase the body returns to normal functioning. It often includes a sense of both well-being and fatigue.

Men usually experience a *refractory period,* a period of time when they are not immediately able to respond to stimulation with an erection and may actually find continued stimulation unwelcome, or even painful. Most women do not experience a refractory period and may be able to immediately return to the plateau stage, allowing for the possibility of multiple orgasms.

Alternative Models of Sexual Response

Masters and Johnson's research has not gone unchallenged. Among the many sex researchers who have proposed alternative models of sexual response, one of the earliest was sex educator and feminist Shere Hite, who in 1976 challenged Masters and Johnson's proposal that orgasm via intercourse alone was "normal." Her research revealed that, for women, this was an atypical response: Only 30% of the women she studied could achieve orgasm by intercourse alone. She moreover found that nearly all women could achieve orgasm easily by masturbation.[25] Then, in 1979, psychiatrist Helen Singer Kaplan proposed a three-phase model of sexual response including desire, arousal, and orgasm.[26]

In the intervening decades, sex researchers have continued to question the relevance of both the Masters and Johnson and the Kaplan models, especially for women. One of the newest models of sexual response in women acknowledges that, unlike most men, many women don't frequently think about sex or hunger for sexual activity. Instead, emotional intimacy, relationship satisfaction, and sexual stimulation all contribute to prompting a woman's desire in a roundabout way. And once desire arises in women, it can easily be dampened by any of several factors, from a distraction in the environment to a careless remark by the partner.[26]

The take-home message? We're not robots acting according to a preset program. Sex is a shared experience that unfolds between two different and highly complex individuals. For a mutually satisfying experience, each partner must discover, respect, and accommodate the other's needs.

plateau The second phase of the sexual response cycle, characterized by intense excitement, rapid heartbeat, genital sensitivity, the secretion of pre-ejaculatory fluid in men, and vaginal swelling in women.

orgasm The peak, or climax, of sexual response, characterized by rhythmic muscle contractions of the genitals and surrounding areas, and ejaculation in men.

resolution The stage of the response cycle in which the body returns to normal functioning.

sexual dysfunctions Problems occurring during any stage of the sexual response cycle.

Sexual Dysfunctions

Sexual dysfunctions are problems that can occur during any stage of the sexual response cycle—curbing desire, interrupting arousal, reducing pleasure, or preventing orgasm. An estimated 43% of women and 31% of men report having had at least one symptom of sexual dysfunction at some point in their life.[27]

Female Sexual Dysfunctions

A variety of problems can keep a woman from enjoying sex. These include painful intercourse, low level of sexual desire, and inability to achieve orgasm:[28]

- **Painful intercourse.** Up to 20% of women experience episodes of pain just before, during, or after intercourse.[29] Often the pain occurs only under certain circumstances, such as when the penis first enters the vagina or during vigorous thrusting. In other cases, the woman experiences a general burning or aching sensation. The causes vary with the type of pain reported, but some of the most common are insufficient vaginal lubrication, prior injury, infection, inflammation, or another underlying disorder, an allergic reaction to a birth control product such as a spermicide or a latex condom, or an anatomical variation called a tipped (or tilted) uterus, in which the uterus, which is normally in a vertical position, is tilted toward the woman's back. Emotional factors such as stress, low self-esteem, or a history of sexual abuse occasionally play a role. Often, simply a change in position or the use of a commercial water-based lubricant can correct the problem. Underlying infection or other disorders should also be treated. In some cases, hormonal medications or therapy can help.
- **Low level of sexual desire.** About 5–15% of women experience a persistently low sex drive.[30] Common physical causes include fatigue, medication side effect, alcohol abuse, pregnancy, breastfeeding, and menopause. In addition, psychological problems and unresolved issues within the relationship can be factors. Lifestyle changes such as regular exercise and stress management can help, as can couples counseling. Hormonal therapy is also available. Finally, some women find that *Kegel exercises*—tightening the pelvic floor muscles as if stopping the flow of urine, holding for a few seconds, and releasing—can help put them back in touch with their sexual anatomy and their sex drive.
- **Inability to achieve orgasm.** About 1 in 5 women worldwide have difficulty experiencing orgasm.[31] The problem can occur as a side effect of prescription medications, including certain antidepressants. Medical problems, relationship problems, embarrassment, or a his-

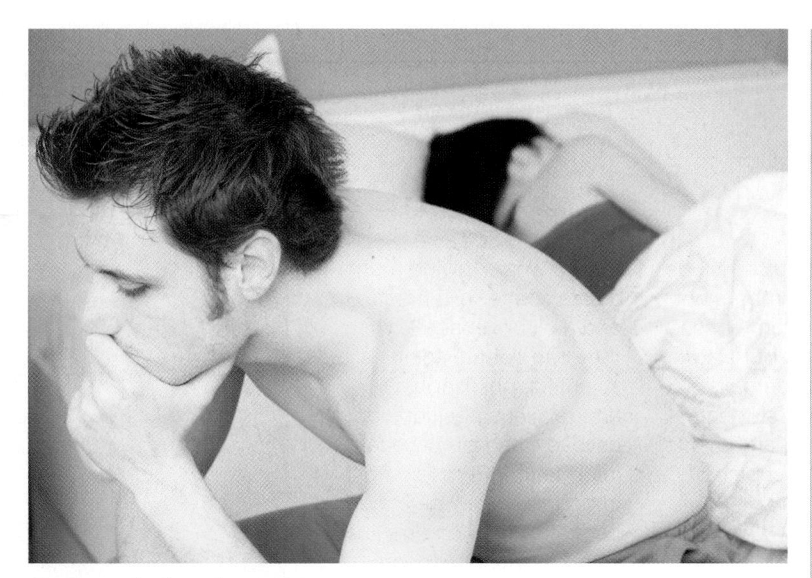

Sexual dysfunctions can occur in both men and women.

tory of sexual abuse or rape can also prevent some women from reaching orgasm. However, one common factor is simply insufficient stimulation of the clitoris. Switching sexual positions can produce more clitoral stimulation during intercourse. Masturbation or use of a vibrator during sex can also help.[31]

Male Sexual Dysfunctions

Being unable to perform sexually can be damaging to a man's self-esteem and place stress on the relationship. Problems related to male sexual function include the following:

- **Erectile dysfunction (ED)** is the inability of a man to get or maintain an erection firm enough for sexual intercourse.[32] The problem is most prevalent among older men. Erectile dysfunction most commonly results from injury or underlying disease, but it can stem from fatigue, stress, depression, use of certain medications, or excessive alcohol or tobacco use. As treatment, a physician may prescribe lifestyle modifications such as weight loss or quitting smoking. Oral medications such as Viagra, Cialis, or Levitra can help by boosting the flow of blood to the penis, enabling an erection to occur; however, they can have serious side effects and are not intended for men with certain underlying health conditions. Surgery may be recommended in cases of underlying injury, and counseling or sex therapy is also an option.
- **Premature ejaculation (PE)** is a condition in which a man ejaculates earlier than he would like to, or than his partner would like him to. In the past, sex researchers and therapists attempted to define PE based on a quantitative time frame (how long it took to ejaculate), whereas today most agree that a male has a problem when poor ejaculatory control interferes with the sexual satisfaction of one or both partners. PE can result from physical factors, but in most cases it is due to psychological factors such as anxiety. In college-aged men it frequently occurs because of lack of experience, intense arousal, and alcohol use.[33] However, hormonal imbalance, infection, nervous system disorders, and other physical causes should be ruled out if PE is chronic. Treatment of any underlying physical problem is important. In many cases, sexual counseling and incorporating into sexual activity a delaying tactic called the "squeeze technique" can resolve the problem.[34]

erectile dysfunction (ED) The inability of a male to obtain or maintain an erection.

premature ejaculation (PE) A condition in which a male ejaculates earlier than he would like to.

abstinence The avoidance of sexual intercourse.

For more information on the "squeeze technique," visit the Mayo Clinic website at www.mayoclinic.com/health/premature-ejaculation/DS00578/DSECTION=treatments-and-drugs.

Sex Therapy

For problems that persist despite following medical advice, an individual's primary care provider may recommend sex therapy, a specialized branch of psychotherapy that addresses concerns directly related to human sexuality. In most states, sex therapy is not licensed separately; however, the American Association of Sexuality Educators, Counselors, and Therapists (AASECT) certifies therapists who have met rigorous standards for the profession.[35]

The process of sex therapy is similar to that used in other branches of psychotherapy, and typically involves an initial interview, development of a treatment plan, and regularly scheduled counseling sessions. The individual or couple may be given homework such as communication exercises or changes to try during sex, depending on their unique needs.[35]

To locate a sex therapist in your area, click on the map at www.aasect.org/directory_usa.asp.

Sexual Behavior

A wide range of human sexual behaviors and interests are considered "normal." Before biologist Alfred Kinsey's research in the late 1940s and early 1950s, Americans had no basis for determining what was the norm. Kinsey's research provided a basis for social comparison and helped answer a question many people wondered about: "Who's doing what with whom and how often are they doing it?" Since Kinsey, many researchers studying this question have concluded that the continuum of "normal" sexual behavior in our society is broad and varied.

Abstinence and Celibacy

Abstinence refers to the avoidance of sexual intercourse. Whether it is by active choice or as a matter of circumstance, many people find themselves abstaining from sexual activity for extended periods of time. This long-term abstinence is referred to as *celibacy*. Some choose celibacy for religious or moral reasons; others out of a desire to avoid becoming pregnant or developing a sexually transmitted infection.[36] The **Spotlight** box takes a closer look at abstinence and celibacy among young adults.

Non-Intercourse Sexual Activity

There are a number of ways people experience sexual pleasure without actually engaging in sexual intercourse. Among them are masturbation, sexual fantasies, kissing, "outercourse," and oral sex.

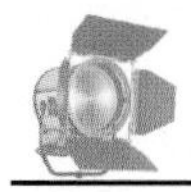

SPOTLIGHT

Celibacy: The New Sexual Revolution?

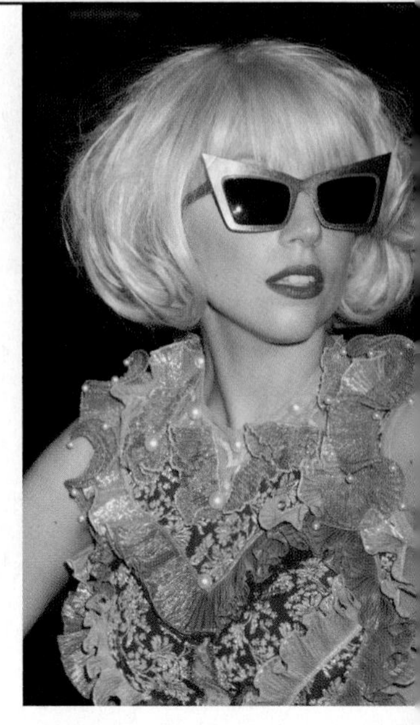
Lady Gaga

Fans worldwide were stunned in the spring of 2010, when pop star Lady Gaga announced in an interview that—despite her steamy MTV image—she was celibate. Moreover, she encouraged her fans to choose celibacy, too: "I can't believe I'm saying this—Don't have sex. It's not really cool anymore to have sex all the time. It's cooler to be strong and independent. It's okay not to have sex. It's okay to get to know people. I'm celibate. Celibacy's fine."[1]

Young people do seem to be waiting longer before having sex. The largest and most reliable government survey on sexuality in America has noted a steady decline in vaginal intercourse among never-married teens since 1988.[2] And the percentage of Americans aged 15 to 24 who said they had never had any type of sexual contact rose in the past decade from about 22% to about 28%.[2] These findings hold up among college students specifically: A national survey of college students conducted in spring 2011 found that just over 30% had never engaged in vaginal sex, and over 27% had never engaged in oral sex.[3]

At the same time, celibacy programs are increasingly visible on college campuses. The campus newspaper at the Lutheran Gustavus Adolphus College in Minnesota recently ran an article titled "Celibacy: The New Hipster Trend?" It proposed that, "On a campus where condoms are handed out like candy . . . celibacy is becoming as hip as organic coffee." But Christian colleges are not alone in reporting the trend: A 2008 *New York Times Magazine* article reported on the emergence of "abstinence clubs" at Ivy League schools, including the Anscombe Societies at Princeton University and MIT, and True Love Revolution at Harvard. The clubs include among their members not only students from conservative religions, but also so-called "new feminists" and philosophy students who use ethical arguments to ground their choice of celibacy.[4]

Not everyone agrees that celibacy is compatible with feminism—or a superior ethical choice for single adults. The movement has drawn a fair amount of controversy, with opponents claiming that the clubs perpetuate gender stereotypes that value women who are virgins and denounce those who are not. Some have accused the clubs of manipulating statistics about unplanned pregnancies and sexually transmitted infections to frighten students into celibacy.

Still, even opponents admit that the clubs provide a valuable service to students who want to abstain from sexual behavior during their college years, giving them a safe space—via meetings and a club website—where they can debate social, scientific, philosophical, and religious positions on celibacy, and simply share information. Perhaps most importantly, they give members a circle of companions who know and respect their choices. And that can mean—as Lady Gaga herself might put it—that they won't get caught in a bad romance.

References: **1.** "Lady Gaga Joins the List of Celibate Stars," by Kate Torgovnick, April 13, 2010, CNN Entertainment, retrieved from http://www.cnn.com/2010/SHOWBIZ/04/12/pro.abstinence.celebs.tf/index.html. **2.** "Sexual Behavior, Sexual Attraction, and Sexual Identity in the United States: Data from the 2006–2008 National Survey of Family Growth" by the U.S. Centers for Disease Control and Prevention (CDC), 2011, *National Health Statistics Report, 36*, March 2011, retrieved from http://www.cdc.gov/nchs/data/nhsr/nhsr036.pdf. **3.** "American College Health Association-National College Health Assessment (ACHA-NCHA II) Reference Group Executive Summary, Spring 2011" by the American College Health Association, 2011, retrieved from http://www.achancha.org/docs/ACHA-NCHA-II_ReferenceGroup_ExecutiveSummary_Spring2011.pdf. **4.** "Students of Virginity" by Randall Patterson, March 30, 2008, *New York Times*, retrieved from http://www.nytimes.com/2008/03/30/magazine/30Chastity-t.html.

Fantasy and Masturbation

Sexual fantasies are sexual or romantic thoughts, daydreams, and imagined scenarios that can be very detailed and explicit, featuring fictional characters or actual people. They may reflect a person's unconscious desires, allowing the person to imagine sexual experiences that they may not feel comfortable acting out in real life.

Masturbation is the manipulation of one's own genitals for sexual pleasure. Masturbation is a healthy and common expression of sexuality. Research indicates that 92% of male college students and nearly half (48%) of female college students have masturbated.[37]

"Outercourse" and Oral Sex

Although the definition can vary, **outercourse** generally refers to sexual intimacy without penetration of the vagina or anus. Outercourse includes everything from kissing and "making out" to manual stimulation of the genitals and mutual masturbation. Because no semen enters the vagina during outercourse, there is no risk of pregnancy. The risk of sexually transmitted infections is also minimized, although infections like herpes and HPV can still spread through simple skin-to-skin contact of the genitals.

masturbation Manipulation of one's own genitals for sexual pleasure.

outercourse Sexual intimacy without penetration of the vagina or anus.

oral sex Stimulation of the genitals by the tongue or mouth.

fellatio Oral stimulation of the penis.

cunnilingus Oral stimulation of the vulva or clitoris.

Oral sex is the stimulation of the genitals by the tongue or mouth. **Fellatio** is oral stimulation of the penis, and **cunnilingus** is oral stimulation of the vulva or clitoris. Some couples use oral sex as *foreplay,* stimulation that is erotic and is intended to increase arousal prior to sexual intercourse. Others engage in oral sex in place of sexual intercourse. Still others avoid the practice. Although oral sex does not result in pregnancy, it is not necessarily "safe" sex. Unprotected oral sex can leave a partner vulnerable to the transmission of herpes, syphilis, hepatitis B, and gonorrhea. Using a condom or dental dam during oral sex can help prevent the spread of sexually transmitted infections.

"Sexting"

Sexting is the use of cell phones or similar electronic devices to send sexually explicit text, photos, or videos. In a recent study, 20% of teens and 33% of young adults reported sending or posting nude or semi-nude photos or videos of themselves. In addition, 39% of teens and 59% of young adults reported they are sending or posting sexually suggestive messages. One-third of male teens and one-fourth of female teens report receiving nude or semi-nude images that were originally meant to be private.[38]

Sexting most frequently occurs in one of three circumstances:

- Exchanges of images only between two romantically involved partners.
- Exchanges between partners and shared outside the relationship.
- Exchanges involving people who are not in a relationship, but at least one of them hopes to be.[39]

Many states are enacting legislation to regulate sexting. Arizona passed a bill in March 2010 making it a class two misdemeanor for minors to possess or send sexually explicit text messages to another minor.[40] This law sets an important precedent because it is specific to the offense. Before its passage, prosecutors could only use child pornography laws, which were written long before the development of wireless technologies and were thus difficult to apply. It is likely that the new bill will prompt more research into and regulation of sexting among minors.

Do you have questions about sex that you are afraid to ask? *Go Ask Alice* is a website sponsored by Columbia University that answers many frequently asked questions: www.goaskalice.columbia.edu.

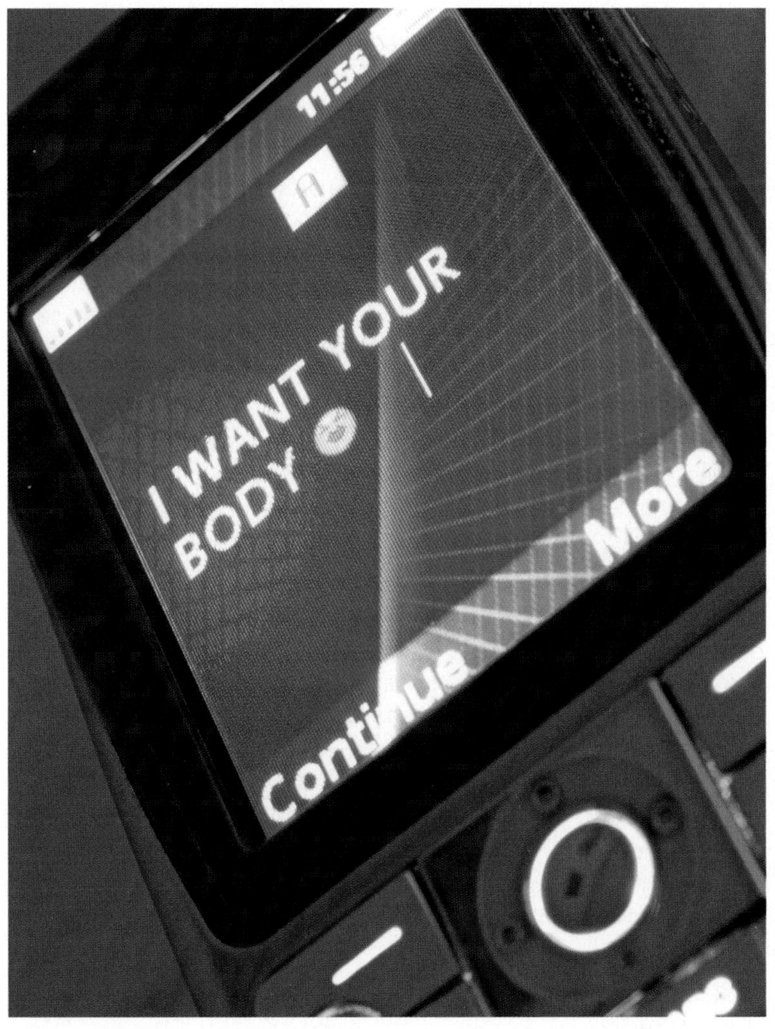

"Sexting" can leave you vulnerable to privacy breaches and embarrassment.

Sexual Intercourse

Sexual intercourse, or *coitus,* is sexual union involving genital penetration. For many heterosexuals, the term is synonymous with **vaginal intercourse,** the insertion of the penis into the vagina. Unless they are trying to conceive, couples engaging in vaginal intercourse are encouraged to practice "safe sex." The use of condoms is advised to avoid unintended pregnancy while reducing the couple's risk for sexually transmitted infection.

Long considered a taboo in U.S. society, **anal intercourse** has increasingly become accepted, especially among younger generations. About 32% of men and 30% of women aged 20–24 have had anal sex with a partner of the opposite sex.[1] The practice involves penile penetration of the anus and rectum. Because the tissues lining these organs are thinner and more fragile than those of the vagina, anal intercourse is the riskiest sexual behavior in terms of both injury and transmission of infectious disease. It represents one of the primary risk factors for acquiring HIV, the virus that causes AIDS, and is also associated with the spread of syphilis and gonorrhea. Latex condoms should be used, but they are more likely to tear during anal sex.

Paraphilias

What happens in the bedroom between consenting adults—as long as it doesn't involve physical or emotional harm—is their private concern. Many couples enjoy experimenting with sexual massage, erotic videos, vibrators and other sex toys, role-playing (nurse-patient, teacher-student, etc.), cross-dressing, story-telling, and other behaviors. Such experimentation is normal, and can even enhance intimacy between the partners. In contrast, **paraphilias** are psychiatric disorders in which individuals have sexual fantasies or urges or engage in sexual behaviors involving objects, nonconsenting adults, or children, or experiences involving suffering or humiliation.[41] People with paraphilias find it difficult or impossible to become sexually excited in the absence of their chosen stimulus. Of the following examples, many constitute criminal behavior:

- *Fetishism* involves looking at, touching, or smelling an object (called a *fetish*) while masturbating. Commonly the fetish is a woman's undergarment or pair of shoes, which a consenting adult agrees to wear during sex.

sexting The use of cell phones or similar electronic devices to send sexually explicit text, photos, or videos.

vaginal intercourse Intercourse characterized by the insertion of the penis into the vagina.

anal intercourse Intercourse characterized by the insertion of the penis into a partner's anus and rectum.

paraphilia Any of a variety psychiatric disorders in which the individual's sexual fantasies, urges, or behaviors involve objects, nonconsenting adults, children, or experiences involving suffering or humiliation.

- *Voyeurism* is, essentially, spying on someone for sexual gratification. The vulnerability of the person being observed, the likelihood that he or she would experience humiliation if the spying were discovered, and the potential for being caught in the act increase the individual's excitement. Ogling a sunbather on a beach would not be considered criminal conduct; however, voyeurism is a criminal act if it occurs in a place where the person being observed would have a reasonable expectation of privacy.
- *Exhibitionism* is exposure of the individual's genitals to an unsuspecting stranger. Sometimes the individual masturbates during the act. Commonly called "flashing," exhibitionism is a form of indecent exposure, and is illegal.
- *Masochism* is the achievement of sexual gratification by engaging in fantasies or acts that involve being humiliated or abused. In contrast, *sadism* is the achievement of sexual gratification by causing psychological or physical suffering to another. Although it can sometimes occur in sex games between consenting adults, at its most extreme, sadism can involve abuse, rape, torture, or even murder.
- *Pedophilia* is sexual contact—whether voyeurism, fondling, or sexual intercourse—with children. Any form is a criminal act. About two-thirds of victims are girls.[41]

Of the variety of treatments for paraphilias, none has proven highly successful; however, clinicians may prescribe drugs that reduce the individual's sex drive, antidepressants, or other medications, as well as psychotherapy.[41]

Sex for Sale

The commercial sex industry presents a fundamental paradox: Its billions of dollars in annual sales suggest widespread popularity, yet its legal status and ethics are the subject of continual and intense debate. Commercial sex includes stripping, lap dancing, phone sex, computer sex (called cyber sex), and other enterprises; however, here we focus on pornography and prostitution.

Pornography

Pornography is explicit sexual material that is used for sexual excitement and erotic stimulation. The pornography industry is big business: In 2006 alone, the revenues topped $96 billion. Porn can be found in a host of media, including sculpture, painting, books, magazines, photos, animation, film, and video games; however, the two top revenue generators are video sales and rentals, and Internet sites. Of all websites, approximately 12% (4.2 million) are pornographic, and 25% of all search engine requests (68 million) are related to pornography.[42]

A study conducted by East Carolina University found that 43% of college students reported looking at pornography at least once or twice a week. Almost 32% of college men reported viewing pornography three to five times per week, whereas less than 4% of women reported doing so. The findings from this study also suggest that the Internet is the primary source of pornography for college students.[43]

Along with commercial pornography websites, there has been an increase in noncommercial sites where visitors can post their own photos and videos. Some of these sites are devoted to college students and are referred to as "dorm porn." Some experts contend that both sexting and noncommercial pornographic websites reflect a larger trend toward digital self-exploitation.[44]

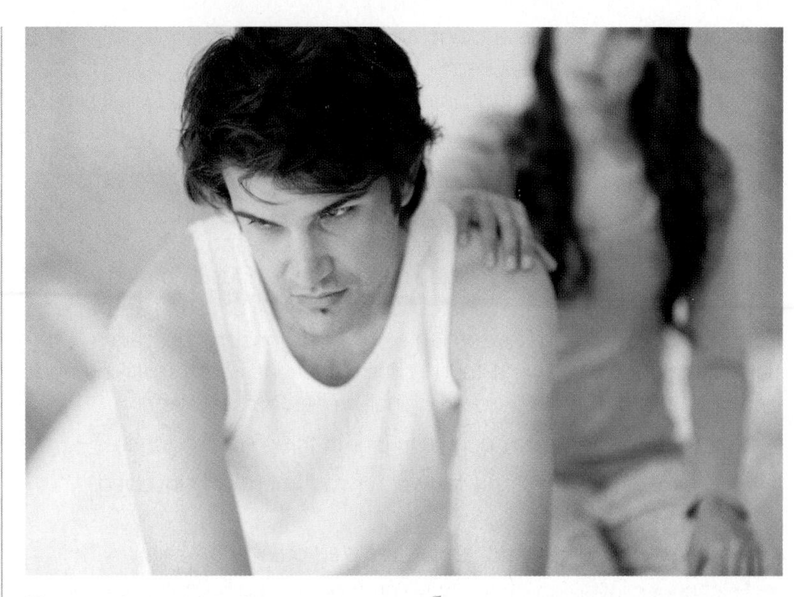

Excessive use of **pornography** can interfere with relationships in real life.

In the East Carolina University study, men expressed greater approval of pornography, and women reported feeling more threatened by it. Is there anything behind these concerns? Here are some observations from a 2005 Senate Judiciary Committee hearing on pornography.[45]

Effects on Users

Looking at porn wastes time: Studies are delayed or cut short, work is interrupted, and relationships are put on hold. It also wastes money: Once users become "acclimated" to free sites, they move to expensive services. Porn has addictive elements, claiming increasing amounts of time and money, interfering with activities of daily living, goals, and relationships, and involving a sense of compulsion. Particularly on the Internet, users find themselves turning more and more often to increasingly violent and shocking images, including those involving torture or children. Many users report feeling increasingly debased by their porn use; images that once would have disgusted them come to seem "routine," and ever harder-core porn becomes a requirement for sexual arousal.

Effects on Relationships

Porn is essentially a form of voyeurism, involving looking at but not interacting with the model or actor. As such, it elevates the physical—body parts and acts—while ignoring all other qualities that make us human. Viewers learn to relate to others as objects rather than to form and maintain relationships with them. Not surprisingly, porn reduces the viewer's ability to be close to others—including their current partner. Many find that their sex lives deteriorate and their relationships collapse. In a 2004 poll, one in four divorced respondents said Internet pornography and chat had contributed to the breakup. Some psychologists view pornography use as a hallmark of disconnection and a risk factor for developing a true intimacy disorder.

pornography Explicit sexual material used for sexual excitement and erotic stimulation.

prostitution (also called *sex work*) The act of engaging in sexual activity for payment.

Prostitution

Prostitution (sex work) is the act of engaging in sexual activity for payment—typically money, but sometimes drugs or other goods. Like porn, it is a global industry with a varying legal status. In the United States, prostitution is legal only in certain counties in Nevada, which employ approximately 1,000 prostitutes. In addition, an estimated 200,000 to 300,000 U.S. and foreign-born children are trafficked as prostitutes in the United States.[46] These children typically have been abandoned by or have run away from abusive families, or are recruited into prostitution by forced abduction, pressure from parents, or deceptive agreements between parents and traffickers. The average age at which girls first become victims of prostitution is 12–14.[46]

Increasing evidence points to involvement in the sex industry among college students.[47] In the past decade, media reports have surfaced about student sex work in American and European colleges and universities. A 2010 study of undergraduates at a London university gathered data on the students' financial and employment circumstances and their views on participation in sex work. Results suggested not only a widespread awareness of student sex work, but also an understanding that those who engaged in it did so because of their financial situation. Despite the enormous risks—rape, beating, torture, and murder, as well as sexually transmitted infection, unplanned pregnancy, and psychologic stress and trauma—a relatively high proportion of students (16.5%) indicated that they would be willing to engage in sex work to pay for their education.[47]

Should sex work be legalized? Proponents argue that legalization removes the criminal element and thus protects women and children. Opponents of legalization point out that, in countries where prostitution is legal, sex industries are larger and create a demand for more prostitutes, thereby acting as a magnet for traffickers. Indeed, legalization can actually promote the growth of a parallel illegal sex industry fed by women and children who have been abducted or deceived into it. For example, since 1999, there have been reports that at least 80% of women in Dutch legal prostitution had been trafficked. In 2009, the Dutch government closed approximately two-thirds of the legal brothels in Amsterdam because of its inability to control traffickers and other organized crime.[48]

Sexual Orientation and Gender Identity

At a very early age, humans begin to develop their **sexual orientation,** their romantic and physical attraction toward others. Experts believe that our natural tendency to be attracted to men or women—or both—is shaped by a confluence of biological, environmental, and cognitive factors, with sexual orientation being neither a conscious choice nor something that can be readily changed.

Sex researcher Alfred Kinsey theorized that sexual orientation could be delineated on one basic continuum, broken down into seven parts. At one end of the Kinsey Scale are **heterosexuals,** "straight" people sexually attracted to or engaging in sexual relations with a member of the opposite sex. On the other end are **homosexuals,** *gays* or *lesbians* who are attracted to or engaging in sexual relations with people of the same sex. In the middle are **bisexuals,** individuals who are attracted to or engaging in sexual relations with members of their own sex as well as the opposite sex. Recently, the term *multisexual* has emerged among people who refuse to identify themselves as straight, gay, or bisexual.

sexual orientation Romantic and physical attraction toward others.

heterosexuals People who are sexually attracted to partners of the opposite sex.

homosexuals People who are sexually attracted to partners of the same sex.

bisexuals People who are attracted to partners of both the same and the opposite sex.

homophobia The irrational fear of, aversion to, or discrimination against homosexuals or homosexuality.

Heterosexuality

Throughout the world, the majority of people describe themselves as heterosexual. This is true in the United States as well: Almost 94% of women and 96% of men aged 18–44 identified themselves as heterosexual in a 2011 government survey.[1] Intriguingly, the same survey found that only 82.4% of women and 91.7% of men reported they are attracted exclusively to members of the opposite sex; many who are strictly heterosexual in their behavior report being attracted "mostly" but not exclusively to members of the opposite sex.

Heterosexuality is the only sexual orientation that receives full social and legal legitimacy in most countries, including the United States. As a result of this and other cultural factors, homosexuals and bisexuals can be subjected to "heterosexism," a system of negative attitudes, bias, and discrimination in favor of heterosexual relationships. Those with a heterosexist view think that their orientation is the only "normal" one.

Homosexuality

In 2011, 11.7% of females and 4.3% of males aged 15 to 44 reported having had at least one same-sex partner in the past year. However, only 1.4% of women and 1.8% of men say they are attracted mostly or only to members of the same sex.[1] These statistics may be artificially low, due to under-reporting of same-sex attraction because of fear of stigmatization.

Homosexuality is deep-rooted in many world cultures, having been an accepted practice in some parts of the ancient world. In other regions it has been and is still shunned. For example, in some countries, homosexuality is considered a mental illness, and in many others, it is a crime punishable by imprisonment or even death.

The American Psychiatric Association removed homosexuality from its manual of psychiatric disorders in 1973, in response to a growing understanding of homosexuality as an entirely normal sexual orientation. Correspondingly, there has been an increasing acceptance of homosexuality in U.S. culture. For example, in a 1973 survey, 70% of people in the United States reported believing that homosexual relations are always sinful; but in 2009, only 49% expressed this belief.[49] In 1992, only one Fortune 500 company offered health insurance benefits to domestic partners. By 2006, that number had grown to 253.[50]

Still, many gays and lesbians continue to face discrimination and harassment in the United States, a fact acknowledged by 64% of the population.[49] **Homophobia** is the irrational fear of, aversion to, or discrimination against homosexuals or homosexuality. The harassment often begins at an early age. In one survey of Massachusetts youths, researchers found that twice as many homosexual and bisexual students as heterosexual students reported being threatened or injured with a weapon at their public high school that year.[51] They were also twice as likely to have skipped school in the previous

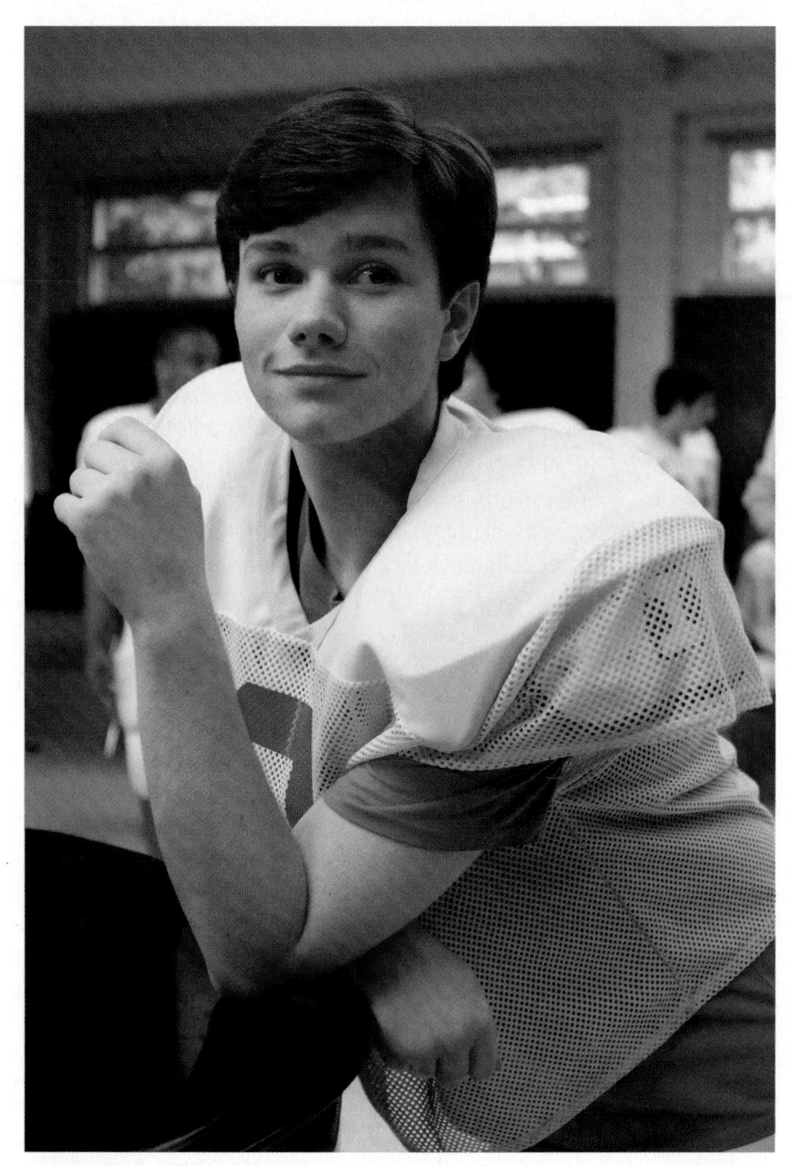

On the hit show **Glee,** the character of Kurt is an openly gay teen. Gay characters on TV reflect the increasing acceptance of homosexuality in the United States.

month out of a concern for their own safety. In another study, 92% of homosexual and bisexual students in middle and high school said they frequently were subjected to homophobic remarks and slurs, with some of the derogatory expressions even being uttered by faculty or staff.[52] Homophobia sometimes erupts into criminal violence: In 2008, the FBI reported more than 1,200 incidents of hate crimes against homosexuals.[53]

Bisexuality

One rigid definition of bisexuality is having romantic or sexual relations with people of the same and opposite gender. Yet some bisexuals choose not to act on their innate impulses, while others have not had the opportunity to do so. A better gauge of bisexuality is having an attraction to both men and women. In the United States, 15.3% of women and 4.9% of men report such attraction.[1]

The intensity of bisexual attraction can fluctuate over time, but bisexuality should not be seen as a "phase" that a person is going through. In one long-term study of bisexual women, the subjects reported being attracted to both sexes throughout the 10-year study period.[54] Bisexuality, the experts wrote, is a "stable identity" rather than a "transitional stage."

Transgenderism and Transsexuality

Whereas the term *sex* refers to an individual's biological status as male or female, *gender* includes the ways people act, interact, and feel about themselves. **Transgenderism** is the condition in which someone's *gender identity* (sense of him- or herself as male or female) or gender expression is different from his or her *assigned sex*. Sex assignment occurs at birth—as long as a baby is born with typical male or female external genitalia. The term *transgenderism* is not used in cases when an infant is born with ambiguous genitalia. This condition is known as a *disorder of sexual development*, and in such cases, sex assignment is delayed until genetic and hormonal testing is conducted.

Once assigned, sex usually becomes a profound component of a growing child's gender identity. But for some people, the sex they have been assigned and the gender they identify with differ. The American Psychological Association states that "Anyone whose identity, appearance, or behavior falls outside of conventional gender norms can be described as transgender. However, not everyone whose appearance or behavior is gender-atypical will identify as a transgender person."[55]

Transsexuals are transgender individuals who live, usually full time, as the gender opposite to their assigned sex. Female-to-male (FTM) transsexuals are biological females who now live as males, while male-to-female (MTF) transsexuals are the opposite. Some choose to have hormonal treatments and surgical procedures to complete the physical transformation from one sex to the other. Others may *cross-dress*, adopting the clothing, hairstyle, and other aspects of appearance of the opposite sex. That said, cross-dressers, also known as *transvestites*, are a diverse group; many people who engage in cross-dressing identify with their assigned gender.

Watch videos of lesbian, gay, bisexual, and transgender individuals struggling with acceptance—or upload a video of your own—at the international It Gets Better website at www.itgetsbetter.org.

Change Yourself, Change Your World

Healthy sexuality requires not only caring for your reproductive system, but also accepting and supporting your sexual orientation, preferences, and values—and those of your peers.

Personal Choices

We've presented a lot of facts about sexuality—but how do you integrate cold facts with the complex desires you feel every day of your real life? And how do you make sure that the decisions you make about whether, when, and with whom to have sex are aligned with your goals and your dreams?

Know What You Want

The first step is to clarify what you want—and that requires you to distinguish your own values from

transgenderism The state in which someone's gender identity or gender expression is different from his or her assigned sex at birth.

transsexual A transgendered individual who lives as the gender opposite to her or his assigned sex.

SELF-ASSESSMENT

Take this self-assessment online at www.pearsonhighered.com/lynchelmore.

Are You and Your Partner Ready for Sex?

Maybe you've only been on two dates. Maybe you've been "just friends" for two years. But sooner or later, the question is going to demand an answer: Are the two of you ready for your relationship to become sexual? Here are some questions that can help you decide.

1. Is your decision to have sex completely your own? (that is, you feel no pressure from others, including your partner)
   yes no
2. Is your decision to have sex based on the right reasons? (The **wrong reasons** are peer pressure, a need to fit in or make your partner happy, or a belief that sex will make your relationship with your partner better, or closer. If you decide to have sex, it **should be** because you feel emotionally and physically ready and your partner is someone you love, trust, and respect.)
   yes no
3. Do you feel your partner would respect any decision you made about whether to have sex or not?
   yes no
4. Do you trust and respect your partner?
   yes no
5. Are you able to comfortably talk to your partner about sex and your partner's sexual history?
   yes no
6. Do you know how to prevent pregnancy and STIs?
   yes no
7. Are you and your partner willing to use contraception to prevent pregnancy and STIs?
   yes no
8. Have you and your partner talked about what both of you would do in the event of pregnancy or if one of you were to develop an STI?
   yes no
9. Do you feel completely comfortable with the idea of having sex with this partner?
   yes no

HOW TO INTERPRET YOUR SCORE

If you answered **No** to **any** of these questions, you are not really ready for sex. If you think you should have sexual intercourse because others want you to or everyone else is doing it, these are not the right reasons. You should only decide to have sex because you trust and respect your partner, you know the possible risks, you know how to protect yourself against the risks, and most importantly, because you know that you are ready!

Source: "Quiz: Are You Ready for Sex?" © 2010 by the Center for Young Women's Health at Children's Hospital, Boston. All rights reserved. Used with permission. www.youngwomenshealth.org.

those of the people around you. Start by listing every question you can think of related to sexuality: whether or not to be sexually active, types of behaviors to engage in, sexual orientation, use of contraception, etc. Now ask yourself: What do your parents think? What does your religion (if any) teach? What do college administrators say? The media? Your peers? Your closest friends? How do these messages differ, and is there a way to negotiate those differences? Finally, write down a response that feels most authentically your own.

This process of clarification may take some time, but any important decision in life deserves careful consideration. What's more, thinking through your values now—and putting them in writing—will help you avoid impulsive behavior that you may regret tomorrow.

What if the most urgent question in your mind right now is whether or not you're ready for a current friendship to become sexual? For help coming up with an answer, see the **Self-Assessment: Are You and Your Partner Ready for Sex?**

Communicate

Once you've clarified your sexual values and preferences for yourself, the next essential step is to communicate them . . . ideally, way before becoming sexually involved. So how do you get up the nerve to talk candidly about sex? See **Practical Strategies for Health: Communicating Effectively About Sex.**

Protect Yourself

Each year, there are more than 15 million sexually transmitted infections (STIs) among people in the United States, and well over 1 million terminations of unintended pregnancies.[56] Given these statistics, it seems obvious that—if you're sexually active—you should consistently practice safe sex. If you engage in sexual activity, insist on using a condom and—whether you're male or female—learn how to use it properly. See your health-care provider at least annually and make sure to fully discuss your sexual activity, method of birth control, and measures for protecting against STIs. If you're a woman, make sure you follow your health-care provider's advice on how often to have a pelvic exam with a Pap test.

If you drink alcohol, avoid intoxication. As we noted earlier, intoxication dramatically increases your chances of having a sexual encounter you'll later regret—including one leading to pregnancy or an STI.

STUDENT STORY

Pressured into Sex

"Hi, I'm Monique, and yes, I have been pressured into having sex and it's really, really stressful, especially if you have someone that you really like and he's telling you 'well you should do it now' and 'if you really like me . . .' It causes you to be in a position where you don't want to lose this person, you really want him to like you as much as you like him, but it's really not the best idea. It gets you into other situations that you might think you're ready for, but you're really not, as far as pregnancy or if you don't know how to use condoms, you can contract an STI. To a student who may feel pressured to have sex, I say wait until you're really ready and make sure you have all the information you need."

1: What would you say if someone were trying to pressure you into sex and you didn't feel ready for it?

2: What type of information would you need before you had sex with someone for the first time?

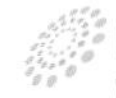

Do you have a story similar to Monique's? Share your story at www.pearsonhighered.com/lynchelmore.

Practical Strategies for Health

Communicating Effectively About Sex

If you're thinking about beginning a sexual relationship with someone, it's important to be able to communicate effectively about topics like sexual history, sexual health, contraceptive preferences, and how comfortable you each are with different types of sexual activity. If you aren't ready to talk honestly with a prospective partner about sex, take that as a sign that you're not ready for sex. If you are ready to have the conversation, here are some strategies:

- **Do some preparation.** Jot down thoughts, concerns, and questions in advance (see the **Choosing to Change Worksheet** at the end of the chapter). For instance, it's important to know your partner's sexual history. What can you do to feel more comfortable asking about it? Rehearsing the words in advance doesn't commit you to following a script, but it can help you frame your message in the moment with greater ease, clarity, and sensitivity.
- **Agree on a time and place to talk.** Once you're secure about the content of the conversation you want to have, set aside a time when you're both relaxed and not distracted, and a place that's comfortable and private. You might want to tell your partner that there are some things you'd like to talk about, and suggest that the two of you go for a walk together.
- **Express your questions, concerns, and desires from a personal perspective.** Use "I" statements consistently, as in, "I'd like to know about your sexual history, and I will be honest in sharing mine." Pay attention to your partner's responses. Take in not only the words used, but your partner's body language as well.
- **Near the end of the conversation, recap any decisions you've mutually made.** Include steps that you'll take, such as, "Okay, so tomorrow we'll both schedule appointments at the campus health center to get screened for STIs."

Source: Adapted from *Tips to Talk to Your Partner About Sex* by the Society of Obstetricians and Gynaecologists of Canada, 2006, retrieved from http://www.sexualityandu.ca/adults/tips-1.aspx#.

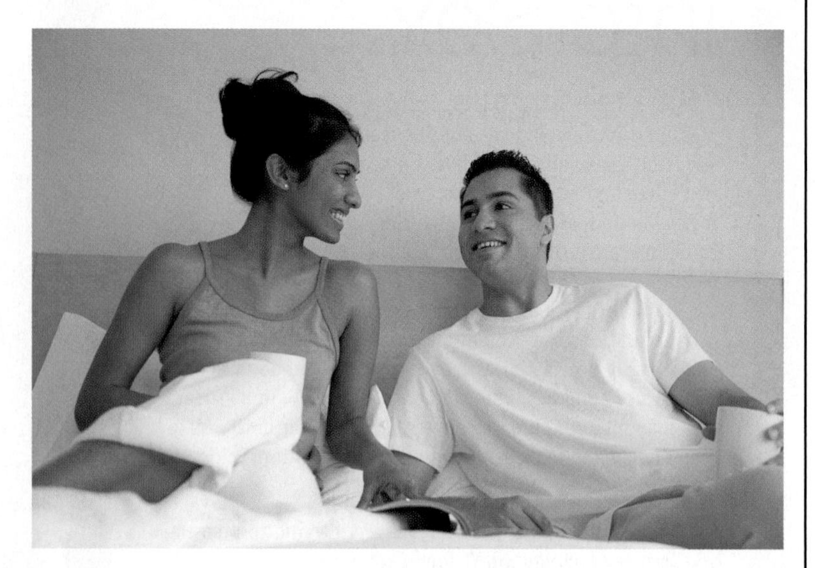

Campus Advocacy

"I've always felt that sexuality is a really slippery thing. In this day and age, it tends to get categorized and labeled, and I think labels are for food. Canned food." –Michael Stipe, lead vocalist for the rock band R.E.M.

How can we avoid the trap of labeling ourselves or others based on our sexual histories, desires, behaviors, or orientation? How can we develop tolerance in ourselves and promote tolerance among others in our community? Different methods have arisen on different college campuses across the United States. Here are just a few ideas:

- Over 200 U.S. colleges and universities have programs fostering alliances among heterosexual and LGBT students. These programs typically have names such as Safe Zone, Safe Space, Safe Harbor, and Safe On Campus. The hallmark of these "Safe" programs is the public identification of "allies" by placing a "Safe" symbol—usually a pink triangle or a rainbow—on doors or walls of offices or living spaces.
- Campus Tolerance was founded in 2002 to combat anti-Semitism on college campuses. Subsequently, its mission broadened to fight all intolerance on campus, including anti-women, anti-gay, and other forms. Among many activities, they've established a Tolerance Rating for Universities. Find out more at the organization's Facebook page.
- CollegeTown is a diversity immersion program modeled after the National Conference for Community and Justice's (NCCJ) AnyTown high school program. In this four-day/three-night retreat, students explore issues of discrimination, including racism, sexism, and homophobia, as well as ways to build community. CollegeTown graduates return to their campuses empowered to act as leaders, promoting respect for all. To see how it works, check out the CollegeTown group at Arizona State University, Tempe, on Facebook.

Watch videos of real students discussing sexuality at www.pearsonhighered.com/lynchelmore.

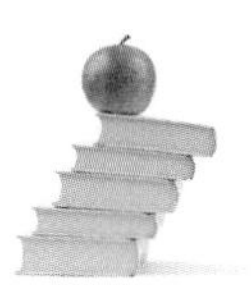

Choosing to Change Worksheet

To complete this worksheet online, visit **www.pearsonhighered.com/lynchelmore.**

A *sexual relationship* involves two people who mutually consent to participate in sexual acts such as kissing, stroking, rubbing, or intercourse. Such relationships can be sources of pleasure, happiness, and joy, or of pain, sadness, disappointment, and health risks. No respectful partner uses pressure or force to engage in sexual relationships. According to the National Guidelines Task Force, a *sexually healthy relationship* is consensual, nonexploitative, honest, mutually pleasurable, safe, and protected from unwanted pregnancy, STIs, and other harm. In a sexually healthy relationship, both partners have a right to be fully informed and a responsibility to be fully honest when it comes to making choices about sexual activity.

Directions: Fill in your stage of behavior change in Step 1 and then complete the step that applies to your stage of change.

Step 1: Your Stage of Behavior Change. Please check one of the following statements that best describes your current behavior when it comes to participating in a sexual relationship.

_____________ I do not intend to participate in a sexual relationship in the next 6 months. (Precontemplation)

_____________ I might participate in a sexual relationship in the next 6 months. (Contemplation)

_____________ I am prepared to participate in a sexually healthy relationship in the next month. (Preparation)

_____________ I have been in sexually healthy relationship for less than 6 months. (Action)

_____________ I have been in a sexually healthy relationship for more than 6 months and want to maintain it. (Maintenance)

Step 2: Precontemplation or Contemplation Stages. If you are currently abstaining from sex, you may be happy with this choice at this stage in your life. This is perfectly normal, healthy, and smart. However, to avoid peer pressure, it may be important to clarify and communicate why you are abstaining. Many college women and men abstain from sex for various reasons, including preventing pregnancy and STIs; waiting until they're ready or waiting to find the right partner; focusing on school, career, or extracurricular activities; and for personal, moral, or religious beliefs and values. Write down all the reasons you are currently abstinent.

____

____

____

____

It also helps to understand your own values. Based on your reasons for being abstinent, compare your answers with (1) what your parents and family think, (2) what your close friends and peers think, (3) what your health-care providers and educators think, and (4) what is depicted by the mass media. What level of influence does each of these four groups have on your reasons?

____

____

____

____

Step 3: Preparation Stage. If you are currently in an intimate, mature relationship and wondering whether or not you're ready for it to become sexual, take the Self-Assessment on page 429. If you answered **No** to any of the nine questions, you and your partner are *not* ready for a sexual relationship. If you answered yes to each of the questions, then it is important to talk to your partner in advance, even if you think you already know how each other feels. Write down your answers to the following questions:

What's important for you to talk about before you have sex?

____

How do you think your relationship might change if you and your partner have sex?

____

What are your feelings about wanting to be sexually exclusive with your partner versus having multiple sexual partners?

____

What do you think about the different birth control methods available to you?

____

What do you think about how partners share costs and responsibilities related to birth control?

____

Share your answers from Step 3 with the person with whom you are in an intimate, mature relationship and discuss them. How do your feelings compare or differ?

____

____

____

Step 4: Action or Maintenance Stages. If you are currently in a sexual relationship, is the relationship healthy, based on the definition stated at the beginning of this Worksheet? If yes, describe why you feel this way. If not, describe why you feel this way and how you plan to deal with this concern.

____

____

____

____

____

____

____

____

Chapter Summary

- Students engage in sexual activity for physical and emotional reasons, as well as insecurity and goal achievement. Intoxication is strongly associated with the decision to have sex and to participate in risky sex, and significantly increases the risk of unplanned pregnancy or a sexually transmitted infection.
- Male and female sexual anatomy includes both external and internal organs. Among the female organs are the paired ovaries, one of which releases an egg cell monthly, and the uterus, where a fertilized egg implants and grows. Among the male organs are the paired testes, which constantly manufacture sperm—the male reproductive cells—that travel through a series of ducts to contribute to the man's semen.
- Puberty is a 2–3-year period of transition from childhood to adolescence, during which reproduction becomes possible.
- The menstrual cycle is an approximately monthly series of events in a nonpregnant woman of childbearing age. These events, which include the buildup and shedding of the uterine lining, are controlled by hormones, which simultaneously coordinate the maturation and release of an egg cell from a woman's ovary.
- Sex research suggests that, even today, sexual attraction is powerfully influenced by the evolutionary drive to reproduce.
- The Masters and Johnson model of human sexual response consists of a series of four phases including excitement, plateau, orgasm, and resolution. Its relevance, particularly for women, has been challenged by researchers who suggest that a woman's response is typically more indirect and complex.
- Sexual dysfunction is fairly prevalent in the United States, with a sizable portion of men and women having difficulty enjoying sex at some point in their lives.
- Abstinence is the avoidance of sexual intercourse.
- Sexual behavior includes much more than just sexual intercourse, with hugging, kissing, masturbation, and other forms of non-intercourse sexual activity all being a healthy part of a sexually active lifestyle.
- Pornography is viewed at least weekly by 43% of college students; however, its use costs time and money, can become addictive, and is a form of voyeurism that can be emotionally damaging to the user and to his or her relationships.
- In the United States, prostitution is illegal except in certain counties of the state of Nevada; however, hundreds of thousands of children are illegally trafficked as prostitutes, and—despite a variety of serious risks—some college students engage in sex work to pay for their education.
- Most researchers believe that sexual orientation is neither a conscious choice nor something that can be readily changed. In the United States, about 1.4% of women and 1.8% of men say they are attracted mostly or only to members of the same sex (homosexuality); another 15.3% of women and 4.9% of men report attraction to both men and women (bisexuality).
- Healthy sexuality requires that you know what you want, communicate your values to others, and protect yourself from unintended pregnancy and sexually transmitted infections.
- Across the United States, students are working to promote tolerance on issues of gender and sexual orientation and expression.

Test Your Knowledge

1. Fertilization of a woman's ovum with a man's sperm typically occurs in the
   a. vagina.
   b. ovary.
   c. fallopian tube.
   d. uterus.

2. What is a woman's first period called?
   a. menstruation
   b. ovulation
   c. menarche
   d. menopause

3. Which of the following structures manufactures sperm?
   a. glans penis
   b. epididymis
   c. vas deferens
   d. testes

4. What is the name for the last phase of the Masters and Johnson model of sexual response?
   a. finality
   b. resolution
   c. conclusion
   d. climax

Get Critical

What happened

On September 22, 2010, 18-year-old Tyler Clementi leapt to his death from the George Washington Bridge connecting New York and New Jersey. Clementi, a talented violinist, was a freshman at Rutgers University. Shortly before his death, Clementi learned that his roommate and another classmate had secretly used a webcam to watch him having a sexual encounter with another man and Tweeted about it, inviting friends to watch a future encounter live over the Internet. The case received national attention, sparking debates about online privacy and the social pressures felt by gay teens. Clementi's roommate was convicted of a hate crime for his actions.

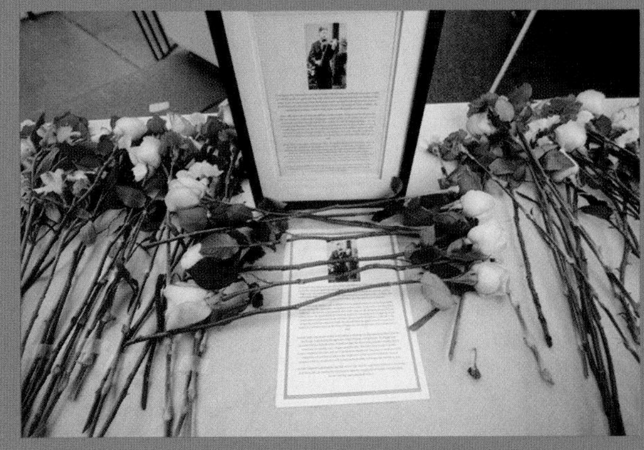

A memorial for Tyler Clementi.

What do you think?

- What can communities do to provide more support for gay, bisexual, or questioning teens?
- Do you consider Clementi's classmates' actions a hate crime? Why or why not?

5. Which of the following statements about oral sex is true?
   a. It is a form of safe sex.
   b. It is a form of outercourse.
   c. It is a form of masturbation.
   d. It is a form of sexual intercourse.

6. The act of spying on someone for sexual gratification is called
   a. voyeurism.
   b. fetishism.
   c. exhibitionism.
   d. sadism.

7. Which of the following is true about prostitution?
   a. It is illegal throughout the United States.
   b. Most prostitutes first engage in the activity around age 18–20.
   c. It is a victimless crime.
   d. Legalization can increase trafficking of women and children into illegal sex work.

8. In the United States, the percentages of people who say they are sexually attracted to both men and women are
   a. about 5% of women and 1.5% of men.
   b. about 10% of women and 3% of men.
   c. about 15% of women and 5% of men.
   d. about 20% of women and 7.5% of men.

9. Which of the following describes a transgender individual?
   a. a person whose assigned sex differs from the gender he or she identifies with
   b. a person born with both male and female genitalia
   c. a person who is about equally attracted to both males and females
   d. a person who adopts the clothing and other aspects of appearance of the opposite sex

10. Which of the following is important in protecting your sexual health?
   a. Avoid intoxication.
   b. Have regular health-care exams.
   c. Practice safe sex.
   d. Do all of the above.

Get Connected

Mobile Tips!

Scan this QR code with your mobile device to access additional tips about healthy sexuality. Or, via your mobile device, go to **http://mobiletips.pearsoncmg.com** and navigate to Chapter 15.

Health Online Visit the following websites for further information about the topics in this chapter:

- Planned Parenthood
  www.plannedparenthood.org
- WomensHealth.gov
  www.womenshealth.gov
- StayTeen.org: Waiting
  www.stayteen.org/waiting
- Go Ask Alice (advice about sexuality and sexual health)
  www.goaskalice.columbia.edu

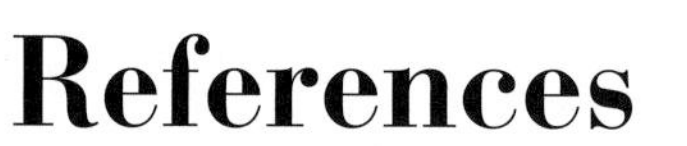

Website links are subject to change. To access updated web links, please visit ***www.pearsonhighered.com/lynchelmore***.

References

i. U.S. Centers for Disease Control and Prevention (CDC). (2011, March). Sexual Behavior, Sexual Attraction, and Sexual Identity in the United States: Data from the 2006–2008 National Survey of Family Growth. *National Health Statistics Report*, 36. Retrieved from http://www.cdc.gov/nchs/data/nhsr/nhsr036.pdf.

ii. National Campaign to Prevent Teen and Unplanned Pregnancy and CosmoGirl.com. (2009). *Sex and tech: Results from a survey of teens and young adults*. Retrieved from http://www.thenationalcampaign.org/sextech/PDF/SexTech_Summary.pdf.

1. U.S. Centers for Disease Control and Prevention (CDC). (2011, March). Sexual Behavior, Sexual Attraction, and Sexual Identity in the United States: Data from the 2006–2008 National Survey of Family Growth. *National Health Statistics Report*, 36. Retrieved from http://www.cdc.gov/nchs/data/nhsr/nhsr036.pdf.

2. American College Health Association. (2011, spring). *American College Health Association-National College Health Assessment (ACHA-NCHA II) Reference Group Executive Summary, Spring 2011.* Retrieved from http://www.achancha.org/docs/ACHA-NCHA-II_ReferenceGroup_ExecutiveSummary_Spring2011.pdf.

3. Cooper, M. L. (2002, March). Alcohol use and risky sexual behavior among college students and youth: Evaluating the evidence. *J Stud Alcohol Suppl 14*, 101–117.

4. American Medical Association. (2006, March 8). Sex and intoxication more common among women on spring break, according to AMA poll. Robert Wood Johnson Foundation. Retrieved from http://www.rwjf.org/pr/product.jsp?id=21831.

5. Meston, C. M., & Buss, D. M. (2007). Why humans have sex. *Archives of Sexual Behavior, 36,* 477–507. Retrieved from http://homepage.psy.utexas.edu/homepage/group/MestonLAB/Publications/WhyHaveSex.pdf.

6. Medline Plus. (2009, February 27). Adolescent development. *National Library of Medicine*. Retrieved from http://www.nlm.nih.gov/medlineplus/ency/article/002003.htm.

7. American Cancer Society. (2010). *Learn about cancer: Cervical cancer.* Retrieved from http://www.cancer.org/Cancer/CervicalCancer/DetailedGuide/cervical-cancer-risk-factors.

8. National Cancer Institute. (2008). *What you need to know about prostate cancer*. Retrieved from http://www.cancer.gov/cancertopics/wyntk/prostate/page4.

9. National Women's Health Information Center. (2009). *Menstruation and the menstrual cycle.* Retrieved from http://www.womenshealth.gov/faq/menstruation.cfm#f.

10. American Congress of Obstetricians and Gynecologists. (2008). *Premenstrual syndrome*. Retrieved from http://www.acog.org/publications/patient_education/bp057.cfm.

11. Dickerson, L. M., Mazyck, P. J., & Hunter, M. H. (2003). Premenstrual syndrome. *American Family Physician, 67* (8), 1743–1752. Retrieved from http://www.aafp.org/afp/20030415/1743.html.

12. National Women's Health Information Center. (2010). *Premenstrual syndrome: Frequently asked questions*. Retrieved from http://www.womenshealth.gov/faq/premenstrual-syndrome.cfm.

13. American Congress of Obstetricians and Gynecologists. (2006). *Dysmenorrhea*. Retrieved from http://www.acog.org/publications/patient_education/bp046.cfm.

14. French, L. (2005). Dysmenorrhea. *American Family Physician, 71* (2), 285–291.

15. American Congress of Obstetricians and Gynecologists. (2008). *Endometriosis*. Retrieved from http://www.acog.org/publications/patient_education/bp013.cfm.

16. National Women's Health Information Center. (2009). *Menstruation and the menstrual cycle.* Retrieved from http://www.womenshealth.gov/faq/menstruation.cfm#e.

17. Farley, D. (1991, October). On the teen scene: TSS—Reducing the risks. *FDA Consumer*.

18. Cable News Network. (2009, April 13). The laws of sexual attraction. Retrieved from http://articles.cnn.com/2009-04-13/living/o.laws.of.sex.attraction_1_attraction-mhc-testosterone-levels?_s=PM:LIVING.

19. Hughes, S. M., Dispenza, F., & Gallup, G. G., Jr. (2004). Ratings of voice attractiveness predict sexual behavior and body configuration. *Evolution and Human Behavior, 25*, 295–304.

20. Gangestad, S. W., Thornhill, R., & Garver-Apgar, C. E. (2010). Men's facial masculinity predicts changes in their female partners' sexual interests across the ovulatory cycle, whereas men's intelligence does not. *Evolution and Human Behavior, 31*, 412–424.

21. Cohn, D., and Fry, R. (2010, January 19). Women, men, and the new economics of marriage. Pew Research Center. Retrieved from http://pewsocialtrends.org/2010/01/19/women-men-and-the-new-economics-of-marriage.

22. Planned Parenthood. (2011). *Understanding sexual pleasure.* Retrieved from http://www.plannedparenthood.org/health-topics/sex-101/understanding-sexual-pleasure-23902.htm.

23. Hughes, S. M., Harrison, M. A., & Gallup, G. G. (2007). Sex differences in romantic kissing among college students: An evolutionary perspective. *Evolutionary Psychology*, *5* (3), 612–631.

24. Masters, W. H., & Johnson, V. E. (1966). *Human sexual response*, 1st ed. New York: Bantam.

25. Hite, S. (1976, 1981, 2004). *The Hite report: A nationwide study of female sexuality*, rev. 2004. New York: Seven Stories Press.

26. Association of Reproductive Health Professionals. (2008). What you need to know: Female sexual response. *ARHP Factsheets*. Retrieved from http://www.arhp.org/factsheets.

27. American Society for Reproductive Medicine. (2008). *Patient fact sheet: Sexual dysfunction and infertility.* Retrieved from http://www.asrm.org/FactSheetsandBooklets.

28. MedlinePlus. (2010). *Female sexual dysfunction.* Retrieved from http://www.nlm.nih.gov/medlineplus/sexualproblemsinwomen.html.

29. Mayo Foundation for Medical Education and Research. (2009). *Painful intercourse (dyspareunia).* Retrieved from http://www.mayoclinic.com/health/painful-intercourse/DS01044.

30. Mayo Foundation for Medical Education and Research. (2009). *Low sex drive in women.* Retrieved from http://www.mayoclinic.com/health/low-sex-drive-in-women/DS01043.

31. Mayo Foundation for Medical Education and Research. (2009). *Anorgasmia*. Retrieved from http://www.mayoclinic.com/health/anorgasmia/DS01051/DSECTION=symptoms.

32. National Kidney and Urologic Diseases Information Clearinghouse. (2005). *Erectile dysfunction* (NIH Publication No. 06-3923). Retrieved from http://kidney.niddk.nih.gov/kudiseases/pubs/impotence.

33. MedlinePlus. (2008). *Premature ejaculation.* Retrieved from http://www.nlm.nih.gov/medlineplus/ency/article/001524.htm.

34. Mayo Foundation for Medical Education and Research. (2009). *Premature ejaculation*. Retrieved from http://www.mayoclinic.com/health/premature-ejaculation/DS00578/DSECTION=alternative%2Dmedicine.

35. American Association of Sexuality Educators, Counselors, and Therapists. (2004). What is sex therapy? Retrieved from http://www.aasect.org/faqs.asp#What_is_ST.

36. Rosenbaum, J. E. (2009). Patient teenagers? A comparison of the sexual behavior of virginity pledgers and matched nonpledgers. *Pediatrics, 123* (1), 110–120.

37. Higgins, J. A., Trussell, J., Moore, N. B., & Davidson, J. K. (2010). Young adult sexual health: Current and prior sexual behaviors among non-Hispanic white U.S. college students. *Sexual Health, 7* (1), 35–43.

38. National Campaign to Prevent Teen and Unplanned Pregnancy and CosmoGirl.com. (2009). *Sex and tech: Results from a survey of teens and young adults.* Retrieved from http://www.thenationalcampaign.org/sextech.

39. Lenhart, A. (2009). *Teens and sexting.* Retrieved from http://www.pewinternet.org/Reports/2009/Teens-and-Sexting.aspx.

40. Newman, A. (2010, March 23). Senate passes Arizona sexting law. *Arizona Daily Wildcat.* Retrieved from http://wildcat.arizona.edu/news/senate-passes-arizona-sexting-law-1.1276167.

41. Comer, R. J. (2010). *Abnormal psychology*, 7th ed. New York: Worth Publishers, 435–440.

42. Brigham Young University. (2010). *National pornography statistics.* Retrieved from https://wsr.byu.edu/pornographystats.

43. O'Reilly, S., Knox, D., & Zusman, M. E. (2007, June). College student attitudes toward pornography use. *College Student Journal*, *41*, 402–404.

44. Jaishankar, K. (2009, January–June). Editorial: Sexting: A new form of victimless crime? *International Journal of Cyber Criminology, 3* (1), 21–25.

45. United States Senate. (2005, November 10). Why the government should care about pornography. Senate Judiciary Committee: Testimony of Pamela Paul. Retrieved from http://judiciary.senate.gov/hearings/testimony.cfm?id=1674&wit_id=4824.

46. United States Department of Justice. (2009). *Domestic sex trafficking of minors.* Retrieved from http://www.justice.gov/criminal/ceos/prostitution.html.

47. Sanders, T., Myers, E., & Smith, D. (2010, May). Participation in sex work: Students' views. *Sex Education: Sexuality, Society and Learning, 10* (2), 145–156.

48. Farley, M. (2009, March). Myths & facts about legalized prostitution. *Prostitution Research & Education*. Retrieved from http://www.prostitutionresearch.com/laws/000234.html.

49. Pew Research Center. (2009). *Majority continues to support civil unions*. Retrieved from http://pewforum.org/Gay-Marriage-and-Homosexuality/Majority-Continues-To-Support-Civil-Unions.aspx#4.

50. Joyce, A. (2006, June 30). Majority of large firms offer employees domestic partner benefits. *Washington Post*. Retrieved from http://www.washingtonpost.com/wp-dyn/content/article/2006/06/29/AR2006062902049.html.

51. Massachusetts Department of Education. (2001). *2001 Massachusetts Youth Risk Behavior Survey results.* Retrieved from http://www.doe.mass.edu/cnp/hprograms/yrbs/01/results.pdf.

52. Kosciw, J. G. (2004). *The 2003 National School Climate Survey: The school-related experiences of our nation's lesbian, gay, bisexual and transgender youth*. New York: GLSEN.

53. Federal Bureau of Investigation. (2009). *2008 hate crime statistics.* Retrieved from http://www.fbi.gov/ucr/hc2008/data/table_01.html.

54. Diamond, L. M. (2008). Female bisexuality from adolescence to adulthood: Results from a 10-year longitudinal study. *Developmental Psychology, 44* (1), 5–14.

55. American Psychological Association. (2010). *Answers to your questions about transgendered individuals and gender identity*. Retrieved from http://www.apa.org/topics/sexuality/transgender.aspx.

56. American Pregnancy Association. (2010). *Statistics.* Retrieved from http://www.americanpregnancy.org/main/statistics.html.

16 Sexually Transmitted Infections: Protecting Your Health and Fertility

- About 19 million people in the United States each year contract a sexually transmitted infection.[i]

- Each year, sexually transmitted infections cause about 24,000 American women to become infertile.[i]

- Approximately 20% of the people in the United States infected with HIV do not realize it.[ii]

LEARNING OBJECTIVES

IDENTIFY the most common risk factors for sexually transmitted infections (STIs).

DESCRIBE the stages of HIV infection and its progression to AIDS.

DISCUSS the current treatment options for someone infected with HIV.

IDENTIFY the potential long-term effects of three common viral STIs.

COMPARE three common bacterial STIs, their signs and symptoms, and treatment.

EXPLAIN the relationship between STIs, pelvic inflammatory disease, and infertility.

IDENTIFY three common STIs transmitted by parasites.

EXPLAIN how to reduce your risk of acquiring an STI.

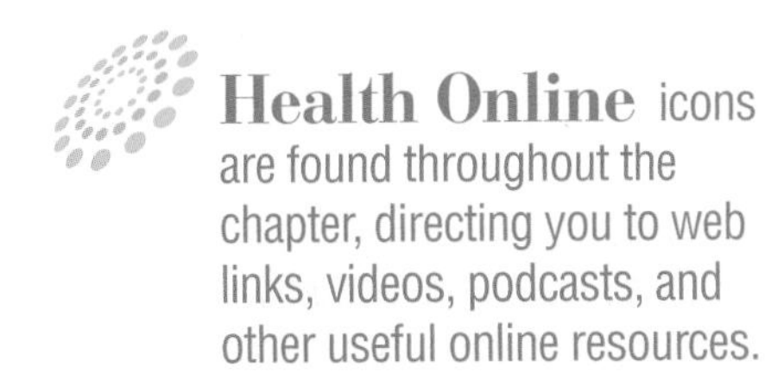
Health Online icons are found throughout the chapter, directing you to web links, videos, podcasts, and other useful online resources.

It makes no difference if you're rich or poor, naive or worldly, in love or virtual strangers—

if you're sexually active, you risk infection. Some sexually transmitted infections are mild and can be cured with medication. Others are incurable, erupting again and again for the rest of your life. A few are deadly. So whether you have multiple partners, are in a committed relationship, or even if you've chosen celibacy for now, it's important to learn the facts about sexually transmitted infections, how they're spread, and what can be done to prevent them.

An Overview of Sexually Transmitted Infections

By definition, a **sexually transmitted infection (STI)** is any infection for which the primary mode of transmission is sexual contact. Another term you may be familiar with is *sexually transmitted disease (STD)*; however, we think of a *disease* as a condition that causes signs and symptoms, whereas some people infected with certain STIs may not develop any apparent health problems—or not for a period of time. Still, the person is capable of transmitting the infection to a partner, who may quickly develop pain, blisters, or other indications of disease. Because some STIs have this capacity to remain latent (undetected), we use the term *STI* throughout this chapter.

sexually transmitted infections (STIs) Infections transmitted mainly through sexual activity, such as vaginal, anal, or oral sex.

STIs by the Numbers

It's estimated that, worldwide, nearly a million people acquire an STI *every day*.[1] This includes more than 50,000 new cases a day in the United States alone. That translates into approximately 19 million new cases of STIs among Americans annually, draining the U.S. health-care system of more than $16 billion each year.[2]

The CDC estimates that, whereas 15- to 24-year-olds represent only 25% of the sexually active population, they account for nearly 50% of all new STI cases.[3] Among sexually active U.S. teens, the STI prevalence is 40% and those with three or more partners have a prevalence of more than 50%. Even among girls aged 14 to 19 reporting only one lifetime partner, approximately 20% have at least one STI.[4] See the **Diversity and Health** box on the next page for more information on rates of STIs in different populations.

Chain of Infection

The first link in the chain of infection is a pathogen. There are more than 30 different sexually transmissible viruses, bacteria, and parasites.[1] We'll look at some of the most common later in this chapter.

STI pathogens are typically transmitted from one partner to another in blood, semen, or the secretions of the mucous membranes of the male or female genitals, the anus, or the

DIVERSITY & HEALTH

Rates of STIs for Different Sexes, Ages, Races, and Sexual Orientations

STIs may affect people of different sexes, ages, races, and sexual orientations differently. Certain groups are at higher risk for particular STIs or STIs in general.

Sex

- Women are biologically more susceptible to becoming infected with STIs than men are. Young women, especially, are at high risk because the cells lining the cervix are more immature and vulnerable to infection.

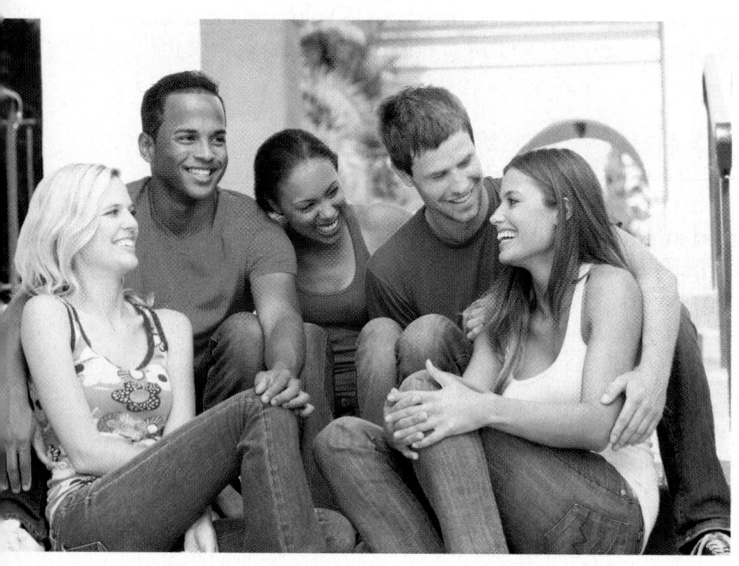

Young people are one of the groups at elevated risk for STIs.

- Women are less likely than men to experience symptoms of STIs, which can postpone detection and treatment.
- Women are more likely than men to experience long-term, severe side effects of STIs, such as infertility and cervical cancer.
- Women report 2.8 times as many cases of chlamydia as men.[1]
- Men accounted for 74% of new HIV/AIDS cases in 2007; women accounted for 26%.[2]
- Men reported 5.1 times as many cases of syphilis as women.[1]

Age

- People aged 15 to 24 have five times the reported rate of chlamydia as people aged 25 and older.[1]
- People aged 15 to 24 have four times the reported rate of gonorrhea as the rest of the population.[1]
- People aged 20 to 29 made up 25% of new HIV/AIDS cases in 2007.[2]

Race

- African Americans continue to experience an epidemic of HIV/AIDS, comprising 46% of the people living with HIV in the United States.[2]
- African Americans—especially young African American women—are at disproportionately high risk for other STIs as well.
- Hispanics are disproportionately affected by HIV/AIDS, gonorrhea, chlamydia, and syphilis.[1] Although Hispanics make up 15% of the U.S. population, they comprise 18% of new HIV/AIDS cases in the United States.[2]
- Native Americans/Alaska Natives are at a disproportionately high risk for gonorrhea and chlamydia.[1]
- Asian and Pacific Islander groups are experiencing growing rates of HIV/AIDS in the United States.[2]

Sexual Orientation

- Both homosexual and bisexual men who have sex with men are at high risk for HIV infection, syphilis, and other STIs. Women who have sex with these men share this increased risk.
- The risk of female-to-female HIV transmission is low but possible, especially if one or both partners have sores on their genitals, if partners share sex toys, or if they participate in rough sex. Women can pass other STIs to one another as well.

Data from *STD Health Disparities*, by the Centers for Disease Control and Prevention, 2010, retrieved from http://www.cdc.gov/std/health-disparities/default.htm; *HIV/AIDS*, by the Centers for Disease Control and Prevention, 2010, retrieved from http://www.cdc.gov/hiv.

mouth. Kissing is not risk free: Some viruses, including the herpes virus, can be transmitted via kissing. Some viruses and parasites can be transmitted merely with intimate skin-to-skin contact. Nonsexual modes of transmission are via shared needles, whether for IV drug use, tattoos, or body piercings, or transmission from a pregnant woman to her fetus.

Anyone who is sexually active qualifies as a susceptible host for STI pathogens. Beyond that, certain factors can increase your vulnerability:

- Being infected with one STI increases your risk for others, often because blisters or sores are present that serve as portals of entry.
- Chemical irritation to the mucous membranes—typically from vaginal douching or from use of a spermicide—can increase your susceptibility to STIs. The active ingredient in all over-the-counter (OTC) spermicides sold in the United States is nonoxynol-9 (N-9). The lubricant in some condoms also contains N-9. Although N-9 immobilizes sperm, clinical trials have shown that it not only fails to protect against STIs, but also irritates the partners' tissues and actually increases the risk of STIs.[5]
- Mechanical irritation, whether from aggressively flossing your teeth before oral sex or from engaging in "rough sex," can also increase your susceptibility. Mechanical irritation is one reason that anal sex carries a much higher risk of STI transmission than either vaginal or oral sex. Whereas the tissues of the vaginal wall are specialized to accommodate friction, the tissues lining the rectum are delicate and easily tear. Because the blood vessels supplying these tissues are very close to the surface, such tears allow any STI pathogens that may be present to pass easily into the bloodstream. Not only the receiving partner, but the partner who inserts his penis into an infected partner is at risk because pathogens can enter the opening at the tip of the penis, or can seep into scratches, cuts, or sores on the penis.[6]

Avoiding Transmission

Although you may have heard that having sex in a hot tub reduces your risk of acquiring an STI, it's not true. Other common myths are that "female contraceptives" like a cervical cap, diaphragm, contraceptive sponge, or IUD offer protection. They don't. Douching after sex, urinating after sex, and bathing after sex also are useless—and douching can actually propel pathogens deeper into the reproductive tract. So what does work? Abstinence from all forms of sexual activity provides the best protection from STIs. If you choose to have sex, the following practices can help you avoid transmission.

Mutual Monogamy

The safest sex is between two mutually monogamous partners who have been tested and are uninfected. *Mutual monogamy* means that both partners are engaged in a long-term commitment to having sex only with the other. This is not the same as *serial monogamy*, in which a person has one exclusive relationship after another, none of which lasts for long. Many STIs have a latency period of days, weeks, or even months before testing can detect antibodies or other evidence of infection. This means that a person who has recently left a relationship, even if it was monogamous and followed by negative STI tests, cannot be considered uninfected. If either partner has recently had sex with someone else, it is considered high risk to have sex without a condom.

Condom Use

Clinical trials over decades have shown that, when used correctly and consistently, from start to finish, every time, condoms significantly reduce transmission of most STIs. Still, they are not 100% effective. Lambskin condoms, for example, do not offer any protection against STIs. Latex condoms do block the transmission of STIs in genital secretions; however, herpes, genital warts, and infestations with parasites can be transmitted during latex condom use because the microbes are commonly present in unprotected areas.[7] Most importantly, latex condoms don't provide any protection when they're left in the nightstand drawer. People who assume that sex without a condom is okay "once in a while" are mistaken: Many STI pathogens are remarkably efficient in moving from reservoir to host. The bacterium that causes gonorrhea, for example, will be transmitted from an infected male not wearing a condom to a female 70–80% of the time in a single act of vaginal intercourse.[8]

Does using a latex condom make anal sex safe? Respected public health authorities, including the United States Surgeon General, have concluded that, even with a condom, anal intercourse is a dangerous practice.[5] Here's why:

- Condoms are more likely to break during anal intercourse than during other types of sex because of the greater amount of friction and other stresses involved.
- Oil-based lubricants such as petroleum jelly damage condoms, increasing the likelihood that they will tear. And although many public health advisories suggest using water-based lubricants during anal sex, even these lubricants can contain substances that are toxic to rectal lining cells, prompting the chemical irritation that makes it easier for an STI to gain access to a new host. A recent study found that partners who use lubricants during anal sex are *more* likely to be infected with an STI than partners who do not, and 76% of the study participants reported using water-based lubricants.[9] Another study identified specific chemicals in several popular water-based lubricants that disrupt the lining cells.[9]

Are condoms necessary during oral sex? Although the risk of transmitting an STI during oral sex is lower than during anal or vaginal sex, numerous studies have shown that HIV, herpes, genital warts, and several other STIs are transmissible during all forms of unprotected oral sex. A latex condom should be used during oral-penile sex and a dental dam (a thin sheet of latex originally used in dentistry) or cut-open condom during oral-vaginal sex.[10]

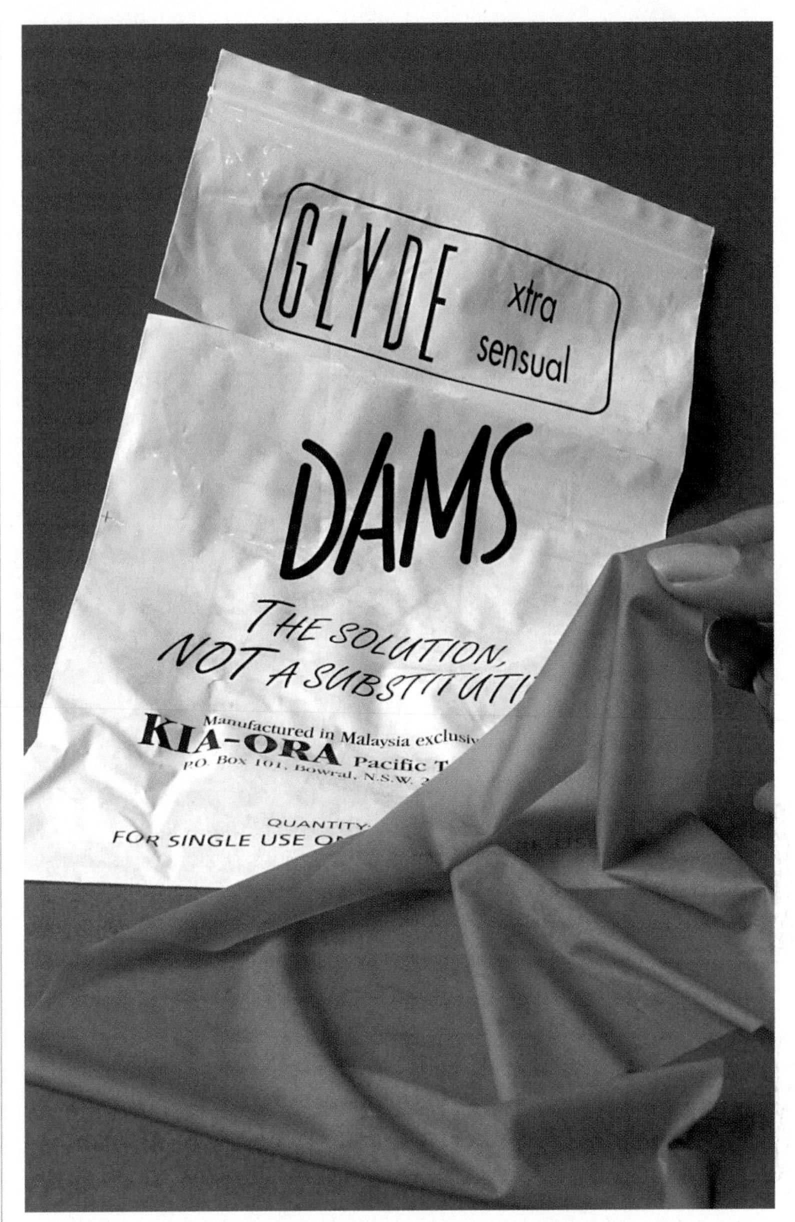

A **dental dam** helps make oral sex safer.

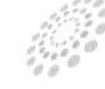 This interactive tutorial gives an overview of STIs: www.nlm.nih.gov/medlineplus/tutorials/sexuallytransmitteddiseases/htm/_yes_50_no_0.htm.

Risk Factors for STIs

We just noted that young people represent only a quarter of the sexually active population, but acquire nearly half of all STIs. What makes these years so risky? The CDC cites a combination of biological, behavioral, and cultural factors:[3]

- Adolescent females may have a physiologically increased susceptibility to infection with certain STI pathogens because of instability of the immature cells of their cervix.

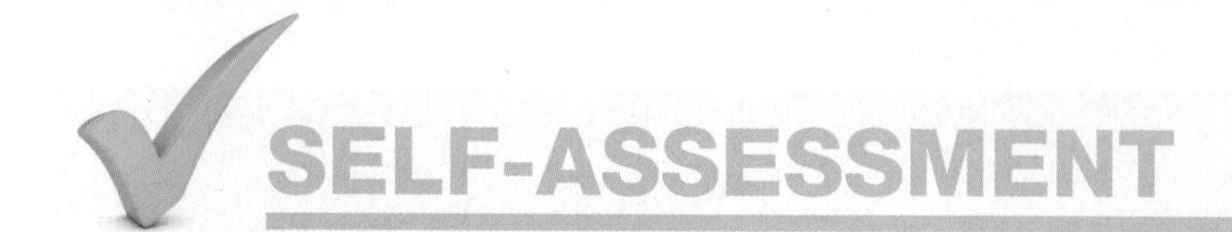

Take this self-assessment online at www.pearsonhighered.com/lynchelmore.

Are You at Risk for an STI?

If you engage in sexual activity, then you are at risk for contracting an STI. However, your level of risk depends on certain behaviors.

"Sex" includes oral, vaginal, or anal sex, and a sexual partner is somebody with whom you have had oral, vaginal, or anal sex.

1. In the past 12 months, have you been diagnosed with any STI?*
   ☐ yes ☐ no
2. In the past 12 months, have you had more than one sexual partner?
   ☐ yes ☐ no
3. In the past 12 months, do you think your sexual partner(s) had any other partners?
   ☐ yes ☐ not sure ☐ no
4. In the past 12 months, have you had sex with a new partner?
   ☐ yes ☐ no
5. Are you currently planning on having sex with a new partner?
   ☐ yes ☐ not sure ☐ no
6. In the past 12 months, how often have you used condoms during vaginal or anal intercourse or latex barriers during oral sex?
   ☐ always ☐ some of the time ☐ most of the time ☐ never
7. Do you discuss sexual history and testing with your partner(s)?
   ☐ always ☐ sometimes ☐ never

HOW TO INTERPRET YOUR SCORE

If you answered "yes" or "not sure" to questions 1–5, you may be at higher risk for STIs. If you answered anything other than "always" to questions 6 and 7, you may be at higher risk for STIs.

Consider making an appointment at your campus health center for STI screening and/or to discuss prevention strategies.

*Having had an STI recently may put you at higher risk for other STIs.

Source: Adapted from *UC Berkeley Sexually Transmitted Infection (STI) Risk Assessment*, by the UC Berkeley University Health Services Tang Center, no date, retrieved from http://uhs.berkeley.edu/students/pdf/Patient%20Self-assessment.pdf.

- Young people may face multiple barriers to accessing quality health care, including lack of insurance or other ability to pay, lack of transportation, discomfort with facilities and services designed for adults, and concerns about confidentiality.
- Young people often belong to overlapping social networks—such as campus departments, clubs, or societies—within which they form couples, split up, and form new couples. STIs within such networks are likely to spread broadly.
- As a group, young people have a tendency to underestimate their risk of infection. Many studies conducted among college students have found that, despite the high prevalence of high-risk sexual behaviors, a majority—as much as 86.8% in one study—did not perceive themselves to be at risk.[11]

No matter how old you are, your likelihood of contracting an STI depends primarily on your behaviors. Activities that increase your risk include:

- Having oral, vaginal, or anal sex without using a latex condom
- Having sex with multiple partners, especially strangers, and not discussing STIs before sex
- Exchanging sex for drugs or money
- Participating in sex while drunk or high on drugs
- Coming into direct skin-to-skin contact with someone who has infections such as HPV, herpes, pubic lice, or scabies
- Injecting substances with dirty needles or syringes—or having unprotected sex with someone who has
- Sharing needles for tattoos or body piercings—or having unprotected sex with someone who has
- Failing to be vaccinated against hepatitis B (HBV) or human papillomavirus (HPV)

Are you at risk for a sexually transmitted infection? Take the **Self-Assessment** on this page to find out.

HIV and AIDS

In the summer of 1981, physicians in Los Angeles, San Francisco, and New York began reporting cases of similar rare illnesses in young homosexual males. The disorders—a type of fungal pneumonia and a form of skin cancer—were essentially unknown except in people with a compromised immune system. Within weeks, more cases of these disorders were reported in patients who injected illicit drugs, and then in a patient with hemophilia (a blood-clotting disease) who had received blood transfusions. Researchers soon recognized that the underlying problem was a deficiency (shortage) of immune cells, and theorized that a viral infection was to blame. By 1984, the virus responsible for this immune deficiency had been identified, and in 1986 it was named the *human immunodeficiency virus* (*HIV*).

Accounting for an estimated 30 million deaths worldwide since its discovery, HIV is the most serious of all sexually transmitted pathogens.[12] There are more than 33 million people living with HIV, with infection rates in sub-Saharan Africa—at 5% of the adult population—especially high **(Figure 16.1).** In the United States, an estimated 1.2 million people live with HIV infection. Men who have sex with other men are disproportionately infected, as are sex workers and intravenous drug users. By race, African Americans face the most severe HIV burden.[13]

Researchers believe that HIV infections in humans can be traced back to chimpanzees in West Africa. It is thought that the virus jumped from primates to people when hunters seeking monkeys as bush meat came into contact with the infected blood of their prey. The virus spread across Africa and then to other parts of the world.

Transmission of HIV

Like other STI pathogens, HIV is transmitted in blood, semen, and other body fluids. Once infected with HIV, people can transmit it to others even if they have not experienced any symptoms. About 9 out of 10 infections are sexually transmitted **(Figure 16.2).** If you already have

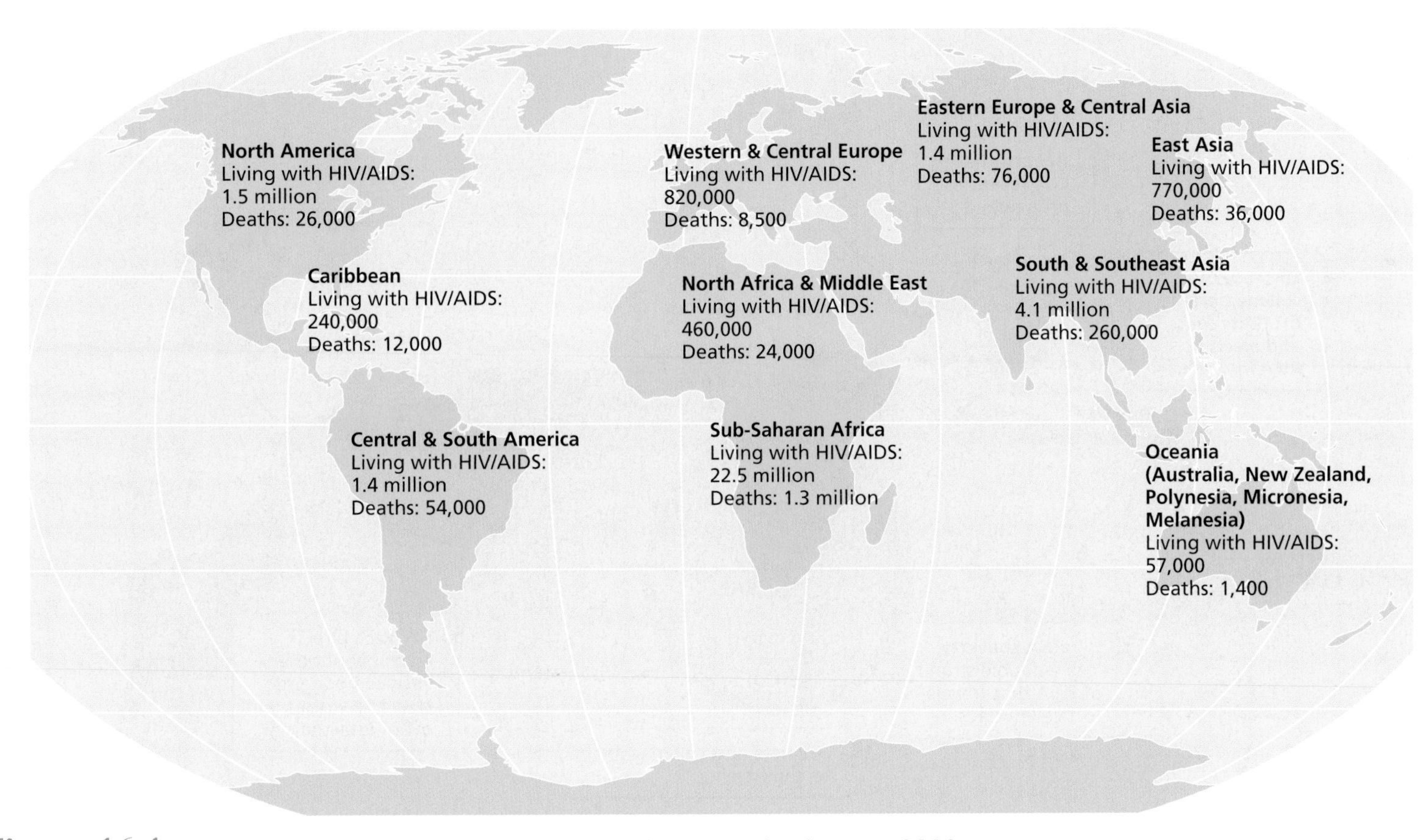
North America
Living with HIV/AIDS:
1.5 million
Deaths: 26,000
Western & Central Europe
Living with HIV/AIDS:
820,000
Deaths: 8,500
Eastern Europe & Central Asia
Living with HIV/AIDS:
1.4 million
Deaths: 76,000
East Asia
Living with HIV/AIDS:
770,000
Deaths: 36,000
Caribbean
Living with HIV/AIDS:
240,000
Deaths: 12,000
North Africa & Middle East
Living with HIV/AIDS:
460,000
Deaths: 24,000
South & Southeast Asia
Living with HIV/AIDS:
4.1 million
Deaths: 260,000
Central & South America
Living with HIV/AIDS:
1.4 million
Deaths: 54,000
Sub-Saharan Africa
Living with HIV/AIDS:
22.5 million
Deaths: 1.3 million
Oceania
(Australia, New Zealand, Polynesia, Micronesia, Melanesia)
Living with HIV/AIDS:
57,000
Deaths: 1,400

Figure 16.1 HIV/AIDS around the world. Deaths shown are for the year 2009.

Data from *2010 UNAIDS Report on the Global AIDS Epidemic*, by the Joint United Nations Programme on HIV/AIDS (UNAIDS), 2010. Available at http://www.unaids.org/globalreport/Global_report.htm.

another STI, such as herpes or syphilis, your risk of becoming infected with HIV increases significantly. Having intercourse while high on drugs is also risky, as you are less likely to think clearly and practice safe sex. In contrast, you cannot catch the virus through sneezing, handshakes, sharing food, or any other type of casual contact.

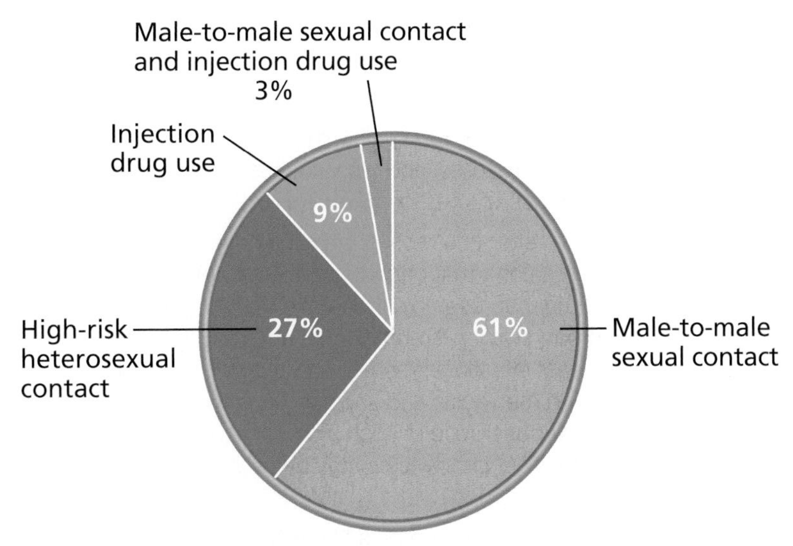

Figure 16.2 Transmission categories for new HIV/AIDS cases in adolescents and adults

Source: HIV/AIDS in the United States, by the U.S. Department of Health and Human Services, Centers for Disease Control and Prevention, November 7, 2011, *HIV in the United States*, retrieved from www.cdc.gov/hiv/resources/factsheets/us.htm.

Intravenous drug users are at very high risk of contracting HIV if they share needles or syringes with other users. Efforts to sterilize equipment, including washing with bleach, are not always successful at killing HIV. Sharing needles for tattoos or body piercing is also risky. In the past, HIV was occasionally transmitted to recipients of blood transfusions; however, due to reforms, all donated blood in the United States is now screened for the virus and is considered safe. Although strict precautions are mandated in health-care facilities to protect workers from contact with contaminated body fluids or medical waste such as used needles, HIV transmission from patients to clinicians has occurred.

Infected mothers are at risk of giving the virus to their infants, which is called *mother-to-child transmission* (MTCT). This can occur during pregnancy, childbirth, and breast-feeding. Although this mode of transmission is rare in the United States, the World Health Organization estimates that worldwide, 430,000 children are newly infected each year, 90% through MTCT.[14] Treatment of the mother greatly reduces transmission to the fetus. Untreated, approximately 50% of infected children will die before age 2.

This interactive tutorial discusses HIV infection and AIDS: www.nlm.nih.gov/medlineplus/tutorials/aids/htm/index.htm.

Replication of HIV

HIV is like any other pathogen in that the initial infective "dose" cannot cause significant harm unless it has a means to *replicate*—that is, to make exact copies of itself. For a mere virus, HIV has an astonishingly

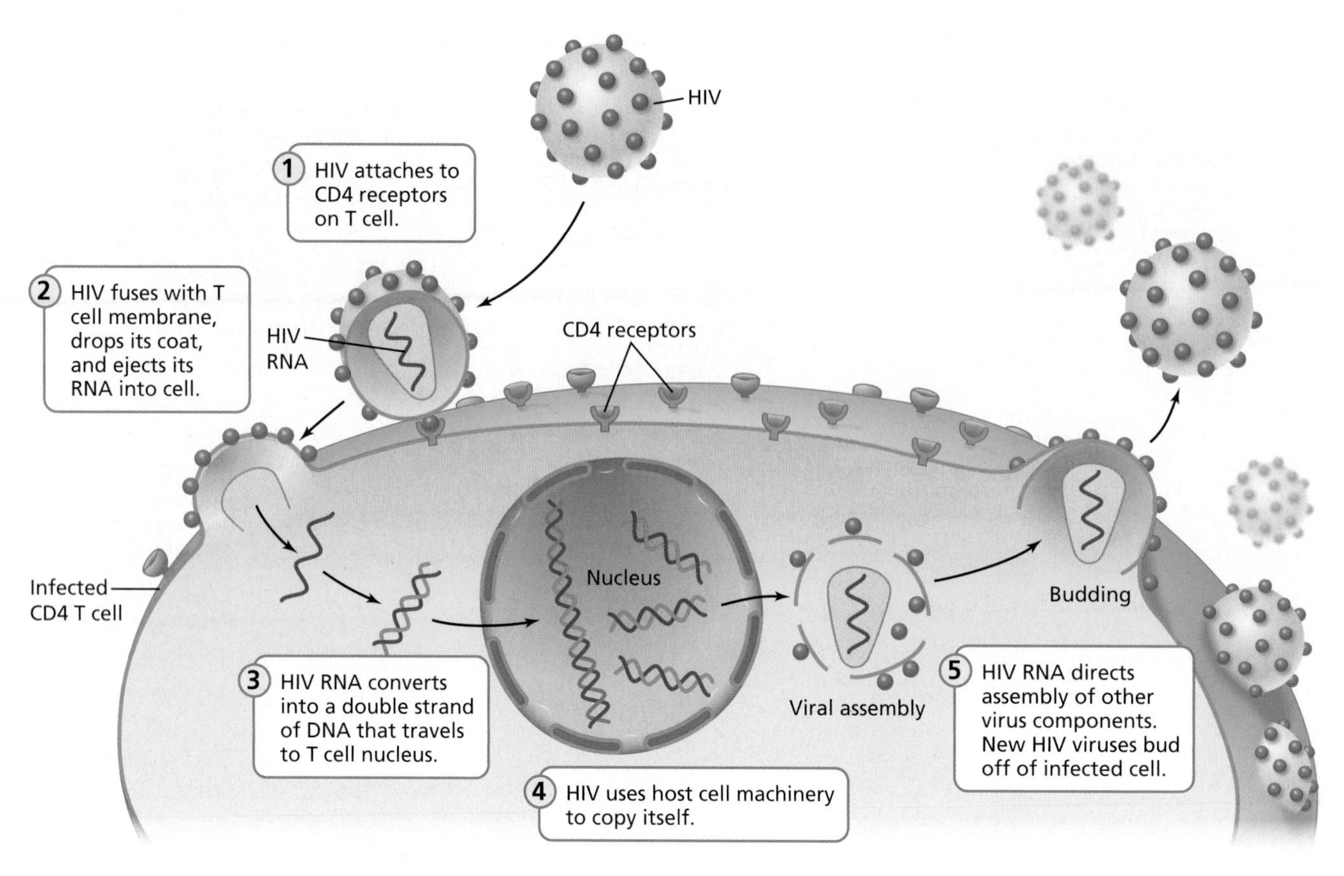
HIV
1 HIV attaches to CD4 receptors on T cell.
2 HIV fuses with T cell membrane, drops its coat, and ejects its RNA into cell.
HIV RNA
CD4 receptors
Infected CD4 T cell
Nucleus
Budding
Viral assembly
3 HIV RNA converts into a double strand of DNA that travels to T cell nucleus.
4 HIV uses host cell machinery to copy itself.
5 HIV RNA directs assembly of other virus components. New HIV viruses bud off of infected cell.

Figure 16.3 **Stages of HIV replication**

sophisticated mechanism for replication. The steps in this process are depicted in **Figure 16.3:**

1. HIV happens to have an outer envelope studded with particular proteins that fit perfectly into the CD4 receptors on helper T cells (CD4 T cells), which are important players in the body's immune response. (See Chapter 13.) After gaining entry into the bloodstream, HIV soon encounters circulating CD4 T cells. When it does, it uses these proteins to attach to their receptors.
2. The HIV envelope fuses with the CD4 T cell membrane. This allows the inner, pathogenic portion of the HIV to then enter the T cell. Once inside the T cell, the HIV sheds its inner coat, freeing its genetic material, a single strand of a compound called RNA.
3. The HIV uses an enzyme to transcribe (convert) its single strand of RNA into a double strand of DNA, the genetic "template" used by human cells to manufacture proteins. This viral DNA then moves into the T cell's nucleus.
4. There, it may hide out for days or years, inactive and undetected by the infected person's immune system. But sooner or later, it uses the host cell to assemble new, immature copies of itself.
5. Huge numbers of these new viruses bud from the T cell membrane into the bloodstream, where they mature into potent viruses. The T cell membrane becomes so punctured by the budding viruses that it cannot hold its contents, and self-destructs. In the meantime, the new viruses go on to infect more CD4 T cells and the replication process begins all over again.

The immune system mounts a vigorous response to the initial infection. B cells multiply and produce HIV antibodies. CD4 T cells also multiply and secrete cytokines, and CD8 T cells (cytotoxic T cells) directly destroy many virally infected T cells. This stops the progression of the initial infection; however, the virus continues to replicate at low levels, and the immune system continues to fight it. After many years or decades, CD4 T cell counts begin to decline more sharply, the immune system becomes increasingly weakened, and the body loses its ability to fight off infections and cancers.

Progression of HIV Infection

Now that you understand how HIV hijacks the immune system, you can appreciate the signs, symptoms, and diseases the body experiences during each of the stages of infection **(Figure 16.4).**

The first few weeks after contracting the virus are called the *primary infection stage.* During that period, most—but not all—people experience symptoms that resemble those of a bad flu. Fatigue, fever, headache, sore throat, swollen lymph glands, and muscle aches are reported. Diarrhea, yeast infections, rashes, and mouth sores also sometimes occur, and even meningitis and shingles. From the initial exposure to the virus to the disappearance of such symptoms, this stage may last from 2 to 3 months. Antibody tests may be negative for HIV during much or all of this stage.

The primary infection is followed by a stage of *clinical latency*, when the person typically experiences no significant symptoms and the virus is reproducing only at low levels. This period may last up to 8 years, and in some people even longer.[15] Eventually, however, HIV replication begins to exceed the immune system's ability to fight it.

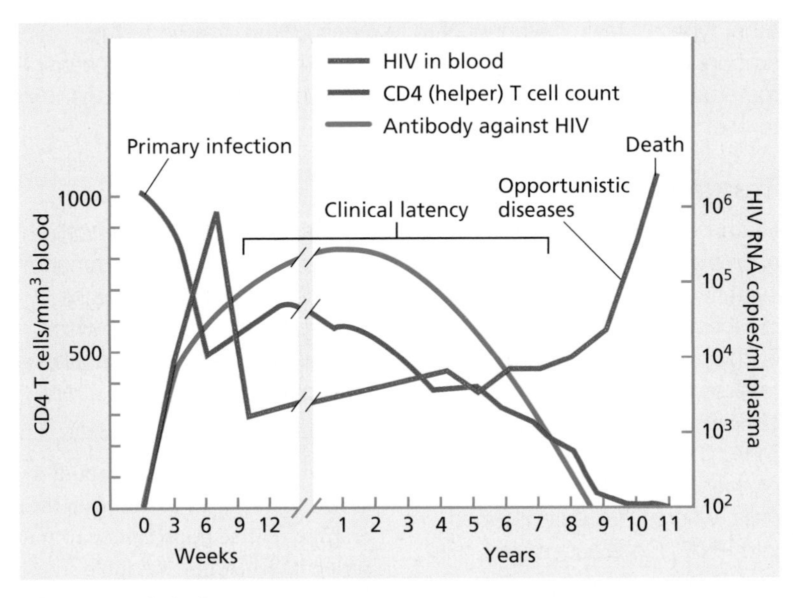

Figure 16.4 Characteristic course of HIV infection, from primary infection to AIDS. After the primary infection, there is typically a lengthy period of latency before the individual develops AIDS.

Source: Adapted from Bauman, R. *Microbiology with Diseases by Taxonomy,* 3rd ed., Fig. 25.25, p. 723. © 2012. Reproduced by permission of Pearson Education, Inc.

As the loss of CD4 T cells accelerates, the person becomes increasingly vulnerable to **opportunistic diseases**—infections and cancers that take advantage of a weakened immune system. These include the fungal pneumonia, called *Pneumocystis jiroveci*, and the skin cancer, called *Kaposi's sarcoma*, that were seen in the first patients in the early 1980s. They also include tuberculosis, which is responsible for 1 in every 4 deaths from HIV infection, as well as meningitis, eye infections, yeast infections, parasite infections, and other types of cancer. An HIV-positive person is diagnosed with **acquired immunodeficiency syndrome (AIDS)** when at least one opportunistic disease has developed or when that person's CD4 T cell count drops below 200 cells per microliter of blood (a healthy CD4 count is between 500 and 1,600 cells per microliter).[15] As the CD4 T cell count drops below 100, additional complications can arise, including severe diarrhea, weight loss, and dementia.

A small percentage of HIV-positive people never develop AIDS. Called *nonprogressors*, they appear to have genetic differences that prevent the virus from damaging their immune cells. The vast majority of HIV infections do, however, progress to AIDS. Without treatment, AIDS is invariably fatal, usually within about 3 years of diagnosis.[16]

Diagnosis of HIV

The Centers for Disease Control and Prevention (CDC) estimates that, of the 1.2 million people in the United States infected with HIV, about one-fifth do not realize it.[13] Between 2007 and 2010, the CDC implemented an HIV testing initiative in which more than 2.7 million HIV tests were conducted among people aged 13 to 64 during routine health-care visits. More than 1 out of every 100 tests (1.1%) turned out to be positive for HIV, and 62% of the people who tested positive reported that they had been unaware of their infection.[17] As noted earlier, primary HIV infection can have no symptoms or be mistaken for the flu, so HIV screening is critical. Early diagnosis allows prompt treatment and enables people to avoid transmitting the infection to others.

opportunistic diseases Infections and cancers that develop almost exclusively in people with a weakened immune system.

acquired immunodeficiency syndrome (AIDS) The final stage of infection with the human immunodeficiency virus (HIV), which attacks the immune system, leaving the patient vulnerable to various infections and cancers.

If you're ever tempted to believe that only males need to worry about HIV/AIDS, log onto www.womenshealth.gov/hiv-aids/share-your-story. There, you can read the postings of HIV-positive women of all ages, and their loved ones.

The standard HIV screening test is the *enzyme-linked immunoassay* (abbreviated *ELISA* or *EIA*). This test looks for the presence of antibodies to the virus rather than for the virus itself: If B cells are producing antibodies to HIV, then HIV is present in the body. A vial of blood is drawn and sent to a lab for analysis. Falsely positive results are common, so if the test is positive, it is immediately followed by a second ELISA test using the same blood sample. If this second test is also positive, then the laboratory will conduct a more sophisticated and time-consuming test called the *Western blot*. This test can determine whether or not the blood sample contains certain proteins characteristic of HIV. Only if all three tests are positive is a diagnosis of HIV infection made. It can take several days or longer before the results of these tests are available.

Fortunately, several rapid screening tests are now available that can provide results in as little as 20 minutes. Like the ELISA test, these rapid tests screen for antibodies to HIV. They are minimally invasive, requiring only that a clinician swab the inside of your mouth or obtain a drop of blood from your fingertip. Rapid tests are not available everywhere, however, and a positive result requires confirmatory tests.

Both the ELISA and the rapid tests only work after a person's immune system has begun to develop antibodies to HIV. Most people show a detectable level of antibodies in about 3 weeks; however, it can take up to 6 months in some people.[18] Therefore, any results from tests conducted too soon after potential exposure to the virus are unreliable. In some areas, however, patients can request one of two types of early detection tests. These include a test that can detect genetic material produced by the HIV as early as 6 days after infection, and a test that can identify an HIV protein one to 4 weeks after infection. However, these tests are more expensive than the ELISA or rapid tests, and are not available everywhere.[19]

The CDC recommends that all people between the ages of 13 and 64 be tested for HIV at least once during a routine doctor's visit. People at high risk for HIV (intravenous-drug users, people engaging in unprotected sex or with multiple sex partners) should be tested annually, and pregnant women should be tested as part of their routine prenatal care. Despite these recommendations, only 25% of college students report having ever been tested for HIV.[20] Privacy and confidentiality are concerns that keep many people—especially young people—from getting tested. Is at-home testing the answer? See the nearby **Consumer Corner** and find out.

In people who test negative for HIV, retesting is recommended if there was any potential exposure (unprotected sex or shared needle use) within the past three months. In people who test positive for HIV,

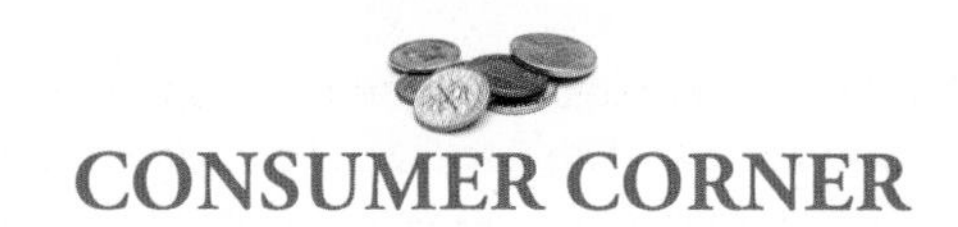

CONSUMER CORNER

Pros and Cons of HIV Testing at Home

Although there are several "FDA-approved" HIV test kits, only two are approved for at-home use.

The Home Access HIV-1 Test System can be purchased over the counter from most drug stores. It requires that you collect from your fingertip several drops of blood and, using a PIN number, mail the blood sample anonymously to a lab.[1] You then phone in for the results, which you access via your PIN. The Home Access System offers consumers pre- and post-test counseling. As with all HIV tests, any positive result must be followed up with a more sensitive test.

A newer test, approved by the FDA in 2012, provides same-day results at home. Called the OraQuick Test, it requires only that you take a swab of oral fluids at the gum lines, and place the swab in a developer vial. The results are provided in less than an hour. The test is considered highly accurate in identifying those who do not have the virus; that is, only 1 in 5000 uninfected people will have a result falsely indicating that they have the virus. However, 1 out of 12 infected people will have a falsely negative result.[2] The OraQuick Test also offers consumers pre- and post-test counseling.

If you're trying to decide whether or not at-home testing is right for you, consider the following:

- **Urgency with accuracy.** If you feel you can't wait for results, and are uncomfortable with the OraQuick Test's rate of false negatives, then visit your health-care provider.
- **Anonymity.** At-home tests provide privacy and anonymity. The pre- and post-test counseling is also anonymous and confidential.
- **Cost.** Depending on your health insurance status and your provider, home testing can be more or less expensive than clinical testing.

No matter what type of test, bear in mind that "morning after" testing is useless. It takes, on average, two to 8 weeks after infection or, in rare cases, 6 months, to develop detectable antibodies.[3]

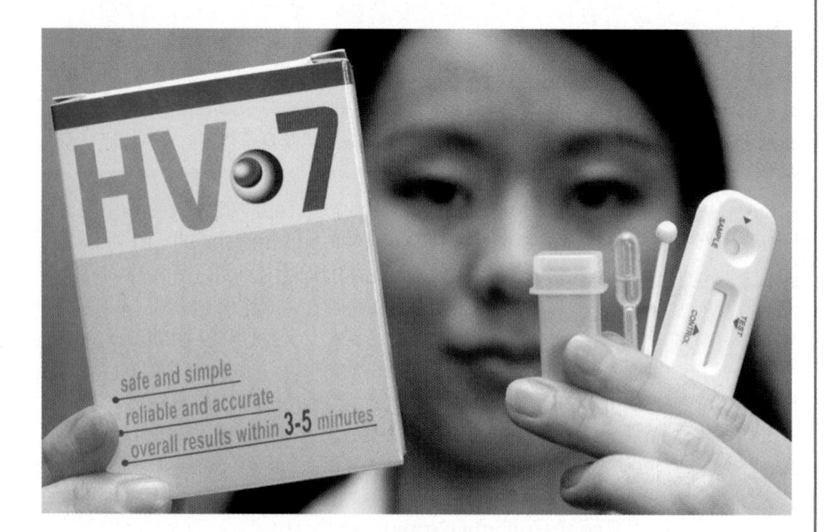

HV7
safe and simple
reliable and accurate
overall results within 3-5 minutes

References: **1.** "HIV Testing Basics for Consumers," by the U.S. Centers for Disease Control and Prevention, April 9, 2010, available at http://www.cdc.gov/hiv/topics/testing/resources/qa/index.htm. **2.** "FDA approves first over-the-counter home-use rapid HIV test," by the U.S. Food and Drug Administration, July 3, 2012, available at http://www.fda.gov/NewsEvents/Newsroom/PressAnnouncements/ucm310542.htm. **3.** "Vital Facts About HIV Home Test Kits," by the U.S. Food and Drug Administration, April 16, 2012, available at http://www.fda.gov/ForConsumers/ConsumerUpdates/ucm048553.htm.

other types of tests are conducted to measure the *viral load*—the amount of HIV in the blood. This information helps the physician predict the progression of the disease and decide which treatment options to use.

Treatment

HIV and AIDS are not curable, but they are treatable. Treatments called *antiretroviral therapies* can slow the deterioration of a person's immune system, and are responsible for a dramatic decrease in AIDS deaths in recent years. The term *antiretroviral* reflects the nature of HIV, which is classified as a **retrovirus;** that is, a virus that uses an enzyme called *reverse transcriptase* to transcribe its genetic material—a single strand of RNA—into double-stranded DNA. (This is the *reverse* of what happens in the nucleus of human cells, where DNA is transcribed into RNA.) Once assembled, this viral DNA inserts itself into the CD4 T cell nucleus and uses its DNA to replicate.

retrovirus A virus that contains a single strand of RNA and uses the enzyme reverse transcriptase to transcribe its RNA into a double strand of DNA.

There are several classes of antiretroviral drugs, each of which acts in a unique way to interrupt a step in the replication process:[21]

- *CCR5 antagonists* work by blocking a so-called *CCR5 co-receptor* that, without the drug, would signal the CD4 T cell's main receptor to accept the HIV. The drug thereby keeps the HIV from binding to a CD4 T cell in the first place.
- *Fusion inhibitors* work by impairing the ability of the HIV envelope to fuse with the CD4 T cell's membrane.
- *Reverse transcriptase inhibitors* (*RTIs*) work by disrupting the function of reverse transcriptase, thereby preventing the HIV from making the necessary change from RNA to DNA. There are two classes of RTIs.
- *Integrase strand transfer inhibitors* disable the enzyme integrase, which HIV manufactures to assist its integration into the DNA of infected cells.
- *Protease inhibitors* work by blocking the activity of an enzyme called protease, which the HIV uses to separate long protein molecules into smaller proteins with which it assembles new viruses.

These medications are frequently prescribed in combinations of three or four in a regimen often referred to as a *highly active antiretroviral therapy*, or HAART. For many HIV-positive people, HAART has changed their condition from a terminal illness to a chronic, manageable disease. With HAART, the average life expectancy of people newly diagnosed with HIV has been steadily increasing. Recent projection models suggest that a 39-year-old entering HIV care can expect to live until age 63.[22]

However, HIV drugs are very expensive, have toxic side effects, and do not work for everyone. For some, they may work for only a limited period of time. This is mainly because, when HIV replicates, genetic mutations occur with unusual frequency. Drugs developed for one version of HIV may not work on mutated versions.

Along with antiretroviral therapies, physicians may also prescribe medications such as antibiotics and antifungals in an effort to prevent opportunistic infections like pneumonia, toxoplasmosis, or tuberculosis.

Is there any "morning after" treatment for people who have had unprotected sex and are concerned that they might have been exposed to HIV? As early as the 1990s, health-care workers who had needlestick injuries or had been splashed with body fluids from an HIV-positive patient were given antiretroviral drugs to reduce their HIV risk. One study has suggested that this practice (generally referred to as *post-exposure prophylaxis*) might reduce the risk of acquiring HIV by as much as 85%.[23] Currently, post-exposure HAART is recommended not only for health-care workers exposed to HIV, but for anyone who has engaged in sexual intercourse or needle sharing with high-risk individuals. Victims of sexual assault are also routinely offered HAART. Animal studies suggest that treatment is most effective when initiated within 36 hours, and should last for 28 days.[23]

These podcasts discuss HIV testing and prevention: www.cdc.gov/hiv/resources/podcasts/index.htm.

The Future of AIDS Prevention

As with smallpox, polio, and other infectious diseases, a vaccine would offer the best long-term strategy for halting the worldwide spread of HIV. Since 1987, more than 30 vaccines have been tested, but none has yet been shown to effectively protect against HIV.[24] The effort is challenging for many reasons, primarily because there are so many subtypes of HIV virus, each of which mutates frequently. Developing a single vaccine against so many variants has not been possible. Moreover, vaccines are typically developed after intense study of the physiologic mechanisms by which people recover from an infection spontaneously. No one recovers from infection with HIV. Still, advances in vaccine research continue. In 2011, for example, researchers in Madrid announced success in an initial early trial of a new HIV vaccine made up of a combination of four HIV genes. And many other vaccine trials are under way.

Microbicides—chemicals that kill microorganisms—are another branch of HIV research slowly yielding results. For example, a vaginal gel that substantially reduces the risk of HIV infection is undergoing clinical trials, and researchers are developing a topical microbicide that coats the HIV and prevents it from binding to CD4 cells.[25, 26]

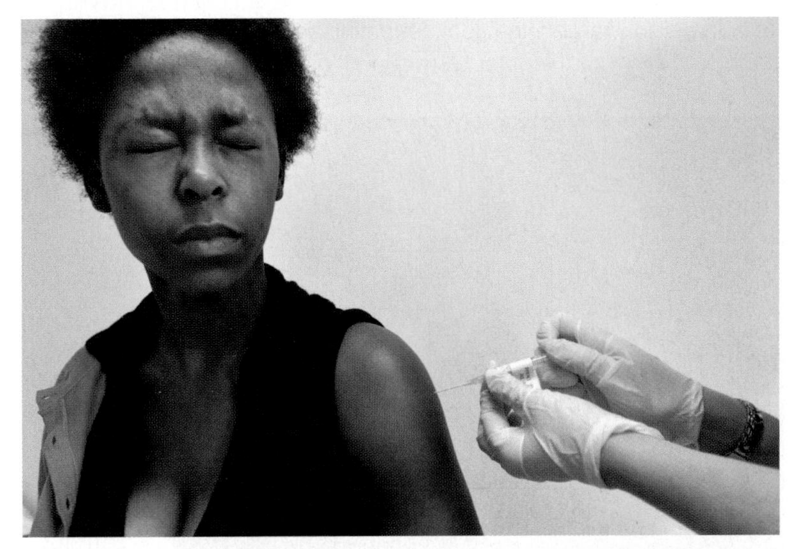

HIV vaccine trials are under way all over the world, but so far an effective vaccine has not been found. This woman has volunteered for a vaccine trial taking place in Cape Town, South Africa.

For people known to be at significant risk for HIV infection, including HIV-negative partners of HIV-positive men and women, the U.S. Food and Drug Administration (FDA) approved in 2012 a new medication that reduces the risk of transmission. Called Truvada, it is an oral medication taken in tablet form. In clinical trials, Truvada taken once daily in combination with safer sex practices reduced infection rates by 42% among gay and bisexual men and by 75% among heterosexual couples.[27]

Other Viral STIs

Like HIV, other viral STIs cannot be cured, although some can be conquered naturally by your immune system, and others can be controlled with prompt medical treatment. Here, we discuss hepatitis B, herpes, and human papillomavirus.

Hepatitis B

Hepatitis is inflammation of the liver. Multiple types exist, not all of which are due to infection. Hepatitis B is liver inflammation due to infection with the hepatitis B virus (HBV). As many as 1.4 million people in the United States currently live with a chronic hepatitis B infection.[28]

Modes of Transmission

HBV is more than 50 times as infectious as the virus that causes HIV, and is most commonly spread through unprotected sex.[28] It can also be transmitted through sharing toothbrushes, nail clippers, razors, or needles or other drug paraphernalia with an infected person. MTCT of HBV can also occur during childbirth.

Signs and Symptoms

People infected with HBV may experience no symptoms at all, or the symptoms may not appear for several months. They include muscle and joint pain, loss of appetite, nausea, vomiting, weakness and fatigue, and jaundice (yellow skin) and dark urine due to liver dysfunction. Although these initial symptoms usually go away on their own, in about 5% of infected adults, HBV remains in the body, slowly damaging the liver. Both cirrhosis of the liver—which leads to liver failure—and liver cancer are long-term complications of chronic infection.[29]

Diagnosis and Treatment

Infection is diagnosed with a test to detect the presence of HBV core antigen. This is important to distinguish someone with HBV infection from someone who has had an HBV vaccination, but it cannot distinguish a recent infection from one that occurred in the past. Another test for an HBV surface antigen indicates active infection.

There is no medical treatment for active hepatitis B, though the physician will monitor a patient's liver function with blood tests. Because HBV stresses the liver, anyone with an active or chronic infection should avoid alcohol and all medications, including OTC drugs and herbal supplements. Chronic HBV can be treated with antiviral medications, but if HBV progresses, a liver transplant may be the only option.

If you know you have been exposed to hepatitis B, contact your doctor right away. Passive immunization with hepatitis B immune globulin (antibodies specific for HBV) within 24 hours of exposure may reduce your risk of developing hepatitis B. In 1991, pediatricians began to routinely immunize children against hepatitis B. Since then, infection rates have dropped by an estimated 80%. However, a recent study

> *"Most infected people do not realize they have genital herpes because they don't have symptoms or their symptoms are mild . . ."*

found that 25% of college students immunized as children no longer showed immune memory to HBV, and needed booster shots.[30]

Genital Herpes

Genital herpes is an STI caused by either of two types of herpes simplex virus, designated as HSV-1 and HSV-2. Both strains are also capable of causing oral herpes. (See Chapter 13.)

Modes of Transmission

Both herpes strains are extremely contagious. They are typically transmitted during direct skin-to-skin contact, usually through vaginal, oral, or anal sex. HSV-1 infection is very common: 50–80% of people in the United States have it, and as many as 90% of people have it by age 50.[31] People are typically exposed in childhood, through nonsexual kisses by family members or friends. HSV-2 is less common, found in about 16.2% of adults in the United States.[32] Almost twice as many women as men are infected with HSV-2. Oral sex can pass both types of herpes virus back and forth between the mouth and the genitals. Oral transmission may help to explain why, although HSV-2 is much more commonly the culprit in genital herpes within the adult population overall, some studies have found that, among college students, HSV-1 is responsible for more cases.[33]

Signs and Symptoms

Most infected people do not realize they have genital herpes because they don't have symptoms or their symptoms are mild or mistaken for something else, such as jock itch, a yeast infection, or even insect bites. However, when symptoms occur, they can be very painful. The hallmark of genital herpes is small, itchy, burning blisters or sores in the genital or anal area **(Figure 16.5).** The first outbreak usually occurs within 2 weeks of infection, is accompanied by flulike symptoms, and takes about 3 weeks to heal. Several less severe outbreaks tend to occur during the first year after the initial episode, after which outbreaks typically become less frequent over time. However, the virus usually remains in the body for life, lying dormant in nerve cells until the next recurrence. Stress, illness, poor diet, inadequate rest, and friction in the genital area can trigger outbreaks. In some women, outbreaks are associated with menstruation.

Herpes is most infectious when blisters or sores are present on an infected person. However, the virus can be shed and passed on to others even when a person has intact skin and is experiencing no other signs or symptoms. If you have ever had an outbreak of genital herpes, you should consider yourself contagious even if you have not had an outbreak for years. It is important to tell any potential partners that you have genital herpes.

Genital herpes can leave the body vulnerable to other sexually transmitted infections. The risk to a herpes patient of becoming infected with HIV if exposed to it is two to three times that of people who do not have herpes.[31] It can also make people with an HIV infection more infectious. In a pregnant woman with an active genital herpes infection, MTCT is possible during vaginal birth, so a cesarean section is typically performed. HSV infection can be fatal in a newborn. Also, a recent study suggests that, in males, genital herpes may double the risk for prostate cancer.[34]

Diagnosis and Treatment

To diagnose herpes, a doctor takes a swab from a blister within the first 48 hours after it appears. If there is a sufficient amount of virus in the blister it is possible to distinguish it as either HSV-1 or HSV-2. Tests are also available that look for antibodies to the herpes virus in the blood. Many of the older tests cannot differentiate between

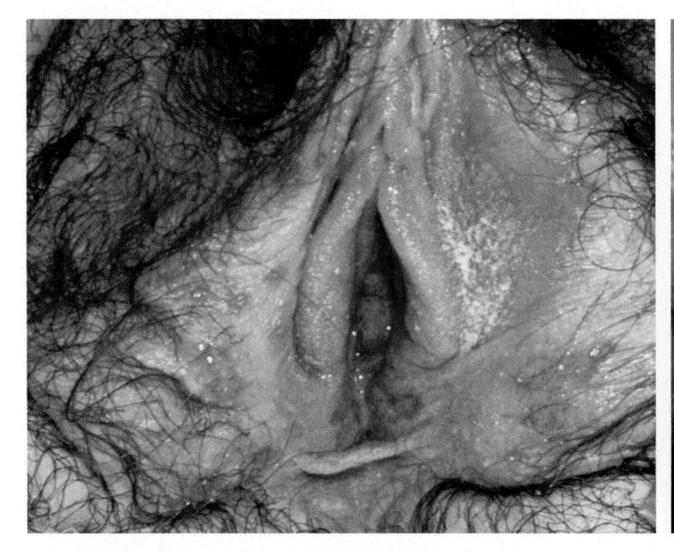

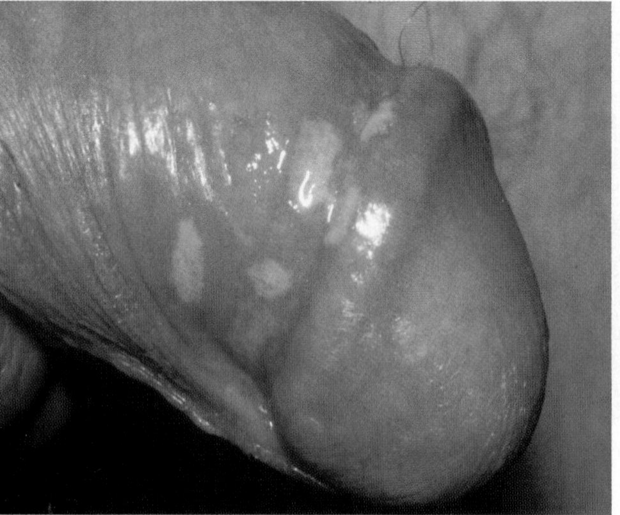

Figure 16.5 Genital herpes sores

infection with HSV-1 or HSV-2, but newer blood tests are much more accurate.

Treatments for genital herpes are targeted toward alleviating symptoms. Antiviral medications such as acyclovir can reduce the pain and hasten the healing of the sores. For patients who are experiencing frequent outbreaks, physicians may prescribe daily use of acyclovir to suppress recurrences and viral shedding, and reduce the risk of transmitting herpes to a sexual partner.

Condoms or dental dams should always be used if a partner has genital herpes, whether or not sores are present and whether or not the infected partner is taking an antiviral medication. They are not foolproof, however, as areas not covered by the barrier may shed the virus. Sex should be avoided entirely when one partner has visible herpes sores.

Human Papillomavirus

Human papillomavirus (HPV) causes all types of warts, wherever they may be on your body. There are over 100 types of HPV, although only four are responsible for most genital HPV infections. Genital HPV infection is the most common STI, and about half of all sexually active Americans will develop it at some point in their lives.[35] HPV is also the most reported STI on college campuses. An estimated 20 million people in the United States are currently infected, and an additional 6 million develop HPV infection every year.[35]

Modes of Transmission

The infection is spread through skin-to-skin contact, usually during vaginal, oral, or anal sex. Transmission can occur even when no signs or symptoms are present. Rarely, MTCT can occur during vaginal birth.

Signs and Symptoms

Most people infected with HPV don't experience any signs or symptoms. In about 90% of cases, the body's immune system overcomes an HPV infection naturally within about 2 years.[35] However, some infections result in genital warts, which are typically painless bumps so small that they may go unnoticed. Warts can be raised or flat, pink or flesh-toned, and there may be only a single one or multiple clusters **(Figure 16.6).** Warts can develop not only in the genital region, but also in the throat.

Some strains of HPV cause changes in cells that can lead to cancer. The types of HPV that cause cancer of the throat, cervix, vagina, penis, and anus are called "high-risk" strains. These strains do not cause warts and can only be detected with clinical testing.

Diagnosis and Treatment

Each year, about 400 men are diagnosed with HPV-associated penile cancer. HPV transmission during oral sex is also thought to account for an increase over the past two decades of cancers of the tonsils, tongue, and throat. However, of all HPV-related cancers, cervical cancer is the most significant public health concern: Each year, more than 12,000 American women are diagnosed with cervical cancer and more than 4,000 die.[36]

All of these cancers begin when infection with high-risk HPV causes a precancerous change in cells called *dysplasia*. When detected early, cells affected by dysplasia can be excised—often by laser surgery—with relatively minor pain and bleeding. But when left undetected, dysplasia can progress to cancer. That is why the Pap test, which is used to screen for cervical dysplasia, is a critical test for sexually active women. (For precise screening guidelines, see Chapter 12.) A woman's health-care provider may also recommend a separate test for high-risk strains of HPV. Currently there is no test for HPV in men.[37]

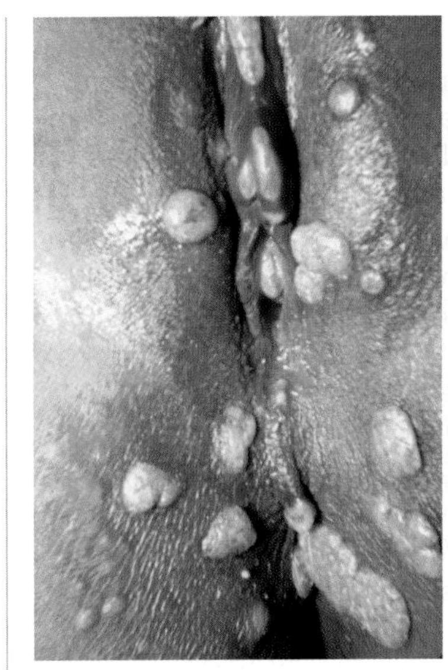
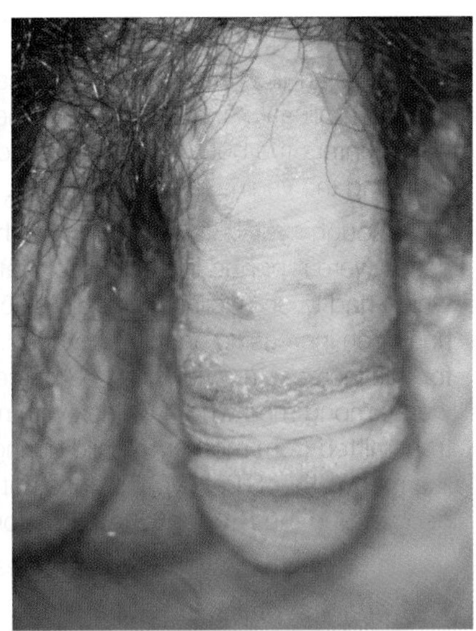

Figure 16.6 Genital warts

Genital warts can be treated with topical medications that are applied directly to the skin. They can also be frozen off through cryotherapy, burned off through electrocauterization, or removed by laser surgery. Warts can return, however, because these treatments do not cure the underlying HPV infection.

The FDA has approved two vaccines to protect against HPV in females up to age 26. These are Gardasil® and Cervarix®. Both vaccines protect against the two types of HPV associated with high-risk cervical cancer (types 16 and 18), but only Gardasil® also protects against the types of HPV commonly associated with cancers of the vulva, vagina, anus, and throat, as well as genital warts. The FDA has also approved the use of Gardasil® for the prevention of genital warts and HPV-associated cancers in males up to age 26.[38]

The vaccine is licensed for use in boys and girls as young as age 9, and the CDC recommends vaccination of all children—male and female—by age 11 or 12.[39] Virginia and Washington, DC, mandate the vaccine for middle-school girls.[40] But since HPV is sexually transmitted, many parents, politicians, and even some physicians are asking why preteens should be vaccinated. Concerns include research suggesting that protection lasts for only about 5 years, leaving adolescents needing a booster shot by the time they are 16 or 17, an age when they are far more likely to be sexually active and perhaps less likely to be getting regular health care. Even some pediatricians who support the vaccine do not believe that states should require it—or at least not until long-term studies confirm its safety and effectiveness.[40]

Bacterial STIs

STIs transmitted by bacteria can almost always be successfully treated with antibiotics if detected early. However, if they are allowed to progress, the complications can be severe and sometimes even fatal.

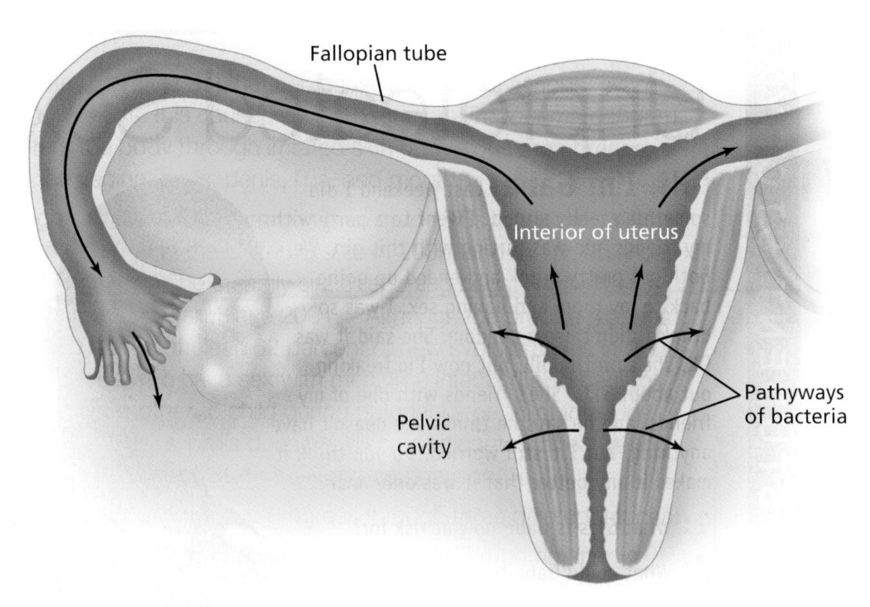

Figure 16.8 Pelvic inflammatory disease. PID occurs when bacteria spread from the vagina and cervix into the uterus, fallopian tubes, and/or peritoneum.

structures. This can lead to infertility or even death. PID affects an estimated 750,000 women in the United States every year, causing infertility in about 10–15%.[46]

How PID Develops

PID can result from infection with any of a variety of microorganisms, but the two most common culprits are *Neisseria gonorrhoeae* and *Chlamydia trachomatis*. With PID, bacteria can spread into the uterus, fallopian tubes, or even to the peritoneum, the membrane that lines the abdominal cavity and covers most of the abdominal organs **(Figure 16.8).** When bacteria infect the fallopian tubes, the resulting inflammation can cause the development of scar tissue. This can block a fertilized egg from moving into the uterus, leaving it to burrow into the tube lining, causing an ectopic pregnancy. As an ectopic pregnancy grows, it can rupture the tube, causing internal bleeding and even death. If the tubes are completely blocked by scar tissue, sperm cannot reach the woman's egg, and she will be infertile.[46]

Signs and Symptoms

Women may have no idea that they have PID, even as their reproductive system is being damaged. But symptoms do commonly occur, including chronic abdominal or pelvic pain, fever, irregular menstrual bleeding, painful intercourse, painful urination, or a foul-smelling vaginal discharge. The condition often goes unrecognized by patients and physicians alike.

Diagnosis and Treatment

No single test detects the presence of PID. Doctors typically perform a pelvic examination and test for chlamydia and gonorrhea. However, an abdominal ultrasound and even laparoscopy (minimally invasive surgery) may be needed to confirm the diagnosis. Antibiotics can cure the infection, but cannot undo any of the damage already done to a woman's reproductive organs. For that reason, prompt treatment is always critical. A woman's sex partners also should be treated—even if they have no symptoms—to keep from transmitting the bacteria back and forth. In some cases, a woman may need surgery to reduce the scarring. However, she may still remain infertile.

Avoiding sexually transmitted infections—or getting immediate medical care should one occur—will help protect women from developing PID. Because gonorrhea and chlamydia often have no noticeable symptoms, sexually active women should undergo regular pelvic examinations and annual chlamydia testing. Sexually active women under the age of 25 have a higher risk of PID because their cervix is not fully mature, increasing their susceptibility to the infections that prompt PID. In addition, women increase their risk of PID by douching, having recently had an IUD for birth control inserted, and having multiple sex partners.

Learn more about PID at www.livestrong.com/video/1804-pelvic-inflammatory-disease-health-byte.

Parasitic STIs

The most common sexually transmitted parasites are pubic lice and scabies, which are multicellular creatures, and *Trichomonas vaginalis*, a single-celled parasite.

Pubic Lice and Scabies

Pubic lice, or *Pthirus pubis*, are tiny six-legged creatures that infest pubic hair **(Figure 16.9).** Commonly known as "crabs," they can also attach themselves to eyebrows, eyelashes, beards, mustaches, or chest hair. Scabies is caused by tiny, eight-legged mites that burrow into the top layer of a person's skin and lay eggs. Scabies generally occurs in and around folds of skin, but can affect other parts of the body as well. Pubic lice and scabies are usually transmitted through sexual contact but occasionally are spread through contact with clothing, towels, sheets, or toilet seats that have been used by an infected person. They can be transmitted during sex even when a condom is used, because they can infest areas not covered by the condom.

The most common symptom of pubic lice and scabies is itching, especially during the night. In some instances, the infested area also becomes inflamed, and scabies can sometimes cause allergic reactions.

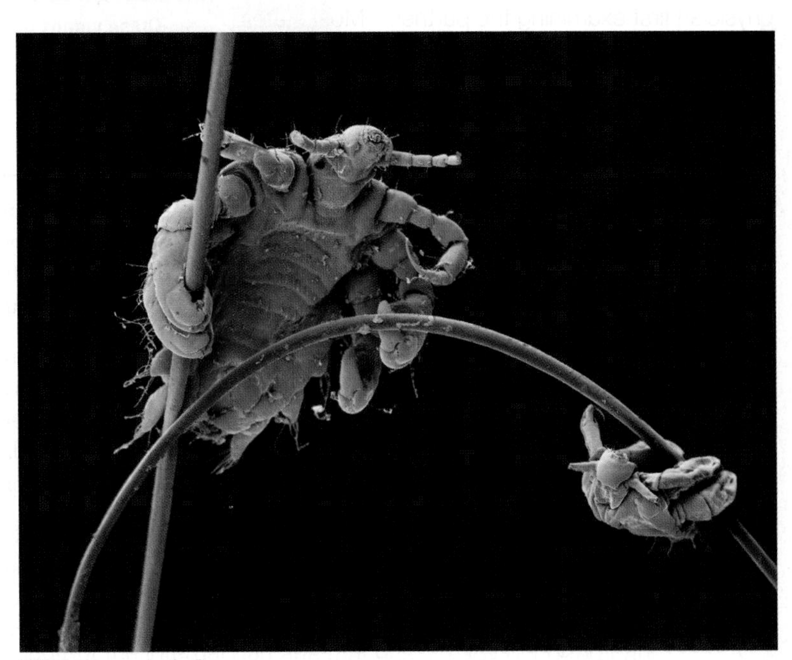

Figure 16.9 Pubic lice

The pests themselves do not spread disease, but excessive scratching of the skin can cause a bacterial infection.

A pubic lice or scabies infestation can be easily diagnosed with a doctor's visit. Prescribed creams or lotions can usually clear up these conditions, although an oral medication may be used for cases that are harder to treat.

Trichomoniasis

Trichomoniasis, or "trich," is caused by a protozoan called *Trichomonas vaginalis*. It is the most common curable STI in young women, although a recent study shows that the incidence is even higher in women over the age of 40.[47] Men can be infected as well. More than 7.4 million infections occur annually in the United States.[48]

The most common route of transmission is vaginal-penile intercourse. However, an infected woman can transmit *T. vaginalis* to a female sex partner during vulva-to-vulva contact. Fortunately, women often experience symptoms, typically within 5 to 28 days, so they seek medical treatment. Symptoms include painful urination, pain during intercourse, vaginal itching and irritation, and a greenish-yellow, strong-smelling vaginal discharge. Men often do not experience symptoms, but if they do they include irritation inside the penis and slight discharge. Infected women are at increased risk for HIV infection, and are more likely to pass HIV to a partner. Studies also suggest that infected men and women are at increased risk for infertility.

Trich in women is diagnosed with laboratory analysis of a vaginal swab. In women, a pelvic exam will reveal small red sores on the vaginal wall or cervix. Infection can be cured with oral antimicrobial drugs, usually metronidazole. Both partners must be treated, and must avoid sex until treatment is finished and all symptoms have cleared.

Change Yourself, Change Your World

If you're thinking about getting sexually involved with someone, reading this chapter has probably been a sobering experience. Warts and blisters, foul-smelling discharge, pain, infertility, death.... The picture of STIs can be gruesome, but now that you've got the facts, you're ready to make choices to protect yourself and your partner.

Personal Choices

Protection starts with a few simple actions. See the **Practical Strategies for Health** for a summary of steps you can take to reduce your STI risk.

Get Vaccinated

After vaccination, your body needs time to build up antibodies to protect you from active infection. So the ideal time to get vaccinated is before your first sexual experience. If you're already sexually active, vaccination can help protect you in future relationships.

Although hepatitis A is not primarily transmitted through sexual contact, the CDC recommends that men who have sex with men receive the hepatitis A vaccine. All people need immunization against hepatitis B. We noted earlier that a quarter of students entering college with a history of childhood hepatitis B immunization no longer showed immune memory to HBV. So check with your health-care provider about getting an HBV booster vaccine. And if you weren't vaccinated as a child, do it now.

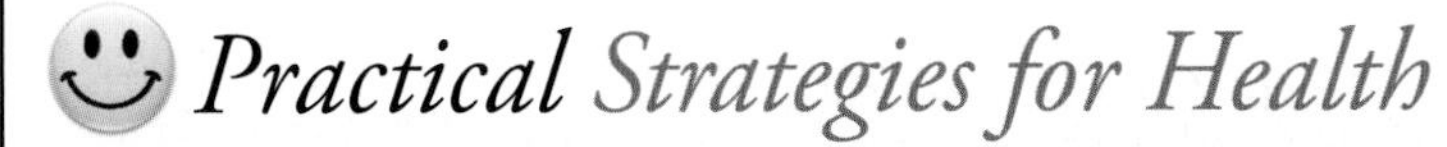

Reducing Risk of STIs

A few simple steps can dramatically reduce your risk of contracting an STI.

- **Consider abstinence.** Abstinence from sexual intercourse is the most effective method of avoiding STIs.
- **Explore non-intercourse sexual activity.** Share fantasies, kisses, and mutual masturbation.
- **Get vaccinated.** Before you become sexually active, ask your doctor about vaccines for HPV and hepatitis B. Men who have sex with other men should be vaccinated for hepatitis A as well.
- **Be faithful.** If you decide to have sex, do it with one uninfected partner who is not having sex with others, has not had sex with others for several months, and has tested negative for STIs, including HIV.
- **Get tested.** If you are sexually active, the only way to know for sure whether you have an infection is to be tested by a health practitioner. Many STIs have no noticeable symptoms and can go undetected for years, when treatment may be too late. It is important that both partners get tested before beginning a new sexual relationship.
- **Use a condom or latex barrier.** Use latex or polyurethane condoms correctly and consistently for all vaginal or anal sexual encounters. Condoms, dental dams, or latex squares should be used for oral sex.
- **Get annual checkups.** Annual checkups are a good time to discuss your sexual practices with your doctor.
- **Be alert to symptoms.** Should you develop any signs of an STI, get checked out by a physician right away. Prompt treatment can make all the difference between an effective treatment and long-term problems.
- **Be picky.** Limit the total number of sex partners you have in your lifetime.

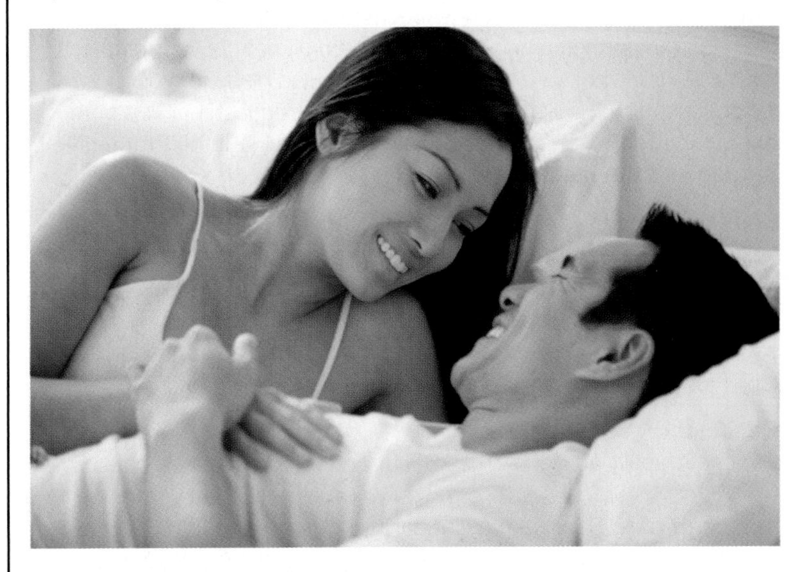

The CDC also recommends vaccination against HPV for both males and females aged 9 to 26. If you haven't received the HPV vaccine, or if more than 5 years have passed since your vaccination, make an appointment with your health-care provider or your campus health services and ask for it.

Practical Strategies for Health

Talking About Safer Sex

If you're not ready to talk about your sexual experiences or STIs with a new partner, you're not ready to have sex. It may feel awkward or embarrassing, but it's essential. Before you have sex with a new person, ask him or her the following questions:

- Do you have an STI or any symptoms that might be due to an STI?
- Have you ever had an STI?
  - If so, how long ago was this?
  - What did you do about it?
  - If you were treated, have you been tested since treatment? Were you positive or negative?
- Have you ever had unprotected sex?
  - If so, have you been tested for STIs since then? Were you positive or negative?
  - If not, have you ever been tested for STIs? Were you positive or negative?
- Are you prepared to use a condom?
- Are there any other safe sex measures you want to take?

Be prepared to answer these questions yourself as well. In many cases, you will find that your partner is concerned about these issues too. If your partner is unwilling to discuss safe sex or does not want to participate in the same level of safe sex that you do, reconsider sex with that person.

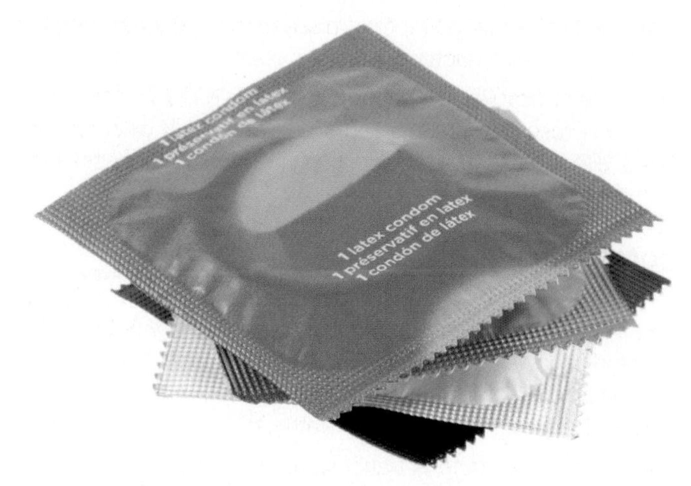

Condoms. Using them correctly and consistently is one of the most important ways to protect against STIs.

Talk About It

Before a relationship gets physical, ask yourself what you expect from your partner. Your answers might range from values such as honesty and commitment to practical measures like STI testing and condom use. Once you've clarified your expectations, it's time to communicate them to your partner, offering your own commitment to your partner's health as well. Choose a "no pressure" time and place for your conversation, such as on a weekend afternoon, and suggest that you both turn off your cell phones. For talking points, check out the **Practical Strategies for Health** above.

Use Condoms

One of the most important ways to protect yourself from STIs is to use latex condoms correctly and consistently—with every sex act. Always use a new condom. Never use an unapproved lubricant such as massage oil or petroleum jelly. Follow all manufacturer's instructions carefully. (For more information about condom use, see Chapter 17.)

Get Tested

If you're sexually active, discuss STI testing with your health-care provider at each routine visit. Even if you've never noticed any signs or symptoms of an STI, you may be harboring one. Especially if you're considering getting involved with someone new, get tested. If you don't have a regular health-care provider, visit your campus health center, which may offer free or low-cost testing.

Bear in mind that it can take weeks or even months for antibodies to certain STIs to show up in lab tests. Because of this, you need to allow a short period of time to elapse between your suspected exposure and testing. On the other hand, prompt treatment is important, so don't wait any longer than necessary for testing. If you're concerned about high-risk exposure to HIV, see your physician immediately! A course of treatment with HAART can significantly reduce your risk for developing an active infection.

The CDC recommends HIV testing at least once between ages 13 and 64 for people at low risk. If you're at high risk—for instance, if you have sex with more than one partner or are a male who has sex with males—then you should have an HIV test annually.[49]

Sexually active women should talk with their physician about how often they need a Pap test and whether or not they should have a test for specific high-risk strains of HPV. All sexually active women aged 25 or younger should have annual testing for chlamydia and gonorrhea, and women over 25 should have testing if starting a new relationship.

If you find out that you've tested positive for any STI, tell your current partner and anyone you've had sex with during the past year. Encourage them to seek testing, too. If you're uncomfortable revealing your test results, talk with your health-care provider. Most states require that certain STIs be reported to public health authorities, who can then notify partners, anonymously and confidentially, about exposure to STDs. Some public health departments now use email notification.[50]

To find a local clinic where you can be tested for STIs, just type in your zip code at http://hivtest.cdc.gov/STDTesting.aspx.

Get Treated

We've discussed treatment for each specific STI. In general, viral STIs are not curable, but antiviral medication can suppress herpes outbreaks, and HAART can keep HIV infection in check for many years. Both herpes and HIV can be transmitted while the person is taking medication, so condom use is still essential.

Bacterial STIs are usually curable with antibiotics, sometimes in a single dose. Trichomoniasis can also be cured with drug therapy. Taking the entire course of prescribed medication is essential, as is partner treatment. You must both avoid sex until the treatment is finished and you no longer have any sores or other symptoms.

Campus Advocacy

Earlier we noted that STIs tend to spread in small networks—such as on college campuses. It makes sense, then, that the actions you take to reduce your own STI risk will ripple out, benefiting many others in your campus community. But there's more you can do. Ongoing programs are in place on many college campuses to reduce the spread of STIs. Consider volunteering to assist in these efforts. Or if there's not much happening on your campus, talk with your health instructor or campus health services staff about getting any of the following STI prevention activities off the ground:

- **STI awareness event.** Work with faculty and administration to organize an STI awareness event to include speakers, films, CDC fact sheet distribution, condom giveaways, health screenings, games, and other events. Invite nearby bars and restaurants to give out free condoms and STI prevention brochures.
- **Open house.** Work with your campus health services center to schedule an open house offering walk-in STI testing, free condoms, and prevention information.
- **Fund-raising.** Sell T-shirts or other merchandise, organize a walk or run, or sponsor a benefit concert. Donate proceeds to a community STI prevention program.
- **Information.** Write an article or editorial for the campus paper, club newsletter, or email bulletin. Schedule interviews with STI experts on campus radio stations. Insert on your campus website links to sites with STI information, such as www.cdc.gov/std.

Need some inspiration? Check out Get Yourself Tested (GYT), a collaborative effort from MTV, the Kaiser Foundation, the CDC, and other national partners. At the GYT website, you can order T-shirts, buttons, videos, posters, and other materials, organize a testing event, or sign up to become a GYT campus ambassador. Visit www.itsyoursexlife.com/gyt/gytnow.

Want to get involved in a larger arena? CrowdOutAIDS is a collaborative online project by and for young adults. Sponsored by the United Nations' UNAIDS, its goals are to connect young adults online to share knowledge and find solutions to check the spread of HIV. Make your voice heard. Sign up at www.crowdoutaids.org.

Watch videos of real students discussing STIs at www.pearsonhighered.com/lynchelmore.

STUDENT STORY

Talking Honestly About STIs

"Hi, I'm Abbey. I absolutely think that people have a responsibility to tell someone if they have a sexually transmitted disease before they have sex. That is definitely something that their partner should know ahead of time, and it's deceitful to hide that from them. If someone asked me if I had an STI right before sex, I would answer honestly. I wouldn't be put off. I would understand why they would want to know that, and respect that they want to be safe and responsible with their body. How would I ask someone if they had an STI? I would just straightforwardly ask them."

1: Why is it so important to discuss sexual histories and exposure to sexually transmitted infections with a new partner prior to sex?

2: Why is it risky for sexually active individuals to skip regular medical checkups?

Do you have a story similar to Abbey's? Share your story at www.pearsonhighered.com/lynchelmore.

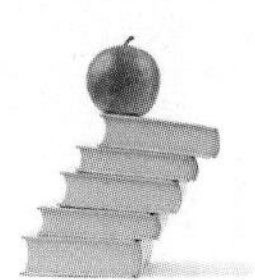

Choosing to Change Worksheet

To complete this worksheet online, visit www.pearsonhighered.com/lynchelmore.

Your likelihood of contracting an STI depends primarily on your behaviors. To reduce your risk of contracting an STI, follow the steps below.

Directions: Fill in your stage of change in Step 1 and complete Steps 2, 3, or 4, depending on which one applies to your stage of change.

Step 1: Your Stage of Behavior Change. Please check one of the following statements that best describes your readiness to reduce your STI risk.

_____________ I do not intend to reduce my STI risk in the next 6 months. (Precontemplation)

_____________ I might reduce my STI risk in the next 6 months. (Contemplation)

_____________ I am prepared to reduce my STI risk in the next month. (Preparation)

_____________ I have been reducing my STI risk for less than 6 months. (Action)

_____________ I have been reducing my STI risk for more than 6 months. (Maintenance)

Step 2: Precontemplation and Contemplation Stages. Increasing your knowledge of the risk factors for contracting an STI can help motivate you to change. If you answered "Yes" or "Don't Know" to any of the 10 items below you may be at a higher risk for STIs.

1. I have had oral, vaginal, or anal sex without using a latex condom.	Yes	No	
2. I have had sex with multiple partners and not discussed STIs before having sex.	Yes	No	
3. I have had sex after consuming alcohol.	Yes	No	
4. I have had sex while under the influence of illegal drugs.	Yes	No	
5. I have exchanged sex for drugs or money.	Yes	No	
6. I have come into direct contact with someone who has infections such as HPV, herpes, pubic lice, or scabies.	Yes	No	Don't Know
7. I have injected substances with dirty needles or syringes—or have had unprotected sex with someone who has.	Yes	No	Don't Know
8. I have shared needles for tattoos or body piercings—or have had unprotected sex with someone who has.	Yes	No	Don't Know
9. I have not been vaccinated against hepatitis A, hepatitis B, or human papillomavirus.	Yes	No	
10. I have had sex while infected with an STI.	Yes	No	Don't Know

What might be some barriers holding you back from taking action on reducing your STI risk factor(s) and how could you overcome them?

Barrier	Strategy for Overcoming Barrier
Example: My partner doesn't want to wear a condom.	*I will explain to him why it is important to wear one and how I feel about his lack of wanting to use one.*

Step 3: Preparation and Action Stages. For each of the risk reduction guidelines listed below, indicate one action you can take (or have already taken) to meet that guideline in your own life. Be specific.

Reducing Your Personal STI Risk

STI Risk Reduction Guideline	Specific Action to Meet Guideline
Become more educated about the risks, symptoms, treatment, and prevention of STIs.	*Example: Talk to my nurse practitioner about safer sex practices and/or any STI symptoms I should watch out for.*
For STIs with an available vaccine (HPV and hepatitis B), get vaccinated.	
Be alert for signs or symptoms of STIs.	
Get tested.	
Communicate with sexual partners about your sexual histories, including histories of STIs.	
Don't impair your judgment before participating in sexual activity by using drugs or alcohol.	
Always use a latex condom from start to finish.	
Practice safe oral sex by using condoms, dental dams, or latex squares.	
Limit your number of sexual partners.	

Write down a specific **goal** for reducing your STI risk, including a timeline, below.

Step 4: Maintenance Stage. Your goal is to stay focused and maintain your commitment to preventing STIs. What benefits of practicing STI prevention are most important to you and why?

How easy has it been to practice STI prevention? Is it truly a habit or do you need to expend some effort to do it? How can you keep yourself on track?

Chapter Summary

- Although 15- to 24-year-olds represent only one-fourth of the sexually active population, they account for nearly half of all new STI cases.
- STI pathogens are typically transmitted from one partner to another in blood, semen, or the secretions of the mucous membranes of the male or female genitals, the anus, or the mouth. Anal sex carries a much higher risk of STI transmission than either vaginal or oral sex.
- Mutual monogamy is second only to abstinence in offering the best protection against acquiring an STI. Mutual monogamy requires long-term commitment and is not the same as serial monogamy.
- Many STIs have a latency period of weeks to months before testing can detect antibodies or other evidence of infection. If either partner has recently had sex with someone else, it is considered high risk to have sex without a condom.
- Although genital herpes, genital warts, and infestations with parasites can be sexually transmitted even when partners use a latex condom, clinical trials over decades have shown that, when used correctly and consistently, condoms significantly reduce transmission of most STIs.
- HIV is the most serious of the sexually transmitted pathogens. It targets and destroys the CD4 T cells of the immune system, leaving the host vulnerable to a variety of opportunistic infections and cancers characteristic of acquired immunodeficiency syndrome (AIDS).
- Diagnosis of HIV infection requires multiple tests, typically the ELISA followed by the Western blot. Early detection is important because prompt treatment with highly active antiretroviral therapy (HAART) can significantly prolong life. Left untreated, AIDS typically leads to death within about 3 years.
- Three other viral STIs are common. These include hepatitis B, genital herpes, and human papillomavirus (HPV).
- Hepatitis B infection lingers in the body in a small percentage of infected people, gradually destroying liver cells and leading to liver failure or liver cancer.
- Genital herpes produces outbreaks of itchy blisters that may recur throughout a person's lifetime. There is no cure, but antiviral medication can help suppress outbreaks.
- Certain strains of HPV cause genital warts, whereas high-risk strains promote cancers of the reproductive system, including cervical cancer in women and penile cancer in men. High-risk HPV transmitted during oral sex is associated with throat cancer, and high-risk HPV transmitted during anal sex is associated with anal cancer.
- Common bacterial STIs include syphilis, gonorrhea, and chlamydia. Regular screening for these infections is important for anyone who is sexually active, because they may not produce obvious signs or symptoms, and they can be cured if antibiotics are administered early, but they have long-term complications if left untreated.
- Gonorrhea and chlamydia are the STIs most commonly responsible for pelvic inflammatory disease, which can result in infertility or a life-threatening ectopic pregnancy.
- Pubic lice, scabies, and trichomoniasis are common sexually transmitted parasitic infections. They cause itching and other symptoms, and are readily cured with treatment.
- Abstinence is the best means of preventing sexually transmitted infections. If you're sexually active, you can reduce your risk by getting the appropriate vaccines, talking about STIs with potential partners prior to becoming sexually involved, limiting your number of sexual partners, and using latex condoms correctly and consistently. You should also have regular STI testing, and if you are diagnosed with an STI, get prompt treatment.
- Every step you take to protect yourself from STIs will also benefit your current and future sex partners, and their partners. You can also assist or support STI prevention efforts on campus and in your community.

Test Your Knowledge

1. Which of the following activities is associated with the lowest risk for acquiring an STI?
   a. unprotected vaginal sex with someone who ended a monogamous relationship 2 weeks ago
   b. unprotected anal sex with someone who has no signs or symptoms of an STI
   c. vaginal sex using a latex condom
   d. anal sex using a latex condom

2. Latex condoms
   a. are 100% effective against all STIs.
   b. offer greater protection against STIs when they are lubricated with a spermicide.
   c. can be reused.
   d. offer protection against many STIs during oral-penile sex.

3. Which of the following viruses has an envelope studded with proteins that fit the CD4 receptors on helper T cells?
   a. HIV
   b. HBV
   c. HSV-2
   d. HPV

4. The first couple of weeks after being infected with HIV is called the
   a. asymptomatic stage.
   b. primary infection stage.
   c. pre-infection stage.
   d. inactive stage.

5. Antibiotics are appropriate treatments against
   a. genital warts.
   b. gonorrhea.
   c. scabies.
   d. all of the above.

6. The most commonly reported sexually transmitted infection among college students is
   a. HPV.
   b. genital herpes.
   c. syphilis.
   d. HIV/AIDS.

7. Pelvic inflammatory disease
   a. is most commonly caused by HIV or HSV-2.
   b. typically spreads to the urethra.
   c. is a potential complication of gonorrhea in both men and women.
   d. can result in an ectopic pregnancy.

8. Cervical cancer is caused by
   a. hepatitis B (HBV).
   b. chlamydia.
   c. human papillomavirus (HPV).
   d. gonorrhea.

9. *Trichomonas vaginalis*
   a. does not infect males.
   b. is a type of protozoan.
   c. cannot be cured, but can be managed with antimicrobial drugs.
   d. is commonly spread by contact with sheets, towels, and clothing.

10. Which of the following practices will reduce your risk of contracting an STI?
    a. purchasing a package of condoms
    b. avoiding partners who look sick
    c. limiting your number of partners
    d. all of the above

Get Critical

What happened:

In the summer of 2011, the entertainment blogs buzzed with the news that an unnamed male celebrity "of substantial fame internationally" had been sued for transmitting genital herpes to an unidentified sex partner who had been assured by the celebrity that he was "STD free." The case was allegedly settled for five million dollars. This was just one of many such court cases in which plaintiffs have sued sex partners—usually ones with deep pockets—for lying about their sexual health history and transmitting an incurable STI, typically herpes or HIV.

Such cases may seem straightforward, but in reality they're notoriously difficult to win. First of all, plaintiffs must have the money to pursue legal action in the first place. Second, if the plaintiff has had more than one sex partner, he or she might not be able to prove conclusively that the accused was responsible for the STI. Third, the plaintiff must be able to show that the accused knew that he or she was infected. This can be difficult, because many STIs don't produce symptoms in everyone who is infected. Even when plaintiffs are awarded a financial settlement, they may still feel inadequately compensated for such a violation of their trust, and in the case of viral STIs, one that has left them with an incurable disease.

What do you think?

- Consent to engage in sexual intercourse requires that the person giving consent have the information necessary to make intelligent decisions. If one person is concealing an STI from the other, is consensual sex possible?
- In your view, should people convicted of lying to a potential partner about an incurable STI get off by paying a fine, or should they serve jail time?
- When someone lies about his or her sexual health history, how can sex partners protect themselves from an STI?

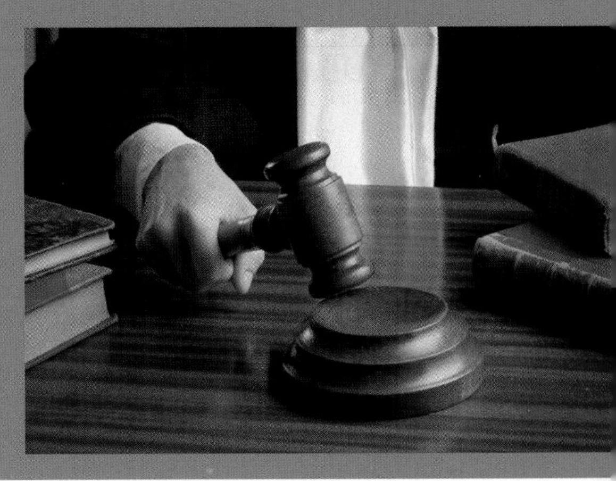

Get Connected

Mobile Tips!

Scan this QR code with your mobile device to access additional tips about reducing your risk for STIs. Or, via your mobile device, go to **http://mobiletips.pearsoncmg.com** and navigate to Chapter 16.

Health Online Visit the following websites for further information about the topics in this chapter:

- Medline Plus
  www.nlm.nih.gov/medlineplus
- American Social Health Association
  www.ashastd.org
- Planned Parenthood, Sexually Transmitted Diseases
  www.plannedparenthood.org/health-topics/stds-hiv-safer-sex-101.htm
- Center for Young Women's Health, College Health: Sexual Health
  www.youngwomenshealth.org/collegehealth10.html
- The Body: The Complete HIV/AIDS Resource
  www.thebody.com
- Smartersex.org
  www.smartersex.org
- Go Ask Alice
  http://goaskalice.columbia.edu

Website links are subject to change. To access updated web links, please visit ***www.pearsonhighered.com/lynchelmore.***

References

i. Centers for Disease Control and Prevention. (2010). *Trends in sexually transmitted diseases in the United States: 2009 National data for chlamydia, gonorrhea, and syphilis.* Retrieved from http://www.cdc.gov/std/stats09/trends.htm.

ii. Centers for Disease Control and Prevention. (2011, November 7). *HIV in the United States*. Retrieved from http://www.cdc.gov/hiv/resources/factsheets/us.htm.

1. World Health Organization. (2007). *Global strategy for the prevention and control of sexually transmitted infections: 2006–2015. Breaking the chain of transmission.* Geneva, Switzerland: WHO Press.

2. Centers for Disease Control and Prevention. (2010). *Sexually transmitted disease surveillance, 2009.* Retrieved from http://www.cdc.gov/std/stats09/default.htm.

3. Centers for Disease Control and Prevention. (2010). *Sexually transmitted disease surveillance, 2009: STDs in adolescents and young adults.* Retrieved from http://www.cdc.gov/std/stats09/adol.htm.

4. Forhan, S. E., Gottlieb, S. L., Sternberg, M. R., Fujie, X., Datta, S. D., McQuillan, G. M., . . . Markowitz, L. E. (2009). Prevalence of sexually transmitted infections among female adolescents aged 14 to 19 in the United States. *Pediatrics, 124* (6), 1505–1512. doi: 10.1542/peds.2009-0674.

5. Food and Drug Administration. (2010, July 22). *Condoms and sexually transmitted diseases.* Retrieved from http://www.fda.gov/ForConsumers/byAudience/ForPatientAdvocates/HIVandAIDSActivities/ucm126372.htm#should.

6. Centers for Disease Control and Prevention. (2010, March 25). *HIV transmission*. Retrieved from http://www.cdc.gov/hiv/resources/qa/transmission.htm.

7. Centers for Disease Control and Prevention. (2011, September 13). *Condoms and STDs: Fact sheet for public health personnel.* Retrieved from http://www.cdc.gov/condomeffectiveness/latex.htm.

8. Mayo Foundation. (2011, February 24). Sexually transmitted diseases. Retrieved from http://www.mayoclinic.com/health/sexually-transmitted-diseases-stds/DS01123.

9. Microbicides 2010 (International Conference on Microbicides). (2010, May 25). Use of lubricants with anal sex could increase risk of HIV. *ScienceDaily*. Retrieved from http://www.sciencedaily.com-/releases/2010/05/100525094900.htm.

10. Centers for Disease Control and Prevention. (2009, June 3). *Oral sex and HIV risk*. Retrieved from http://www.cdc.gov/hiv/resources/factsheets/oralsex.htm.

11. Inungu, J., Mumford, V., Younis, M., & Langford, S. (2009). HIV knowledge, attitudes and practices among college students in the United States. *Journal of Health and Human Services Administration, 32* (3), 259–277.

12. Joint United Nations Programme on HIV/AIDS (UNAIDS). (2010). *The 2010 UNAIDS report on the global AIDS epidemic.* Retrieved from http://www.unaids.org/documents/20101123_FS_Global_em_en.pdf.

13. Centers for Disease Control and Prevention. (2011, November 7). *HIV in the United States.* Retrieved from http://www.cdc.gov/hiv/resources/factsheets/us.htm.

14. World Health Organization. (n.d.). *Mother-to-child transmission of HIV.* Retrieved from http://www.who.int/hiv/topics/mtct/en/index.html.

15. U.S. Department of Health and Human Services. (2010, October 12). *Stages of HIV.* AIDS.gov. Retrieved from http://aids.gov/hiv-aids-basics/diagnosed-with-hiv-aids/hiv-in-your-body/stages-of-hiv.

16. U.S. National Library of Medicine. (2011, June 9). *AIDS.* PubMed. Retrieved from http://www.ncbi.nlm.nih.gov/pubmedhealth/PMH0001620.

17. Centers for Disease Control and Prevention. (2011, June 24). Results of the expanded HIV testing initiative—25 jurisdictions, United States, 2007–2010. *MMWR, 60* (24), 805–810. Retrieved from http://www.cdc.gov/mmwr/preview/mmwrhtml/mm6024a2.htm.

18. Food and Drug Administration. (2012, April 16). *Vital facts about HIV home test kits*. Available at http://www.fda.gov/ForConsumers/ConsumerUpdates/ucm048553.htm.

19. Mayo Foundation. (2009, December 3). HIV testing. Retrieved from http://www.mayoclinic.com/health/hiv-testing/MY00954/DSECTION=what-you-can-expect.

20. American College Health Association. (2012). *American College Health Association National College Health Assessment II: Reference group executive summary, fall 2011*. Linthicum, MD: American College Health Association.

21. Department of Health and Human Services, Panel on Antiretroviral Guidelines for Adults and Adolescents. (2011, October 14). *Guidelines for the use of antiretroviral agents in HIV-1-infected adults and adolescents*. Retrieved from http://www.aidsinfo.nih.gov/ContentFiles/AdultandAdolescentGL.pdf.

22. World Health Organization. (2009). Love in the era of HAART. *HIV/AIDS Prevention and Care Newsletter, 2* (1), 1. Retrieved from http://www.wpro.who.int/NR/rdonlyres/48B1DC54-F2CC-4704-8199-1E7FBEA002EA/0/ARVnewsletter_vol2issue1_July2009.pdf.

23. Landovitz, R. J., & Currier, J. S. (2009, October 29). Postexposure prophylaxis for HIV infection. *New England Journal of Medicine,* 361, 1768–1775. Retrieved from http://www.nejm.org/doi/full/10.1056/NEJMcp0904189.

24. Ross, A. L., Brave, A., Scarlatti, G., Manrique, A., & Buonaguro, L. (2010, May). Progress towards development of an HIV vaccine: Report of the AIDS vaccine 2009 conference. *The Lancet—Infectious Diseases*, 10.

25. Keller, D. M. (2010, July 21). Tenofvir vaginal gel first microbicide to prevent HIV, HSV infections. AIDS 2010: XVIII International AIDS Conference: Abstract TUSS0504. Presented July 19, 2010. *Medscape Medical News*. Retrieved from http://www.medscape.com/viewarticle/725583.

26. Mahalingam, A., Geonnotti, A. R., Balzarini, J., & Kiser, P. F. (2011). Activity and safety of synthetic lectins based on benzoboroxole-functionalized polymers for inhibition of HIV entry. *Molecular Pharmaceutics*, 110831135436035 DOI: 10.1021/mp2002957.

27. U.S. Food and Drug Administration. (2012, July 16). FDA Approves First Medication to Reduce HIV Risk. Retrieved from http://www.fda.gov/ForConsumers/ConsumerUpdates/ucm311821.htm

28. Centers for Disease Control and Prevention. (2009). *Hepatitis B FAQs for the public.* Retrieved from http://www.cdc.gov/hepatitis/B/bFAQ.htm.

29. U.S. National Library of Medicine. (2010, November 23). *Hepatitis B.* Retrieved from http://www.ncbi.nlm.nih.gov/pubmedhealth/PMH0001324.

30. Jan, C. F., Huang, K. C., Chien, Y. C., Greydanus, D. E., Davies, D., Chiu, T. Y., . . . Chen, D. S. (2010). Determination of immune memory to hepatitis B vaccination through early booster response in college students. *Hepatology*, *51* (5), 1547–1554.

31. American Social Health Association. (n.d.). *Treatment for oral herpes.* Retrieved from http://www.ashastd.org/herpes/herpes_learn_treatment.cfm#2.

32. Centers for Disease Control and Prevention. (2010). *CDC study finds U.S. herpes rates remain high* [Press release]. Retrieved from http://www.cdc.gov/nchhstp/Newsroom/hsv2pressrelease.html.

33. Horowitz, R., Alerstuck, S., Williams, E. A., & Melby, B. (2010). Herpes simplex virus infection in a university health population: Clinical manifestations, epidemiology, and implications. *Journal of American College Health, 59* (2) 69–74.

34. Jancin, B. (2011, April). Genital herpes may double prostate cancer risk. *Skin & Allergy News: Infectious Diseases*, *42*, (4), 28.

35. Centers for Disease Control and Prevention. (2011, November 7). *CDC fact sheet: Genital HPV infection.* Retrieved from http://www.cdc.gov/std/hpv/stdfact-hpv.htm.

36. American Cancer Society. (2012). *Cancer facts and figures 2012.* Retrieved from http://www.cancer.org/acs/groups/content/@epidemiologysurveilance/documents/document/acspc-031941.pdf.

37. Centers for Disease Control and Prevention. (2011, August 25). *HPV and men: Fact sheet*. Retrieved from http://www.cdc.gov/std/hpv/stdfact-hpv-and-men.htm.

38. U.S. Food and Drug Administration. (2009, October 16). *FDA approves new indication for Gardasil to prevent genital warts in men and boys* [News release]. Retrieved from http://www.fda.gov/NewsEvents/Newsroom/PressAnnouncements/ucm187003.htm.

39. Centers for Disease Control and Prevention. (2011, October 25). *Press briefing transcript: ACIP recommends all 11–12-year-old males get vaccinated against HPV*. Retrieved from http://www.cdc.gov/media/releases/2011/t1025_hpv_12yroldvaccine.html.

40. Knox, R. (2011, September 19). HPV vaccine: The science behind the controversy. *National Public Radio*. Retrieved from http://www.npr.org/2011/09/19/140543977/hpv-vaccine-the-science-behind-the-controversy.

41. Centers for Disease Control and Prevention. (2010, November 22). *Sexually transmitted diseases surveillance, 2009: Syphilis.* Retrieved from http://www.cdc.gov/std/stats09/syphilis.htm.

42. Mayo Clinic. (2009). *Gonorrhea.* Retrieved from http://www.mayoclinic.com/print/gonorrhea/DS00180.

43. Centers for Disease Control and Prevention. (2011, September 13). *Expedited partner therapy.* Retrieved from http://www.cdc.gov/std/ept/default.htm.

44. American Social Health Association. (n.d.). *Chlamydia: Questions and answers.* Retrieved from http://www.ashastd.org/learn/learn_chlamydia.cfm.

45. Centers for Disease Control and Prevention. (2011, August 17). *CDC fact sheet: Chlamydia.* Retrieved from http://www.cdc.gov/std/chlamydia/stdfact-chlamydia.htm.

46. Centers for Disease Control and Prevention. (2011, March 25). *CDC fact sheet: Pelvic inflammatory disease.* Retrieved from http://www.cdc.gov/std/PID/STDFact-PID.htm.

47. Ginocchio, C. C., Chapin, K., Smith, J. S., Aslanzadeh, J., Snook, J., Hill, C. S., & Gaydos, C. A. (2011, July). Prevalence of *Trichomonas vaginalis* and coinfection with *Chlamydia trachomatis* and *Neisseria gonorrhoea* in the USA as determined by the aptima *Trichomonas vaginalis* nucleic acid amplification assay. *Sexually Transmitted Infections, 87* (1), A72–A73.

48. Centers for Disease Control and Prevention. (2011, November 11). *CDC fact sheet: Trichomoniasis.* Retrieved from http://www.cdc.gov/std/trichomonas/stdfact-trichomoniasis.htm.

49. Centers for Disease Control and Prevention. (2007, January 22). *HIV testing: Questions and answers for the general public.* Retrieved from http://www.cdc.gov/hiv/topics/testing/resources/qa/qa_general-public.htm.

50. Tuller, D. (2009, January 19). After hook-ups, e cards that warn, 'get checked.' *The New York Times*. Retrieved from http://www.nytimes.com/2009/01/20/health/20partners.html.

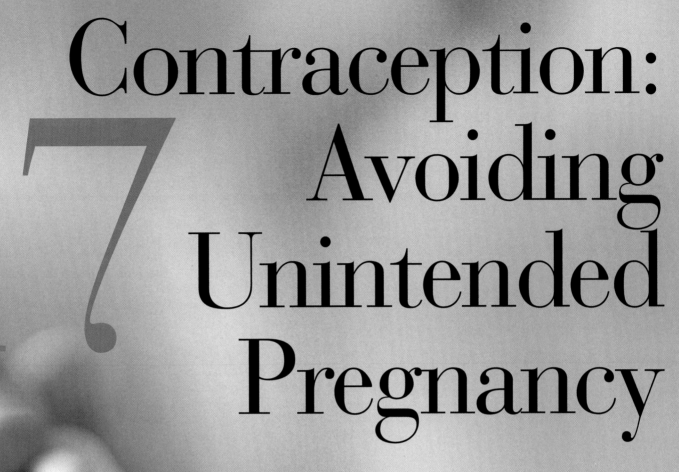

17 Contraception: Avoiding Unintended Pregnancy

- Among unmarried women in their 20s, 7 out of 10 pregnancies are unintended.[i]

- More than 75% of unmarried sexually active adults aged 18 to 29 say that it is very important to avoid pregnancy in their lives right now.[i]

- About half of these adults admit that they don't use contraceptives every time they have sex.[i]

LEARNING OBJECTIVES

EXPLORE the variety of reasons that young adults are at high risk for unintended pregnancy.

IDENTIFY the physiologic events involved in conception.

DESCRIBE the fertility awareness method of contraception.

COMPARE and contrast different over-the-counter methods of contraception.

IDENTIFY the benefits and drawbacks of the prescription methods of contraception.

DESCRIBE the surgical methods for preventing pregnancy.

DISCUSS the laws and politics of abortion, the medical and surgical abortion methods, and potential complications.

IDENTIFY the key choices you can make to avoid unintended pregnancy.

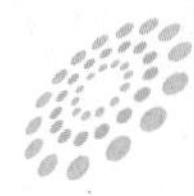

Health Online icons are found throughout the chapter, directing you to web links, videos, podcasts, and other useful online resources.

On screen, romantic partners don't plan to have sex.

The music swells, the lights dim, and . . . slow fade to rumpled sheets. The problem with such scenes is, they're rarely followed by ones depicting consequences . . . like an unintended pregnancy. So we get the message that unplanned sexual encounters are normal, desirable—even "the way it should be." And because we fail to plan for sex, we fail to plan for pregnancy. About half of all pregnancies in the United States are unintended, and among unmarried women in their 20s, fully seven out of ten pregnancies are not planned.[1]

Unintended Pregnancy in the United States

unintended pregnancy A pregnancy that is either mistimed or unwanted at the time of conception.

The U.S. Centers for Disease Control and Prevention (CDC) defines an **unintended pregnancy** as a pregnancy that is either mistimed or unwanted at the time of conception. Unintended pregnancy is associated with delayed prenatal care, which increases the risk of harm to both the mother and the fetus.[2] Moreover, women with unintended pregnancies are more likely to delay or entirely fail to make certain lifestyle changes—such as eating a more nourishing diet, avoiding alcohol, and quitting smoking—that are critical to their own and their baby's health.

More than 75% of sexually active unmarried adults aged 18 to 29 report that it is very important for them to avoid pregnancy. Yet half of this same population also report that they fail to use contraception consistently.[1] Although you might assume that college students would be highly motivated to avoid pregnancy, in a recent survey, only 53.7% of sexually active college students reported using contraception the last time they had vaginal intercourse.[3] Why the mismatch? In 2009, the National Campaign to Prevent Teen and Unplanned Pregnancy published the results of a survey suggesting that the following factors contribute significantly to unintended pregnancy among sexually active unmarried Americans aged 18 to 29:[1]

- **Economic factors.** Disparities in access to quality health care make contraceptives—especially the most reliable forms such as the birth control pill—less available to some young adults. Economic factors also affect access to quality education, including sex education, as well as opportunities for young women to envision life choices other than motherhood.
- **Lack of knowledge.** Many young adults know little about contraceptive methods. For instance, 30% say they know little or nothing about condoms, and 56% say they have never even heard of hormonal implants.
- **Unwarranted fears.** More than 25% of women believe that using birth control pills for an extended period of time will directly cause a serious disease such as cancer even in healthy, nonsmoking women. Also, 30% believe it's quite likely that using an IUD will cause an infection.
- **False beliefs.** Over 40% of young adults believe that even highly effective contraceptive methods such as birth control pills are unreliable. Moreover, a surprising 59% of women believe it's at least slightly likely that they are infertile (the actual rate is just over 8%).
- **Values.** About 13% of young adults view contraception as morally wrong.

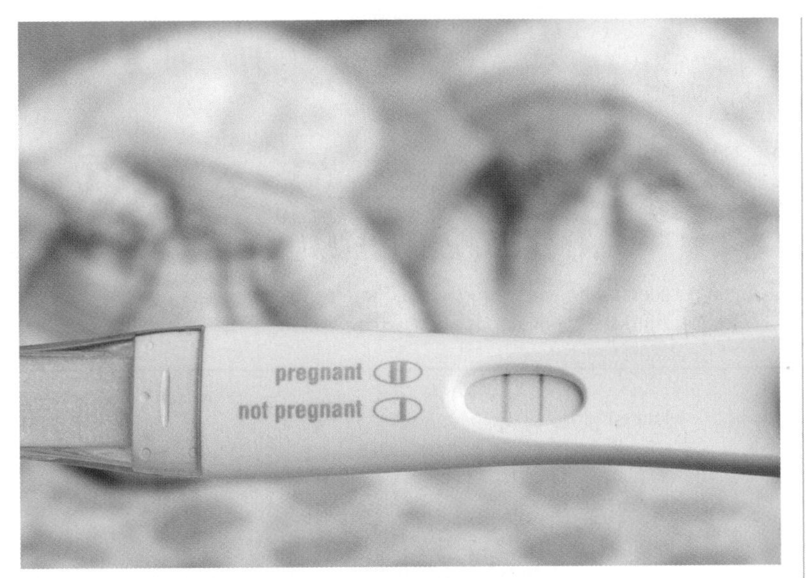
pregnant
not pregnant

Unintended pregnancies can result if you don't use birth control consistently and correctly every time.

- **Ambivalence.** Even among those who say it's important to them to avoid pregnancy, 20% of women and 43% of men say that they would be at least a little pleased if they found out that they or their partner were pregnant.

Notice how many of these issues reflect lack of information or misinformation. If you're not really sure exactly how pregnancy happens, or how the different contraceptives work, or how effective they are, then you're less likely to use them correctly and consistently. And you or your partner is more likely to end up pregnant. That's where this chapter comes in.

Watch an animation of ovulation at www.mayoclinic.com/health/ovulation/MM00108.

Conception and Contraception

Conception is the combination of the genetic material (DNA) of a woman's ovum (egg cell) and a man's sperm cell. It is the initial event in pregnancy, but researchers estimate that more than half of all conceptions end spontaneously before a woman even knows she is pregnant.[4] Strictly speaking, **contraception** is a behavior or product intended to oppose (*contra-* means "against") conception. Some methods broadly referred to as contraception, however, prevent pregnancy in other ways, such as by causing a woman's uterus to expel the conception. We therefore define contraception as any method used to prevent pregnancy.

How Does Conception Occur?

At birth, a female's ovaries are filled with more than 1 million ovarian follicles, each containing an immature ovum; most of these are absorbed into the ovary during childhood, but about 400,000 are still present when she has her first menstrual period. After puberty, a woman's body prepares itself for pregnancy approximately once each month by ovulating—releasing one mature ovum **(Figure 17.1).** Meanwhile, a man's testes are constantly creating sperm, millions of which are released into the woman's vagina during ejaculation. The vast majority of these sperm will never find their way to their target—millions will leak from the woman's vagina, be trapped in its thick mucus, or be destroyed in its acidic environment. The sperm that do reach the ovum—typically while it is still within the fallopian tube—next face the difficult task of penetrating its thick outer capsule. Thousands of sperm secrete enzymes that dissolve a region of this capsule. As soon as a minute portion of the ovum is exposed, the next sperm that approaches will be able to make contact with it and will be pulled into the ovum interior. The ovum will then undergo a chemical change that will block any further sperm from penetrating its membrane. The "winning sperm" then travels to the egg's nucleus, where conception—also called fertilization—occurs.

Even then, pregnancy is not guaranteed. The fertilized egg, now called a **zygote,** must travel through the fallopian tube toward the uterus. It's a perilous journey: Any scar tissue within the tube can "snag" the zygote so that it attaches to the wall of the tube, where it cannot grow. In successful pregnancies, the zygote travels unimpeded through the tube, dividing repeatedly along the way. The initial fertilized cell becomes two, then four, and so on, creating a little ball of cells called a **blastocyst.** About 4 to 5 days after conception, the blastocyst emerges into the uterus and burrows into the endometrium (see Figure 17.1, step 4). This event is called **implantation.** In some

conception The combination of the genetic material (DNA) of a woman's ovum and a man's sperm.

contraception Any method used to prevent pregnancy.

zygote A fertilized ovum.

blastocyst Early stage of embryonic development in which multiple cell divisions have produced an initial cell mass.

implantation The lodging of a blastocyst in the endometrium of the uterus.

3 Zygote (fertilized egg) undergoes rapid cell division as it travels toward uterus, developing into blastocyst
Zygote
2 Fertilization: Egg is fertilized by a single sperm cell in the fallopian tube
Fallopian tube
Sperm
Ovary
Uterus
1 Ovulation: Egg is released from ovary
Ovum
4 Implantation: Blastocyst arrives at uterus and implants into the uterine lining

Figure 17.1 Events required for pregnancy. The process includes ovulation, fertilization, and implantation.

Source: Adapted from Thompson, J., Manore, M., and Vaughan, L., *The Science of Nutrition*, 2nd ed., p. 380, Fig. 10.17. © 2011 Pearson Education.

cases the blastocyst will make it into the uterus but fail to implant, and the entire process from menstruation to ovulation will begin all over again.

What Methods of Contraception Are Available?

Contraceptive options differ in technique, price, effectiveness, and side effects, but they all have the same goal: to prevent pregnancy. They do this in a number of ways:

- *Natural methods* involve no pills or devices and are therefore always available and cost free.
- *Barrier methods* work to prevent sperm from reaching an egg.
- *Hormonal methods* deliver hormones to a woman. Most of these medications prevent ovulation: If no egg is released, it can't be fertilized. Some block implantation, or promote contractions of the uterus that expel the endometrium and its implanted blastocyst.
- *Surgical methods* are available for women and for men, and are the most permanent of options.

Which Method Is Best?

The answer to this question depends on each individual couple. When deciding which type of birth control to use, couples should consider how comfortable they are with the method, how many side effects it has, the woman's health history, how well the method works, the cost, and how likely they are to use it correctly and consistently. Every method has a published **failure rate** indicating the percentage of women who typically get pregnant after using that method for one year. However, the figures are a bit misleading. That's because failure rates indicate pregnancy rates if the method is used exactly as directed, a concept known as "perfect use." In reality, couples do not always use birth control perfectly. Women forget to take their pills. Men put condoms on improperly. The end result is what is known as "typical use," which has substantially higher pregnancy rates. For example, the failure rate for condoms with perfect use—correctly and consistently during every act of intercourse—is only 2 to 3 pregnancies per 100 women per year. But the typical use failure rate ranges as high as 15 per 100 women per year.[5]

Another critical factor is the **continuation rate,** or the percentage of couples who continue to practice that form of birth control. Often, couples will stop using one method and, before choosing a new method, will have unprotected sex. Certain public health strategies, such as decreasing the cost or increasing the availability of over-the-counter (OTC) contraceptives, or teaching physicians to prescribe a greater number of birth control pill packs per prescription, can improve continuation rates and reduce unintended pregnancies.[6]

Table 17.1 summarizes different forms of contraception, organized into four general categories: cost-free methods, methods available over the counter, methods requiring a prescription, and surgical methods. As we take a closer look at these methods, take note of differences in availability, cost, effectiveness, ease of use, and whether or not the method provides protection against sexually transmitted infection. Meanwhile, the **Student Stats** box illustrates the most popular forms of contraception reported by college students.

failure rate The percentage of women who typically get pregnant after using a given contraceptive method for one year.

continuation rate The percentage of couples who continue to practice a given form of birth control.

STUDENT STATS

Top Contraceptives among College Students

Among students who engaged in vaginal intercourse and used contraception, the top methods are listed below.

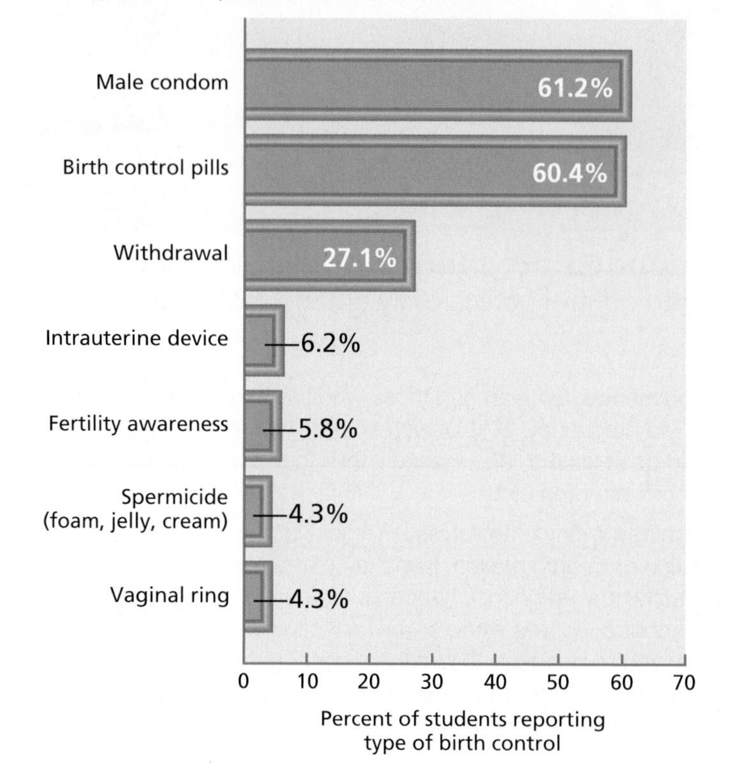

Data from *American College Health Association-National College Health Assessment (ACHA-NCHA II) Reference Group Executive Summary, Fall 2011*, by the American College Health Association, 2012, retrieved from http://www.acha-ncha.org.

Cost-Free Methods of Contraception

Four methods of contraception are always available, and are cost free. They include abstinence and intimacy without intercourse, which are 100% reliable with consistent commitment. The fertility awareness and withdrawal methods are not highly reliable.

Intimacy Without Intercourse

Some couples who desire a sexual relationship yet want to avoid the risks of pregnancy and sexually transmitted infections opt for non-intercourse sexual activities like kissing, "making out," manual stimulation of the genitals, and mutual masturbation. Because intercourse doesn't occur, the chance of pregnancy or sexually transmitted infection is theoretically zero. However, in reality, this method requires a high level of commitment, self-discipline, and mutual cooperation and trust.

Table 17.1: A Summary of Contraceptive Options

Method	Description	Advantages	Disadvantages	Failure Rate*	Average Cost
Cost-Free Methods					
Intimacy without intercourse	Engaging in sexual or sensual behavior without vaginal penetration	Prevents pregnancy and STIs	Requires mutual commitment, trust, and self-control	No statistics available	No cost
Fertility awareness (rhythm or calendar method)	Understanding the monthly menstrual cycle and avoiding intercourse on fertile days	No cost	No protection against STIs; not as effective if cycle is irregular; high possibility of failure	1–25	No cost
Withdrawal	Withdrawing the penis before ejaculation	No cost	No protection against STIs; high risk of pregnancy; requires physical and psychological control and awareness	19	No cost
Over-the-Counter Methods					
Male condom	Very thin sheath that fits over an erect penis to prevent semen from entering vagina	No medical exam required; side effects are uncommon; latex condoms protect against many STIs	Only about 80–94% effective at preventing pregnancy; if not used correctly, unintended pregnancies can occur; requires planning	2–15	$0.50–$3.00 each use
Female condom	A thin sheath with a soft outer ring and a pliable inner ring; the condom covers the inside of the entire vagina	Protects against STIs	Some users may have difficulty inserting the condom correctly	5–21	$0.50–$3.00 each use
Contraceptive sponge	A round, soft foam sponge containing spermicide with a nylon loop for removal	Easy to obtain, no medical exam required; easy to carry; can be left in place for up to 30 hours	No protection against STIs and increases risk of STIs and other infections; may cause irritation in some women	9–16	$9–$15 for a packet of three sponges
Spermicides	Chemical compounds that immobilize sperm	Easy to obtain, no medical exam required; variety of forms for convenience	May leak; high failure rate if used alone; doesn't protect against STIs; increases risk of some STIs	18–29 if used alone, but spermicides increase protection when used with other barrier methods	$0.50–$3.00 each use
Emergency contraception (EC) (Also known as the "morning-after pill")	A single pill or two pills containing a synthetic form of progesterone which can suppress ovulation and disrupt implantation	Effective when used within 72 hours after unprotected intercourse to prevent pregnancy, although it is most effective within the first 24 hours following intercourse	Not effective if woman has already ovulated prior to using; begins to lose effectiveness 24–72 hours after intercourse; does not protect against STIs	No statistics available	$35–$60
Methods Requiring Prescriptions					
Diaphragm	A soft dome-shaped cup with a flexible rim that is filled with spermicide and fits inside the vagina, covering the cervix	Does not require the ingestion of hormones; may be left in place for up to 24 hours	No protection against STIs; cannot be used during menstruation; some women find insertion difficult; may become dislodged; requires an exam and fitting by a health-care provider; may cause urinary tract infection or vaginal irritation in some users	6–16	$100–$200 for device, fitting, and spermicide
Cervical cap	A pliable cup filled with spermicide that fits inside the vagina, covering the cervix	Does not require the ingestion of hormones; may be left in place for up to 48 hours	No protection against STIs; cannot be used during menstruation; some women find insertion difficult; may become dislodged; requires an exam and fitting by a health-care provider; may cause urinary tract infection or vaginal irritation in some users	6–16	$100–$200 for device, fitting, and spermicide
Intrauterine Device (IUD)					
ParaGard	A small T-shaped plastic device that releases copper	No action necessary before, during, or after sex; can be left in place for 10–12 years	No protection against STIs; in rare cases, may cause infections or the device may slip out	Less than 1	$200–$300
Mirena	A small T-shaped plastic device that releases progestin	No action necessary before, during, or after sex; may lessen periods or they may cease; can be left in place for up to 5 years	No protection against STIs; in rare cases, may cause infections or the device may slip out	Less than 1	$200–$300
Birth control pills *A variety of combination pills are available.*	Pills containing the hormones estrogen and progestin, which prevent pregnancy; one pill should be taken at the same time each day	Convenient; helps protect against cancer of the ovaries and uterus; some women have lighter periods and milder cramps	No protection against STIs; requires taking a pill each day, which may be hard to remember; refills must be on hand; requires ingesting artificial hormones; adverse effects possible; consultation with health-care provider is essential	1–8	$20–35 per month

(continued)

Table 17.1: **A Summary of Contraceptive Options** (continued)

Method	Description	Advantages	Disadvantages	Failure Rate*	Average Cost
Emergency contraception (EC)/ella	A "morning-after pill" that can be taken up to 5 days after sexual intercourse to suppress ovulation and prevent pregnancy	Unlike OTC EC, can be taken up to 5 days after sexual intercourse and still be effective	Not effective if woman has already ovulated prior to using; does not protect against STIs; requires a prescription	No statistics available	No information available at press time
"Mini-pill"	Pills containing the hormone progestin, which prevents pregnancy	Convenient; helps protect against cancer of the ovaries and uterus; some women have lighter periods and milder cramps; better choice for women who are at risk for developing blood clots	No protection against STIs; requires taking a pill each day, which may be hard to remember; refills must be on hand; requires ingesting artificial hormones; several adverse effects possible; consultation with health-care provider is essential	1–8	$20–35 per month
Transdermal patch	A thin plastic patch that is placed on the skin, which releases the hormones estrogen and progestin slowly into the body	Convenient—woman does not have to remember to take a pill every day; may reduce risk of endometrial cancer and other cancers, relieve PMS and menstrual cramping, and improve acne	No protection against STIs; may cause bleeding between periods, breast tenderness, or nausea and vomiting; may cause skin irritation at patch site; may alter a woman's sexual desire; may be less effective in women who weigh more than 198 pounds; several long-term adverse effects possible; consultation with health-care provider is essential	1–8	$25–30 per month
Vaginal ring	A small flexible ring that releases the hormones estrogen and progestin slowly into the body	Convenient—woman does not have to remember to take a pill every day; may reduce risk of endometrial cancer and other cancers, relieve PMS and menstrual cramping, and improve acne	No protection against STIs; may cause bleeding between periods, breast tenderness, or nausea and vomiting; may increase vaginal discharge and lead to irritation or infection; may alter a woman's sexual desire; several long-term adverse effects possible; consultation with health-care provider is essential	1–8	Cost of initial health-care appointment plus $15–$50 per month
Monthly injections	An injection containing the hormones estrogen and progestin	Convenient, may help reduce risk of certain cancers and promote lighter, shorter periods	No protection against STIs; requires monthly visit to health-care provider; side effects may include bloating/weight gain, headaches, vaginal bleeding, and irregular periods; women over the age of 35 or who smoke or have certain health conditions are at risk for serious adverse effects	1–3	$30–$35 month
Quarterly injections	An injection containing the hormone progestin	Convenient; requires only one injection four times a year; helps protect against endometrial cancer; reduces monthly bleeding and anemia; in most cases, women stop having their periods	No protection against STIs; side effects may include amenorrhea, headaches, depression, loss of interest in sex, and bone loss; fertility may be delayed for many months after discontinuing; not advised for women who want less than a year of birth control	1–3	$60–$75 for 3 months
Implant	A thin plastic rod containing the hormone progestin	Convenient; lasts for 3 years; helps protect women from endometrial cancer	No protection against STIs; insertion and removal of implants requires a small cut in the skin, and scarring may occur; if implants fail, there is a greater chance of ectopic pregnancy; side effects may include acne, headaches, weight gain	1	$450–$750 for 5 years
Surgical Methods					
Tubal ligation	The fallopian tubes are surgically tied or otherwise sealed	Convenient; no hormonal effect; permanent solution to birth control	No protection against STIs; invasive; permanent	Less than 1	$1,500–$6,000
Hysterectomy	Surgical removal of a woman's uterus, sometimes along with her ovaries and fallopian tubes	May be necessary to treat health conditions such as excessive menstrual bleeding or tumors	Irreversible	No statistics available	No information available
Vasectomy	A minor surgical procedure performed at a hospital or clinic in which the vas deferens is tied off and cut on both sides of the scrotum	Convenient; procedure does not affect sexual desire or hormone levels; male may resume sex as soon as it is comfortable; permanent solution to birth control	No protection against STIs; after the procedure the male will still have viable sperm for a period of time; sterilization is considered permanent	Less than 1	$350–$1,000, including sperm count

*Number of women out of 100 likely to become pregnant during the first year of use. Number ranges indicate perfect versus typical use.

Data from: *Comparing Effectiveness of Birth Control Methods*, by Planned Parenthood (n.d.), retrieved from http://www.plannedparenthood.org/health-topics/birth-control/birth-control-effectiveness-chart-22710.htm.

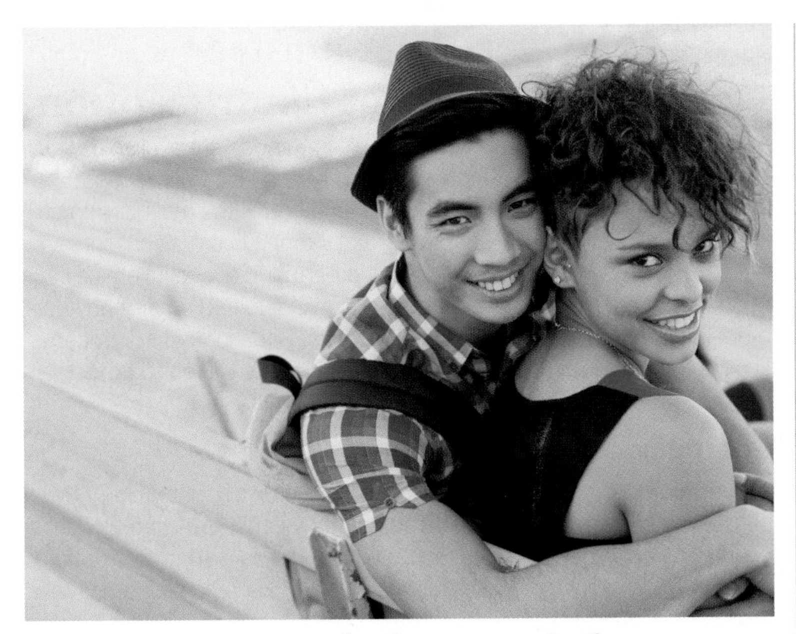

Couples who practice **abstinence** or **intimacy without intercourse** greatly reduce their risks of both pregnancy and STIs.

Fertility Awareness Methods

Fertility-awareness methods (FAM) include several techniques requiring the woman to understand and monitor the changes that occur in her body during her monthly ovulatory and menstrual cycles. Because most women's cycles vary somewhat from month to month, it's essential that a woman using FAM track her cycles for several months (a full year is ideal) before relying on it. The Institute for Reproductive Health at Georgetown University, which has been studying FAM, reports that, when used by women with very regular 28–32-day cycles, it is 95% effective with correct use, and 88% effective with typical use.[7] Women with irregular cycles should rely on other methods of contraception.

fertility awareness methods (FAM) Any of a variety of methods of avoiding pregnancy that require tracking of changes that occur in a woman's body throughout her monthly cycle, with periods of abstinence when the woman is fertile. Also known as natural family planning.

There are three basic fertility awareness methods, but an approach combining two or all three is more effective. **Figure 17.2** provides an example of fertility tracking over the course of a month.

- **Calendar method.** In this method, which is also called the *standard days method*, a woman tracks on a calendar the day her menstrual period begins each month. The day before her period begins again is the last cycle day. Using the data from several months, the woman next calculates her average cycle length (for example, 28 days, 32 days, etc.). Next, the woman estimates the cycle days on which she is fertile. In doing so, two key facts come into play: First, variations in cycle length typically occur in the first half of the cycle, prior to ovulation. The second half of the cycle, from ovulation to the start of the next period, tends to last 14 days. A second key fact is the survival time of sperm and ovum: Sperm can survive for 5 days in the vagina—possibly more—and an ovum may be viable for up to 2 days after ovulation. This means that a woman might become pregnant if she has unprotected intercourse as many as 5 days before she ovulates, or as many as 2 days afterward. However, to allow for cycle variability, women should avoid intercourse for 7 days prior to the estimated day of ovulation, the day of ovulation itself, and for 4 days afterward. Thus, a woman practicing the calendar method would mark her calendar to indicate these 12 "unsafe" days.
- **Cervical mucus method.** Under the influence of reproductive hormones, a woman's cervical mucus changes in quality and quantity. A discharge of copious, slippery cervical mucus indicates that she is fertile—this "wet" mucus occurs as ovulation approaches. The woman should avoid intercourse from the first day that she notices this wet mucus until 4 days after it peaks, which is estimated to be the day she ovulates. During this period of wet mucus, she should also be on the watch for a sharp pain, something like a runner's stitch, in one side of her lower abdomen. This mid-cycle pain indicates ovulation and may last for several minutes to several hours. A minority of women experience this mid-cycle pain, but those who do are able to precisely note the day on which they ovulated.
- **Temperature method.** Some women also track their body temperature, which typically rises slightly after ovulation. However, because the temperature increase is so slight—usually less than 1 degree—and must be recorded at the same time every morning before getting out of bed, many women do not have success with this method.

Recently, some electronics manufacturers and software developers have been offering fertility awareness computers and apps to help women who want to become pregnant determine the range of days on which they are most fertile. Although research supports the use of these products to help women achieve pregnancy, they have not been adequately studied for effectiveness in preventing pregnancy.

In addition to the careful planning required, the fertility awareness method requires couples to abstain from sexual intercourse for 12 days out of each

Sunday	Monday	Tuesday	Wednesday	Thursday	Friday	Saturday
1	2	3	④ Start of period	5	6	7
8	9	10 ✕	11 ✕	12 ✕	13 ✕	14 ✕
15 ✕ Cervical mucous spotted	16 ✕	17 ✕ Sharp pain, ovulation?	18 ✕	19 ✕	20 ✕	21 ✕
22	23	24	25	26	27	28
29	30	① Start of period	2	3	4	5

Start of period: ○ Avoid sex: ✕

Figure 17.2 Fertility awareness tracking. Jotting down key events in the menstrual and ovulatory cycles can help couples identify the dates on which to avoid intercourse.

cycle. If couples also abstain during the first few days the woman is having her period, this can eliminate half of all days each month. During that time, the couple can use other forms of contraception, or engage in non-intercourse sexual activity. Also note that when the couple does engage in unprotected intercourse, both partners may be at risk for sexually transmitted infection.

Withdrawal

Also called *coitus interruptus,* the **withdrawal** method requires the man to withdraw his penis from his partner's vagina before he ejaculates. Because the man is frequently unable to do this, withdrawal is associated with a very high failure rate (see Table 17.1). Even if the man can exert the required self-control, pregnancy can still occur because the pre-ejaculate fluid may contain sperm. This method also provides no protection against sexually transmitted infection, and can be unsatisfying for both partners.

withdrawal The withdrawal of the penis from the vagina before ejaculation.

spermicide A substance containing a chemical that immobilizes sperm.

Over-the-Counter Methods of Contraception

Over-the-counter (OTC) methods are available without a prescription or examination. The most commonly used OTC method is the male condom: In 2008, about 93% of women in a national survey said that they'd had a partner use one.[8] Female condoms, the contraceptive sponge, spermicides, and emergency hormonal contraceptives are other OTC options. For a look at contraceptive use by age and race, see the nearby **Diversity & Health** box.

Spermicides

A **spermicide** is any substance containing chemicals that prevent pregnancy by immobilizing sperm so that they cannot reach a woman's ovum. The only such chemical approved for use as a spermicide in the United States is nonoxynol-9. Spermicides are available as foams, gels,

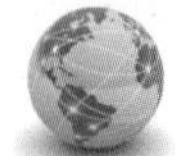

DIVERSITY & HEALTH

Differences in Contraception by Age and Race

A 2010 report from the National Center for Health Statistics revealed the following results from a survey of American women:

Overall

- 99% had used some form of contraception at some time, and 62% were currently using contraception.
- Among the 38% not currently using contraception, some were not currently sexually active, others were pregnant or trying to conceive, and still others were infertile. However, the remaining women—7.3% of all women surveyed—reported that they were currently sexually active, and did not desire pregnancy, but were not using contraception.

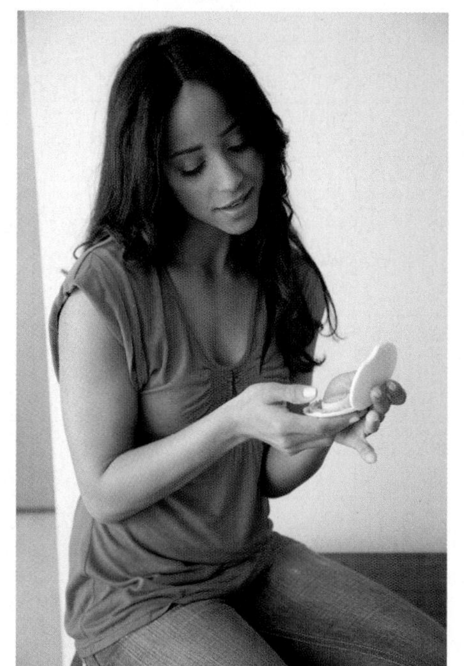

Age

- 28% of girls aged 15 to 19 and 55% of women aged 20 to 24 use contraceptives.
- The most popular method of contraception in women under age 30 is the birth control pill. Popularity of the pill declines with age: 48% of women aged 20 to 24 use the pill, but only 11% of women aged 40 to 44.
- In women over age 30, the most popular method is female sterilization. Half of women using contraception at age 40 to 44 rely on female sterilization.

Race/Ethnicity

- White women are more likely than other ethnic groups to report that they currently use or have ever used birth control pills for contraception: 21% of white women currently use the pill and 89% have used it at some time. Only 11% of blacks and Hispanics currently choose this method, and just 78% of black women, 68% of Hispanic women, and 56% of Asian women have ever used the pill.
- In contrast, black women are more likely to have used injectable contraceptives (Depo-Provera): 30% versus 26% of Hispanic women and 19% of white women.
- White women are more likely than other groups to have a partner who has had a vasectomy: 8% versus just 2% of Hispanics and 1% of blacks.
- Black women were more likely than women of other races to be at risk for unintended pregnancy because of failure to use a method of contraception: 16% were at risk versus 9% of Hispanic, Asian, or white women.

Data from *Use of Contraception in the United States, 1982–2008,* by W. D. Mosher and J. Jones, 2010, National Center for Health Statistics, *Vital Health Statistics 23* (29).

film, and suppositories. They are inserted deep in the vagina, against the cervix, where they block the entrance to the uterus and immobilize sperm. The woman needs to insert the spermicide at least ten minutes before intercourse. It remains effective for up to one hour.

Spermicides are inexpensive and convenient, but they are not very effective in preventing pregnancy (see Table 17.1). They also fail to prevent sexually transmitted infection when used alone. In fact, frequent use of spermicides can irritate the lining cells of either partner's tissues and actually increase their risk for a sexually transmitted infection.[9]

Male Condom

The **male condom** is a thin sheath, typically made of latex, which is unrolled over the erect penis prior to vaginal penetration. It acts as a barrier to keep semen, blood, and other body fluids from being passed from one partner to another during sexual intercourse. If used correctly and consistently, it offers excellent protection against pregnancy and sexually transmitted infection. Either can occur, however, if the condom tears, breaks, or comes off during sex.

Lambskin condoms are effective contraceptives, and many people find them more comfortable than latex; however, they do not reliably protect against infection, including HIV infection. The U.S. Food and Drug Administration advises that, unless you or your partner is allergic to latex, you should shop for latex condoms with packaging that clearly states that the condoms prevent infection and pregnancy. For those allergic to latex, polyurethane condoms are available and effective; however, they are slightly more likely than latex condoms to break or to slip off during sex. A variety of "novelty condoms" are also available. If the package does not say anything about either disease prevention or pregnancy prevention, then you should assume that they are intended only for sexual stimulation, not protection.[10] Also check the package expiration date. Condoms should not be purchased or used after that date.

condom (male condom) A thin sheath typically made of latex that is unrolled over the erect penis prior to vaginal penetration and serves as a barrier to conception.

At home, store condoms in a cool, dry place away from direct sunlight. Don't keep one in your wallet or pocket for more than a few hours. If a condom feels either dried out or gummy when you remove it from the package, don't use it. And check the expiration date on stored condoms periodically. Discard them if the date has passed.

Some condoms come prelubricated. For those that are not, apply a water-based lubricant to prevent tissue irritation and reduce the risk of the condom tearing. Never use an oil-based lubricant such as petroleum jelly, massage oil, body lotions, or baby oil, as these can break down the latex.

Some condoms come lubricated with spermicides containing nonoxynol-9, the active ingredient in all spermicides sold in the United States. As noted earlier, although nonoxynol-9 is a moderately effective contraceptive, it produces tissue irritation that actually increases the risk of transmission of sexually transmitted infections and therefore should be avoided.

To use a condom, tear open the package gently. Don't use scissors or your teeth. When the penis is erect, squeeze the air out of the tip of the condom and place it over the glans (head) of the penis **(Figure 17.3),** leaving space at the tip to collect semen. Roll the condom down over the shaft of the penis as far as possible. After ejaculation, but before the penis has become flaccid (soft), grasp the condom at the base of the penis and withdraw. Failing to grasp the base of the condom during withdrawal may allow semen to spill into the vagina. Pull the condom off gently, making sure semen doesn't spill out. Wrap the condom in tissue and throw it away in the trash. Do not flush it down the toilet. Use a new condom for every act of intercourse.

Some men feel that wearing a condom decreases their level of stimulation and pleasure. Some women find that condoms produce irritation. Experimenting with different sizes, types, and brands, as well as using a water-based personal lubricant, may help.

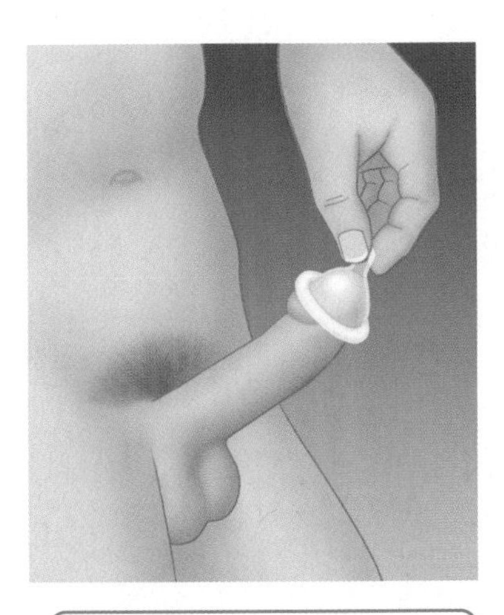

(1) Pinch the tip of the condom to expel any air.

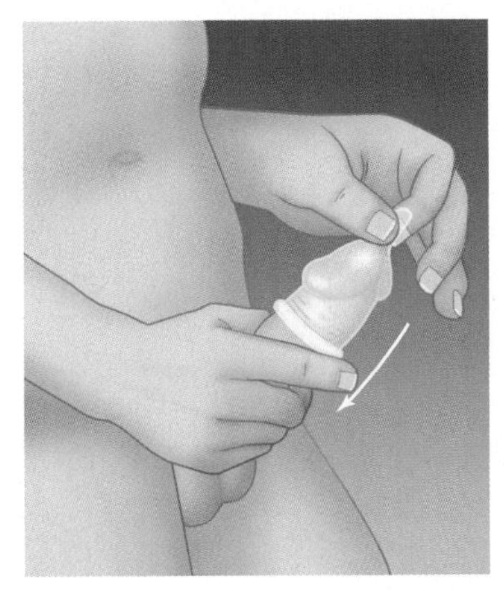

(2) Keep the tip pinched with one hand. Use the other hand to roll the condom onto the penis.

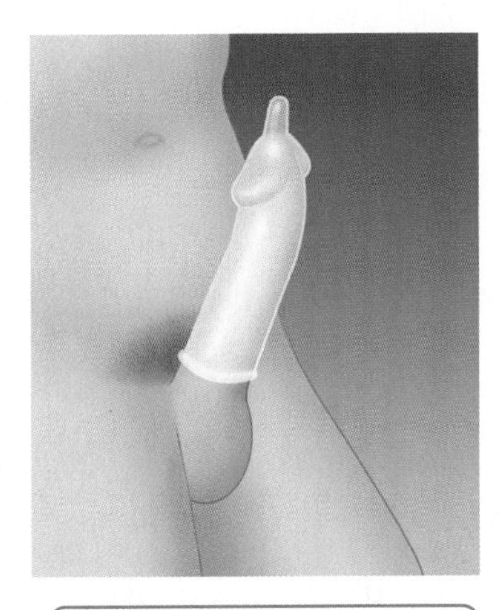

(3) Make sure the condom smoothly covers the entire penis.

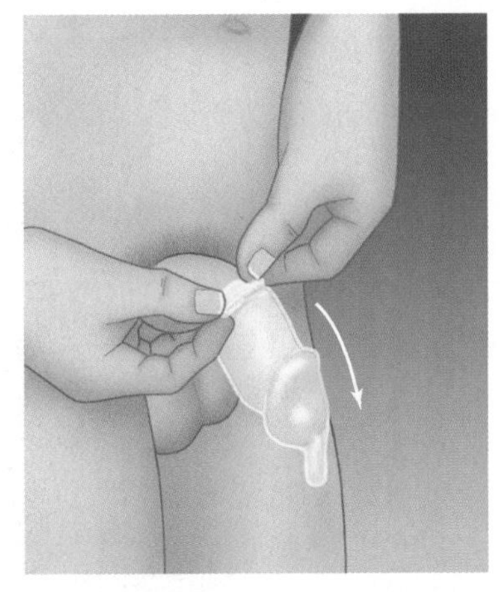

(4) After ejaculation, hold on to the base of the condom as you withdraw. Remove the condom carefully so that semen does not spill.

Figure 17.3 **Applying a male condom.**

Female Condom

In 1993, the FDA approved the first **female condom** (FC), a lubricated polyurethane sheath with flexible rings on either end **(Figure 17.4).** Because it was expensive, the female condom wasn't widely used. But in 2009, the FDA approved a new, less costly female condom called FC2. This version is similar to the original in design, but made with synthetic latex.

The female condom can be inserted several hours before sex. It can be awkward to insert, so new users should practice a few times until they feel confident that it is correctly placed. After washing her hands, the woman squeezes the inner ring at the closed end of the tube and, spreading the labia, inserts the ring into the vagina, pushing it past the pubic bone until it rests against the cervix. The outer ring and about one inch of the sheath remain outside the body, partly covering the labia. This provides protection for the labia against certain infections, such as genital herpes and genital warts.

During intercourse, the woman holds the outer ring in place so that it does not slip upwards into the vagina. After her partner has ejaculated, the woman should squeeze and twist the outer ring of the condom to keep the fluids inside, then remove it carefully before sitting or standing up. The condom should be wrapped in tissues and thrown away.

Female and male condoms should not be used together. Doing so increases friction and may result in tearing.

Some women find that the outer ring of the female condom provides extra stimulation during sex, whereas others find the female condom uncomfortable. It can also get pushed upward into the vagina, and can leak, break, or slip. Finally, it is associated with a higher pregnancy rate than is the male condom (see Table 17.1).

For more information, including a video on the FC2, go to www.fc2.us.com/howtousefc2.html.

female condom A thin sheath with flexible rings that is inserted into the vagina prior to vaginal penetration and serves as a barrier to conception.

contraceptive sponge A flexible foam disk containing spermicide that is inserted in the vagina prior to sex.

Contraceptive Sponge

A soft, flexible foam disk about two inches in diameter **(Figure 17.5),** the **contraceptive sponge** is another convenient OTC contraceptive option for women. It not only works as a physical barrier, blocking the entrance of the cervix, but also contains spermicide that immobilizes sperm.

The sponge can be inserted up to 24 hours before intercourse. The woman washes her hands and moistens the sponge with a small amount of water, then squeezes it. This activates the spermicide. She then pinches the rim of the sponge closed and inserts it into the vagina until it rests against the cervix. When correctly placed, the woman can feel the nylon loop on the bottom of the sponge with her fingertip. The sponge must be left in place for at least 6 hours after intercourse. To remove it, the woman simply tugs the nylon loop at the base of the sponge and pulls it out slowly and gently. The sponge should be wrapped in tissue and thrown away.

Many women like using the sponge because it can be purchased for low cost without a prescription, can be worn for as long as 30 hours, can't usually be felt by either partner, and contains no hormones. The sponge can cause irritation, however, as well as dryness. It does not protect against sexually transmitted infection; in fact, the spermicide it contains slightly increases the risk of contracting one. The sponge is associated with an increased risk for a urinary tract infection, vaginal infection, and toxic shock syndrome.

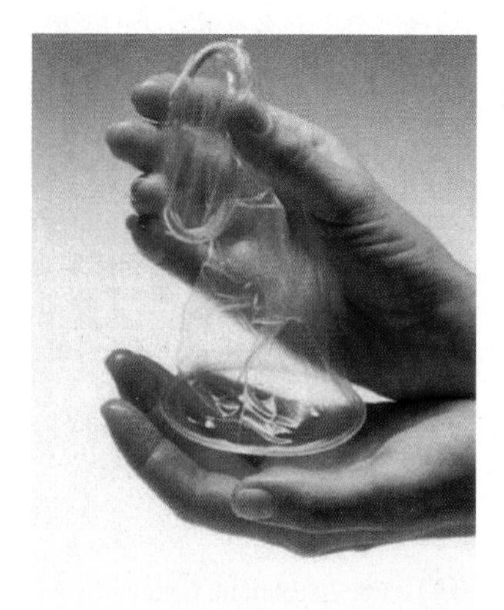

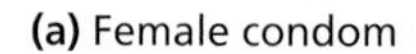

(a) Female condom

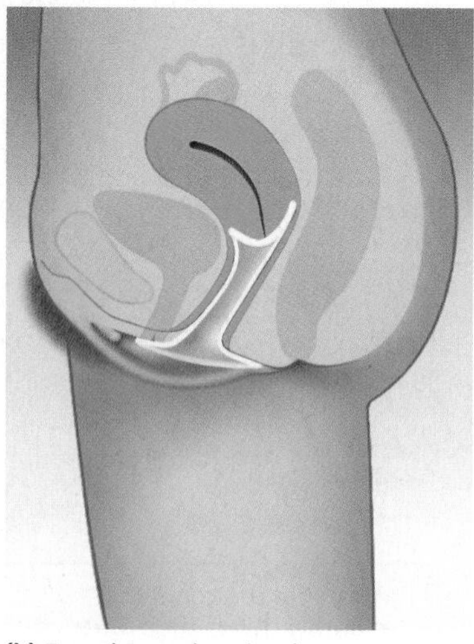

(b) Female condom in place

Figure 17.4 **The female condom. a)** The FC2 is made of a synthetic latex. **b)** A female condom properly inserted.

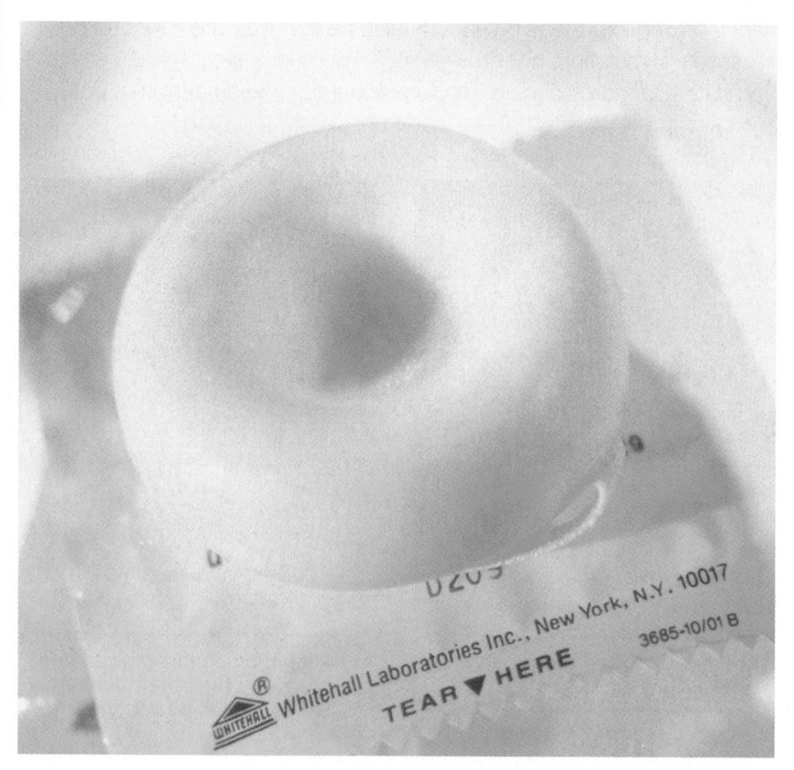

Figure 17.5 **A contraceptive sponge.**

OTC Emergency Contraception (EC)

Also called the "morning-after pill," **emergency contraception (EC)** is currently available to consumers age 17 or older without a prescription under the brand name Plan B and a less expensive generic version called Next Choice. Both consist of pills containing a synthetic version of the female reproductive hormone progesterone, which is also found in a lower dose in birth control pills. The effectiveness of EC varies according to how soon it is used after unprotected sex. Although it can reduce the likelihood of pregnancy for up to 72 hours, it is most effective when taken within the first 24 hours after intercourse.[11]

EC prevents pregnancy by delaying or inhibiting ovulation. If ovulation has just occurred, EC will have no effect. It should not be confused with *RU-486,* the so-called "abortion pill." If a woman is already pregnant, EC will not end the pregnancy.

EC has been used by millions of women for over a decade and in 2008, 10% of women reported having used it at least once.[8] EC is considered very safe; however, about 1 in 4 women experiences side effects such as nausea and vomiting, abdominal pain, fatigue, vaginal bleeding, headache, or dizziness. Also, the woman's next period may be heavier or lighter than normal. EC should not be used as a regular method of contraception, as doing so can disturb a woman's normal ovulatory and menstrual cycle. It is also much more expensive than other OTC methods (see Table 17.1).

EC is available by prescription for teens aged 16 and younger. Also, as we discuss shortly, a form of EC that can be effective up to 120 hours after intercourse is now available by prescription.

Prescription Methods of Contraception

Many more sophisticated methods of contraception are available by prescription. These include barrier methods and a variety of prescription hormone products. Notice that all of these options are for women. Research into such methods for males is ongoing.

Barrier Methods Available by Prescription

Prescription barrier methods include the diaphragm, cervical cap, and IUD.

Diaphragm

The **diaphragm** is a shallow, flexible cup made of either silicone or latex with a spring in the rim. The woman fills the cup with spermicide and inserts it into the vagina until it covers the cervix **(Figure 17.6).** It therefore acts as both a barrier and a chemical contraceptive. Because of anatomical differences in women's reproductive structures, a diaphragm must be fitted by the woman's health-care provider, and a new size might be needed if a woman gives birth, gains weight, or has a miscarriage, abortion, or pelvic surgery. Diaphragms are not expensive devices, however, and they typically last up to 2 years. A woman should check her diaphragm periodically by holding it up to the light and looking for tears or holes.

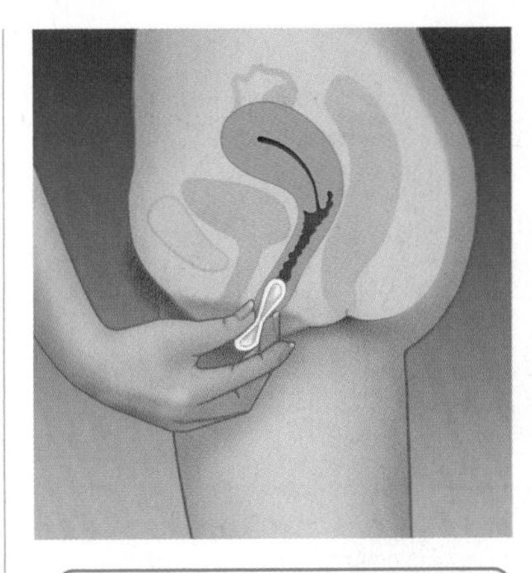

1 After filling the diaphragm with spermicide, hold it dome-side down and squeeze the opposite sides of the rim together.

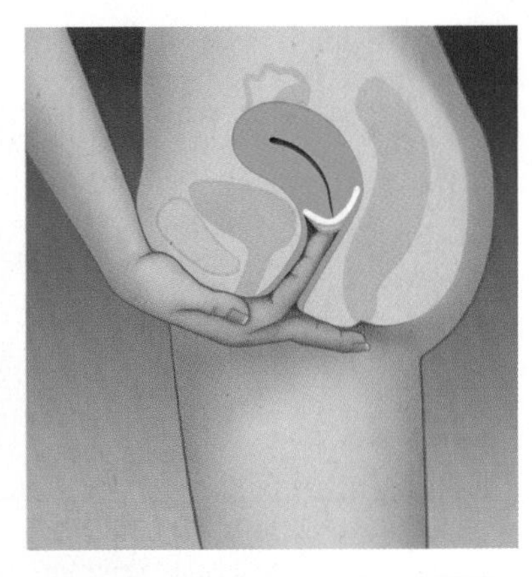

2 Insert the diaphragm into the vagina, pushing it along the vaginal floor as far back as it will go. Make sure the diaphragm completely covers the cervix (the bump at the back of your vagina). Tuck the front rim of the diaphragm up against your pelvic bone.

Figure 17.6 **Inserting a diaphragm.**

After washing her hands, the woman applies spermicide to the diaphragm, including the rim, folds it to contain the spermicide, and inserts it into the vagina. The diaphragm should be tucked behind the pubic bone, covering the cervix (see Figure 17.6). It must be left in place for at least 6 hours following intercourse, and may be left in place for up to 24 hours.

The diaphragm can be inserted hours ahead of time, is convenient, and usually cannot be felt by either partner. However, it is not as effective as many contraceptives, in part because it can be dislodged during sex. Moreover, because it requires application of spermicide, it increases the risk for sexually transmitted infection. It is also associated with an increased risk of urinary tract infection and toxic shock syndrome in the woman.

Cervical Cap

Sold under the brand name FemCap, the **cervical cap** is a small, flexible cup made of silicone **(Figure 17.7).** Like the diaphragm, it requires the application of spermicide, and therefore increases the risk for sexually transmitted infection. Moreover, it must be fitted by a clinician. However, it is designed to conform to the wearer's anatomy and adjust to changes during intercourse. Its insertion, effectiveness, cost, and durability are similar to those of a diaphragm (see Table 17.1). It can be left in place for up to 48 hours, and is removed by tugging on the device's removal strap.

Intrauterine Device (IUD)

An **intrauterine device (IUD)** is a plastic, T-shaped device that is inserted by a health-care provider into

emergency contraception (EC; morning after pill) A pill or pills containing a synthetic form of the hormone progesterone and used to prevent pregnancy after unprotected sex.

diaphragm A flexible shallow cup with a spring in the rim; it is filled with spermicide and inserted in the vagina prior to sex to prevent pregnancy.

cervical cap A flexible silicone cap that is filled with spermicide and inserted in the vagina prior to sex to prevent pregnancy.

intrauterine device (IUD) A plastic, T-shaped device that is inserted in the uterus for long-term pregnancy prevention.

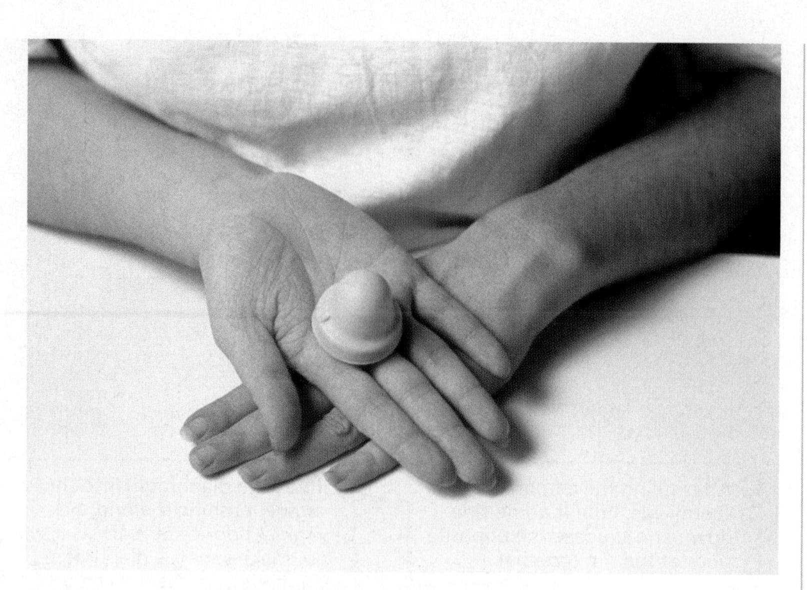

Figure 17.7 The cervical cap.

the uterus for long-term pregnancy prevention **(Figure 17.8).** It is one of the most highly effective methods of contraception available: fewer than 1 in 100 women will become pregnant after a year of use. Two types are available:

- The ParaGard copper IUD continually releases copper, which works either by preventing sperm from reaching the fallopian tubes, or by preventing implantation of a fertilized egg, should conception occur. It can be effective for up to 12 years. ParaGard can also be used for emergency contraception if inserted within 5 days of unprotected intercourse. Side effects include cramps, nausea, severe menstrual pain, anemia due to heavier menstrual bleeding, and painful sex.[12]
- The Mirena hormonal IUD releases progestin, which works either by thickening the cervical mucus—blocking sperm transit—or by suppressing ovulation. It can be effective for up to 5 years. A beneficial side effect is lighter menstrual periods. Adverse side effects include weight gain, acne, headaches, ovarian cysts, and abdominal pain.[13]

Women who use either ParaGard or the Mirena IUD have a higher risk for an ectopic pregnancy; however, because either device prevents most pregnancies, women who use it are at lower risk of having an ectopic pregnancy than women who are not using contraception.

Neither of these devices guards against sexually transmitted infection, and both can be expelled from the uterus. Also, women who currently have a pelvic infection, or who have had a pelvic infection within the past 3 months, are not candidates for an IUD. Although the initial cost of insertion is significant, use of an IUD is much less expensive over time than the regular purchase of birth control pills, and is at least comparable to use of a diaphragm or cervical cap, which require more frequent replacement.

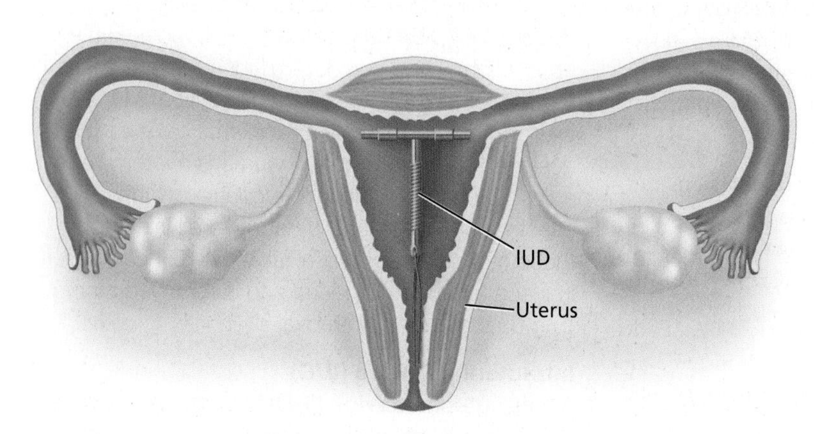

Figure 17.8 An intrauterine device in place.

Hormonal Methods Available by Prescription

Prescription hormonal methods are available in various delivery methods, including pills, a skin patch, and others. Bear in mind that, although all of the hormonal methods are convenient and highly effective at preventing pregnancy, they do not protect against sexually transmitted infection; thus, use of a latex condom is still important. Women who smoke have a significantly increased risk for heart disease and using a hormonal method of contraception increases that risk. Women who use a hormonal method of contraception are strongly advised to quit smoking.[14] Also, a few antibiotics and other medications can interfere with the action of some hormonal methods. As always, it's important to tell your health-care provider about all of the medications and supplements you're currently taking.

Because the hormonal methods work by releasing reproductive hormones into the body, they can provoke symptoms that mimic those of early pregnancy, including nausea, breast tenderness, and moodiness. Side effects that most women welcome include reduced menstrual cramps and lighter menstrual periods. Some hormonal methods stop menstruation completely. Typically, periods resume within a few months of discontinuing the method.

Birth Control Pills

Synthetic versions of the reproductive hormones estrogen and progesterone (called progestin) are combined in **birth control pills,** typically referred to simply as "the pill." A progestin-only "mini-pill" is also available for women who—usually for health reasons—cannot take synthetic estrogen. Both forms are highly effective contraceptives (see Table 17.1). They work by suppressing ovulation, causing changes in the woman's cervical mucus that make it inhospitable to sperm, and making the endometrium thinner and unsuitable for implantation. In 2008, 82% of women reported that they had used the pill at some time, and 17% reported currently using it.[8]

birth control pills Pills containing combinations of hormones that prevent pregnancy when taken regularly as directed.

Rarely, women who have taken the pill for several months or years experience long-term adverse effects. These include increased blood pressure and a slightly increased risk of cardiovascular disease, including heart attacks and strokes. This cardiovascular risk is more significant in women who have pre-existing high blood pressure, diabetes, or high cholesterol, and in women who smoke, are obese, or are over age 35. Women with any history of a blood clotting disorder should not use hormonal contraceptives. Long-term use can also increase a woman's risk for cervical and liver cancer. The mini-pill is associated with a lower risk of these serious side effects; however, it commonly causes minor breakthrough bleeding (or "spotting") between menstrual periods. Finally, either type of pill may alter a woman's level of sexual desire.

> *"The bottom line is, generally healthy, nonsmoking women can rely on birth control pills for years and even decades."*

On the upside, pill use can decrease a woman's risk for ovarian and endometrial cancer. The relationship between pill use and breast cancer is not clear.[15] The pill is also associated with a reduction in acne and PMS and, because of lighter or missed periods, a decreased risk for iron-deficiency anemia (some iron is lost in the normal menstrual flow). The bottom line is, generally healthy, nonsmoking women can rely on birth control pills for years and even decades. Still, anyone considering this method of contraception should discuss the risks and benefits with her health-care provider.

Birth control pills typically come in 21-day, 24-day, or 28-day packs **(Figure 17.9).** The 24- and 28-day packs contain some inactive pills that help a woman maintain the habit of taking a pill each day. She experiences a light menstrual period during the days she is not taking any pills or is taking inactive pills. Extended-cycle pills typically contain 84 active and 7 inactive pills; thus, the woman experiences only four menstrual periods a year.

Combination pills can be *monophasic*, with each pill containing the same dose of hormones, or *multiphasic*, with varying doses of hormones in each active pill. Other types are used on longer schedules.

STUDENT STORY

Deciding to Get on the Pill

"Hi, I'm Betty. I discussed contraceptives with my mom because she works in maternal health care. She gave me so many options; she had this huge planner out and was like 'this is a female condom and this is this and that'—and it was just like, I don't even want to know all the other stuff. I didn't want an IUD and I didn't want a female condom or anything like that . . . I was like, let me go to the simplest form. That way if I decide 'OK, if I don't want to take this anymore, then I can get rid of it.' I ended up deciding to get on the pill. The pros are that you always know when your period is going to arrive, it lessens PMS and cramping, and you won't get pregnant. The cons—you have to continuously stay on it. You have to keep it as a ritual: like, get in the shower, brush your teeth, and before you brush your teeth, take your pill. Sometimes it can make you nauseous. That's another con, but other than that, it's great."

1: Given what you've learned in this chapter, do you think birth control pills alone are enough to protect you (or your partner) against pregnancy? How about STIs? Explain your answer.

2: Betty was able to turn to her mom for advice on what contraceptive was right for her. Think about the resources available to you. Where will you go to learn more about contraceptive options and decide which one is right for you?

Do you have a story similar to Betty's? Share your story at www.pearsonhighered.com/lynchelmore.

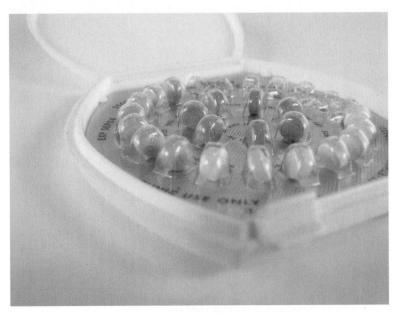

Figure 17.9 **A typical pack of birth control pills.**

The woman's physician will advise her on how to use the particular brand prescribed. With all brands, however, it's important to take the pill at the same time each day. The makers of birth control pills advise that women use another contraceptive method during at least the first month on the pill; however, because birth control pills offer no protection from sexually transmitted infection, a latex condom should always be used in addition to the pill.

Transdermal Patch

Estrogen and progestin can also be delivered via a patch that sticks to the skin (called a *transdermal patch*). Sold by the brand name OrthoEvra, the patch is skin-colored and only about the size of a large postage stamp **(Figure 17.10).** The patch is replaced weekly for 3 weeks, followed by a patch-free week. The patch works in the same manner as birth control pills, can prompt the same side effects, and is associated with the same health risks, including lack of protection against STIs. It may also prompt some local skin irritation. The patch also offers the same benefits of other hormonal methods, including reduced acne, PMS, and menstrual cramps, and lighter periods.

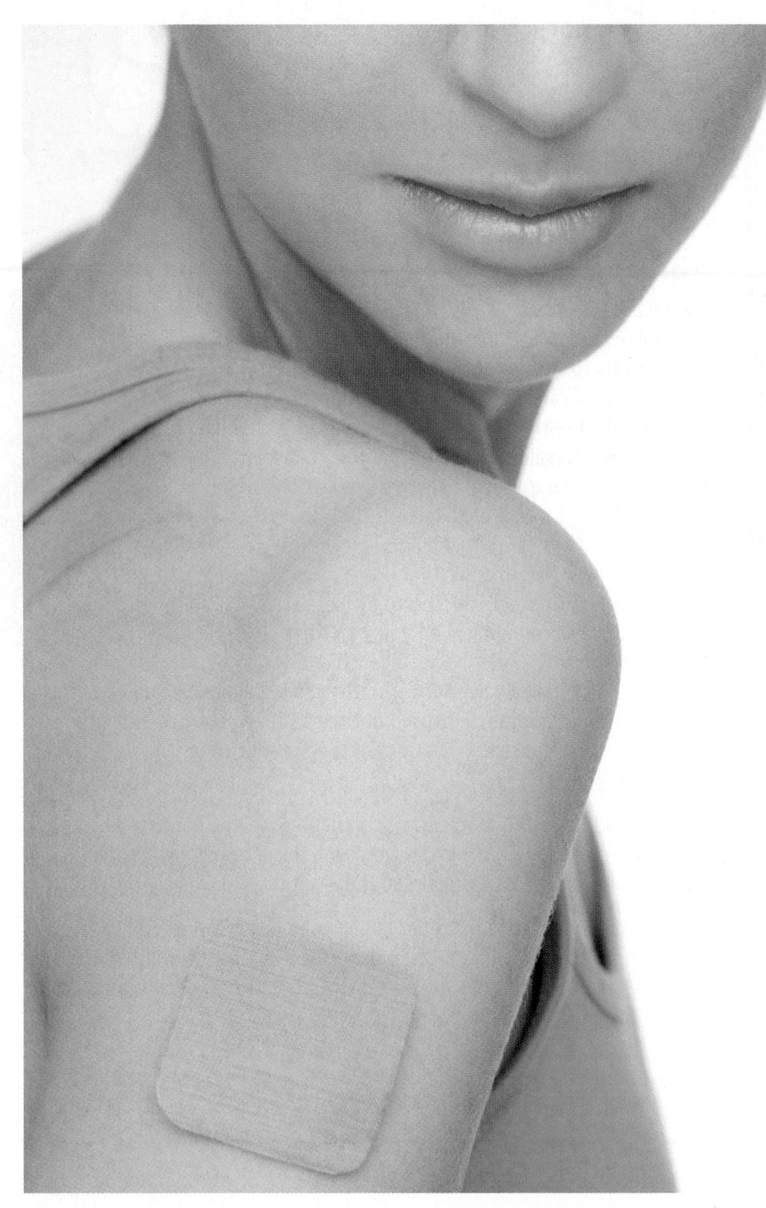

Figure 17.10 A transdermal patch.

The woman applies the patch to a clean, dry area on her upper outer arm, upper back, lower abdomen, or buttocks, pressing for ten seconds to make sure it adheres. She should check the patch daily to make sure it is not coming loose. On the same day of the following week, she should remove the patch, fold it so that it sticks together, and throw it away. Unless it is her patch-free week, she should then apply a fresh patch. During her patch-free week, the woman will usually have her period.

Vaginal Ring

Sold under the brand name NuvaRing, the vaginal ring is a small, flexible ring that releases estrogen and progestin **(Figure 17.11).** It is as effective as birth control pills, and is associated with the same side effects, risks, and benefits. However, it is also associated with a moderately increased risk of vaginal infections.

To insert it, the woman presses the sides of the ring together and guides it into the vagina. The precise position of the ring is not important—unlike barrier contraceptives, it does not need to encircle the cervix. Like the transdermal patch, the vaginal ring is used for 3 weeks followed by a week without the device. After 3 weeks, the woman hooks one finger beneath the ring and gently removes it. One week later, she inserts a new ring.

Hormonal Implants and Injections

Another hormonal alternative is an under-the-skin implant marketed under the name Implanon. Made of a flexible plastic, it is smaller than a matchstick and is inserted in the upper arm **(Figure 17.12).** Insertion typically takes only a few minutes and is done by the woman's health-care provider during an office visit. Once in place, Implanon releases progestin. It therefore has effects, benefits, and risks similar to those of the mini-pill. In addition, in cases in which Implanon fails to prevent conception, there is an increased risk that the zygote will implant in one of the fallopian tubes, resulting in an ectopic pregnancy.

Although the health-care exam, device, and insertion require an initial investment of several hundred dollars, Implanon is effective for up to 3 years. It has also proven to be one of the most reliable forms of contraception.

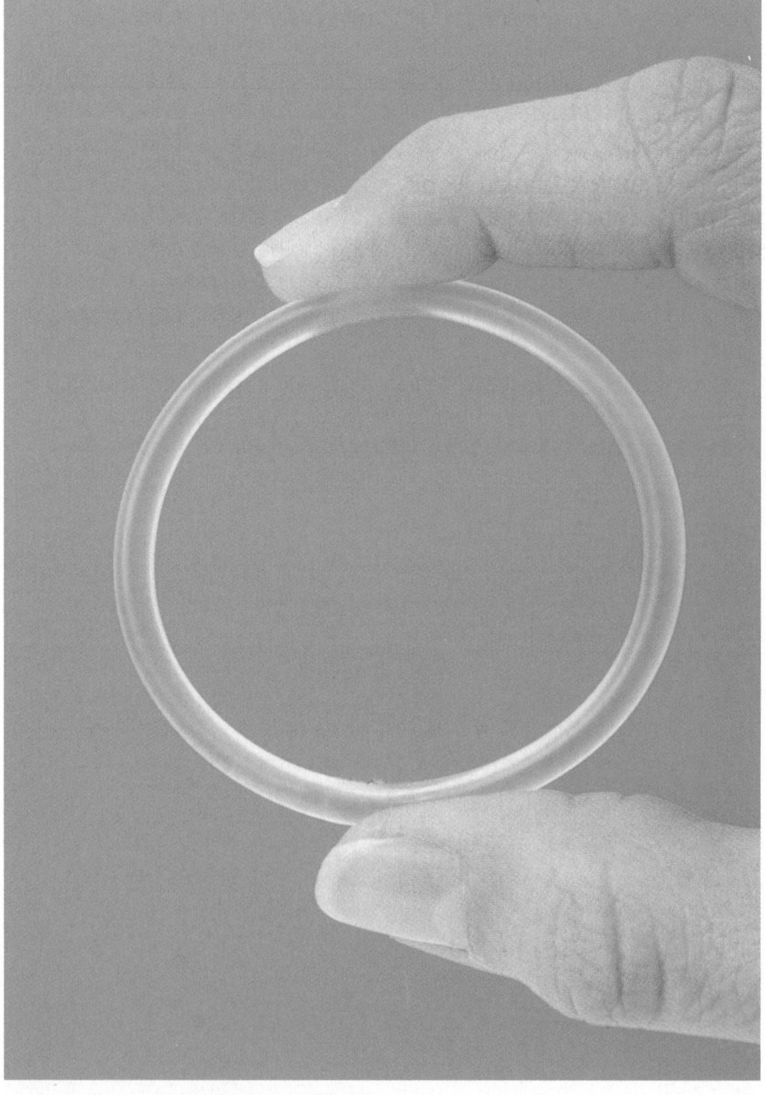

Figure 17.11 A vaginal ring.

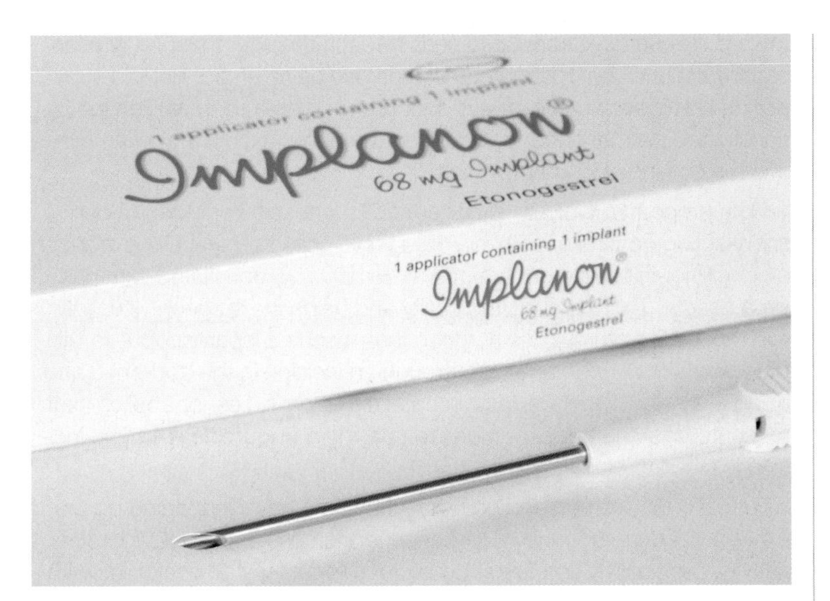

Figure 17.12 **A hormonal implant.**

Progestin can also be delivered via injections—commonly referred to as "birth control shots" or by the brand name Depo-Provera. Each injection costs about $60 to $75, but is effective for 3 months. (A less expensive estrogen-progestin injection is also available, but because it has to be administered monthly, it is not often chosen.) Because it may take up to one year for regular menstrual periods to resume after using Depo-Provera, it's not a sensible method for women who might want to become pregnant soon. In addition to the side effects and risks associated with other progestin delivery methods, Depo-Provera can prompt a gradual loss of bone mineral density in users. This loss of bone mass increases the longer the woman uses this method. Fortunately, the condition slowly reverses in the months after the woman stops using it.

Prescription Emergency Contraception (ella)
In 2010, the FDA approved a new emergency contraceptive (EC) pill called *ella*. At this date, it is available only by prescription. Whereas OTC EC contains a version of progestin, ella contains the medication ulipristal acetate (UPA), which is not a reproductive hormone, but rather works to change the way cells respond to progesterone. The effect is similar to that of progestin: ella strongly suppresses ovulation. Although it may also cause some thinning of the endometrium, the effect is not thought to be strong enough to prevent implantation if a developing blastocyst is already present. In other words, ella is not an "abortion pill," and is not prescribed for women who are pregnant.

Unlike the OTC versions of EC, which begin to lose effectiveness within 24 hours after sexual intercourse, ella is effective for up to 120 hours (5 days) after unprotected sex, and its effectiveness does not diminish within this time. In a study of nearly 1,700 women comparing the OTC hormonal EC with ella, the overall reduction in pregnancy was somewhat better with ella: 15 pregnancies among women who used ella versus 22 among those who used the synthetic progesterone. However, among the 203 women who were given EC between 72 and 120 hours after unprotected sex, there were no pregnancies in those who used ella versus three among the hormonal EC users.[16]

The possible side effects associated with ella include abdominal pain, headache, nausea, dizziness, and menstrual discomfort at the next period.

Surgical Methods for Preventing Pregnancy

The surgical methods discussed here are classified as *sterilization;* that is, they permanently prevent conception by involving surgical manipulation of the reproductive organs. Therefore, these methods are appropriate only for people who already have children and don't want any more, or for people who have made a reasoned decision that they do not want ever to have children. Couples should consider possible life changes such as divorce, remarriage, or death of children, in which case pregnancy may be desired.

Before scheduling any of the following procedures, the health-care provider will usually meet with the candidate—and his or her partner if the candidate is in a committed relationship—to assess their readiness to make the choice for permanent contraception. If the individual or couple requesting the procedure are young or appear psychologically conflicted, or if the relationship seems unstable, the provider may advise them to choose a reversible form of contraception.

Couples who have decided to pursue permanent contraception next need to decide—him or her? As we explain below, the male procedure, vasectomy, is less invasive, takes less time to perform, and costs less money than the comparable female procedure, tubal ligation. Vasectomy also avoids general anesthesia, has a shorter and more straightforward recovery period, and is associated with a lower risk for long-term complications.

Vasectomy

vasectomy Form of permanent surgical sterilization that seals off the vas deferens, preventing sperm from reaching ejaculate.

A **vasectomy** is a surgical procedure in which a man's vas deferens is sealed off on both sides of the scrotum. This makes it impossible for sperm—which are manufactured in the testes—to make their way upward and into the semen. The man typically notices no difference in the quantity of semen he ejaculates, and since the procedure has no effect on his testosterone levels, there are no changes in his secondary sex characteristics or libido.

The surgery is done on an outpatient basis and takes only 20–30 minutes. The area is numbed so the man is awake throughout, and an incision or tiny puncture is made in the scrotum. The surgeon locates the vas deferens, cuts it, and seals it with ties, clips, or heat **(Figure 17.13).** The incision is stitched closed (the puncture technique requires no closure).

Immediately afterward, the man commonly experiences swelling, bruising, and discomfort, which may last for a few days. Ice, rest, and scrotal support is the only treatment necessary. The man needs to avoid vigorous physical activity, including sex, for about a week. Viable sperm will be present in his ejaculate for several weeks, so another form of birth control needs to be used until his physician determines that his semen is clear of sperm. Long-term complications of vasectomy are rare.

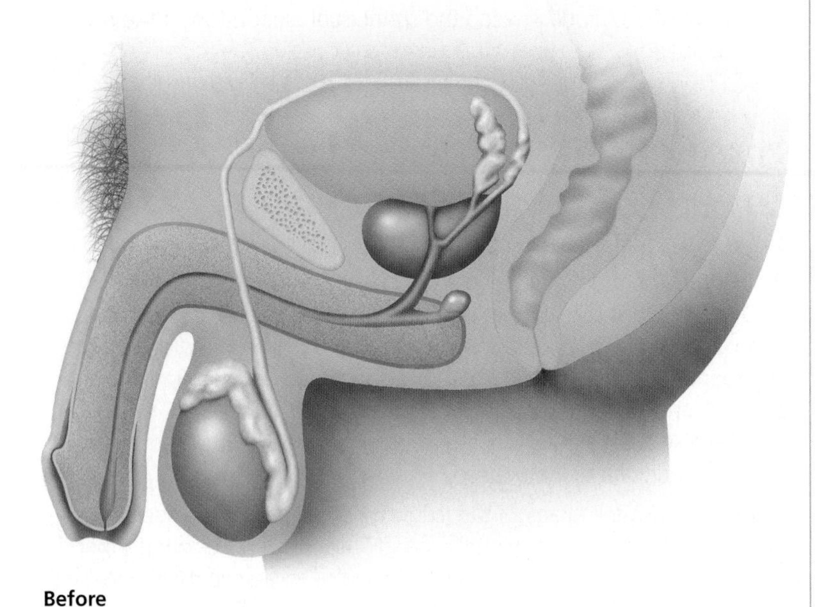

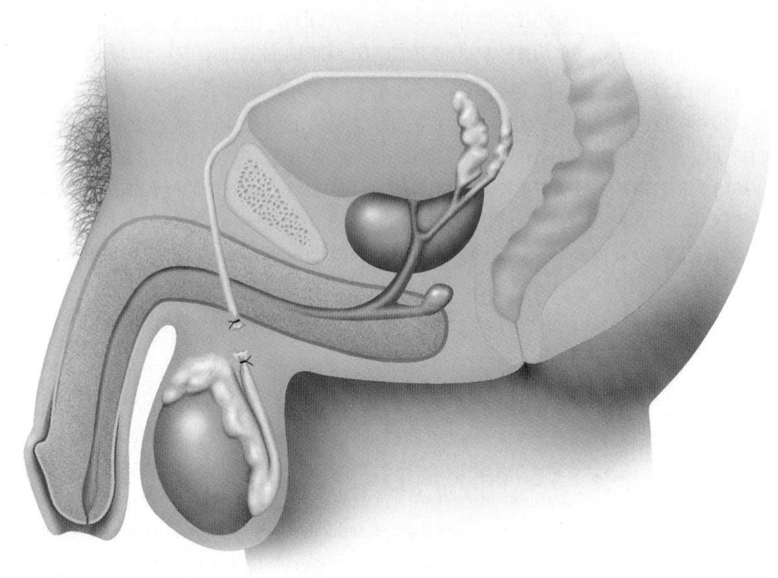

Figure 17.13 **Vasectomy.** Surgical cutting and sealing of the vas deferens prevents sperm from reaching semen and is a highly effective, permanent form of contraception.

Vasectomy is nearly 100% effective at preventing pregnancy; however, it is difficult to reverse. Thus, men who choose it should consider the procedure permanent.[17]

Surgical Options for Women

tubal ligation Form of permanent surgical sterilization that seals off the fallopian tubes, preventing sperm and ovum from making contact.

Women commonly refer to **tubal ligation** as "having their tubes tied." In this surgical procedure, the fallopian tubes are ligated—tied off or otherwise sealed—to prevent the egg from traveling toward the uterus. Sperm also cannot reach the egg; thus, fertilization cannot occur. Tubal ligation can sometimes be reversed, but the surgery is complex and not always successful. Therefore, tubal ligation is considered permanent and should not be undertaken if a woman thinks she may change her mind.

The procedure typically is performed in a hospital or clinic, under short-acting general anesthesia or regional anesthesia (such as a spinal block). Prior to the procedure, the abdomen may be inflated with gas via a needle. This expands the cavity and helps the surgeon visualize the various structures. The surgeon then inserts a laparoscope—a thin tube with a light and camera—through an incision in the abdomen and, using a variety of surgical instruments, either clips, ties, or applies heat to (cauterizes) the fallopian tubes to seal them **(Figure 17.14).** The incision is stitched closed.

Usually, the woman can go home the same day. Depending on the exact procedure, she may experience tenderness and pain. Vigorous activity, especially lifting, must be avoided for at least 3 weeks. As with any surgery, potential complications include excessive bleeding, infection, and damage to nearby organs.

Another permanent surgical option for women is *hysteroscopic tubal occlusion*. *Hystero-* is a word root meaning "uterus," and to occlude is to block. In this procedure, the surgeon accesses the uterus with a hysteroscope, a tube similar to a laparoscope but inserted through the cervix specifically for viewing the uterus. Next, an implant is placed in the tubes at their juncture with the uterus. Scar tissue forms as a result, blocking the tubes. As this method is much less invasive than tubal ligation, the risk of complications is lower and the recovery time faster than for pelvic surgery.

A *hysterectomy* is a procedure in which a woman's uterus is surgically removed, sometimes along with her ovaries and fallopian tubes. It is considered a method of permanent, absolute, irreversible sterilization and is not an option for women who merely desire contraception. However, if a woman has other factors, such as excessive menstrual bleeding, or benign or malignant tumors in the uterus, and she desires to permanently cease childbearing, then a hysterectomy may be considered. Although removal of the reproductive organs cancels the woman's risk for cancer in these organs, the ovaries secrete reproductive

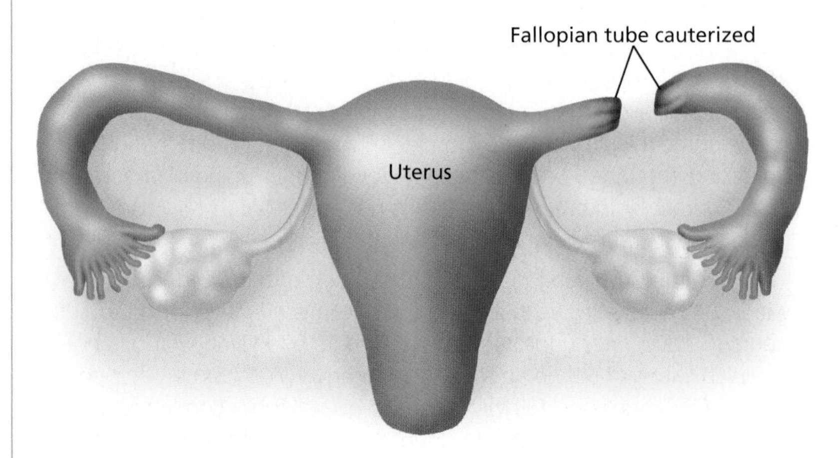

Figure 17.14 **Tubal ligation.** In this procedure, both fallopian tubes are surgically sealed. This prevents ovum and sperm from making contact and is a highly effective, permanent form of contraception.

hormones, and their removal prompts immediate menopause. This increases the woman's risk for osteoporosis and cardiovascular disease, and hormone replacement therapy may be advised.

Which contraceptive method is right for you? To find out, log onto www.plannedparenthood.org/all-access/my-method-26542.htm and take the MyMethod quiz. It's written for women, but men can take it as well, by answering the questions from the perspective of their partner.

Abortion

Birth control failure—and the failure to use birth control—combine to create about 3 million unintended pregnancies in the United States every year.[18] Many women experiencing an unplanned pregnancy decide to keep their baby. Some—typically fewer than 2%—maintain the pregnancy but relinquish the baby for adoption. About 14% miscarry, and about 42% choose abortion each year.[19] **Abortion** is a medical or surgical procedure used to terminate a pregnancy, and involves removing the embryo or fetus from the uterus.

abortion A medical or surgical procedure used to terminate a pregnancy.

In 2008, the U.S. abortion rate reached its lowest level since 1974. Still, more than 825,000 legal abortions were reported to the CDC in 2008.[20] Looked at another way, for every 1,000 live births, there were 234 abortions. Of every 1,000 women aged 15 to 44 years, 16 had had an abortion; however, women 20 to 29 years old accounted for the great majority.[20]

Abortion rates also vary by race and income. White women have 36% of all abortions, followed by black women at 30% and Hispanic women at 25%. Women living at or below the federal poverty level account for 42% of all abortions, and women living just above the poverty level account for another 27%. Fully 75% of women seeking an abortion report that they are doing so because they cannot afford to have a child.[21]

Laws and Politics of Abortion

Abortion has long been a contentious issue in the United States. Despite largely being legal during the nation's founding years, both abortion and contraception gradually fell out of favor. The Federal Comstock Act of 1873 criminalized the distribution or possession of devices, medication, or even information used for abortion or contraception. For a century, many women who wanted to terminate an unwanted pregnancy resorted to "back-alley" abortions, often performed in unsterile environments by untrained personnel using rudimentary instruments. Others resorted to abortifacients, substances (usually herbs or minerals) used to induce an abortion. These procedures were dangerous, resulting in hemorrhage, infection, poisoning, and other crises, and many women died attempting to end an unwanted pregnancy.

In 1973, the U.S. Supreme Court made a landmark decision in the case of *Roe v. Wade* that all women had a constitutional right to an abortion in the first 6 months of their pregnancy. The legislation trumped all state laws limiting women's access to an abortion, and stipulated that individual states could only ban abortions during the final 3 months of pregnancy, considered the period of *fetal viability*, when a fetus would have a chance at surviving outside the womb. From the fourth through the sixth month of pregnancy, however, states could regulate the abortion procedure in the interest of maternal health.

The *Roe v. Wade* ruling sparked a national debate on abortion ethics that has only intensified in recent decades. Some of the main arguments commonly advanced for and against abortion rights are listed in Table 17.2.

The issue of so-called *late-term* and *partial-birth abortions* has become a matter of intense political, religious, and ethical contention. Although no standard definition of these terms has emerged, some define a late-term abortion as one that takes place between 14 and 24 weeks' gestation, and a partial-birth abortion as one that takes place after 22 weeks, or during the period of fetal viability. Even many who support abortion rights in general oppose such abortions. In considering this

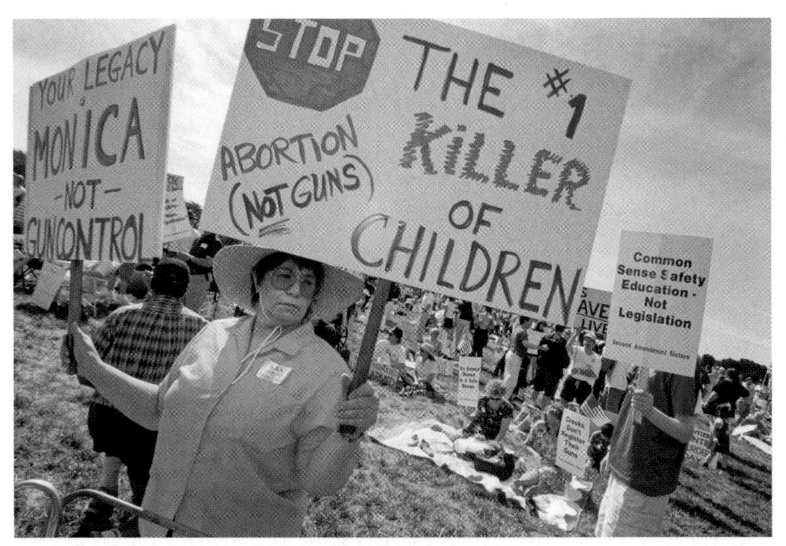
YOUR LEGACY
MONICA
-NOT-
GUN CONTROL
STOP
ABORTION
(NOT GUNS)
THE #1
KILLER
OF
CHILDREN
Common
Sense Safety
Education -
Not
Legislation

Abortion became legal in the United States in 1973 but remains a controversial issue.

Table 17.2: Arguments in Opposition and Support of Abortion Rights

Arguments in Opposition to Abortion Rights	Arguments in Support of Abortion Rights
Life begins at conception, and abortion is therefore murder.	Legal abortion is performed when the embryo or fetus is not capable of sustaining life independently, and is therefore not murder.
Performing an abortion violates medical ethics, which require health-care providers to promote and preserve life.	If safe clinical abortions were no longer legal, women would again resort to "back-alley" abortions, resulting in cases of permanent infertility, serious disease, and death.
Abortion exposes girls and women to significant risk of physical and psychological harm.	Carrying an unwanted pregnancy to term exposes girls and women to significant risk of physical and psychological harm.
Women with an unwanted pregnancy should relinquish their baby for adoption, because many people are on waiting lists to adopt a child.	Carrying an unwanted pregnancy to term and then relinquishing the newborn for adoption can promote physical and emotional harm.
Highly reliable forms of contraception are readily available. Abortion should not be available as a form of birth control.	Among sexually active couples, no method of contraception is 100% reliable. Although the rate of unintended pregnancies can be reduced, some are inevitable, and women should not be forced to carry them to term.

issue, it's important to keep in perspective how few abortions take place after the first 3 months of pregnancy: In 2008, more than 90 percent of abortions were performed at or before 13 weeks' gestation, and more than 60 percent were performed at or before week 8.[20] Studies have revealed a social factor influencing late-term abortions: Teens aged 15 and under, minority women, and women with a low level of education are disproportionately represented in those seeking late-term abortion.[22]

Abortion continues to be legal in the United States, but a number of state rulings have chipped away at *Roe v. Wade,* placing new restrictions on who can get an abortion, and when. More than 30 states now require that minors notify their parents before getting an abortion, often needing parental permission to continue with the procedure. Others impose a mandatory waiting period on women, requiring them to read information on alternatives to abortion before being allowed to terminate their pregnancy. The U.S. Congress has also blocked the use of federal Medicaid funds to pay for elective abortions except when a pregnancy would endanger a woman's life, or in cases of rape or incest. Moreover, a national movement is under way to pass a Constitutional amendment to ban abortion, and many politicians—from President Ronald Reagan in the 1980s to contenders in the most recent political campaigns—have endorsed it.

More than legislation can limit a woman's access to abortion. The total number of abortion providers in the United States has declined over the past three decades for a number of reasons: Older physicians with personal experience of the complications and deaths of illegal abortions prior to *Roe v. Wade* have retired or passed away. Over the same period, fear of violence against abortion providers has caused fewer medical residents to seek certification in the procedure. Currently 86% of counties in the United States have no abortion services. [23]

suction curettage A method of surgical abortion characterized by vacuum aspiration; typically used in the first 6 to 12 weeks of pregnancy.

Methods of Abortion

There are two types of procedures for terminating a pregnancy: medical and surgical abortion. *Medical abortion,* which involves the administration of medications (via pill or injection) to end a pregnancy, has been gaining in popularity since its approval by the U.S. Food and Drug Administration in 2000. Over 14% of women who underwent an abortion in 2008 used the medical method, up from 1% just a few years before.[20] *Surgical abortion* has a much longer history in the United States, and remains the prevailing option.

Which method is advised? The World Health Organization has stated, "There is little, if any, difference between medical and surgical abortion in terms of safety and efficacy. Thus, both methods are similar from a medical point of view and there are only very few situations where a recommendation for one or the other method for medical reasons can be given."[24]

Medical Abortion

Medical abortions are intended for women in the earliest stages of pregnancy, within 7 weeks of the start of their last menstrual period (9 weeks of pregnancy). There is no surgery, and no anesthesia. The medical route is recommended if the woman has health risks that make surgery unadvisable, such as obesity or uterine malformations.

Some women opt for surgical abortion because the medical method is more time consuming. The process starts with the administration—either by pill or injection—of the medication *mifepristone,* also known as *RU-486.* The medication blocks progesterone, which is needed to support a pregnancy. Two days later, the woman takes a pill containing the drug *misoprostol,* which causes the uterus to contract and expel the fertilized egg along with the endometrial lining. The pregnancy usually terminates within hours after the second drug is ingested, but sometimes can take up to 2 days. Two weeks after the process is initiated, women are instructed to return to their physician's office for a follow-up exam. The procedure successfully terminates pregnancy in more than 96% of cases.[25] If the pregnancy was not successfully terminated, a surgical abortion is then recommended.

The expulsion of the pregnancy from the uterus can cause severe cramping pain, nausea, heavy bleeding, fever, and diarrhea. Nevertheless, many women choose medical abortion because it allows them to end an unwanted pregnancy in privacy at home, and without the trauma of an invasive surgical procedure.

Surgical Abortion

Suction curettage, or vacuum aspiration, is the surgical abortion method most commonly chosen. Typically used in the first 6 to 12 weeks of pregnancy, it involves an injection to numb the cervix, followed by the insertion of a series of rods of increasing thickness to dilate (widen) the opening of the cervix. Once the cervix is adequately dilated, the physician inserts a hollow tube through the cervix into the uterus. The tube is attached to a pump, which generates suction to remove tissue from the uterine walls **(Figure 17.15).** Usually performed in a doctor's office or outpatient clinic, suction curettage is a relatively quick procedure, often taking just minutes to complete.

Manual vacuum aspiration is similar to suction curettage, but can be performed much earlier in the pregnancy. Doctors use thin flexible

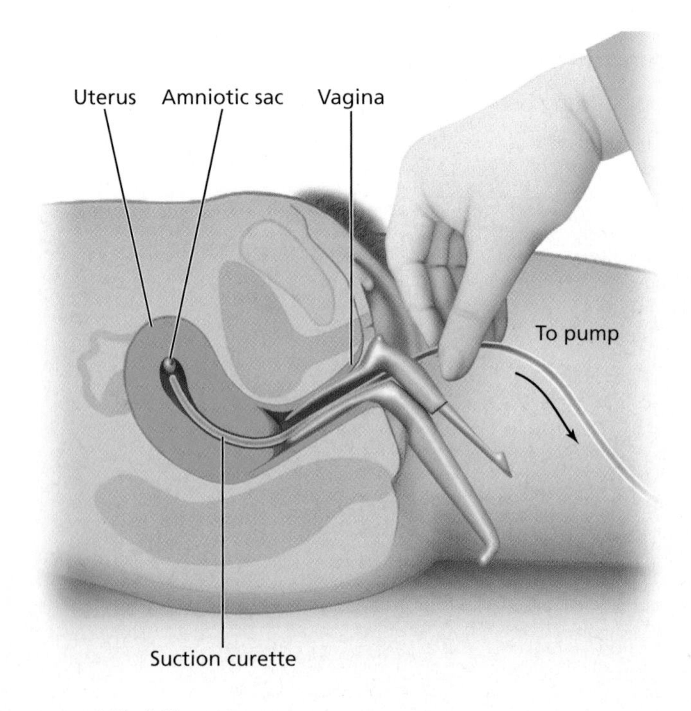

Figure 17.15 **Suction curettage abortion.** A hollow tube is inserted into the uterus and a pump generates suction to remove tissue from the uterine walls, aborting the pregnancy.

tubing attached to a handheld syringe and insert it through the cervix into the uterus. The syringe—rather than a machine—creates enough suction to strip the uterine lining and terminate the pregnancy.

For pregnancies that have progressed beyond 12 weeks, **dilation and evacuation (D&E)** may be performed. This procedure requires multiple trips to the health-care provider. During the first visit, the health-care provider performs an ultrasound scan to determine the status of the pregnancy and eligibility for the procedure. Then, 24 hours before the surgery, the cervix is numbed and a medication administered that will dilate it slowly. At the final appointment, either at a clinic or a hospital, the woman is given a local anesthetic, or in some cases spinal or general anesthesia, and the physician uses instruments and suction to remove the pregnancy. The procedure can produce pain and heavy bleeding, and is associated with a variety of possible complications. Follow-up care is important.

dilation and evacuation (D&E) A multistep method of surgical abortion that may be used in pregnancies that have progressed beyond 12 weeks.

Complications of Abortion

The earlier an abortion is performed, the lower the risk of complications; however, at every gestational stage, abortion is safer than carrying the pregnancy to term.[26] Serious complications of abortion are extremely rare, but may include hemorrhage, fever, adverse effects from anesthesia, perforation of the uterus, injury to the bladder or the intestines, infection, and a disorder characterized by coagulation within the blood vessels. In some abortions, the embryo or fetus is not completely removed from the uterus and the procedure must be done again.

Deaths due to abortion are also very rare. For example, of the more than 800,000 legally induced abortions performed in the United States in 2007, there were 6 known fatalities.[20] Of these, only one was related to a medical abortion, and five followed surgical abortions.

As you have seen, for the vast majority of women who get an abortion, physical complications are not an issue. But what about psychological ones? Does having an abortion cause significant psychological distress—or even a mental breakdown? See the nearby **Myth or Fact?** box and find out.

Change Yourself, Change Your World

Unintended pregnancy costs the U.S. health care system more than $11 billion annually.[27] So when you decide to take responsibility for your fertility, you help not only yourself and your partner, but everybody else in your world.

MYTH OR FACT?

Does Having an Abortion Cause Mental Health Problems?

Abortion critics have argued that women who undergo an abortion are at risk for a constellation of mental health problems they call *postabortion traumatic stress syndrome*.

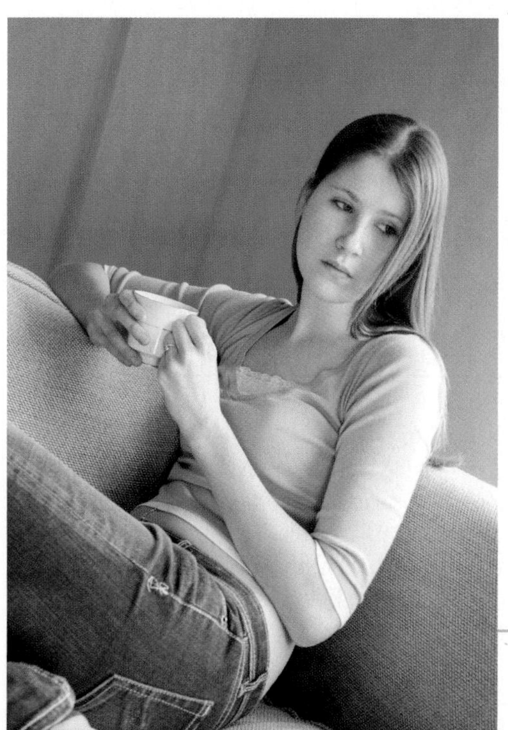

Yet this is not recognized as a legitimate mental health condition by either the American Psychological Association or the American Psychiatric Association. Still, recognizing that abortion can be stressful for some women, causing feelings of sadness or guilt, the American Psychological Association convened a task force on abortion and mental health. In 2008, it concluded that there is no credible evidence that terminating a single unwanted pregnancy creates mental health problems for adult women. The risk, they found, was no greater than if the women had opted to give birth.[1]

The report also noted that poverty, exposure to violence, and other social factors increase a woman's risk of experiencing both unwanted pregnancy and mental health problems after a pregnancy, no matter whether the woman has an abortion or carries the pregnancy to term.

Moreover, a study of more than 13,000 women in England and Wales concluded that those who had ended their unwanted pregnancy with abortion and those who had carried their unwanted pregnancy to term had the same risk for subsequent mental health problems. Similar studies in other countries have produced similar results.[2] In short, despite many studies involving thousands of women over decades, no conclusive evidence has emerged to support the claim that having an abortion increases a woman's risk for subsequent mental health problems.

References: **1.** "Report of the APA Task Force on Mental Health and Abortion," by the American Psychological Association Task Force on Mental Health and Abortion, 2008, Washington, DC: APA Public Interest Government Relations Office, retrieved from www.apa.org. **2.** "Abortion and Mental Health: Myths and Realities," by S. A. Cohen, 2006, *Guttmacher Policy Review, 9* (3), retrieved from http://www.guttmacher.org/pubs/gpr/09/3/gpr090308.html.

SELF-ASSESSMENT

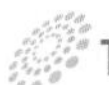 Take this self-assessment online at www.pearsonhighered.com/lynchelmore.

"I Can't Get Pregnant"—True or False?

Take the quiz below to see if you can tell truth from fiction concerning pregnancy and birth control.

1. I can't get pregnant if it's the first time. ___ True ___ False
2. I can't get pregnant if he doesn't "come" inside me. ___ True ___ False
3. I can't get pregnant if I'm breast-feeding. ___ True ___ False
4. I can't get pregnant if I douche after sex. ___ True ___ False
5. I can't get pregnant if I'm having my period. ___ True ___ False
6. I can't get pregnant if I only have anal sex. ___ True ___ False

HOW TO INTERPRET YOUR SCORE

1. **FALSE!** Without birth control, it's possible to get pregnant any time you have sex, including the very first time.
2. **FALSE!** "Pulling out" is not an effective birth control method. It's hard for a man to withdraw at just the right time. Also, a small amount of semen—enough to get you pregnant!—is released during sex even before a man ejaculates.
3. **FALSE!** It is true that breast-feeding lowers the risk of pregnancy for some women. But breast-feeding is not a reliable birth control method (whether your period has started again or not). To prevent pregnancy, use a birth control method that's safe for breast-feeding moms.
4. **FALSE!** Douching (flushing the vagina) does not prevent pregnancy. And douching can be harmful—it makes it easier to get vaginal infections and sexually transmitted infections (STIs).
5. **FALSE!** The monthly release of an egg from the ovaries isn't always regular. Although extremely unlikely, it is possible to ovulate even during your period. And if you don't use birth control, you could get pregnant.
6. **That's true.** But you can get HIV and other sexually transmitted infections! To protect yourself and others against HIV and other STIs, always use a new latex male condom (or a female condom) every time you have sex—vaginal, anal, or oral—no matter what kind of birth control you use.

If you're sexually active, the only way to prevent pregnancy is to choose an effective birth control method, and to use it correctly and consistently.

No matter what form of birth control you choose, always use latex or polyurethane condoms to prevent HIV and other sexually transmitted infections.

Source: Adapted from *"I Can't Get Pregnant"—True or False?* by the The New York City Department of Health and Mental Hygiene, retrieved from http://www.nyc.gov/html/doh/downloads/pdf/csi/contrakit-pt-getpregnant-fact.pdf.

Personal Choices

Here's a sobering statistic: A young, healthy couple has a 20% chance of pregnancy in just a single month of unprotected sex.[28] That risk continues each month so that, by the end of a year, 85% of couples engaging in unprotected sex will be confronted with a pregnancy. This chapter has identified each of the current common and reliable forms of contraception. Here we explore a few ways you can take responsibility for your reproductive choices.

- **Examine your knowledge, beliefs, and values.** If you're sexually active, have you examined your thinking for any myths, misconceptions, or ambivalence you might be holding about avoiding—or achieving—parenthood? Earlier, we said that half of sexually active adults of college age report that they fail to use contraception consistently. Which half do you belong in—and why? Take the **Self-Assessment** above and find out.
- **Choose the best option available.** The best option is the one that has the lowest failure rate and that you can and will use correctly and consistently, every time. It should also offer protection against STIs. Women should also consider their health history and the interaction of any medications they might be taking. For example, a couple may combine a hormonal method with male condoms for protection against sexually transmitted infections. Or if sex is infrequent, an OTC method such as male or female condoms—which protect against STIs—might be more suitable.
- **Use it correctly and consistently.** No method is reliable if it's used incorrectly or only occasionally. Do the research on the right way to use your method. Read the package insert, go to the online product website, and practice if necessary. If you leave the learning until you're "in the moment," you're very likely to make a mistake. Don't forget that, if you're choosing condoms, you should check the package to make sure they protect against both pregnancy and STIs, and that the expiration date hasn't passed.
- **Have a back-up plan.** When the condom slips off or the diaphragm dislodges, it's important to have a back-up method of contraception ready. This might mean a container of spermicide, or one of the OTC emergency contraceptives, Next Choice or Plan B.
- **What if pregnancy happens anyway?** If you and your partner face an unintended pregnancy, your options are to allow the pregnancy to continue and either keep or relinquish the newborn for adoption, or to have an abortion. How can you decide which option is best for you? The Child Welfare Information Gateway from the U.S. Department of Health and Human Services advises that you consult a licensed therapist or clinical social worker who doesn't stand to gain financially from whatever decision you make. Your campus health services center should be able to make a referral to a reliable, unbiased provider. When you go, here are some questions to ask:[29]
  - What are our options for this pregnancy?
  - Can you help us explore our feelings about this pregnancy as well as about our own goals and plans?
  - As expectant mother and father, what are our different rights and responsibilities?
  - Whether we decide to end the pregnancy, relinquish the baby for adoption, or parent the baby ourselves, how can you help us?

Want to chat with an expert about your unintended pregnancy? Get the advice you need at www.childwelfare.gov/pubs/f_pregna/f_pregna1.cfm. Click the "Questions" button at the left on your screen.

Campus Advocacy

Imagine a world where every child is cherished. Where no abortion debate exists because there is no need for abortion. Where everyone learns about and has access to reliable forms of contraception, and uses them correctly and consistently. Whether you're sexually active right now, or not, you can take steps to help create such a world.

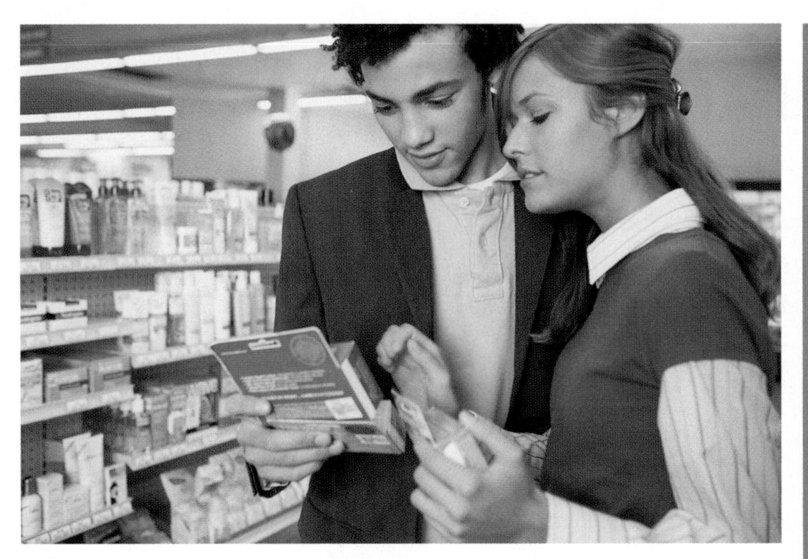

Choose a contraceptive with your partner and make sure you both understand how to use it.

STUDENT STORY

Choosing a Contraceptive

"Hi, I'm Paul. My girlfriend and I are in love and sexually active. We use condoms, but, I don't really think it feels as good with a condom. My girlfriend doesn't want to take the pill and have all those hormones in her, so I'm wondering if we could try withdrawal and how effective it really is. We're both really concerned about pregnancy, so I don't want to try anything that could lead to that, but I'm hoping that there's something other than condoms that we could use."

1: How effective is withdrawal? Do you think that's a good option for Paul and his girlfriend?

2: What other options do Paul and his girlfriend have, if she doesn't want to take hormonal contraceptives? Are any as effective as a properly used condom? What could they do to reduce the risk of pregnancy as much as possible?

3: What other concerns should Paul and his girlfriend take into account when choosing a contraceptive?

Do you have a story similar to Paul's? Share your story at www.pearsonhighered.com/lynchelmore.

First, visit your campus health services center and confirm that it offers a variety of low-cost contraceptives. If it doesn't offer low-cost hormonal methods, meet with the health center director and find out why not. In 2009, Congress reinstated a program enabling college health centers to purchase and sell prescription medications, including hormonal contraceptives, at a discounted rate.[30] Make sure your campus health center is taking advantage of this program.

If you meet resistance, organize students on your campus to demonstrate in support of low-cost birth control: Hold a teach-in on contraception, circulate petitions, and meet with administrators. Some important facts to share include:[30]

- About 8.5 million women in the United States do not have access to affordable contraception.
- Low-income women (and that includes many college students) are more than four times more likely than affluent women to have an unintended pregnancy.
- For every $1 spent on family planning services, the government saves $4 in Medicaid expenses.

You can also consider supporting free condom distribution on your campus. The Great American Condom Campaign (GACC) is a youth-led grassroots movement. Each year, GACC members give out 1,000,000 male condoms on college campuses across the United States, educate their peers about sexual health, and organize to improve the policies that affect young people's health and lives. Find out more about GACC at **www.amplifyyourvoice.org/gacc**. While you're at the site, sign the online petition to support no-cost birth control, then share the petition via Facebook or Twitter.

If activism isn't your thing, you can still make individual choices to promote tolerance and respect for different reproductive choices. If someone's on the opposite side of the abortion issue from you, for instance, take a moment to dialogue about what values you hold in common—responsible sexual decision-making, for instance, or a secure and loving home for every child. Best-selling author, former monk, and psychotherapist Thomas Moore reminds us that refusing polarization doesn't mean agreeing with the other person's views, but rather making a connection, and keeping it open, by focusing on our common humanity.[31]

Watch videos of real students discussing contraception at www.pearsonhighered.com/lynchelmore.

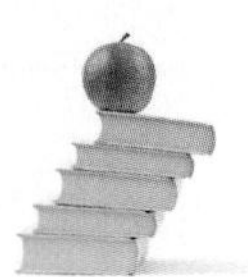

Choosing to Change Worksheet

To complete this worksheet online, visit www.pearsonhighered.com/lynchelmore.

Each birth control method has its pros and cons. Keep in mind that even the most effective birth control methods can fail. But your chances of getting pregnant are lowest if the method you choose always is used correctly and consistently every time you have sex.

Directions: Fill in your stage of change in Step 1 and complete Steps 2, 3, or 4 depending on which ones apply to your stage of change.

Step 1: Your Stage of Behavior Change. Please check one of the following statements that best describes your readiness to follow your selected birth control method correctly and every time you have sex. Keep in mind that abstinence and intimacy without intercourse are forms of birth control.

_____________ I do not plan to use birth control consistently and correctly in the next 6 months. (Precontemplation)

_____________ I might use birth control consistently and correctly in the next 6 months. (Contemplation)

_____________ I am prepared to begin using birth control consistently and correctly in the next month. (Preparation)

_____________ I have been using birth control consistently and correctly for less than 6 months. (Action)

_____________ I have been using birth control consistently and correctly for 6 months or longer. (Maintenance)

Step 2: Precontemplation and Contemplation Stages. What is holding you back from using birth control correctly and consistently every time?

____

____

If a pregnancy were to occur due to inconsistent or incorrect birth control use, what would be the effects on you and your partner? Think of emotional, financial, school, and family effects.

____

____

Even if you don't think you're ready, what could you do to move toward using birth control correctly and consistently?

____

____

Step 3: Preparation, Action, and Maintenance Stages. *Correct use:* Read the packaging of the birth control method you are using. Or, for cost-free methods, re-read the section on these methods. Are you using the birth control method correctly? If not, what have you been doing incorrectly or what are you confused about? How can you begin to use the method correctly?

____

____

Consistent use: If you are in the preparation stage, what is your plan for using this method consistently every time? If you are in the action or maintenance stages, how are you making sure you use the method consistently every time?

Write down your specific **goal** for correct and consistent birth control use, including a timeline.

Step 4: Maintenance Stage. What motivates you to continue practicing correct and consistent birth control?

Are there obstacles you face in using birth control correctly and consistently? If so, how are you dealing with them?

Chapter Summary

- About half of all pregnancies in the United States are unplanned, despite the wide variety of contraceptive options available.
- Factors that contribute to the high rate of unintended pregnancy among young adults include economic disparities, lack of knowledge, unwarranted fears, false beliefs, a value system in which contraception is seen as wrong, and ambivalence about parenthood.
- Successful pregnancy requires ovulation, fertilization, transport of the zygote through the fallopian tube, and implantation. Methods of contraception work by disrupting one or more of these events.
- A contraceptive's failure rate ranges from a lower number indicating perfect use (correctly and consistently) to a higher number indicating typical use.
- Cost-free methods of contraception include abstinence, intimacy without intercourse, fertility awareness methods in which a woman tracks her menstrual cycle lengths and, ideally, changes in her cervical mucus indicating the approach of ovulation, and withdrawal.
- Over-the-counter methods include spermicides, the male and female condom, the contraceptive sponge, and two OTC emergency hormonal contraceptives, Next Choice and Plan B.
- Barrier methods available by prescription include the diaphragm, cervical cap, and IUD. Of these, the IUD is the most effective method.
- Hormonal methods available by prescription include birth control pills, a transdermal patch, a vaginal ring, and hormonal implants and injections.
- Ella is a prescription emergency contraceptive that can be effective as long as 5 days after unprotected intercourse.
- Sterilization permanently prevents conception via surgical manipulation of the reproductive organs. Methods of sterilization include vasectomy in males and tubal ligation and hysteroscopic tubal occlusion in females. Hysterectomy, the removal of the uterus, is an option for women who want to permanently cease childbearing and have other factors, such as uterine tumors, that would be relieved by the procedure.
- Among the choices in contraceptive methods, only male and female condoms provide protection against sexually transmitted infections.
- About 42% of unintended pregnancies end in abortion. More and more women each year opt for medical abortion via administration of oral medication, which is available during the first 9 weeks of pregnancy.

Test Your Knowledge

1. On average, what percentage of pregnancies are unintended in the United States each year?
   a. 20%
   b. 30%
   c. 40%
   d. 50%

2. A fertilized egg is called a(n)
   a. ovum.
   b. zygote.
   c. blastocyst.
   d. embryo.

Get Critical

What happened:

On March 23, 2010, the federal government created the Personal Responsibility Education Program (PREP), which provided states with funding for comprehensive sexuality education. However, the legislation also reauthorized the abstinence-only-until-marriage program, which had expired on June 30, 2009. States now may choose to apply for comprehensive sexuality education funds, abstinence-only funds, or both. In response, some legislators called for the repeal of funding for abstinence-only programs. They argue that:[1]

- Since 1996, the United States has spent more than $1.5 billion on abstinence-only programs that have failed to reduce STIs or unintended pregnancies among adolescents. No study in a professional journal has found abstinence-only programs to be broadly effective. A recent national study found that abstinence education was not only ineffective in preventing teenage pregnancy but may actually be contributing to the high teenage pregnancy rates in the United States.[2]
- In contrast, there is strong evidence that comprehensive approaches do help young people both to withstand the pressures to have sex too soon and to have healthy relationships when they do become sexually active. The research in support of comprehensive sex education programs includes a review of 83 studies worldwide, which found strong evidence that comprehensive programs do reduce rates of STIs and unintended pregnancy.[3]

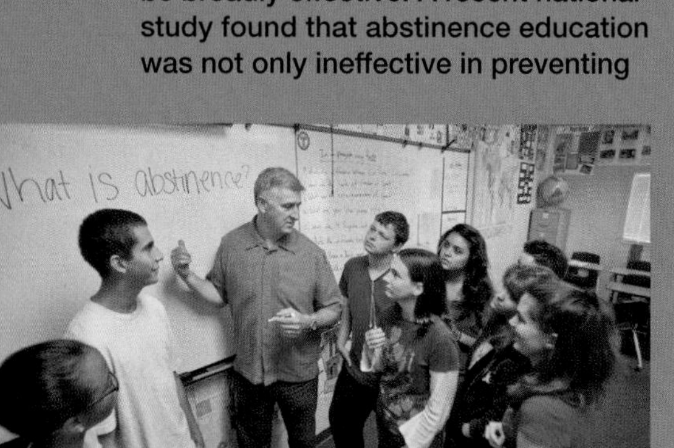

What do you think?

- Did you have "sex ed" in middle school or high school? If so, what type: abstinence-only or comprehensive? Do you think it had a positive effect on you and your peers? If so, in what ways?
- How could it have been improved?
- Do you think that states should have access to federal funding for social programs that research has not shown effective? Why or why not?

References: **1.** "Fact Sheet: End Funding for the Failed Title V Abstinence-Only-Until-Marriage Program; Support Comprehensive Sex Education," by the Sexuality Education and Information Council of the United States, April, 2011, retrieved from http://www.siecus.org/index.cfm?fuseaction=Page.ViewPage&PageID=1271. **2.** "Abstinence-Only Education and Teen Pregnancy Rates: Why We Need Comprehensive Sex Education in the U.S.," by K. F. Stanger-Hall & D. W. Hall, 2011, *PLoS ONE 6* (10), p. e24658. doi:10.1371/journal.pone.0024658. **3.** "Impact of Sex and HIV Prevention Programs on Sexual Behaviors of Youth in Developing and Developed Countries [*Youth Research Working Paper, No. 2*]"by D. Kirby, B. A. Laris, & L. Rolleri, 2005, Research Triangle Park, NC: Family Health International, retrieved from http://www.fhi360.org//NR/rdonlyres/ea77gewes4v3axgiyrnkrpmixaph6cmaesuz3nccrodokejfmerwzi5lsgvvmwl3yfegftswh5m5gc/sexedworkingpaperfinal.pdf.

3. Where must a fertilized egg implant in order to survive and thrive?
   a. ovary
   b. fallopian tube
   c. endometrium
   d. cervix

4. Which of the following methods of contraception is the most permanent?
   a. natural methods
   b. barrier methods
   c. hormonal methods
   d. surgical methods

5. Which of the following statements about male condom use is true?
   a. You should either purchase condoms already lubricated with a spermicide, or apply a spermicide as a lubricant when using.
   b. When the woman is using a female condom, the man should still use a male condom to further reduce the risk of pregnancy and sexually transmitted infection.
   c. If either partner is allergic to latex, the couple should use polyurethane condoms.
   d. Lambskin condoms are more effective than polyurethane condoms in preventing pregnancy and STIs.

6. Depo-Provera is
   a. a hormonal injection.
   b. a hormonal IUD.
   c. a transdermal patch.
   d. a hormonal implant.

7. Of the following methods of birth control, which provide(s) protection against sexually transmitted infection?
   a. diaphragm
   b. spermicides
   c. vasectomy
   d. none of the above

8. What is the approximate chance of getting pregnant in any given month for young, healthy couples who are having unprotected sex?
   a. 5%
   b. 10%
   c. 20%
   d. 30%

9. Which of the following statements about abortion is true?
   a. In 2008, the U.S. abortion rate reached its highest level since 1974.
   b. In 2008, 9 out of 10 abortions were performed during the first 13 weeks of pregnancy.
   c. American women choose medical abortion slightly more often than surgical abortion.
   d. Currently 86% of counties in the United States have abortion services available.

10. Which of the following statistics is true?
   a. Low-income women are more than four times more likely than affluent women to have an unintended pregnancy.
   b. Unintended pregnancy costs the U.S. health care system more than $11 million annually.
   c. For every $1 spent on family planning services, the government saves $2 in Medicaid expenses.
   d. All of the above are true.

Get Connected

Mobile Tips!

Scan this QR code with your mobile device to access additional tips about contraception. Or, via your mobile device, go to **http://mobiletips.pearsoncmg.com** and navigate to Chapter 17.

Health Online **Visit the following websites for further information about the topics in this chapter:**

- Planned Parenthood
  www.plannedparenthood.org
- Womenshealth.gov Birth Control Fact Sheet
  www.womenshealth.gov/publications/our-publications/fact-sheet/birth-control-methods.cfm
- Abstinence
  www.stayteen.org/waiting
- Go Ask Alice (advice about sexuality and sexual health)
  http://goaskalice.columbia.edu

Website links are subject to change. To access updated web links, please visit ***www.pearsonhighered.com/lynchelmore.***

References

i. Kaye, K., Suellentrop, K., & Sloup, C. (2009). *The fog zone: How misperceptions, magical thinking, and ambivalence put young adults at risk for unplanned pregnancy*. Washington, DC: The National Campaign to Prevent Teen and Unplanned Pregnancy. Retrieved from http://www.thenationalcampaign.org/fogzone/PDF/FZ_summary.pdf.

1. Kaye, K., Suellentrop, K., & Sloup, C. (2009). *The fog zone: How misperceptions, magical thinking, and ambivalence put young adults at risk for unplanned pregnancy.* Washington, DC: The National Campaign to Prevent Teen and Unplanned Pregnancy. Retrieved from http://www.thenationalcampaign.org/fogzone/PDF/FZ_summary.pdf.

2. U.S. Centers for Disease Control and Prevention. (2010, April 30). *Unintended pregnancy prevention: Home.* Retrieved from http://www.cdc.gov/reproductivehealth/unintendedpregnancy.

3. American College Health Association. (2012). *American College Health Association-National College Health Assessment (ACHA-NCHA) reference group executive summary, fall 2011*. Retrieved from http://www.acha-ncha.org/reports_ACHA-NCHAII.html.

4. McConnell, T. H., & Hull, K. L. (2011). *Human form, human function*. Baltimore: Lippincott Williams & Wilkins.

5. Go Ask Alice. (2009, March 27). Condoms: An explanation of condom failure rates. Columbia University. Retrieved from http://www.goaskalice.columbia.edu/2219.html.

6. White, K. O., & Westhoff, C. (2011, September). The effect of pack supply on oral contraceptive pill continuation: A randomized, controlled trial. *Obstetrics & Gynecology, 118* (3), 615–622.

7. Institute for Reproductive Health. (n.d.). *Overview of fertility awareness-based methods.* Retrieved from http://www.irh.org/?q=overview_fam.

8. Mosher, W. D., & Jones, J. (2010). *Use of contraception in the United States, 1982–2008*. National Center for Health Statistics. *Vital Health Statistics 23* (29).

9. U.S. Food and Drug Administration. (2009, June 18). *New warning for nonoxynol-9 OTC contraceptive products re: STDs and HIV/AIDS*. Retrieved from http://www.fda.gov/ForConsumers/ByAudience/ForPatientAdvocates/HIVandAIDSActivities/ucm124023.htm.

10. U.S. Food and Drug Administration. (2010, July 22). *Condoms and sexually transmitted diseases*. Retrieved from http://www.fda.gov/ForConsumers/byAudience/ForPatientAdvocates/HIVandAIDSActivities/ucm126372.htm#guar.

11. McGuire, L. (2010). *New emergency contraceptive.* Mayo Foundation for Medical Education and Research. Retrieved from http://www.mayoclinic.com/health/emergency-contraceptive/MY01365.

12. Mayo Foundation for Medical Education and Research. (2012, January 21). *ParaGard (copper IUD)*. Retrieved from http://www.mayoclinic.com/health/paragard/MY00997/DSECTION=risks.

13. Mayo Foundation for Medical Education and Research. (2012, January 21). *Mirena (hormonal IUD).* Retrieved from http://www.mayoclinic.com/health/mirena/MY00998.

14. American Heart Association. (2012). Go red for women: Understand your risks. Retrieved from http://www.goredforwomen.org/understand_your_risks.aspx.

15. Mayo Foundation for Medical Education and Research. (2011, May 21). *Birth control pill FAQ: Benefits, risks and choices.* Retrieved from http://www.mayoclinic.com/health/birth-control-pill/WO00098/NSECTIONGROUP=2.

16. Glasier, A. F., Cameron, S. T., Fine, P. M., Logan, S. J. S., Casale, W., Van Horn, J., . . . Gainer, E. (2010, February 13). Ulipristal acetate versus levonorgestrel for emergency contraception: A randomised non-inferiority trial and meta-analysis. *The Lancet, 375* (9714), 555–562. DOI: 10.1016/S0140-6736(10)60101-8.

17. Mayo Foundation for Medical Education and Research. (2011, February 10). *Vasectomy: Risks*. Retrieved from http://www.mayoclinic.com/health/vasectomy/MY00483/DSECTION=risks.

18. National Campaign to Prevent Teen and Unplanned Pregnancy. (2010). *National data.* Retrieved from http://www.thenationalcampaign.org/national-data/default.aspx.

19. National Campaign to Prevent Teen and Unplanned Pregnancy. (2008). *Policy brief: Thoughts for elected officials about teen and unplanned pregnancy.* Retrieved from http://www.thenationalcampaign.org/resources/pdf/Briefly_PolicyBrief_Thoughts_Elected_Officials.pdf.

20. U.S. Centers for Disease Control. (2011, November 25). *Abortion surveillance—United States, 2008. Morbidity and Mortality Weekly Report, 60* (15).

21. Jones, R. K., Finer, L. B., & Singh, S. (2010). *Characteristics of U.S. abortion patients, 2008*. New York: Guttmacher Institute.

22. Grimes, D. A. (1998, August). The continuing need for late abortions. *Journal of the American Medical Association, 280*, 747–750.

23. Trupin, S. R. (2012, January 31). *Elective abortion*. Medscape Reference. Retrieved from http://emedicine.medscape.com/article/252560-overview.

24. World Health Organization. (2006). *Frequently asked clinical questions about medical abortion.* Retrieved from http://whqlibdoc.who.int/publications/2006/9241594845_eng.pdf.

25. Jones, R. K., Zolna, M. R. S., Henshaw, S. K., & Finer, L. B. (2008). Abortion in the United States: Incidence and access to services, 2005. *Perspectives on Sexual and Reproductive Health, 40* (1), 6–16.

26. Raymond, E. G., & Grimes, D. A. (2012, February). The comparative safety of legal induced abortion and childbirth in the United States. *Obstetrics & Gynecology, 119* (2 Pt 1), 215–219.

27. Sonfield A., Kost, K., Gold, R. B., (2011, June). The public costs of births resulting from unintended pregnancies: National and state-level estimates. *Perspectives on Sexual and Reproductive Health, 43* (2), 94–102. Available from http://www.guttmacher.org/pubs/psrh/full/4309411.pdf.

28. American Society for Reproductive Medicine. (2003). *Age and fertility: A guide for patients*. Retrieved from http://www.reproductivefacts.org/uploadedFiles/ASRM_Content/Resources/Patient_Resources/Fact_Sheets_and_Info_Booklets/agefertility.pdf.

29. U.S. Department of Health and Human Services, Child Welfare Information Gateway. (2007). *Factsheets for families: Are you pregnant and thinking about adoption?* Retrieved from http://www.childwelfare.gov/pubs/f_pregna/f_pregna1.cfm.

30. Feminist Majority Foundation. (2010). *Birth control access campaign*. Retrieved from http://www.feministcampus.org/act/birthcontrol/bcaxCampusHealthCtrs.pdf.

31. Moore, T. (2011, December 19). How to avoid polarizing others. *The Huffington Post*. Retrieved from http://www.huffingtonpost.com/thomas-moore/how-not-to-polarize_b_778137.html.

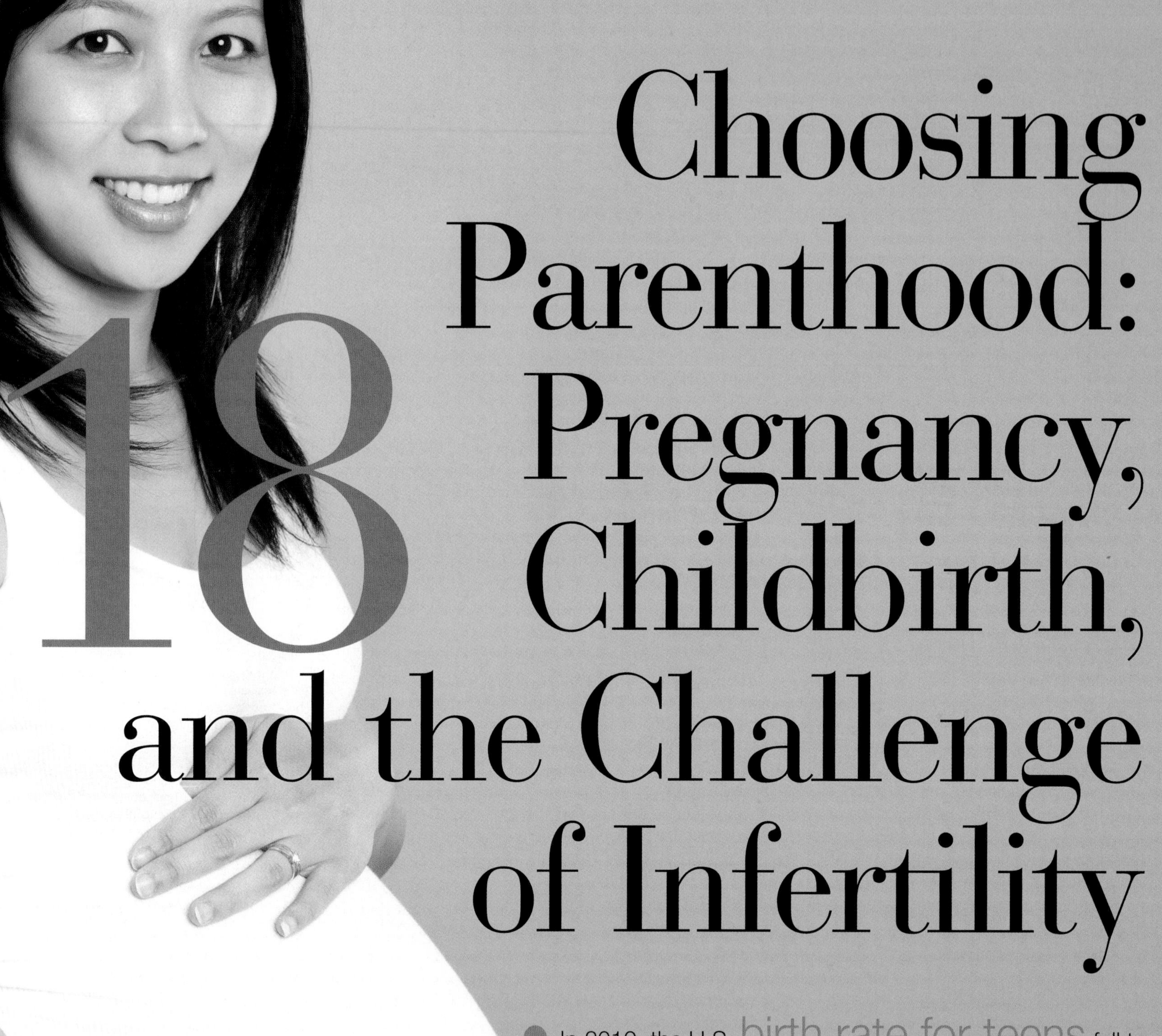

18 Choosing Parenthood: Pregnancy, Childbirth, and the Challenge of Infertility

- In 2010, the U.S. birth rate for teens fell to 34 per 1,000, the lowest rate ever reported.[i]
- Nearly one-third of all U.S. births are by cesarean section.[i]
- About 10% of American women are infertile.[ii]

LEARNING OBJECTIVES

DISCUSS the issues to consider before trying to conceive a child.

DESCRIBE the stages of pregnancy.

IDENTIFY several health concerns that may arise during the prenatal period.

COMPARE and contrast birth options, including the setting and management of pain.

IDENTIFY the stages of labor and birth.

DESCRIBE cesarean birth.

DISCUSS common challenges of the postpartum period.

IDENTIFY the most common causes of infertility, as well as options for infertile couples.

DISCUSS the stresses faced by college students who are pregnant or have young children.

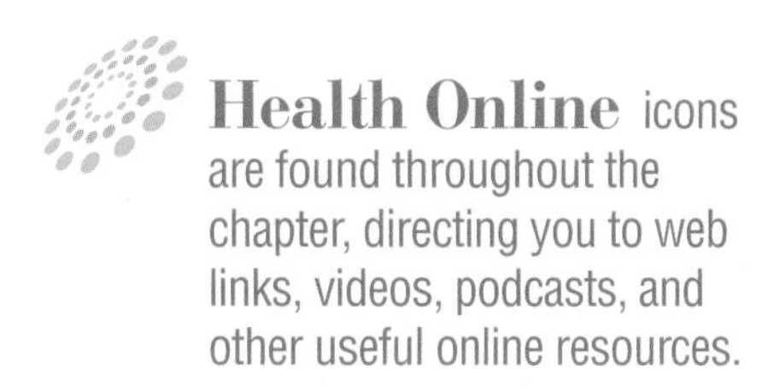

Health Online icons are found throughout the chapter, directing you to web links, videos, podcasts, and other useful online resources.

One of humanity's most commonly shared dreams is that of parenthood.

In a recent survey of more than 5,000 single men and women ages 21 to 34, 51% of males and 46% of females said they wanted to have a child someday.[1] Almost a quarter of American undergraduates already do.[2] But even if that "someday" seems a long way away, there are steps you can take right now to start preparing for parenthood. A first step is to get informed—about pregnancy, birth, and adjustment to a newborn, as well as your options should your dream of becoming a parent be challenged by infertility.

Preparation for Parenthood

Imagine a wail of hunger waking you up in the middle of the night—for the third time. Or being informed by your pediatrician that your child has a serious health problem. Or getting a phone call from the police that your son or daughter has been charged with drunk driving. Although many people describe parenthood as their most deeply satisfying role, few would deny that the challenges it entails can sometimes feel overwhelming. So how can you decide whether or not you're ready to take it on?

Getting Your Life in Order

Before attempting to conceive a child, it is important to develop a *fertility plan,* in which you not only determine whether you want children, and if so how many, but you also completely think through how you will prepare yourself for starting a family. Here are some aspects of your life that should be in order before you have a child:[3]

- As an individual, you've worked through significant emotional issues, whether major conflicts with your own parents, past traumas, addictions, or low self-esteem. If you haven't done this work, these issues are likely to surface quickly when you're faced with the stresses of parenthood.
- As an individual, you're fulfilling your current roles. You're handling your career or academic commitments, nurturing your relationships, and serving your community. Of course you'll experience changes in these roles. But before you choose to take on the demands of parenthood, you should feel satisfied in the roles you currently have.
- As a couple, your relationship is functioning and supportive, and you're committed to each other and to having a family. If this isn't the case, any instability in the relationship is likely to intensify once you're facing parenthood.
- Your finances are sound. You don't have to be wealthy to be a parent, but you should be able to afford the costs of food, clothing, shelter, health care, and the myriad of items from baby gear to hockey skates that your child will require as he or she grows. The U.S. Department of Agriculture projects that, for middle-income families, the average cost of raising a child born in 2010 through high school will top $226,900.[4] Bear in mind that this is just an average, and that every couple's circumstances are unique. On the other hand, this figure doesn't allow for inflation and doesn't include the costs of college! For more on the high cost of parenting in America, see the nearby **Consumer Corner.**

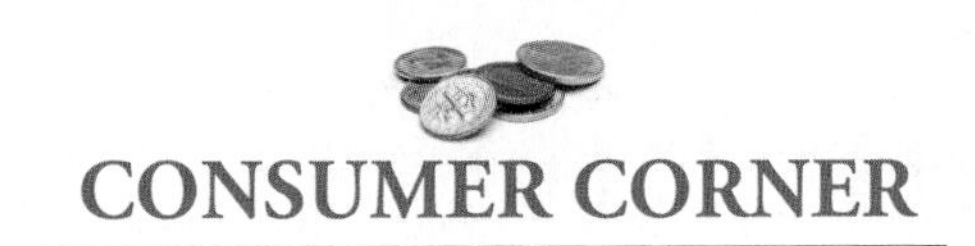

CONSUMER CORNER

The High Costs of American Parenthood

On the lunch menu was white fish in dill sauce, with a side of organic potatoes à l'anglaise. But this wasn't a fancy French bistro. It was a state-run day-care center in France.[1] The support French parents receive for child-rearing begins during pregnancy with national health care, and continues throughout the early years with national paid maternity and paternity leave, subsidies for nannies, and free preschool.

In contrast, the United States is one of only three countries across the globe that clearly have no national law requiring paid leave for new parents. The other two are Swaziland and Papua New Guinea.[2] Moreover, 50 countries offer paid leave not only to new moms but also to new dads. In the United States, workers in companies that have fewer than 50 employees—half the U.S. workforce—are not even guaranteed *unpaid* maternity leave. In other words, pregnant women can be fired if they take time off from their job to give birth.

When it's time to go back to work, how much does day care cost? According to a 2011 report, the average annual cost of full-time infant care varies in the United States from a low of $4,650 in Mississippi to a high of $18,200 in the District of Columbia. Costs for toddler care peak between $11,000 and $14,000 depending on the setting.[3] And when families have more than one child, child care costs go up as well. This high cost places an especially heavy burden on low-income families. A 2010 study of day care costs throughout the United States found that impoverished working families with young children pay 32% of their monthly family income on child care, nearly five times more than families living at 200% of the poverty rate or higher.[4] Although state child care subsidies can ease this burden, in 2009, 19 states had a waiting list.

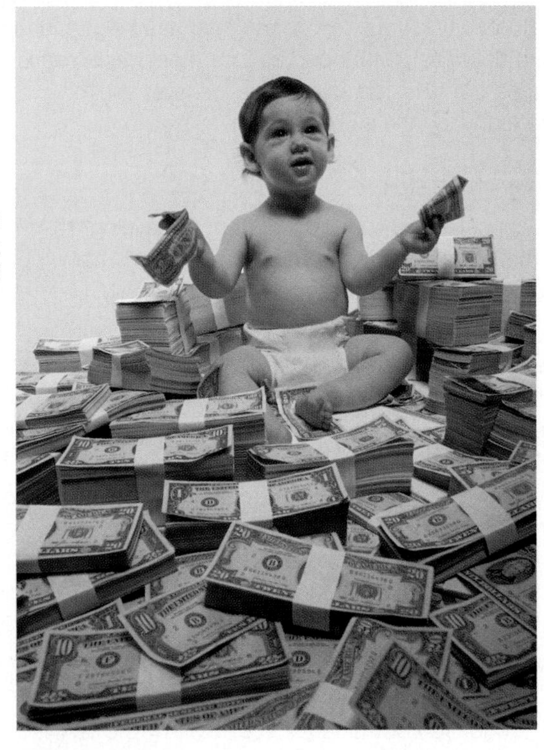

References: **1.** "Raising the Perfect Child, With Time for Smoke Breaks," by S. Meadows, February 7,2012, *The New York Times*, retrieved from http://www.nytimes.com/2012/02/08/books/bringing-up-bebe-a-french-influenced-guide-by-pamela-druckerman.html?scp=7&sq=having%20children&st=cse **2.** "Failing Its Families: Lack of Paid Leave and Work-Family Supports in the U.S.," by Human Rights Watch, February 2011, summary retrieved from http://www.hrw.org/sites/default/files/reports/us0211_brochure_web.pdf. **3.** "Child Care in America: 2011 State Fact Sheets," by the National Association of Child Care Resource & Referral Agencies, July 2011, retrieved from http://www.naccrra.org/sites/default/files/default_site_pages/2011/childcareinamericafacts_2011_final.pdf. **4.** "Low Income and Impoverished Families Pay More Disproportionately for Child Care," by K. Smith & K. Gozjolko, Winter 2010, Carsey Institute, retrieved from http://www.aecf.org/~/media/Pubs/Topics/Economic%20Security/Family%20Economic%20Supports/LowIncomeandImpoverishedFamiliesPayMoreDispro/PB_Smith_LowIncomeChildCare1.pdf.

- You want to give unconditional love. Even if you never experienced it from your own parents, you're not seeking unconditional love for yourself by having a child. Instead, you're deeply committed to providing it to your child.

The costs of raising a child vary according to your geographic location and other factors. So how much would it cost *you* to raise a child? Find out by using the USDA's calculator at www.cnpp.usda.gov/calculatorintro.htm.

Understanding Age-Related Challenges

Although you can't change your age, you can recognize the effects of age on parenting. In the United States, the average age of both fathers and mothers at the birth of their first child is 25.[5] Although there's no perfect age to become a parent, adolescents and adults over age 35 face unique challenges.

Risks for Adolescent Parents

The most significant psychological risk to adolescents who choose parenthood is interruption in the progress of their own developmental tasks, including establishing an identity, gaining autonomy, maintaining an intimate relationship, and developing a sense of achievement.[6] Physically, pregnant teens are at increased risk for iron-deficiency anemia, hypertension, and sexually transmitted infection. They are also more likely to give birth to newborns who are premature or of low birth weight. Social risks include family conflict, loss of peer relationships, and dropping out of high school or college. As a result, teen parents are more likely to experience poverty and to hold unsatisfying, low-paying jobs. Relationship conflict is significant: The majority of teens who marry end up divorced, and up to half of teen mothers experience domestic violence either before or during their pregnancy or shortly after giving birth.[7]

Trusting family relationships, health education from middle school through college, and regular, quality health care can help teens recognize and avoid these risks of pregnancy. (For more information on unintended pregnancy, see Chapter 17.)

Risks for Older Parents

Because they have usually completed their education, are established in their careers, and are more likely to be in stable relationships, older adults contemplating parenthood usually face fewer psychosocial risks than teens. However, fertility in both men and women over age 35 declines somewhat, so it may take an older couple more time to conceive.[8] Also, women over age 35 are more likely than younger women to experience physical problems during pregnancy, including pregnancy-related hypertension, gestational diabetes, and certain other complications, and are more likely to experience miscarriage. The risk of conceiving a child with Down syndrome, a developmental disorder characterized by mental retardation, also increases sharply as a mother enters her 30s.[8] Older fatherhood isn't risk free either: Several recent studies have concluded that children born to fathers over age 35 are somewhat more likely to suffer a mental disorder such as schizophrenia, bipolar disorder, or autism, and to have slightly lower scores on IQ tests.[9]

Taking Charge of Your Health

Most of us recognize that health care throughout pregnancy is important for mother and child. We're less likely to recognize the value of *pre-conception care*, initiated before a couple has even gotten

"Most of us recognize that health care throughout pregnancy is important for mother and child. We're less likely to recognize the value of pre-conception care, initiated before a couple has even gotten pregnant."

pregnant. **Obstetricians**—physicians who specialize in the medical care of women during pregnancy, childbirth, and the first few months after birth—typically work with couples who want to start a family to address any health problems or behaviors that could affect their fertility or maternal or fetal health.

Pre-Existing Conditions

Some of the pre-existing conditions that most commonly affect pregnancy include:

- **Overweight and obesity.** Women who are overweight or obese are more likely to experience infertility, miscarriage, and pre-term birth, as well as pregnancy-related hypertension and gestational diabetes. Their babies are more likely to have a birth defect, be injured during birth, and to be overweight as children. Weight loss before attempting to become pregnant is advised.[10]
- **Chronic diseases.** Pregnancy can exacerbate certain pre-existing disorders, including asthma, diabetes, epilepsy, hypertension, and depression and other mental disorders. The care provider may recommend a change in the management of these conditions before the couple attempts conception.
- **Medication use.** The effects of any over-the-counter or prescription medications on a fetus must be discussed, and different drugs may be prescribed. For example, the prescription acne medication isotretinoin (commonly sold under the brand name Accutane) is capable of causing severe birth defects, and its use must be discontinued before attempting pregnancy. Phenytoin, an antiseizure medication, and lithium, used for bipolar disorder, are other common medications that are harmful to a fetus.
- **Sexually transmitted infections (STIs).** As a result of certain STIs, scar tissue can develop in the woman's fallopian tubes, impairing her fertility. Moreover, some STIs, including genital herpes, are incurable and can harm the fetus if there is an active outbreak at the time of childbirth. Both partners are tested for HIV infection, which can be transmitted from a pregnant woman to her fetus.[6]

Vaccinations

Certain vaccine-preventable diseases, including chicken pox and rubella, can harm a fetus if the mother has an active infection during pregnancy. If a woman isn't sure whether or not she has immunity to these diseases, whether through having had the disease itself or through vaccination, she should request screening. If she needs a shot, she should wait at least 3 months after getting it before attempting to conceive.[11]

Genetic Screening

All couples planning pregnancy are offered screening for a variety of disorders that are due to genetic defects. Even partners who are unaware of any personal history of genetic disease are encouraged to undergo screening. To understand why, let's review some basic genetics.

A gene is a distinct segment of a long, threadlike compound called DNA found within the nucleus of almost all of our body cells **(Figure 18.1).** There, DNA is wound into 46 bundles called chromosomes, which are paired: A person inherits one set of 23 chromosomes from each parent. Every chromosome contains lots of DNA for which the function isn't known, as well as many genes, tiny segments of DNA that code for specific body proteins. You can think of genes as "recipes" for assembling the proteins that form the body's tissues and functional chemicals. Just as a bread recipe that omits the yeast or doubles the flour will cause us to bake a batch of "bad" bread, a gene that is defective will cause cells to assemble useless or harmful proteins.

Because we inherit two copies of every chromosome (one copy from our mother and one from our father), we also inherit two copies of every gene on those chromosomes. As shown in Figure 18.1, the only exceptions are the genes on the male's sex chromosomes, one X and one Y, which are unpaired. (Females have two X chromosomes—a pair.) In many genetic diseases, both copies of the same gene have to be defective for the disorder to produce symptoms. That's because a normal gene in a pair will compensate for a defect on the other gene in that pair. Such disorders are said to be recessive: They "recede" in the presence of one normal gene. But this also means that anyone may be a **carrier** of a recessive genetic defect—that is, a person with no genetic disease who nevertheless has one defective copy of a gene. When two carriers mate, there is a 1 in 4 chance that their offspring will inherit a defective gene from *both* parents, and actually manifest the disorder **(Figure 18.2).** Cystic fibrosis, a disorder affecting the respiratory and gastrointestinal systems, is an example.

Not all genetic disorders are recessive. Some, called dominant disorders, manifest even if only one copy of a gene is defective. That gene "dominates" the normal copy in the pair. An example is Huntington's disease, a very rare but fatal neurological disorder that begins to manifest in adulthood, frequently after the affected person has already passed the gene on to a child.

Finally, a few genetic disorders are "sex-linked." These arise when there is a defect on a gene that is on the sex chromosomes—the X or Y

obstetrician A physician who specializes in the medical care of women during pregnancy, childbirth, and the first few months after birth.

carrier In genetics, a person with no genetic disease who has one normal copy and one defective copy of a gene associated with a recessive genetic disorder.

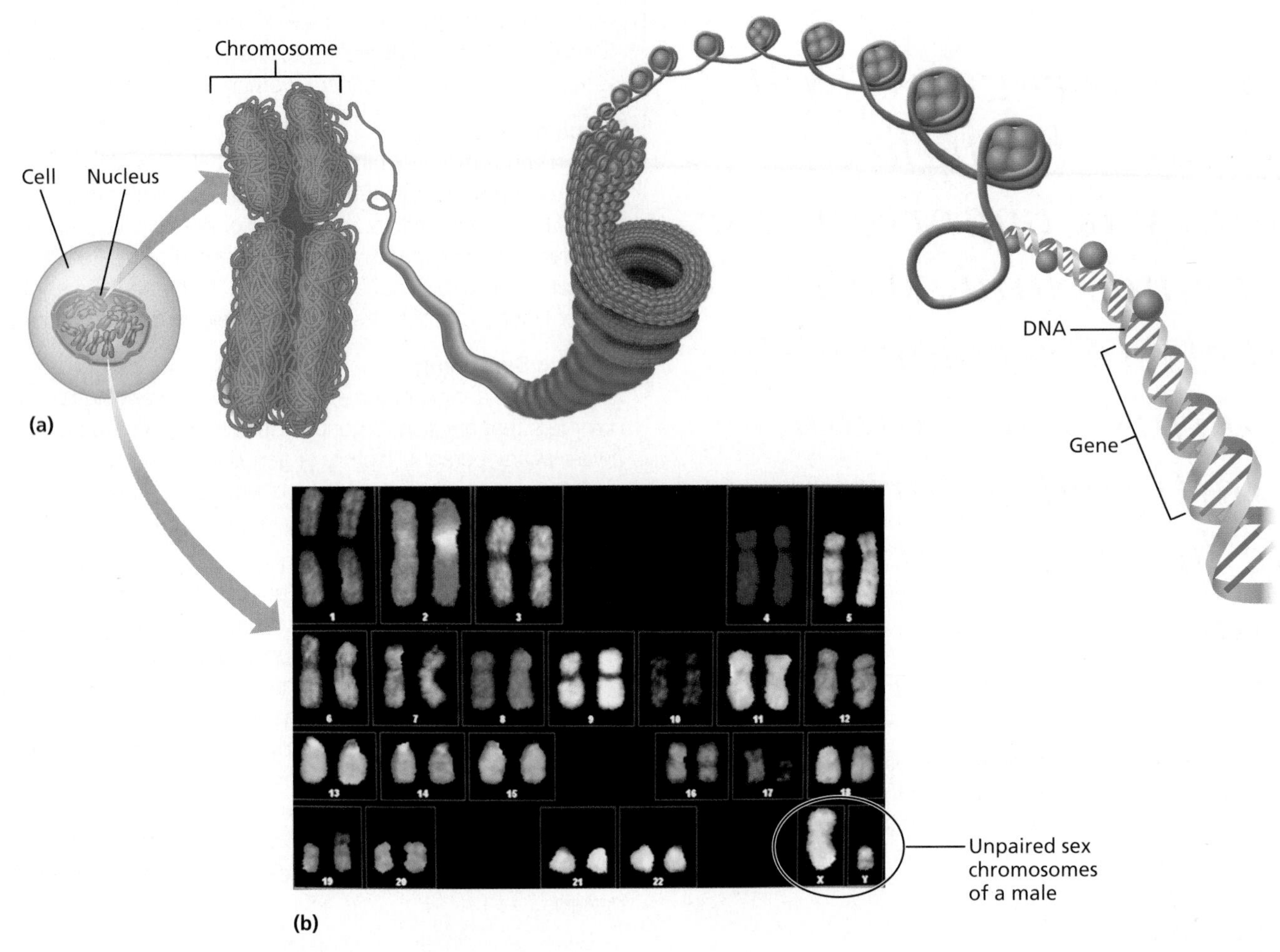

Figure 18.1 Genetic inheritance. (a) DNA is wound into 46 chromosomes packed into the nucleus of cells. A gene is a minute region of DNA that codes for the assembly of a body protein. (b) Chromosomes can be arranged into 23 matched pairs. You inherit one chromosome of each pair from each parent. The last pair are the sex chromosomes. Females have two X chromosomes in this pair, whereas males have an unpaired X and Y.

Source: Adapted from Donatelle, R., *Access to Health*, 12th ed., Fig. 1, p. 474. © 2011. Pearson Education.

chromosomes that cause us to develop into females or males. Females inherit two X chromosomes, one from each parent. Males inherit one X (from their mother) and one Y (from their father). Because males inherit only one X and one Y, any genetic defect on these chromosomes will be unopposed. This is the case, for example, with hemophilia, a disorder of blood clotting. Males inherit the defective gene from their mother's X chromosome. Because they inherit a Y chromosome from their father, the defective gene is unopposed and hemophilia manifests. The gene for hemophilia is recessive; therefore, a girl could be born with hemophilia only if she inherited the defective gene from both her mother and her father.

Pre-conception genetic screening can reveal whether or not the partners are carriers of any genetic defects. For example, if one partner is of French Canadian, Cajun, or Ashkenazi Jewish descent, both partners will be offered screening for Tay Sachs disease, a neurological disorder that is more common in these ethnic groups and is invariably fatal in early childhood. When screening results provide evidence of a genetic defect, a genetic counselor typically meets with the couple to explore the implications and their options for parenthood.

Substance Use

A variety of substances can cause harm to a developing fetus, and some can reduce fertility:

- **Caffeine.** Drinking more than two cups of coffee a day has been linked to reduced fertility.[12] Also, pregnant women who drink a cup and a half of coffee a day may double their risk of having a miscarriage.[13] Other potential adverse effects of caffeine use during pregnancy have been studied, but study results have been inconclusive.[14] Women considering pregnancy should decrease their caffeine consumption, for instance by switching to decaffeinated beverages after their first morning cup of coffee, or by drinking tea, which averages about half the caffeine per cup. They should also avoid energy drinks and caffeinated sodas.
- **Tobacco.** Smoking impairs fertility in both men and women. Nicotine affects the endocrine system, and alters the production of reproductive hormones in both men and women. Moreover, men show a lower sperm count, reduced sperm motility, and increased abnormalities in sperm shape and function. These affect fertility, potential for a miscarriage, and potential for birth defects.[15] In women, smoking appears to damage the ovaries and prompt early meno-

Autosomal recessive

Carrier father

Carrier mother

Affected
Unaffected
Carrier

Affected child
Carrier child
Carrier child
Unaffected child

Figure 18.2 Inheritance of recessive disorders. When two healthy carriers of a gene coding for the same recessive disorder have a child, the probability that the child will be born with the disorder is 1 in 4 for each birth.

STUDENT STORY

Genetic Testing

"Hi, my name is Hannah. My uncle had cystic fibrosis and even though neither of my parents have it, my mom thinks I should get tested for it before I have a baby. It's a little freaky to think there might be some genetic problem with having a kid, but I guess as long as both me and the dad don't have that gene, it should be fine."

1: Is Hannah right that as long as she and her partner don't both carry the cystic fibrosis gene, they will not risk having a child with cystic fibrosis? If both she and her partner carry the cystic fibrosis gene, will they definitely have a child with cystic fibrosis?

2: Does Hannah even need to worry about getting tested for the cystic fibrosis gene if neither of her parents have the condition? Why or why not?

Do you have a story similar to Hannah's? Share your story at www.pearsonhighered.com/lynchelmore.

pause. Toxins in cigarette smoke also increase the likelihood that a woman's eggs will have a genetic abnormality, and that the woman will experience a miscarriage. Women who smoke during pregnancy also have an increased risk of giving birth prematurely, having a baby who is low birth weight, and having their infant die of sudden infant death syndrome (SIDS).[15] Quitting smoking should be a top priority for couples before they attempt to conceive.

- **Alcohol.** For decades, alcohol has been recognized as capable of causing birth defects. **Fetal alcohol spectrum disorders (FASDs)** is the term now used to describe a range of complications—from physical abnormalities to emotional, behavioral, and learning problems—seen in children whose mothers consumed alcohol during pregnancy. In severe cases, the child dies at or shortly after birth. Despite these grim risks, approximately 12% of pregnant women drink; 2–3% engage in binge drinking; and more than 40,000 babies are born each year with some form of FASD.[16]
- **Illicit drugs.** Illicit drugs, including heroin, cocaine, and many others, can cause prematurity and low birth weight, leading causes of newborn death, as well as withdrawal symptoms, including tremors, irritability, vomiting, diarrhea, seizures, and other problems.[6]

fetal alcohol spectrum disorders (FASDs) A range of complications seen in children whose mothers consumed alcohol during pregnancy.

neural tube defect (NTD) A birth defect prompted by failure of the neural tube—the primitive tissue that eventually forms the spinal cord and brain—to close properly during the first weeks of embryonic development.

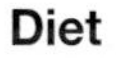

Diet

During a pre-conception visit, the obstetrician may also suggest changes in a woman's diet. A prenatal multivitamin/mineral supplement is often prescribed. It should include adequate iron, zinc, vitamin C, and, perhaps most critically, folic acid (also called folate). Women need at least 400 micrograms of folic acid prior to conception, and at least 600 micrograms throughout pregnancy. Folic acid supplementation is critical because a deficiency of this B vitamin significantly increases the risk that a baby will be born with a **neural tube defect (NTD).** An NTD is a birth defect prompted by failure of the neural tube—the primitive tissue that eventually forms the spinal cord and brain—to close properly **(Figure 18.3).** Mild NTDs often can be surgically repaired with no

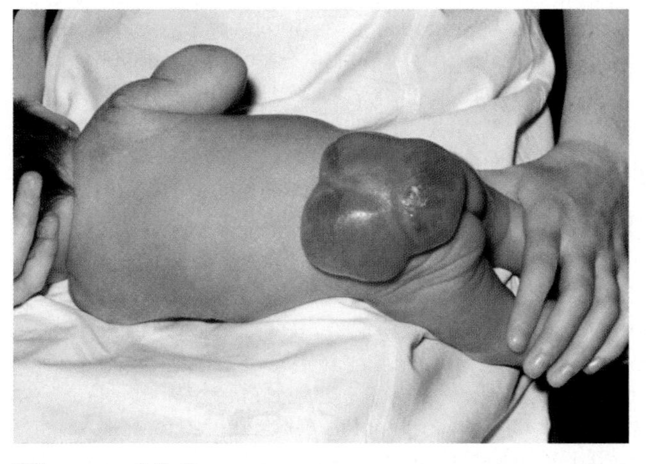

Figure 18.3 Neural tube defect. This infant has spina bifida, a common defect in which failure of the neural tube to completely close allows a portion of spinal cord tissue to protrude at the lower back.

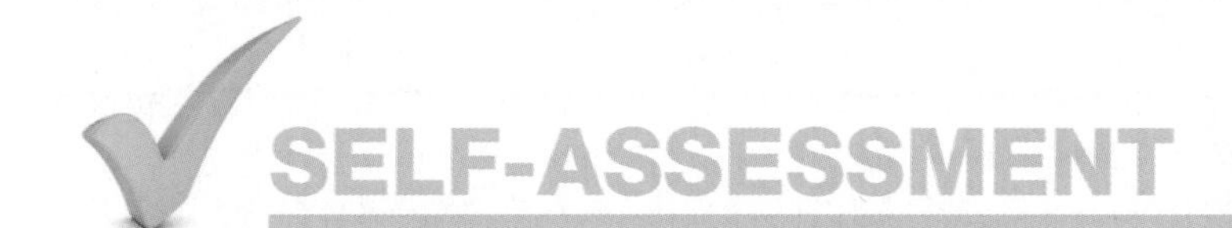

 Take this self-assessment online at www.pearsonhighered.com/lynchelmore.

Pre-Conception Health Quiz

How much do you know about pre-conception health? Take this true/false quiz to find out.

1. Pre-conception health only matters if you have health problems. ____ True ____ False
2. A fertility plan is an agreement a person makes with a doctor. ____ True ____ False
3. Unplanned pregnancies are at greater risk of both pre-term birth and low birth weight babies. ____ True ____ False
4. Only pregnant women need to take folic acid. ____ True ____ False
5. About one in eight babies is born too early. ____ True ____ False
6. Men don't need to worry about pre-conception health. ____ True ____ False
7. Women should make an appointment with their doctors to discuss their pre-conception health at least one month before becoming pregnant. ____ True ____ False
8. It's okay to drink alcohol when you're trying to become pregnant. ____ True ____ False
9. Men can improve their own reproductive health by limiting alcohol use and quitting smoking and/or illegal drug use. ____ True ____ False
10. Knowing about health problems that run in your or your partner's family can help your doctor figure out any genetic risk factors that could affect the health of any children you might have. ____ True ____ False

HOW TO INTERPRET YOUR SCORE

Correct answers:

1. **False.** Pre-conception health matters to all sexually active people. Even if a person's overall health is good, some foods, habits, and medicines can affect an unborn baby.
2. **False.** A fertility plan involves setting goals about having (or not having) children. It also involves knowing what actions you will take to support your goals.
3. **True.** This fact is concerning because half of all pregnancies are not planned. Using an effective birth control every time you have sex is the best way to prevent unplanned pregnancy.
4. **False.** All women who are sexually active should take 400 to 800 micrograms (400 to 800 mcg, or 0.4 to 0.8 mg) of folic acid every day to lower the risk of some birth defects of the brain and spine should pregnancy occur.
5. **True.** Researchers are trying to find out why pre-term births occur and how to prevent pre-term birth. But experts agree that women need to be healthier before becoming pregnant.
6. **False.** Men can take steps to boost their own health and protect the health or their partners. For example, men can be screened and treated for sexually transmitted infections (STIs) to prevent passing an STI to their female partners. STIs can be very harmful to pregnant women and their unborn babies. Also, men who work with chemicals or other toxins can be careful not to expose women to them.
7. **False.** Women should make a pre-conception health visit at least 3 months before pregnancy. And some women need more time to get their bodies ready for pregnancy. Pre-conception care can improve your chances of getting pregnant, having a healthy pregnancy, and having a healthy baby.
8. **False.** The Centers for Disease Control and Prevention recommends that women stop drinking alcohol for at least 3 months before getting pregnant. This way, should you become pregnant, you will avoid potentially harmful exposure of the fetus during the earliest stages of development.
9. **True.** Studies show that men who drink a lot, smoke, or use drugs can have problems with their sperm. This might affect a couple's ability to conceive.
10. **True.** Depending on your genetic risk factors, your doctor might suggest you meet with a genetic professional before or during your pregnancy.

Source: Adapted from *Preconception Health Quiz*, by the U.S. Department of Health and Human Services Office on Women's Health, retrieved from http://womenshealth.gov/pregnancy/mom-to-be-tools/preconception-health-quiz.cfm.

consequence to the child, but severe defects can cause neurological problems, including paralysis. In rare cases, the baby is born without brain tissue and dies at or shortly after birth. Because most women do not learn they are pregnant until several weeks after conception, at which point the neural tube should already have closed, all women of childbearing age, whether or not they intend to become pregnant, should consume the recommended 400 micrograms of folic acid daily. In addition to supplements, enriched breads, cereals, pasta, and other grain products are excellent sources of folic acid, as are green vegetables.

Physical Activity

Women who are not already physically active should establish a regular exercise routine, including aerobic activities and strength training, at least a few months before they attempt to become pregnant. Established exercise habits are easier to maintain throughout pregnancy, and can help elevate mood, improve sleep, prevent excessive weight gain, improve cardiovascular health, increase muscle tone, strength, and endurance, shorten the duration of labor, and help a woman get back to her normal weight after pregnancy.[17]

Pregnancy

Pregnancies are divided into three trimesters, each lasting about 3 months, during which characteristic changes occur in both the mother and the fetus.

What Does the Mother Experience?

Ask a dozen mothers what their pregnancy was like and you're likely to get a dozen very different answers. The signs and symptoms described here are only the most common, and only a few—such as cessation of menstruation—occur in all women.

Early Signs and Symptoms of Pregnancy

When menstruation is expected, but doesn't occur, a woman may find herself wondering, "Am I pregnant?" If she listens closely, her body may tell her the answer. Symptoms suggestive of pregnancy—which can begin to surface even before a woman misses her period—include the following:

- Swollen and unusually sensitive breasts
- Fatigue

- Frequent urination
- Nausea, and sometimes vomiting
- Food aversions or cravings
- Abdominal bloating or pressure
- Dizziness
- Mood swings
- An extremely light "period" known as implantation bleeding that occurs when a fertilized egg implants itself in the uterus

Some women will experience none of these symptoms in the early weeks of their pregnancy. Others may notice a few signs but not right away. Moreover, some symptoms suggestive of pregnancy can also be due to an illness or even impending menstruation. Still, women who suspect they're pregnant can find out for certain with the use of a simple pregnancy test. There are two types on the market: a urine test available over the counter, and a blood test offered only in physicians' offices. Both look for the presence of human chorionic gonadotropin (hCG), a hormone that is only made in the body during pregnancy.

The blood test can detect hCG about a week after ovulation. But many women opt for a home pregnancy test (HPT), which is inexpensive, painless, and private **(Figure 18.4).** Although each HPT brand is different, typically, the woman collects a small sample of urine—ideally when she goes to the bathroom first thing in the morning—and places a test strip in the sample. After a few minutes, a "+" sign or other indicator will appear if the woman is pregnant. The manufacturers of most HPT kits claim that they are able to detect hCG levels about 2 weeks after ovulation—approximately the day a woman's period is due. The accuracy of HPT kits improves, however, when women wait to use them until one week after their period is due.[18]

Because home pregnancy tests are not 100% accurate, women who get a negative result are encouraged to test again 1 week later if they still have not started menstruating.

Changes in a Pregnant Woman's Body

Women typically experience vastly different symptoms during each phase of their pregnancy **(Figure 18.5).** The symptoms just listed are characteristic of the first trimester, but other changes may go unnoticed by the mother-to-be. For example, the heart begins to work harder, and a physician may detect changes in the woman's blood pressure and pulse. These occur because the woman's cardiovascular system gradually becomes responsible for circulating an increasing volume of blood—that of the mother and the developing fetus. Similarly, the kidneys work harder to filter that increasing blood volume, and the mother's breathing patterns change slightly, with breaths becoming deeper and faster to move more oxygen into and wastes out of the increased blood.

The second trimester is sometimes referred to as the "golden age" of pregnancy because women tend to have more energy and fewer of the distressing symptoms of the first trimester, such as nausea. The most

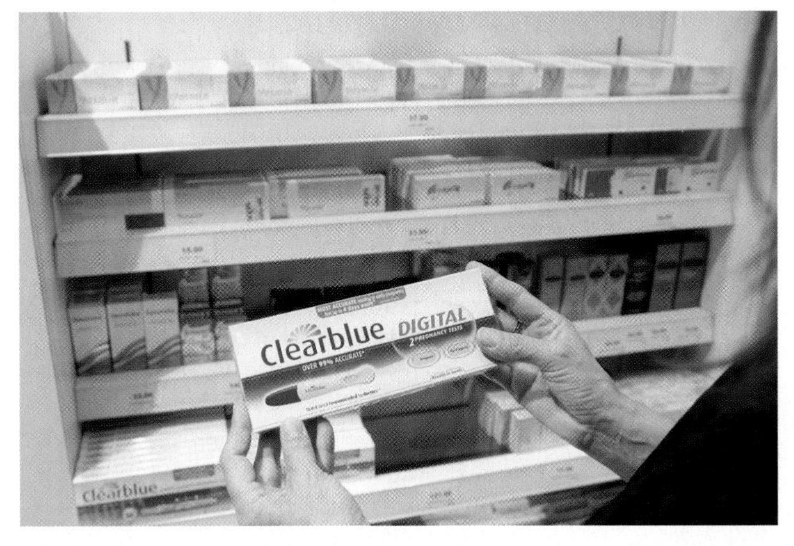

Clearblue DIGITAL

Figure 18.4 Home pregnancy testing. There are many brands of home pregnancy tests, but most work in similar ways.

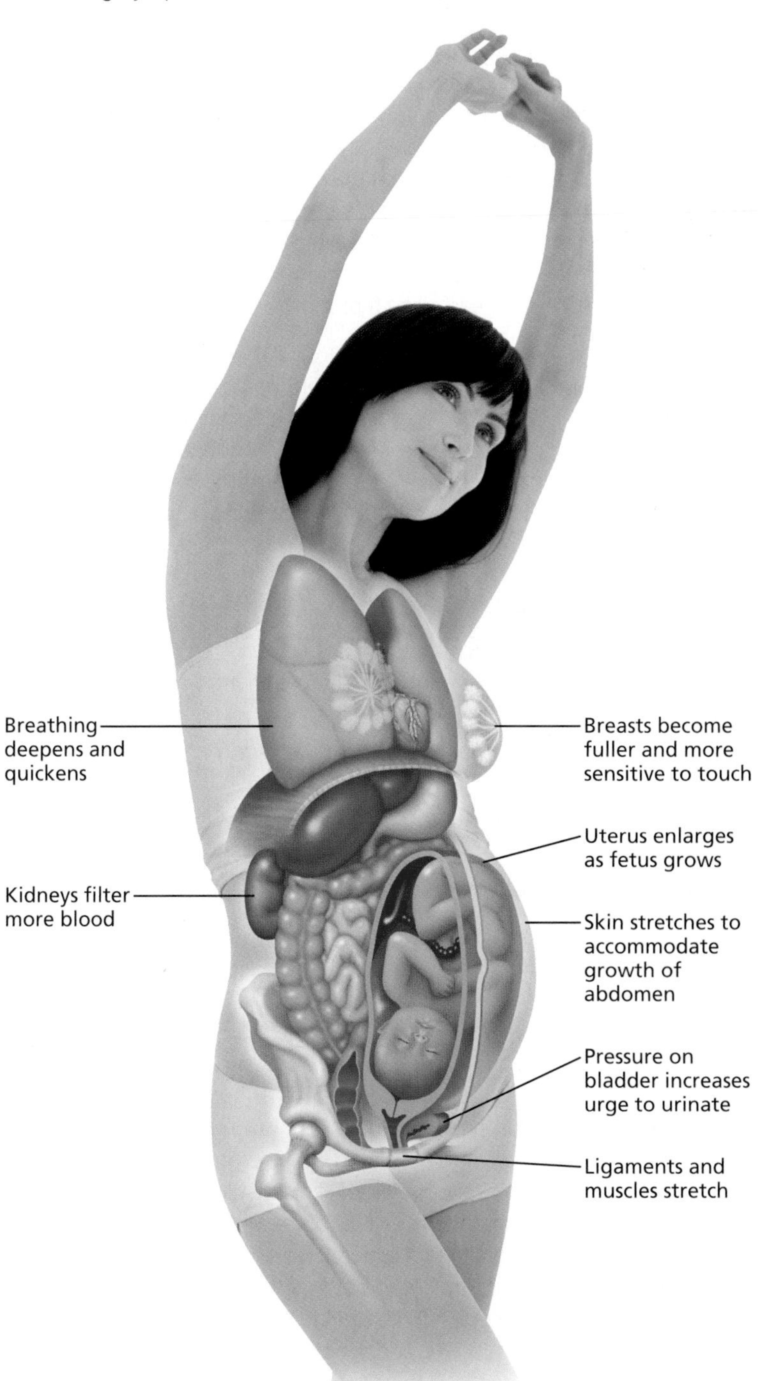

Breathing deepens and quickens
Kidneys filter more blood
Breasts become fuller and more sensitive to touch
Uterus enlarges as fetus grows
Skin stretches to accommodate growth of abdomen
Pressure on bladder increases urge to urinate
Ligaments and muscles stretch

Figure 18.5 Changes in a pregnant woman's body.

noticeable change is weight gain, discussed shortly. Also during this trimester, the woman's ligaments and muscles begin to stretch. Some women notice that they sweat more than they used to, and some experience night sweats. Some women develop acne, even if they never had it before, or develop a characteristic rash on their forehead and cheeks known as the "mask of pregnancy." These changes are due to pregnancy hormones and typically disappear after the baby is born.

In the third trimester, the mother's breasts become fuller and tender to the touch as they prepare for milk production. A fluid called *colostrum* may leak from the breasts. Colostrum is rich in antibodies and continues to be produced for the first few days after birth. Weight gain continues, and the uterus enlarges further, ultimately extending up to the woman's rib cage. The growing uterus presses on the bladder, creating the frequent urge to urinate. It also shifts the woman's center of gravity, exaggerating the curve in her lower back and giving her a characteristic "waddling" walk. The skin stretches to accommodate the growing breasts and abdomen, and sometimes darkens at points on the face and in a thin line near the navel. The cervix secretes a thick "plug" of mucus that seals off the entrance to the uterus, protecting the fetus from bacteria and other potentially harmful agents. Late in pregnancy, the cervix becomes thinner and softer and this plug is expelled, causing a profuse discharge. This is an early sign that the body is preparing for birth.

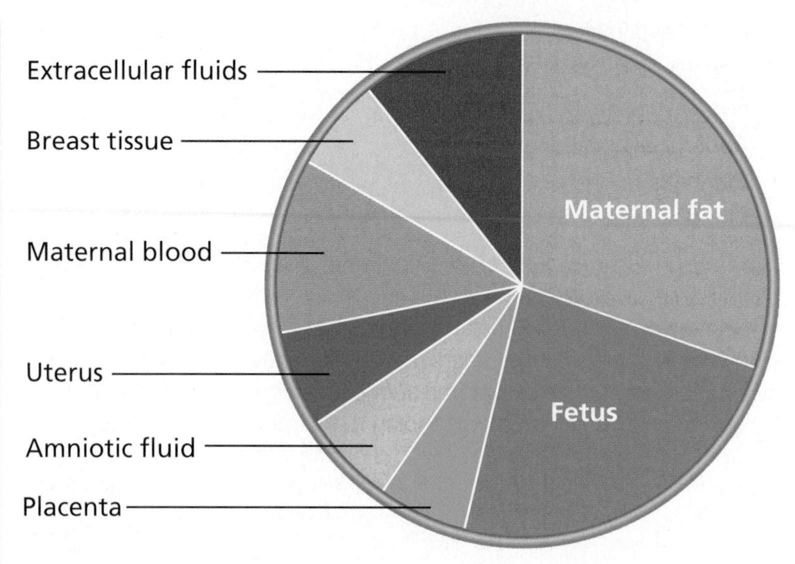

Figure 18.6 Where does the weight go? The weight a woman gains during pregnancy is distributed between her tissues and fluids, her fetus, and the placenta.

Source: Adapted from Thompson, J., and Manore, M., *Nutrition: An Applied Approach*, 3rd ed., Fig. 14.6, p. 508. © 2011. Pearson Education.

Weight Gain

Although it's not uncommon to hear women report that they gained 50 or even 60 pounds during their pregnancy, such a large weight gain is not advised. Gaining too much weight during pregnancy increases the risk that the fetus will be large, and large babies are more likely to experience trauma during birth and to struggle with overweight and obesity in childhood. In addition, the more weight gained during pregnancy, the more difficult it is for the mother to return to her pre-pregnancy weight and the more likely it is that her weight gain will be permanent. National guidelines for weight gain during pregnancy are as follows:[19]

- Women who were underweight prior to pregnancy should gain 28 to 40 pounds.
- Women who were normal weight prior to pregnancy should gain 25 to 35 pounds.
- Women who were overweight prior to pregnancy should gain 15 to 25 pounds.
- Women who were obese prior to pregnancy should gain 11 to 20 pounds.

Women who are pregnant with twins are advised to gain 37 to 54 pounds if they were of normal pre-pregnancy weight, less if they became pregnant while overweight or obese.

Gaining too little weight during pregnancy is also risky. As you might expect, inadequate weight gain increases the risk of having a low birth weight baby. A more surprising finding is that low maternal weight gain and low birth weight are also associated with a significantly increased risk of overweight, obesity, cardiovascular disease, and diabetes if the child has adequate food available as he or she matures. One explanation for this effect is **fetal adaptation.**[20] According to this theory, a fetus deprived of adequate nutrition goes into survival mode. Genetic, hormonal, and other mechanisms are then triggered that favor "hoarding" of any available calories. When food becomes plentiful, these mechanisms can cause children to store excessive body fat, increasing their risk for obesity and its related diseases throughout life.[21] Studies of populations that have endured famine support this theory, as adults born during times of famine have much higher rates of obesity and chronic disease than adults who were born a few years before or after the famine.

fetal adaptation Theory proposing that nutrient deprivation during fetal development may trigger genetic, hormonal, and other mechanisms that favor storage of calories and excessive body fat in childhood and adulthood.

Women should never diet during pregnancy, even if they begin the pregnancy overweight. Instead, women concerned about their weight should eat a nutritious diet within their calorie allowance, in consultation with their obstetrician or a registered dietitian experienced in working with pregnant women.

Where does the weight gained in pregnancy go? About 10 to 12 pounds are accounted for by the fetus itself, the amniotic fluid, and the placenta **(Figure 18.6).** That's why, although a woman may not look or feel lighter immediately after the birth, the scale will show that she has lost about 10 to 12 pounds. The mother's increased blood volume and extracellular fluid account for several more pounds. This resolves within about 2 weeks after birth, allowing most women to shed another 5 to 8 pounds as a result. After that, physical activity can help women lose weight. Also, because the production of breast milk requires a huge number of calories—more than are required during pregnancy!—breastfeeding helps many new mothers shed the remaining pounds.

Common Discomforts of Pregnancy

Given the dramatic physical changes of pregnancy, it's not surprising that many women report experiencing a variety of discomforts. Although no women should anticipate an uncomfortable pregnancy, the following are common.

Many women experience nausea, and some experience vomiting, during the first trimester of pregnancy. Others experience food aversions or crave specific foods. Although these may be distressing, they are due to normal changes in hormones protective of the early pregnancy, and tend to resolve early in the second trimester.[22]

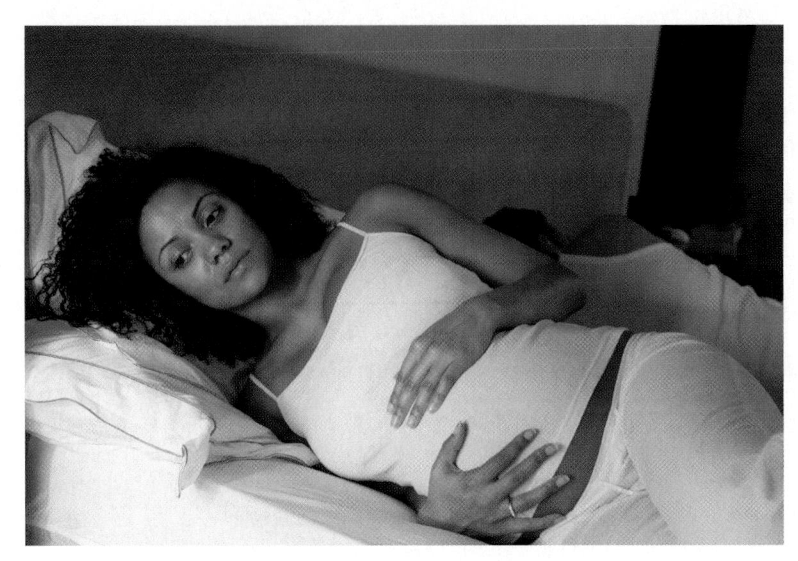

As their bodies change, pregnant women often experience some discomfort or **sleep problems**.

As the uterus expands, it pushes aside the stomach and intestines. At the same time, hormones slow down the transit of food through the gastrointestinal tract. As a result, many pregnant women experience heartburn, indigestion, bloating, and constipation. Both constipation and increased blood volume—which puts more pressure on blood vessels throughout the body—contribute to an increased incidence of hemorrhoids, swollen veins in the rectum. Increased pressure in the veins in the legs can cause swollen and bulging (varicose) veins, and in the blood vessels of the nose, increased pressure can cause frequent nose bleeds.[22]

The expanding uterus also presses downward on the woman's bladder, and the same urge to urinate that she experienced in the first trimester may resume. She may even leak urine when she sneezes, coughs, or laughs.

Dizziness, numbness and tingling, and backache, leg cramps, and other body aches are also common, especially in the third trimester. Fortunately, these discomforts are usually mild and don't signal any underlying disorder, and they tend to resolve as soon as the mother gives birth. That's not the case for two of the most persistent problems of pregnancy—fatigue and disturbed sleep. These typically continue and even worsen in the first few months after the baby is born, usually because of the physiologic strain of childbearing and breast-feeding, and the erratic sleep patterns and feeding demands of the newborn.

What Changes Occur in the Embryo and Fetus?

The fetus also undergoes significant physical changes as it transforms from a microscopic fertilized egg into an average 7.5-pound newborn.

First Trimester

The first trimester, which accounts for the first 13 weeks of pregnancy, is the most critical period of development. At this stage, the fetus is most susceptible to any substances a woman ingests, including illicit drugs, alcohol, and certain medications, and any environmental toxins, from pesticides to the chemicals in cigarette smoke.

Recall that when an egg and sperm combine, they form a single-celled organism known as a zygote. As the zygote makes its way from a woman's fallopian tube to her uterus, it rapidly divides and becomes a cluster of dozens of cells called a blastocyst. The blastocyst, which is no larger than a pinhead, implants itself in the uterine wall, where it begins to receive nourishment. About 2 weeks after fertilization—around the time a woman first misses her period—the growing mass of cells begins to differentiate into distinct tissue layers. The embryonic stage of development has begun, and the organism is now referred to as an **embryo (Figure 18.7).** Three tissue layers develop. One layer folds inward to form the neural tube, which becomes the fetal nerves, brain, and spinal cord. If the mother's diet is deficient in folic acid, a neural tube defect may occur at this stage. The second tissue layer becomes bone, muscle, and skin. The third develops into the fetal respiratory, digestive, and urinary organs.

The growing embryo has a powerful support system. It receives its nutrients and oxygen—and gets rid of its waste products—from the **placenta,** a thick pad of blood vessels and other tissues that develops on the uterine wall and allows the exchange of oxygen, nutrients, and wastes between the mother and baby. The **umbilical cord** also plays a key role: It emerges from the placenta and attaches to the embryo, linking the mother's bloodstream to the embryonic blood vessels. Within the uterus, the embryo is surrounded and protected by **amniotic fluid,** which helps regulate its temperature and allows it to move freely.

By 8 weeks after fertilization, all of the major structures of the human body are in place in at least rudimentary form. The embryo is now called a **fetus,** a term that applies until childbirth. By the time the first trimester comes to a close, the fetus measures 3 to 4 inches in length. Still, it weighs only the equivalent of two dozen paper clips. The bulk of the fetus's growth and maturation of its organs will occur in the trimesters to come.

embryo The growing collection of cells that ultimately becomes a baby.

placenta An organ that develops in the wall of the uterus and allows for the exchange of oxygen, nutrients, and wastes between the mother and the baby.

umbilical cord A vessel linking the bloodstream of the placenta to that of the baby and enabling the exchange of gases, nutrients, and wastes.

amniotic fluid Fluid that surrounds the developing fetus that aids in temperature regulation and allows the baby to move freely.

fetus The term for the developing offspring 8 weeks after fertilization.

Second Trimester

The second trimester is an exciting time for many women as the fetus begins to provide a few signs of the life developing within. The fetal heartbeat can be heard through the obstetrician's stethoscope, and about midway through the second trimester, the woman may begin to feel the fetus moving and kicking. The fetus continues its rapid growth, measuring 13 to 16 inches by the end of the second trimester and weighing around 2 or 3 pounds. All major organs and physiological systems become fully formed, and the fetus might survive if born at the end of this trimester; however, it would require lengthy and intensive hospital care and could suffer long-term health effects.

Third Trimester

During the last 3 months of pregnancy, the fetus gains most of its weight, including a layer of fat needed for insulation during the first weeks of life outside the womb. Its organs continue to mature,

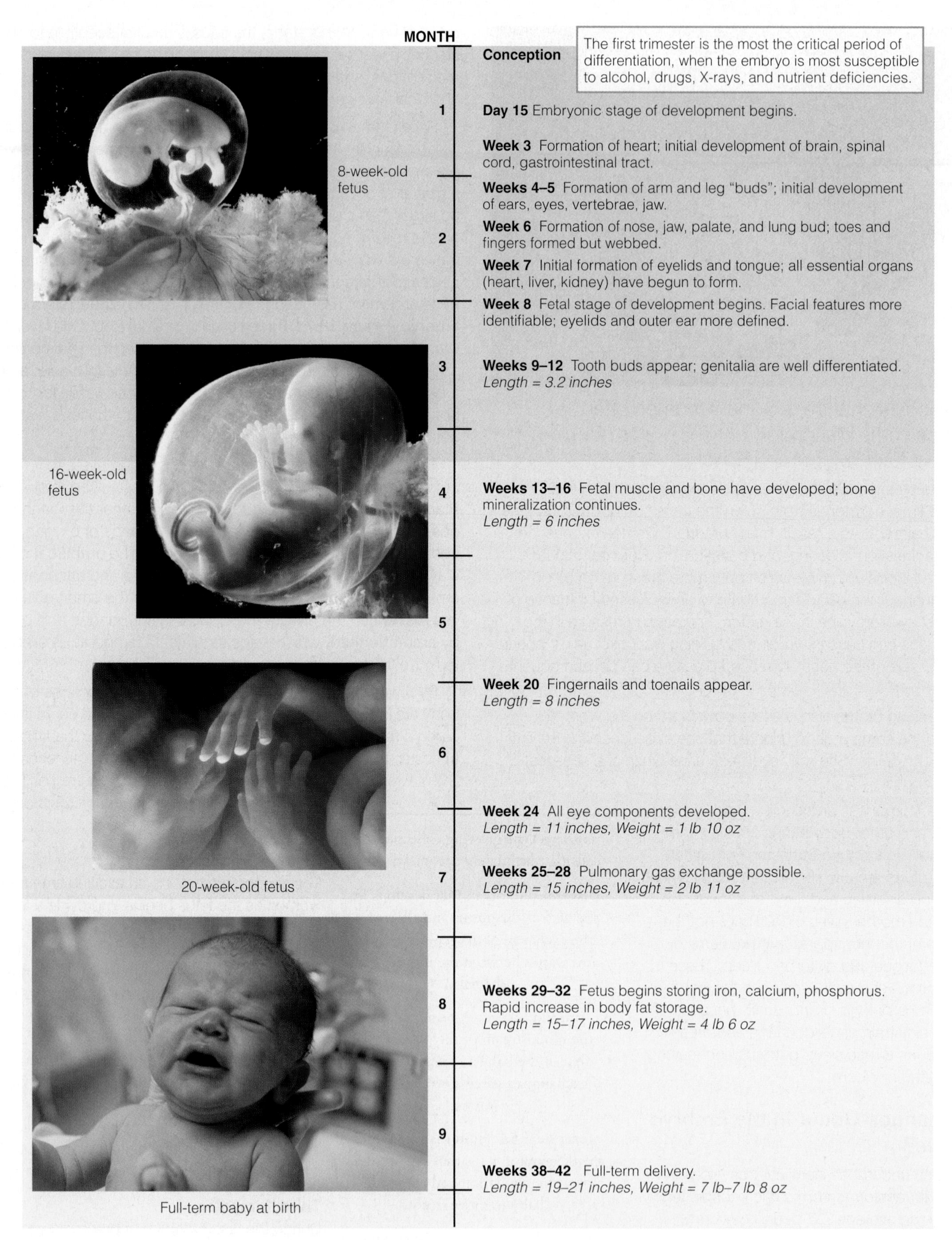

MONTH
Conception
The first trimester is the most the critical period of differentiation, when the embryo is most susceptible to alcohol, drugs, X-rays, and nutrient deficiencies.
1
Day 15 Embryonic stage of development begins.
Week 3 Formation of heart; initial development of brain, spinal cord, gastrointestinal tract.
8-week-old fetus
Weeks 4–5 Formation of arm and leg "buds"; initial development of ears, eyes, vertebrae, jaw.
2
Week 6 Formation of nose, jaw, palate, and lung bud; toes and fingers formed but webbed.
Week 7 Initial formation of eyelids and tongue; all essential organs (heart, liver, kidney) have begun to form.
Week 8 Fetal stage of development begins. Facial features more identifiable; eyelids and outer ear more defined.
3
Weeks 9–12 Tooth buds appear; genitalia are well differentiated.
Length = 3.2 inches
16-week-old fetus
4
Weeks 13–16 Fetal muscle and bone have developed; bone mineralization continues.
Length = 6 inches
5
Week 20 Fingernails and toenails appear.
Length = 8 inches
6
Week 24 All eye components developed.
Length = 11 inches, Weight = 1 lb 10 oz
7
Weeks 25–28 Pulmonary gas exchange possible.
Length = 15 inches, Weight = 2 lb 11 oz
20-week-old fetus
8
Weeks 29–32 Fetus begins storing iron, calcium, phosphorus. Rapid increase in body fat storage.
Length = 15–17 inches, Weight = 4 lb 6 oz
9
Weeks 38–42 Full-term delivery.
Length = 19–21 inches, Weight = 7 lb–7 lb 8 oz
Full-term baby at birth

Figure 18.7 **Stages of embryonic and fetal development.**

and it usually moves into the head-down position that facilitates vaginal birth. Throughout the last trimester, the mother may experience *Braxton Hicks contractions,* irregular movements of the uterus that may be misinterpreted as signs of premature labor. Braxton Hicks contractions, however, are simple tightenings of the uterus, nothing more than false labor.

While a standard pregnancy lasts about 40 weeks, babies are considered full term if they are born between 37 and 42 weeks. Babies born before 37 weeks' gestation are considered pre-term and are at risk for developmental delays and other complications. Babies born after 42 weeks' gestation are post-term and may stop growing in the uterus. In some instances, post-term pregnancies result in stillbirth.

The Compassionate Friends is a nationwide, nondenominational support group for parents who have lost a child at any age from any cause. Visit their website at www.compassionatefriends.org.

Prenatal Health Care

prenatal care Nutritional counseling and regular medical screenings throughout pregnancy to aid the growth and development of the fetus.

The health of the baby depends in part on the health of the mother and the measures she takes during pregnancy to protect them both. **Prenatal care,** which includes regular checkups for pregnancy monitoring and counseling, should be an integral part of every pregnancy. Babies born to mothers who receive no prenatal care are five times more likely to die than those whose mothers do get regular care.[23] As soon as a woman learns she is pregnant, she is encouraged to:

- **Get regular checkups.** Pregnancy providers include obstetricians and certified nurse midwives. If you're pregnant and don't have access to regular health care, visit your campus health center or a community health clinic to learn about the options that are available to you. The initial prenatal visit is followed by regularly scheduled appointments at which the woman is monitored for many factors, including blood pressure, blood sugar, weight gain, and fetal well-being. Although provider recommendations vary, visits are often monthly through the first 28 weeks, then every 2 weeks until week 36, after which the woman is seen weekly until birth.
- **Follow good nutrition advice.** It is commonly said that a pregnant woman is "eating for two," but during pregnancy, the body only needs approximately 400 calories more per day—not exactly a doubling of food.[24] Moreover, that increased need begins only in the second trimester. What is true is that the fetus consumes what the mother consumes, be it fruits, vegetables, lean meats, and whole grains—or cookies, chips, drugs, and alcohol. If you're pregnant, your body has to build a baby while maintaining its own functioning. So to make sure you input the best amounts and types of raw materials, check out the nearby **Practical Strategies for Health: Getting the Nutrients You and Your Baby Need.**

The U.S. Department of Agriculture has a Daily Food Plan for Moms that you can personalize. Find it at www.choosemyplate.gov/supertracker-tools/daily-food-plans/moms.html.

- **Exercise regularly.** Fitness is important to the health of the mother and her growing baby. Exercise can help relieve some of the symptoms of pregnancy and may prevent gestational diabetes. It can also help prepare a woman for labor and childbirth. Although each woman should seek the advice of her health-care provider, in general, regular, moderate exercise such as walking for 30 minutes daily most days of the week is recommended. Special exercises of the pelvic region, called Kegel exercises, are advised for strengthening the muscles of the pelvic floor, which support the uterus and bladder. With Kegel exercises, the woman repeatedly contracts the muscles she uses to stop the flow of urine. Typically she does a set of Kegel exercises a few times each day. Kegel exercises help women reduce their risk of incontinence, a common complaint during and after pregnancy, as well as their risk for a displaced bladder, vagina, and cervix.
- **Avoid all unapproved substances.** We've noted that women anticipating pregnancy should reduce their caffeine use, and completely avoid alcohol, tobacco, and illicit drugs. This is imperative during pregnancy. Women should also consult with their physician about the safety of any prescriptions or over-the-counter

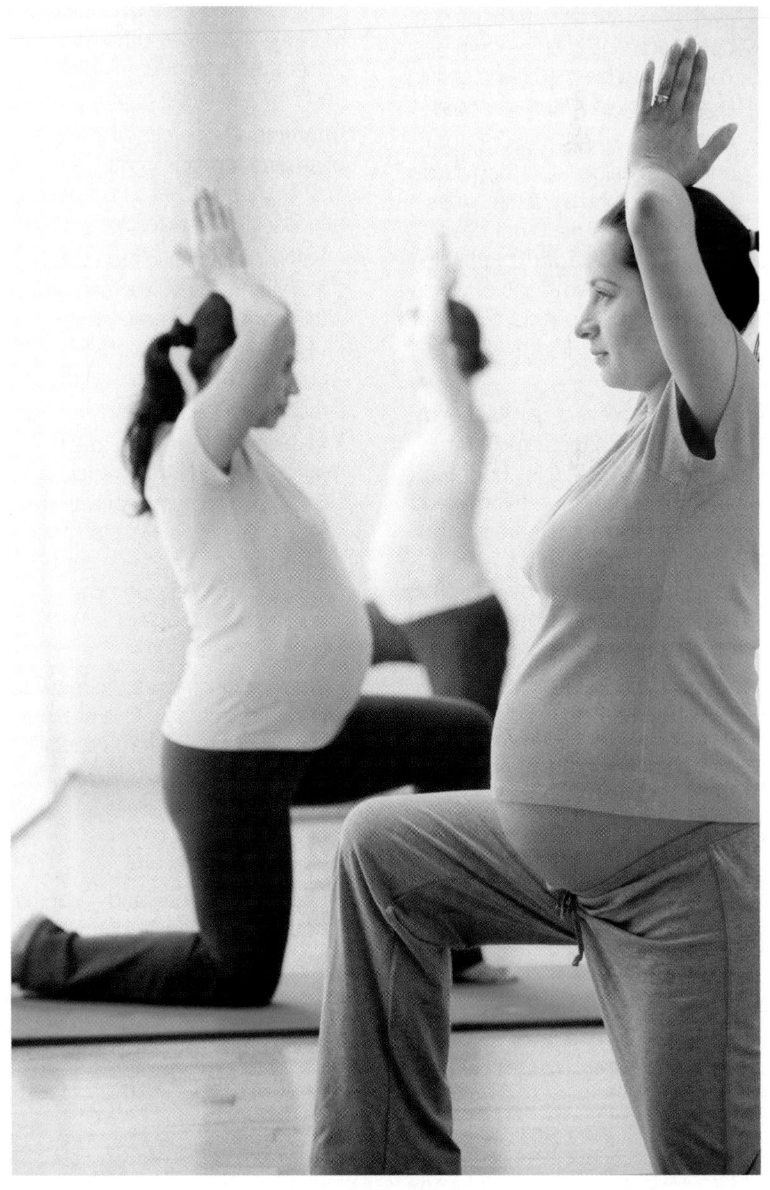

Eating right and following your doctor's **exercise** recommendations are key elements of prenatal care.

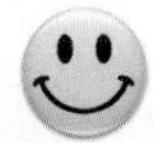 *Practical* Strategies *for* Health

Getting the Nutrients You and Your Baby Need

If you're pregnant, your need for most nutrients increases to support your baby's development and maintain your own health. Let's take a look at the recommendations for specific nutrient groups.

- **Fluids.** Water and other fluids are among the most important nutrients to consume in adequate amounts throughout pregnancy. Without adequate fluid, your blood volume and the amniotic fluid that protects your baby can both decline. Experts recommend you drink at least 10 cups of fluid, including plain water, each day.
- **Calories.** You need about 400 additional calories per day during the second and third trimesters of pregnancy. This is not nearly as much food as you might think! For example, two slices of whole-grain toast with peanut butter and a cup of skim milk provide about 400 calories.
- **Protein.** On average, you need an additional 25 grams of protein each day. This is about the amount of protein in a tuna sandwich on whole-grain bread—but remember, this is in addition to the amount of protein you normally eat. If you weighed 125 pounds prior to pregnancy, your recommended protein intake was 45 grams. So your intake now should be about 70 grams. That's a lot of protein, and you might find it challenging to obtain, especially if you're a vegetarian. For help in planning a diet that meets your protein needs, you may want to consult with a registered dietitian.
- **Carbohydrates.** Try to consume at least 175 grams of carbohydrates a day, and favor carbs that are high in fiber. These include whole-grain foods, legumes and other vegetables, and fruits.
- **Fats.** Your requirement for dietary fat doesn't increase during pregnancy. Choose heart-healthy unsaturated fats and minimize your intake of saturated and *trans* fats. A polyunsaturated fat called DHA is especially important to support the dramatic growth of your baby's brain during the third trimester of pregnancy. Oily fish such as salmon is a good source of DHA, and it is also found in lesser amounts in tuna, chicken, and DHA-enriched eggs.
- **Vitamins.** An increased intake of several vitamins is vital during pregnancy. These increased needs include the following:
  - Folic acid increases to 600 micrograms/day. You can get this from dark green, leafy vegetables, fortified breads and breakfast cereals, and supplements.
  - Vitamin B_{12} increases to 2.6 micrograms/day. This vitamin is available naturally only from foods of animal origin, so if you eat a vegan diet, make sure you're getting enough B_{12} from fortified foods or supplements.
  - Vitamin C increases modestly to 85 milligrams/day. This amount is easy to obtain from vegetables and fruits, including 100% fruit juices.
  - Vitamin A increases modestly to 770 micrograms/day. It's most plentiful in animal foods, but the body converts beta-carotene, which is present in carrots, asparagus, and many other vegetables, into vitamin A, and many breakfast cereals are fortified with vitamin A. It's important not to get too much vitamin A, as consuming just three to four times the recommended amount can result in toxicity, which in turn can cause severe birth defects.
- **Minerals.** Pregnancy creates a significant demand for new red blood cells—not only for the mother's expanding blood volume but also for the fetus, the growing uterus, and the placenta. Therefore, the recommended intake of iron increases by half—from 18 to 27 milligrams a day. As it can be challenging to obtain this level of iron from foods, obstetricians routinely prescribe iron supplements, either as part of or distinct from a prenatal vitamin/mineral supplement. The needs for zinc and iodine also increase modestly. You can obtain zinc from meats and whole-grain foods, including enriched breakfast cereals. Iodine is present in iodized salt.

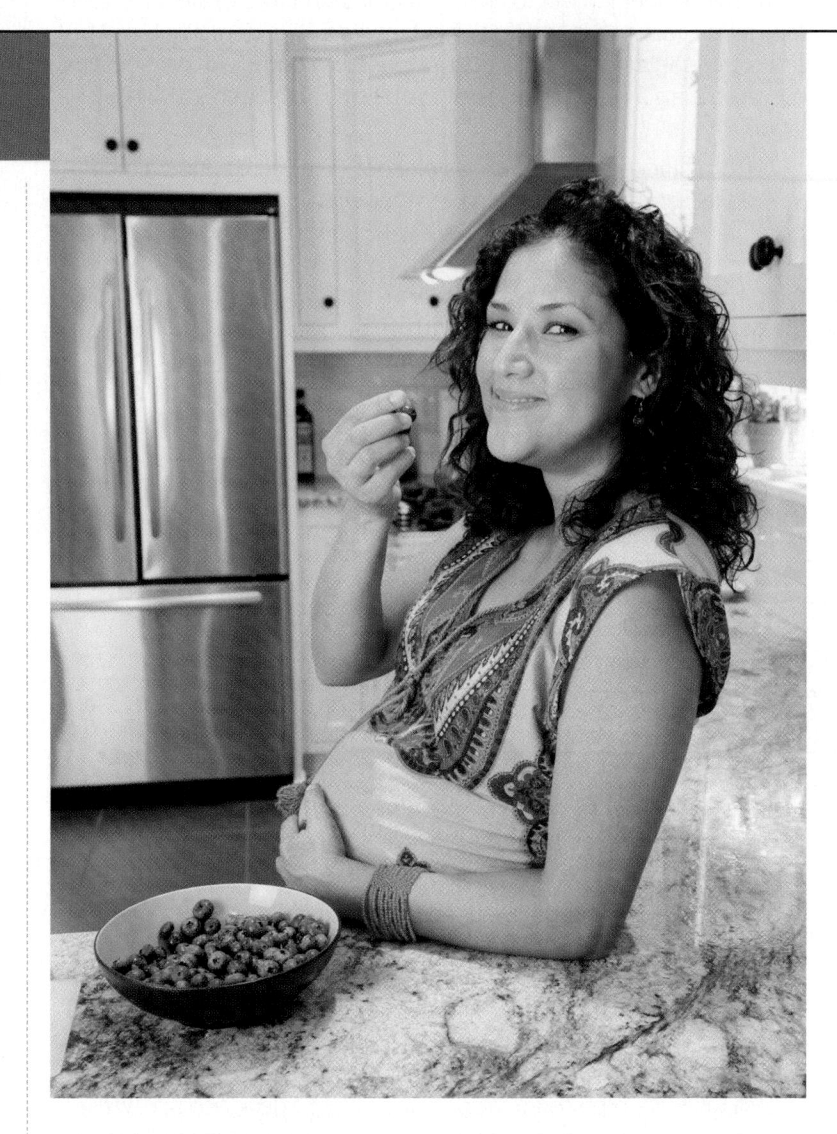

Data from *Nutrition: An Applied Approach*, 3rd ed., by Janice Thompson and Melinda Manore, 2012, San Francisco: Benjamin Cummings, pp. 508–512.

medications they may use. Many women believe that, because herbal supplements are derived from plants, all are safe. This is not true. Some herbs, including blue and black cohosh, goldenseal, and several others, increase the risk of miscarriage or other harm to the fetus. A pregnant woman should always check with her physician before taking any herbal remedies. The same holds true for high-dose vitamin and mineral supplements, unless they have been prescribed.

Prenatal Diagnostic Testing

Earlier we discussed screenings for genetic disorders, which can be conducted when a couple is considering conception. As part of her prenatal care, a pregnant woman will also be offered a variety of diagnostic tests to gather data about the health of the fetus. The most common tests include the following:

- **Ultrasound.** An obstetrician can use ultrasound testing—in which sound waves are generated to produce on a computer screen a black-and-white image of the fetus within the uterus—to help determine the fetus's age, size, and sex, as well as to check for the presence of certain malformations and other birth defects.
- **Maternal blood tests.** The presence of certain hormones and proteins in the pregnant woman's blood suggest an increased risk that her fetus has a chromosomal disorder such as Down syndrome. Whereas genetic disorders occur because of a defect on a specific gene, chromosomal disorders are due to the presence or absence of an entire chromosome or part of a chromosome. For example, children with Down syndrome have three copies of chromosome 21 instead of the normal pair shown in Figure 18.1(b). In some disorders, the structure of a chromosome is misarranged.
- **Amniocentesis.** Using a needle, the obstetrician removes a sample of amniotic fluid from the uterus. The sample is used to detect the presence of Down syndrome and other chromosomal disorders, as well as genetic disorders, metabolic disorders, and neural tube defects. This test is performed between 15 and 20 weeks' gestation.
- **Chorionic villus sampling (CVS).** The chorionic villi are projections of the placenta. A sample of this tissue can reveal the same problems as are detected with amniocentesis, with the exception of neural tube defects. CVS has a higher risk of complications than amniocentesis, but the advantage is that it can be performed a few weeks earlier.

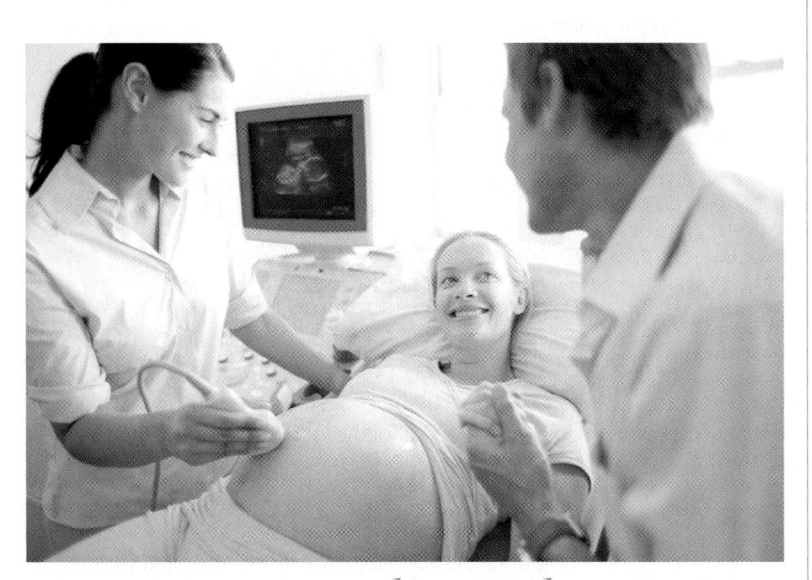

Diagnostic tests, such as **ultrasound,** provide information about the fetus's health.

Prenatal Childbirth Education Classes

A variety of options are available for pregnant women and their partners to learn what they can expect during pregnancy, birth, and the first weeks of parenthood. These classes typically cover the anatomy and physiology of pregnancy, the mother's nutritional needs, the birth process and birth options, breast-feeding, and even newborn care. A list of approved instructors is usually available from prenatal health-care providers.

For more information about options in childbirth education, visit the International Childbirth Education Association at www.icea.org.

Complications of Pregnancy

Most pregnancies progress without a hitch, with the fetus developing properly and the birth being trouble free. For some women, however, there are complications, problems that pose a risk to the health of the mother or baby, or both.

Ectopic Pregnancy

An **ectopic pregnancy** occurs when the zygote implants within one of the fallopian tubes. It can also implant in the cervix or an ovary, although much less frequently. About 2% of all pregnancies in the United States are ectopic.[25]

ectopic pregnancy A pregnancy that occurs when a fertilized egg implants within one of the fallopian tubes instead of the uterus; considered a medical emergency.

As the improperly located embryo begins to grow, the woman may experience severe pain, and the fallopian tube may rupture. An ectopic pregnancy can never develop normally and survive, and is a threat to the mother's life. It is the leading cause of maternal mortality during the first trimester, and accounts for 9% of all maternal deaths. Ectopic pregnancies can also cause scarring in the fallopian tubes, creating future fertility problems: A woman with a history of ectopic pregnancy has a 15% chance of a subsequent pregnancy being ectopic.[25]

Risk factors include smoking, having endometriosis, and having a history of sexually transmitted bacterial infections, especially gonorrhea or chlamydia, which can cause the formation of scar tissue within the tubes. Scar tissue impedes the progress of the zygote through the tube toward the uterus, increasing the chance that it will implant within the tube.

Both medical and surgical approaches to treatment of ectopic pregnancy are available. About a third of women are candidates for the medical approach, which involves administration of an injection of a chemotherapeutic agent called methotrexate. This drug impairs the ability of the implanted cells to multiply, and the pregnancy separates from the site. The mother experiences abdominal pain about 1 to 2 days after the injection. Surgery is necessary for many women, but if the tube has not ruptured, a minimally invasive microsurgery technique can be used that draws the pregnancy out of the tube. In some women, the location of the pregnancy or the tissue damage caused by it makes more radical surgery necessary.[25]

Miscarriage

A **miscarriage,** or *spontaneous abortion,* is a pregnancy that suddenly ends on its own before the 20th week. Most miscarriages occur during the first trimester. An estimated 10–15% of known pregnancies end this way, but because many losses occur before a woman realizes she is pregnant, experts believe the true number could be closer to 40%.[26] Exactly what causes a pregnancy to terminate is not always clear, but the majority of miscarriages are thought to be caused by chromosomal problems in the fetus. The risk is higher in women who are over age 35, have a history of diabetes or thyroid disease, or have a history of miscarriages. Smoking, drinking alcohol, or using illicit drugs while pregnant may also increase a woman's risk of miscarriage.

The American Pregnancy Association describes how you can support a friend who's had a miscarriage: www.americanpregnancy.org/pregnancyloss/mcsupportingothers.html.

Conditions Involving the Placenta

Recall that the placenta is an organ that develops within the uterus to nourish the fetus and remove wastes. Of the many placental problems that can develop, two of the most common are placenta previa, which is typically discovered during mid- to late pregnancy, and a retained placenta, which occurs shortly after birth.

Placenta Previa. In a normal pregnancy, the placenta develops near the top of the uterus. In **placenta previa,** it develops low in the uterus, partially or completely blocking the cervix and therefore interfering with vaginal birth. This happens in about 1 in 200 pregnancies, and is more likely in women who are carrying twins or other multiple fetuses, smoke, have had many children, or are older.[27] The condition is often detected with diagnostic ultrasound, or the woman may experience vaginal bleeding during the second or third trimester. If the fetus is immature, the woman may be hospitalized to try to prolong the pregnancy. Cesarean birth (discussed shortly) is required.

Retained Placenta. In normal births, the placenta is expelled from the mother's uterus within about 30 minutes after birth of the newborn. If this doesn't occur, the mother can experience excessive bleeding and other complications; therefore, the obstetrician will typically attempt to remove a **retained placenta** manually. If manual removal is unsuccessful, surgical removal is necessary. Retained placenta is common, occurring in about 2 or 3 of every 100 births, but manual removal is usually successful. Much more rarely, the placenta is retained because, during pregnancy, it grew into the muscular layer of the uterus. In these cases, referred to as placental adherence, manual removal is impossible, and a hysterectomy (surgical removal of the uterus) may be necessary.[28]

Infection

A variety of infections can harm the pregnancy, especially if the embryo or fetus is exposed during the first trimester, when tissues are differentiating and organs are developing. These include the following.

Toxoplasmosis. The protozoan *Toxoplasma gondii* is transmitted to humans either through consuming undercooked meat or through contact with the feces of an infected cat—whether in soil or in a litter box. The effect of infection on the pregnancy can range from mild to devastating, including blindness, deafness, brain damage, and spontaneous abortion. Pregnant women should wear gloves when gardening, avoid garden areas frequented by cats, and avoid handling a cat's litter box.

Rubella. A mild infectious illness when contracted during childhood or adulthood, rubella can cause deafness, heart defects, mental retardation, and other problems when contracted during pregnancy, especially during the first trimester. Children are routinely vaccinated against rubella, but pregnant women who do not have immunity cannot be vaccinated.

Herpes simplex virus (HSV). A sexually transmitted infection, HSV causes painful blisters in the genital area of both males and females. Both HSV-1 and HSV-2 can cause genital herpes. There is no cure, and outbreaks of the blisters can recur occasionally or frequently throughout the person's lifetime. In women, herpes can also cause blisters on the cervix, and these blisters can infect a fetus during vaginal birth. Infected newborns experience not only the characteristic blisters, but may also have fevers, seizures, vision impairment, and other problems. In women with a history of herpes, the risk of transmitting the infection during vaginal birth is small; however, 30–60% of mothers who experience a herpes infection for the first time close to the end of their pregnancy transmit it to their fetus during vaginal birth.[29] Thus mothers with active infections will need to have a cesarean birth.

Hepatitis B virus (HBV). HBV can be transmitted in a variety of ways, including from mother to fetus. If infection occurs early in pregnancy, the chances are less than 10% that the baby will get the virus. If infection occurs late in pregnancy, there is up to a 90% chance the baby will be infected. Hepatitis infection can be life-threatening in newborns, and those who survive have a high risk (up to 90%) of becoming carriers. When they become adults, these carriers have a 25% risk of dying from cirrhosis or liver cancer; moreover, they can pass the infection on to others.[30]

Human immunodeficiency virus (HIV). HIV infection is as serious a threat to newborns as it is to adults. All pregnant women are offered testing as part of initial prenatal care. Women who test positive will be offered drug therapy beginning after the first trimester, and will be encouraged to have a cesarean birth to avoid exposing the fetus to blood and body fluids that may be contaminated with HIV. Women who receive drug therapy and have a cesarean birth have only a 2% risk of transmitting HIV to their newborn. Babies born to HIV-positive mothers are also given drug therapy for the first 6 weeks of life in order to further reduce their risk of becoming infected. Finally, because HIV can be transmitted via breast milk, HIV-positive mothers need to feed their infants formula.[31]

Hypertensive Disorders

A pregnant woman's blood pressure is normally checked at every prenatal visit to screen for hypertension (high blood pressure), which is the most common medical disorder in pregnancy.[32] If left untreated, hypertension during pregnancy can progress to **preeclampsia,** a serious health condition that can threaten the life of both mother and fetus. Characterized by high blood pressure and protein in the urine, preeclampsia typically develops after the 20th week of pregnancy. Women may begin

miscarriage A pregnancy that suddenly terminates on its own before the 20th week.

placenta previa Development of the placenta low in the uterus, partially or completely blocking the cervix and interfering with vaginal birth.

retained placenta Condition in which expulsion of the placenta does not occur within 30 minutes of childbirth.

preeclampsia A serious health condition characterized by high blood pressure in the pregnant woman.

experiencing headaches, swelling of the hands and face, excessive weight gain, abdominal pain, and even vision changes. Without skilled medical care, preeclampsia can progress to *eclampsia*, a life-threatening condition characterized by seizures and multiple organ failure, as well as fetal death.

About 5–8% of pregnant women develop preeclampsia.[33] Unfortunately, there is no way to prevent it, and the only cure is childbirth. Physicians will often admit a woman with preeclampsia to the hospital so she and her fetus can be closely monitored. Although it can be harmful to the baby to be born prematurely, often it can be even more dangerous for a preeclamptic pregnancy to go full term. The obstetrician may decide to induce labor early in an effort to save both mother and child.

Gestational Diabetes

Gestational diabetes is a form of diabetes that develops in pregnant women with no prior history of diabetes. Women who are overweight and those who are older are at increased risk. Gestational diabetes is a concern for the mother because both hypertension and preeclampsia are more common in women with the condition. These mothers are also more likely to have an unusually large baby and to have a cesarean birth. Although gestational diabetes typically resolves after the woman gives birth, she is at higher than normal risk for acquiring type 2 diabetes later in life. Babies born to women with gestational diabetes may have low blood glucose levels, jaundice, and breathing difficulties, and they too are at increased risk for type 2 diabetes as they grow.[34]

In many women, gestational diabetes is readily controlled with careful attention to diet and regular physical activity. In others, oral medication or insulin injections may be necessary. After birth, both the woman and her child should be tested regularly for type 2 diabetes.

STUDENT STORY

Gestational Diabetes

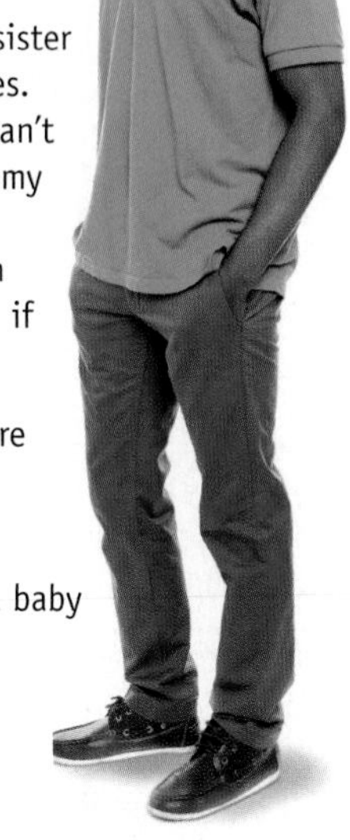

"Hi, I'm Michael. Last year when my sister was pregnant, she developed gestational diabetes. She kept telling me, 'No, I can't eat this. No, I can't eat that.' And she had to take insulin. Now that my nephew is born, she doesn't have the diabetes anymore, but her doctor said she needs to watch out because she might get it again in the future if she doesn't keep her weight and diet in check."

1: What type of diabetes is Michael's sister more likely to develop now that she's had gestational diabetes?

2: What other side effects for both mother and baby can be caused by gestational diabetes?

Do you have a story similar to Michael's? Share your story at www.pearsonhighered.com/lynchelmore.

Pre-Term Birth

Most pregnancies last 37 to 42 weeks. Babies born before 37 weeks are considered **pre-term,** and babies born before 32 weeks are considered early pre-term. In the United States, nearly 12% of births are pre-term.[35] Many factors are associated with an increased risk for pre-term birth, including being underweight, smoking, cocaine use, carrying more than one fetus, and experiencing an infection during pregnancy.

The earlier the baby is born, the more likely that he or she will not survive, or will have serious health problems. For instance, immature fetal lungs do not produce a substance called *surfactant* that helps the lungs recoil with each breath. Thus, pre-term babies often suffer from respiratory distress. They can also experience slowed growth, neurological problems, and other challenges.

Medications called tocolytics may be administered to try to stop labor, and steroid medications may be given to help the fetus's lungs to mature.[36] Many pre-term babies need care in a neonatal intensive care unit (NICU) for weeks or even months after birth.

Low Birth Weight

We noted earlier that the average birth weight in the United States is about 7.5 pounds. Newborns weighing less than 5 pounds, 8 ounces at birth are called **low birth weight** babies and are at risk for serious health problems, including death **(Figure 18.8).** About 1 in every 12 babies (8.1%) born in the United States falls into this category.[35] Pre-term labor is the leading cause, with two out of three low birth weight babies arriving before the 37th week of pregnancy.[35] Low birth weight babies are vulnerable to a

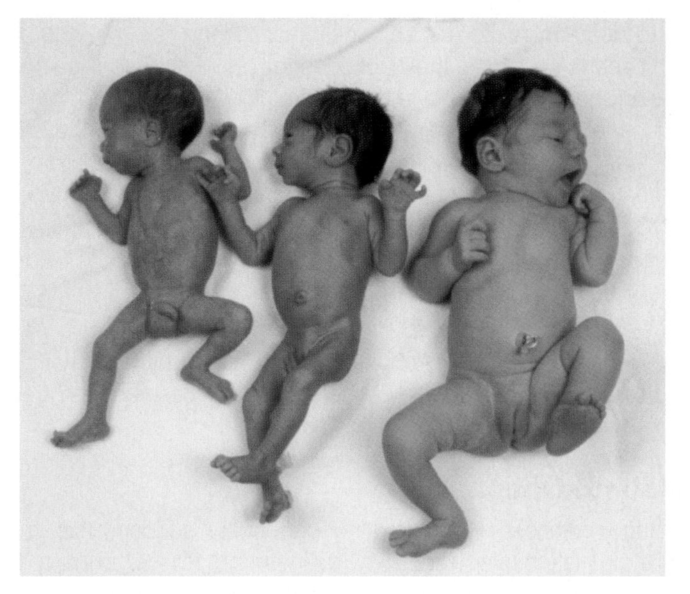

Figure 18.8 **Low birth weight.** This photo shows a term newborn of normal weight on the right, and two term newborns of low birth weight on the left.

gestational diabetes Form of diabetes that develops during pregnancy in women with no prior history of diabetes.

pre-term birth Birth before 37 completed weeks of gestation; births before 32 weeks are considered early pre-term.

low birth weight The term given to birth weights of less than 5 pounds, 8 ounces.

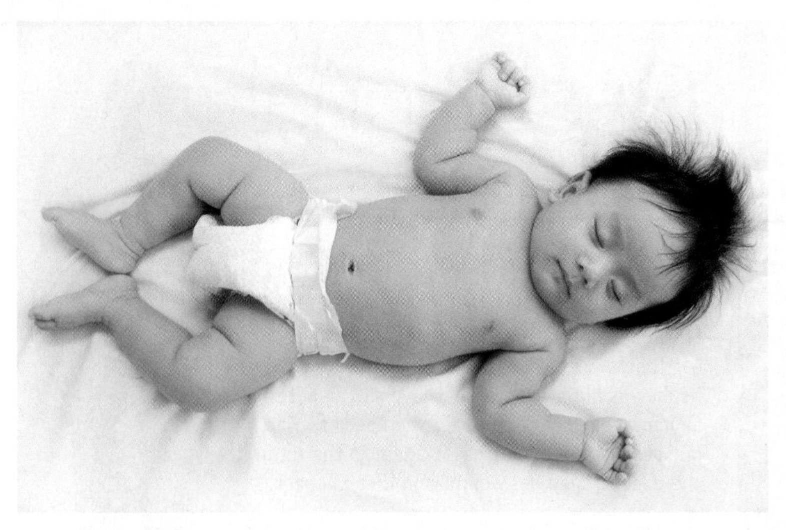

Placing a baby on its back to sleep reduces the risk of **SIDS.**

host of health problems and disabilities, including learning disabilities, cerebral palsy, hearing loss, and vision problems. Women are more likely to have a low birth weight baby if they smoke, drink alcohol, or use illicit drugs during pregnancy.

Infant Mortality

Prematurity and low birth weight are two factors influencing the **infant mortality rate,** a calculation of the ratio of babies who die before their first birthday to those who survive until their first birthday. In 2010, the infant mortality rate in the United States was 6.5 per 1,000 births.[37] Congenital abnormalities, pregnancy complications, and **sudden infant death syndrome (SIDS)** are also to blame. SIDS is the sudden death of a seemingly healthy infant while sleeping. Although researchers still do not entirely understand the phenomenon, they recognize that putting a baby to sleep on its stomach or side increases the risk. In 1992, public health experts and advocates launched the "Back to Sleep" campaign to encourage parents to place babies on their back for sleep. After the first decade of this program, the National Center for Health Statistics noted that SIDS deaths had dropped by more than 50%.[38] And as noted earlier, the infants of mothers who smoke are more likely to die of SIDS.

infant mortality rate A calculation of the ratio of babies who die before their first birthday to those who survive until their first birthday.

sudden infant death syndrome (SIDS) The sudden death of a seemingly healthy infant while sleeping.

Childbirth

In 2009, there were 4,130,665 births in the United States.[39] That's more than 11,300 on an average day. Who's having all these babies? See the nearby **Diversity & Health** box and find out.

Childbirth Options

Once labor begins, a woman and her partner can suddenly feel as if "nature" has taken over. That's why it's important for the couple to have a plan in place, based on choices they've studied and agreed to in advance. Especially important are decisions about health-related aspects of the birth, including the birth setting, attendants, and management of childbirth pain.

Where to Give Birth

Choices in where to give birth range from hospitals to alternative birthing centers to the family's own home. Even with so many choices, 98.9% of women still opt to have their baby in a hospital.[40] Fortunately, many U.S. hospitals today have birthing rooms designed to resemble a bedroom in a home, with comforting wall colors, pictures, a rocking chair, soft lighting, and even music.

Women whose pregnancies are considered high risk because of their age, health problems, or concerns about the health of the baby may be encouraged to give birth in a medical center that has a neonatal intensive care unit. This is also true of women carrying more than one fetus.

Less than 1% of U.S. births in 2009 were home births. Still, a majority of states in the United States have reported an increase in home births in recent years.[40] Supporters point out that home births are more convenient and comfortable, and can cost considerably less than hospital births. In 2011, the American Congress of Obstetricians and Gynecologists (ACOG) issued an opinion on home births, acknowledging that home births involving low-risk mothers are associated with fewer medical interventions than hospital births. ACOG also noted that the risk of newborn death during a home birth is very low. However, that risk is still two to three times higher than during births in hospitals and birthing centers; therefore, ACOG does not support home births.[41]

Birth Attendants

The couple must also decide who will be their primary care provider: a physician, a certified nurse midwife, or a lay midwife. In 2009, more than 92% of births were attended by a physician: 86.7% of births were attended by an M.D., and another 5.4% were attended by a D.O. (Doctor of Osteopathy). Certified nurse midwives, who are registered nurses with advanced training and certification in the care of childbearing families, attended 7.4% of births.[40] Only about 1 in 200 births is attended by a lay midwife. A lay midwife is not a registered nurse; however, some lay midwives pursue specialized training and pass a certification test to become certified midwives (CM).

The couple may also decide to hire a *doula*, a trained but nonmedical care provider (usually an experienced mother) who provides information and support to the woman before, during, and immediately after the birth. Often a close female relative or friend who is a mother fills this role.

Pain Management

About half of all women in labor opt for regional anesthesia, administration of medication that blocks sensation to a body region. Although there are a variety of types and routes of administration, the *epidural block* is the most common anesthetic used in vaginal birth. It involves injection of the medication into the epidural space between the ligaments of the vertebral (spinal) column and the outermost membrane surrounding the spinal cord and lower spinal nerves. Loss of sensation typically occurs within a few minutes. Side effects may include sedation, dizziness, nausea, vomiting, itching, and dry mouth. Some studies suggest that anesthesia can actually prolong the duration of labor, as well as slow the mother's recovery from birth.[6]

Women who opt for so-called "natural childbirth" don't necessarily tolerate pain any better than women who choose anesthesia. Instead,

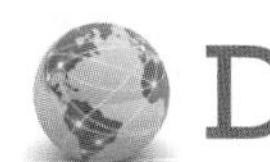

DIVERSITY & HEALTH

Age at First Birth through the Lenses of Geography and Race

Who's having their first baby when, and why is it important to know? Public health researchers track the average age of women when they have their first child. That's because age at first birth influences the total number of births that a woman might have in her life, and this in turn influences population growth. Moreover, the age of the mother, both younger and older, plays a role in incidence of low birth weight babies, multiple births, and babies with birth defects. It also influences the mother's ability to pursue or complete higher education, and build and maintain a career.

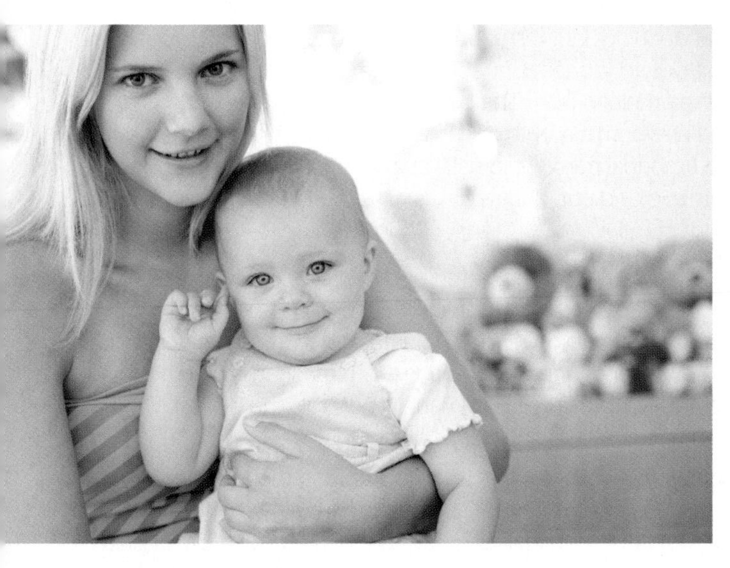

Age overall. About 1 in every 12 first births are to women over age 35. About 1 in 5 are to women under age 20. The rest—at least 75% of births among Americans—are to women between the ages of 20 and 34.

National averages. The national average age at first birth is 25.0. But the state with the oldest first-time mothers is Massachusetts, at 27.7 years old, with Connecticut and New Jersey both close seconds at 27.2. The states with the youngest first-time mothers are all in the Southeast: Alabama, Arkansas, Louisiana, and Mississippi first-time mothers average 20.5 years old or younger.

Global averages. The United States has a younger average age at first birth than any other selected developed nation. Poland, the next youngest, averages almost a full year older, at 25.9. Switzerland, Japan, and the Netherlands have the oldest age at first birth—29 or older.

Race. Among Americans, Asian or Pacific Islander (API) women have the oldest average age at first birth (28.5 years). White women average 26 years, Hispanic women 23.1 years, non-Hispanic black women 22.7 years, and Native American women 21.9 years.

Data from *Delayed Childbearing: More Women Are Having Their First Child Later in Life*, by T. J. Mathews & B. E. Hamilton, August 2009, *National Center for Health Statistics, 29*, pp. 1–18, retrieved from www.cdc.gov/nchs/data/databriefs/db21.htm.

they may view childbirth pain as normal and healthy—a positive sign that their baby is on the way. Many laboring women want to spare their baby any possible adverse effect from pain medications. The pain relief agents used in childbirth do affect the fetus; however, so does a mother's stress response to pain. Therefore, if the mother's pain and anxiety become overwhelming, accepting pain medication may be advisable.[6]

Stages of Labor and Birth

For expectant parents longing to meet their unborn baby, pregnancy and its 40 weeks of waiting can seem like an eternity. The onset of labor is a moment they await with anticipation—and sometimes apprehension—knowing that their lives are about to change forever.

Onset of Labor

Anywhere from several hours to several days before **labor** begins, many women experience a discharge of copious, red-tinged mucus as the plug that has been blocking the cervix throughout the pregnancy is released. This discharge, commonly referred to as the "bloody show," signals that the cervix is beginning to dilate in preparation for labor.

The precise events signaling the onset of labor differ for every woman and every pregnancy. Some women experience vague abdominal cramps and lower back pain that do not go away. Some women begin to experience regular, mild contractions—caused by the release of a hormone called oxytocin—that become more frequent and intense over several hours. Other women don't experience any contractions until their "water breaks"; that is, until the sac holding the amniotic fluid ruptures and amniotic fluid flows out from the vagina. The contractions that follow this event may be delayed and mild, or they may begin immediately and be extremely intense. Despite this variety, the symptoms signal that the woman is experiencing the first of the three stages of the birth process **(Figure 18.9).**

labor The physical processes involved in giving birth.

transition The final phase of the first stage of labor, characterized by the dilation of the cervix and strong, prolonged contractions.

First Stage of Labor

First-time mothers spend an average of 12 to 14 hours in labor, although some progress much more quickly and others more slowly.[42] Those who have already had one vaginal birth tend to experience a faster first stage during subsequent pregnancies.

During the earliest phase of first-stage labor, contractions of the uterus begin to move the fetus toward the birth canal. Contractions also cause the cervix to begin to open—or dilate—and thin out, a process known as *effacement*. Between contractions, the pain typically abates completely and the woman can rest. If the sac holding the amniotic fluid has not already broken, it may do so now.

During active labor, the cervix dilates further and contractions strengthen, lengthen, and become more frequent. Many women request pain medication during this time.

The final phase of this first stage of labor is known as **transition.** Amidst strong and prolonged contractions, the cervix dilates to about 10 centimeters, usually large enough for the baby's head to fit

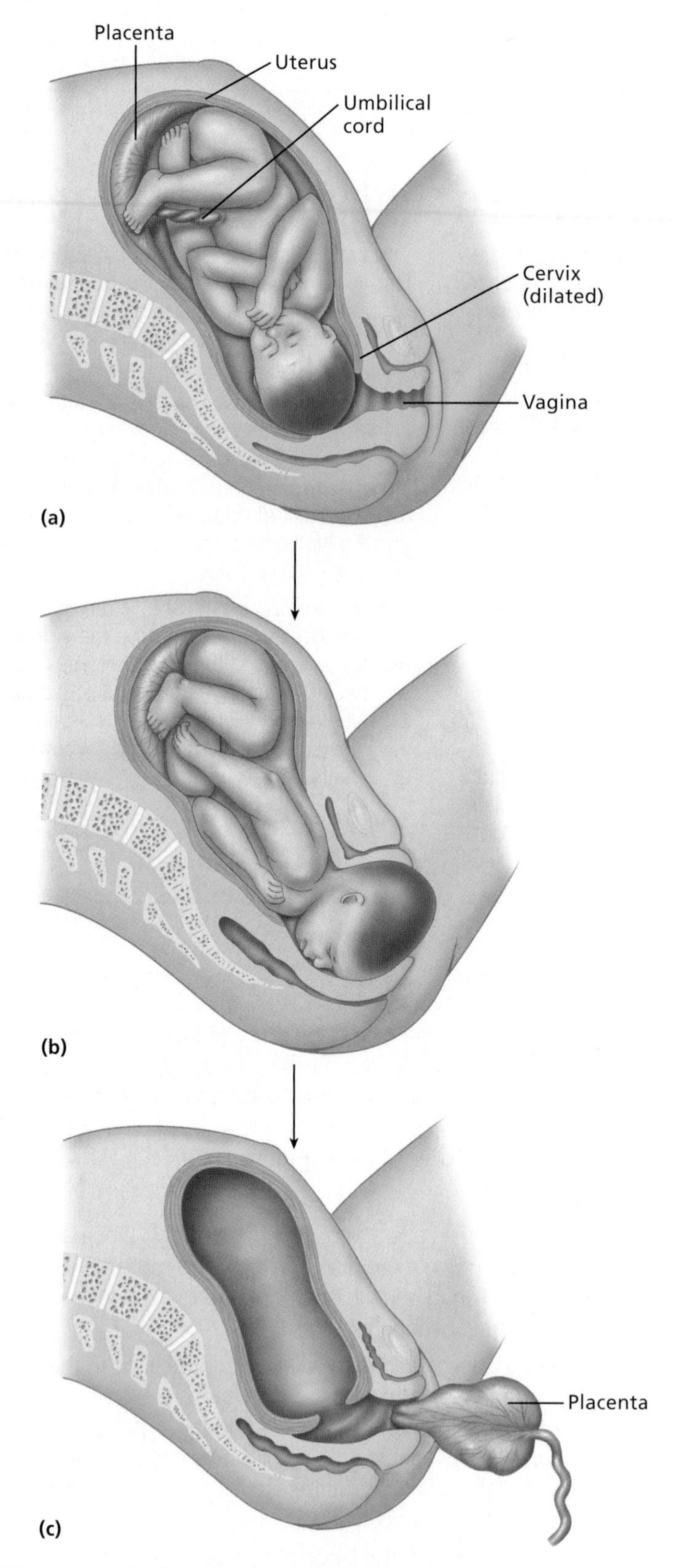

Figure 18.9 Stages of childbirth. (a) The first stage is characterized by cervical dilation and contractions of the uterus that begin to move the baby toward the birth canal. (b) In the second stage, the woman pushes until the baby is born. (c) In the third stage, the placenta is expelled.

Source: Adapted from Stanfield, C., *Principles of Human Physiology,* 4th ed., Fig. 22.24, p. 662. © 2011. Pearson Education.

through. During transition, the woman may begin to feel shaky, sweaty, and weak. Physical and emotional support from care providers and the woman's partner are important during this phase.

Second Stage of Labor

Once the cervix has dilated to 10 centimeters, the woman will be encouraged to help move the fetus further into the birth canal by actively pushing; that is, bearing down with each contraction. Many women find this stage of labor, which can last an average of 30 minutes to 3 hours, more rewarding than the first stage because they can feel that their efforts help the birth to progress.[43] Others, however, view this as the hardest stage of labor. When the baby's head "crowns," or appears at the vaginal opening, labor is almost over. The woman stops pushing, and after one or two further contractions, the baby is born, slick and sticky from the amniotic fluid. The birth attendant removes mucus and fluid from the newborn's mouth and nose, and dries him or her off with a towel. The umbilical cord, which still attaches the newborn to the placenta, is clamped and cut.

Third Stage of Labor

Although the baby has been born, the body still has one important task to do: Expel the placenta. This is typically accomplished by a few more contractions. After expulsion of the placenta, the woman continues to bleed and to experience mild contractions, but massaging the abdomen or breast-feeding the newborn usually controls the bleeding within about 5 to 15 minutes. The final stage of labor is over.

For the baby, the work has just begun. Just one minute after birth, the baby is given its first test, a measurement of how well it tolerated the stresses of birth.[44] This test was developed in 1952 by Dr. Virginia Apgar, and the resulting score, from 1 to 10, is an **Apgar score.** Babies are assessed on five characteristics: their muscle tone, their heart rate, their reflexes, their skin coloration, and their breathing. Five minutes after birth, the test is repeated to see if the baby's score has improved. A final score between 7 and 10 is considered normal. Babies who receive a lower rating may need additional medical assistance.

The birth attendant will also take a sample of blood from the newborn's heel to test for inborn errors of metabolism. The most common of these is phenylketonuria, or PKU, which affects metabolism of the amino acid phenylalanine and allows it to accumulate in brain tissue. Others affect the metabolism of carbohydrates or other amino acids. If detected early, inborn errors of metabolism can be successfully controlled by altering the newborn's diet; however, they can cause mental retardation or even death if left undiagnosed.

Cesarean Birth

A **cesarean birth** (also known as a **c-section**) is a surgical birth. Prior to the procedure, the woman is typically given a *spinal block*, a form of anesthesia that is delivered into the space between the membranes covering the spinal cord and the spinal cord itself. The surgery involves making an incision in the woman's abdominal and uterine walls through which the baby is removed. The rate of c-sections doubled between 1996 and 2009, according to national statistics.[40] Nearly one in three babies, 32.8%,

Apgar score A measurement of how well a newborn tolerated the stresses of birth, as well as how well he or she is adapting to the new environment.

cesarean birth (c-section) Birth of an infant through a surgical incision in the mother's abdominal and uterine walls.

are now delivered via c-section, a statistic that has troubled critics, some of whom argue that the increase is caused by financial incentives and fear of malpractice suits rather than concern for patients. And indeed, failure to perform a cesarean birth is one of the most common malpractice claims in obstetrics.[45]

postpartum The period of approximately 6 weeks during which the mother adjusts physically as well as psychologically to the birth of her child.

Cesarean birth is often necessary when complications arise during the final weeks of pregnancy or during labor. These might include placenta previa, an active genital herpes infection, or an excessively large fetus. Another common reason is a breech presentation; that is, the fetus is not head downward in the uterus, and attempts to turn the fetus have not been successful. Cesarean birth may also be necessary if the mother is obese or is experiencing hypertension or another systemic disorder. Also, women who have had a prior cesarean birth may be encouraged to have one during subsequent pregnancies to avoid the small but serious risk of uterine rupture. An emergency c-section may also be warranted if labor is not progressing, if the fetus appears to be in distress during labor, or if there is a problem with the umbilical cord that cannot be corrected manually. Any of these situations could put the baby's life in jeopardy. Finally, some women elect cesarean birth for convenience, fear of labor, or concern about tearing or other damage to their body.[46]

Although cesarean birth is relatively safe, it has a higher rate of complications, including maternal infection and hemorrhage, and women who have cesarean birth have four times the risk of death compared with women who give birth vaginally.[47] Cesarean birth also involves a longer recovery time for mothers than vaginal birth.

The Postpartum Period

The **postpartum** period is one during which the mother adjusts physically as well as psychologically to the birth of her child. It begins immediately after the birth and lasts about 6 weeks.

Physical Changes

During the first few days postpartum, the uterus sheds lining cells, bacteria, and other debris in a discharge called *lochia*, which gradually decreases over several days. The cervix closes, and the uterus contracts gradually until reaching little more than its pre-pregnant size by the end of the postpartum period.

Mothers tend to experience a level of fatigue that can range from mild to severe, especially if they had a long or otherwise difficult birth, or cannot get daytime rest. Naps during the day are important because new mothers typically wake several times during the night to feed their newborn. Sleep deprivation can develop quickly.

The mother loses about 10 to 12 pounds immediately after birth, and a few more pounds in the following days because of profuse sweating and other fluid loss. If the woman's weight gain didn't exceed recommendations, she typically loses the remaining pounds within the next several weeks. The body's production of breast milk requires more calories than pregnancy itself: an estimated 700 to 800 extra calories per day![24] That's why many women who breast-feed find that they lose their pregnancy weight gain easily, and will continue to lose weight unless they make a conscious effort to eat more.

Breast-Feeding

For about the first 2 days postpartum, the woman's breasts continue to produce colostrum rather than mature milk. This "first milk" is rich in vitamins, minerals, proteins, and antibodies that help protect the newborn from infection. It also contains substances that help the newborn to expel the first, sticky stool, and to establish "friendly" bacteria in the newborn's gastrointestinal tract.[24]

Usually within 2 to 4 days, the mother begins producing mature milk. Antibodies and immune cells in mature milk continue to protect the infant from infections and allergies. Moreover, the amounts and types of nutrients in breast milk are uniquely matched to infants' needs. The composition of the mother's milk changes according to the age of her infant, and even during the course of each feeding, with a more watery milk released initially to quench the baby's thirst, and a progressively more fatty milk produced subsequently to satiate the baby's hunger. The American Academy of Pediatrics recommends breast-feeding exclusively for the first 6 months of life. After 6 months, the mother should continue breast-feeding, while beginning to introduce the infant to other fluids

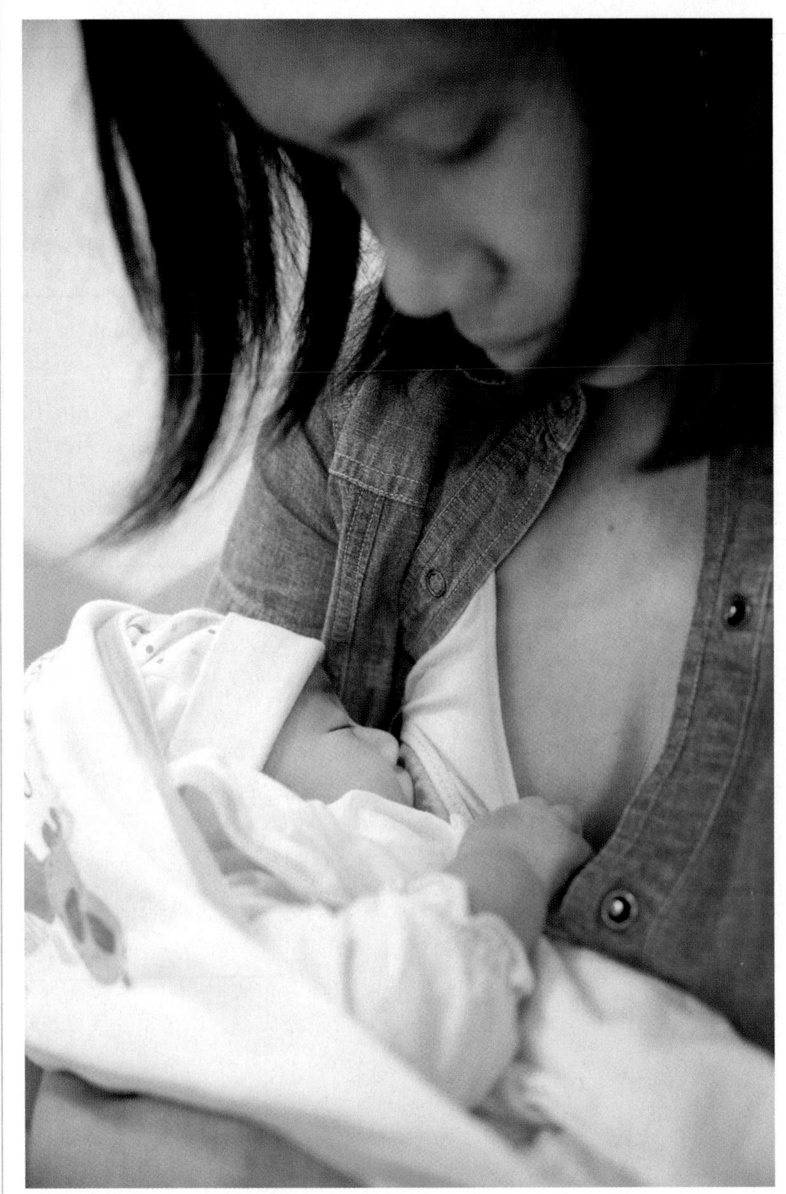

Breast-feeding is recommended for the first six months of life.

and solid foods. If acceptable to the family, breast-feeding should continue as part of the toddler's nourishment into the second year.[48]

The return of the mother's fertility is tied to whether or not she breast-feeds, how much, and for how long. Breast-feeding is often referred to as "natural contraception," because the hormones released during feeding suppress ovulation and menstruation. Exclusive breast-feeding—in which the infant receives only breast milk—reduces the risk of pregnancy. However, it is not considered a reliable form of birth control.

Although breast-feeding is a natural activity, it doesn't always feel natural to first-time mothers. Discomfort, embarrassment, and worries about the quality and quantity of their breast milk discourage many mothers. Fortunately, postpartum nurses are usually trained to provide assistance with breast-feeding. Also, even before their baby is born, mothers who plan to breast-feed can begin to attend meetings of their local chapter of La Leche League International (LLLI), which was founded to promote the benefits of breast-feeding and support women who wish to breast-feed their infants. Mothers can call or visit their local LLLI members for assistance and advice.

For a list of LLLI podcasts offering breast-feeding tips and parenting advice, go to www.llli.org/podcasts.html?m=0,0,8#bf.

Psychological Challenges

New parents—both mother and father—face enormous challenges in adjusting to their new roles and developing **attachment,** an enduring bond of love, for their newborn. Parent-newborn attachment is influenced by many psychological factors, including childhood history, level of self-esteem, and current interpersonal, financial, and other stressors. It can be fostered by social support, not only from extended family members but also from friends who are themselves parents. Membership in a new-parent support group helps many bewildered moms and dads with answers to questions, practical advice, and listening.

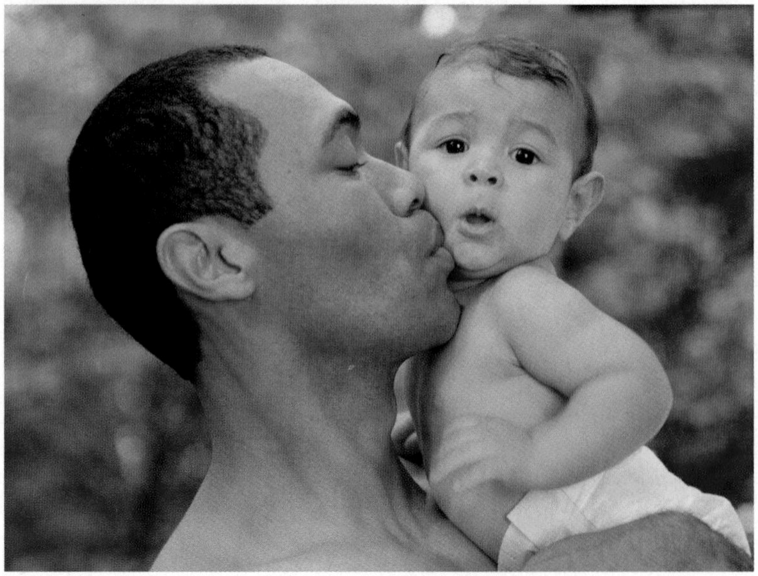

Dads can foster attachment with their baby through holding, playing with, or caring for the baby.

attachment An enduring bond of love for another.

postpartum depression (PPD) A serious mental disorder that develops in the postpartum period and is characterized by persistent feelings of sadness that interfere with daily life.

"One recent study found that 10% of fathers experience PPD, most often in the first 3 to 6 months after the birth of their child."

Breast-feeding promotes mother-infant attachment, but fathers don't need to be left out! They can rest their newborn on their chest between feedings, rock their newborn to sleep, and bottle-feed their newborn with breast milk that mom has pumped. Even tasks like bathing the newborn or changing diapers can be opportunities to foster father-infant attachment.

Another potential challenge is depression. A brief period of so-called *postpartum blues* develops in as many as three-fourths of all mothers, and is characterized as an overall sense of contentment interrupted by brief bouts of depression.[49] Postpartum blues is thought to stem from the tremendous challenges of new motherhood, especially sleep deprivation, combined with rapid fluctuations in reproductive hormones.

In contrast, **postpartum depression (PPD)** is a serious mental disorder that develops in about 13% of women postpartum at some point during the first year after the birth. It is characterized by persistent feelings of sadness, emptiness, hopelessness, guilt, and/or anxiety that interfere with the woman's day-to-day life. She withdraws from family members and friends, feels no enjoyment in formerly pleasurable activities, and may experience headaches, stomachaches, or other physical problems that don't go away. She may even have thoughts of harming herself or her baby.

As with postpartum blues, PPD is thought to be due in part to sleep deprivation and other challenges of motherhood as well as fluctuations in reproductive hormones, especially a dramatic drop in levels of estrogen.[50] A personal or family history of depression increases the risk. Apparently, so does obesity. A recent study followed more than 1,000 first-time mothers through the postpartum period. The incidence of PPD in women of normal weight was 14%, but in obese women, the incidence was 40%.[51] Treatment of PPD includes psychotherapy and often antidepressant medications.

PPD is also increasingly being recognized in fathers. One recent study found that 10% of fathers experience PPD, most often in the first 3 to 6 months after the birth of their child.[52] The father's risk for depression was increased if the mother was depressed.

Postpartum Support International has many resources to help new parents, from DVDs to brochures to live chats. Check them out at www.postpartum.net.

Infertility

Many couples attempt to get pregnant only to find that, month after month, nothing happens. An estimated 10% of women in the United States—about 6.1 million—experience **infertility,** or the inability to conceive or sustain a pregnancy after trying for one year.[53] The problem becomes more prevalent with age, and so doctors recommend that a woman in her 30s get checked for underlying health issues if she has been trying unsuccessfully to get pregnant for more than 6 months. But infertility isn't just a woman's problem. A government study found that 7.5% of all sexually active men in the United States had at some time consulted a physician for help with having a child. Of these men, 18% were diagnosed as infertile.[54] Fortunately, there are many treatment options available, and about two-thirds of couples who have difficulty conceiving ultimately go on to have their own biological children.[55]

Causes of Infertility

Roughly one-third of infertility cases are due to health problems in the woman; another third are due to problems in the man; and the final third are either caused by problems in both partners or simply cannot be explained.[53]

For women, the most common causes of infertility are:

- A failure of ovulation prompted by hormonal problems, advanced age, premature menopause, or scarred ovaries. Women with *polycystic ovary syndrome*, for example, have abnormally high levels of estrogen and testosterone. They are infertile because their ovaries contain many small cysts and they fail to ovulate. Their menstrual flow is typically scanty and can even be absent. Although the cause of polycystic ovary syndrome is not known, obesity is a primary risk factor.
- Blocked fallopian tubes, stemming from endometriosis, a prior ectopic pregnancy, surgery, or, most commonly, an untreated sexually transmitted infection such as chlamydia or gonorrhea that caused scarring in the fallopian tubes and/or progressed into pelvic inflammatory disease (PID).
- A deformed uterus, which can disrupt implantation or lead to miscarriage.
- Uterine fibroids and other noncancerous growths, which can obstruct both the uterus and the fallopian tubes.

The most common causes of infertility in men include:

- A low sperm count, defined as less than 10 million sperm per milliliter of semen.
- Incorrectly formed sperm, which are not able to penetrate the egg.
- Poor sperm motility, or the inability of sperm to move quickly and effectively.

A number of factors can, in turn, increase the man's risk for these problems. Lifestyle factors include smoking cigarettes or marijuana, abuse of alcohol or other drugs, wearing constrictive clothing, and even exposure to excessive heat—for example, from frequent hot baths. Medical factors include certain chronic diseases, certain medications, and certain infections. Contracting mumps during adulthood is a common culprit. Sexually transmitted infections such as gonorrhea can also cause scarring that hinders sperm movement. Finally, environmental exposure to pesticides, lead, and other substances that disrupt hormones can lead to abnormalities in sperm.

For both women and men, prevention of many of these problems is possible. Although couples in their late teens and early 20s are usually more interested in avoiding pregnancy, they should also take steps to preserve their fertility for the years to come. Practicing safe sex can reduce the spread of sexually transmitted infections, which are among the most common causes of infertility. Getting timely treatment for a sexually transmitted infection is also important. Because fertility drops and the risk of birth defects and miscarriages rises when a woman is in her 30s, couples who want to have a child are encouraged to start their family planning before the woman turns 35.

Options for Infertile Couples

Options for infertile couples include medical procedures, surrogate childbearing, and adoption.

Medical Procedures

The type of medical treatment ultimately used by couples to get pregnant depends to a large degree on the root cause of their troubles. These include:

- Surgery to repair blocked fallopian tubes, remove scarring or uterine growths, or treat endometriosis in women. Occasionally, surgery may be indicated if there is a problem with a man's sperm.
- Fertility drugs, which promote ovulation in women. Side effects can include headaches, nausea, hot flashes, and breast tenderness. Because the medications can spur the body to release more than one egg at a time, couples using fertility drugs have a higher chance of having twins or other multiple births.
- Intrauterine insemination, to boost the odds that an egg will be fertilized. Sperm are collected from a woman's partner or a donor and processed in a laboratory, enabling a higher concentration of sperm to be injected into the vagina or uterus through a syringe.
- *In vitro fertilization (IVF),* a procedure that dramatically transformed the field of fertility treatment when the first "test-tube baby" was born in 1978. Egg and sperm are retrieved from a woman and a man and combined in a laboratory dish (*in vitro* means "in glass"), where fertilization may occur. If eggs do become fertilized, they are implanted in the uterus. When multiple fertilized eggs are transferred, multiple births may occur.
- *Gamete intrafallopian transfer (GIFT),* a process similar to IVF. The egg is not fertilized in a laboratory, however. Instead, sperm and several eggs are placed in a woman's fallopian tube. There is no guarantee, though, that the sperm will penetrate at least one of the eggs.
- *Zygote intrafallopian transfer (ZIFT),* fertilization of an egg or eggs in a laboratory setting. Unlike IVF, however, the fertilized eggs are transferred to a fallopian tube rather than the uterus.
- *Intracytoplasmic sperm injection (ICSI),* the direct injection of a single sperm into an egg. The fertilized egg is then implanted in the uterus through normal IVF technology. ICSI may be considered when men have low sperm counts or when fertilization failed to occur in previous IVF attempts.

Surrogate Childbearing

Not all couples choose medical treatment, and in some couples, the procedures are not effective. These couples may consider **surrogate childbearing.** This is a complex legal procedure requiring an agreement with a third party—a fertile woman—to

infertility The inability to conceive or sustain a pregnancy after trying for at least a year.

surrogate childbearing A complex legal arrangement in which a fertile woman agrees to carry a pregnancy for another, usually infertile, woman.

carry a pregnancy to term. Immediately following the baby's birth, the surrogate mother relinquishes the infant. In some cases the surrogate's egg is fertilized through intrauterine insemination with the prospective father's sperm. In other cases, she is impregnated through IVF with the couple's embryo.

adoption The social, emotional, and legal process in which children who will not be raised by their birth parents become full and permanent legal members of another family.

In an altruistic surrogacy arrangement, the woman is not paid a fee, although she is typically reimbursed for medical expenses and other reasonable costs. In a commercial surrogacy arrangement, the woman is paid for her service to the couple above and beyond her expenses. Commercial surrogacy is banned in many states, and several states ban or void all contracts involving surrogate childbearing.[56]

Adoption

Adoption is the social, emotional, and legal process in which children who will not be raised by their birth parents become full and permanent legal members of another family.[57] Many couples as well as single adults pursue adoption, either domestically or internationally. In 2008, there were 136,000 adoptions in the United States.[58] This represents a 15% increase since 1990. Of these adoptions, 41% were from public child welfare agencies, and 13% were international. Private agencies, attorneys, and other sources also facilitate adoptions, and of course stepparents and other family members often pursue legal adoption.

If you think adoption is just for rich people, think again. It's true that adoptions using private agencies can be very expensive. Whether domestic or international, these can cost as much as $20,000 to $30,000 and take several years. But adoptions from foster-care agencies typically cost very little or are free of charge. Children enter foster care when, through no fault of their own, they have to be removed from abusive or neglectful homes. In 2009, there were more than 114,500 American children in public foster care waiting to be adopted.[59] And every year, about 20,000 children "age out" of the system without having been adopted.

Watch real children in foster care share their story. Visit Adopt Us Kids at www.adoptuskids.org/meet-the-children.

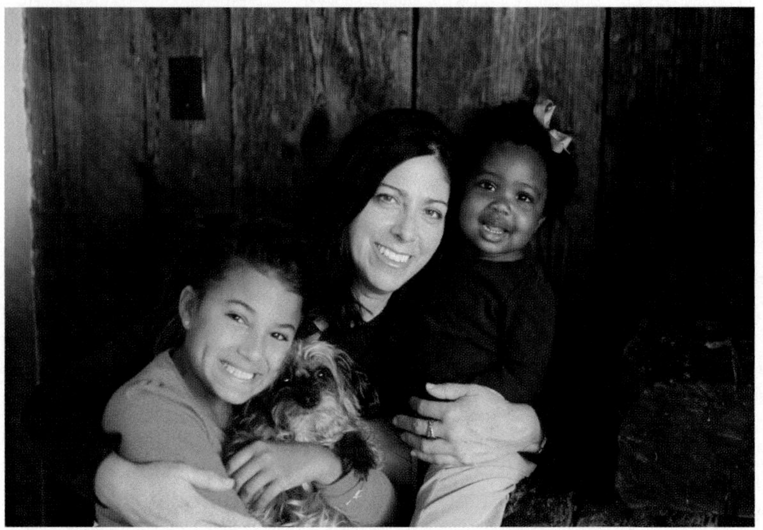

Adoptions are increasing in the U.S.

For anyone considering adoption, a good place to begin research is at the Child Welfare Information Gateway from the U.S Department of Health and Human Services at **www.childwelfare.gov.** The adoption pages explain the laws governing adoption in each state, requirements for adoptive parents, options for adopting, and what applicants can expect once the process begins.

Just as with biological children, bringing home an adopted child is just the first step of a lifelong journey filled with joys and challenges. Having realistic hopes and expectations for their child can help parents achieve attachment, as can a forgiving attitude toward their own mistakes. Fortunately many post-adoption services are available to help, from short-term "respite care" to give parents a brief break from their responsibilities, to financial assistance, to training and support groups.

Change Yourself, Change Your World

In 2010, 9 out of every 100 women aged 20 to 24 gave birth.[35] Many of these new mothers were college students, and many dropped out. One national study found that, among community college students who give birth, 61% abandon their studies.[60] Still, of the 17 million undergraduates in America, nearly one-fourth—3.9 million students—are parents, and about half of these are single parents.[61] So what can you do if you're pregnant and want to finish your degree, or if you want to support other students who are juggling pregnancy or parenthood? Here are some ideas.

Personal Choices

If you find yourself pregnant, and decide to keep your baby and stay in school to finish your college degree program, the good news is that you can do it! But it'll take determination, resourcefulness, and social support. Here's some advice from Linda Bates Parker, a career development advisor at the University of Cincinnati:[62]

- Every day, first thing before you start your day, take a moment to make an affirmation or say a prayer of gratitude for your life and health and that of your baby. Say it out loud so that your baby gets used to hearing your voice.
- Investigate every resource, on and off campus, that might be available to you. These might include campus or community health clinics, childbirth classes, social services organizations, churches, and breast-feeding and new-mother support groups, as well as friends, extended-family members, faculty, and staff members who believe in you. Say yes to any offers that you believe can help you meet your goals.
- Show up for all of your appointments for prenatal care, and follow through on your care provider's advice.
- Make a time line plotting realistic goals for finishing your degree program, launching your career, and flourishing in your first years of motherhood. For instance, you might decide to reduce the number of courses you enroll in each semester, or take only night classes for a semester so that a friend or family member who works days can care for your baby.
- Start saving for and recruiting help to meet your medical and other childbearing expenses now.

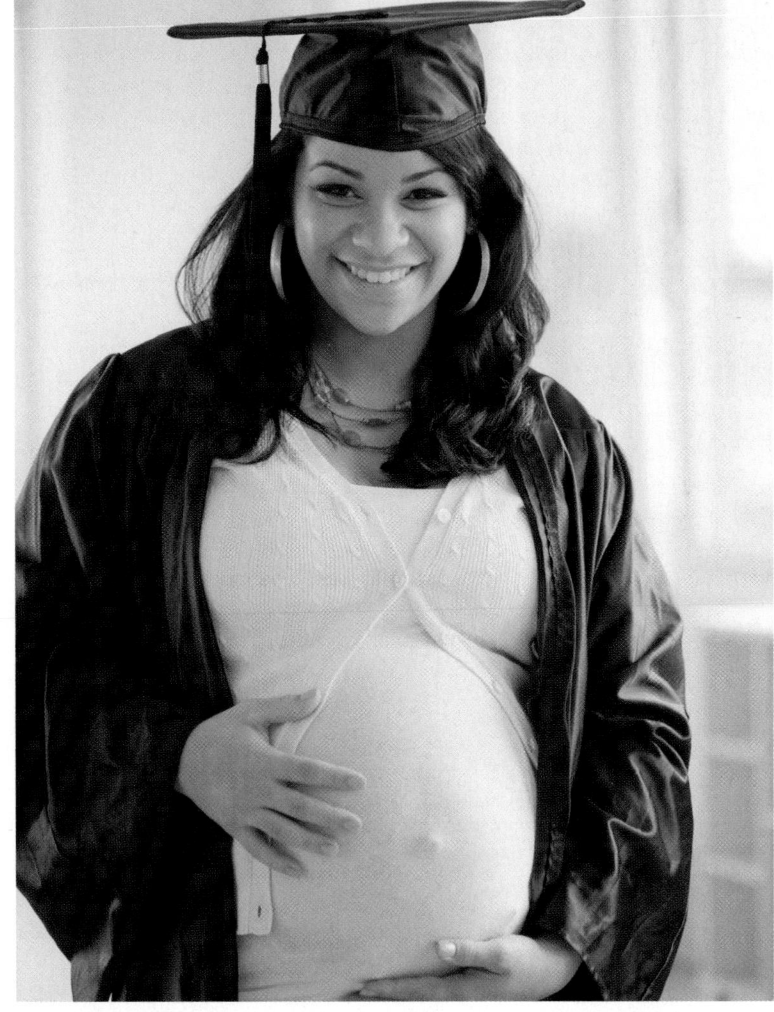

It's a good idea to **make a plan** if you are having a child while finishing your degree.

- Explore your options for affordable infant care on or near campus, and for any state child care subsidies you might qualify for. Often these programs have long waiting lists, so get listed now.
- Finally, reexamine the choices you made that brought you this challenge. Evaluate the wisdom of these choices, and resolve to make future decisions that are in the best interests of you and your baby.

Supporting a Partner or Friend Who Is Pregnant

Your pregnant partner or friend is juggling all of the tasks and challenges of her pre-pregnant life, plus growing her baby. She's likely to experience bursts of energy and elation, as well as fatigue, sadness, and even fear as she sees her old life fading . . . and wonders what's next. Here are some practical ways, large and small, that you can help her.

- Watch your language. Don't tell her she looks tired or huge, and don't comment on her latest acne flare-up. Don't offer advice, unless she asks you for it, or question her morning coffee, or suggest names for the baby. Do tell her she glows, and that you're there to listen if she needs it.
- Clean, cook, and otherwise cater. If you offer to help her clean her apartment or dorm room, she might take that as an insult. So just surprise her by doing it while she's in class or out for a walk or napping. If you have the time and resources, fix her a nutritious meal as well.
- Offer to accompany her on one of her prenatal care appointments. She might appreciate having someone to "download" to afterward. Or go with her to the gym, or the laundromat, or shopping for maternity clothes.
- Give her a present. Maybe a journal or scrapbook where she can keep thoughts, photos, and other mementos of her pregnancy, or a basket of nutritious snacks or personal care items. Or plan a surprise baby shower and invite all her friends. If you can afford it, book her a massage or other spa service.
- Give her hugs. Especially when she's fatigued or cranky, a silent hug can remind her that you care.

Campus Advocacy

Child care is one of the most effective ways that a college or university can help support students with young children, yet only about half of public 2- and 4-year colleges and universities, and less than 10% of private colleges and universities, offer child care.[63] Even those that do have on-campus child care often do not offer infant care, or have so few openings that the majority of students are not served. By offering high-quality, affordable, accessible child care services, campuses could help to ensure the success of one of their most vulnerable populations. How can you help?

If you're not a parent yourself, start by talking to some of your classmates who are. Find out what they know about on-campus child care and other support services, ask them to share their needs, concerns, and frustrations, and offer to get involved. Then do it: Raise the issue with faculty or staff members who've been supportive of other student initiatives. Use your social networking pages to raise awareness of the problem. Visit your campus day care center—if there is one—and talk to the staff. With staff and parent permission, photograph one of the children, and write up a profile of the family for your campus news service.

Other resources for college students who are parents include the Student Parent Success Initiative at **www.iwpr.org/initiatives/student-parent-success-initiative.** The initiative's goals are to increase awareness of the needs of student parents, improve public policies and resources for low-income student parents, and share information about successful programs that support student parents. Also check out the U.S. Department of Education's Child Care Access Means Parents in School Program (CAMPISP) at **www2.ed.gov/programs/campisp/index.html.**

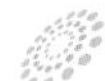 **Watch videos of real students discussing reproductive choices at www.pearsonhighered.com/lynchelmore.**

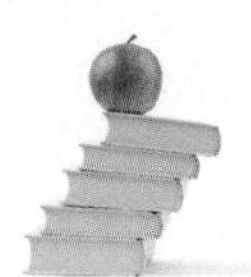

Choosing to Change Worksheet

To complete this worksheet online, visit www.pearsonhighered.com/lynchelmore.

Directions: Fill out Parts I and II.

Part I: Creating a Fertility Plan

Even if pregnancy is not a goal for you right now, it's important to be aware of whether or not you want children and to determine how you will prepare for children should you want them.

1. Which one of the following options describes your feelings about having children? Circle the appropriate response.

I don't want children	I don't want children right now but I want one or more someday	I'm not sure if I want children
I currently want to have a child	I have at least one child and I'm not sure if I want any more	I have at least one child and I want more

Write down why you answered the way you did:

____

____

____

2. If you desire to have a child now or in the future, what do you think you need to do to prepare for having one? Consider each topic below:

Your individual emotional status (Are you emotionally mature and healthy enough to have a child?):

____

____

Your school and career goals (What do you want to achieve before having a child?):

____

____

Your relationships with your partner or other people close to you:

____

____

Your finances:

____

____

Your physical health and health habits (Are any preexisting conditions under control, are you fully vaccinated, will you choose to participate in genetic screening, are you avoiding substances that can impact fertility or affect a fetus, is your diet healthy, and do you participate in regular physical activity?):

____

____

3. If you are unsure as to whether you want to have a child, write down the pros and cons of starting a family below.

Pros	Cons
______________________	______________________
______________________	______________________
______________________	______________________
______________________	______________________

After listing the pros and cons, does that alter your feelings about having a child? Which pros and cons feel the most significant to you?

____

4. If you know you do not want children, what will you do to prevent pregnancy? Do you think you may ever change your mind about having children?

____

____

Part II: Managing Your Fertility

Infertility is defined as the inability to conceive a child despite trying for one year. The condition affects over 5 million Americans, or nearly 1 in 10 individuals of the reproductive age population. Below are some risk factors that may increase your risk of infertility.

Risk Factors for Infertility in Women and Men

Women	Men
Excess alcohol use	Heavy alcohol use
Smoking cigarettes	Smoking cigarettes
Poor diet	Illicit drug use
Unmanaged stress	Unmanaged stress
Older than age 35	Older than age 45
Being overweight or underweight	Certain medications, such as anabolic steroids
Sexually transmitted infections, such as chlamydia and gonorrhea	Exposure to environmental toxins, including pesticides and lead
Athletic or overtraining	Radiation treatment and chemotherapy for cancer
Health problems that cause hormonal changes, such as polycystic ovary syndrome and primary ovarian insufficiency	Health problems such as mumps, serious conditions like kidney disease, or hormone problems

Source: Adapted from *Risk Factors for Infertility in Women and Men,* by the Centers for Disease Control and Prevention, 2012, retrieved from http://www.cdc.gov/reproductivehealth/Infertility/index.htm.

Do you have any of the risk factors for infertility listed on the previous page?

If so, what will you do to manage them and promote your fertility in the case that you want to have a child?

How can you prevent developing risk factors in the future?

Chapter Summary

- Experts suggest that couples preparing for parenthood resolve any emotional, identity, relationship, or financial issues, take steps to reduce any age-related risks, seek pre-conception health care, including vaccinations and genetic screening, and change any behaviors that could adversely affect the pregnancy.
- Pregnancy involves three trimesters, each with unique stages of development for a fetus and physical effects for the mother.
- Although a variety of signs and symptoms suggest pregnancy, reliable tests include an over-the-counter home pregnancy test (HPT) of urine and a blood test available from a health-care provider. Both check for the presence of human chorionic gonadotropin (hCG), a hormone made in the body during pregnancy.
- Guidelines for weight gain during pregnancy vary according to the woman's weight before she became pregnant. Women who were normal weight prior to pregnancy should gain 25 to 35 pounds. Those who were underweight or overweight should gain a few pounds more or less.
- Among the common discomforts of pregnancy, first-trimester nausea, indigestion, an urge to urinate, fatigue, and disturbed sleep are especially common.
- The first trimester of pregnancy is the most critical period of development, when tissues are differentiating into organs. The embryo is most susceptible to alcohol, infectious microorganisms, and other harmful agents at this time.
- The growing embryo receives nutrients and oxygen and eliminates wastes through the placenta, an organ that develops on the inner wall of the uterus.
- During the second trimester, all major organs and systems become fully formed.
- During the third trimester, the fetus gains most of its weight. The third trimester ends, on average, between 37 and 42 weeks.
- Regular prenatal care can lead to a healthier pregnancy and a healthier baby. Diagnostic tests commonly performed as part of prenatal care include ultrasound and blood tests. The couple may opt for amniocentesis or chorionic villus sampling to help detect chromosomal and other abnormalities.
- A common complication of early pregnancy is an ectopic pregnancy, which is the implantation of the blastocyst in the fallopian tube. Miscarriage, also called spontaneous abortion, is a pregnancy that ends spontaneously, usually during the first trimester.
- Later in the pregnancy, the woman may develop a placental problem, an infection, hypertension, or gestational diabetes.
- Babies born between 32 and 37 weeks are considered pre-term. The average birth weight in the United States is about 7.5 pounds. Newborns weighing less than 5 pounds, 8 ounces are low birth weight babies. Both pre-term and low birth weight babies are at increased risk for health problems.
- Almost 99% of women opt to give birth in a hospital, and more than 92% of births are attended by a physician. About 7% of births are attended by certified nurse midwives.
- The first stage of labor is characterized by uterine contractions and cervical dilation. The fetus descends into the birth canal. During the second stage, the woman bears down with each contraction until the baby is born. The third stage of labor is expulsion of the placenta.
- A cesarean birth is a surgical birth. A variety of complications before or during birth may make a cesarean birth necessary; however, cesarean births have a higher risk for maternal death than vaginal births, and recovery of the mother is usually prolonged.
- During the postpartum period, the mother adjusts physically and psychologically to the birth of her child. She loses several pounds of her pregnancy weight, her body produces breast milk, and she faces emotional tasks, such as developing attachment to her child.
- Postpartum depression (PPD) is a serious mental disorder that develops in about 13% of women postpartum. It is thought to be influenced by fluctuations in reproductive hormones, sleep deprivation, and a variety of stressors. PPD can also occur in men.
- Fertility declines with increasing age. Health problems in males and females contribute about equally to fertility problems in couples. Options for infertile couples include medical procedures, surrogate childbearing, and adoption.
- Pregnancy and new parenthood are common reasons that students drop out of college. Access to affordable on-campus child care helps parents complete their degrees.

Test Your Knowledge

1. Neither of the parents of a son born with cystic fibrosis has the disease. Which of the following is true?
   a. Cystic fibrosis is a dominant disorder.
   b. Cystic fibrosis is a sex-linked disorder.
   c. Both parents must be carriers of the defective gene.
   d. One parent must be a carrier of the defective gene but the other parent could have two normal genes.

2. Consuming alcohol during pregnancy increases the risk that the child will experience which of the following?
   a. learning disabilities
   b. behavioral problems
   c. physical abnormalities
   d. all of the above

3. Deficiency in the mother of which of the following nutrients is associated with an increased risk for giving birth to a child with a neural tube defect?
   a. folic acid
   b. vitamin A
   c. iron
   d. protein

4. A pregnant woman needs
   a. to go on a weight-loss diet if she is obese at the start of her pregnancy.
   b. to consume approximately 400 additional calories per day in the second and third trimesters of her pregnancy.
   c. to gain approximately 15–25 pounds if she is of normal weight at the start of her pregnancy.
   d. to achieve the majority of her pregnancy weight gain during the first trimester.

5. What is the developing offspring called after the first 8 weeks of pregnancy?
   a. embryo
   b. blastocyst
   c. fetus
   d. zygote

6. Vaccination prior to pregnancy can protect the woman's fetus from
   a. toxoplasmosis.
   b. rubella.
   c. herpes simplex virus.
   d. human immunodeficiency virus.

7. A baby born at 35 weeks' gestation and weighing 6 pounds, 2 ounces is considered
   a. pre-term and normal birth weight.
   b. pre-term and low birth weight.
   c. full term and normal birth weight.
   d. full term and low birth weight.

8. The childbearing mother is encouraged to actively push during
   a. the first stage of labor.
   b. transition.
   c. the second stage of labor.
   d. the third stage of labor.

9. Breast-feeding provides
   a. antibodies and immune cells that help protect the infant from infections and allergies.
   b. reliable contraception as long as the mother does not supplement with formula.
   c. all of the nutrients an infant needs for at least the first full year of life.
   d. all of the above.

10. Which of the following infertility treatments involves placing sperm and several eggs in a woman's fallopian tube, rather than accomplishing fertilization in the lab?
    a. ZIFT
    b. ICSI
    c. GIFT
    d. IVF

Get Critical

What happened:

In November 2011, the National Center for Health Statistics released some good news. The teen birth rate had fallen 9% in 2010, to 34 per 1,000, the lowest ever recorded. In response, the National Campaign to Prevent Teen and Unplanned Pregnancy gave credit to health and educational programs, as well as increased media attention to the issue—including from MTV, the producer of the popular reality TV shows *16 and Pregnant* and *Teen Mom*. MTV was quick to capitalize on the endorsement. On the *MTV Remote Control Blog* page, spokesperson Lisa Chudnofsky explained that, by focusing its efforts on showing "the harsh truths about unplanned parenthood," MTV's teen pregnancy programming was making a real difference in discouraging teen birth.[1]

Not everyone agrees. Critics suggest that, by making the teens into celebrities solely because they got pregnant at age 16, the shows glamorize and actually encourage teen pregnancy and motherhood. Although a dedicated fan of the program, one college student observed, "Young girls go through pregnancies every day. They don't make it onto the covers of magazines. That is not reality."[2]

What do you think?

- Have you seen *16 and Pregnant* or *Teen Mom*? If so, has watching these programs had any effect on your thoughts about becoming a parent? If so, how?
- In addition to reality TV shows, what other factors—social, political, economic, technological, etc.—might be influencing the rate of teen births in the United States?

References: **1.** "Kick-Ass New Stat: U.S. Teen Birth Rate Down 9 Percent," by L. Chudnofsky, November 21, 2011, *MTV Remote Control Blog*, retrieved from http://remotecontrol.mtv.com/2011/11/21/teen-birth-rate-down-9-percent. **2.** "For Some Students, 'Teen Mom' Isn't a Cautionary Tale," by K. C. Grant, October 14, 2010, *ABC News*, retrieved from http://abcnews.go.com/Entertainment/teen-moms-celebs-campus/story?id=11872306#.TzFK_5iNo20.

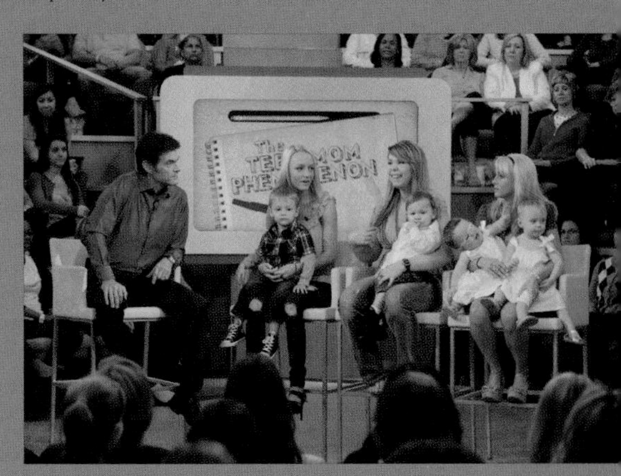

Several "Teen Moms" on The Dr. Oz Show.

Get Connected

Mobile Tips!

Scan this QR code with your mobile device to access additional tips about pregnancy and parenthood. Or, via your mobile device, go to **http://mobiletips.pearsoncmg.com** and navigate to Chapter 18.

Health Online **Visit the following websites for further information about the topics in this chapter:**

- American Pregnancy Association
  www.americanpregnancy.org
- National Women's Health Information Center
  www.womenshealth.gov
- American Fertility Association (AFA)
  www.theafa.org
- Child Welfare Information Gateway (advice about adoption)
  www.childwelfare.gov

Website links are subject to change. To access updated web links, please visit ***www.pearsonhighered.com/lynchelmore***.

References

i. Hamilton, B. E., Martin, J. A., & Ventura, S. J. (2011). Births: Preliminary data for 2010. *National Vital Statistics Reports* web release *60* (2). Hyattsville, MD: National Center for Health Statistics.

ii. U.S. Centers for Disease Control and Prevention. (2011, June 28). *Infertility FAQs*. Retrieved from http://www.cdc.gov/reproductivehealth/Infertility/#2.

1. Luscombe, B. (2011, February 3). Debunking the myth of the slippery bachelor. *Time*. Retrieved from http://www.time.com/time/magazine/article/0,9171,2046035,00.html.

2. Miller, K., Gault, B., & Thorman, A. (2011, March). Improving child care access to promote postsecondary success among low-income parents. *Institute for Women's Policy Research, Perspectives on Sexual and Reproductive Health*, 1–64. Retrieved from http://www.iwpr.org/blog/2011/05/03/college-students-with-children-need-campuses-with-child-care.

3. National Healthy Marriage Resource Center. (2012). Are you ready for a child? Retrieved from http://www.twoofus.org/educational-content/articles/are-you-ready-for-a-child/index.aspx.

4. U.S. Department of Agriculture. (2011, June 9). *Expenditures on children by families*. Retrieved from http://www.cnpp.usda.gov/Publications/CRC/2010CRCPressRelease.pdf.

5. Martinez, G. M., Chandra, A., Abma, J. C., Jones, J., & Mosher, W. D. (2006). Fertility, contraception, and fatherhood: Data on men and women from cycle 6 (2002) of the National Survey of Family Growth. National Center for Health Statistics. *Vital Health Statistics, 23* (26).

6. Davidson, M., London, M., & Ladewig, P. (2012). *Maternal-newborn nursing and women's health across the lifespan,* 9th ed. Upper Saddle River, NJ: Pearson Education.

7. National Coalition Against Domestic Violence. (2007). *reproductive health and pregnancy: Why it matters.* Washington, DC: NCADV Public Policy Office.

8. March of Dimes. (2009, May). Pregnancy after 35. Retrieved from http://www.marchofdimes.com/pregnancy/trying_after35.html.

9. Carey, B. (2012, August 22). Father's age is linked to risk of autism and schizophrenia. *The New York Times*. page A1. Available on line at http://www.nytimes.com/2012/08/23/health/fathers-age-is-linked-to-risk-of-autism-and-schizophrenia.html?_r=1&nl=todaysheadlines&emc=edit_th_20120823.

10. March of Dimes. (2011). Overweight and obesity during pregnancy. Retrieved from http://www.marchofdimes.com/pregnancy/complications_obesity.html.

11. Centers for Disease Control and Prevention. (2012, May 1). *Clinical care for women: Immunization*. Retrieved from http://www.cdc.gov/preconception/careforwomen/immunization.html.

12. Practice Committee of the American Society for Reproductive Medicine in collaboration with the Society for Reproductive Endocrinology and Infertility. (2008). Optimizing natural fertility. *Fertility and Sterility*, *90* (5 Suppl), S1–S6.

13. Weng, X., Odouli, R., & Li, D. (2008). Maternal caffeine consumption during pregnancy and the risk of miscarriage: A prospective cohort study. *American Journal of Obstetrics & Gynecology*, *198* (3), 279e1–279e8.

14. Bakker, R., Steegers, E. A., Obradov, A., Raat, H., Hofman, A., & Jaddoe, W. V. (2010). Maternal caffeine intake from coffee and tea, fetal growth, and the risks of adverse birth outcomes: The generation R study. *American Journal of Clinical Nutrition, 92* (5), 1691–1698.

15. U.S. Department of Health and Human Services. (2010). *How tobacco smoke causes disease: The biology and behavioral basis for smoking-attributable disease: A report of the Surgeon General.* Retrieved from http://www.surgeongeneral.gov/library/tobaccosmoke/report/index.html.

16. Olson, H. C., Ohlemiller, M. M., O'Connor, M. J., Brown, C. W., Morris, C. A., Damus, K., & the National Task Force on Fetal Alcohol Syndrome and Fetal Alcohol Effect. (2009, March). *A call to action: Advancing essential services and research on fetal alcohol spectrum disorders – A report of the National Task Force on Fetal Alcohol Syndrome and Fetal Alcohol Effect*. Retrieved from http://www.cdc.gov/ncbddd/fasd/documents/calltoaction.pdf.

17. American Congress of Obstetricians and Gynecologists. (2011, August). Exercise during pregnancy. Retrieved from http://www.acog.org/~/media/For%20Patients/faq119.ashx?dmc=1&ts=20120202T1522575907.

18. Mayo Foundation. (2010, October 30). Home pregnancy tests: Can you trust the results? Retrieved from http://www.mayoclinic.com/health/home-pregnancy-tests/PR00100.

19. Institute of Medicine. (2011, August 30). *Weight gain during pregnancy: Reexamining the guidelines*. Retrieved from http://www.iom.edu/Reports/2009/Weight-Gain-During-Pregnancy-Reexamining-the-Guidelines.aspx.

20. Kaijser, M., Bonamy, A. K. E., Akre, O., Cnattingius, S., Granath, F., Norman, M., & Ekbom, A. (2009). Perinatal risk factors for diabetes in later life. *Diabetes, 58*, 523–526.

21. Jaddoe, V. W. V. (2008). Fetal nutritional origins of adult diseases: Challenges for epidemiological research. *European Journal of Epidemiology, 23,* 767–771.

22. U.S. Department of Health and Human Services. (2010, September 27). *Pregnancy: Body changes and discomforts.* Retrieved from http://womenshealth.gov/pregnancy/you-are-pregnant/body-changes-discomforts.cfm#j.

23. U.S. Department of Health and Human Services, Health Resources and Services Administration, Maternal and Child Health Bureau. (2009). *A healthy start: Begin before baby's born.* Retrieved from http://mchb.hrsa.gov/programs/womeninfants/prenatal.htm.

24. Thompson, J., & Manore, M. (2012). *Nutrition: An applied approach*, 3rd ed. San Francisco: Benjamin Cummings.

25. Sepillian, V. P. (2011, March 8). Ectopic pregnancy. *Medscape Reference*. Retrieved from http://emedicine.medscape.com/article/258768-overview.

26. March of Dimes. (2009). Miscarriage. Retrieved from http://www.marchofdimes.com/professionals/14332_1192.asp.

27. National Library of Medicine. (2011, September 12). *Placenta previa.* Retrieved from http://www.ncbi.nlm.nih.gov/pubmedhealth/PMH0001902.

28. Cunningham, F. G., Leveno, K. J., Bloom, S. L., Hauth, J. C., Gilstrap, L. C., & Wenstrom, K. D. (2010). *Williams obstetrics*, 23rd ed. New York: McGraw-Hill.

29. American Congress of Obstetricians and Gynecologists. (2011, May). Genital herpes. Retrieved from http://www.acog.org/~/media/For%20Patients/faq054.ashx.

30. American Congress of Obstetricians and Gynecologists. (2011, August). Hepatitis B in pregnancy. Retrieved from http://www.acog.org/~/media/For%20Patients/faq093.ashx.

31. American Congress of Obstetricians and Gynecologists. (2011, August). HIV and pregnancy. Retrieved from http://www.acog.org/~/media/For%20Patients/faq113.ashx.

32. American Congress of Obstetricians and Gynecologists. (2011, August). High blood pressure during pregnancy. Retrieved from http://www.acog.org/~/media/For%20Patients/faq034.ashx.

33. Kuklina, E. V., Ayala, C., & Callaghan, W. M. (2009). Hypertensive disorders and severe obstetric morbidity in the United States. *Obstetrics & Gynecology*, *113* (6), 1299–1306.

34. American Congress of Obstetricians and Gynecologists. (2011, December). Gestational diabetes. Retrieved from http://www.acog.org/~/media/For%20Patients/faq177.ashx.

35. Hamilton, B. E., Martin, J. A., & Ventura, S. J. (2011). Births: Preliminary data for 2010. *National Vital Statistics Reports* web release *60* (2). Hyattsville, MD: National Center for Health Statistics.

36. American Congress of Obstetricians and Gynecologists. (2011, May). Preterm labor. Retrieved from http://www.acog.org/~/media/For%20Patients/faq087.ashx.

37. World Bank. (2011). *Mortality rate, infant (per 1,000 live births).* Retrieved from http://data.worldbank.org/indicator/SP.DYN.IMRT.IN.

38. U.S. Department of Health and Human Services. (2004). *Birth, infant mortality, and life expectancy, 1980–2002.* Retrieved from http://www.hhs-stat.net/scripts/topic.cfm?id=738.

39. National Center for Health Statistics. (2011, November 30). *Births and natality.* Retrieved from http://www.cdc.gov/nchs/fastats/births.htm.

40. Martin, J. A., Hamilton, B. E., Ventura, S. J., Michelle, M. A., Osterman, J. K., Kirmeyer, S., Mathews, T. J., & Wilson, E. (2011, November). Births: Final data for 2009. *National Vital Statistics Reports, 60* (1). Retrieved from http://www.cdc.gov/nchs/data/nvsr/nvsr60/nvsr60_01.pdf.

41. American Congress of Obstetricians and Gynecologists. (2011, January). The American Congress of Obstetricians and Gynecologists issues opinion on planned home births. Retrieved from http://www.acog.org/About_ACOG/News_Room/News_Releases/2011/The_American_College_of_Obstetricians_and_Gynecologists_Issues_Opinion_on_Planned_Home_Births.

42. American Congress of Obstetricians and Gynecologists. (2007). You and your baby: Prenatal care, labor and delivery, and postpartum care. Retrieved from http://www.acog.org/publications/patient_education/ab005.cfm.

43. U.S. Department of Health and Human Services. (2009, March 6). *Depression during and after pregnancy fact sheet.* Retrieved from http://www.womenshealth.gov/publications/our-publications/fact-sheet/depression-pregnancy.cfm#b.

44. MedlinePlus. (2009). *APGAR.* Retrieved from http://www.nlm.nih.gov/medlineplus/ency/article/003402.htm.

45. American Congress of Obstetricians and Gynecologists. (2009, May 21). Catch 22 for New York's obstetricians: Failing state insurance system leaves OBs no options. *ACOG News*: Press Release. Retrieved from http://mail.ny.acog.org/website/Catch22NYOB.pdf.

46. Michaluk, C.A. (2009, May–June). Cesarean delivery by maternal request: What neonatal nurses need to know. *Neonatal Network, 28* (3), 145–150.

47. Lothian, D. (2006). The cesarean catastrophe. *Journal of Perinatal Education*, *15* (1): 42–45.

48. American Academy of Pediatrics, Section on Breastfeeding. (2005). Policy statement: Breastfeeding and the use of human milk. *Pediatrics, 115* (2), 496–506.

49. Beck, C. T. (2008). State of the science on postpartum depression: What nurse researchers have contributed. *MCN: American Journal of Maternal-Child Nursing*, *33* (3), 151–156.

50. Sacher, J., Wilson, A. A., Houle, S., Rusjan, P., Hassan, S., Bloomfield, P. M., Stewart, D. E., & Meyer, J. H. (2010). Elevated brain monoamine oxidase a binding in the early postpartum period. *Archives of General Psychiatry, 67* (4), 468–474.

51. LaCoursiere, D., Barrett-Connor, E., O'Hara, M., Hutton, A., & Varner, M. (2010). The association between prepregnancy obesity and screening positive for postpartum depression. *BJOG: An International Journal of Obstetrics & Gynecology, 117*, 1011–1018.

52. Paulson, J. F., & Bazemore, S. D. (2010). Prenatal and postpartum depression in fathers and its association with maternal depression. *Journal of the American Medical Association, 303* (19), 1961–1969.

53. U.S. Centers for Disease Control and Prevention. (2011, June 28). *Infertility FAQs.* Retrieved from http://www.cdc.gov/reproductivehealth/Infertility/#2.

54. Anderson, J. E., Farr, S. L., Jamieson, D. J., Warner, L., & Macaluso, M. (2009). Infertility services reported by men in the United States: National survey data. *Fertility and Sterility, 6*, 2466–2470.

55. MedlinePlus. (2009). *Infertility*. Retrieved from http://www.nlm.nih.gov/medlineplus/infertility.html.

56. Center for American Progress. (2007, December 17). Guide to state surrogacy laws. Retrieved from http://www.americanprogress.org/issues/2007/12/surrogacy_laws.html.

57. Child Welfare Information Gateway. (2012). *Introduction to adoption.* Washington, DC: U.S. Department of Health and Human Services, Children's Bureau. Retrieved from http://www.childwelfare.gov/adoption/intro.cfm.

58. Child Welfare Information Gateway. (2011). *How many children were adopted in 2007 and 2008?* Washington, DC: U.S. Department of Health and Human Services, Children's Bureau. Retrieved from http://www.childwelfare.gov/pubs/adopted0708.pdf.

59. Child Welfare Information Gateway. (2010, August). *How many children are waiting for adoption?* Washington, DC: U.S. Department of Health and Human Services, Children's Bureau. Retrieved from http://www.acf.hhs.gov/programs/cb/stats_research/afcars/waiting2009.pdf.

60. National Campaign to Prevent Teen and Unplanned Pregnancy. (2009, November). *Unplanned pregnancy and community colleges.* Retrieved from http://www.thenationalcampaign.org/resources/pdf/briefly-unplanned-pregnancy-and-community-colleges.pdf.

61. Miller, K., Gault, B., & Thorman, A. (2011, March). Improving child care access to promote postsecondary success among low-income parents. *Institute for Women's Policy Research, Perspectives on Sexual and Reproductive Health*, 1–64.

62. Parker, L. B. (2003). THE BLACK COLLEGIAN Magazine. Second semester super issue 2003. Retrieved from http://www.black-collegian.com/study/campus_advisor/advisor2003-2nd.shtml.

63. Garcia, E. (2011, May 3). College students with children need campuses with child care. *Institute for Women's Policy Research*. Available online at http://www.iwpr.org/blog/2011/05/03/college-students-with-children-need-campuses-with-child-care.

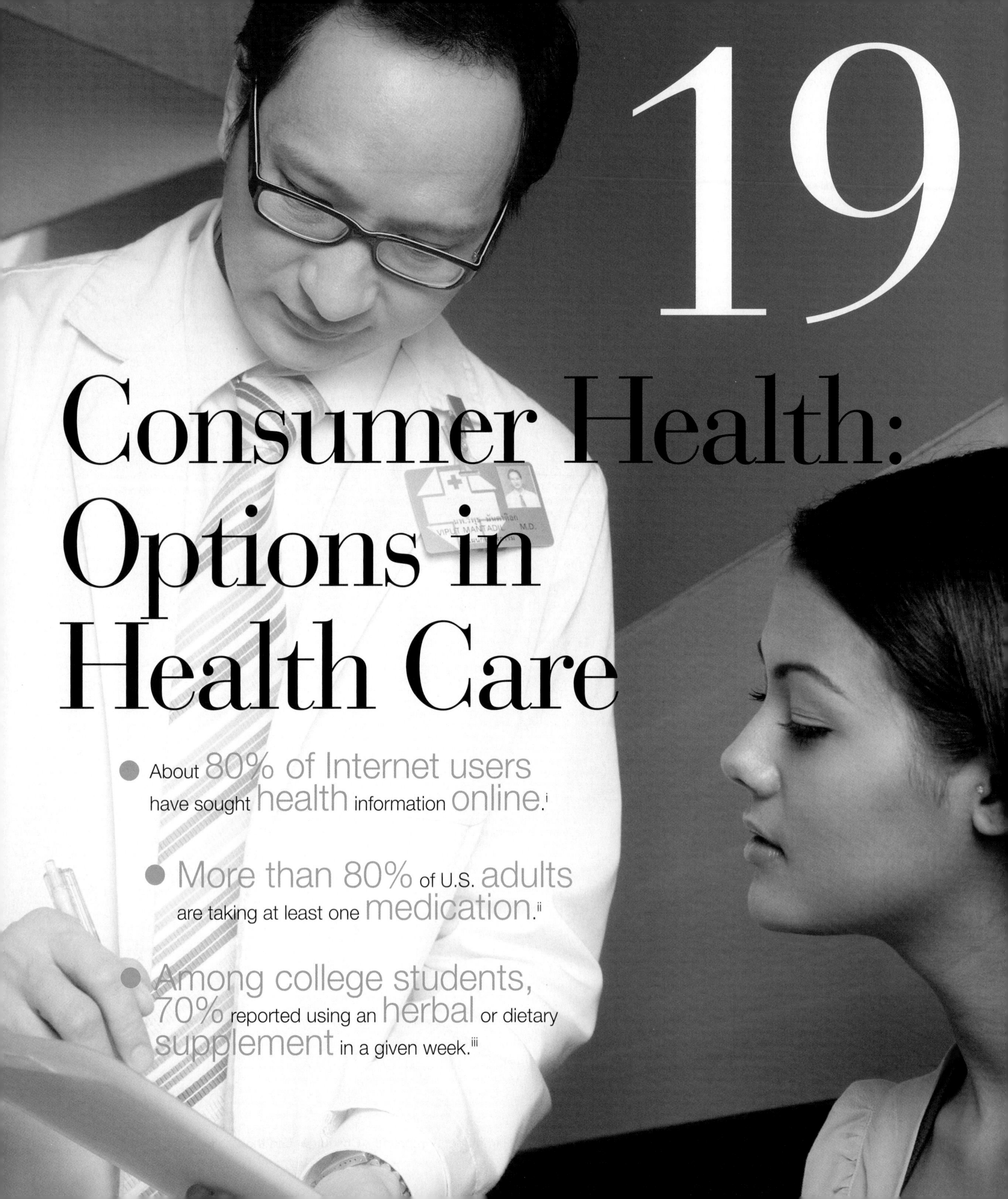

19

Consumer Health: Options in Health Care

- About 80% of Internet users have sought health information online.[i]
- More than 80% of U.S. adults are taking at least one medication.[ii]
- Among college students, 70% reported using an herbal or dietary supplement in a given week.[iii]

LEARNING OBJECTIVES

DESCRIBE different aspects of *self-care*.

IDENTIFY factors indicating that it's time to seek professional health care.

DISCUSS strategies for being a smart health-care consumer.

DESCRIBE the differences between *conventional medicine, complementary medicine,* and *alternative medicine*.

IDENTIFY multiple methods of paying for health care.

DISCUSS the genomic revolution and the future of personal health.

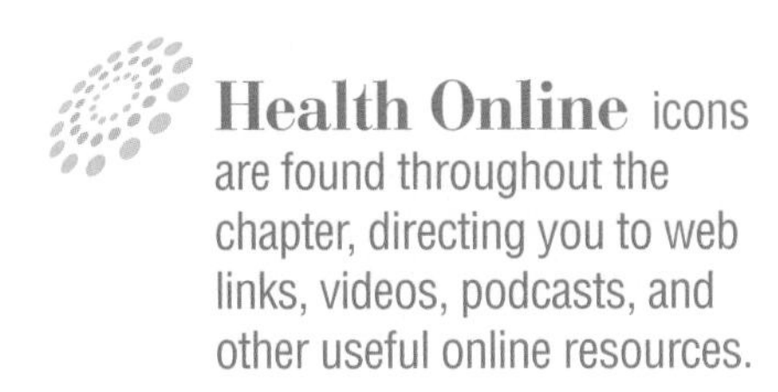

Health Online icons are found throughout the chapter, directing you to web links, videos, podcasts, and other useful online resources.

It's near the end of the semester, and you've been feeling physically run-down.

Things got worse this morning, when you woke up with a bad sore throat, a fever, and—most troubling—a skin rash. What should you do?

Maybe you'll go online and do a search on your symptoms to decide whether they are serious enough to seek professional help. You might take an over-the-counter medicine for the sore throat and fever, and ask a parent or friend for advice about the rash. If you decide to consult a doctor, things can quickly get complicated: Should you visit the student health center? What if there isn't one? Should you call your doctor at home? What if you don't have a regular physician? How will you pay for the health care? What if you don't have health insurance?

These are all examples of questions related to **consumer health.** In the United States today, we have more tools and options for taking care of our health than ever before. The Internet makes an unprecedented amount of health information available at our fingertips. We can purchase a wide range of over-the-counter drugs and medications. We can choose to seek care at a traditional hospital, at a drugstore clinic, or at a campus health center. We can try alternative therapies like acupuncture or chiropractic, and select from a broad array of health-care professionals and insurance plans.

But this growing world of health choices also requires active and informed decision-making. Increasingly, the burden is on you to research information, critically evaluate it, and make educated decisions that are best for you. You need to be a smarter health consumer than ever before. This chapter will help!

Choosing Self-Care

There are many things you can do on your own to stay healthy. As you've learned throughout this book, some of the most important health behaviors are preventive, aimed at promoting your overall wellness and reducing the likelihood that you will get sick in the first place. Maintaining basic wellness behaviors, learning how to critically evaluate health information (especially online), educating yourself about over-the-counter medications and supplements, using home health tests, and knowing when it's time to seek professional help are all examples of **self-care.**

Practicing Prevention

Preventive begins with the basic wellness behaviors you've learned about in this book, such as eating nutritiously, exercising, and refraining from unhealthful behaviors like smoking or excessive drinking. Regularly brushing your teeth and flossing, making sure you get enough sleep, keeping your stress level under control, and maintaining good relationships with your friends and loved ones are additional aspects of self-care

consumer health An umbrella term encompassing topics related to the purchase and consumption of health-related products and services.

self-care Actions you take to keep yourself healthy.

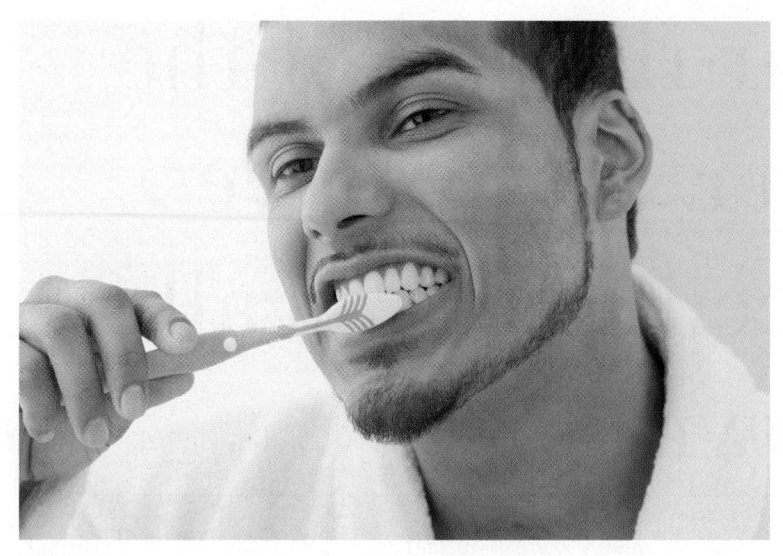

Figure 19.1 **Self-care includes basic wellness habits such as regularly brushing your teeth.**

(Figure 19.1). Common-sense preventive behaviors—such as wearing a seat belt inside a car, wearing a helmet while riding a bike, or practicing safe sex—can protect you from serious injuries and illnesses. Similarly, the simple act of regularly washing your hands with soap and hot water can protect you from contracting infectious diseases.

Prevention also means staying on top of regular health checks, including physicals and dental visits. When you are in college, these visits can be easy to skip amid a busy schedule, or harder to organize because you may be away from your regular doctor or dentist at home or unsure how you'll pay for care. Later in this chapter, we'll look at resources that make it easier for students to get the health care they need.

Finding Accurate Health Information

If you are living away from home for the first time, you also have new responsibilities for making your own decisions about your care. Some

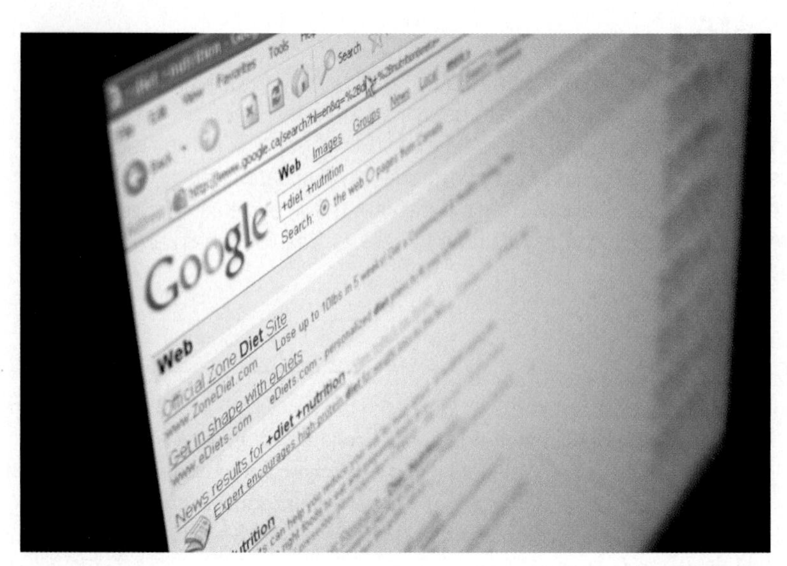

The **Internet** is increasingly the first place people turn for health information.

may be relatively simple, such as thinking about a new nutrition plan or choosing a bottle of seasonal allergy pills at the drugstore. Others, such as considering a new weight-loss supplement, thinking about contraception, or choosing a doctor, are more complex. Making any health-related decision intelligently starts with the ability to analyze health information for yourself.

Evaluating Health Information and Tools

About 79% of all U.S. adults and about 95% of college-age Americans use the Internet.[1] More than 80% of Internet users between the ages of 18 and 65 have sought health information online. Using the Internet as a health resource has become so common that some health professionals jokingly gripe that they've been replaced by "Dr. Google." Yet going online doesn't necessarily mean that one knows what to do with the health information found there. One study of college students found that, in general, the understanding of online health information is "generally sub par."[2]

As you may recall, in Chapter 1, we introduced some basic strategies for evaluating online information. (See **Spotlight: Evaluating Health Information in the Media** in Chapter 1.) But the online world represents only one facet of all the health information you are likely to encounter each day. You may hear about new scientific studies on news programs, or see ads for health-related products in magazines. A friend might recommend a new health-related software program, or "app," for your phone. Regardless of where you find your health information, you will be able to evaluate it better if you get answers to a few basic questions:

- What is the source? Is the information provider a health expert, or a group of such professionals? What are the source's credentials?
- What does the source have at stake? Is the information provider relatively unbiased, or does the source have a stake in how the information might be used? Will anyone benefit financially from how the information is perceived or used? If you are using a mobile app, does it have a one-time cost, or ongoing fees?
- Is the information or tool supported by facts? Are those facts stated clearly, with supporting evidence to establish their credibility?
- Does the information or tool come with a "time stamp"? Does the site or app say when its underlying information was published or last updated? If it relies on scientific studies, are those relatively recent or somewhat dated? A site or app with relatively recent information is preferable, assuming that other criteria for quality information are met.
- Is the information presented in a balanced manner? Does it include and discuss other options or points of view, or pretend they don't exist?
- Does the information or tool offer something that sounds too good to be true? Achieving good health and wellness is a rewarding but ongoing process. Simplistic quick fixes may be of little actual substance.
- Does the site carry HONcode certification? The HONcode is a code of ethics for health and medical websites that guides site developers in setting up good-quality, objective, and transparent medical information. Sites with HONcode certification carry a HONcode label.

For more information about the HONcode, visit www.hon.ch/HONcode.

In addition to using these questions to evaluate health information in the news and other media, you can also watch for these "red flags," identified by health experts at the University of California, San Francisco:[3]

- The information is anonymous.
- There is a conflict of interest.
- The information is one-sided or biased.
- The information is outdated.
- There is a claim of a miracle or secret cure.
- No evidence is cited.
- The grammar is poor and words are misspelled.

Much of the health information and tools you'll find online or in the media claim to rely on scientific research studies. The Internet has made these studies more accessible than ever before, and you don't need to be a scientist to read them. Next, we'll look at how you can make sense of scientific findings.

Understanding Research Studies

Reliable health information is supported by **evidence-based medicine**—practices that are based on systematic, scientific study. The process that supports quality research is called the "scientific method," and includes the following steps: First, the researcher makes an observation that prompts one or more questions about the factor observed. The researcher then formulates an educated guess (or hypothesis) that attempts to answer one or more of the original questions, and conducts an experiment to test that educated guess. The experiment generates data that either challenges the hypothesis or supports it. Scientists typically share the results of their experiments with other researchers in the form of published research studies.

evidence-based medicine Health-care policies and practices based on systematic, scientific study.

over-the-counter (OTC) medication A medication available for purchase without a prescription.

If a health-related research claim is based on a credible study grounded in the scientific method, that integrity will be apparent in its published research findings. But not all studies are equally reliable. To evaluate the validity and reliability of such studies, consider the following questions:

- Is the description of this research specific and detailed? Credible research claims should include who conducted the study and their credentials, the research institutions involved, the question the study was trying to answer, and the dates the research was conducted and/or published.
- Who published this research? Quality science is published in *peer-reviewed journals,* publications where experts screen and evaluate all submissions. Research findings are also sometimes presented at meetings of scientific societies.
- Who were the study participants? Was the research done on animals or people? Studies conducted on people usually have the greatest medical validity.
- How many people participated? The larger the pool of participants, the more significant the results. Especially significant studies often involve tens of thousands of people over several years.
- What were the profiles of the participants? How similar were they to you? The results of a health study of breast cancer prevention in 10,000 postmenopausal women may not be relevant to you if you are a woman in your 20s.
- Is the study the first of its kind? Scientific findings carry more weight if they have been replicated by other researchers.
- Do the people behind the study have any conflicts of interest? Credible studies disclose who paid for the research and whether the scientists involved have any financial or other interest in the outcome.

Credible health information sites highlight this type of scientific information or make it relatively easy to find. If you have trouble finding answers to these types of questions when researching health information or products, think twice about the believability of the information you are viewing.

Options for Self-Care

In addition to practicing prevention and finding good health information, self-care means being your own caregiver from time to time. You may want to take an over-the-counter medication, consider a new vitamin, or give yourself a home health test. Or, you may find yourself responsible for managing a chronic health condition, such as asthma or diabetes. First, we'll look at a common form of self-care—the medications you can easily buy off the shelf.

Evaluating Over-the-Counter Medications

In any given week, more than 80% of U.S. adults are taking at least one type of medication.[4] The most readily available are **over-the-counter (OTC) medications,** which do not require a doctor's prescription. The U.S. Food and Drug Administration (FDA) regulates both prescription and OTC medications. The FDA defines OTC medications as those that:

- Have benefits outweighing their risks
- Have low potential for misuse
- Consumers can use for self-diagnosed conditions
- Can be adequately labeled
- Do not require consultation with health practitioners for safe and effective use of the product[5]

About 74% of college students take at least one OTC drug a week, with pain relievers the most common.[6] (See the **Student Stats** box on page 518.)

Many OTC drugs are effective, and are often more affordable than prescription medications. One analysis showed that brand-name prescription drugs can cost over 10 times more than OTC medications.[7] But even though they are widely available, OTC medications can still carry risks and side effects. It is important to read labels carefully, to not exceed the recommended dosage, to use the medications for their intended purposes, and to talk to your doctor or pharmacist if you have any questions. (See **Consumer Corner: Using an Over-the-Counter Medication Safely** on page 519.)

Medicines in My Home at www.accessdata.fda.gov/videos/cder/mimh/index.cfm is an interactive presentation on how to choose and use OTC medications safely.

Evaluating Dietary Supplements

Do you regularly take dietary supplements? According to a survey of college students, about 70% used an herbal or dietary supplement in a given week.[5] Although supplements are popular, they are not without risk. Supplements are not legally regulated in the same ways as OTC or prescription medications, and research into the benefits of their use remains controversial and inconclusive.

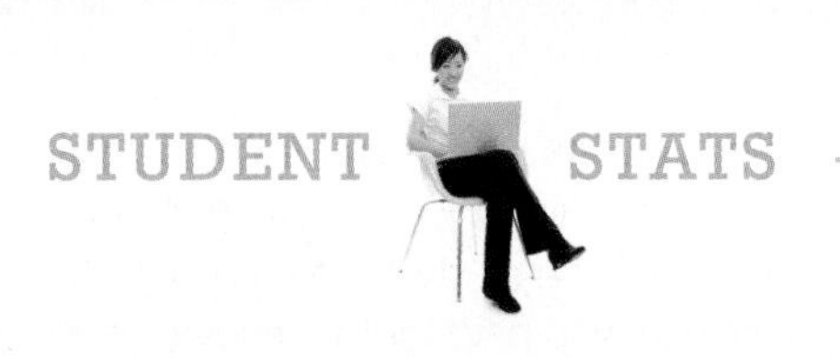

Top Over-the-Counter Medications and Supplements Used by Students

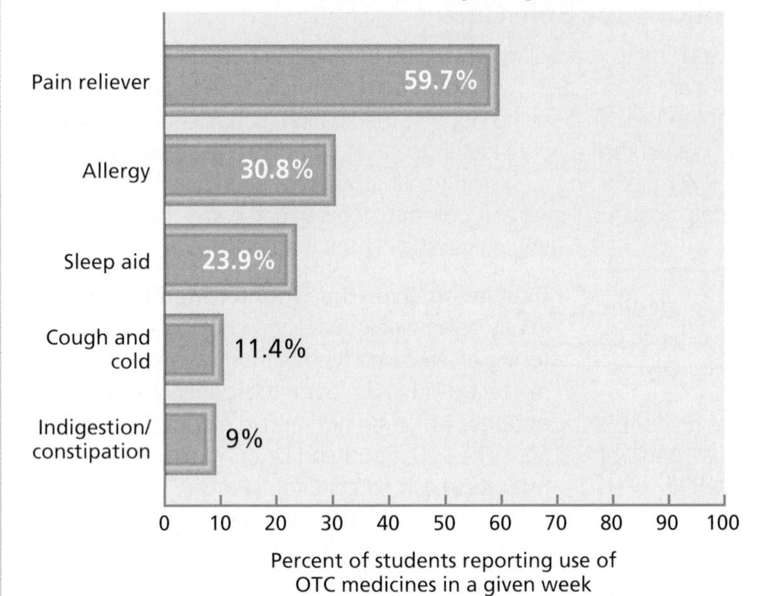

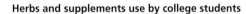

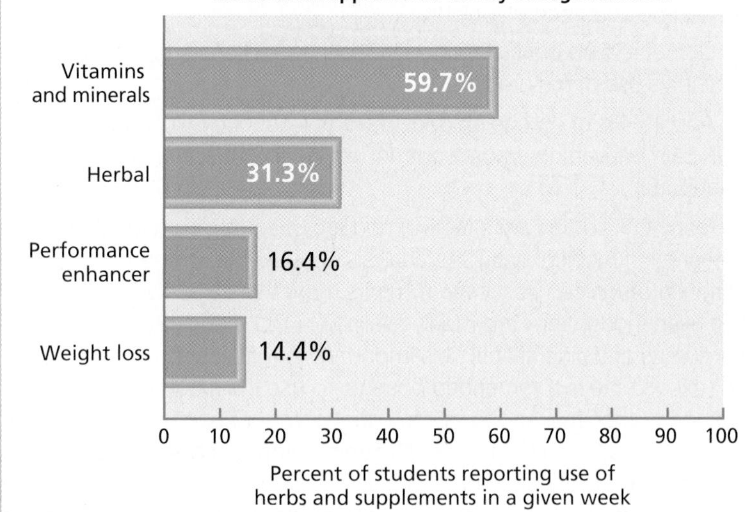

Data from "Over-the-Counter Medication and Herbal or Dietary Supplement Use in College: Dose Frequency and Relationship to Self-Reported Distress" by M. Stasio, K. Curry, K. Sutton-Skinner, & D. Glassman, 2008, *Journal of the American College Health Association, 56* (5), pp. 535–547.

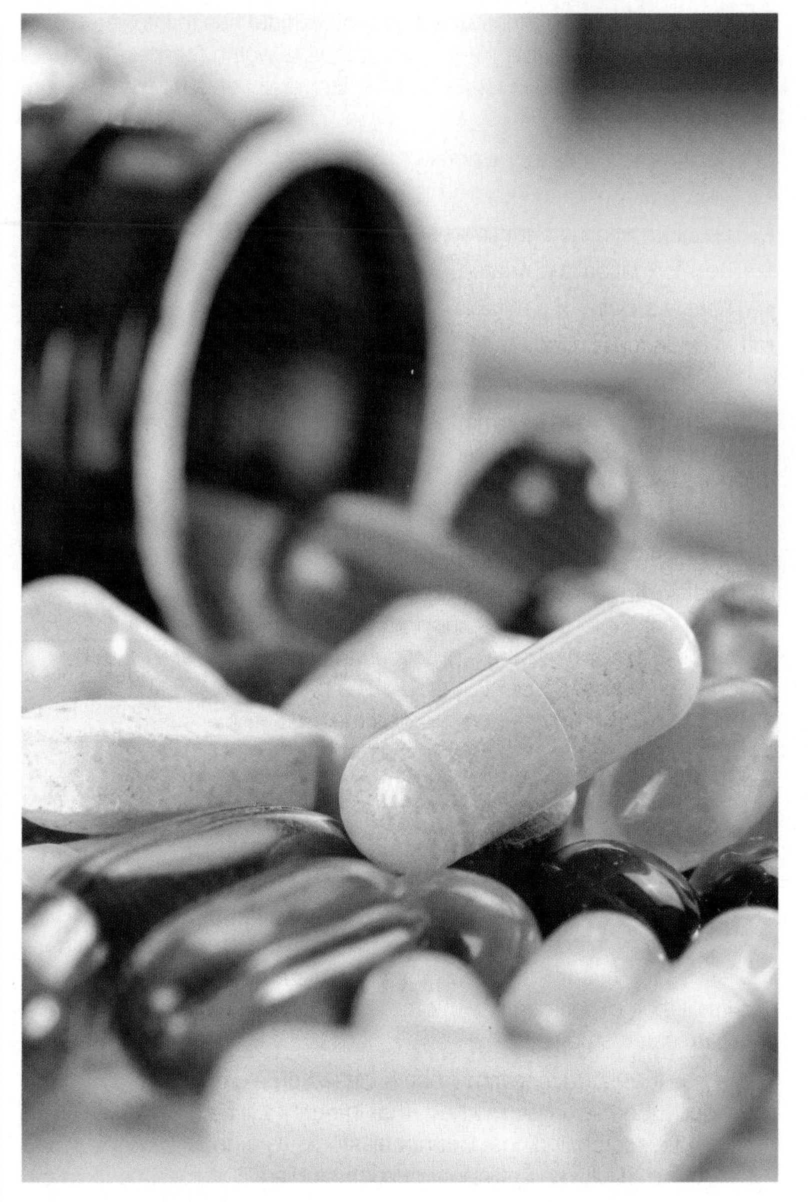

Figure 19.2 Dietary supplements are popular, but there is no scientific consensus about their health benefits.

Dietary supplements are products taken by mouth that include ingredients such as vitamins, minerals, amino acids, herbs, botanicals, or other compounds that could supplement the diet **(Figure 19.2).** They are generally not administered by a doctor. Whereas the FDA requires extensive evaluations of a prescription or OTC drug's safety and efficacy before it can be sold, supplements do not get this same screening. Federal laws bar supplement advertisements from making specific claims about supplement benefits that haven't been proven (supplement advertisements, for example, cannot promise to cure a particular type of cancer). But there are no regulations for the general claims these ads can make. You may commonly come across supplement advertisements featuring vague statements or leading questions such as "Stay healthy!" or "Need more energy?" There may be no scientific research to back up such language. Also, be aware that a supplement may tout itself as free of one risky ingredient, but that doesn't mean it is free of other harmful substances.

Before taking any dietary supplements, consider these guidelines:

dietary supplements Products taken by mouth that include ingredients such as vitamins, minerals, amino acids, herbs, botanicals, or other compounds that could supplement the diet.

Where to Find Conventional Health Care

Conventional medicine was once offered primarily through doctors' offices and hospitals, but its availability has since expanded to better meet the needs of patients. The following are examples of facilities that offer conventional care:

- **Student health centers** serve students on university campuses. Some focus on basic primary care and student health needs, such as minor illnesses and contraception. Others feature a wider range of care, including substance abuse counseling, vision care, pharmacy, and dental services. Few offer emergency services. If a center doesn't offer a particular type of care, staff will usually provide referrals to off-campus care providers. On many campuses, student health centers are available to all enrolled students and most of the costs are covered by fees paid as part of student enrollment.
- **Primary care facilities** are the backbone of the health-care system. These facilities meet everyday medical needs, seeing patients for checkups, screenings, and minor ailments and providing referrals to more specialized care if needed. Costs are often covered by patient health insurance or a combination of insurance and patient payments.
- **Nonprofit clinics** provide primary care for free or at a reduced cost. They often focus on underserved communities and groups who would otherwise have little access to primary care.
- **Corporate wellness centers** provide care to employees. A few offer a full range of services, but most focus on efforts to help employees live more healthfully by offering programs such as smoking cessation, fitness, or weight loss.
- **Retail clinics,** also known as convenient care clinics or drugstore clinics, operate out of large stores and pharmacies **(Figure 19.5).** These clinics are designed to provide basic primary care, such as screenings and treatment of minor ailments, in a timely manner for people who don't have a primary care doctor, can't wait for an appointment at a primary care facility, and/or lack health insurance. Costs are lower than they would be at most traditional doctors' offices, and are often paid directly by the patient or through insurance.

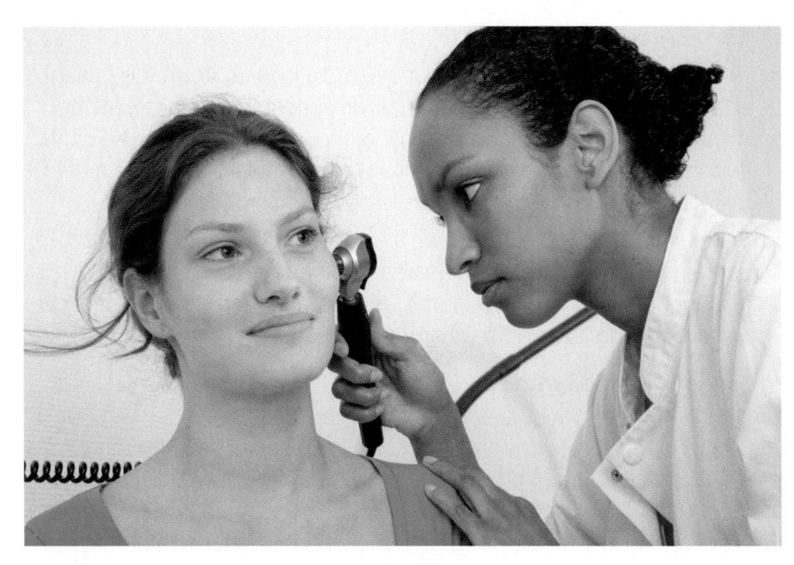

Figure 19.4 Nurse practitioners are an example of conventional health-care providers.

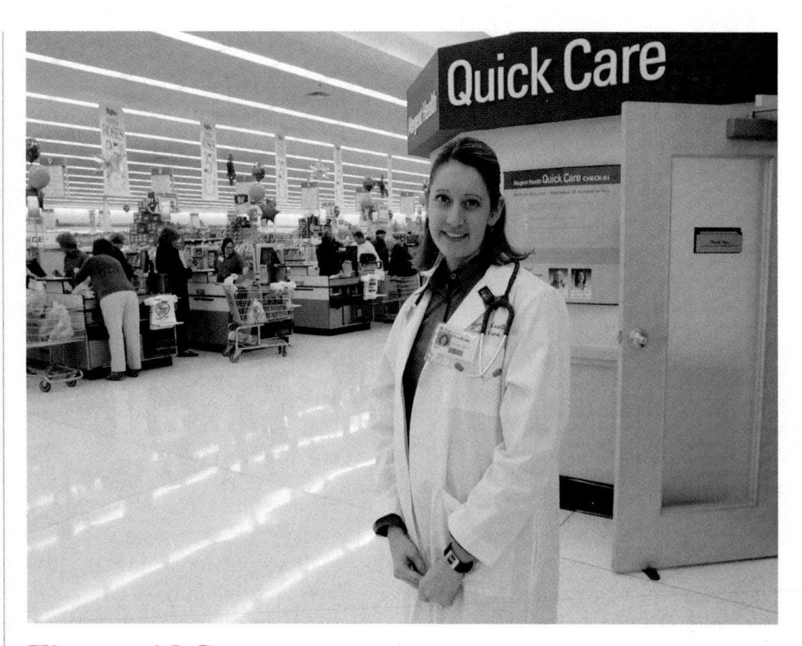

Figure 19.5 Health services are sometimes offered through large retail stores.

- **Urgent care centers** typically see patients with illnesses that need immediate attention but don't require the full resources of a hospital emergency department. These centers often see many patients on evenings and weekends, when primary care centers are closed. Though not as expensive as emergency rooms, urgent care centers often charge a premium for their services, which can either be covered by insurance or paid directly by the patient.
- **Specialist centers** provide specific categories of medicine, such as obstetrics, cardiac care, or oncology. Most patients access specialists through referrals from a primary care center. Specialty care is an important part of the medical system, but can be quite costly to patients if not covered by insurance.
- **Hospitals** provide the highest level of care. Hospitals handle everything from emergencies to surgeries to complex screenings and cancer treatment. Patients can be seen on an *outpatient* basis, in which they visit the hospital but don't stay overnight, or on an *inpatient* basis, where care is provided for an extended period of time and overnight stays are included.

Choosing a Provider

If you are the age of a traditional college student, you probably haven't had much say in the past over who served as your care provider. Your family probably chose a pediatrician when you were younger, and if you attend your campus health center now, you probably see the first provider with an available appointment.

But at some point, you'll choose your own primary care provider, either a physician, nurse practitioner, or physician assistant who serves as your everyday contact with the health care system. Your primary care provider will see you for checkups and most screenings, answer your basic health questions, treat minor ailments, write prescriptions, and provide referrals for more complex health concerns. Because your primary care provider will also provide most of your preventive care, it's important to find one before you get sick.

Living Without Health Insurance

STUDENT STORY

"My name is Holly. I am 45 years old. I was a single parent for about 12 years. I could not afford insurance for myself—it just wasn't in my budget. My kids always came first. If I got sick, I stayed at home and took care of myself. One time I had really bad abdominal pain and did not go to see the doctor because I didn't have any insurance. It got so bad that I couldn't stand up. I had to go to the emergency room and they did emergency surgery on me. My gallbladder had ruptured and the poison from that went through my system. I ended up being in the hospital for 5 days because of that. If I had gone to the doctor sooner, they would have caught it sooner. My doctor's bill ended up being a little over $12,000. That's a lot of money for a single mom."

1: Holly is a nontraditional-aged college student. What are some health-care options that may be available to her, despite her lack of health insurance?

Do you have a story similar to Holly's? Share your story at www.pearsonhighered.com/lynchelmore.

To get started, check two resources: your insurance plan and your friends and family. If your health insurance limits the providers you can see, start with those on the plan's list. Then ask your friends and family for their recommendations.

Once you have a list of providers to contact, start by calling their offices and ask a few questions of a nurse or other office staff:

- Is this provider accepting new patients?
- What insurance plans does this office accept?
- If a physician, is this doctor *board-certified,* meaning that he or she has undergone extra training after medical school to specialize in an area such as family practice?
- How does the office handle lab work? Is there a lab in-house or nearby, or will you have to travel to a different location for a procedure such as a blood test?
- Is this a group practice? If so, will you mostly see your provider, or all the providers in the group? If so, how many of them are there and what are their specialties?
- Who will care for you if your doctor is unavailable?
- Is this medical practice affiliated with any particular hospitals or specialty centers?
- Does this practice offer newer methods of contacting your provider, such as email?

When you meet your provider in person, make sure that he or she listens to you, encourages you to ask questions, answers your questions completely, and treats you with respect. If you don't feel comfortable with a provider, shop around until you do.

Conventional Medical Tests and Treatments

Conventional health-care providers do much more than just prescribe medicines. Your care team may also recommend certain tests to identify the cause of a health issue, offer physical interventions such as surgery or physical therapy, or even provide more holistic care through options such as psychiatric counseling or medically supervised exercise programs.

Medical Tests

A medical test provides evidence suggesting the presence, absence, or progression of disease. Some medical tests are *diagnostic*, meaning care provider uses them to determine whether or not a particular problem or disease exists when the patient shows signs or symptoms of the disease.[10] *Screening* tests are used to detect or predict the presence of disease when the patient shows no symptoms.[10] *Monitoring* tests examine the progression of a disease or the success of treatment over time.

Medical tests may rely on physical samples taken from a patient's body, such as blood or urine, or images taken of a patient's body, such as an X-ray. The results of medical tests are often used to either choose a treatment or see if a particular treatment is effective. Common types of medical tests include:

- Blood tests, in which a blood sample is analyzed to see if it contains certain substances or pathogens, and if so, at what levels. Blood tests are widely used to evaluate a large number of conditions, ranging from blood glucose to cholesterol levels to levels of toxins such as lead.
- Urine tests, or *urinanalysis,* in which a urine sample is studied for levels of certain substances or pathogens. Urine tests can be used to detect everything from sexually transmitted infections to pregnancy.
- Imaging tests, in which a "picture" of a part of a patient's body is taken to see if particular conditions can be detected. X-rays, ultrasounds, CT (or computerized tomography) scans, MRI (magnetic resonance imaging), and PET (positron emission tomography) scans are just some examples of medical imaging technologies. Imaging can be used to study both hard tissues, such as bone, and soft tissues, such as the brain or the heart and its surrounding blood vessels **(Figure 19.6).**
- Microbial culture, in which a tissue sample is taken from the patient, and then placed in a nutrient-rich environment to see if it contains microbes responsible for an infection and, if so, what type. If you've ever had the back of your throat swabbed to see if you have a strep infection, for example, you've undergone a microbial culture.
- Genetic tests, in which a person's DNA is extracted from a blood, saliva, or tissue sample and analyzed to see if it contains any significant health-related genetic differences. We'll look more closely at genetic testing later in this chapter.

Prescription Medications

Prescription medications are those that can only be obtained after authorization from a medical provider. Over the last decade, the number of Americans who took at least one prescription drug in a given month increased from 44% to 48%.[11] Spending on prescription drugs reached $307.4 billion in 2010, which reflects a somewhat slower rate of spending growth than in previous years but is still more than double the amount spent in 1999.[11,12]

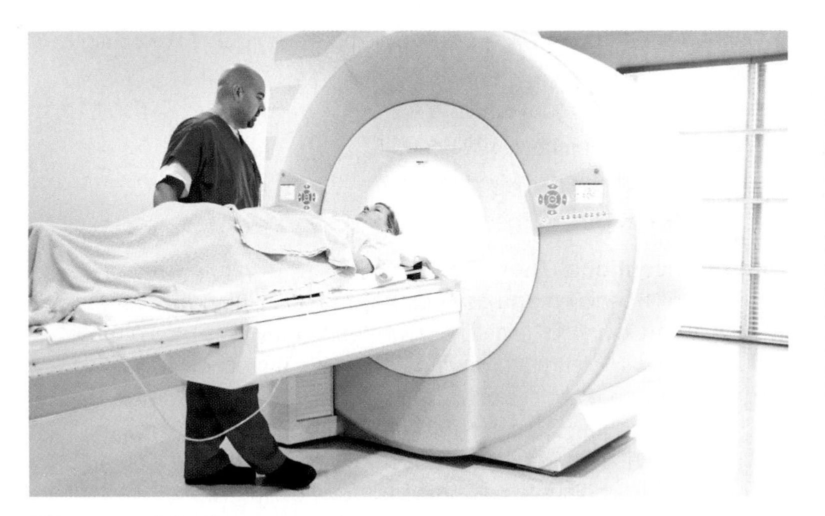

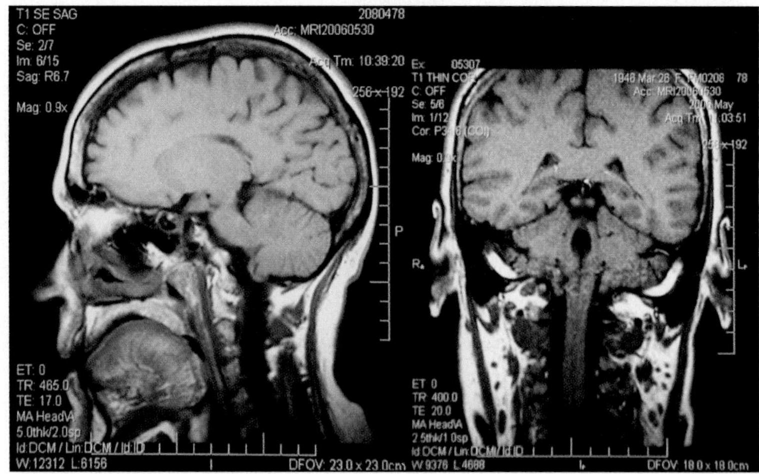

Figure 19.6 Magnetic resonance imaging (MRI) is a medical test that can study hard and soft tissues in the body. At left, the MRI machine. At right, MRI images of the head.

Development and Approval. Like OTC drugs, prescription medications are regulated by the FDA, which reviews and approves new drugs before they are available to doctors and patients. There are several steps in the development and approval process, and each drug requires a unique pathway.[13] The entire process often takes years, although some drugs for serious or life-threatening conditions that have few existing treatment options may receive accelerated approval.[13]

One of the most important elements of the drug development and approval process is the **clinical trial** stage. Clinical trials are tests of proposed new drugs using human subjects, and often occur in three phases.[13] Phase 1 trials are usually performed on healthy volunteers with the goal of determining the drug's safety, most frequent side effects, and how the body metabolizes and excretes the drug.[13] If Phase 1 trials show the drug to be safe, Phase 2 trials begin to determine the drug's effectiveness on people who have the disease or condition for which the drug is intended.[13] If the drug is shown to be both safe and effective in the earlier two phases, Phase 3 trials of a larger group of subjects (from several hundred to several thousand) gather more information about safety and effectiveness among differing populations and using different doses and combinations with other drugs.[13]

Brand-Name vs. Generic Drugs. When a new prescription drug first goes on the market, it is usually protected by a patent that allows only the drug's developer to manufacture it. These patent-protected prescription drugs are usually referred to as **brand-name drugs,** and they often carry a higher cost. But after a drug developer's patent expires, usually within 14 years, other manufacturers may also make and sell a copy of the same drug. These copies, known as **generic drugs,** are required by law to contain the same active ingredients as the brand-name drugs they replicate. However, they often cost much less than the brand-name version—sometimes just a fraction of the brand-name's price tag. If your doctor recommends a prescription drug, ask about generic equivalents to save money.

clinical trials Tests of proposed new drugs using human subjects.

brand-name drugs Patent-protected prescription drugs that can only be manufactured by one drug company and which usually carry a higher cost.

generic drugs Copies of brand-name drugs that can be created by other drug companies after a drug developer's patent expires. These drugs are required by law to contain the same active ingredients as the brand-name drugs they replicate.

surgery A procedure that treats injuries, disease, or disorders by physically cutting into and manipulating the body.

elective surgery A nonessential surgery. The patient can decide when and if to undergo the procedure.

Adverse Drug Events. Although prescription drugs are common, they are not always safe. According to one groundbreaking examination of errors related to prescription drugs, about 1.5 million discrete problems, or *adverse drug events,* occur in the United States each year.[14] For tips on how to protect yourself from prescription drug–related errors, see the **Consumer Corner** on page 526.

Not all problems related to prescription drugs are accidental: These medications are sometimes deliberately misused. (See Chapter 8 for a review of the issues surrounding the misuse of prescription drugs.)

Surgeries

Surgeries are procedures that treat injuries, disease, and disorders by physically cutting into and manipulating the body. About 95 million surgeries are performed in the United States each year, including about 48 million *inpatient* procedures performed in hospitals and 47 million *outpatient* procedures performed in ambulatory surgical centers, facilities located outside hospitals.[15,16] Outpatient surgeries can also be performed in hospitals. If you have an outpatient procedure at a hospital, you will likely be released and can go home in the same day. If you have an inpatient procedure, you may need to stay in the hospital to recover for a certain period of time as determined by your doctor.

While some surgeries are necessary to save lives, such as in repairing physical trauma from a car crash, many are **elective,** meaning the patient can decide when and if to undergo the procedure. If your doctor recommends surgery, or refers you to a surgeon for further discussion, here are some questions that federal health-care quality experts recommend asking and considering before agreeing to the procedure:[17]

- Are there alternatives to surgery?
- What are the benefits of having the surgery?
- What are the risks of having the surgery?
- What will happen if I don't have this surgery?
- Where can I get a second opinion?

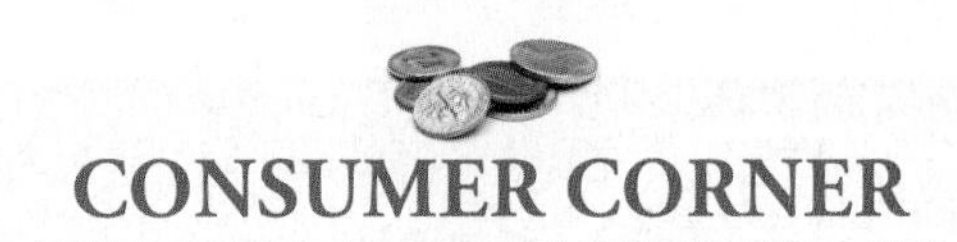

CONSUMER CORNER

How You Can Prevent Medication Errors

At best, medication errors will delay your recovery from an illness. At worst, they can cause significant harm or even death. Here are a few basic steps you can take to protect yourself.

At home and during medical appointments:

- Keep a list of all your medications, including prescription drugs, over-the-counter medications, and supplements.
- Bring your list to your medical appointments, or better yet, bring your medications. This will give your health-care providers a clear view of what you take and at what dose.
- Make sure your health-care provider knows about any prior medication allergies or adverse reactions.
- If your health-care provider hands you a written prescription, make sure you can read it. For electronic or phone-delivered prescriptions, get the name of the medication in writing so that you know you are getting the right drug later.
- Don't keep or take expired medications. They may no longer be effective past their expiration date, or may work differently than expected.

At the pharmacy:

- Make sure the name of the drug (brand or generic) and the directions for use received at the pharmacy are the same as those written down by the prescriber.
- Ask for written information about the medication if it isn't provided automatically.
- Talk to your pharmacist about your medication. Including how to take it properly, side effects, and what to do if you experience side effects.
- Be sure you understand your medication labels. For example, ask if "four times daily" means taking a dose every six hours around the clock or just during regular waking hours.

In the hospital:

- Ask what drugs you are being given at the hospital, or have someone (such as a friend or relative) ask for you and inform your care team about your medication history.
- Do not take a drug without being told the purpose for doing so.
- Most hospitals now have patients wear a barcode bracelet or other temporary identification tag. Don't let anyone give you medication without first checking your identification tag and making sure the medicine is truly meant for you.
- Prior to surgery, ask whether there are medications, especially prescription antibiotics, that you should take or any that you should stop taking preoperatively.
- When you leave the hospital, make sure you understand not only any new medicines you should be taking, but how doses or use guidelines for prior medications might have changed. This can get confusing, so ask to talk to your health-care provider or pharmacist about your list of medications in detail.

Sources: Adapted from *20 Tips to Help Prevent Medical Errors. Patient Fact Sheet,* by the Agency for Healthcare Research and Quality, September 2011, AHRQ Publication No. 11-0089, retrieved from http://www.ahrq.gov/consumer/20tips.htm; *Recommendations and Safety Tips: How to Prevent Medication Errors,* by the Institute for Safe Medication Practices, 2004, retrieved from www.ismp.org/pressroom/Patient_Broc.pdf; and *Fact Sheet: What You Can Do to Avoid Medication Errors,* by the Institute of Medicine, Committee on Identifying and Preventing Medication Errors, July 2006, retrieved from http://www.iom.edu/~/media/Files/Report%20Files/2006/Preventing-Medication-Errors-Quality-Chasm-Series/medicationerrorsfactsheet.pdf.

- What has been your experience in doing the surgery? How many have you performed?
- Where will the surgery be done?
- What kind of anesthesia will I need?
- How long will it take me to recover?
- How much will the surgery cost?

Other Conventional Therapies

Conventional medicine also goes far beyond tests, pills, and surgeries. If you have an injury, for example, your doctor may prescribe a medication but also recommend **physical therapy,** a practice in which a trained health-care professional called a *physical therapist* treats the injured area with remedies such as massage, targeted exercise, and application of heat or cold to the affected area. If you have a chronic condition such as diabetes or a food allergy, you may be referred to a professional dietitian who can help you develop and follow a medically supervised diet to help keep you healthy. In a growing number of conventional medicine centers, you'll also increasingly see the use of unconventional practices. In many cancer care centers, for example, it's increasingly common to find meditation classes offered alongside appointments for chemotherapy. This combination of conventional care and alternative therapies is known as *integrative medicine,* an area we will look at more closely a little later in this chapter.

physical therapy A practice in which a physical therapist treats an injured area with remedies such as massage, targeted exercise, and application of heat or cold.

Health Insurance Portability and Accountability Act (HIPAA) Legislation that protects your medical privacy.

Being a Smart Patient

Once you've chosen a doctor, you'll often find that your first visit starts with a pile of paperwork. Though it's tempting to rush through the forms, it's worth your time to review them. Many of these documents explain your rights and protections as a patient. While the types of documents you receive will vary from practice to practice, common policies and disclosures include:

- **How your privacy will be protected.** A set of federal rules called the **Health Insurance Portability and Accountability Act,** or **HIPAA,** protects your medical privacy, and reputable care providers comply with HIPAA.
- **What treatments and care you are authorizing.** In *informed consent* documents, you should find care options and procedures explained thoroughly, along with their risks and benefits and any available alternatives. While routine care, such as a checkup, doesn't usually require an informed consent, procedures that carry more risk often do.
- **Who is responsible for paying for your care.** Make sure you understand any paperwork related to costs and payment responsibilities before your appointment begins.

Once you are comfortable with the paperwork, your visits will be more productive if you think of your care provider as a partner. He or she has the expertise to help you improve your health, but his or her work will be more safe and effective if you are actively and constructively engaged in the process. Although most medical providers are conscientious, dedicated professionals, mistakes and medical errors often occur. One study found that among patients treated in hospitals, about 1 in 3 will experience some type of medical error, and that the cost of such errors totals more than $17 billion in the United States each year.[18]

Here are some suggestions from the American Academy of Family Physicians, a leading group representing primary care doctors, for how to get the most out of a medical appointment and help your care team avoid medical errors:[19]

- ***Talk* to your care provider.** Be sure to tell your care provider about any past or current health issues or concerns, even if they are embarrassing. Many medical appointments are only 15 minutes long, so effective communication is key to letting your care provider treat you.
- **Ask questions.** Let your care provider know if you don't understand something. If you need more time to discuss an issue, be vocal about it. If your appointment ends before all your questions have been answered, you can follow up with someone else in the office or schedule another appointment to discuss the issue further.
- **Take information home with you.** Take notes during your appointment, ask your care provider for handouts, or ask the office to supply background or reference materials.
- **Follow up with your care provider.** Follow the instructions you receive, such as getting additional tests or seeing a specialist. If you've been given a new medication and feel worse or have problems with the drug, let your care provider know right away. If you took a test and haven't received the results, let your care provider's office know.
- **Prevent medical errors through active communication.** This step is key, and requires continuous, active participation on your part. Let your care provider know all the medicines, supplements, and other substances you may be taking (including alcohol) to help prevent risky drug interactions. Be proactive about sharing information with all members of your medical team, especially if you have more than one caregiver; if you have surgery, for example, your care team may include a dozen professionals. Make sure you understand the side effects of any medication you are prescribed. If you are being discharged from care, make sure you understand any follow-up treatments to be done at home.

Ask your doctor **questions** to be sure you understand your care needs.

Complementary and Alternative Medicine (CAM)

Conventional medicine can be very effective, but for a growing number of people, it's not the only answer. Conventional medicine's focus on physical ailments after they arise may sometimes overlook preventive steps and care that could have warded off illness. Some people are uncomfortable with the way that conventional medicine often treats normal parts of life, such as childbirth or death in old age, as problems that require heavy medical management. Others are interested in health practices that take a broader, more holistic approach, looking beyond the body to include the mind and spirit as well.

complementary and alternative medicine (CAM) Health practices and traditions not typically part of conventional Western medicine, either used alone (alternative medicine) or in conjunction with conventional medicine (complementary medicine).

These interests have led to the growth of **complementary and alternative medicine (CAM).** The term *alternative medicine* is used to refer to those practices and traditions not typically part of conventional Western medicine, including everything from herbal remedies and meditation to chiropractors and traditional Chinese medicine. *Complementary medicine*, also sometimes referred to as *integrative medicine*, refers to care combining conventional and alternative medicine. Many of us routinely practice complementary medicine without realizing it, perhaps trying an herbal remedy to treat a cold but seeing a traditional doctor for a serious injury.

Alternative medicine has become such a common part of our approach to health that federal health officials now discuss and study it in a scientific way, and many states now require some CAM practitioners to be licensed. The National Center for Complementary and Alternative Medicine (NCCAM) groups CAM into five major domains: whole medical systems, mind–body medicine, natural products, manipulative and body-based practices, and energy and movement therapies.[20]

Whole Medical Systems

Whole medical systems are built on theories and systems encompassing the totality of a person's health. Under these approaches, the whole person is evaluated and treated, not just an isolated set of problems or symptoms. These traditional health systems have typically evolved apart from and earlier than conventional Western medicine, although several, such as homeopathy, developed in Western cultures. While traditional whole-body medicine is found all over the world, several types are now common in the United States, including traditional Chinese medicine, homeopathy, naturopathy, and Ayurveda.

Traditional Chinese Medicine

Traditional Chinese medicine is a sophisticated system of remedies that, while complex, is primarily concerned with understanding and adjusting flows of energy in the body to maintain balance and health. This ancient system revolves around the concept of the free flow of chi

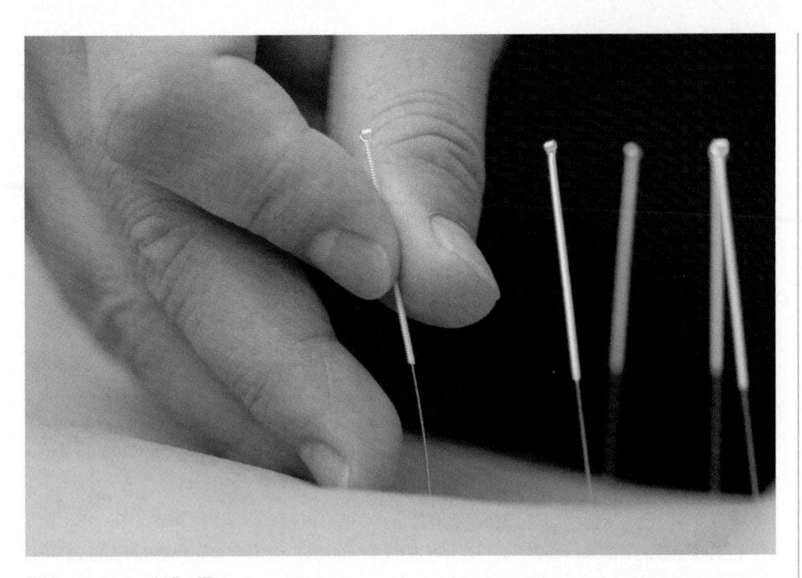

Figure 19.7 **Acupuncture, a type of traditional Chinese medicine, is an example of alternative health care.**

(sometimes spelled *qi*) (pronounced *chee*), or energy, through the body. Illness is believed to occur when chi is blocked or disrupted. Practitioners restore and rebalance chi not only to treat illness but also to prevent it, and to increase overall energy.

Herbal remedies figure prominently in this system, as do the practices of acupuncture and acupressure **(Figure 19.7).** In acupuncture, thin needles are inserted at key points in the body to balance or restore the flow of chi. A related technique, acupressure, uses firm touch at key energy points. In addition to being a common part of overall traditional Chinese care, acupuncture has also been used in Western settings for everything from pain relief to reducing nausea during cancer treatment.

Acupuncture appears to have relatively few side effects, although problems can arise when needles are not used or sterilized correctly. Acupuncture appears to be effective in treating chronic pain, in treating women's health disorders such as PMS or painful periods, and in easing side effects of cancer care.[21]

Homeopathy

Homeopathy, a Western alternative medicine system, is based on the assumption that "like cures like." That is, a substance that produces symptoms or illness is thought to cure or alleviate symptoms of that same illness, when administered in highly diluted quantities. Homeopathy is used in an attempt to treat common health problems such as nausea, sinus infections, and fever, and it is increasingly common to find homeopathic remedies for colds and flu alongside conventional medicine products on drugstore shelves.

Given the very diluted levels at which homeopathic substances are usually used, few side effects have been reported. However, many health-care providers debate homeopathy's usefulness. A large analysis of more than 100 homeopathy studies found that the practice offered no significant effect.[22]

Naturopathy

Also largely developed in Western cultures, the practice of naturopathy incorporates traditional therapies and techniques from all over the world, from herbs to dietary changes and exercise, with an emphasis on supporting health rather than treating disease. Naturopathy is especially popular with some people interested in an overall health approach that promotes wellness and prevents illness. The practice has become widespread enough to merit its own credentialing program. Care providers called *naturopaths* who have received 4 years of training and passed a licensing exam may add the credentials of "N.D." (Naturopathic Doctor) to their professional titles.

However, questions remain about naturopathy. Some treatments, such as herbs, interact in an adverse way with prescription drugs, or produce other adverse effects. According to NCCAM, scientific studies of the effectiveness of naturopathy are still preliminary.[23]

Ayurveda

Ayurveda, one of the world's oldest medical systems, originated in India. It aims to integrate and balance the body, mind, and spirit to help prevent illness and promote wellness. Ayurvedic medicine uses a variety of products and techniques, including yoga, herbal remedies, modified diets, and massage, to cleanse the body and restore balance. People who use Ayurveda, either on its own or in conjunction with conventional medicine, often choose it in the belief that it will help cleanse their body of harmful substances and energies and help restore balance, vitality, and overall health.

Some of the herbal remedies used in Ayurveda can interact adversely with prescription medications. In addition, an Ayurvedic therapy called *colonic irrigation*, which is meant to cleanse the digestive tract, can have adverse effects. One NCCAM study of Ayurvedic medications found that some contained toxins such as mercury or lead.[24] According to NCCAM, scientific studies of the effectiveness of Ayurveda are still preliminary and more research is needed.[25]

Mind–Body Medicine

This form of CAM uses techniques designed to boost the mind's capacity to affect the body. Some of these techniques, such as patient support groups, are now considered part of Western medicine. Others, such as prayer or meditation, are still considered CAM.

Mind–body practices rely on the connection between the mental and physical realms and seek to create a more positive interaction between the two. Guided imagery, hypnotherapy, and meditation are popular forms of mind–body medicine. Mind–body techniques are used to help prevent illness by reducing factors such as stress, and to help treat disorders such as depression, anxiety, and insomnia. These therapies are also sometimes used to support cancer patients by reducing patient anxiety, isolation, and stress.

Most mind–body therapies are considered relatively safe. Some studies show some benefit, but most scientists caution that that research is still preliminary. One study of the efficacy of meditation as a treatment for a variety of illnesses found some benefit, but cautioned that more research remains to be done.[26]

Natural Products

Natural products practices, also known as *biologically based practices,* rely on substances found in nature, such as vitamins and herbs. These practices focus on using herbs, other plant-derived medicines called botanicals, dietary supplements, and sometimes even beneficial microbes to treat disorders ranging from the common cold to serious conditions such as depression and cancer. Echinacea, or coneflower, for example, is popularly used to treat colds and upper respiratory infections. Natural products are also sometimes used to try to maintain wellness and prevent illness. But just because these therapies are "natural" does not make them safe. As with any medication, natural remedies may have side effects or dangerous interactions with other medicines, especially when taken in large amounts. First, we'll look at some types of natural products, and then discuss risks and safety considerations.

Nutrient Supplements

Supplements, a type of CAM now widely available, include vitamins, minerals, metabolites, and enzymes. While a balanced diet can provide all of these substances at a basic level, some CAM practices may recommend high levels of specific substances when trying to prevent or treat an illness. It is increasingly common, for example, to find the mineral zinc sold as a lozenge or throat spray to treat a cold. Or, many Americans now reach for daily fish oil supplements and the omega-3 fatty acids they contain to address a wide range of health problems, including unhealthful levels of certain fats in the blood, heart disease, and menstrual pain.

Medicinal Herbs

Herbal remedies, derived from plants, form a foundation for CAM and conventional medicine alike. Many of the pharmaceutical medications we use today are based on plants and herbs used to treat illnesses around the world for centuries. Along with echinacea, the herb taken as a cold remedy, some herbs now commonly used include:

- Black cohosh, taken to reduce symptoms of menopause
- Flaxseed and flaxseed oil, taken for a wide variety of conditions, including the prevention of heart disease and cancer
- Ginkgo, or ginkgo biloba, taken to improve circulation and memory and slow the progression of age-related dementia
- Ginseng, taken to improve immune function and memory
- St. John's wort, taken to treat depression **(Figure 19.8)**

Probiotics

These beneficial organisms help maintain the natural balance of healthful bacteria, or *microflora*, in the intestines. A healthy person's gut contains hundreds of types of beneficial bacteria, believed to help with everything from general digestion and digestive illnesses to warding off infections.[27] But certain influences, including the foods you eat and the use of antibiotics, may disrupt your bacterial balance. Probiotic supplements, usually taken in the form of a liquid, powder, or capsule, may help restore this balance. Certain foods, such as some types of naturally cultured yogurt, are also high in probiotics.

Probiotics may also grow and thrive in the body more effectively when prebiotics—carbohydrates that probiotics consume as food—are present. Prebiotics are commonly found in certain raw greens and vegetables, such as Jerusalem artichokes and onions, whole grains, and bananas.

Important Considerations about Natural Products

Natural products may not be as highly processed as pharmaceutical medications, but they are still medicines. This group of alternative therapies is among the most risky, as these substances have the potential for harm if taken in high doses or for long periods of time, or if they interact badly with conventional drugs. For example, one botanical, ephedra, is now banned in the United States because of its harmful side effects. Using natural products requires asking the same questions you'd consider when given a new prescription medication from your doctor:

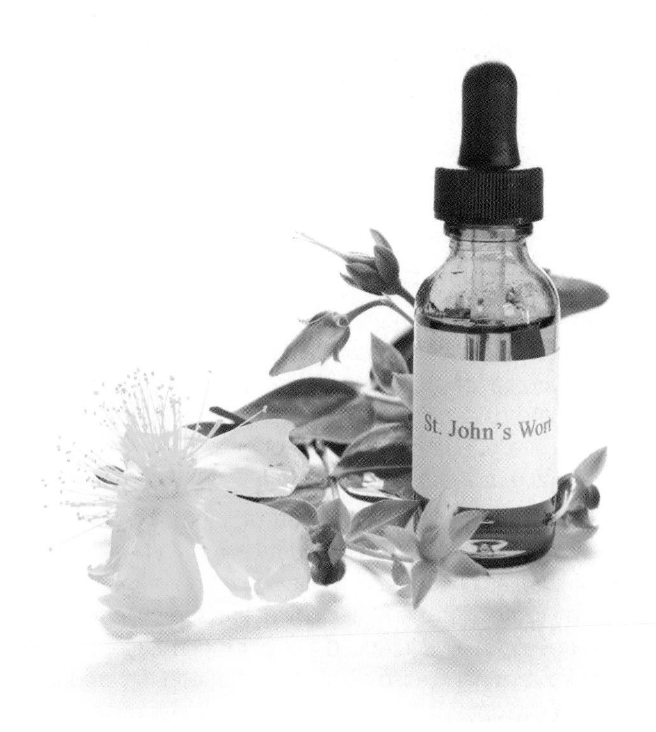

Figure 19.8 St. John's wort is a medicinal herb that can be used to help depression, but users should talk to their health-care provider before taking it.

- **Is it effective?** Whereas research has found some natural products to be effective, efficacy depends on the remedy in question and the condition it is being used to treat. Studies of the use of St. John's wort to treat depression, for example, have been mixed: One large analysis found that the herb offered benefits equal to prescription antidepressants in cases of minor depression, but minimal benefit in cases of major depression.[28] In the case of fish oil, studies have found clear benefits in addressing unhealthful levels of certain fats in the blood, but no efficacy for other conditions, such as type 2 diabetes.[29] For many natural products, research on efficacy remains inconclusive or preliminary.[25]
- **Is it safe?** As with any medicine, natural products have the potential to interact with other drugs you may be taking or even the foods you eat. St. John's wort, for example, has been found to limit the effectiveness of some prescription medications, including birth control pills and blood thinners.[28] As is true for any medicine, dose also matters. Some vitamins, such as A and D, for example, are less easily flushed from the body, and high doses have the potential to accumulate and be harmful. Even something as "natural" as fish oil, taken in doses of more than three grams per day, may be harmful by limiting the blood's ability to clot.[29] You can also review the information on evaluating supplements discussed earlier in this chapter.
- **Is it right for me?** Just because a supplement or herb seemed to help a friend doesn't mean it will be helpful for you. Your health is complex and highly personal. You might be taking a prescription medication, for example, that has the potential for harmful interactions with certain herbs. Talk to your primary care provider or student health center about natural products you are considering. Too often,

people try to manage this aspect of their care on their own: One national study of more than 22,000 adults found that of those taking supplements to support cognitive health and brain function, almost 40 percent did not discuss their supplement use with their doctor.[30] Communicating with your care team can help you make informed personal decisions about natural medicines.

Manipulative and Body-Based Practices

These therapies focus on moving, stretching, or realigning sections of the body, with a focus on restoring overall wellness by correcting parts of the body that are out of alignment. These techniques are often used to treat stiffness and pain, but may also be used to address other conditions, including stress, emotional issues, or overall healing after physical trauma such as a car accident.

Chiropractic medicine, which focuses on structure and connections of joints and muscles, is an especially popular form of this type of CAM. Practitioners, known as chiropractors, often focus on proper alignment and health of the spine, back, and neck. Credentialed chiropractors must undergo training in an accredited 4-year program after college and receive a professional license before they can add the credentials "D.C." (Doctor of Chiropractic) to their title. Another discipline, osteopathic medicine, also requires substantial training. Osteopathic doctors, (D.O.s) focus on building health through manipulation of the bones and muscles, and face educational and licensing requirements similar to conventional doctors.

Another common form of body-based practices is massage therapy. Massage relies on application of pressure to the skin, muscles, and bones. While popular as a form of stress reduction and relaxation, massage can also relieve pain, restore motion to parts of the body, and improve posture. Many health-care providers, from physical therapists to osteopaths, incorporate some form of massage into their practices.

When administered correctly, chiropractic medicine has been shown to be effective for joint and bone pain, such as low back pain.[31] Lighter forms of manipulative and body-based therapies are generally safe. But any intense physical manipulation of the body, especially of the spine, can be very dangerous, especially if a practitioner lacks training.

Energy and Movement Therapies

These forms of treatment center on the idea that manipulating energy in or entering the body will build wellness or restore health. These CAM practices either focus on fields of energy originating within the body (biofields) or from external sources (electromagnetic fields). Changing or increasing the flow of the fields of energy, practitioners say, can have a variety of health benefits, including stress reduction, pain relief, and improvement of cardiac health.

Qigong and tai chi are movement-based components of traditional Chinese medicine, which combine gentle movements, breathing, and meditation to adjust the body's chi. Many people around the world practice qigong or tai chi daily to build and maintain wellness. Magnet therapy, in which strong magnets are placed near injured or painful areas of the body, and Reiki, in which the practitioner's hands are placed on or near a patient's body in certain positions to adjust the body's energy flows, are other examples of energy treatments.

The health risks of energy therapies appear to be relatively minor. But their effectiveness remains unclear. Most of the research done to date is either preliminary or inconclusive. One large analysis of the efficacy of qigong in reducing high blood pressure, for example, found some encouraging evidence, but cautioned that further study is needed.[32]

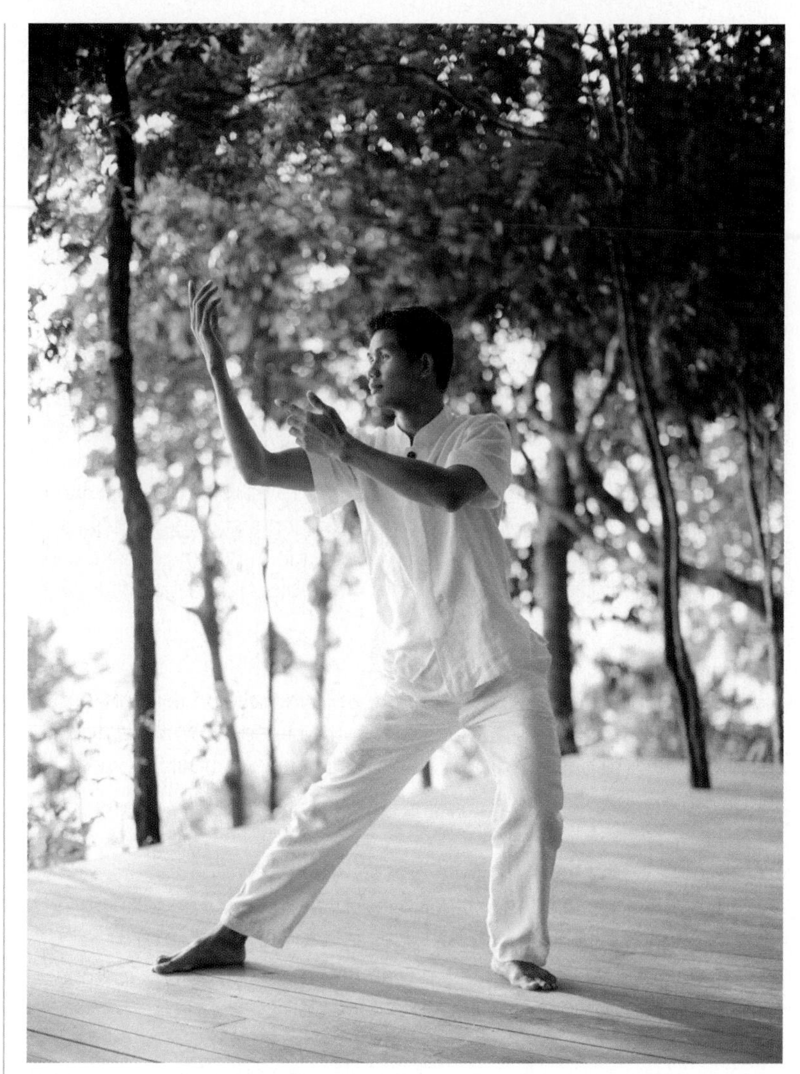

Qigong is a movement therapy that may promote physical wellness, but more research needs to be done.

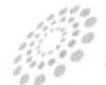 **To see qigong and tai chi in action, go to http://nccam.nih.gov/video/taichidvd-3 and http://nccam.nih.gov/video/taichidvd-4.**

Evaluating Complementary and Alternative Therapies

The effectiveness of many CAM therapies is still being studied, and research is inconclusive for many of these practices. If you are considering a CAM therapy, either on your own or through a practitioner, NCCAM offers the following suggestions:

- Take charge of your health by being an informed consumer. Find out what the scientific evidence is about any therapy's safety and effectiveness.
- Be aware that individuals respond differently to treatments, whether conventional or CAM. How a person might respond to a CAM therapy depends on many things, including the person's state of health, how the therapy is used, or the person's belief in the therapy.

what the **Affordable Care Act** means for you

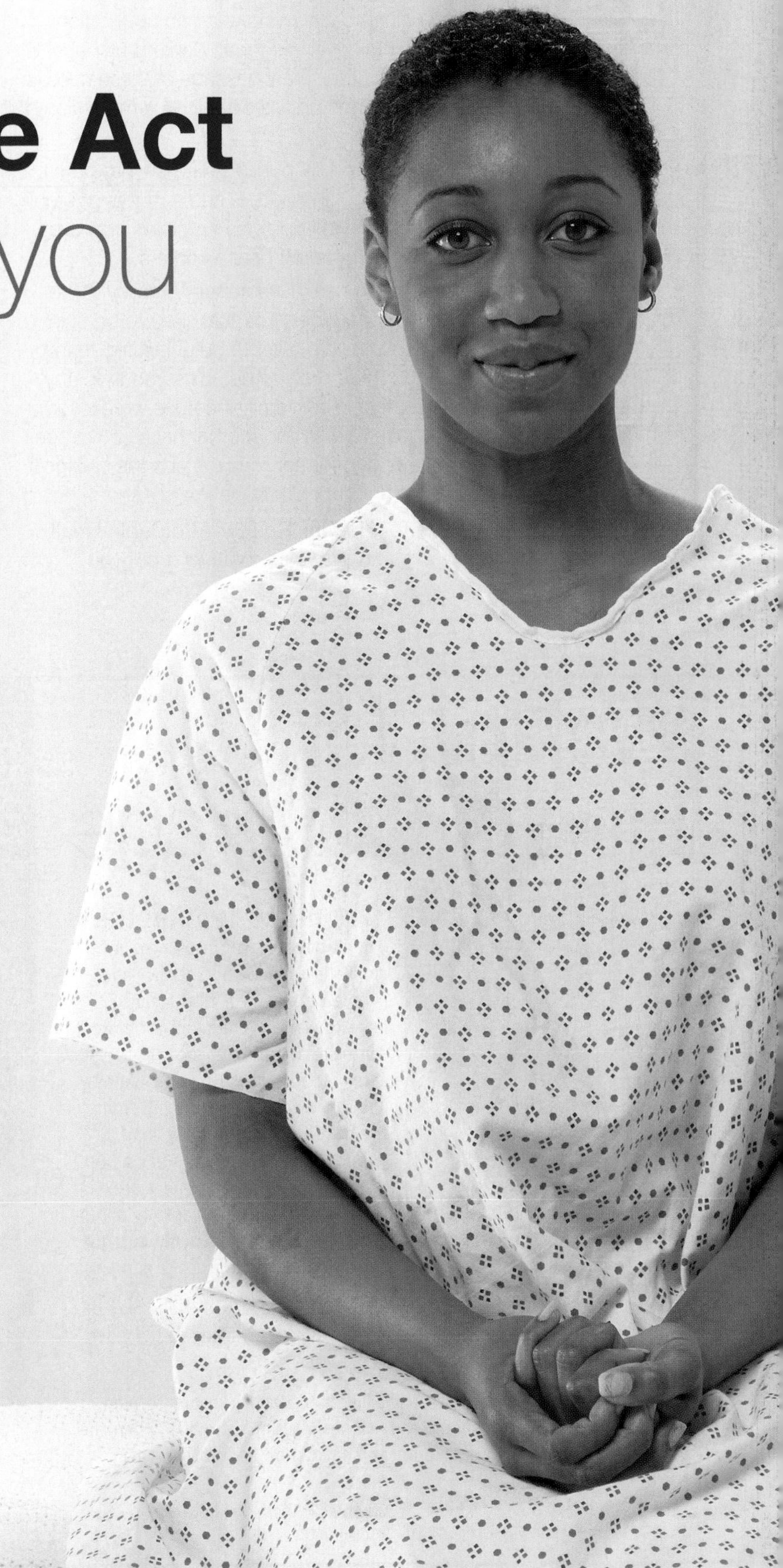

In 2012, health insurance made big headlines as the Supreme Court upheld as Constitutional key provisions of the Affordable Care Act of 2010, which was designed to increase health-care access for millions of Americans. Many of the reforms don't take effect until 2014 or later, and may face delays in some states. Others are already in place, and can make a real difference to students and young people. Here are some highlights:

- **A new requirement that many Americans be insured or pay a penalty.** This feature of the law, known as the "individual mandate," requires Americans to have at least minimal health insurance to cover emergencies and serious conditions. The penalty for not having coverage is planned to be fully in place by 2016.
- **New health insurance "exchanges."** In order to help Americans afford the cost of the insurance being required by the individual mandate, these insurance marketplaces are intended to create large pools of insured individuals and small businesses, enabling them to compare health plans and enroll at a lower cost than possible if they sought insurance independently. Individuals and small companies have typically faced higher prices and other restrictions in the insurance market, and the exchanges are intended to reduce disparities and improve access to affordable coverage. Exchanges should be available in some states as early as 2014.
- **Better protections for people with pre-existing conditions.** Children insured through private insurance plans, such as those offered through an employer, cannot be denied coverage because of pre-existing conditions. This protection has already taken effect. In 2014, adults will also be protected from discrimination based on pre-existing conditions. In the meantime, these adults can join a national "high risk pool," a group that provides consumers with immediate options for purchasing coverage.
- **Get sick, stay insured.** Health plans cannot cut off coverage if a person becomes sick, a practice known as rescission. This protection has already taken effect.
- **No lifetime limits.** Insurers can no longer place a lifetime cap on the insurance benefits you receive.
- **For young people, the magic number is 26.** You can now stay on a parent's insurance plan until your 26th birthday, if your parent so chooses.
- **Guaranteed coverage for women's health.** Eight preventive health services for women, including FDA-approved contraceptives, mammograms, and well-woman checkups, must now be offered to women in newly created health plans without any out-of-pocket cost. Under the new health-care law, women will also be shielded from having to pay more for insurance than men.

Learn more about the Affordable Care Act, including details about how the reforms affect you, at **www.healthcare.gov.**

Sources: 1. *Taking Health Care into Your Own Hands,* by HealthCare.gov (publication date not available), retrieved from www.healthcare.gov. 2. *Affordable Health Care for America: Key Provisions That Take Effect Immediately,* from the Office of Speaker Nancy Pelosi, May 3, 2010, retrieved from http://docs.house.gov/energycommerce/IMMEDIATE_PROVISIONS.pdf.

of plans receive the same protections as other Americans under the Affordable Care Act.[41] Under the proposals, insurers could no longer impose yearly dollar limits on the amount they spend on health benefits (starting in 2014), could not drop coverage when a student gets sick because of an unintentional mistake on an application, and could not deny or exclude coverage for students under age 19 because of a pre-existing condition. Final passage of these rules is increasingly likely, but still depends on the overall implementation of the Affordable Care Act.

- About 6% of students are covered by public insurance programs, such as Medicaid, for low-income individuals and families, or Medicare, for students with long-term disabilities. Recipients may also receive some care through their student health centers.
- About 20% of students have no health insurance. Among 18- to 23-year-olds, those aged 22 and older are more likely to be uninsured. Students of color are far more likely to be uninsured than white students, with Latinos more likely to be uninsured than any other group. Students reporting lower family incomes were also more likely to be without coverage. Without other health coverage, a student's only affordable option for services may be the college's student health center.

See **Practical Strategies for Health: Tips for Affordable Health Care** for ideas about how to find health care that won't put you in debt.

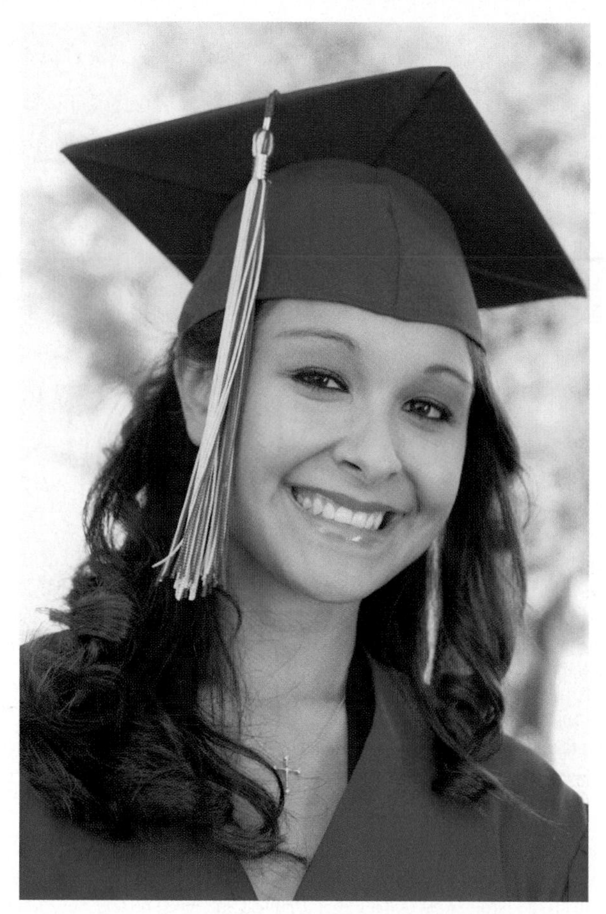

Will you still have **health insurance** when you graduate? If you're not sure, find out.

STUDENT STORY

Waiting for Health Coverage

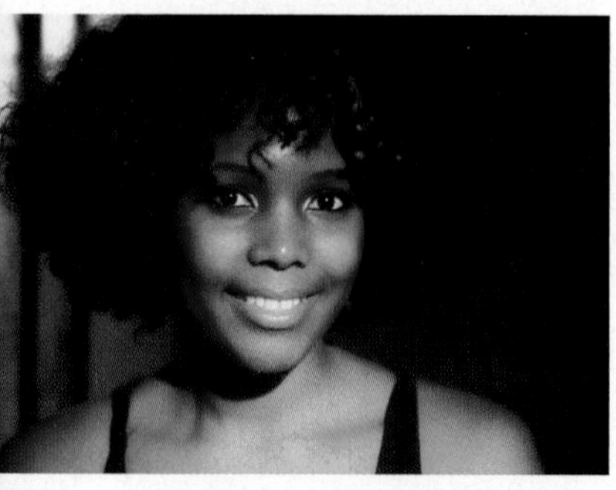

"My name is Anuella. I don't have health insurance. My mom's insurance only lets her add people once a year. That means I have to wait several months before I can have anything checked out—an ear infection, or if I break a bone—unless I want a really big bill from the hospital coming in the mail. Nobody has the money to pay a $500 bill just to get your ear checked out by a doctor. And even for a prescription, it's like $100. When I had health insurance, it was only about $20 to fill a prescription. Now it costs way more than it should cost for just a couple of little pills."

1: As a college student, what other sources of health coverage may be available to Anuella? What are her options besides waiting to be added to her mother's insurance plan?

2: Assume Anuella gets added to her mother's health insurance plan. What kinds of questions should she ask her insurance provider when she graduates from college? How long can she stay on her mother's plan?

Do you have a story similar to Anuella's? Share your story at www.pearsonhighered.com/lynchelmore.

What Happens When I Graduate?

When it's time to get your diploma, add one more task to your "to-do" list: Find out what happens to your health insurance. Students going straight to graduate school or a job offering health insurance may have little or no gap in their coverage. But if you will be going without coverage for any length of time, you'll need to take steps to protect yourself.

If you have insurance through your parents, that coverage can continue until you reach the age of 26. If you have health insurance through your school, that coverage often ends around the time of your graduation. In some cases, policies literally stop the day you graduate. In others, you may have a couple of months of coverage before you are no longer eligible. If you are covered through a public program, your insurance is less likely to be tied to your student status, but find out for sure.

When your coverage ends, you'll likely have options to extend it, but at a high price. College and university policies can often be extended, but the cost will likely be at least double the cost of the original premium. For example, if your campus policy cost $1,200 per year, you'd pay at least $2,400 per year for the extension. You may be able to extend your coverage under your family or campus policy through a program called *COBRA*, but such policies often cost at least $300 or more a month, for a yearly bill of $3,600 or more.

You may also choose to purchase a policy on the individual insurance market. For younger people who are less likely to get sick, these are often more affordable than programs such as COBRA, usually carrying premiums of about $100 to $200 a month. Many of these

Practical Strategies for Health

Tips for Affordable Health Care

No form of health-care coverage will pay for every penny of your health-care costs. To help ensure you don't wind up with medical bills that you can't afford, keep these strategies in mind:

- If you have your own insurance, make sure you understand the basic limits of the policy. How much do you have to pay in deductibles? What other out-of-pocket payments or co-pays are you responsible for? Does your insurance restrict your care geographically? Does it have a separate prescription plan? What services or providers are excluded? Does it stop covering you when you reach a certain age? What are the rules on visiting a hospital in an emergency? Make sure you keep a current copy of your insurance card, which you'll need to show medical providers when you receive care.
- Learn about what services are offered at your college's student health center. If a service isn't provided, ask about discount programs the center may have with other providers. Student health centers may have discount arrangements with local pharmacies, dentists, and other types of health providers.
- If you are uninsured or if your campus doesn't have a health center, ask your health instructor about local resources that provide free or low-cost care. Your campus or community may offer low-cost health coverage. Your campus may also offer health discount programs with local providers. There may be a nonprofit clinic nearby, or a retail clinic available at your local pharmacy.
- If you do need care, avoid heading to the emergency room or calling an ambulance unless you truly require emergency attention. Although emergency rooms are required to treat all patients who enter their doors seeking help (even patients with minor illnesses who don't have insurance), the care they provide is expensive, and you'll be billed directly. For less serious ailments, you can often receive the care you need at a much lower price from a community or retail clinic.
- Take care of your health preventively, which will help reduce the amount and cost of medical care you may need.

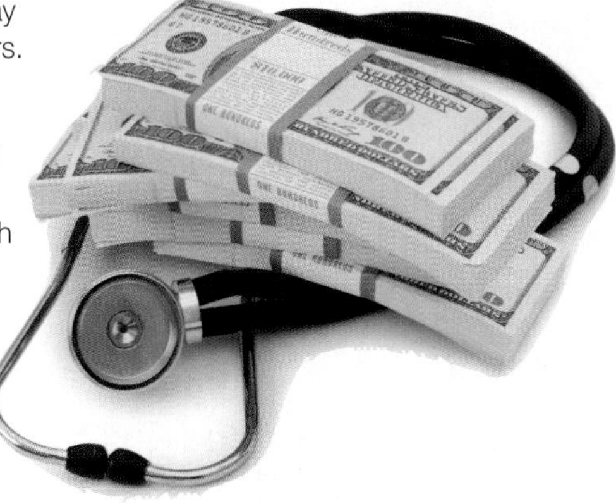

policies, however, currently offer the type of "mini-med" coverage described earlier in this chapter. Many types of services probably won't be included. Make sure you understand the limits of your policy, and purchase one that gives you as much flexibility and coverage as possible. If you'll be graduating after 2014, you may also have access to a more comprehensive individual policy through the Affordable Care Act and your state's insurance exchange. You can track the progress of creating insurance exchanges in your state at **www.healthcare.gov.**

Want to comparison shop between two health insurance policies? Visit www.money-zine.com/Calculators/Insurance-Calculators/Health-Care-Insurance-Cost-Calculator.

"Personalized Medicine" and the Future of Consumer Health

New medical advances against major diseases such as cancer are made each year. In the coming years, however, few advances will have as much potential to fundamentally reshape how you think about your health as personal **genomics.** Defined broadly as the study of the human **genome** (the biological code that "builds" a human being), genomics once seemed largely confined to science fiction. But with the decoding of the human genome completed in 2003, our understanding of this "code of life" has made it possible for us to examine our own genomes and understand some of the information they hold about our health. The goal of this effort is **personalized medicine,** or health care based on the idea that because your individual DNA is unique, your health is as well, and your care and treatments should be tailored to you.

genomics The study of genomes and their effects on health and development.

genome The genetic material of any living organism.

personalized medicine Health care based on the idea that because your individual DNA is unique, your health is as well, and your care and treatments should be tailored to you.

A Short Course in Genetics and Genomics

Genomics sounds complex—and it is—but to get a basic understanding of your own genome, you only need to know a few key concepts:

- **DNA** (deoxyribonucleic acid) is the material that carries the biological instructions that "build" us. These instructions are *genetic*, meaning that they are inherited from our parents and ancestors. For example, your DNA is genetic information because you inherited it from your mother and father, who passed their DNA on to you when you were conceived. If you have a genetic disorder, it means you have a health condition passed on in the DNA you inherited from someone in your family.
- **Genes** are packets of DNA that carry the code for specific building blocks in your body.
- **Chromosomes** are packets of genes and supporting DNA that make up your genome.
- **Your genome** is your entire collection of DNA, coiled in a tight double spiral. Copies of your genome are found in almost every cell in your body. Although all human beings share mostly the same DNA, everyone's genome contains a few unique differences, or *genetic variants*. Your variants make you distinct in many ways, including in some of the ways your health may develop.
- **Your genome is not your destiny.** Though DNA is powerful, it is not the only factor that determines who you are or how healthy you may be. Environment and behavior choices are also powerful forces that can shape your health.

Uses of Genomic Information

As our understanding of the human genome evolves, this information is rapidly transforming health care. In the past, health has often been discussed in terms of "one size fits all" or "one size fits many." But genomic information increasingly enables people, either on their own or through their care providers, to find approaches more likely to work for them on an individual basis. Here are some of the ways genomic understanding is reshaping health.

family health history A detailed record of health issues in one's family that presents a picture of shared health risks.

whole-genome scanning A form of genetic testing that looks for variants within a person's genome.

genome sequencing The full decoding of an entire genome.

Family Health Histories

Federal health officials now encourage everyone in the United States to create a basic **family health history,** or a record of health conditions that have appeared in a family over time. Health histories used to be reserved for families with rare genetic conditions, such as the blood clotting disorder hemophilia. Now, however, genomic research has revealed that many common health conditions, such as type 2 diabetes, high cholesterol, and heart disease, have a genetic component. Creating a family health history enables you and your relatives to look for patterns of illness that might indicate genetic risk. If you find that you are at greater risk for a disease, you can then take steps early to minimize your risk by making healthier choices, such as improving your diet or seeking out certain screening tests earlier or more frequently.

You can find information on creating a family health history at www.hhs.gov/familyhistory.

Single-Gene Testing

If you or your care provider think you are at risk for a genetic illness, you may opt to have genetic testing, or analysis of a certain gene or section of a particular chromosome. Such *single-gene testing* can tell you whether you carry DNA variants known to be linked to particular health conditions. Some women with particular family backgrounds, for example, choose to be tested for breast cancer–related variants in genes called *BRCA1* and *BRCA2*. If they find that they are at increased genetic risk, they may opt for medical treatments that reduce their risk.

These tests are powerful, but they are also expensive and emotionally complex. Most such genetic testing is usually conducted with the help and support of a *genetic counselor*, a medical professional who helps patients understand genetic testing, assess their own feelings and beliefs about such testing, decide whether they want testing, and determine how they will respond to the results. As genomics becomes a larger part of our health system, the number of genetic counselors is growing rapidly.

Whole-Genome Scanning and Sequencing

Other genetic technologies enable you to read your whole genome at once and see what it says about your risk for a variety of health conditions. In some cases, this form of testing only looks at specific points on your genome, a process called **whole-genome scanning.** Scientists can also decode and spell out every point on your genome, a process called **genome sequencing.** Scanning is simpler and cheaper, and is thus more widely available. Full-genome sequencing remains far too costly for most people.

Although assessment of your whole genome holds great promise for providing a broad look at what your genome says about your health, this form of testing remains controversial. Proponents say that whole-genome assessment is now ready for widespread use. Critics counter that our understanding of health-related genetic risks is still too new for the information to be of much practical medical use, and that related ethical considerations can be complicated. For example, if you discovered that you carried a particular genetic mutation related to an increased risk of cancer, would it change how you lived your life? Would you want health insurance companies to know? What and when would you tell your children about their own possible risk?

If you find yourself thinking about any form of DNA testing, consider speaking with a genetic counselor first to help you find options that are right for you. These health-care professionals are experts in explaining genetic options and helping people sort through personal values as they consider genetic testing or personalized medicine.

DNA Tests and Medical Choices

In addition to providing information about risks for certain illnesses, DNA information can sometimes help us decide how to treat them. Each of us, for example, carries DNA variants that affect how our

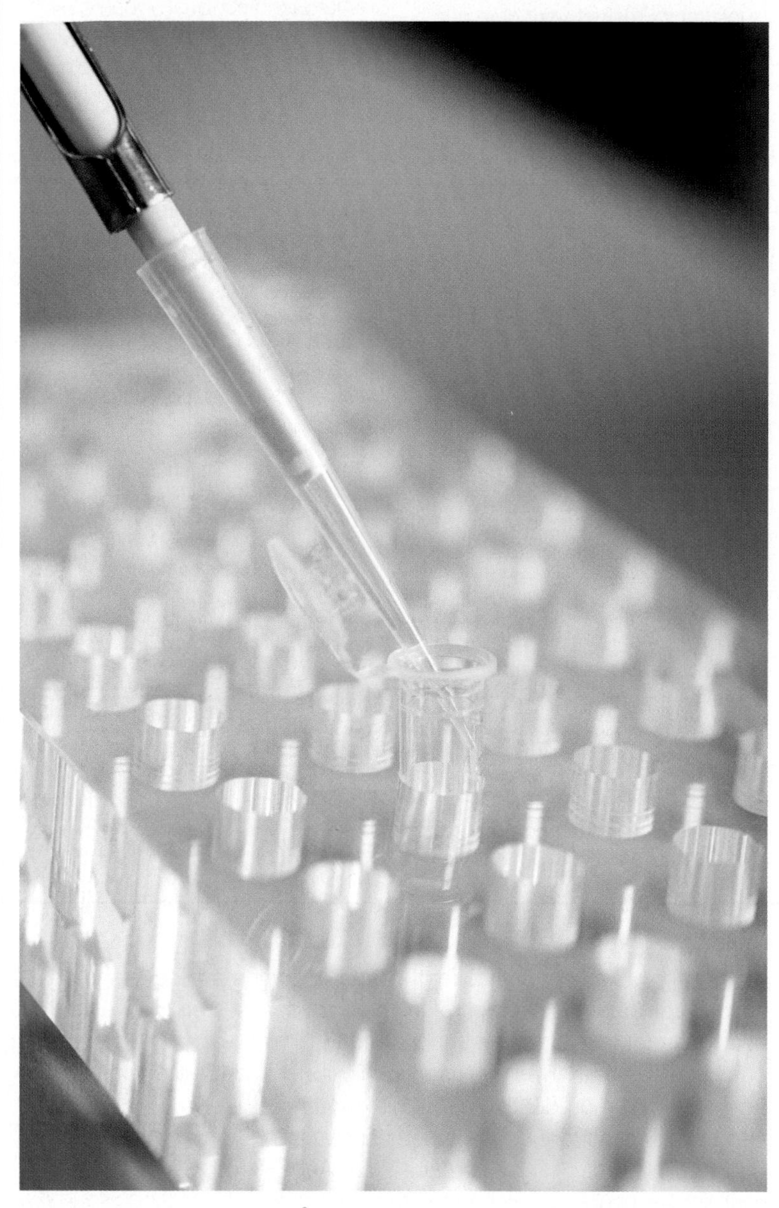

Advances in **genomics** are resulting in high-tech options for personalized health care.

bodies process certain medications. The study of this DNA–drug interaction, called **pharmacogenomics,** has already changed the way doctors prescribe certain blood thinners and other medications. In the case of some cancers, doctors can now analyze the DNA of tumors to determine which treatments might best stop them.

Ethical, Social, and Legal Implications of Genomic Advances

Genomic advances can enable you to take a more personal approach to your health. But for many, it also raises doubts and fears. What about privacy? Will others use your genetic information to discriminate against you? Will DNA differences that you carry appear in medical records that can be used to justify higher insurance premiums?

These questions are already shaping new laws designed to help build a lifetime of better health in the genomic era. In 2008, after more than a decade of debate, U.S. lawmakers enacted the *Genetic Information Nondiscrimination Act*, or *GINA*. This law strengthens the privacy of personal DNA information and prohibits genetic discrimination in health insurance and employment.

Still, other questions remain. Should genetic discrimination also be barred in other types of insurance, such as disability insurance? How widely should personal DNA information be shared? Will DNA knowledge make people feel more empowered about their health, or more hopeless? These and other important questions will continue to spur discussion and regulation as the genomic revolution unfolds.

Change Yourself, Change Your World

"Be a smart patient? My own best health-care advocate? I'm just trying to get through this term!" The idea of being an active health consumer may feel a little daunting, but paying attention to just a few basic steps on a regular basis will go a long way.

pharmacogenomics The use of DNA information to choose medications and make prescribing decisions.

Personal Choices

Investing a little time in these five areas will pay off, now and in the long run:

- **Practice prevention.** Use the information you've gained from this course and this book to build and maintain wellness. Take the **Self-Assessment** to see if you're practicing prevention enough.
- **Make informed choices.** Spend time learning about any new health option. If you don't have the information you need, ask. Make sure you get all the details.
- **Find the right care before you need it.** Don't wait until you are sick to find a doctor. Learn about care providers on campus and in your community. That knowledge will make everything easier when you do need care.
- **Know when you need help.** When you have the busy schedule of a student, it's easy to push health issues aside for later. But waiting can mean complications. Taking an hour to visit the student health center might make the difference between resting for a day or two and losing a bigger chunk of time to illness. If you have questions or concerns about your health, get help early.
- **Know how you'll pay.** Few surprises can be as bad as a big medical bill that you didn't expect. Before you get sick, understand your health insurance, what it covers, and what costs it leaves in your hands. If you have an HSA or FSA, stay on top of your balance.

Campus Advocacy

You don't have to wait for federal health-care reform to help your fellow students get the care they need. Across the country, groups of students are working to bring insurance reform and more affordable coverage to their campuses.

At Tufts University in Massachusetts, for example, students formed the Students Health Organizing Coalition (SHOC) in 2008 to help address the needs of their peers with little or no insurance coverage and sizable amounts of medical debt. The group first met with campus officials, and then expanded its reach to state regulators and legislators, demanding insurance reform.

SHOC's work led to a state report that exposed larger profit margins for student insurers, even if they offered less coverage than other types of health insurance. The state of Massachusetts then decided to offer improved insurance coverage to state residents at most state schools. SHOC representatives later testified on a panel before the U.S. Senate as federal lawmakers considered student insurance reform.

To help improve insurance coverage for students on your campus, start by asking friends and classmates about their insurance experiences. Host a roundtable discussion, or set up an online forum where fellow students can post their stories. You are likely to find that many of your fellow students face insurance dilemmas. Once you know the nature of such issues on your campus, you and other concerned students can speak with your campus administrators and health center about possible changes that help get everyone on your campus the coverage—and health care—they need.

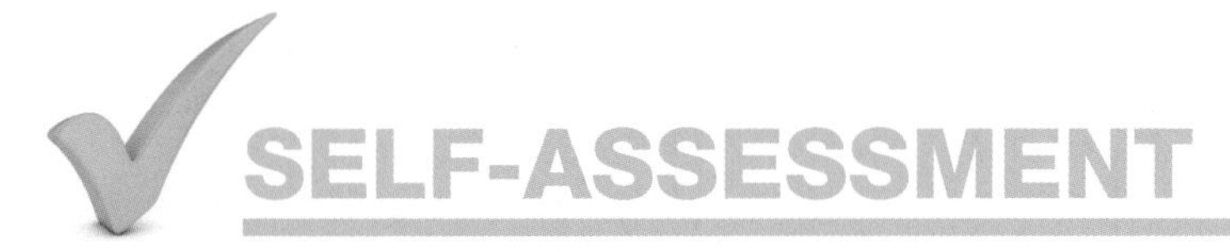

How Proactive Are You About Preventive Health Care?

1.	Have you visited a doctor for a physical exam in the past year?	yes	no
2.	If female, have you had a gynecological exam (including a Pap test) in the past year?	yes	no
3.	Do you regularly brush your teeth and floss?	yes	no
4.	Have you visited a dentist in the past 6 months?	yes	no
5.	Have you had a general vision exam in the past 2 years?	yes	no
6.	Have you received a tetanus/diphtheria booster shot in the past 10 years?	yes	no
7.	Have you received an influenza vaccination in the past year?	yes	no
8.	Have you received a meningococcal vaccine in the past 5 years?	yes	no
9.	If female and under 26, have you ever received an HPV vaccination?	yes	no
10.	Do you have health insurance?	yes	no

HOW TO INTERPRET YOUR SCORE

The more "yes" responses you gave, the more proactive you are about preventive health care. See Table 19.1 for a list of recommended health screenings.

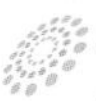
Take this self-assessment online at www.pearsonhighered.com/lynchelmore.

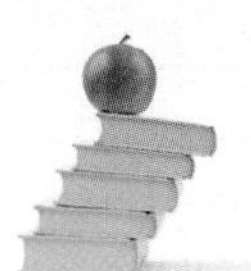

Choosing to Change Worksheet

To complete this worksheet online, visit www.pearsonhighered.com/lynchelmore.

It's easy to be passive about health care, and to not worry about preventive care or having health insurance until you get sick or injured. But a little planning and action in advance can greatly pay off down the line by reducing the risks of developing an illness and by offering you protection if or when you do need medical care.

Directions: Fill in your stage of change in Part I and complete the rest of the Part with your stage of change in mind. Regardless of your stage of change, everyone should complete Part II.

Part I: Becoming Proactive about Preventive Care

Step 1: Your Stage of Behavior Change. Check one of the following statements that best describes your readiness to be proactive about your healthcare.

_____________ I do not plan to take part in preventive care in the next 6 months. (Precontemplation)

_____________ I might take part in preventive care in the next 6 months. (Contemplation)

_____________ I am prepared to begin taking part in preventive care in the next month. (Preparation)

_____________ I have been taking part in preventive care for less than 6 months. (Action)

_____________ I have been taking part in preventive care for 6 months or longer. (Maintenance)

Step 2: Response to Self-Assessment. Complete the Self-Assessment on page 539.

1. Which questions did you answer "No" to? Based on this Self-Assessment, what can you do to be more proactive about your preventive care?

____

____

____

2. What concerns or obstacles, if any, do you have about the preventive care behaviors described in this chapter? Write down who you could contact to ask questions about your concerns or how you could overcome these obstacles.

Example: I am concerned that having an eye exam will cost a lot of money. I could visit the campus health center to see if there are any low-cost programs for optometrist visits.

____

____

____

3. Regardless of your stage of change, what do you think the benefits of practicing proactive care are? What are the drawbacks?

Benefits: ____

Drawbacks: ____

Part II: Scheduling Preventive Care Appointments

Use this worksheet to start becoming more proactive about your health.

	Past Behavior	Future Behavior
Physical exam	When was the last time you had a physical exam? ______________	When will you schedule your next exam? ______________
Gynecological exam with Pap test (for females)	When was the last time you had a gynecological exam? ______________	When will you schedule your next exam? ______________
Dental care	When was the last time you visited a dentist? ______________	When will you schedule your next exam? ______________
Vision care	When was the last time you had a general vision exam? ______________	When will you schedule your next exam? ______________
Tetanus/diphtheria booster shot	When was the last time you received a tetanus/diphtheria booster shot? ______________	If it's been over 10 years since your last booster, when will you schedule your next vaccination? ______________
Protection from influenza	When was the last time you received an influenza vaccination? ______________	If it's been over a year since your last vaccination, when will you schedule your next one? ______________
Health insurance	Do you have health insurance? ______________	If you do not have health insurance, when will you investigate the options available to you? ______________

Chapter Summary

- Our health system is increasingly one in which individuals have an abundance of choices, but also the responsibility of researching information, critically evaluating it, and making educated decisions.
- Self-care includes maintaining basic wellness habits, evaluating health information critically, using over-the-counter medications properly, exercising caution when taking dietary supplements, using home health tests properly, and knowing when it is time to see a doctor.
- Preventive care, such as periodic screenings and checkups, can help prevent health problems or catch them early when they are often easier to treat.
- Conventional medicine is characterized by a focus on the physical aspects and treatment of disease; the presence of discernible, defined symptoms; the maintenance of public health; and the use of scientific evidence and the scientific method.
- Conventional care is now available from a wide variety of facilities and providers, ranging from hospitals to student health centers to retail clinics.
- When choosing a primary care provider, find out whether he or she is covered by your insurance plan, and ask friends and family for recommendations. When you attend an appointment with your provider, make sure he or she listens to you, answers your questions completely, and treats you with respect. Be vocal and honest with your provider about all aspects of your health.
- Complementary and alternative medicine (CAM) encompasses therapies and practices outside those of conventional medicine. CAM practices often look beyond the physical aspects of disease to issues that connect mind, body, and spirit.
- Examples of CAM include traditional Chinese medicine, biologically based practices such as the use of herbs and botanicals, mind–body therapies, manipulative therapies, and energy therapies.
- CAM is popular, but many CAM practices have not been proven effective, and some have not been proven safe. Research any CAM therapy or provider before starting care, and make sure both your CAM and conventional practitioners know the full range of care you are receiving as well as your health history and habits to make sure you are being treated safely.

- Options for paying for health care include discount health programs, health insurance, health savings accounts, and flexible spending accounts.
- The Affordable Care Act, a set of national health-care reforms upheld as Constitutional by the Supreme Court in 2012, already offers greater insurance options and protections for many people, and intends to make it easier for individuals and small businesses to buy affordable insurance beginning in 2014.
- Health insurance policies come in many forms, including managed-care plans, fee-for-service plans, and public plans. Under the Affordable Care Act, policies will be available through state-run exchanges beginning in 2014. Under this system, many Americans will be required to purchase health insurance or pay a penalty beginning in 2016.
- Genomics is the study of the human genome. Genomic research is spurring the development of personalized health care based on an individual's DNA.
- Examples of genomic applications in health care include prenatal testing, testing for single-gene disorders, whole-genome scanning, and genome sequencing.

Test Your Knowledge

1. What is NOT an example of preventive care?
   a. eating nutritiously
   b. wearing a seatbelt
   c. scheduling regular physicals
   d. taking cold medication correctly

2. What are the typical characteristics of credible health-related research?
   a. publication in a peer-reviewed journal
   b. a large pool of study participants
   c. results that have been replicated by other scientists
   d. all of the above

3. Which of the following is true about dietary supplements?
   a. There is scientific consensus about their health benefits.
   b. They are extensively evaluated for safety by government agencies before they can be sold.
   c. They may not be appropriate for certain populations.
   d. There are regulations governing the general marketing claims they can make.

4. Which of the following is NOT considered a practitioner of conventional medicine?
   a. medical doctors
   b. acupuncturists
   c. nurse practitioners
   d. dentists

5. Screening tests are
   a. used to analyze certain genes or segments of a chromosome.
   b. used to monitor the progress of a disease.
   c. used to identify a disease when symptoms are present.
   d. used to identify a disease when symptoms are not present.

6. What is acupuncture an example of?
   a. alternative medicine
   b. conventional medicine
   c. energy therapy
   d. naturopathy

Get Critical

What happened:

Actress Christina Applegate has enjoyed a long and varied career as a comic actress in film and television. While the roles she plays usually tend to be more light-hearted, she has weathered a serious health crisis in her private life: breast cancer at the age of 36. Because she developed the disease at such a young age, Applegate decided to undergo genetic testing for *BRCA* mutations. The test revealed that she carries a *BRCA1* mutation, greatly elevating her lifetime risk of breast cancer. Applegate responded by undergoing a double mastectomy to prevent her cancer from returning.[1] Since her diagnosis and surgery in 2008, her work on stage and screen has continued steadily, she has created Right Action for Women—a foundation to help other young women with breast cancer—and she gave birth to her first child, a baby girl, in 2011.

What do you think?

- **Have you or has anyone in your family undergone genetic testing?**
- **If not, would you consider it? Under what circumstances?**
- **Would you make major medical or life decisions based on the results of a genetic test? What resources would you turn to in helping you make those decisions?**
- **If you did undergo genetic testing, your results may also have relevance for your biological relatives—would you feel obligated to share your results with them? What might be the pros and cons of sharing your genetic information with your family?**

Reference: 1. "Applegate Has Double Mastectomy," by the British Broadcasting Corporation, August 19, 2008, retrieved from http://news.bbc.co.uk/2/hi/entertainment/7570211.stm.

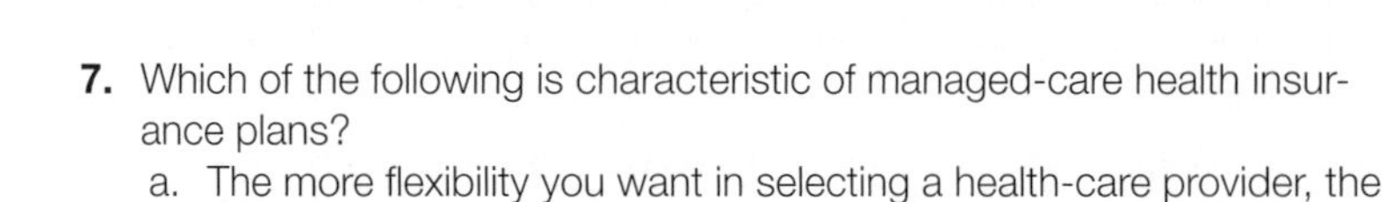

7. Which of the following is characteristic of managed-care health insurance plans?
   a. The more flexibility you want in selecting a health-care provider, the more the insurance will cost.
   b. They don't cover medication.
   c. There are no out-of-pocket fees associated with them.
   d. They offer no flexibility for medical care outside of the plan's approved providers.

8. One provision of the Affordable Care Act is that young people can stay on a parent's insurance plan until what maximum age?
   a. 18
   b. 21
   c. 26
   d. 30

9. Analyzing a person's DNA to assess his or her risk of developing a single-gene disorder is an example of
   a. whole-genome scanning.
   b. single-gene testing.
   c. genome sequencing.
   d. genetic variation.

10. The study of DNA–drug interactions is called
   a. pharmacogenomics.
   b. chemogenomics.
   c. genetic polypharmacy.
   d. carrier testing.

Get Connected 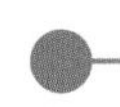

Mobile Tips!

Scan this QR code with your mobile device to access additional tips about consumer health. Or, via your mobile device, go to **http://mobiletips.pearsoncmg.com** and navigate to Chapter 19.

Health Online **Visit the following websites for further information about topics in this chapter:**

- The Medical Library Association's Top 100 List: Health Websites You Can Trust
  http://caphis.mlanet.org/consumer/index.html
- Evaluating Health Information on the Internet (from the National Cancer Institute)
  www.cancer.gov/cancertopics/cancerlibrary/health-info-online
- Agency for Healthcare Research and Quality (AHRQ)
  www.ahrq.gov
- National Center for Complementary and Alternative Medicine
  http://nccam.nih.gov
- The Human Genome Project
  www.ornl.gov/sci/techresources/Human_Genome/home.shtml

Website links are subject to change. To access updated web links, please visit ***www.pearsonhighered.com/lynchelmore***.

References 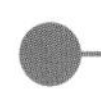

i. Pew Internet & American Life Project. (2011). *Health topics*. Retrieved from http://pewinternet.org/Reports/2011/HealthTopics.aspx.

ii. Slone Epidemiology Center at Boston University. (2006). *Patterns of medication use in the United States: A report from the Slone survey*. Retrieved from http://www.bu.edu/slone/SloneSurvey/AnnualRpt/SloneSurveyWebReport2006.pdf.

iii. Stasio, M., Curry, K., Sutton-Skinner, K., & Glassman, D. (2008). Over-the-counter medication and herbal or dietary supplement use in college: Dose frequency and relationship to self-reported distress. *Journal of the American College Health Association, 56* (5), 535–547.

1. Pew Internet & American Life Project. (2010). *Generations 2010*. Retrieved from http://pewinternet.org/Reports/2010/Generations-2010.aspx.

2. Stellefson, M., Hanik, B., Chaney, B., Chaney, D., Tennant, B., & Chavvaria, E. (2011). eHealth literacy among college students: A systematic review with implications for eHealth education. *Journal of Medical Internet Research, 13* (4), e102.

3. University of California, San Francisco. (2012). *Evaluating health information.* Retrieved from http://www.ucsfhealth.org/education/evaluating_health_information/index.html.

4. Slone Epidemiology Center at Boston University. (2006). *Patterns of medication use in the United States: A report from the Slone survey*. Retrieved from http://www.bu.edu/slone/SloneSurvey/AnnualRpt/SloneSurveyWebReport2006.pdf.

5. U.S. Food and Drug Administration, Center for Drug Evaluation and Research. (2009). *Regulation of nonprescription products*. Retrieved from http://www.fda.gov/cder/Offices/otc/default.htm.

6. Stasio, M., Curry, K., Sutton-Skinner, K., & Glassman, D. (2008). Over-the-counter medication and herbal or dietary supplement use in college: Dose frequency and relationship to self-reported distress. *Journal of the American College Health Association, 56* (5), 535–547.

7. Kittinger, P., & Herrick, D. (2005). Patient power: Over-the-counter drugs. *National Center for Policy Analysis, Brief Analysis, 524.* Retrieved from http://www.ncpa.org/pub/ba524.

8. American Academy of Family Physicians. (2010). *When should I go to the emergency department?* Retrieved from http://www3.acep.org/patients.aspx?id=26018.

9. Porter, R. S. (ed.). (2007). *The Merck manual of medical Information—Home edition.* Whitehouse Station, NJ: Merck & Co., Inc. Available at http://www.merck.com/mmhe.

10. Kanchanaraksa, S. (2008).) *Evaluation of diagnostic and screening tests: Validity and reliability.* PPT lecture notes, Johns Hopkins Bloomberg School of Public Health. © The Johns Hopkins University and Sukon Kanchanaraksa. Retrieved from http://ocw.jhsph.edu/courses/fundepi/PDFs/Lecture11.pdf.

11. Gum, Q., Dillon, C., & Burt, V. (2010). Prescription drug use continues to increase: U.S. prescription drug data for 2007–2008. *NCHS Data Brief, 42*. Retrieved from http://www.cdc.gov/nchs/data/databriefs/db42.htm.

12. Berkot, B. (2011, April 19). U.S. drug spending slows; hits $307 bln in 2010: Report. *Reuters*. Retrieved from http://www.reuters.com/article/2011/04/19/us-drug-spending-idUSTRE73I4G920110419.

13. U.S. Food and Drug Administration. (2012). *The FDA's drug review process: Ensuring drugs are safe and effective.* Retrieved from http://www.fda.gov/Drugs/ResourcesForYou/Consumers/ucm143534.htm.

14. Aspden, P., Wolcott, J., Bootman, J., & Cronenwett, L. (2007). Preventing medical errors: Quality chasm series. Washington, DC: The National Academies Press.

15. Centers for Disease Control and Prevention. (2012). Inpatient surgery (FastStats). Retrieved from http://www.cdc.gov/nchs/fastats/insurg.htm.

16. Hollingsworth, J., Krein, S., Ye, Z., Kim, H., & Hollenbeck, B. (2011).) Opening of ambulatory surgery centers and procedure use in elderly patients. *Archives of Surgery. 146* (2),187–193.

17. Agency for Healthcare Research and Quality. (2002). *Quick tips when planning for surgery.* Retrieved from http://www.ahrq.gov/consumer/quicktips/tipsurgery.htm.

18. Van Den Bos, J., Rustagi, K., Gray, T., Halford, M., Ziemkiewicz, E., & Shreve, J. (2011). The $17.1 billion problem: The annual cost of measurable medical errors. *Health Affairs, 30* (4), 596–603.

19. American Academy of Family Physicians. (2009). *Tips for talking to your doctor*. Retrieved from http://familydoctor.org/online/famdocen/home/patadvocacy/healthcare/837.html; American Academy of Family Physicians. (2010). *Medical errors: Tips to help prevent them*. Retrieved from http://familydoctor.org/online/famdocen/home/healthy/safety/safety/736.html.

20. National Center for Complementary and Alternative Medicine. (2007). CAM basics: What is CAM? Retrieved from http://nccam.nih.gov/health/whatiscam/overview.htm.

21. Park, J., Linde, K., Manheimer, E., Molsberger, A., Sherman, K., Smith, C., . . . Schnyer, R. (2008). The status and future of acupuncture clinical research. *Journal of Complementary and Alternative Medicine, 14* (7), 871–881.

22. Shang, A., Huwiler-Müntener, K., Nartey, L., Juni, P., Dörig, S., Sterne, J., Pewsner, D., & Egger, M. (2005). Are the clinical effects of homoeopathy placebo effects? Comparative

study of placebo-controlled trials of homoeopathy and allopathy. *The Lancet, 366* (9487), 726–732.

23. National Center for Complementary and Alternative Medicine. (2009). *Backgrounder: An introduction to naturopathy.* Retrieved from http://nccam.nih.gov/health/naturopathy.

24. National Center for Complementary and Alternative Medicine. (2009, May). *Backgrounder: Ayurvedic medicine: An introduction.* Retrieved from http://nccam.nih.gov/health/ayurveda/introduction.htm.

25. National Center for Complementary and Alternative Medicine. (2009). *Backgrounder: Herbs at a glance.* Retrieved from http://nccam.nih.gov/health/herbsataglance.htm.

26. Arias, A., Steinberg, K., Banga, A., & Trestman, R. (2006.) Systematic review of the efficacy of meditation techniques as treatments for mental illness. *Journal of Alternative and Complementary Medicine, 12* (8), 817–832.

27. Weichselbaum, E. (2010.) Potential benefits of priobiotics – main findings of an in-depth review. British Journal of Community Nursing, 15(3), 110-114.

28. National Center for Complementary and Alternative Medicine. (2012).) *Get the facts: St. John's wort and depression.* Retrieved from http://nccam.nih.gov/health/stjohnswort/sjw-and-depression.htm.

29. National Library of Medicine. (2012). *MedlinePlus: Fish oil.* Retrieved from http://www.nlm.nih.gov/medlineplus/druginfo/natural/993.html.

30. Laditka, J., Laditka, S., Tait, E., & Tsulukidze, M. (2012, February 8). Use of dietary supplements for cognitive health: Results of a national survey of adults in the United States. *American Journal of Alzheimer's Disease & Other Dementias.*

31. Chou, R., Qaseem, A., Snow, V., Casey, D., Cross, J., Shekelle, P., Owens, D., the Clinical Efficacy Assessment Subcommittee of the American College of Physicians, & the American College of Physicians/American Pain Society Low Back Pain Guidelines Panel. (2007). Diagnosis and treatment of low back pain: A joint clinical practice guideline from the American College of Physicians and the American Pain Society. *Annals of Internal Medicine, 147*, 478–491.

32. Lee, M., Pittler, R., Guo, M., & Ernst, E. (2007.) Qigong for hypertension: A systematic review of randomized clinical trials. *Journal of Hypertension, 25* (8), 1525–1532.

33. National Center for Complementary and Alternative Medicine. (2009). *CAM basics: Are you considering complementary and alternative medicine?* Retrieved from http://nccam.nih.gov/health/decisions/consideringcam.htm.

34. National Center for Complementary and Alternative Medicine. (2009). *CAM basics: Selecting a complementary and alternative medicine practitioner.* Retrieved from http://nccam.nih.gov/health/decisions/practitioner.htm.

35. World Health Organization. (2008). *World health statistics: Global health indicators*. Retrieved from http://www.who.int/entity/whois/whostat/4.xls.

36. California Healthcare Foundation. (2012). *Healthcare costs 101.* Retrieved from http://www.chcf.org/publications/2012/08/health-care-costs-101.

37. Kaiser Family Foundation. (2011). Employer health benefits 2011 annual survey. Retrieved from http://ehbs.kff.org/?CFID=192542357&CFTOKEN=12627353&jsessionid=6030ad11146e96c8e8fd352f1477544d1283.

38. U.S. Government Accountability Office. (2008). *Health insurance: Most college students are covered through employer-sponsored plans, and some colleges and states are taking steps to increase coverage.* Report GAO-08-389. Retrieved from http://www.gao.gov/new.items/d08389.pdf.

39. Jost, T. (2008). Access to health care: Is self-help the answer? *Journal of Legal Medicine, 29,* 23–40.

40. Collins, S. (2008). Consumer-driven health care: Why it won't solve what ails the United States health system. *Journal of Legal Medicine, 28,* 53–77.

41. U.S. Department of Health and Human Services. (2011). *New rule ensures students get health insurance protections of the Affordable Care Act.* Retrieved from http://www.hhs.gov/news/press/2011pres/02/20110209a.html.

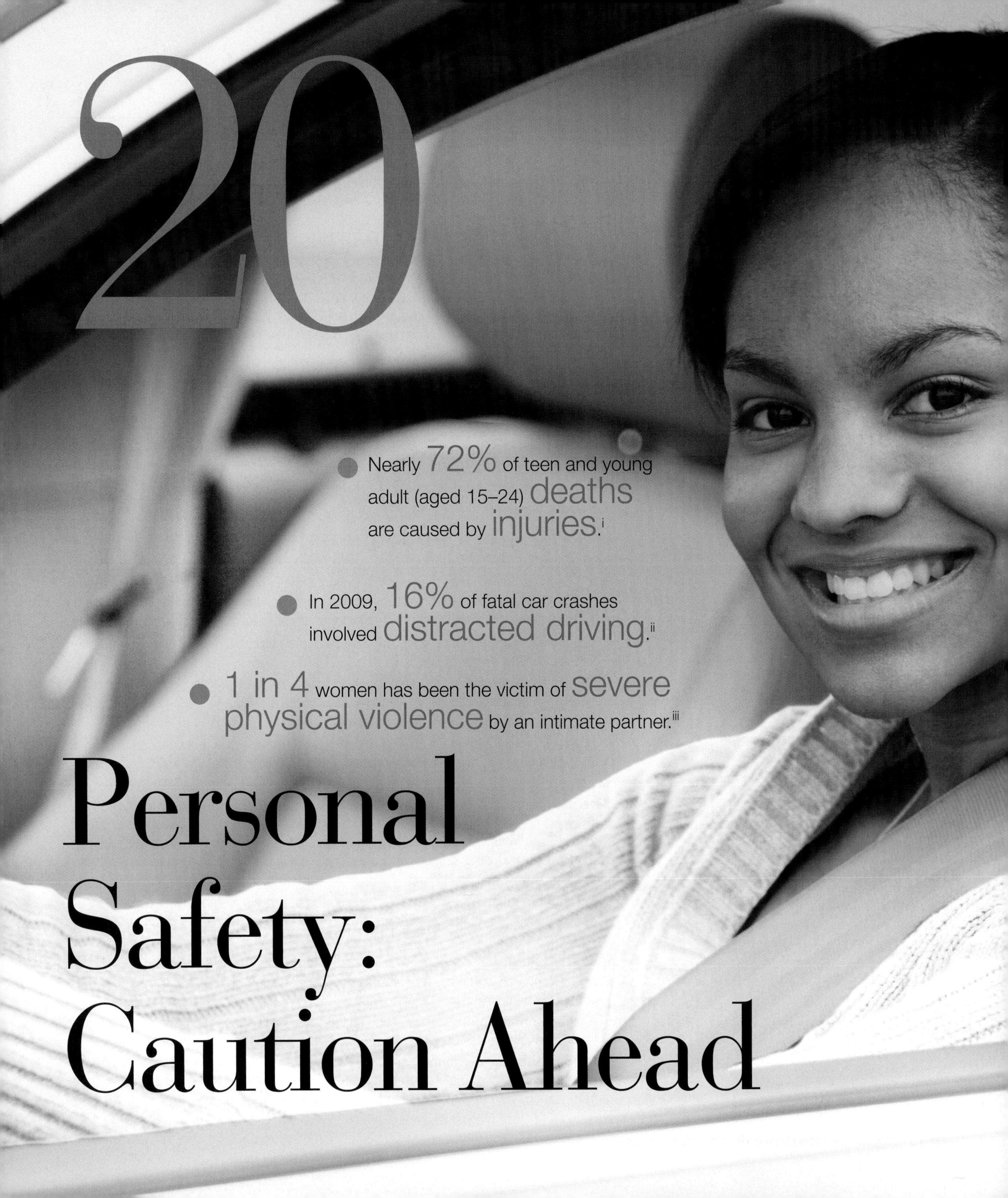

20

- Nearly 72% of teen and young adult (aged 15–24) deaths are caused by injuries.[i]
- In 2009, 16% of fatal car crashes involved distracted driving.[ii]
- 1 in 4 women has been the victim of severe physical violence by an intimate partner.[iii]

Personal Safety: Caution Ahead

Stay out of trouble!

LEARNING OBJECTIVES

IDENTIFY the most common unintentional injuries and contributing factors.

DISCUSS ways you can reduce your risk of motor vehicle accidents.

EXPLAIN how to reduce your risk of poisonings, drownings, falls, and fires.

DEMONSTRATE proper body mechanics for typing, texting, lifting, and wearing a backpack.

DISCUSS violence within communities, including school and campus violence.

DEFINE and **DESCRIBE** intimate partner violence, including the factors that keep victims in abusive relationships.

IDENTIFY strategies for preventing sexual violence.

EXPLAIN how you can help improve campus safety.

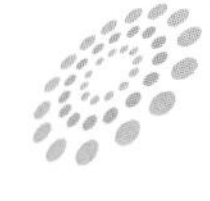

Health Online icons are found throughout the chapter, directing you to web links, videos, podcasts, and other useful online resources.

Did your parents ever shout this warning as you headed out the door? And if so, what did it mean to you? Driving within the speed limit? Staying sober at parties? In this chapter, we use the term **personal safety** to describe anything people do to stay out of trouble. Specifically, it's the practice of making decisions and taking actions that reduce your risk of injury and death.

Injuries are the number-one killer of Americans between the ages of 1 and 44.[1] They cause more deaths among people in this age group than all types of diseases—heart disease, cancer, infections, etc.—put together. According to national estimates, injuries cost our economy over 400 billion dollars each year in direct medical costs and productivity losses.[2] The good news is that a handful of simple choices can help you significantly reduce your injury risk.

Injuries fall into two main categories. An **unintentional injury** is any bodily damage not deliberately inflicted. Common examples are injuries sustained in motor vehicle accidents, falls, and fires. **Intentional injuries,** on the other hand, are purposefully inflicted through physical or sexual violence. Note that self-inflicted injuries and suicide are considered intentional injuries.

personal safety The practice of making decisions and taking actions that reduce your risk of injury and death.

unintentional injury (accidents) Bodily damage that is not deliberately caused.

intentional injury Physical harm that is purposefully inflicted through violence.

Overview of Unintentional Injuries

Unintentional injuries, or those that occur without intent to cause harm, send more than 28 million people to emergency rooms in the United States each year.[3] In 2010, they caused over 118,000 deaths among Americans of all ages.[1] The National Safety Council (NSC) ranks the leading causes of unintentional injury death as follows:[4]

- Motor vehicle accidents caused over 35,000 deaths in 2010, making them the primary cause of unintentional deaths.[1]
- Unintentional poisonings, including drug overdose, rank a close second, killing about 30,000 Americans annually.[5]
- Falls, which account for about 25,000 deaths annually, are third.[5]
- Choking, drowning, and fires are the fourth to sixth most common causes of unintentional injury deaths. Together they account for about 10,000 deaths each year.[5]

We tend to think of unintentional injuries as *accidents*, happening by chance without any perceptible cause. However, public health officials point out that unintentional injuries typically involve one or more contributing factors such as intoxication, fatigue, and distraction. For this reason, many unintentional injuries are considered preventable. Although every type of unintentional injury has unique circumstances, as a group they have some risk factors in common:

- **Substance abuse.** Heavy alcohol consumption or other substance abuse increases the risk of many types of unintentional injuries. Alcohol is a factor in 60% of fatal burn injuries and drownings and 40% of fatal motor vehicle accidents and falls.[6]
- **Sex.** Males account for almost two-thirds of the deaths attributed to unintentional injuries.[5]
- **Age.** Compared with other age groups, young people (aged 15 to 29) account for the largest proportion of overall injury death.
- **Environmental factors.** Factors such as increased traffic volume or poor weather conditions can increase risk of automobile, motorcycle, bicycle, or recreational injury.
- **Divided attention.** Performing any type of potentially dangerous activity without completely focusing on the task at hand increases the risk of injury. This includes everything from texting while driving to surfing the Internet while cooking.

STUDENT STATS

Top Five Causes of Death in the United States among People Aged 15–24

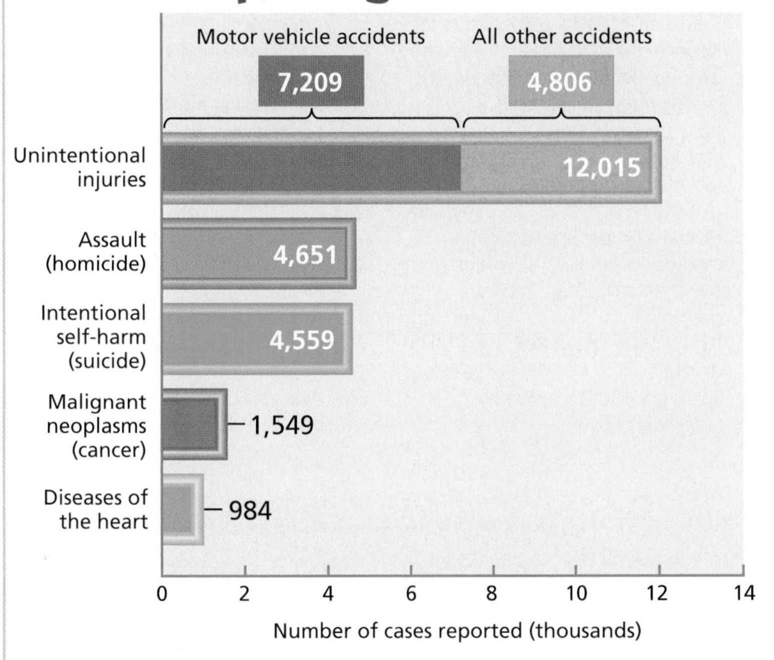

Source: Data from *Deaths: Preliminary Data for 2010,* by S. L. Murphy, J. Q. Xu, & K. D. Kochanek, January 11, 2012, *National Vital Statistics Reports 60* (4), Hyattsville, MD: National Center for Health Statistics, retrieved from http://www.cdc.gov/nchs/data/nvsr/nvsr60/nvsr60_04.pdf.

- **High-risk activity.** Certain activities are at least moderately risky no matter what precautions are taken. Skiing and snowboarding cost an average of 40 lives each year in the United States, and mountaineering fatalities average about 25 per year.[7,8] Many sports, from soccer to competitive diving, can lead to injury.

Motor Vehicle Accidents

On average each year, more than 2 million people in the United States are injured in a motor vehicle accident (MVA); in 2010, more than 35,000 died.[1] About one-quarter of all deaths among people between the ages of 15 and 24 are due to MVAs.[1] No other single cause of death claims more young lives.

What Factors Increase the Risk for Motor Vehicle Accidents?

The National Safety Council identifies the following as key factors contributing to MVAs.

Distracted Driving

Talking on your phone, sending a text message, or fiddling with your stereo while you drive dramatically increases your chance of getting into a car accident. Consider these statistics:

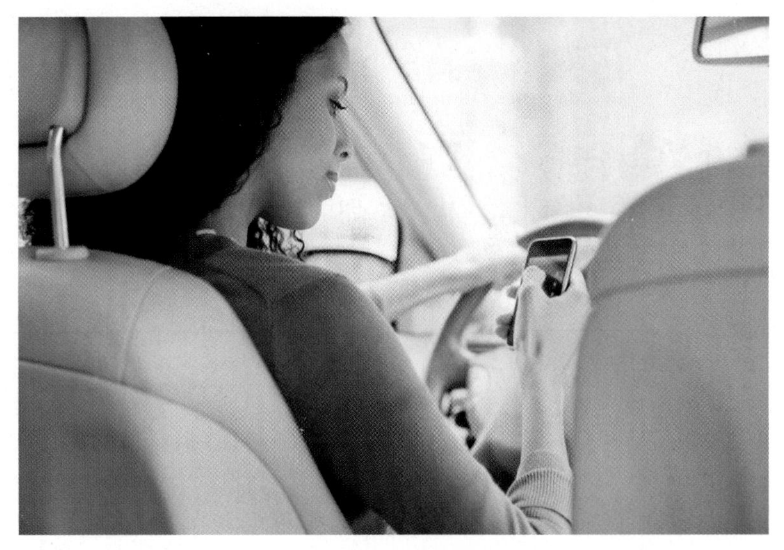

Texting while driving is incredibly dangerous.

- In 2009, 5,474 people were killed in MVAs involving distracted driving. These crashes represented 16% of all fatal MVAs that year. Nearly 20% of them involved cell phone use.[9]
- The risk of getting into a car accident that causes injury goes up fourfold when a driver is speaking on a cell phone.[10] Studies have found that even if you are speaking on a hands-free cell phone, you are just as distracted, and one study indicated that you may be just as impaired as a legally intoxicated driver.[11,12,13]
- The risk of an MVA goes up eightfold when texting while driving.[10] It's hardly surprising, then, that texting while driving has been outlawed in 35 states and the District of Columbia.[14] In 2012, a Massachusetts court found a teen guilty of vehicular homicide for causing a fatal car crash by texting while driving. The teen was sentenced to 4 years in prison. Sentences in upcoming texting-while-driving fatality cases are expected to be similar.

Despite the dangers of distracted driving, a 2011 study found that a startling 91% of college students admit to texting while driving.[15] Another study found that 92% of college students read text messages while driving, and that 70% even initiate messages while driving.[16]

 **Try the *New York Times* game that tests how distracted you become while trying to text message while driving: www.nytimes.com/interactive/2009/07/19/technology/20090719-driving-game.html.**

Impaired Driving

Impaired driving includes driving after you've been drinking or using drugs, as well as driving while drowsy. All forms are extremely dangerous.

Driving with a blood alcohol concentration of 0.08% or higher is illegal in all 50 states. But drinking even a small amount of alcohol impairs your vision, motor control, and coordination, impedes your ability to do two things at the same time, and reduces your judgment and alertness—all necessary for driving. In 2009, 32% of all MVA deaths were linked to a driver who'd been drinking.[17]

Drugs other than alcohol, such as marijuana or cocaine, are also a factor in MVAs, as are some prescription and over-the-counter

SELF-ASSESSMENT

Take this self-assessment online at www.pearsonhighered.com/lynchelmore.

Are You an Aggressive Driver?

Do you have aggressive habits that could threaten your safety or the safety of others on the road? Circle yes or no for each question.

Do you . . .

1. Overtake other vehicles **only** on the left? yes no
2. Avoid blocking passing lanes? yes no
3. Yield to faster traffic by moving to the right? yes no
4. Keep to the right as much as possible on narrow streets and at intersections? yes no
5. Maintain appropriate distance when following other vehicles, bicyclists, or motorcyclists? yes no
6. Provide appropriate distance when cutting in after passing a vehicle? yes no
7. Use headlights in cloudy, raining, or low-light conditions? yes no
8. Yield to pedestrians? yes no
9. Come to a complete stop at stop signs or before a right turn at a red light? yes no
10. Stop for red traffic lights? yes no
11. Approach intersections and pedestrians at slow speeds to show your intention and ability to stop? yes no
12. Follow right-of-way rules at four-way stops? yes no
13. Drive below posted speed limits when conditions warrant? yes no
14. Drive at slower speeds in construction zones? yes no
15. Maintain speeds appropriate for conditions? yes no
16. Use turn signals for turns and lane changes? yes no
17. Make eye contact and signal intentions where needed? yes no
18. Acknowledge intentions of others? yes no
19. Use your horn sparingly around pedestrians, at night, around hospitals, and at other times? yes no
20. Avoid unnecessary use of high beam headlights? yes no
21. Yield and move to the right for emergency vehicles? yes no
22. Refrain from flashing headlights to signal a desire to pass? yes no
23. Drive trucks at posted speeds, in the proper lanes, using nonaggressive lane changing? yes no
24. Make slow, deliberate U-turns? yes no
25. Maintain proper speeds around roadway crashes? yes no
26. Avoid returning inappropriate gestures? yes no
27. Avoid challenging other drivers? yes no
28. Try to get out of the way of aggressive drivers? yes no
29. Refrain from momentarily using High Occupancy Vehicle (HOV) lanes to pass vehicles? yes no
30. Focus on driving and avoid distracting activities (e.g., smoking, use of a cell phone, reading, shaving)? yes no
31. Avoid driving when drowsy? yes no
32. Avoid blocking the right-hand turn lane? yes no
33. Avoid taking more than one parking space? yes no
34. Avoid parking in a disabled space (if you are not disabled)? yes no
35. Avoid letting your door hit the car parked next to you? yes no
36. Avoid using the cell phone while driving? yes no
37. Avoid stopping in the road to talk with a pedestrian or other driver? yes no
38. Avoid inflicting loud music on neighboring cars? yes no

HOW TO INTERPRET YOUR SCORE

0–3 "no" answers: Excellent
4–7 "no" answers: Good
8–11 "no" answers: Fair
12–38 "no" answers: Poor

Source: Adapted from *Are You an Aggressive Driver or a Smooth Operator?* by the New Jersey Office of the Attorney General, Division of Highway Traffic Safety, retrieved from http://www.state.nj.us/lps/hts/SO_Quiz.pdf.

medications. Sleep medications as a factor in MVAs have been the focus of intense media coverage; however, pain medications, anti-anxiety medications, and even over-the-counter cold remedies can also affect driving skills. A total of 19 states have strict laws that forbid any presence of a prohibited substance in the blood of drivers.[18]

Research studies have consistently found that drowsiness is a factor in about 1 out of 6 fatal MVAs.[19] Fatigue slows your reaction time and reduces your attention level, ability to process information, and the accuracy of your short-term memory, all of which impair your driving and your ability to avoid an accident. Yet more than 40% of drivers admit to having fallen asleep behind the wheel. As of 2010, New Jersey was the only state with a law specifically prohibiting driving while drowsy; however, prosecutors in various parts of the United States have won convictions of drivers involved in fatal MVAs who got behind the wheel knowing they were drowsy.

Watch a video on the dangers and legal consequences of drowsy driving at www.youtube.com/watch?v=GO1cvqYMExo.

Skipping Seat Belts

Almost all states require that drivers and passengers use seat belts and, if they are young children, child safety seats. Yet about 17% of vehicle occupants don't consistently use these proven lifesavers.[20] Seat belt use is lowest among people between the ages of 16 and 24; however, college students do better than their peers. In a national survey, less than 4% stated that they don't wear a seat belt consistently—or ever.[21]

The benefits of seat belts are unrivaled. Some people fail to buckle up in the belief that airbags provide sufficient crash protection, but it's just not true: Seat belts are the single most effective prevention against injury or death in a car crash.[22] Between 2004 and 2008, seat belts saved 75,000 lives. One benefit of seat belts is that they prevent you from being thrown from the car—an event that is five times more deadly than if you remain in the car during an accident.[23]

Speeding and Other Forms of Aggressive Driving

Aggressive driving is defined by the National Highway Traffic Safety Administration as the operation of a motor vehicle in a manner that endangers or is likely to endanger people or property. Examples of aggressive driving include speeding, driving too quickly for road conditions, cutting off other vehicles, tailgating, and abruptly changing lanes. Aggressive driving is estimated to be a factor in more than 55% of fatal car crashes.[24]

Speeding—driving at a rate above the posted speed limit—reduces the amount of time you have to react to conditions in the road in front of you, increases the distance needed to stop in an emergency, and reduces the effectiveness of safety devices like seat belts and airbags. On average, 1,000 drivers a month are killed in speed-related accidents.[25]

How Can You Reduce Your Risk for Motor Vehicle Accidents?

Proven risk-reduction strategies include making wise decisions before and during your trip, and maintaining a safe vehicle.

Practice Prevention

Your first line of defense is prevention. Don't get behind the wheel if you've been drinking—even a small amount—or using any other drugs. Pick a designated driver, use your campus's SafeRides program, or call a cab. Never get in a car with a driver who is impaired. If possible, take away the keys of someone who has been drinking or using drugs and wants to get behind the wheel. One bad decision can kill you or others.

Don't drive if you haven't had adequate sleep. You might not feel sleepy, but many drivers in drowsy-driving MVAs report that they did not feel sleepy before they nodded off.

Don't set off if you haven't allowed enough time for your trip. If you can't get where you want to go by the time you want to get there, stay home, call, and reschedule.

Another preventive strategy is to brush up on your driving skills. Consider taking a defensive driving course. The National Safety Council offers these courses for novice and experienced drivers in communities, state programs, and via online self-study. Find out more at www.nsc.org.

Finally, before you set off, buckle up. It only takes a second. And in most states, it's the law.

Drive Defensively

Once you get on the road, the following actions can help you avoid being involved in an MVA.

- **Stay within speed limits.** Driving fast reduces your ability to adjust to driving conditions and avoid accidents.
- **Slow down when the weather is bad.** Poor weather conditions mean it may take longer to stop the car on a wet surface, vision could be reduced, or roads could be icy.
- **Don't tailgate.** Tailgating, or following too closely to the car in front of you, increases your chances of an accident by reducing the amount of time and distance you have to react to events in front of you. Use the 3-second rule when following: Make sure you are following at such a distance that it takes at least 3 seconds for your car to cross a fixed reference point after the car in front of you crosses it. When driving at higher speeds, on slippery roads, or when you are being followed by a tailgater, increase your distance even more.
- **Follow the rules of the road.** Signal before turning or changing lanes, look both ways before entering an intersection, check your blind spot, make a full stop at all stop signs, and obey traffic signals.
- **Don't text or otherwise distract yourself.** Put your phone out of reach before you get in the car. If you must talk or text, pull over to the side of the road. Set up your music before you start driving. Don't try to eat, shave, or put on make-up, even if you are stopped in traffic or at a stoplight.
- **Stay aware of other drivers.** If you notice someone ahead driving erratically, he or she may be intoxicated or drowsy. Increase the distance between your cars, such as by slowing down or changing lanes. You may even decide that your safest bet is to pull over and call 9-1-1.
- **Take a break if you start to feel sleepy.** If you get drowsy, pull fully off the road into a lighted parking lot or rest area. If possible, drink a cup of coffee or another caffeinated beverage, then roll up your windows and lock your doors, and take a short nap—about 15 to 20 minutes. By the time you wake up, the caffeine will have had a chance to get into your system. Leave the car for a few minutes of fresh air and exercise before getting back behind the wheel. On long drives, take a break every 2 hours or 100 miles to get out of the car, stretch, and check your level of fatigue.

STUDENT STORY

Car Accident

"Hi, my name is Caleb. When I was 16 years old, I got in my very first car accident. I've been in other car accidents since then, but this was by far the worst. I was in a rush one day, and I was going through an intersection that I thought was a four-way stop and just stopped at the stop sign, didn't really look either way and continued going. Well, it turns out it was a two-way stop and there was a guy going about 40 miles an hour, and all I heard was just the blare of his horn. Within an instant the guy hit me. I was able to keep control of the car and I was wearing my seat belt, so I wasn't hurt at all, but my back left passenger door was just obliterated. The window was shattered out. The door was dented in beyond repair. I know if I hadn't been wearing my seat belt, any number of injuries could have happened."

1: What personal and environmental factors increased Caleb's risk of getting into a car accident?

2: What could Caleb have done to prevent that car accident from occurring?

 **Do you have a story similar to Caleb's? Share your story at www.pearsonhighered.com/lynchelmore.**

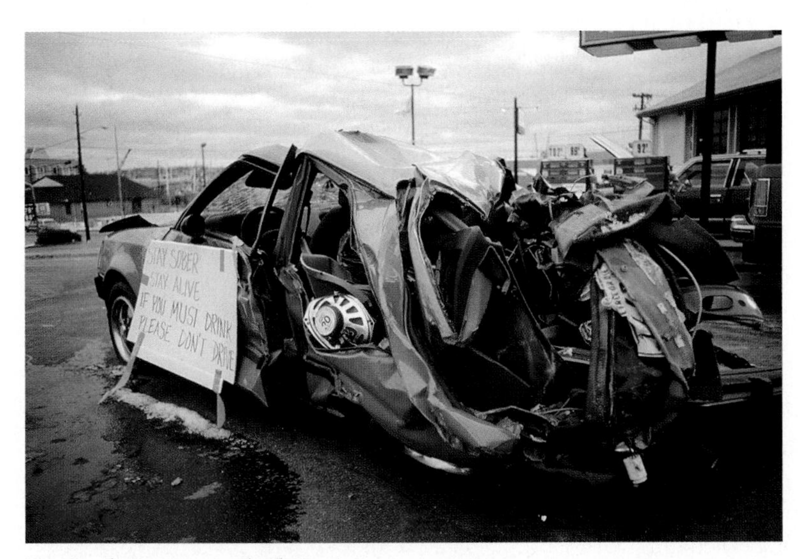
STAY SOBER
STAY ALIVE
IF YOU MUST DRINK
PLEASE DON'T DRIVE

Drinking and driving can kill you or others.

Maintain a Safe Vehicle

You can also keep yourself safer on the road by keeping your car in good condition and choosing and using additional safety features whenever possible. Make sure you have enough gas to get where you're going, and that your oil and windshield-washer fluid levels are adequate. Check the air pressure in your tires. And make sure that your headlights—both high and low beams—and wipers are in working order.

When you are looking at a new car, consider some of the following safety features.

Airbags. Airbags inflate in a fraction of a second after an accident, protecting you from impact against the car's interior or outside objects. As soon as a crash begins, sensors determine the severity of the crash, and deploy the airbags if it's serious enough. Driver and passenger airbags are required by law for all new passenger cars, SUVs, and light trucks. Some cars also offer optional side-impact airbags, which provide added protection during a sideways collision.

Although airbags provide protection during an accident, they are designed to be used with seat belts, and adults and children should always wear seat belts whenever they are in a car.

View just how quickly an airbag deploys at www.iihs.org/video.aspx/info/static_airbag.

Child safety seats. Car crashes are the leading cause of death for children in the United States.[26] Parents should use rear-facing car seats for infants until they reach the height or weight limit for the seat, at least until the child is 1 year old or 20 pounds. Although state laws vary, most require that children over a year old sit in forward-facing child safety seats until they are at least 4 years old or 40 pounds. Once children outgrow safety seats, parents should use booster seats to ensure that seat belts are positioned properly against the child—lap belt against the upper thighs and shoulder belt crossing the chest. Once a child is 4 feet, 9 inches tall, the booster seat can be removed.

Antilock brakes. Most new vehicles offer antilock brakes, which provide more traction in emergency braking situations, such as on slippery roads or when you brake suddenly. If you don't have antilock brakes, you can still prevent them from locking up by not "slamming on the brakes." Instead, apply the brakes with a pumping motion.

Electronic stability control. One new technology that greatly reduces the risk of accidents is electronic stability control (ESC). ESC uses sensors and computers in the car to recognize what the driver is doing. If the driver suddenly turns the steering wheel, a move that can lead to a spin-out or a rollover, ESC will make automatic shifts in speed or direction to reduce the risk of loss of control. Studies show that ESC can reduce fatal single-car accidents by 51% and fatal multi-car accidents by 19%, a safety benefit so dramatic that beginning with 2012 models, all cars, SUVs, pickups, and minivans are required to be equipped with standard ESC.[27]

Other Traffic Injuries

Accidents while walking, jogging, or cycling on roadways can also cause injuries, one of the more common of which is **traumatic brain injury (TBI).** TBI is caused when the head is jolted or hit, or when an object pierces the skull, resulting in a sudden injury that damages the brain. While many TBI patients recover quickly, a significant number face a lifetime of disability, and some die. Each year, about 1.7 million Americans sustain a TBI.[28] Spinal cord injuries, fractures, and internal injuries are also common in MVAs involving pedestrians and cyclists.

traumatic brain injury (TBI) An injury that disrupts normal functioning of the brain, caused by a jolt or blow to the brain or a penetrating head wound.

Accidents Involving Pedestrians and Cyclists

In 2009, just over 4,000 pedestrians were killed in traffic accidents, and 59,000 were injured.[17] The majority of these accidents occurred in the twilight and evening hours. Although the primary factor was improper crossing of a roadway, more than 10% occurred because the pedestrian was not visible to the driver. Thus, it's important to wear reflective clothing whenever you go out for an evening walk or run. Unlike cyclists, pedestrians should always travel on the side of the road opposite the direction of traffic, so that you're facing oncoming vehicles, and wherever there are sidewalks, use them.

Overall, the number of MVA injuries, while still significant, has been declining—except among motorcycle riders. The rate of motorcyclists injured in crashes almost doubled from 1998 to 2008.[29] In 2009 about 84,000 motorcycle riders and passengers were injured and, of those, nearly 4,600 died.[17] Over half the motorcyclists injured in crashes are involved in "single-vehicle crashes," meaning that no other motorcycle or car was a factor. According to traffic safety statistics, motorcyclists are about six times more likely than those riding in a car to die in a crash.[17] Even though motorcycles are known to be more dangerous than cars, fewer than half of all states require that adults wear a helmet when riding a motorcycle, a factor that contributes to injuries and deaths.[17]

Bikes may not pack the force or speed of a car or motorcycle, but riding one still carries risks. According to national statistics, about half a million people—mostly boys and younger men—wind up in emergency rooms because of bike crash injuries each year in the United States, with about 50,000 of these involving motor vehicles. In 2009, 630 died.[30]

Although cars need to make room on the road for bikes, bike riders are responsible for road safety as well. In one study of bike crashes, cyclists were found to be at fault about half the time, mostly due to unsafe riding habits such as riding against traffic and running stop signs.[31] Unlike pedestrians, cyclists should always travel in the same direction as the flow of vehicular traffic.

As with motorcycles, varying helmet laws contribute to the injury statistics. Though many states have laws requiring bike helmets for teens and children who ride, more than a dozen do not, and in most states, helmets are optional for adults. Even if it is not legally required in your area, wearing a proper helmet while on a bike is essential for reducing the risk of TBIs. In a national survey, 68% of college students who ride a bike said they only sometimes, rarely, or never wear a bike helmet.[21]

Safety Tips for Pedestrians and Cyclists

The likelihood of being in an accident can be reduced if you follow these simple guidelines.

- **Follow the rules of the road.** Pedestrians and cyclists may be more nimble than cars, but avoid the temptation to bend the rules. When on foot, cross in designated crosswalks, and travel against the flow of traffic. When cycling,

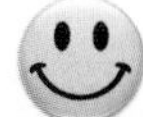

Practical Strategies for Health

Preventing RSI When Working on a Computer

Knowing how to set up your computer for optimal posture can help you avoid RSI.

- Keep your neck in a neutral position by using a laptop stand, monitor risers, books, or packages of paper to raise the top of the screen to about eye level.
- Angle the screen to avoid bending your head forward.
- Use a document holder to position documents you are typing from vertically, rather than bending your head to look at them.
- Allow for good hand and wrist posture by placing your keyboard and mouse on an adjustable keyboard tray that can be moved up or down. Keyboard and mouse should be positioned slightly at or below elbow height. If a laptop is your main computer, set up a work station with a regular-size external keyboard and mouse attached to it.
- When typing, don't bend and twist your hand to reach awkward key combinations. If you need to hit multiple keys at once, use a separate hand for each key, rather than contorting your hand to reach both keys with the same set of fingers.
- Keep your wrists straight. Don't rest your palms on the keyboard so that your hands are angled up from your wrists. Your wrists should be straight and your fingers should reach down slightly to find the keys.
- Use a chair that supports a comfortable upright or slightly reclined posture. Prop your feet up to maintain a comfortable trunk-thigh angle, if needed.
- Position the screen at a right angle to windows to reduce glare. Use a desk lamp or laptop light that plugs into a USB port for extra light, if needed.
- Clean your screen frequently with computer-safe antistatic cleaning material. Dust on the screen can make it difficult to read and increase eyestrain.
- Stop and stretch every 30 to 45 minutes.
- When carrying a laptop, use a wheeled case or a backpack with wide, padded straps, rather than a bag that places all the weight on one shoulder.

Adapted from *Ergonomic Tips for Laptop Users*, by U.C. Berkeley's Ergonomics Program for Faculty and Staff, 2007, retrieved May 2010 from http://uhs.berkeley.edu/facstaff/pdf/ergonomics/laptop.pdf.

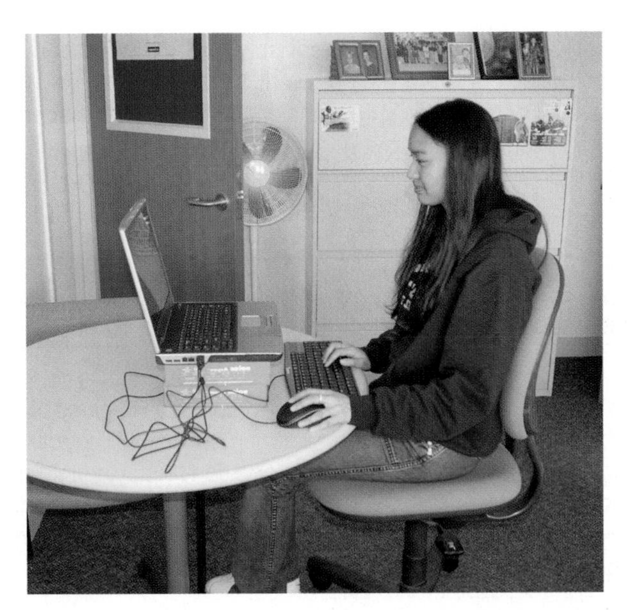

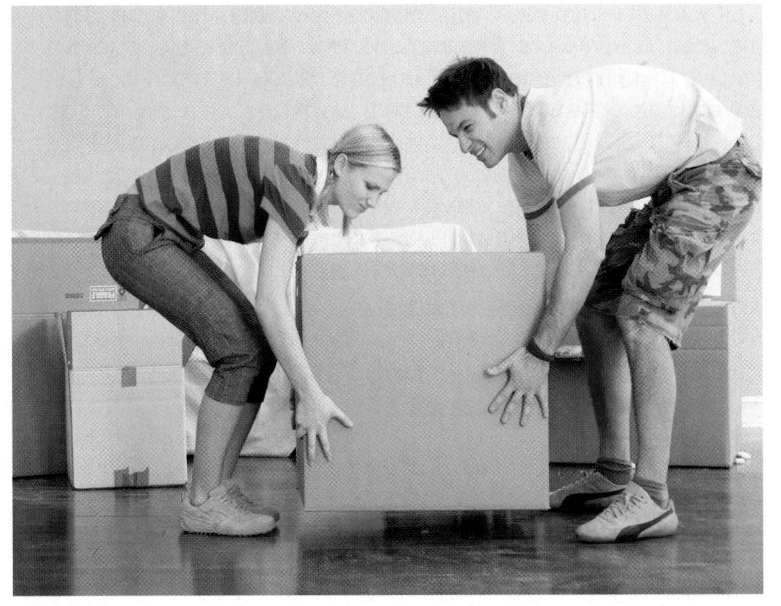

(a) The wrong way to lift

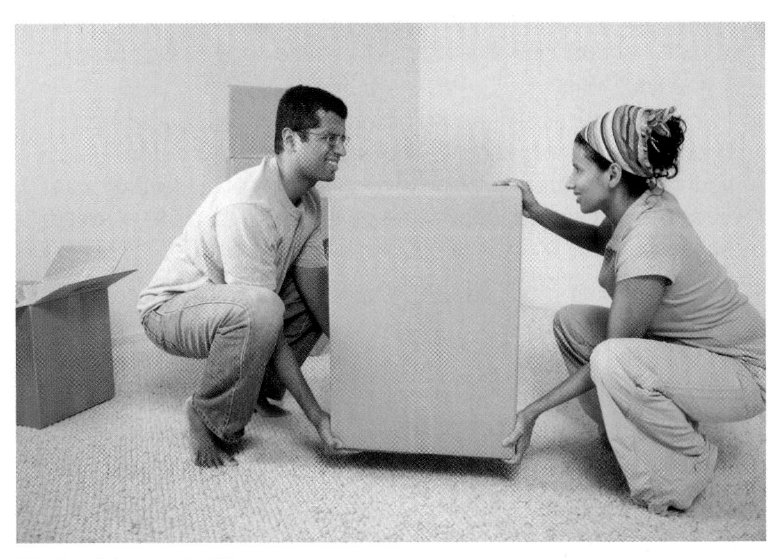

(b) The right way to lift

Figure 20.2 Proper lifting. Rather than (a) bending over the object to be lifted, (b) stand near it, then bend your knees and hips. Bring the object as close as possible to your body, then hold onto it as you rise.

Back Injuries

Lifting heavy objects is a leading cause of injury on the job.[52] If you've got a heavy box or other object to pick up and carry, start by making sure your balance is good. Then keep your back straight and crouch down to the object by bending at the knees and hips; do not bend at the waist **(Figure 20.2).** Once you've picked up the item, lift by straightening your legs. Keep the object close to your body by holding your elbows close to your body. This helps keep strain off your spine. Don't twist your body while carrying the load; if you need to change directions, change your foot placement. To release the object, lower it down by bending your knees, not your back. If you need to lift something that weighs more than 50 pounds or is an awkward shape, get another person to help you, or use a hand truck or other lifting and carrying device.

If you suffer from back pain, but don't have a job that requires lifting, your backpack might be to blame. How do you know? Pack it as you would for an average day, then put it on your bathroom scale. If it weighs more than 15% of your body weight, it's too heavy. You can also tell it's too heavy if you find yourself having to lean forward to carry it, or struggling to get it on or off. If that sounds like you, lighten the load. Before you leave for classes each morning, sort through the stuff in your backpack, and keep only what you need for that day. Here are some more options for protecting your back:

- Use a pack with wide, padded straps, and multiple compartments in which to distribute the contents. Never use a messenger bag or other shoulder bag for heavy loads.
- Place the heaviest items in the main compartment closest to your back. Use side compartments to help distribute the weight of lighter items.
- Use proper lifting technique to put on your backpack. Lower your body by flexing at your hips and knees, pick it up, and put it over your shoulders. Then straighten up. Never bend over and sling your backpack onto one shoulder.
- When you've got it on properly, your pack should rest evenly between your shoulders against your upper back **(Figure 20.3).** The shoulder straps should be snug, so that the pack doesn't hang below your waist.
- If you have to stand for a long period of time wearing your backpack—such as while waiting at a bus or subway stop—check your posture. Avoid slouching, and take some of the load off your back by resting one foot at a time on a step, curb, or other raised surface.
- If you can't limit your load to 15% or less of your weight, consider using a rolling backpack.
- Exercise regularly. Aerobic, flexibility, and strength-training exercises will help improve your stamina, alignment, and muscle conditioning and reduce your risk for back injury.
- Maintain a healthy weight. Carrying extra weight, especially in the abdominal area, strains your lower back. Losing weight can reduce that stress, and relieve the pain.

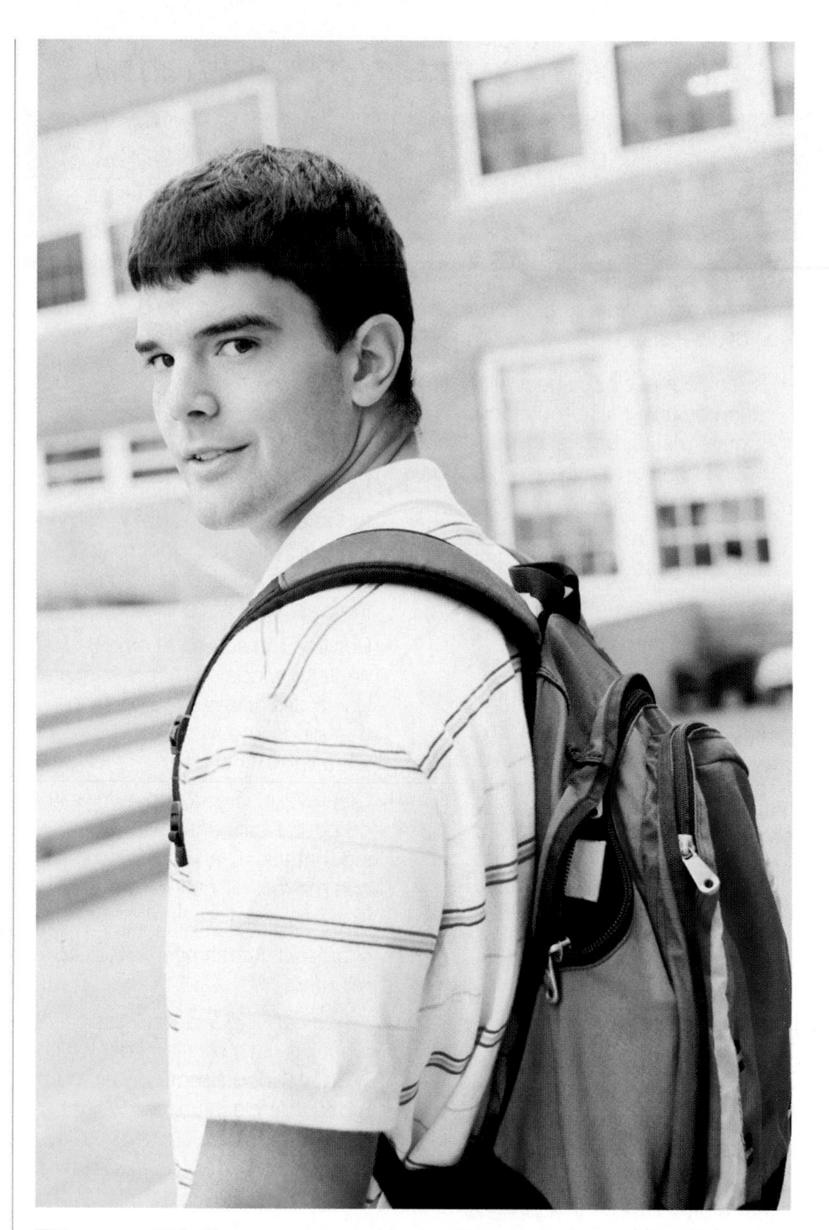

Figure 20.3 **The right way to wear a backpack.**

Weather-Related Injuries

We don't normally think of tornadoes touching down in Maine, or blizzards blasting Texas, but from time to time, most areas of the United States experience a wide range of weather-related emergencies. To stay safe, preparation is key. When possible, local media outlets give advance notice of potentially dangerous weather, but it's essential to know how to interpret the information they provide. To do that, you need to understand the difference between a weather watch, warning, and advisory.

- **Watch.** The National Weather Service (NWS) issues a "watch" when the conditions are in place for dangerous weather, but either an event hasn't yet happened or it hasn't reached your region. In short, a watch tells you to stay informed and get prepared.
- **Warning.** The NWS issues a "warning" when dangerous weather is present in your area; however, the action you need to take for each type of warning differs. A tornado warning, for instance, means that you should be ready to take shelter immediately, whereas a winter storm warning means to stay off the roads.
- **Advisory.** The NWS issues an "advisory" when a weather event is likely to occur, but is not likely to be as severe as those for which there would be a warning. For instance, a "winter weather advisory for snow" means that between 4 and 7 inches of snow is expected to fall within the next 12 hours. In contrast, a heavier snowfall would prompt a winter storm warning.

The National Weather Service offers "weather radio" 24 hours a day from the NWS station nearest you. To find out where to tune in, go to www.nws.noaa.gov/nwr/nwrbro.htm and click on your state.

Most colleges and universities also have systems in place to alert students to weather events and other emergencies. Find our what your campus's system is, and use it. In addition to staying informed, preparedness requires that you have a plan in place for responding in weather emergencies, and an emergency supply kit. For more information, see the nearby **Practical Strategies for Health.**

Practical Strategies for Health

Prepare for Home Emergencies

Whether you live in a dorm, an apartment, shared housing, or at home with your family, the U.S. Department of Homeland Security recommends taking a few basic safety precautions to prepare yourself for a natural disaster, house fire, or some other type of emergency:

- Be informed about the different types of emergencies that could occur in your area and their appropriate responses.
- Have an emergency plan. If you live on campus, your school has probably developed such plans for student housing. Find out about yours.
- Keep an emergency supply kit on hand.

Here is a list of basic items to stock in your emergency supply kit. Consider adding other items based on your individual needs.

- Water, one gallon of water per person per day for at least 3 days, for drinking and sanitation
- Food, at least a 3-day supply of nonperishable food
- Battery-powered or hand-crank radio and a NOAA (National Oceanic and Atmospheric Administration) Weather Radio with tone alert, and extra batteries for both
- Flashlight and extra batteries
- First aid kit
- Whistle to signal for help
- Dust mask, to help filter contaminated air, and plastic sheeting and duct tape to create a shelter in place
- Moist towelettes, garbage bags, and plastic ties for personal sanitation
- Wrench or pliers to turn off utilities
- Can opener for food (if kit contains canned food)
- Local maps
- Cell phone with chargers

Source: Adapted from *Ready,* by the U.S. Department of Homeland Security Ready Campaign, retrieved from http://www.ready.gov.

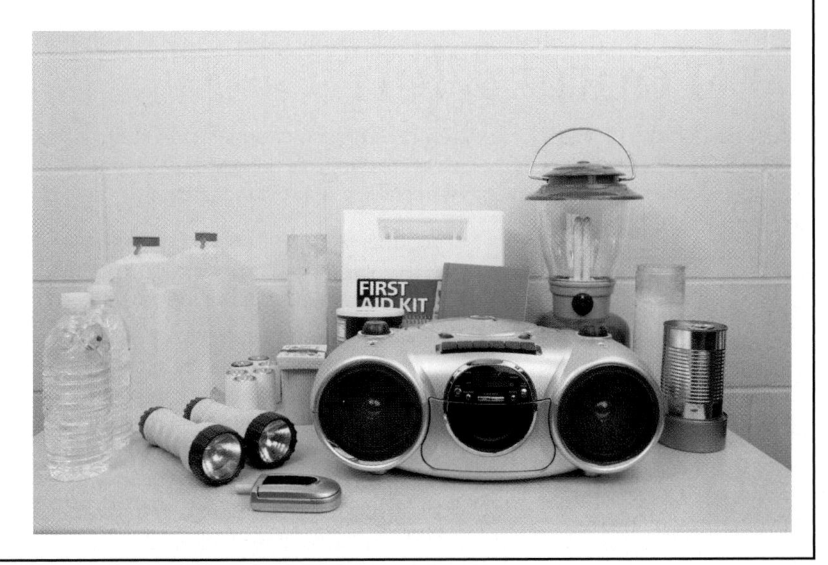

Overview of Intentional Injuries and Violence

Recall that intentional injuries are purposefully inflicted through **violence,** the use of force—threatened or actual—with the intent of causing harm. Violence is a serious health concern, especially for young people. Injuries caused by violence accounted for more than 2.5 million emergency room visits in 2008, and about half of all injury-related visits are from people between the ages of 15 and 44.[3]

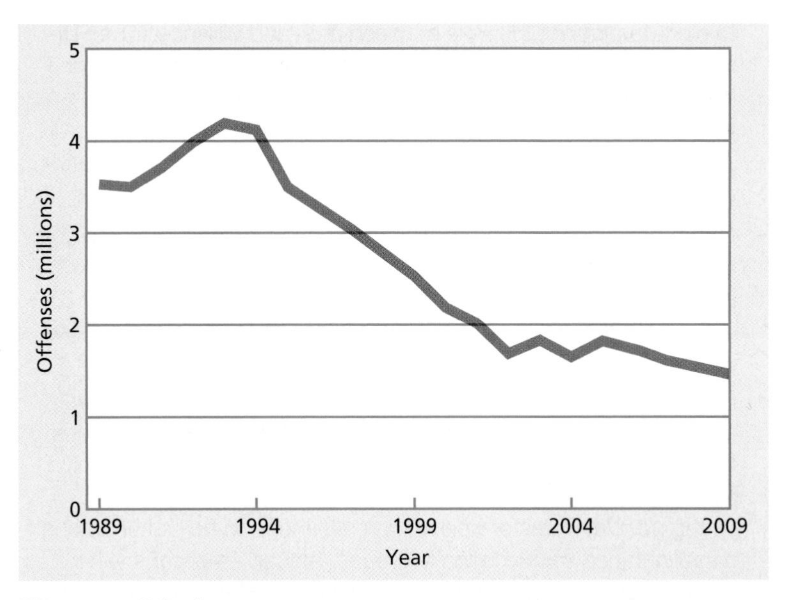

Figure 20.4 Violent crime rates over the last 20 years. The serious violent crimes included are murder, rape, robbery, and aggravated assault. Rates include estimates for crimes not reported to the police.

Data from "Four Measures of Serious Violent Crime" in *Key Facts at a Glance* by the Bureau of Justice Statistics. Retrieved August 7, 2012 from http://bjs.ojp.usdoj.gov/content/glance/cv2.cfm.

The Federal Bureau of Investigation (FBI) defines **violent crime** as one of four offenses involving force or the threat or force: murder and non-negligent manslaughter, forcible rape, robbery, and aggravated assault. Although levels of violent crime in the United States have fluctuated in recent years, the overall number of violent crimes has dropped in the last two decades **(Figure 20.4).**[53] Still, in 2009, more than 1.4 million violent crimes were committed in the United States—more than 3,800 a day.[54] Of these attacks:

- About 61% were aggravated assault, or an attack intended to cause serious injury, often involving a weapon.
- About 31% were robberies, or the taking of or attempt to take anything of value from a person by violence and/or by putting the victim in fear.
- Almost 7% were forcible rapes.
- Just over 1% were murders.

Many attacks have underpinnings in complex webs of personal, family, community, and social factors, including:

- **Sex.** Most violent crime is committed by men. Of more than 550,000 arrests for murder, rape, robbery, and assault in 2010, 80% of those taken into custody were men. Men are also more often victims—about 77% of all people murdered in the United States in 2010 were male.[55] Crime experts continue

violence Use of physical force—threatened or actual—with the intent of causing harm.

violent crime One of four offenses involving force or the threat or force: murder and non-negligent manslaughter, forcible rape, robbery, and aggravated assault.

to work to pinpoint the links between men and violence.[56] See **Diversity & Health: Injuries and Violence: Special Concerns for Young Men** for more possible reasons men are at higher risk than women.

- **Age.** Teens and young adults experience the highest rate of violent crime.
- **Guns.** The United States continues to have a high murder rate compared with other industrialized countries, and many experts link this phenomenon to the easy availability of firearms. In 2010, about 67% of the nation's murders, 41% of robberies, and 21% of aggravated assaults were committed with the use of a gun.[54]
- **Poverty.** Regions that are lower in income and status consistently see more crime. Communities that are distressed, with poor housing, high crime rates, high unemployment, and limited community services, often have higher rates of violence, especially among young people. Rates of violent crime also tend to be higher among disadvantaged socioeconomic groups. African Americans, who make up about 13% of the U.S. population and are more likely to live in poverty, comprise almost half of all murder victims.[55]
- **Interpersonal relationships.** Many crime victims know their attackers. Women are especially vulnerable to criminal acts at the hands of an acquaintance, friend, intimate partner, family member, or spouse.[57]
- **Drugs and alcohol.** Substances that disrupt judgment and impair your ability to control your emotions consistently emerge as a factor in violence. One landmark study of violent crime in the United States found that alcohol was a factor in almost 40% of all cases.[58] In another study that looked at drinking on college campuses over 2 years, more than 600,000 students reported being hit or assaulted by another student who'd been drinking.[59] The use of drugs, or their sale, is also a factor in many types of crime.
- **Childhood environment.** Researchers have consistently noted that children raised in violent surroundings are more likely to grow up to be violent adults.[60]
- **Violence in the media.** From TV shows, movies, video games, and song lyrics, most children and teenagers are exposed to thousands of violent messages each year. Although crime researchers continue to debate the exact level of influence media violence has on personal violence and crime, most agree that violence in the media contributes to an increased level of aggressive behavior and a perception that violence is normal.[61]
- **Personal and cultural beliefs.** In some cases, personal values or religious beliefs may be interpreted in ways that justify the use of violence. Violence can also be targeted against people of one religious group by those of a different faith.
- **Stress.** Think about the last time you were under a great deal of stress, and how you were quicker to anger than you might have been otherwise. People who are consistently under stress are more likely to react violently, especially if they are prone to anger easily.

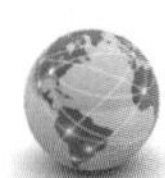

DIVERSITY & HEALTH

Injuries and Violence: Special Concerns for Young Men

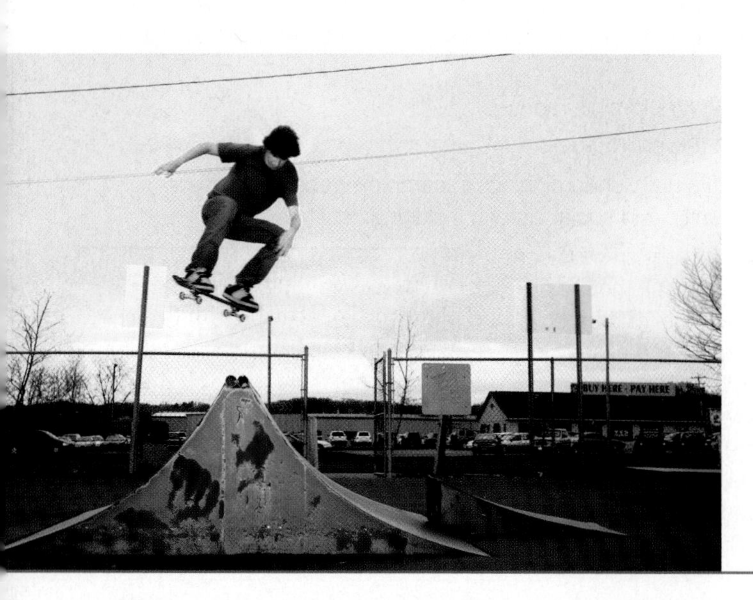

Two of the biggest risk factors for injury and death due to accidents or violence are things none of us can control: age and sex. If you are young, and you are male, your risk for getting hurt or killed in an accident or attack is almost always higher than that of women or any other age group. Sexual assault is one of the few situations where women are in more danger, but for most other types of violence and injuries, young men are at higher risk.

The reasons for these higher risks are widely debated among researchers. Some suggest that the influence of the male hormone testosterone leads to more aggression, anger, and risk taking. Some point to gender roles that encourage men, especially young men, to be tough, aggressive, risk taking, or confrontational. Others say that a mix of these factors often puts young men in harm's way.

Reducing the risk of injury doesn't mean taking all the fun out of your life. Instead, experts suggest, channel your energies in ways less likely to get you hurt or killed. Here are just a few suggestions:

- Your car is no place for an adrenaline rush. Find thrills in sports, video games, or anywhere but behind the wheel.
- Watch how much you drink. As discussed throughout this chapter, alcohol is a significant risk factor for unintentional and intentional injuries. Whether you are the aggressor or the victim, you don't want to wind up a drinking-related statistic. For more information on alcohol and its effects, see Chapter 9.
- Anger can't help you solve problems. It's natural to get angry, but anger can quickly escalate a conflict into violence. Learning to manage anger and find other ways to resolve problems is one of the manliest things you can do. For more information about managing anger and stress, see Chapters 2 and 3.

Violence within Communities

Over the past decade, several studies have reported similar findings on the role of the media in the cultivation of fear of crime. In essence, the studies have found that media reports of crime wildly exceed actual rates of crime, and that exposure to these crime-saturated television and print news reports greatly increases people's perception of their own vulnerability to crime and their concern about crime within society—even though the actual rate of crime has been declining dramatically for many years.[62, 63] As you read the following discussion, keeping this research in mind might help you maintain a realistic perspective. Although even one violent crime is too many, our society has been making progress in reducing this threat. At the end of this chapter, we'll discuss ways you can get involved in these efforts.

Assault

Assault, a physical attack or threat of attack on another person, is one of the leading categories of violent crime. **Aggravated assault** is an assault committed with the intent to cause severe injury, or an assault or threatened attack with a weapon or other means likely to cause death or major injury. Although most aggravated assaults do involve a weapon, 27% of cases in 2010 were committed with fists or feet. Although nearly 779,000 aggravated assaults were committed in 2010, this number represents a 14.3% decline from 2001.[64] More effective prevention programs and tougher law enforcement appear to have helped reduce the number of assaults.

aggravated assault An attack intended to cause serious physical harm, often involving a weapon.

murder The act of intentionally and unjustifiably killing another person.

gang An economic or social group that forms to intimidate and control members and outsiders through threats and violence.

Murder

Murder is the willful (not negligent) killing of another person. The FBI includes in this category non-negligent manslaughter, which is the willful killing of another "without malice aforethought"—in other words, without having previously planned to do so. The category does not include justifiable homicide, an example of which could be self-defense.

Murder is second only to unintentional injuries as the leading cause of death in the United States among people between the ages of 15 and 24. As noted earlier, the great majority of murder victims and perpetrators are male. Two-thirds of murders involve firearms.[65] Mass murders, such as the murder of 14 people at a Colorado movie theatre in the summer of 2012, often involve assault rifles. Private possession of these semiautomatic weapons, which were developed for military and law enforcement use, is not banned in all states.

Nationwide, 14,748 people were murdered in 2010. This was an 8% decrease from 2001.[66] About 43% of these victims were murdered by someone they knew.[67] As with assault, prevention program and law enforcement efforts appear to be helping to reduce the U.S. murder rate.

Gang Violence

Many violent criminals don't act alone. **Gangs,** or economic and social groups that form to intimidate and control both their members and outsiders through threats and violence, are responsible for many acts of violent crime. According to the FBI, about 1 million gang members belonging to more than 20,000 gangs are criminally active in the United States, and commit as much as 80% of the crime within some communities.[68] They are major factors in the drug trade, and some also participate in armed robbery, assault, auto theft, extortion, fraud, home invasion, weapons dealing, and human trafficking. More and more women are joining gangs, and gangs are also increasing their range, becoming more active in suburban and rural areas.[68] With their sense of inclusion and camaraderie, gangs can seem appealing, especially in distressed neighborhoods where regular jobs are few and families and schools are strained. But once inside, gang members often find themselves caught in a culture of intimidation and crime that is difficult to escape.

School and Campus Violence

When two students went on a murderous rampage at Columbine High School in 1999, many Americans began to fear that going to school amounted to putting one's life at risk. Subsequent incidents, most recently the February 2012 murder of three high school students sitting at a cafeteria table in Chardon, Ohio, have reinforced this fear. Yet despite these high-profile tragedies, overall levels of crime on elementary, middle, and high school campuses have dropped in the past decade. Moreover, a national analysis found that students are much more likely to be seriously hurt or killed off campus than while at school. During the 2008–2009 school year, for example, there were 17 homicides of school-aged children within American schools, but 1,562 homicides of school-aged children within their homes and communities.[69]

What Columbine means to high schools, Virginia Tech has come to mean for colleges and universities. In the horrifying 2007 mass shooting, a student killed 32 others and himself. In response to the tragedy, U.S. colleges and universities have developed new emergency response plans and procedures, upgraded communication systems, and implemented new safety techniques and services. At the same time, some are finding their policies in conflict with state laws allowing students with permits to carry a concealed weapon on campus. For example, in March 2012, the Colorado Supreme Court struck down the University of Colorado's ban

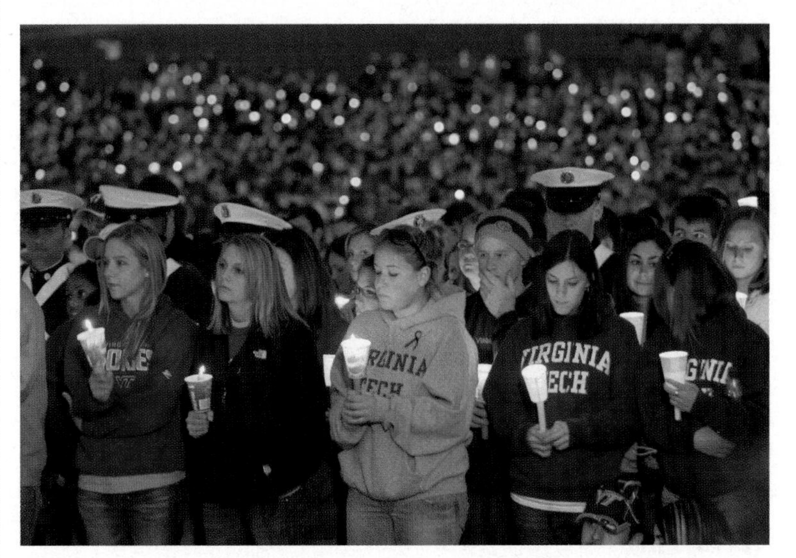

The Virginia Tech shootings in 2007 prompted colleges to reevaluate their safety and alert procedures.

on carrying a concealed weapon on campus. This followed an Arizona ruling the month before allowing students with state permits to carry concealed weapons onto Arizona college campuses. Six states now allow guns on campus.[70] Some proponents of so-called "concealed carry laws" say these rulings will make campuses safer, because students will be less likely to pull out a gun if they know that other students might also have guns. Others disagree, pointing to research suggesting that the availability of weapons increases rates of murder and unintentional deaths.

Other types of violent crime occur on campus as well. In 2010, law enforcement officials reported 15 murders, over 2,900 forcible sex offenses, about 1,800 robberies, and more than 2,500 aggravated assaults on 2- and 4-year campuses in the United States.[71] All U.S. universities are required to disclose statistics about the crimes reported on and near their campuses. The legislation that mandates this disclosure is the Clery Act, named after Lehigh University student Jeanne Clery, who in 1986 was beaten, raped, and murdered in her dorm room when dormitory security doors were propped open, allowing a perpetrator to enter. Unfortunately, many campus crimes still go unreported, with victims often too embarrassed, ashamed, or afraid to step forward. Reporting a crime is the first step toward addressing the problem and making a campus safer for everyone.

Another common problem on college campuses is **hazing,** a set of initiation rituals for fraternities, sports teams, or other groups that are typically humiliating, degrading, or abusive and can result in injury or death. Hazing is dangerous because peer pressure or other power dynamics induce those being hazed to participate in high-risk activities that they wouldn't perform otherwise. About 55% of college students involved in clubs, teams, and organizations experience hazing.[72] According to one expert on hazings, a total of 27 deaths were attributed to hazing in the decade between 2002 and 2011. Alcohol poisoning and physical abuse are usually the causes of death.[73]

Hate Crimes

Certain crimes are fueled by bias against another person's or group's race or ethnicity, religion, national origin, sexual orientation, or disability. Any acts—whether physical assaults or vandalism against property—due to such prejudice have been classified as **hate crimes.** More than 6,600 incidents involving such offenses were reported to the FBI in 2010. Of these, almost half were driven by bias against the victim's race, whereas religious bias and sexual orientation bias were each involved in 20% of hate crimes.[74] Over 10% of these hate crimes occurred in schools or on college campuses.[74]

Hate crimes tend to reflect prevalent social and cultural biases. Hate crimes against Muslims in the United States, for example, jumped after the terrorist attacks of September 11, 2001. In recent years, hate crimes fueled by ethnicity or national origin bias have been committed against Hispanics in increasing numbers, a phenomenon experts attribute to the ongoing debate over immigration.[75]

Terrorism

Terrorism is premeditated, politically motivated violence against nonmilitary people by subnational groups or clandestine agents, usually in an effort to influence a larger audience. The year 2001 saw more terrorism on U.S. soil than had ever before been seen. The dangerous bacterium that causes anthrax was deliberately dispatched through the U.S. postal system and more than 3,000 people died in the September 11 attacks. Since then, the numbers of deaths and injuries due to terrorism in the United States have dropped greatly, but the effects remain. Terrorism is a crime that operates on many levels: It can maim or kill, but it also alters everyday life by cultivating fear.

As a result, fighting terrorism requires both physical force and psychological finesse. In response to the terrorist attacks in 2001, the U.S. government created the Department of Homeland Security, a government agency tasked with defending the nation against terrorism and other threats. Other agencies, such as the FBI, CIA, the U.S. military, and state and local law enforcement also guard against terrorism. Ongoing efforts work not just to disarm, catch, or kill terrorists, but to discredit their tactics, diminish the perception of threats, and reduce their abilities to win public support and new recruits.

These efforts matter both on U.S. soil and abroad. In 2010, more than 11,500 terrorist attacks occurred in 72 countries, causing over 13,000 deaths. In the Western Hemisphere, there were 340 attacks in 2010, with 279 deaths.[76] Muslim extremists were responsible for more than 60% of all terrorist attacks in 2010, and civilians in Muslim countries were most often the victims. More than 15% of the dead were police and other peace officers.[76]

Cyber Crime

If you're like many college students, you love your wired and wireless gadgets and networks. You might even feel that you couldn't survive without them! But do you know how to protect your online connections from being used to commit crime? **Cyber crime** (also called *high-tech crime*) is broadly defined as any criminal activity using a network or computer, including those involving your laptop, cell phone, the ATM at your bank, and those you access every time you swipe your card to pay for groceries, a meal, or gas.

Cyber crime is typically behind identity theft and financial scams. The Department of Justice (DOJ) defines identity theft as unauthorized use of credit cards and other accounts such as checking accounts, as well as misuse of personal information to obtain new accounts or loans or to commit other crimes. DOJ estimates suggest that about 3% of households in America experience identity theft involving at least one member each year. Households headed by people aged 18 to 24 are the most likely to experience identity theft.[77] Identity thieves typically obtain your information by:

- Hacking into the computer systems of financial and retail organizations
- Obtaining credit reports by posing as a landlord or employer
- "Skimming" your credit card number as your card is being processed
- Rummaging through your trash
- Stealing your wallet or purse, smartphone, or mail
- "Phishing" or "vishing": sending you a letter, email, or voice or text message claiming to be

hazing Initiation rituals to enter a fraternity or other group that can be humiliating, hazardous, or physically or emotionally abusive, regardless of the person's willingness to participate.

hate crime A crime fueled by bias against another person's or group's race or ethnicity, religion, national origin, sexual orientation, or disability.

terrorism Premeditated, politically motivated violence against noncombatant individuals, usually as a means of influence.

cyber crime Any criminal activity using a network or computer.

from a legitimate business you deal with, and asking you to update or validate your account information.

How can you protect yourself? Here are some suggestions from the FBI:[78]

- Don't respond to emails, automated voice messages (whether via a land line or cell phone), or text messages from unknown sources.
- Never click on links or attachments within unsolicited messages. Don't download anything unless you trust the source.
- When buying online, use a legitimate payment service and a credit card, because unauthorized charges can be disputed. Check each seller's rating and feedback. Be wary of those with a 100% positive score, with a low number of feedback postings, or with all feedback posted around the same date.
- Review your bank account and credit card statements as soon as they arrive in the mail, or more frequently if you use an online account system.
- Use and maintain anti-virus software and a firewall. Buy a security program such as SmrtGuard for your smartphone and use it.

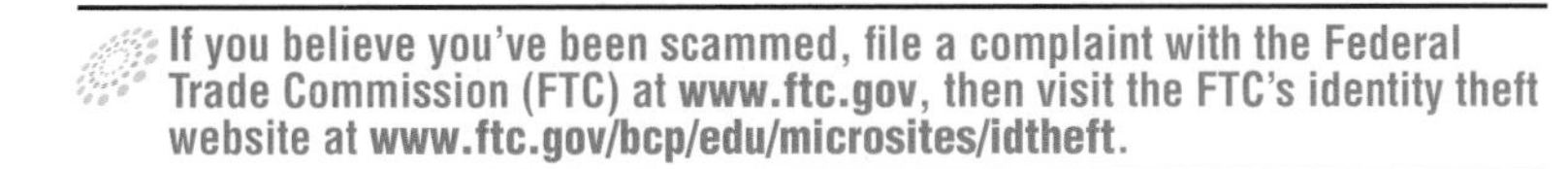

If you believe you've been scammed, file a complaint with the Federal Trade Commission (FTC) at www.ftc.gov, then visit the FTC's identity theft website at www.ftc.gov/bcp/edu/microsites/idtheft.

STUDENT STORY

Abusive Relationship

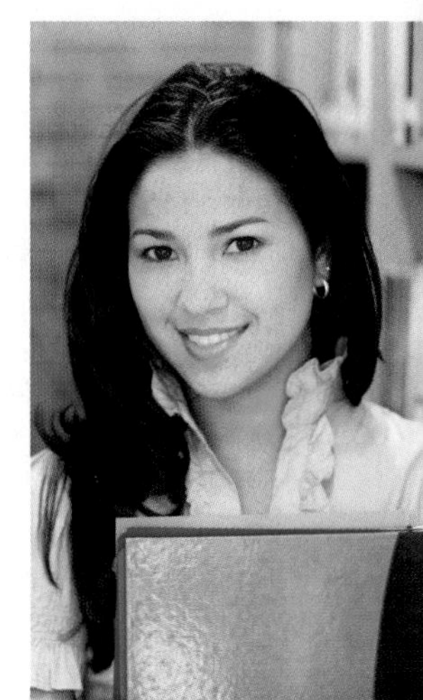

"Hi, I'm Jenny. I was dating a guy for a few months who I really liked and everything seemed great at first, but he slowly started to get more and more controlling. First he didn't want to go out with my friends, then after a while he didn't want *me* to go out with my friends. He got really jealous any time he saw me talking to another guy and he started making me check in with him every day to let him know my schedule. He even checked my cell phone to see who I was talking to. One day we got into a fight about it and he grabbed me and pushed me into a wall. I got really scared and left immediately. I broke up with him by text and I've avoided him ever since."

1: What could have happened if Jenny had stayed with her abusive boyfriend?

2: What else could Jenny have done in response to her boyfriend's behavior along with breaking up with him?

3: Was Jenny right to break up with him with a text or should she have met up with him to explain?

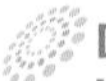

Do you have a story similar to Jenny's? Share your story at www.pearsonhighered.com/lynchelmore.

Violence within Relationships

We all desire relationships that are grounded in mutual support, respect, and affection, but sometimes we find ourselves in relationships characterized by abuse. In a phenomenon known as **domestic violence,** one or more members of a household experience physical, psychological, or sexual harm from another member. When the abuse is perpetrated by a current or former partner or spouse, it is known as **intimate partner violence (IPV).** Forms of IPV include physical and emotional abuse, and sexual violence, such as rape, when it occurs between intimate partners. We discuss sexual violence later in this chapter.

Intimate Partner Violence

Victims of intimate partner violence can be married or not married, heterosexual, gay or lesbian, living together, separated, or dating. Many cases go unreported, so the exact scope of this problem is hard to pin down. The CDC estimates that 12 million Americans experience IPV each year.[79] Women are disproportionately affected:

- 1 in 4 women has been the victim of severe physical violence by an intimate partner versus 1 in 7 men.
- Nearly 1 in 5 women has been raped versus 1 in 71 men.[79]
- Women make up 70% of all deaths due to IPV, versus 30% for men.[80]

Some experts believe that moving away from home to college can increase a teen's vulnerability to IPV, in part because of the decrease in parental monitoring and support and the desire to fit in.[81]

At its core, abuse in an intimate relationship arises from the abuser's need for control. That effort at control may take the form of abusing others psychologically, through comments and actions that try to erode the other person's confidence, independence, and sense of self-worth. Withholding money, keeping a partner from contacting family or friends, stopping a partner from getting or keeping a job, and constant putdowns are all characteristics of emotional abuse. Physical forms of abuse include any type of physical assault or use of physical restraint. In most cases, emotional abuse and controlling behaviors accompany physical abuse when it is present in a relationship.

Some people who find themselves the victim of an episode of abuse end the relationship and leave immediately. But other abuse victims, especially women, stay, and may find themselves subject to further and more severe abuse. Most such domestic and intimate partner abuse captures the victim in a situation that is difficult to escape, identified as *the cycle of violence*:

- **Tension building.** A phase in which relatively minor abuse occurs, and the victim responds by trying to please the abuser and avoid provoking another attack.
- **Acute battering.** A phase in which the abuser lashes out more forcefully, no matter how accommodating or conciliatory the victim has been.
- **Remorse.** A phase in which the abuser may feel shock and denial over the abuse and swear it will never happen again. Over time, however, the tensions and need for control that started the cycle resurface, and abuse starts anew, often more seriously than before.

domestic violence An abusive situation in which a family member physically, psychologically, or sexually abuses one or more other family members.

intimate partner violence (IPV) An abusive situation in which one member of a couple or intimate relationship may physically, psychologically, or sexually abuse the other.

Victims stay in abusive relationships for a variety of reasons. Some are financially dependent on their partners, or have children and don't want to break up their family. Some come from belief systems or cultures that forbid family separation or divorce. Some may still love their abuser. Others may lack the self-confidence to take action, or don't know where to go. Some may be afraid of what their partner might do to them if they try to leave.

A variety of organizations provide counseling and shelter to victims of IPV. One annual survey of domestic violence groups found that on a given day, more than 65,000 adults and children received shelter, housing, legal counseling, emotional counseling, or other types of support related to family and intimate violence.[82] More than 9,000 others seeking such help had to be turned away for lack of adequate services.

IPV persists, in part, because of a broad lack of understanding of how and why it occurs. In one survey of college students, more than half agreed with IPV myths such as that some instances are caused by women picking physical fights with their partners, or that most women can get out of an abusive relationship if they really want to.[83] College men taking the survey were more likely to agree with these myths than college women.

For an interview from CNN that explores the myths surrounding sexual assault, watch www.cnn.com/video/#/video/living/2011/04/06/rape.and.sex.abuse.myths.hln.

Stalking and Cyber Stalking

Stalking is a pattern of harassment or threats directed at a specific person that is intended to cause intimidation and fear, often through repeated, unwanted contact. According to a national survey, more than 5 million women are stalked each year in the United States.[84] Women were about three times as likely to be stalked as men, and men make up the majority of stalkers. Overall, 1 in 6 women has been stalked in her lifetime, versus 1 in 19 men.[80]

stalking A pattern of harassment and threats directed at a specific person that is intended to cause intimidation and fear, often through repeated, unwanted contact.

In one survey of college women, about 20% reported having been stalked while in college, and the overwhelming majority of their stalkers were men the victim knew, including acquaintances, classmates, and boyfriends or ex-boyfriends.[85] The same pattern is true for the general public—only about 1 in 8 stalking incidents involves a stranger.[84]

Common stalking behaviors include:

- Making unwanted phone calls
- Sending unwanted letters, emails, or text messages
- Following or spying
- Showing up at places where the victim would be, with no legitimate reason
- Waiting for the victim, with no legitimate reason
- Leaving unwanted items or presents for the victim
- Posting information or spreading rumors about the victim online, in a public place, or by word of mouth

Stalking may also take the form of contact through digital and online communications, a phenomenon called *cyber stalking*. Although both traditional stalkers and cyber stalkers are motivated by an obsession with having power and control over their victims, cyber stalkers are more likely to avoid detection, using tactics such as creating a variety of screen names at different sites to maintain their anonymity.[86]

If you are being stalked, don't try to reason with your stalker. Stalking is not rational behavior. Instead, start by letting the stalker know that the attention is unwelcome. Have someone else deliver this message for you—this thwarts the stalker's goal of trying to force contact with you. Vary your routines, change your typical routes, and avoid being alone as much as possible. Stop "checking in" at places, posting information about your location, or publicly revealing your whereabouts through GPS locator apps, or on any social media sites you use. Keep a record of all contacts with the stalker. Get a new phone number, but leave the old one active. Ask a friend to screen and keep a record of calls to the old number. If the stalker persists, get help from your resident advisor, campus health center, campus security, or law enforcement.

Child Abuse

Unfortunately, children are not immune from domestic violence. Child protective services (CPS) agents estimated that 772,000 American children were victims of maltreatment in 2008. Almost 60% of these cases involved child neglect, such as failure to provide basic food, shelter, medical care, or education. The remainder of cases were physical, sexual, and emotional in nature. More than 1,700 of these children died.[87] Four out of five of these victims were less than 4 years old.[87] The rates of abuse are highest for children from birth to age 3.[88]

Factors that lead to child abuse include psychological issues in the adult caregiver such as low self-esteem, feelings of being out of control, poor impulse control, depression, anxiety, and anti-social behavior. Substance abuse, single parenthood, poverty, the presence of other domestic violence in the home, negative attitudes about childhood behavior or child development, and teen parenthood also increase the risk of child abuse. In addition, children who are physically, cognitively, or emotionally disabled are almost twice as likely to experience abuse. About a third of children who are abused will go on to abuse their own children.[88]

Elder Abuse

Elder abuse is the physical, emotional, psychological, financial, sexual, or verbal abuse, neglect, or exploitation of someone over the age of 60. It can occur in the home, in a nursing home, a hospital, or elsewhere. It is believed that more than 500,000 older adults suffer from such maltreatment each year.[89] However, it is a largely hidden crime: Experts estimate that only 1 in 6 cases is reported.[90] Victims may not inform others because they are physically or mentally unable to do so, or because they fear the loss of their caregiver, whom they rely on and may care for deeply. Elder abuse occurs across socioeconomic classes, cultures, and races. Women, elders at more advanced ages, those with dementia or mental health issues, and elders who are physically or socially isolated are at higher risk.

Often, the stress of caregiving is a factor in elder abuse, especially if the elder has lost bladder or bowel control or is confused or combative. Other risk factors include a high level of stress, depression, lack of social support, substance abuse, and simple lack of training in how to care for an older adult. Finding an adult day care program or hiring a home health aide for a few hours a week can help.

Addressing Violence within Relationships

If you find yourself attracted to someone, is there any way to tell—before you get in too deep—if the person has the potential for violence? Although there's no such thing as an IPV profile, the CDC has gathered a list of risk factors. They include:[91]

- Low self-esteem
- Low academic achievement
- A history of aggressive or delinquent behavior
- A history of having been abused as a child
- Alcohol or other substance abuse
- Anger and hostility
- Depression and social isolation
- Belief in strict gender roles
- Desire for power and control

What if you're already in a relationship that's causing you to feel unsafe, or you've experienced one or more episodes of IPV? What if you're frightened by something you see in the relationship of a friend? Don't wait for things to "get better": Contact your student health center or the National Domestic Violence Hotline at 1-800-799-SAFE (7233) or at TTY ("text telephone" for the hearing impaired) 1-800-787-3224, or visit **www.thehotline.org**.

If you have children or plan to some day, and were abused yourself as a child, you are at risk of continuing that cycle of abuse. Health and child wellness centers around the country offer classes and counseling in positive parenting skills that help prevent child maltreatment. If you suspect that a child you know is being neglected or abused, seek help. Contact the National Child Abuse Hotline at 1-800-4-A-CHILD (1-800-422-4453).

If you suspect that an elderly family member or close friend is being maltreated in some way by a caregiver, you have a few options. Initially, you might try offering to visit for a few hours a week to give the caregiver some relief. You might also work with other loved ones to set up a group visitation schedule. If you are very concerned about the elder, call the National Elder Abuse Hotline at 1-800-677-1116.

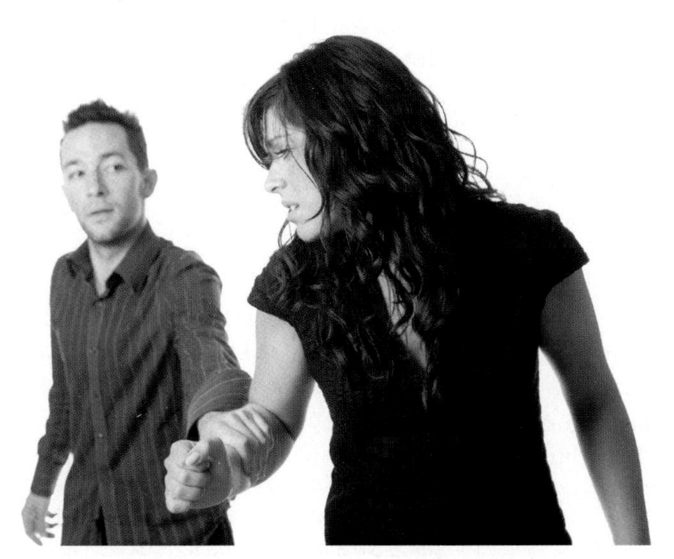

If you are in an **abusive relationship,** you can find help to get out.

Sexual Violence

Although no standard definition of the term has emerged, **sexual violence** encompasses several forms of nonconsensual sexual activity, including noncontact sexual abuse, such as voyeurism or verbal harassment, unwanted touching, attempted but uncompleted sex acts, and completed sex acts. The common factor in all of these is the lack of consent of the victim, either because he or she refused consent, or was threatened, coerced, intoxicated, underage, developmentally disabled, or otherwise legally incapable of either giving or refusing consent. Sexual violence is often referred to as sexual assault.

Risk Factors for Sexual Violence

Factors that increase the risk for sexual violence include:

- **Negative attitudes about women.** Men who report hostility toward women or who hold low opinions of women are more likely to show higher levels of sexual aggression and to believe in myths like "When she says 'no,' she really means 'yes.'"
- **Rape-tolerant attitudes.** Several studies of college students have confirmed that college men are more likely to hold attitudes that are tolerant of rape, such as "Some women ask to be raped" or "It's all right to get a woman drunk just to have sex with her."[92]
- **Gender role stereotypes.** Outdated social perceptions hold that men should always insist on sex, and that women who decline are just playing "hard to get."
- **Alcohol and drugs.** People who have consumed alcohol to excess, either voluntarily or involuntarily, or who have used or been given a drug, are more vulnerable to sexual assault. Many college women reporting an assault said they were incapacitated at the time, often by alcohol.[93] In one study, about 15% of men reported having used some form of alcohol-related coercion, and 20% admitted having friends who'd gotten a woman drunk or high to have sex with her.[92]
- **"No" isn't always heard as "No."** Studies have found that some young men have problems understanding a young woman's sexual refusals. Less direct refusals, such as body language that displays a lack of interest, or attempts at polite rejection such as "I don't think it's a good idea," were misinterpreted by some young men as agreeing to sex.[94]

sexual violence Any form of nonconsensual sexual activity.

sexual harassment Unwelcome language or contact of a sexual nature that explicitly or implicitly affects academic or employment situations, unreasonably interferes with work or school performance, or creates an intimidating, hostile, or offensive work or school environment.

Sexual Harassment

Unwanted language or contact of a sexual nature that occurs in school or workplace settings is considered **sexual harassment** when it explicitly or implicitly affects a person's job or academic situation, work or school performance, or creates an intimidating, hostile, or offensive environment. Sexual harassment is a form of discrimination that violates federal civil rights law.

According to legal guidelines, sexual harassment can occur in a variety of circumstances, including but not limited to the following possibilities. In all cases the harasser's conduct must be unwelcome.

- The victim and the harasser may be a woman or man, and the two parties do not have to be of the opposite sex.
- The harasser can be the victim's supervisor (or teacher), an agent of the employer (or school), a coworker (or fellow student), or a nonemployee (or nonstudent).
- The victim does not have to be the person harassed, but can be anyone affected by the offensive conduct.
- Harassment may occur even if the victim suffers no economic injury or stays on the job or at school.[95]

On campus, sexual harassment can take the form of everything from a student making sexually explicit remarks that make others uncomfortable to a professor demanding sexual favors from a student in exchange for a better grade. In one survey of college students, about 60% of all students (male and female) reported having been sexually harassed while enrolled in school. About 80% of those harassed said their harasser was a fellow student. About 50% of college men admitted to having harassed someone, and about 22% said they had done so more than once. Only 10% of those harassed said they had reported the incident to a campus official.[96]

If you are being harassed, the first step is to confront your harasser. State clearly, in person or in writing, that the actions are unwelcome. Be direct: Tell the harasser to stop, and state that you consider these actions to be sexual harassment. If direct communication has no effect, keep a record of all harassing contacts and behavior, and report the problem to campus or workplace supervisors. They are required by law to take your report seriously and investigate.

Rape

Rape is a form of sexual violence involving oral, anal, or vaginal penetration using force, threats, or taking advantage of circumstances that make a person incapable of consenting to sex. Any sexual activity with a person younger than the legally defined "age of consent" is also considered a form of rape called **statutory rape,** regardless of whether any coercion or force was involved.

The FBI refers to the crime of rape as *forcible rape* and defines it more narrowly as "the carnal knowledge of a female forcibly and against her will." In 2010, FBI records showed that nearly 85,000 women in the United States were forcibly raped.[97] However, because males also experience rape, many rapes go unreported, and definitions of what constitute rape vary, estimates of the actual incidence of rape in the United States are much higher. As noted earlier, a large-scale national survey found that about 1 in 5 women and 1 in 71 men in the United States report having been raped at some point in their lives.[79] The same survey found that more than 1 million women had been raped the previous year. Among female victims, 79% of rapes occur before age 25. In one survey of college women, almost 20% said they'd been sexually assaulted during their undergraduate years.[93]

rape Nonconsensual oral, anal, or vaginal penetration by body parts or objects, using force, threats of bodily harm, or taking advantage of circumstances that make a person incapable of consenting to sex.

statutory rape Any sexual activity with a person younger than the legally defined "age of consent," regardless of whether any coercion or force was involved.

date (acquaintance) rape Coerced, forceful, or threatening sexual activity in which the victim knows the attacker.

date rape drugs Drugs used to assist in a sexual assault, often given to the victim without his or her knowledge or consent.

Date Rape

Of rapes documented among college students, many take the form of **date (acquaintance) rape.** This form of coerced sexual activity, in which the victim knows the attacker, can have a severe long-term emotional impact because the victim is attacked by someone who was trusted. Date rape is sometimes preceded by intimate partner violence that escalates to sexual violence. As with other types of sexual assault, many cases of date rape go unreported. Drinking and drug use are factors, and in some instances the victim is unknowingly given a drug to facilitate rape.

Date Rape Drugs

Drugs used to assist in a sexual assault, or **date rape drugs,** are powerful, dangerous, and difficult to detect once they've been slipped into a drink. They can make a victim weak or confused, lower inhibitions, or cause loss of consciousness—all conditions that leave the person unable to refuse sex or fend off an assault. These drugs can also make it difficult for the victim to remember later what happened while he or she was drugged. The most common date rape drugs, which can come in pill, liquid, or powder form, include flunitrazepam (Rohypnol), Ketamine, or GHB (gamma-hydroxybutyric acid).

Under federal law, convicted rapists who use a date rape drug to incapacitate a victim automatically have 20 years added to their sentences.

The following precautions can help you avoid accidentally consuming a date rape drug.

- Bring a trusted friend with you whenever you go to parties or clubs.
- Don't accept drinks, including nonalcoholic ones, from other people. If you're at a club, go up to the bar yourself and watch as the bartender prepares your drink.
- If someone offers to buy you a drink, go with the person to the bar, and carry it back yourself.
- Open drink containers yourself.
- Keep your drink with you at all times. If you've left it unattended, pour it out.
- Don't share drinks, or drink from punch bowls or other open, shared containers.
- If you feel drunk and haven't had any alcohol, or have been drinking but feel that the effects are much stronger than usual, get help from a friend immediately.

Reducing the Risk of Date Rape

Preventing date rape requires effort from both men and women.

For women:

- When dating someone you don't know well, stay in public or go out in a group. Arrange for your own transportation; don't rely on your date for transport.
- Watch out for coercive behavior on a date. If your date tries to pressure you into activities you'd rather avoid, such as drinking heavily, you may face similar pressures for sex as well.
- Trust your instincts. If you feel uncomfortable with someone, respect that feeling and act on it by getting away from the person immediately. You

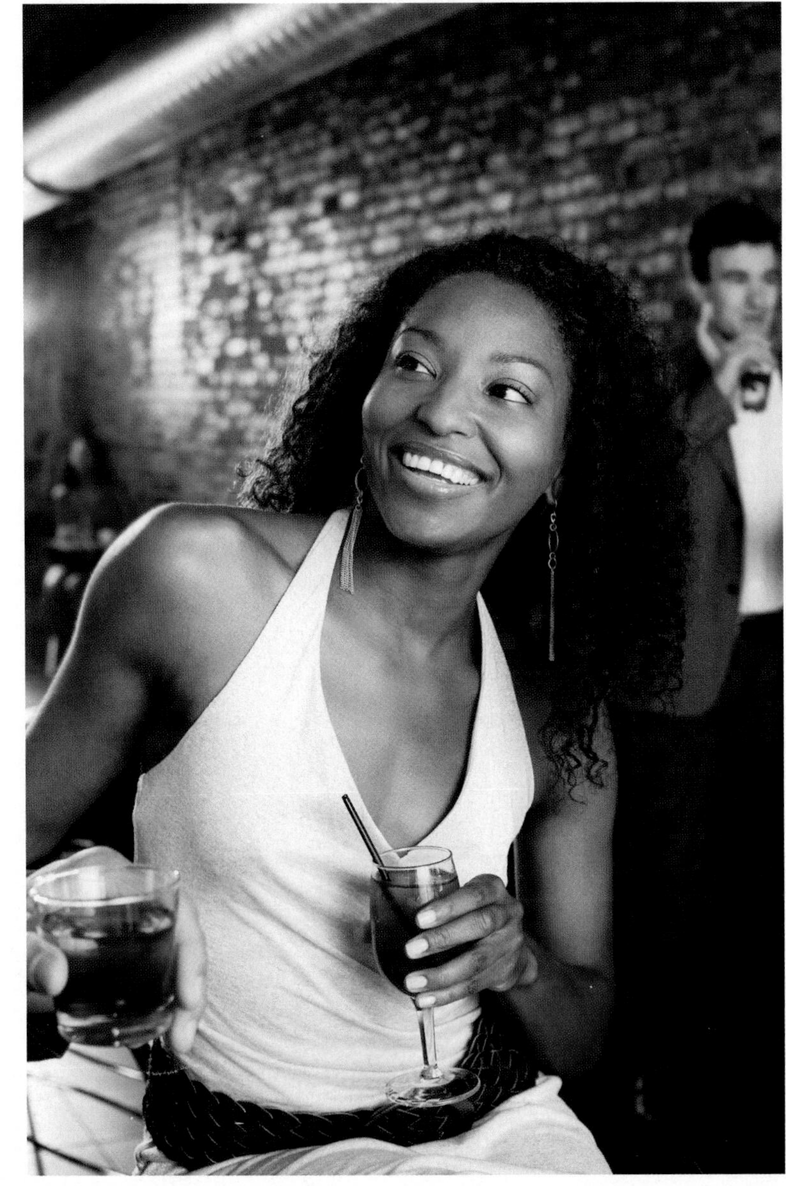

Date rape drugs can be difficult to detect once added to drinks.

have no obligation to protect this person's feelings. Your obligation is to protect yourself.

- Tell others about what is happening to you. If you are being pressured to drink or have sex by someone aggressive at a party, let your friends know and get out of there.
- Keep in mind that drinking and drugs make it harder for you to communicate clearly and set limits about sex.
- Be assertive and direct with both your words and your actions. If you are being pressured for sex and don't want to participate, it's no time to send mixed messages. Say "No!" or "Stop it!" loudly and clearly. If the pressure persists or worsens, tell the other person that he or she is attempting rape. Yell, make a scene, and run away.

For men:

- "No" means "No." Even if you think her outfit means "Yes," or her flirtatious manner means "Yes," pay attention to her reactions and words. When in doubt, back off.
- Women who are intoxicated cannot legally consent to sex. Again, sex with a woman who is drunk or under the influence of drugs is rape.
- Drinking and drugs make it harder for you to communicate clearly and set limits about sex, too.
- Remember what being together offers—and what it doesn't. It offers both of you a chance to get to know each other better in a social setting. It is not an automatic ticket to sex. You both have the right to set limits and refuse any level of sexual activity.

Defending Yourself Against Rape

What if you've followed all the precautions, but still find yourself in a threatening situation? Experts suggest that, unless the assailant is carrying a weapon, immediate action on your part can be effective. Many potential victims think and talk their way out of an attack. For instance, you might say that your roommate is due back any moment, or that you have genital herpes or are HIV-positive, or that your father is a local police officer. You can also try pretending to faint, or crying hysterically, or acting as if you're having a mental breakdown. The simple act of screaming can stop an attack. Scream as loud and as high as you can, and keep screaming as you attempt to run.

If you can't get away, fighting may increase your risk for injury but it will also decrease the chance that the rape attempt will succeed. Rather than wasting your energy flailing about, strike for the attacker's most vulnerable areas: eyes, ears, temples, base of skull, windpipe (Adam's apple), spine, groin, and knees. Because thigh muscles are far more powerful than arm muscles, kicking can be more effective than hitting. Some self-defense experts advise dropping to the floor. This gives you a firm base from which to strike with your legs, and because most men are used to upper-body fighting, this may well take your assailant by surprise. In the split second it takes him to figure out his next move, you'll have an opportunity to kick your assailant's knee joint, roll out of his reach, and run.

Again, if your attacker is armed, you may endanger your life by fighting. Every situation is different, so use your best judgment. Choosing not to resist does not equal consent.

If You Are Raped or Sexually Assaulted

If you are raped or otherwise sexually assaulted, remember that you are not to blame. Sexual violence occurs because the attacker is hostile, not because of something you've said, done, or worn. It is a violent crime, and sex happens to be the weapon.

After an assault, go to a place where you feel safe, and call someone you trust. Write down as many facts about the attack as you can remember. Try not to change your clothes or clean up; you'll destroy physical evidence that may be helpful if you report the attack to the police. Instead, go to a hospital to be treated for any injuries you've received and screened for sexually transmitted infections. If female, you can be monitored for pregnancy and you may be offered emergency contraception. Physical evidence can be collected at that time while you decide whether to report the attack. When you seek medical care, ask for referrals to a counselor who can help you deal with the many emotional and psychological challenges that can arise after a sexual assault.

The decision to report a rape or sexual assault can be difficult. You may be reluctant to talk about the attack publicly. Top barriers to reporting a sexual assault include shame, guilt, and embarrassment;

> *"Sexual assailants tend to repeat their behavior. By reporting a sexual assault, you may prevent another attack in the future."*

concerns about confidentiality; and concerns about not being believed.[98] Moreover, a year-long investigation of sexual assault on college campuses by the Center for Public Integrity revealed that, even when found guilty, perpetrators rarely face tough punishments such as expulsion and criminal proceedings, whereas many victims feel so traumatized that they drop out of school.[99]

Reporting the crime, however, may help restore your sense of power and control. Sexual assailants tend to repeat their behavior. By reporting a sexual assault, you may prevent another attack in the future.

Sexual Abuse of Children

Of the 800,000 cases of child abuse documented in 2007, about 64,000 took the form of sexual abuse.[88] This form of assault covers any type of sexual contact, regardless of the apparent willingness of the child, between an adult and a child below the legal age of consent. It is also a hidden crime that often goes unreported, with actual cases estimated at about three times the number of those documented in police files.[100]

This type of abuse takes many forms, including inappropriate touching, exposure of genitalia to a child, and using a child as a pornography subject. Most abusers are men who know the children they abuse, and about one-third of abusers are related to their victims.[101]

For sexually abused children, the long-term emotional and psychological effects are often devastating. If you think a child you know is being sexually abused, get help immediately.

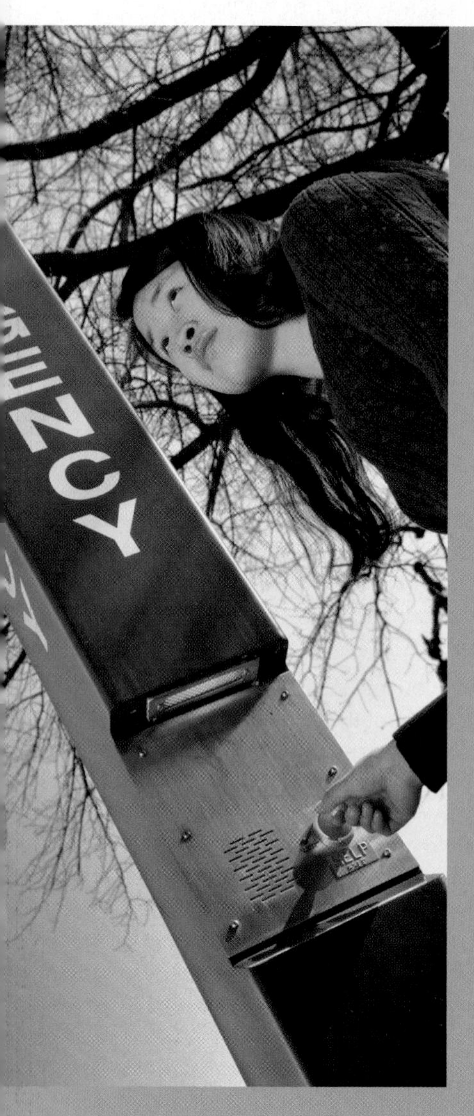

10 Tips for CAMPUS SAFETY

1. Program numbers for campus safety services into your cell phone, because most 911 calls from cell phones go to highway safety dispatchers, not local police. Also program in the direct line for the local police department. Sign up for email alerts from your campus safety services as well.
2. Whether you live in a dorm, group house, or apartment, know where the smoke detectors are and make sure they are working. Know where the emergency exits are and what your fire escape plan is.
3. Keep entryways, stairways, and hallways well-lit and free of clutter. Don't stand on chairs, beds, or shelves to change ceiling lights or swat an insect above your reach. Instead, use a proper footstool or short ladder.
4. Drink in moderation, if at all. Alcohol is a factor in fires, falls, drownings, and many other injury situations, as well as in assaults, date rapes, and other campus crimes.
5. If you make purchases online using your credit card, don't use a shared computer. If you own a smartphone, password-protect it. Also, make sure you know how to remotely lock it and erase personal data. If it's lost or stolen, you'll need to act fast to protect yourself from cyber crime.
6. Keep your doors locked when you're home and when you're out, and don't loan out your keys. Never prop open access doors or let strangers in. If someone has arrived to visit another occupant, they can get the person they are visiting to let them in.
7. Don't travel alone after dark. Take a shuttle, go with a friend, or use the security escorts available on many campuses.
8. Give friends or family your schedule of classes, work, and other activities.
9. Keep your valuables hidden. That's not always easy to do in a small dorm room, but it should still be possible to keep money, ATM cards, jewelry, and other valuables out of plain sight.
10. Know your surroundings and trust your instincts. If something doesn't seem right, get help by calling campus security.

Source: Adapted from *Seven Tips for Campus Safety*, by Security on Campus, Inc., 2008, retrieved from http://www.securityoncampus.org/index.php?option=com_content&view=article&id=1563; *College Student Safety Tips*, by Livesecure.org, 2009, retrieved from http://www.livesecure.org/college-student-safety-tips; *College Safety Tips—Campus Safety Tips*, by Collegesafe.com, 2003, retrieved from http://www.collegesafe.com/campus_safety_tips.htm.

Effects of Sexual Violence

Sexual violence has immediate and long-term consequences on psychological and social health. Following sexual violence, victims often experience depression, increased risk of suicide, substance abuse, sleep disorders, sexual dysfunction, and post-traumatic stress disorder. They may also have decreased capacity to form intimate bonds with partners, strained relationships with loved ones, and, in some groups, sexual abuse can lead to rejection of the victim by partners or family.

Children who are sexually abused often come to suffer from low self-esteem, feelings of worthlessness, and abnormal or distorted views of sex. Among other problems, sexually abused children may also develop distrust of adults, difficulty relating to others except on sexual terms, depression, withdrawal from loved ones, secretiveness, delinquency, and feelings of being "dirty" or "damaged."

Change Yourself, Change Your World

By taking some basic injury-prevention precautions, knowing how to support a friend who has experienced violence, and encouraging others to look for nonviolent ways to resolve conflicts, you can help keep yourself from becoming a statistic and build a safer campus and community.

Personal Choices

Fires, falls, crimes, and abusive relationships unfortunately do occur on college campuses. For general tips on how to reduce your risk for unintentional and intentional injury on campus, see the **Ten Tips for Campus Safety** box on the opposite page.

A 2011 survey of college students nationwide found that nearly 20% had experienced verbal threats, and nearly 10% had been involved in an emotionally abusive intimate relationship in the past year. See the **Student Stats** box for other findings of this survey. Although these statistics on campus violence may be frightening, the problem can be confronted. While in college, you can help by:

- **Knowing your campus safety rules and resources.** Especially since the Virginia Tech shootings, most U.S. college campuses have revised and improved their campus safety rules and resources. Learn what they are and how you can take advantage of them to protect your personal safety.
- **Avoiding substance abuse.** As you've learned in this chapter, alcohol and other substance abuse is closely tied to many types of violent crime. (See Chapters 8 and 9 for ways to get involved in reducing substance abuse on your campus.)
- **Steering clear of social pressures that encourage violence.** You may encounter acquaintances or groups that encourage domination of others, hostility to outsiders, binge drinking, or sexual aggression. Don't play along.
- **Making sure any guns in your residence are handled safely.** Keep them unloaded, out of sight, and securely away from kids. Invest in a lock-and-load indicator, and use it. Also, take a course in gun safety.
- **Reporting crime.** If you see or hear about a crime, let campus security or police know.

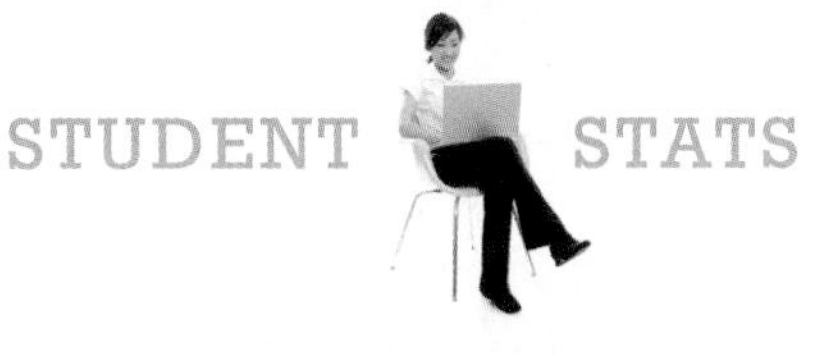

Violent Crime and Abusive Relationships on Campus

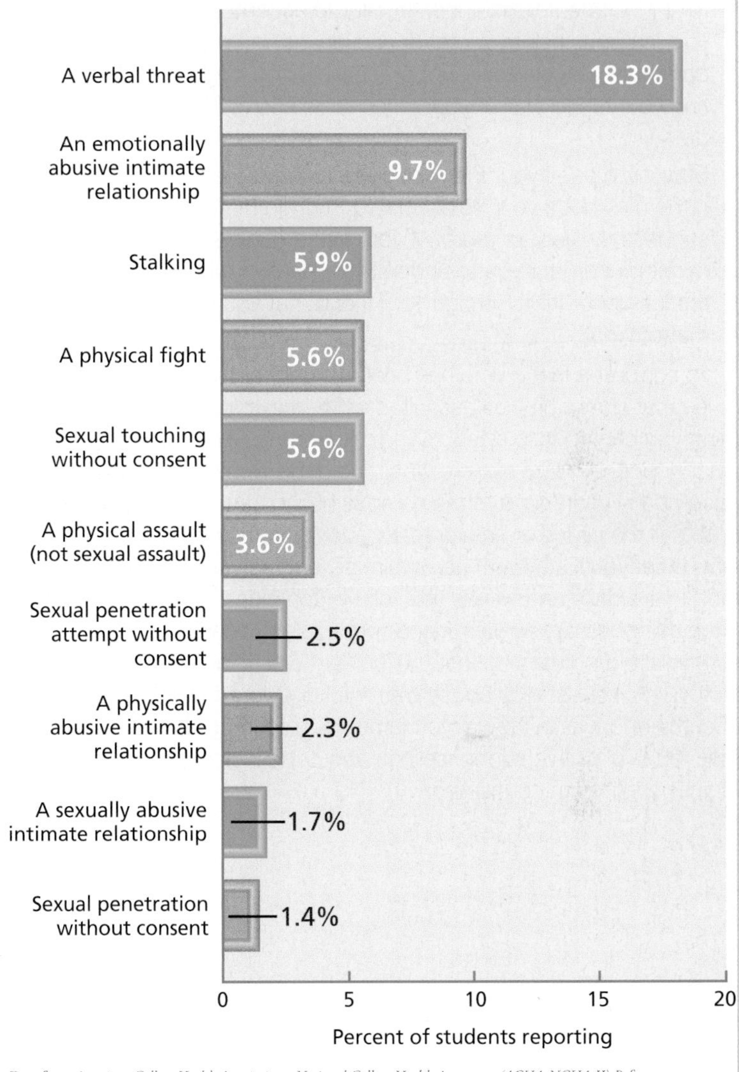

Data from *American College Health Association - National College Health Assessment (ACHA-NCHA II) Reference Group Executive Summary, Fall 2011*, by the American College Health Association, 2012, retrieved from http://www.acha-ncha.org/reports_ACHA-NCHAII.html.

Helping a Friend

Your friend shows up with black-and-blue bruises on both arms. You ask what that's about, and your friend shrugs, saying she had a fight with her boyfriend, and asks that you forget it. Should you forget it? If not, what could you possibly do that might help? The U.S. Department of Health and Human Services offers the following suggestions for helping a friend who's being abused:[102]

- Assuming you're somewhere private and have time to talk without being interrupted, ask your friend to tell you a little more about what she or he has been going through. Listen. Don't interrupt. Keep in mind that it might be very hard for your friend to talk about it. That's especially true for males experiencing abuse.

- Tell your friend you're concerned about her or his safety. Try to help your friend to see that what's going on just isn't right, and that she or he can do something about it and has your support.
- Don't place shame, blame, or guilt on your friend. Don't say, "You just need to break up." Instead, say something like, "I get scared thinking about what might happen to you."
- Offer specific assistance. Help your friend make an action plan. This might include, for instance, an offer to accompany your friend to your campus health center or security office, an IPV agency in your community, or another support service. You might also consider letting your friend stay at your place while she or he figures out what to do.
- Stay involved. If your friend decides to leave the relationship, she or he may need your help working through feelings of loneliness, sadness, anxiety, or regret. If your friend decides to stay, although it might be hard for you to understand, keep in mind that you cannot rescue her or him. Remind your friend that you're always there no matter what.

To support a friend who has been sexually assaulted—or who believes that she or he was assaulted while intoxicated—the most helpful thing you can do is to listen. Give your friend plenty of time to explain what happened, and explore what she or he wants to do next. Offer to accompany your friend to the campus health center or security office, or to call the police or an advocacy agency in the community. Tell your friend that you'll stay with her or him as long as you're needed, and do that. In the days and weeks that follow, continue to listen when and as often as necessary as your friend "processes" what's happened. Make sure to avoid suggesting that the incident was in any way your friend's fault. Even if substance abuse was involved, your friend was a victim of crime and was in no way to blame. It's also important to understand that you might have strong feelings about the incident yourself, and might benefit from counseling.

Campus Advocacy

Although it's easy to feel overwhelmed by issues of campus safety, the good news is that there are many ways you can help. Here are just a few:

- Students Against Violence Everywhere (SAVE) has more than 2,000 chapters in schools and colleges nationwide. SAVE works to promote personal safety and reduce violent crime and victimization. Chapters typically meet one or two evenings per month to organize service projects and awareness campaigns. For more information, check out **www.nationalsave.org**
- The National Organization for Women (NOW) has chapters on campuses across the United States. Founded in 1966, NOW has been working for decades to promote the equality of women. Whether you're male or female, you're invited to join NOW's Campus Action Network. Go to **www.now.org/chapters/campus/signup.html.** While you're on that site, consider downloading the toolkit for preventing and fighting sexual assault on campus, which includes a campus resource quiz, action items, sample letters, flyers, and more resources to help you take action today.
- Join Students Active for Ending Rape (SAFER), the American Association of University Women's student group dedicated to fighting sexual assault on campus. Download the AAUW-SAFER Campus Sexual Assault Program in a Box from **www.aauw.org/act/laf/library/assault_students.cfm** to get started.
- Men often feel as if their gender automatically makes them responsible for the problem of violence, and excludes them from becoming part of the solution. Not so. A national organization called Men Can Stop Rape shifts the responsibility for violence prevention toward men by promoting healthy, nonviolent masculinity, and engaging men as allies in proactive solutions to end violence against women. This organization is operating right now on college campuses across the nation. Find out more about its Campus Men of Strength Clubs at **www.mencanstoprape.org/The-Campus-Men-of-Strength-Club.**

Watch videos of real students discussing personal safety at www.pearsonhighered.com/lynchelmore.

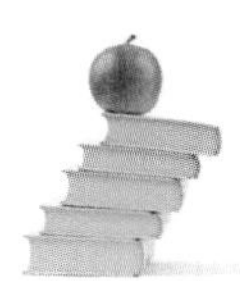

Choosing to Change Worksheet

To complete this worksheet online, visit www.pearsonhighered.com/lynchelmore.

Part I. Understanding Your Risk from Aggressive Driving

You had the opportunity to make observations about whether or not you have aggressive driving habits by completing the "Are You an Aggressive Driver?" Self-Assessment on page 548. List each of your aggressive habits.

____

____

Part II. Avoiding Aggressive Driving

Directions: Fill in your stage of change in Step 1 and complete Steps 2, 3, or 4, depending on which one applies to your stage of change.

Step 1: Your Stage of Behavior Change. Please check one of the following statements that best describe your readiness to make your driving safer.

_______ I do not intend to improve my driving in the next 6 months. (Precontemplation)

_______ I am contemplating improving my driving in the next 6 months. (Contemplation)

_______ I am planning on improving my driving in the next month. (Preparation)

_______ I have been improving my driving for less than 6 months. (Action)

_______ I have been improving my driving for 6 months or longer. (Maintenance)

Step 2: Precontemplation and Contemplation Stages. Consider what you can do to make your driving less aggressive.

What are the advantages of adopting these behaviors to increase driving safety? (List at least three.)

1. ____
2. ____
3. ____

What are some things that might get in the way of your efforts to implement these behaviors? (List at least two.)

1. ____
2. ____

What ideas do you have to overcome these obstacles?

____

____

Step 3: Preparation. How do you expect to benefit from adopting these behaviors and actions to increase driving safety?

____

____

Which of these reasons is most important to you, and why?

____

____

List a specific **goal,** including a timeline, for improving your driving.

____

Step 4: Action and Maintenance. In what ways have you benefited from adopting these behaviors and actions?

____

____

What motivates you the most to continue practicing these behaviors and why?

____

____

How easy are these behaviors and actions to increase safe driving to maintain? Is it truly a habit or do you need to expend some effort to do it?

____

____

Chapter Summary

- Injuries are the leading cause of death among Americans between the ages of 1 and 44.
- One of the most significant risk factors for injuries is substance abuse.
- Motor vehicle accidents claim more lives among Americans aged 15 to 24 than any other single cause of death.
- Distracted driving, impaired driving, poor use of safety features, speeding, and other forms of aggressive driving are risk factors for MVAs.
- Motorcyclists are about six times more likely than those riding in a car to die in a crash. Not all states require motorcyclists to wear a helmet, but each year, helmets save thousands of lives.
- Bicycle injuries send more than half a million people to emergency departments in the United States each year, and cause several hundred deaths. Failure to wear a bike helmet is a top factor in head injuries among cyclists.
- Every day, about 75 Americans die from unintentional poisoning. Many of these deaths are due to overdose of legal and illicit drugs.
- Falls, caused by slippery or unstable flooring, cluttered stairs, or improper use of ladders, are the top culprit in home injuries.
- In adults, eating too fast, without chewing food properly, is the most common factor in choking. Use of the Heimlich maneuver can save the life of someone who is choking.
- Drowning is the second leading cause of unintentional injury death in people aged 10 to 19. Consumption of alcohol is a factor in 60% of drowning deaths.
- Careless handling of lit cigarettes or candles, along with improperly used or maintained cooking and heating equipment, are the causes of most home fires. Alcohol plays a role in about 60% of fire fatalities.
- If there are guns in your home, keep them unloaded, put away, and away from children. Use a safety lock-and-load indicator, and always treat a gun as if it were loaded, even if you think it isn't.
- Both repetitive strain injuries and back injuries are common among college students. Take frequent breaks from typing and texting, and lighten the load in your backpack.
- To avoid weather-related injuries, stay informed and prepared. Stock an emergency supply kit.
- Violence is also a leading cause of death and injury among young people, especially young men.
- Violent crimes include murder, forcible rape, robbery, and aggravated assault. In 2010, there were 15 murders, over 2,900 forcible sex offenses, about 1,800 robberies, and more than 2,500 aggravated assaults on 2- and 4-year college campuses in the United States.
- Most violent crimes are committed by men. Men are more likely to be murdered than women, and women are more likely to be raped. Women are also more likely to be victimized by intimate partner violence.
- The rate of violent crime in the United States has been declining for many years.
- Murder is second only to unintentional injuries as the leading cause of death in the United States among people between the ages of 15 and 24.
- Cyber crime, including identity theft, is a growing problem in the United States.
- Intimate partner violence is experienced by more than 12 million Americans each year. It includes psychological abuse as well as physical and sexual assault. Victims stay in abusive relationships for a variety of reasons.

- Stalking is a pattern of harassment or threats directed at a specific person that is intended to cause intimidation and fear. More than 5 million American women experience stalking each year.
- Sexual violence can take many forms, including unwanted touching, unwanted uncompleted or completed sexual acts, and noncontact violations such as voyeurism or sexual harassment. Many women who are sexually assaulted know their attackers.
- Date rape is a common problem on college campuses. Drinking and drug use is a factor in many cases of date rape, and the problem persists, in part, because of rape-tolerant attitudes and misconceptions about women held by some college men.
- You can greatly reduce your risk for rape by staying sober and communicating your choices firmly and clearly. If you find yourself in a threatening situation, unless the assailant is carrying a weapon, you may be able to talk, act, run, scream, and/or fight your way out of it.
- Declining rates of violent crime show that prevention works, including personal steps such as knowing and respecting campus safety rules, drinking moderately, handling guns safely, encouraging a culture of respect, refusing to remain silent if you witness any aggressive act, and reporting crime. You can help support a friend experiencing violence by listening without judgment, and encouraging practical actions such as using campus resources.

Test Your Knowledge

1. What cause of injury most often kills people in the United States between the ages of 15 and 24?
   a. car crashes
   b. violence, such as a fight or a gunshot
   c. drowning
   d. bike accidents

2. Which of the following is dangerous when you are driving?
   a. feeling drowsy
   b. texting
   c. talking on your hands-free cell phone
   d. all of the above

3. Carpal tunnel syndrome
   a. is a type of repetitive strain injury.
   b. isn't an issue if you mostly use a keypad on a cell phone or PDA.
   c. is due to compression of the carpal bones of the wrist.
   d. is typically prompted when people put out their hands to attempt to break a fall.

4. What is the leading cause of unintentional injuries at home?
   a. drowning in a bathtub or pool
   b. residential fires
   c. gunshots
   d. falls

5. About what percentage of murders are known to have been committed by someone the victim knew?
   a. 18%
   b. 43%
   c. 61%
   d. 84%

6. Which of the following statements about cyber crime is true?
   a. Households headed by people age 65 and older are most likely to experience identity theft.
   b. "Skimming" is the practice of stealing another person's mail.

Get Critical

What happened:

On February 22, 2012, former University of Virginia student George Hughely V was convicted of second-degree murder in the death of his ex-girlfriend, Yeardley Love. The jury decided against a conviction of murder in the first degree, determining that Hughely had not intended to kill Love when he kicked in the door of her apartment on May 2, 2010, and beat her unconscious. He'd been drinking heavily all day in the company of his father and friends, and several witnesses reported recognizing that he was very drunk. Moreover, when interviewed by police the next morning, Hughely expressed shock and grief when informed that Love was dead. Hughely's defense team argued that the death was a "tragic accident," and that their client was guilty only of manslaughter. But jurors didn't buy it. Hughely's prior arrests for intoxication, as well as previous assaults on Love and a trail of threatening emails, convinced them that, although Hughely may not have planned to murder Love that night, he had acted with reckless disregard for her life. In August 2012, he was sentenced to 23 years in prison.

What do you think?

- **Hughely had assaulted Love before, and in at least one email message, said he wished he had killed her. A first-degree murder sentence requires premeditation. Do you think that Hughely was guilty of first-degree murder? Or do you agree with his defense team that his obvious intoxication meant he could not be held responsible for his actions?**
- **Hughely's father and friends knew that he abused alcohol and was prone to violence. In 2007, he'd been charged with underage possession of alcohol and reckless driving, and in 2008, he was arrested for public drunkenness and had to be subdued with a taser. Just 2 months before the murder, a friend had broken up what appeared to be a strangulation attempt on Yeardley Love. To what extent—if any—could Hughely's father and friends have contributed to Love's murder? Does the University of Virginia bear any blame?**
- **If you had a friend who was being threatened by an ex-partner, what would you do?**

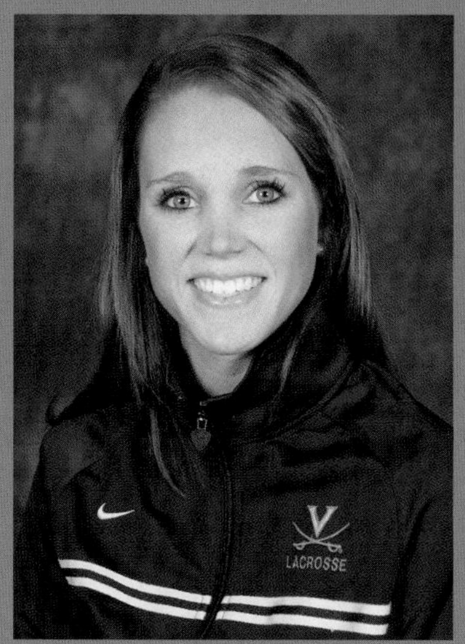

Yeardley Love.

c. It is not safe to respond to text messages from unknown sources.
d. None of the above are true.

7. Which of the following is a common cause of death in hazing incidents?
a. water intoxication
b. alcohol poisoning
c. physical assault
d. both b and c

8. What is a hate crime?
a. a crime driven by dislike of someone personally
b. a crime driven by bias against a person's or group's race, ethnicity or national origin, sexual orientation, or religious beliefs
c. premeditated, politically motivated violence intended to influence a large audience
d. none of the above

9. Sexual harassment
a. occurs in both schools and workplaces.
b. by definition involves loss of employment or academic standing.
c. only affects young women.
d. applies only to the two people involved, not to anyone else around them.

10. Date rape
a. is more likely if one or both people on a date have been drinking.
b. doesn't carry the same legal penalties as other types of rape.
c. is legally known as statutory rape.
d. is all of the above.

Get Connected

Mobile Tips!

Scan this QR code with your mobile device to access additional tips about reducing your risk for intentional and unintentional injuries. Or, via your mobile device, go to **http://mobiletips.pearsoncmg.com**. and navigate to Chapter 20.

Health Online Visit the following websites for further information about the topics in this chapter:

- National Center for Injury Prevention & Control
  www.cdc.gov/injury/index.html
- National Safety Council
  www.nsc.org
- Home Safety Council
  http://homesafetycouncil.org
- American Association of Poison Control Centers
  www.aapcc.org
- Injury Prevention Web
  www.injuryprevention.org
- Motorcycle Safety Foundation
  www.msf-usa.org
- National Domestic Violence Hotline
  www.thehotline.org
- Childhelp National Child Abuse Hotline
  www.childhelp.org
- Rape, Abuse, & Incest National Network (RAINN)
  www.rainn.org
- No Woman Left Behind
  www.facebook.com/NWLBCampaign

Website links are subject to change. To access updated web links, please visit *www.pearsonhighered.com/lynchelmore*.

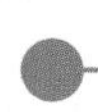

References

i. Murphy, S. L., Xu, J. Q., & Kochanek, K. D. (2012, January 11). Deaths: Preliminary data for 2010. *National Vital Statistics Reports 60* (4). Hyattsville, MD: National Center for Health Statistics. Retrieved from http://www.cdc.gov/nchs/data/nvsr/nvsr60/nvsr60_04.pdf.

ii. National Highway Traffic Safety Administration. (2010, September). *Distracted driving 2009. Traffic safety facts research note.* DOT HS 811 379. Retrieved from http://www.distraction.gov/download/research-pdf/Distracted-Driving-2009.pdf.

iii. Centers for Disease Control and Prevention. (2011). *National intimate partner and sexual violence survey: Highlights of 2010 findings.* Retrieved from http://www.cdc.gov/violenceprevention/nisvs.

1. Murphy, S. L., Xu, J. Q., & Kochanek, K. D. (2012, January 11). Deaths: Preliminary data for 2010. *National Vital Statistics Reports 60* (4). Hyattsville, MD: National Center for Health Statistics. Retrieved from http://www.cdc.gov/nchs/data/nvsr/nvsr60/nvsr60_04.pdf.

2. Centers for Disease Control and Prevention. (2012, January 17). *Injuries and violence are leading causes of death: Key data and statistics.* Retrieved from http://www.cdc.gov/injury/overview/data.html.

3. Centers for Disease Control and Prevention. (2010). *2008 Emergency department summary tables. National hospital ambulatory medical care survey*. Retrieved from http://www.cdc.gov/nchs/data/ahcd/nhamcs_emergency/nhamcsed2008.pdf.

4. National Safety Council. (2012, February 29). *Safety at home*. Retrieved from http://www.nsc.org/safety_home/Pages/safety_at_home.aspx.

5. Centers for Disease Control and Prevention. (2010). CDC WISQARS (Web-based Injury Statistics Query and Reporting System). Atlanta, GA: U.S. Department of Health and Human Services, CDC. Available at http://www.cdc.gov/injury/wisqars.

6. National Institute on Alcohol Abuse and Alcoholism. (2010). *Rethinking drinking: Alcohol and your health.* Retrieved from http://rethinkingdrinking.niaaa.nih.gov/WhatsTheHarm/WhatAreTheRisks.asp.

7. National Ski Areas Association. (2011, September 1). Facts about skiing/snowboarding safety. Retrieved from http://www.nsaa.org/nsaa/press/NSAA-Facts-Ski-SnowB-Safety-9-11.pdf.

8. American Alpine Club. (2012). Accidents in North American mountaineering. Retrieved from http://c535846.r46.cf2.rackcdn.com/anam_2007.pdf.

9. National Highway Traffic Safety Administration. (2010, September). *Distracted driving 2009. Traffic safety facts research note.* Retrieved from http://www.distraction.gov/download/research-pdf/Distracted-Driving-2009.pdf.

10. Austin, M. (2009, June). Texting while driving: How dangerous is it? *Car and Driver.* Retrieved from http://www.caranddriver.com/features/09q2/texting_while_driving_how_dangerous_is_it_-feature.

11. Patten, C. J. D., Kircher, A., Ostlund, J., & Nilsson, L. (2004). Using mobile telephones: Cognitive workload and attention resource allocation. *Accident Analysis and Prevention, 36,* 341–350.

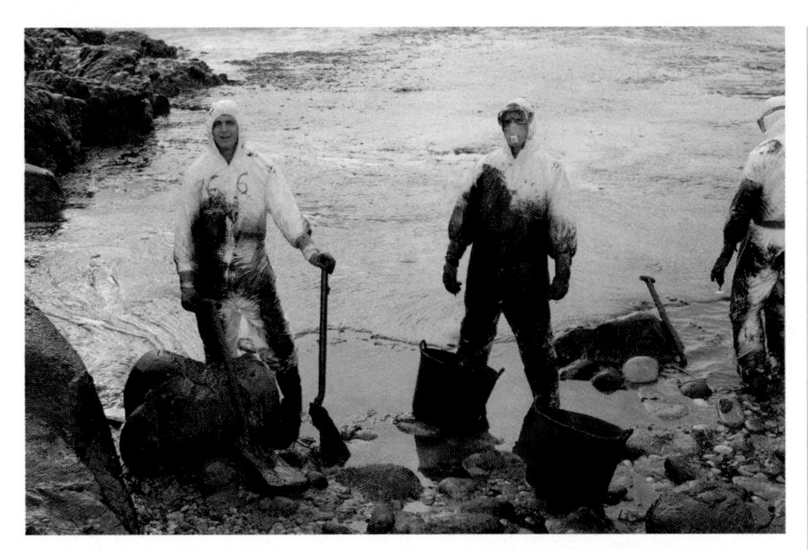

Pollution, such as oil spills, can have long-lasting effects on the health of humans and the environment.

Defining Your Environment

Your environment includes, of course, the features of the natural world that surround you, such as air, water, and soil. It also includes the "built" environment, which encompasses manufactured structures and products; components of transportation networks such as streets and airports; waste management systems; and human alterations to the natural world, such as dams or irrigation systems. Your environment also includes social aspects, including your socioeconomic status and factors in your community such as the level of crime. All of these influence human health. For example, residents of a neighborhood with walking and bike paths, community gardens, and a low-cost health-care clinic are likely to enjoy better health than residents of a neighborhood without such amenities. (To review these factors, see Chapter 1.)

We said earlier that, although we all live in a local ecosystem, all humans share one global environment. This means that we're affected both by local conditions and by conditions many miles away. The fact that we all share one global ecosystem makes environmental health a global issue.

Environmental Health Is a Global Issue

In the United States, it can be easy to think that environmental health relates only to conditions close to home. The U.S. Environmental Protection Agency (EPA) exists to protect human health and to safeguard the natural environment—air, water, and land—upon which life depends.[3] We enjoy environmental policies that curb pollution, provide safe drinking water, and protect open spaces for relaxation and exercise. We also issue public health warnings if air quality is poor or the water at a public beach becomes polluted. So we may think that, if our own immediate ecosystem is protected, then we must be as well.

But our local ecosystem is tied to that of our planet. As a result, no one community or nation can provide an environmental "island of safety." For instance, almost all of us watch for the lowest prices when we shop, and in recent decades, that often means buying goods made in China. This consumer demand has led to an enormous surge in manufacturing in China, a country where environmental enforcement is not as strong as it is in North America and Western Europe. The factories that make the goods we buy, and the coal-burning power plants that fuel them, release large quantities of mercury and other airborne pollutants. These pollutants have profound health effects in China, where air pollution is a leading cause of death.[4] But the damage doesn't end at China's borders. Scooped up by powerful winds, these contaminants blow across the Pacific Ocean and fall upon North America, where scientists have detected them in the air over Los Angeles and in snowfall in Colorado's Rocky Mountains.[5] The affordable flat-screen TVs and digital cameras that we buy here may seem like a bargain, but their effect on the global ecosystem is, in fact, very costly.

The Evolution of Environmental Health

The environmental health movement got its start over a century ago, when advances in microbiology led to broad acceptance of the germ theory of disease. Public health experts came to understand that the diseases responsible for most illness and death were infectious; that is, that they were caused by harmful microbes in people's drinking water, food, and even in the air they breathed. Public health organizations began to develop policies for safe food-handling practices, the management of trash and sewage, and maintenance of a pure public water supply. These efforts paved the way for the broader developments in environmental health that emerged after Word War II.

The improved standard of living in the United States in the postwar years led to an unprecedented population boom. That meant more mouths to feed, which translated into a need for increased agricultural production. Industries in the United States complied by providing a variety of new synthetic fertilizers and pesticides, most notoriously an insecticide called DDT, which began poisoning not just insects, but fish and birds, from the time it was first released for agricultural use in 1945. Then, in 1962, marine biologist Rachel Carson published *Silent Spring,* a book that was to galvanize the environmental movement. In it, Carson warned about the harmful effects of indiscriminate use of DDT and other synthetic pesticides—for example, she asked her readers to consider the effect of pesticides on songbird species, whose extinction might someday lead to a "silent spring."

Skeptics accused Carson of shallow science, but scientists found her research convincing and readers flocked to her cause. In the years that followed, as people in the United States learned about the effects of the defoliation tactics used in jungles during the Vietnam War, they became even more concerned about air, water, and soil pollution. The establishment of the EPA in 1970 was significantly influenced by these pivotal events.[6]

Today, environmental health still encompasses efforts to improve sanitation and reduce the use of harmful pesticides and other pollutants. But since the establishment of the Intergovernmental Panel on Climate Change (IPCC) in 1988, it is increasingly focused on studying the broader effects of global climate change. The IPCC was established by the United Nations Environment Program and the World Meteorological Organization, and thousands of scientists worldwide contribute to its work. One of the IPCC's major activities is the preparation of comprehensive assessment reports on the state of climate change.

An issue as broad as climate change may not seem to have immediate connections to personal health, but a glance at ongoing research shows just how intricately these two issues are related. For example, studies have found that even a slightly warmer planet can lead to more extreme weather events such as hurricanes, more outbreaks of infectious disease, and more food shortages due to altered growing seasons and crop failures.[7] Other potential health effects include increased air pollution and more cases of illnesses carried by insects and rodents.[8] Melting of polar ice means a rise in sea level that threatens coastal communities and could submerge entire islands. According to the World Health Organization, climate change already claims more than 150,000 lives worldwide every year.[9] It's clear, then, why global climate change has become the primary focus of environmental health. We'll look more closely at climate change later in this chapter.

Toward Sustainability

In the last few decades, environmentalists, environmental health experts, and millions of people around the world have taken steps to reverse the effects of environmental damage or prevent further destruction. The concept of **sustainability** is a key aspect of this new movement toward improved environmental awareness and efforts. Sustainability, in very general terms, is the ability to meet society's current needs without compromising future generations' abilities to meet their own needs; it includes policies for ensuring that various aspects of our environment do not become overtaxed, depleted, or destroyed. For example, many programs now exist that allow each of us to *offset,* or counterbalance, the global warming emissions we create. For instance, you may opt to take a long plane flight, and then offset the carbon emissions generated during the flight by contributing a few dollars to a program that sustains forests that absorb and recycle such harmful emissions.

As with any population group, college students vary in their level of concern about pollution and climate change. Check out the **Student Stats** for a look at national trends.

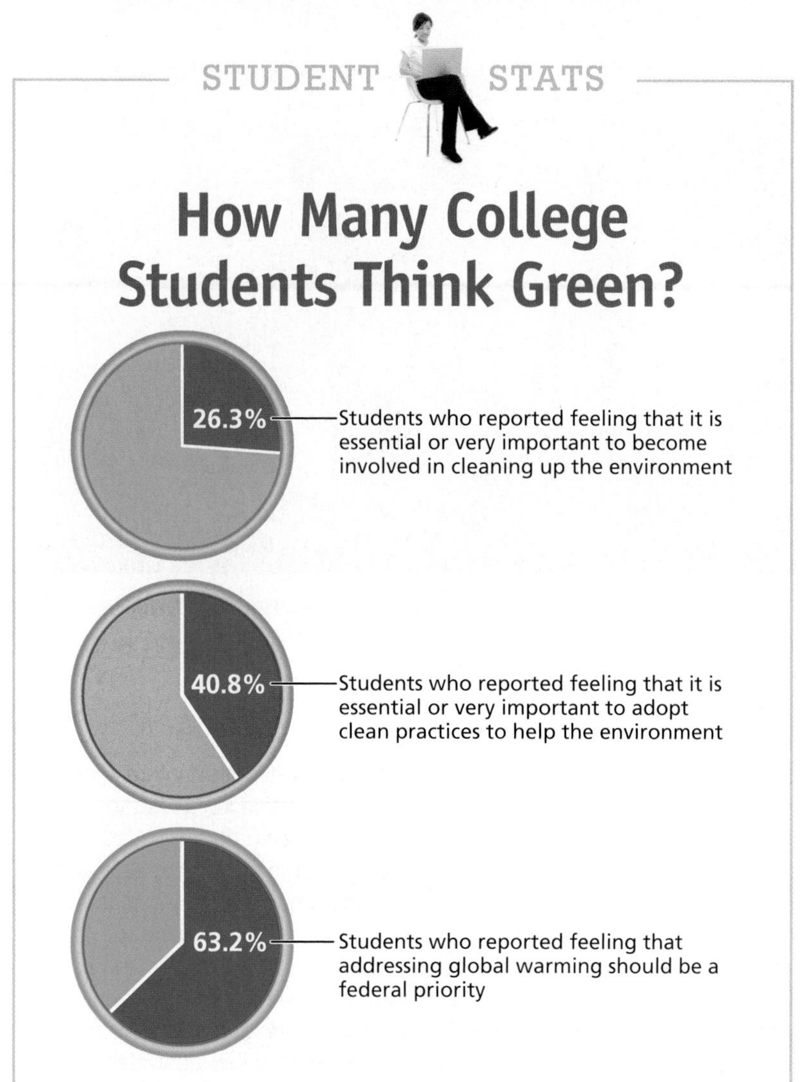

Data from *The American Freshman: National Norms Fall 2011,* by the Higher Education Research Institute, 2011, retrieved from http://heri.ucla.edu/PDFs/pubs/TFS/Norms/Monographs/TheAmericanFreshman2011.pdf.

Overpopulation and Globalization

We share the ecosystem that is Earth with countless other organisms—and none has a greater environmental impact than we do. The demands we place on the environment have skyrocketed in the last two centuries, driven largely by an explosion in the number of people living on our planet. It took all of human history up to the year 1804 for the world's population to reach 1 billion people **(Figure 21.1).** By the end of 2011, it had reached 7 billion, and that number is estimated to exceed 9 billion before 2050. How did the world's population grow so large so fast?

Factors Contributing to Population Growth

A number of factors have driven this trend. Improvements in agricultural production and food storage, preservation, and transportation have made the world's food supply more abundant, accessible, and reliable. A well-nourished population is of course better able to fight disease and will enjoy greater longevity. At the same time, advances in health care, including immunization, antibiotics, and new forms of surgery, have reduced deaths of infants, children, and childbearing women, and at the same time have increased our average life expectancy to just over 78 years.[10] Public health measures such as improved sanitation and infection control, and even campaigns to reduce smoking and other harmful behaviors, have also decreased mortality and increased longevity.

And then there's the sheer mathematics of exponential growth. To understand its contribution to the world's population explosion, let's look at two contrasting examples. Population researchers track population changes by looking at women's **fertility rate,** so we'll do the same.

Let's say that the women in a rural village in the year 1700 each give birth to an average of four children, two sons and two daughters, but because of the high rate of infectious disease in children, on average, only one of the two daughters survives into adulthood to have four children of her own. Even if you were to track this pattern over a dozen generations, you'd have no net growth in population. That's because the village is demonstrating what population researchers refer to as **replacement-level fertility;** that is, the level of fertility at which a population exactly replaces itself from one generation to the next. In our hypothetical village in 1700, where infant and child mortality rates are high, replacement-level fertility is 4.0.

sustainability The ability to meet society's current needs without compromising future generations' abilities to meet their own needs; includes policies for ensuring that certain components of the environment are not depleted or destroyed.

fertility rate Within a given population, the average number of births per woman.

replacement-level fertility The level of fertility at which a population exactly replaces itself from one generation to the next.

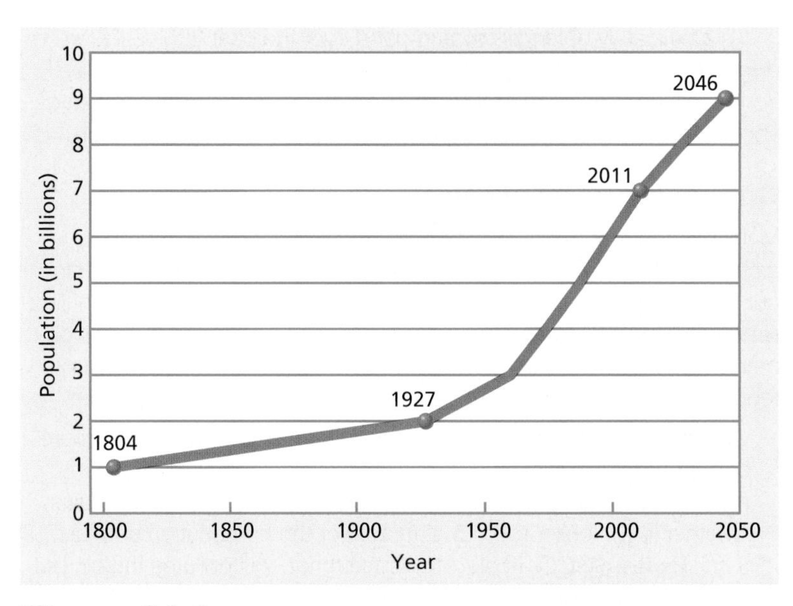

Figure 21.1 World population growth in billions.

Data from *The State of World Population 2011*, by the Population Division of the United Nations Department of Economic and Social Affairs, United Nations Population Fund, 2009, pp. 2–3, retrieved from http://foweb.unfpa.org/SWP2011/reports/EN-SWOP2011-FINAL.pdf.

Because of the technological advances just discussed, in developed countries today, replacement-level fertility averages 2.1 children per woman. So let's imagine what would happen in the same village today if the women have, on average, the same number of children as the women in 1700—two sons and two daughters. These well-nourished, immunized children all survive, typically, to adulthood and the two daughters each give birth to four children of their own. Within just three generations, one grandmother will have produced two daughters and four granddaughters. The population will have quadrupled. Within seven generations, it will have increased 64-fold! You can probably understand now how the world's population grew so large so quickly after 1804 (see Figure 21.1).

Want to find out what the world population stands at today? Go to the World Population Clock: www.census.gov/main/www/popclock.html.

Effects of Overpopulation

To understand the effects of overpopulation, it helps to appreciate the concept of **carrying capacity,** which is the number of organisms of one species—in this case, *Homo sapiens*—that an environment can support indefinitely. Carrying capacity is important because, as a population grows, its demands on its environment increase. Humans need clean air and water, **arable** land on which to grow food, materials for manufacturing, and sources of energy. As countries become more populous, these demands on the environment surge. As a population begins to exceed carrying capacity, food shortages increase, reserves of oil and other sources of energy decline, and the production of air, water, and land pollution overwhelms the environment's capacity for elimination and regeneration.[11] Is this already happening on planet Earth? Consider that 925 million people, more than 13% of the Earth's population, are undernourished.[12] Or that 1.3 billion people, about 20% of the global population, already are without electricity while global demand for energy is expected to increase by one-third over the next 25 years.[13]

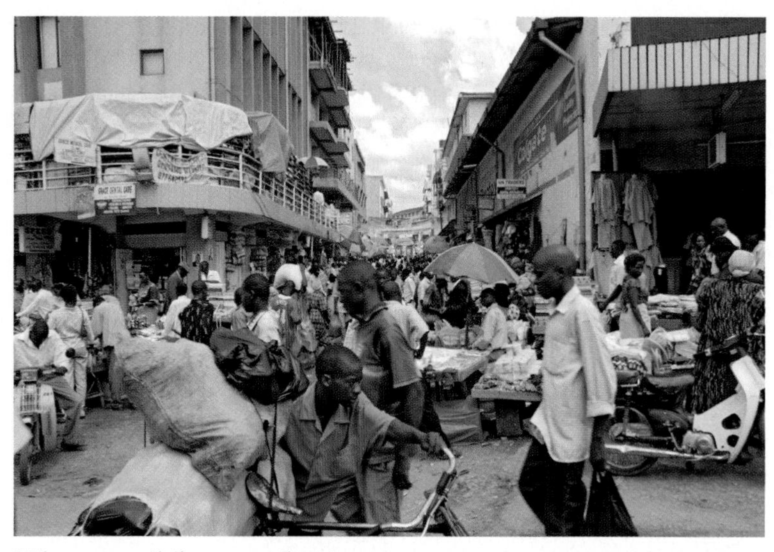

The world population is growing more rapidly than ever, especially in developing countries like Uganda.

Another major factor in global carrying capacity is wealth. More-developed countries enjoy a lifestyle that consumes more resources and generates more waste than that of less-developed countries. For example, although they account for less than 20% of the world's population, industrialized nations contribute roughly 40% of global carbon emissions.[14] The United States has about 5% of the world's people but uses about 22% of its energy.[15] In short, industrialized nations have a larger **ecological footprint.** But as more and more nations transition out of poverty, and their citizens strive to achieve a higher standard of living, their ecological footprint grows. This phenomenon is one aspect of **globalization**—the interaction and integration of regional phenomena such as diets, technologies, arts and entertainment, economies, and other factors, on a global scale. Many of the forces behind globalization have positive aims. But they also carry enormous environmental demands. For example, if more of the world's population drives a gasoline-powered car on a regular basis, the effect is accelerated depletion of oil reserves, more pollution-emitting oil refineries, more tailpipe emissions, and more smog.

carrying capacity The number of organisms of one species that an environment can support indefinitely.

arable Suitable for cultivation of crops.

ecological footprint The collective impact of an entity on its resources, ecosystems, and other key environmental features.

globalization The interaction and integration of regional phenomena globally.

Reversing Population Growth

Within any individual country, several factors contribute to population growth, stability, or decline. These include the ratio of immigration to emigration; life expectancy and mortality; and the fertility rate. For instance, the fertility rate in the United States has hovered at or below replacement level since the mid-1970s, yet the population has continued to grow.[16] The primary reason for this increase is immigration. In countries with a low rate of immigration as well as a low fertility rate, the population may be stable or even in decline. Currently, almost 99% of the world's population growth is taking place in less developed regions.[17] This is in part because, although malnutrition and poor health care increase the replacement-level fertility rate well above 2.1, the fertility rate in some countries in these regions is above 6.[16]

For obvious reasons, then, global efforts at reducing population growth focus on reducing fertility. Probably the most famous—and controversial—of these efforts has been China's "one child policy," instituted in 1979. Couples that adhere to the policy are eligible for financial and other rewards, but those who do not face thousands of dollars in fines. One of the most serious social consequences of the policy has been a growing gender imbalance: Because boys are favored, prenatal sex screening and abortion of female fetuses, as well as infanticide of female newborns, has resulted in China having millions more male children and young adults.

Fortunately, most population control has been achieved by social reforms, especially increasing the availability and affordability of reliable contraceptives, and promoting equal access to education and career opportunities for women. Together, these social factors have helped curb population growth in many regions. Currently, more than 70 nations around the globe have fertility rates below replacement level, and some have rates below 1.5. These include many European and Eastern European countries, as well as a few countries in Asia, including Hong Kong, Singapore, Japan, and others.[16] As a result, these countries have achieved either *zero population growth*—in which a country's number of live births and immigrations is the same as the number of deaths and emigrations—or *negative population growth*—in which a country's population actually declines. Again, these achievements have come about less as a result of governmental mandates than of increased access to contraception, higher education, and professional opportunities for women.[18]

Although there has long been a perception that fertility in Muslim countries is resistant to decline, this is not true. The decline of fertility rates in the Muslim world in the past three decades has been dramatic, averaging 2.6 fewer births per woman between 1975 and 2010, or an average 41% decline. Globally, the average decline in fertility in this period has been 33%.[19]

Within individual nations, negative population growth can present challenges, including an imbalance between retirees and younger people in the workforce; however, a decline in population doesn't necessarily cause a decline in a nation's economy or standard of living.[20] Still, population control is only part of the solution to increasing our environmental health. Industrialized nations must also develop "greener" technologies and services, and share these with the developing world, so that globalization can have a more positive effect on our local and global environments.[21] Developing these greener technologies and services requires an understanding of the scope of the challenges we face. First, we'll look at the air we breathe.

Air Pollution

Close to our planet's surface, air provides the oxygen and carbon dioxide that support human, animal, and plant life. Higher up, in the region of our atmosphere called the stratosphere, a natural layer of gas called *ozone* shields us from excessive sunlight. In between, a mixture of water vapor and other naturally occurring gases, called *greenhouse gases,* occurs. This layer allows solar heat to reach our planet, and retains some of this heat close to Earth's surface. This phenomenon helps keep our planet warm enough to sustain life (Figure 21.3 on page 582 illustrates this process).

It's a delicately balanced system, and over the past 200 years, we've disrupted it, largely through the burning of *fossil fuels,* or fuels derived from decayed organic matter buried underground. In the United States, about 83% of the energy we use is derived from burning fossil fuels.[22]

Common Air Pollutants

Many different pollutants dirty our air, from gases that contribute to global warming to tiny particles of soot and other irritants that damage our lungs. In the United States, environmental regulators have identified almost 200 air pollutants that can harm human health and the environment.[23] Of these, seven pollutants receive close ongoing scrutiny from regulators, health-care researchers, and scientists.[24] These include:

- **Carbon dioxide (CO_2),** a gas naturally found in Earth's atmosphere and, at normal levels, an essential part of life. Carbon dioxide is also a prime ingredient in emissions from the burning of fossil fuels, whether in the boiler room of a factory or the combustion engine of a car. Excessive CO_2 in our atmosphere not only pollutes the air, but serves as a greenhouse gas, trapping heat and contributing heavily to global warming. We'll look more closely at global warming shortly.
- **Carbon monoxide (CO),** also a gas that originates from the burning of fossil fuels. Poisonous to humans, it inhibits the blood's ability to carry oxygen, and excessive exposure can lead to sickness or death. Carbon monoxide can also be a dangerous indoor air pollutant, a facet we'll further address later in this chapter.
- **Sulfur dioxide (SO_2),** a gas that forms when fossil fuels are burned or processed or during metal processing. It is linked to numerous health problems, especially respiratory diseases. SO_2 can also dissolve in water to form acid, and is a primary culprit in the phenomenon of acid rain, discussed shortly.
- **Nitrogen dioxide (NO_2),** a gas also emitted during the burning of fossil fuels. Lower levels can contribute to respiratory illness, and higher levels can be fatal.
- **Ozone (O_3),** a gas composed of three atoms of oxygen, is described by the EPA as "good up high, bad nearby."[25] That is, whereas ozone in the stratosphere is protective, ground-level ozone, which is produced when certain pollutants mix with sunlight, is a harmful com-

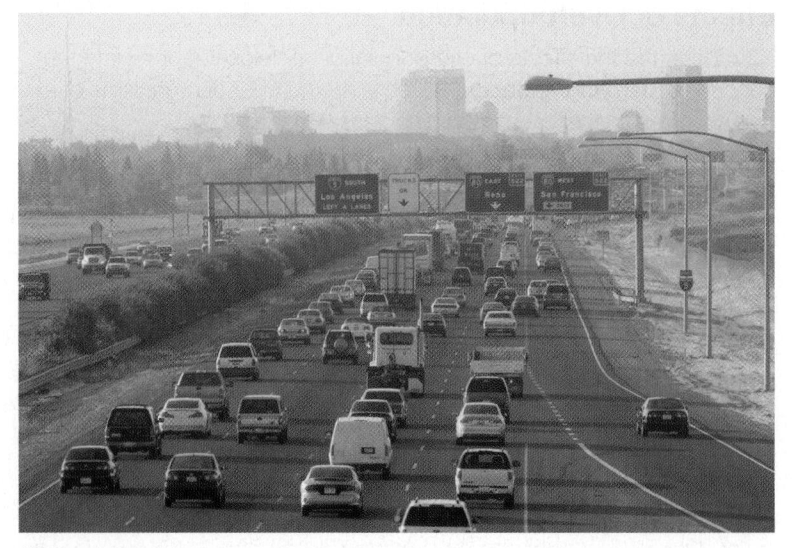

Cars produce many of the emissions that pollute our air.

ponent of smog (discussed shortly). Not only is ground-level ozone a potent respiratory irritant, it also damages crops, trees, and other plant life.

- **Hydrocarbons,** gaseous combinations of hydrogen and carbon that form during the burning of fossil fuels. Hydrocarbons are a precursor to ground-level ozone.
- **Particulates,** minute solid pollutants such as soot that form during the burning of fossil fuels, industrial processes, or the production of almost any kind of smoke, including tobacco smoke. Particulates can lodge in the lungs and trigger or worsen respiratory conditions.

Air Quality Index (AQI) An index for measuring daily air quality according to a list of federal air criteria, published by city or region.

In the United States, environmental health officials have established air quality standards for levels of these pollutants to protect public health. National and local air quality officials regularly monitor the air for these pollutants, and issue health advisories as needed through a tool called the **Air Quality Index (AQI).** When you hear of an air pollution–related health alert on your local radio station, for example, the announcement is usually triggered by a potentially hazardous local score on the Air Quality Index. For a guide to this index, see **Figure 21.2.**

Table 21.1 identifies some of the most common types of outdoor air pollution, their sources, composition, and health effects. Next, we'll take a look at how these pollutants accumulate into some broader environmental phenomena.

When the AQI is in this range:	...air quality conditions are	...as symbolized by this color:
0 to 50	Good	Green
51 to 100	Moderate	Yellow
101 to 150	Unhealthy for sensitive groups	Orange
151 to 200	Unhealthy	Red
201 to 300	Very unhealthy	Purple
301 to 500	Hazardous	Maroon

Figure 21.2 Air Quality Index (AQI).

Source: Air Quality Index (AQI) – A Guide to Air Quality and Your Health, by AIRNow, 2010, retrieved from http://www.airnow.gov/index.cfm?action=aqibasics.aqi.

Environmental Phenomena Associated with Air Pollution

Air pollution increases the risk of asthma and other diseases in humans, and is harmful to animal and plant life. In addition, air pollution causes several broad environmental phenomena, including smog, global warming, thinning of the stratospheric ozone layer, and acid rain.

Look up the air quality in your area at www.airnow.gov.

Table 21.1: Common Types of Outdoor Air Pollution

Pollutant	Source	Description	Health Effects	Who's Most at Risk
Vehicle exhaust	All motorized vehicles and tools powered by fossil fuels, including cars, trucks, lawnmowers, tanker ships, and airplanes. One gallon of gasoline is estimated to produce about 19 pounds of CO_2, as well as many other air pollutants.[1]	A wide range of pollutants and toxins, including CO_2, CO, SO_2, O_3, and hydrocarbons. Particulate matter is also of high concern, especially from older vehicles and engines and locations where vehicle emissions concentrate, such as near freeways.	Breathing difficulties; increased rates of asthma and other lung diseases, cardiovascular disease, and cancer; increased risk of premature death.[2] Particulate matter in the lungs appears to trigger inflammation and can increase a person's risk of death from cardiovascular causes.[3]	People with chronic heart and lung diseases, older adults, those who live near busy freeways and roadways, and children. Levels of ozone and particulate matter are high enough in many parts of the United States to threaten children's health.[4]
Fossil fuel emissions	Power plants, which burn fossil fuels, including coal and natural gas, to generate electricity; office buildings and manufacturing facilities that burn fossil fuels.	A wide range of pollutants and toxins, including CO_2, CO, SO_2, O_3, and hydrocarbons. Particulate matter and mercury are also of concern, especially from power plants and factories that burn coal. Some factory emissions may also contain toxic metals such as lead, cadmium, or copper.	Cardiovascular and respiratory disease; cancer. At coal-burning plants, the health effects of mercury, a powerful neurotoxin, are also of concern. Emissions of toxic metals can cause developmental damage, lung damage, and certain cancers.	People with chronic heart and lung diseases and children may be especially vulnerable.
Smoke	Byproduct of burning both fossil fuels and plant matter, such as wood or tobacco. Can arise from large events like forest fires or small daily sources, such as a home fireplace or even a cigarette being smoked nearby.	Gases from wood smoke include toxins such as benzene. Pollutants include soot and fine particulate matter, which can settle in eyes and lungs.[5] Tobacco smoke releases approximately 4,000 chemicals, including 60 carcinogens.	*Mild:* burning eyes, runny nose, bronchitis. *Severe:* aggravation of chronic heart and lung diseases; increased risk of cancer.[6]	Wood smoke: people with chronic heart or lung diseases, including asthma; older adults; children. Tobacco smoke: both smokers and those who breathe secondhand smoke.
Deforestation and dust	Deforestation leads to soil dehydration and damage and excessive airborne dust. Because trees and plants recycle CO_2, deforestation also increases the levels of CO_2 in our atmosphere.	Fine particulate matter from a variety of sources (soil, vegetation, surface pollutants) in the form of dust; excessive CO_2 in the atmosphere contributes to global warming.	On an individual level, breathing difficulties and reduced lung function; on a public health level, increased risk of certain diseases and dangerous weather events due to global warming.	Given global wind and weather patterns, deforestation and dust affect both those who live near deforested or dust-producing areas and people half a world away.

References: **1.** *Emission Facts: Greenhouse Gas Emissions from a Typical Passenger Vehicle*, by the Environmental Protection Agency, 2005, retrieved from http://www.epa.gov/oms/climate/420f05004.htm. **2.** "Health Effects Associated with Exposure to Ambient Air Pollution," by J. Samet & D. Krewski, 2007, *Journal of Toxicology and Environmental Health, Part A, 70*, 227–242. **3.** "Mortality Effects of Longer Term Exposures to Fine Particulate Air Pollution: Review of Recent Epidemiological Evidence," by C. Pope, 2007, *Inhalation Toxicology, 19*, pp. 33–38. **4.** "Ambient Air Pollution: Health Hazards to Children," by the American Academy of Pediatrics Committee on Environmental Health, 2004, *Pediatrics, 114*, pp. 1699–1707. **5.** "Woodsmoke Health Effects: A Review," by L. Naeher, M. Brauer, M. Lipsett, J. Zelikoff, C. Simpson, J. Koenig, & K. Smith, 2007, *Inhalation Toxicology, 19*, pp. 67–106. **6.** "How Smoke from Fires Can Affect Your Health," in *AIRNOW: Quality of Air Means Quality of Life*, by AIRNow, n.d., retrieved from http://www.airnow.gov/index.cfm?action=smoke.index.

Production of Smog

A term originally coined from the words "smoke" and "fog," smog describes a brown, murky, ozone-laden mixture of pollutants that arises from motor vehicle exhaust, coal burning, and the manufacturing and use of paints, solvents, pesticides, and several other compounds. Weather and geography usually have a role in creating this brew. In valleys where air is trapped by surrounding mountains, a weather phenomenon called a *temperature inversion* can maintain a cooler layer of air under a layer of warmer air. Sunlight then triggers chemical changes in the pollutants suspended in that air, forming ozone-rich smog that lingers until winds blow it away. Smog is most likely to develop during the summer months, when temperature inversions are more likely, and in warmer climates. According to the American Lung Association, almost 60% of the U.S. population lives in areas with unhealthful levels of ozone-rich smog.[26]

global warming A sustained increase in the Earth's temperature due to an increase in the greenhouse effect resulting from pollution.

climate change A change in the state of the climate that can be identified by changes in the average and/or variability of its properties that persist for an extended period.

Global Warming and Climate Change

As discussed earlier in this chapter, Earth supports life, in part, because layers of gases in our atmosphere provide a *greenhouse effect,* allowing the sun's energy to enter and then trapping some of it close to the surface of the planet. At the right levels, the greenhouse effect is necessary to our survival. But human-made air pollution has increased it **(Figure 21.3).** The result is **global warming,** a sustained rise in the planet's atmospheric temperature across geographic regions. Global warming is one aspect of the broader concern about climate change introduced at the beginning of this chapter. The IPCC defines **climate change** as a change in the state of the climate that can be identified by changes in its properties that persist for an extended period, typically decades or longer. Climate change may be due to natural internal processes or to external factors, including human activity.[27] Climate change includes not only temperature increases, but changes in patterns of rainfall, an increase in extreme weather events such as hurricanes, droughts, blizzards, and heat waves, rising sea levels, and disruptions in ecosystems, including losses of entire species. It's also accompanied by a range of negative effects on human health, from food shortages to increases in infectious disease.

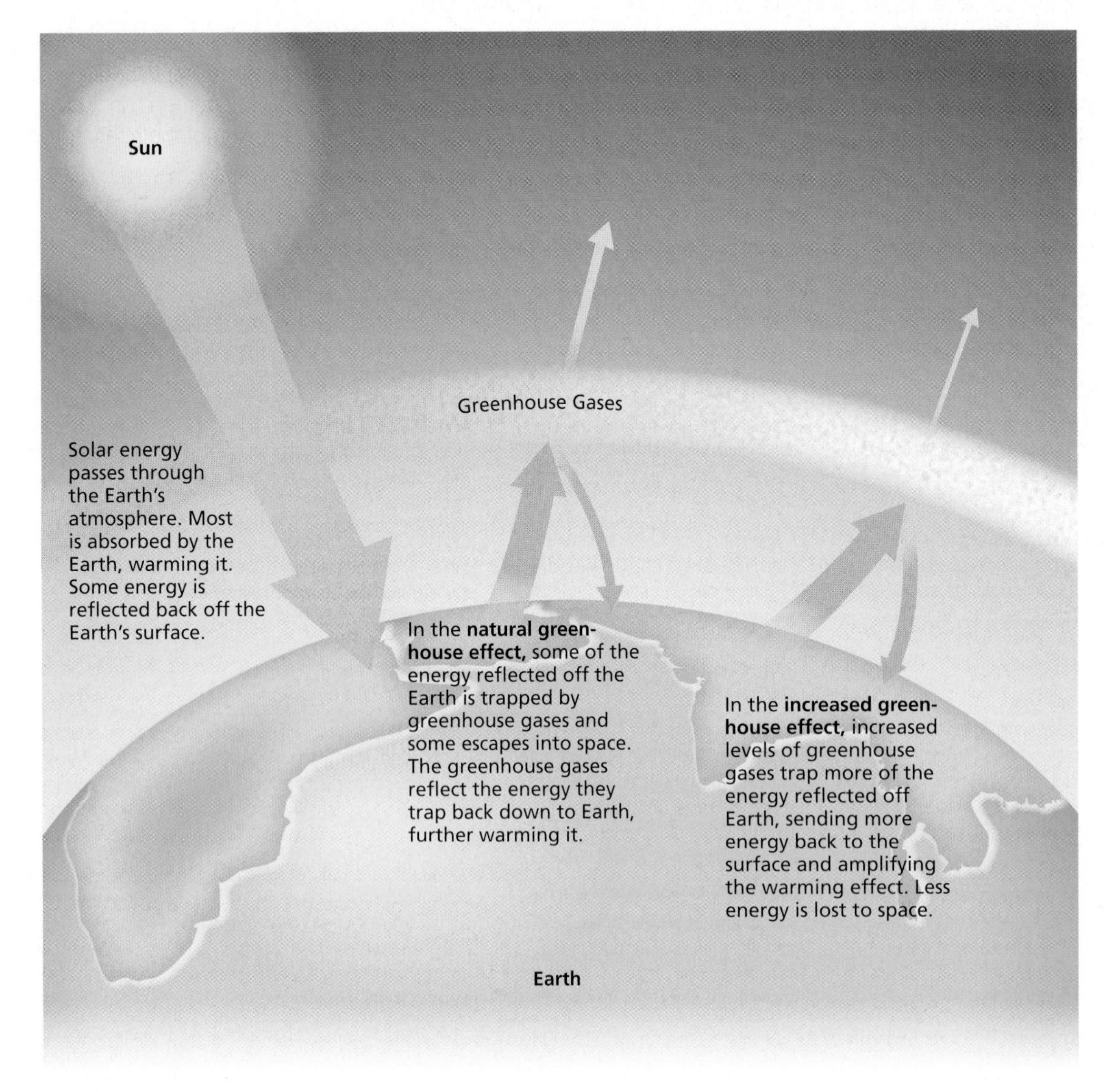

Figure 21.3 **The greenhouse effect.**

What's the evidence for global warming? Here are some sobering statistics:

- The global temperature record shows an average warming of about 1.3°F (0.74°C) over the past century.
- Seven of the eight warmest years on record have occurred since 2001, and 8 of the top 10 years for extreme one-day precipitation events have occurred since 1990.
- Within the past 30 years, the rate of warming across the globe has been approximately three times greater than the rate over the last 100 years.
- The extent of Arctic sea ice in 2009 was 24% below the historical average.
- Past climate information suggests that the warmth of the last half-century is unusual in at least the previous 1,300 years in the Northern Hemisphere.[28, 29]

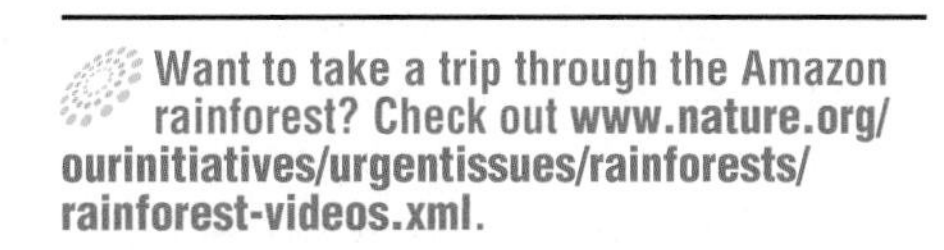

Want to take a trip through the Amazon rainforest? Check out www.nature.org/ourinitiatives/urgentissues/rainforests/rainforest-videos.xml.

In light of this data, the Intergovernmental Panel on Climate Change (IPCC) has concluded that warming of the Earth's climate system is now "unequivocal."[28]

What's the relationship between air pollution and global warming? Many of the gases that produce the greenhouse effect, such as carbon dioxide, methane, and hydrocarbons, are the same as those emitted in vehicle exhaust and other human activities that burn fossil fuels **(Figure 21.4).** The United States is currently the global leader in producing greenhouse gases, responsible for about 21% of all emissions.[30] But while the industrialized world has long led the way in producing greenhouse gases, the developing world is catching up. U.S. environmental regulators estimate that by 2015, emissions produced by developing nations will equal, and then surpass, those produced by more developed countries.[31]

What's your carbon footprint? Find carbon footprint calculators at www.nature.org/greenliving/carboncalculator and www.climatecrisis.net/take_action/become_carbon_neutral.php.

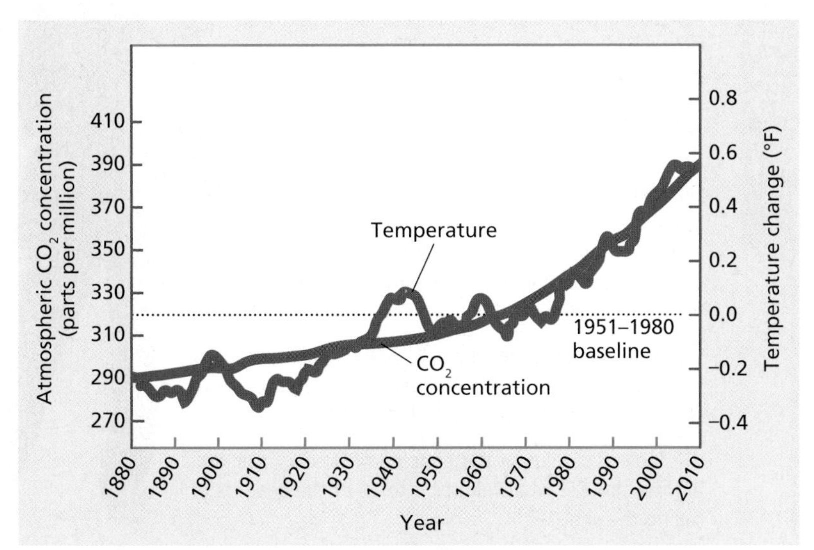

Figure 21.4 Increase in global surface temperature and in atmospheric CO_2 levels, 1880–2010. The increase in temperature and atmospheric CO_2 levels paralells the burning of fossil fuels.

But fossil fuel emissions are not solely responsible for global warming. Two additional, interrelated factors include deforestation and worldwide meat consumption. As you may remember from a discussion of photosynthesis in your high school biology class, plants use energy from sunlight to convert CO_2 and hydrogen into carbohydrates. In the process, they release oxygen as a by-product. The clearing of huge forests—typically rainforests—for residential, agricultural, and industrial use thus deprives us of a natural mechanism for the removal of CO_2 from our atmosphere. The importance of maintaining forested lands is acknowledged internationally; nevertheless, the Nature Conservancy reports that every second of every day, a rainforest area the size of a football field is destroyed.[32]

Often, forests are cut down to clear land for the grazing of cattle and other ruminant animals raised for meat. Moreover, meat production is directly harmful because the digestive tracts of these animals produce methane, a potent greenhouse gas. Cows and other ruminant animals exhale methane with every breath, and excrete it in their wastes. A molecule of methane produces more than 20 times the warming of a molecule of CO_2 and remains in the atmosphere for up to 15 years.[33] The Food and Agriculture Organization of the United Nations estimates that livestock production is responsible for 18% of all greenhouse gas emissions, more than are produced by transportation.[34] Moreover, the fossil fuel consumption required to produce a serving of steak has been estimated to be 16 times higher than that required to produce a serving of rice and vegetables.[35] Still, a blanket recommendation to choose vegetarian meals to help the environment may be overly simplistic, because highly processed soy products also require significant energy to produce. Thus, the content of vegetarian meals matters, with whole foods a superior choice to packaged vegetarian meals.

In addition to choosing three times a day what to eat, you make choices each day about how to get from home to school to work, how to light, heat, and cool your home, whether or not to reuse, recycle, and compost, and what products to buy and avoid. Because each of these choices influences the generation of greenhouse gases, each contributes in a small way to your individual *carbon footprint*—the total greenhouse gas emissions for which you are personally responsible.

Thinning of the Ozone Layer

As you learned earlier in this chapter, the layer of ozone many miles up in the stratosphere is protective, shielding us from excessive solar radiation.

Certain industrial chemicals called *chlorofluorocarbons (CFCs)* can drift into the stratosphere and eat away at this blanket of planetary protection. Although this term may not be familiar, CFCs are actually a part of everyday life. Your refrigerator and air conditioner most likely rely on them, as CFCs are used in coolants. CFCs are also used as foaming agents in some rigid foam products, such as foam-based coffee cups or takeout containers. You can also find them in some spray propellants, some types of fire extinguishers, and some industrial solvents.

Over the last 30 years, CFCs have led to significant **ozone depletion,** a gradual thinning of the

ozone depletion Destruction of the stratospheric ozone layer, which shields the Earth from harmful levels of ultraviolet radiation, resulting from pollution.

ozone layer worldwide, and a more dramatic loss of ozone—referred to as the development of "ozone holes"—over some parts of the world. Ozone depletion poses serious problems because it allows more UV radiation to reach the Earth. This increases your risk for sunburn, skin cancer, and cataracts (cloudy regions that develop over the lens of the eyes).[36] It also disrupts plant reproduction and threatens the survival of microscopic aquatic plant life—called *phytoplankton*—that is the foundation of the marine food chain. Scientists once thought that only regions closest to the poles, especially Antarctica, Australia, and parts of South America, were seriously affected. But research has revealed seasonal ozone thinning over other regions as well, including North America, where ozone levels declined by as much as 10% over the last three decades.[23]

Many countries, recognizing the dangers of CFCs and ozone depletion, have been phasing out their use of these chemicals. As a result, the ozone layer has started to recover. But because CFCs can persist in the atmosphere for decades, the ozone layer likely will only be fully restored decades after these chemicals are no longer released anywhere.

Production of Acid Rain

Some air pollutants do more than burn your eyes or form clouds of smog. They can also dissolve in water, turning the precipitation that nourishes our ecosystem into a hazardous deluge.

When sulfur dioxide and nitrogen oxide are released into the air from the burning of fossil fuels, they can react with other airborne matter to form acidic compounds. These acids then dissolve in rain, snow, or fog, falling to Earth and making waterways and soil more acidic. This phenomenon, commonly called **acid rain,** can harm fish, birds, animals, and vegetation, and even damage human-made structures such as buildings and monuments.

acid rain A phenomenon in which airborne pollutants are transformed by chemical processes into acidic compounds, then mix with rain, snow, or fog and are deposited on Earth.

In the United States, the regions that have been most affected by acid rain include industrial sections of the Northeast, upper Midwest, and Great Lakes area. Although environmental measurements show a reduction in acid deposits in these areas over the last 20 years, many affected waterways still show significant levels of acid, and scientists are working to study the long-term health and environmental effects of this type of pollution.[23]

What Can Be Done to Reduce Air Pollution and Climate Change?

Each day, dozens of decisions you make, large and small, from how long you stay in the shower to whether or not you eat meat at lunch, can help reduce energy use and its resulting emissions and slow climate change. These efforts are important; however, the biggest changes will come about via policy-making, especially at the national and international levels. Let's look at the wide range of options for improving our air.

Personal Choices

To reduce air pollution, reduce your carbon footprint, and improve the quality of the air you breathe, one way to begin is to reduce your energy consumption. For example, vehicle exhaust accounts for about one-half of all air-polluting emissions in the United States.[37] So walking, bicycling, or using public transport can make a big difference. And every time you leave the light burning, you increase your local power plant's use of fossil fuels. To find out how to curb your energy appetite, see **Practical Strategies for Change: Reducing Your Energy Consumption.**

National Policy-Making

The Clean Air Act of 1963 was passed to control air pollution, initially by authorizing research into air quality, and later by authorizing the EPA to develop and enforce regulations to reduce the public's exposure to airborne contaminants. An amendment to the Clean Air Act in 1990, for example, required the EPA to address acid rain and ozone depletion, as well as to set limits on the levels of mercury, arsenic, lead, and other toxic air pollutants in the atmosphere. In early 2012, the EPA released a set of new standards to control hazardous air pollution from coal- and oil-fired power plants, which are the nation's largest source of greenhouse gas emissions. Utilities were given 3 years to fully comply with the requirements. Although industry lobbyists immediately began challenging the new standards, many utility companies are already meeting them.

Also in 2012, the United States Senate Committee on Energy and Natural Resources introduced a new Clean Energy Standards (CES) Act to promote low- and zero-carbon electricity generation and drive clean-energy innovation. The CES Act would

STUDENT STORY

Car vs. Campus Shuttle

"Hi, I'm Toby. Don't get me wrong, I feel like I'm a pretty 'green' person. I recycle and I've even started buying notebooks that are made out of recycled paper. But I grew up in LA where everyone drives, and I'm very attached to my car. There's a free campus shuttle that goes from my apartment complex to school, and some of my friends try to get me to take it, but I don't. I like the freedom that driving gives me—I don't have to wait for the shuttle, I can put my music on the stereo, and I can leave stuff in my car if I want to. It's only a 15-minute drive; I don't think it's really that bad to take my car."

1: What do you think about Toby's decision to drive instead of take the campus shuttle? Would you take the shuttle or drive if you were in his shoes?

2: Toby lists some of the benefits of driving over taking the shuttle; what might be some of the benefits of taking the shuttle?

3: If Toby continues to drive, what could he do to help protect the environment as a driver?

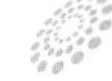
Do you have a story similar to Toby's? Share your story at www.pearsonhighered.com/lynchelmore.

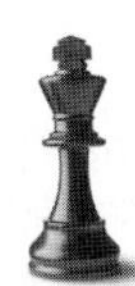

Practical Strategies for Change

Reducing Your Energy Consumption

One way to reduce global warming and the other effects of air pollution is to reduce your consumption of electricity and fossil fuels. The following personal steps can make a real difference:

- **Drive less.** Few choices you make matter more than this when it comes to outdoor air pollution. Walk, cycle, take public transit, or ride-share. You'll get yourself in better shape, and you'll also save money.
- **Take care of your car.** When you do drive, fill your gas tank with cleaner fuels, keep your tires properly inflated, and keep your car tuned up. A better-functioning vehicle releases fewer pollutants and emissions.
- **Don't idle.** If your car is stopped while you wait to pick someone up, turn off the engine and cut your emissions.
- **Limit your use of other gasoline engines.** Do you really need that gas-powered lawn mower or snow blower when a push mower or shovel could do the trick? Many local air quality protection agencies offer incentives to get these polluting devices out of our communities, so find out what options are available to you.
- **Use less electricity.** Every time you turn on an appliance, you increase demand on your local power plant, which then has to burn more fuel. Turn off lights, electronics, and appliances when not in use. Watch out for "energy vampires"—devices such as computers that can stay on indefinitely and drive up energy use and your utility bills. Use power strips with a single on-off switch that let you turn connected electronics (such as your computer, scanner, and printer, or TV, stereo, and DVD player) on and off all at once. And finally, replace incandescent light bulbs with energy-saving LEDs or compact fluorescent bulbs.

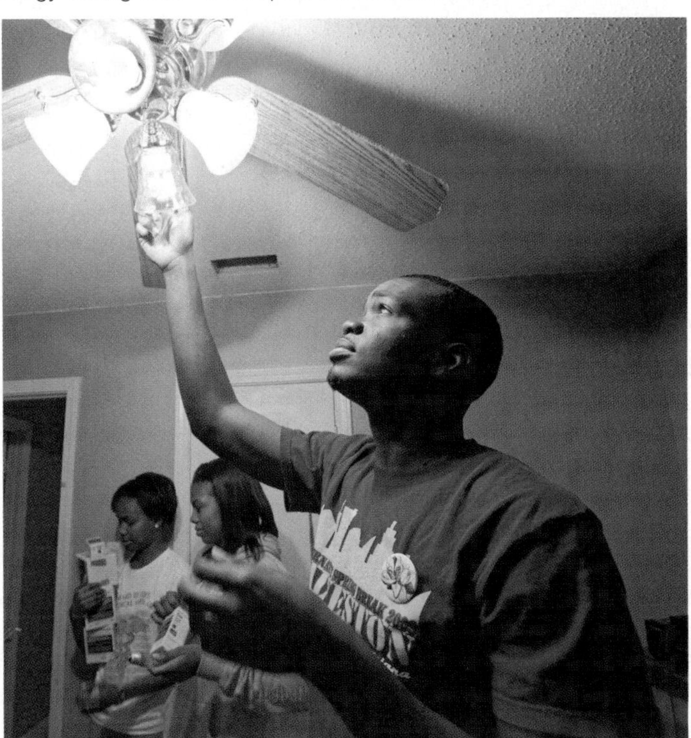

Compact fluorescent light bulbs use about 75% less energy than traditional bulbs.

require America's largest utility companies to sell an increasing percentage of their electricity from clean-energy sources. It is currently awaiting further action.

Along with these legislative measures, the U.S. Department of Energy (DOE) has implemented a variety of strategies in recent years to support green technology and reduce harmful emissions. These include the following:

- *Support for energy science.* The DOE has sponsored million-dollar awards for groundbreaking energy research projects, launched dozens of Energy Frontier Research Centers to accelerate innovation, and established scholarships and internships for college students to study and work in energy-related fields.
- *Residential energy-saving incentives*. DOE grant programs and tax credits have helped hundreds of thousands of American families to improve the energy efficiency of their homes by such measures as installing solar panels, replacing old windows, adding insulation, and switching to energy-efficient appliances.
- *Biofuels*. The Department of Energy (DOE) has also made a commitment to increasing the development of so-called *biofuels;* that is, fuels made from living material such as plants. For example, DOE scientists are working to develop strains of bacteria that can digest switchgrass (a perennial grass native to the United States) into sugars to produce gasoline, diesel, and jet fuels.
- *Smart Grid.* You've probably also heard about the Smart Grid, a DOE project to increase the efficiency of our electrical power transmission in a way that will also contribute to a more healthful environment.

To watch a video on the new SmartGrid, go to www.smartgrid.gov and click on What is the Smart Grid?

Federal regulations have also been implemented to toughen energy standards for vehicle manufacturing to reduce fuel consumption and emissions. In 2012, the EPA announced that 2010 vehicle emissions were the lowest since the Agency began keeping records in 1975, and fuel economy, at an average of 22.6 miles per gallon, was the highest.[38] Contributing to this achievement has been the increasing popularity of hybrid cars. Wondering if they live up to their hype? Check out the **Myth or Fact?** box on the next page and find out.

Want to check out the average miles per gallon of any car on America's roads? Go to www.fueleconomy.gov and enter the year, make, and model of the car you're researching.

International Policy-Making

For two decades, leaders of nations all over the globe have been meeting annually under the auspices of the United Nations Framework Convention on Climate Change (UNFCCC) to discuss climate change and its impacts, and to develop legally binding targets for the reduction of greenhouse gas emissions.[39] One of the most famous treaties to come from these delegations was the Kyoto Protocol, negotiated in Kyoto, Japan, in 1998. It would require developed nations to reduce their emission of greenhouse gases by 5.2%, but would not impose requirements on developing nations, including some with major pollution-generating economies such as China, India, and Brazil. The UNFCCC operates by consensus, meaning that failure of any of the participating countries to agree can delay action. And indeed a small number of countries, including the United States, have failed to accept the Kyoto Protocol, largely because of concerns that it fails to impose requirements on developing nations. The 2011 UNFCCC conference, in Durban, South Africa, advanced implementation of the Kyoto Protocol only marginally. As a result, many countries have now become disillusioned with the slow pace of the process and the fact that the rate of greenhouse gas emissions has only increased since the talks began two decades ago. In fact, global emissions of carbon dioxide jumped by 5.9% in 2010, the largest increase on record.[40]

The American Lung Association publishes an annual ranking of cities in the United States with the best and worst air quality. Find your city's ranking at www.stateoftheair.org.

Frustrated by these data, in 2012, the United States, Canada, four other nations, and the United Nations Environment Program jointly announced a voluntary initiative to reduce the emissions of common pollutants such as soot and methane that contribute to an estimated 30% of global warming. The United States and Canada have pledged several million dollars to help get the program running and recruit other nations to participate.

MYTH OR FACT?

Do Hybrid Cars Merit Their Hype?

Hybrid electric vehicles (HEVs) are cars that can run on two fuel sources: gasoline and electricity.

Although the technology began in the 1970s, the first commercial HEV to hit the road, in 1997, was the Toyota Prius, and it still dominates the market. The Union of Concerned Scientists' 2012 Hybrid Scorecard gives top ranking to the Prius, with an "environmental improvement score"—which measures the smog-forming and global-warming pollution performance of the car against its conventional counterparts—of 9.2 out of 10 possible points.[1] The Department of Energy's fuel economy site identifies an average of 50 miles per gallon for the 2012 Prius.[2]

Still, not everyone is sold on the environmental benefits of hybrid cars. Critics point out that the construction step, not the fuel step, is where the costs to the environment show up.

Let's start with the hybrid's battery, which is made with a variety of metals, including lithium, copper, and manganese, all of which are derived from mining or similar processes that are harmful to the environment.[3] Environmental activists are lobbying for mining companies to clean up their operations, but international regulations will be required. Supporters of HEVs argue, however, that the environmental damage from petroleum production is worse than the damage from mining.

Like the battery in your laptop, an HEV battery loses its storage capacity over time, and eventually will have to be replaced. Models vary, but many have battery warranties of 100,000 miles. When the battery does need to be replaced, what happens to its toxic wastes? Only a few facilities in the United States are currently able to recycle HEV batteries, and only partially; however, the Department of Energy is partnering with car makers and recycling companies to develop technologies for fully recycling them.

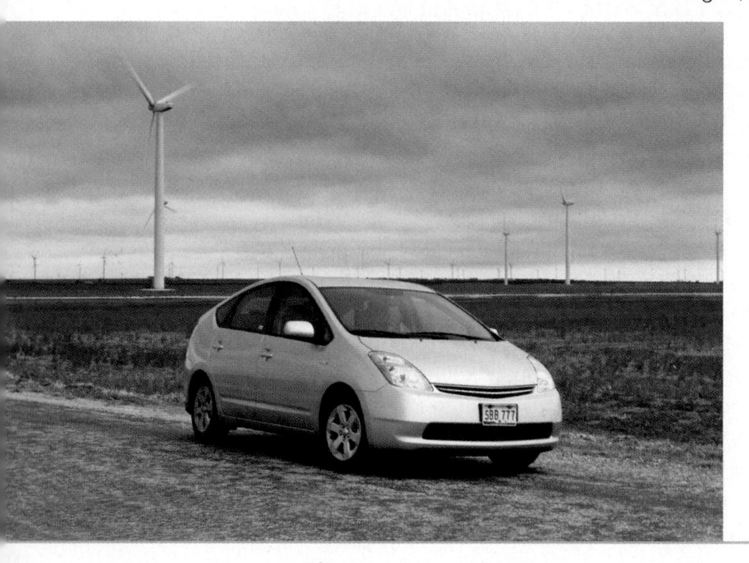

Then there's the manufacture of the car itself, a process powered by fossil fuels. A recent analysis by the National Academies found that the production of HEVs causes greater environmental damage than the manufacture of traditional vehicles, and will continue to do so even with advances in technology until at least 2030.[4]

Once the car is on the road, there's the emissions issue, often referred to as the "long tailpipe." This concern doesn't involve HEVs like the Prius in which the battery recharges as the car brakes. It arises for so-called "plug-ins" like the Nissan Leaf or the Chevy Volt that require the owner to recharge the battery by plugging it in to the same electric power grid you use when you turn on a light. Depending on where you live and what time of day you charge your car, your utility company will be burning coal, nuclear power, or natural gas.[3] Nevertheless, supporters of HEVs point out that, even when recharged on grids burning coal, the cars emit less carbon than conventional vehicles, and as more and more grids switch to solar, wind, and other clean sources of energy, electric power will become cleaner.

One point of agreement between supporters and critics of HEVs is that focusing on engineering obscures the fundamental problem, which is the very concept of the private automobile. Anything that leads to more driving is going to harm the environment. Better environmental strategies are walkable neighborhoods, bicycle infrastructure, and affordable, accessible, and reliable public transportation.[4]

References: **1.** "Hybrid Scorecard," by the Union of Concerned Scientists, 2011, retrieved from http://www.hybridcenter.org/hybrid-scorecard/#UCS_Hybrid_Scorecard. **2.** "Fuel Economy: Compare Side-by-Side," by the U.S. Department of Energy, 2012, retrieved from www.fueleconomy.gov. **3.** "5 Concerns about Electric-Car Batteries," by J. Gordon, 2011, *MSN Autos*, retrieved from http://editorial.autos.msn.com/article.aspx?cp-documentid=1176838. **4.** "Let's Power Down the Hype about Electric Cars," by O. Zehner, March 5, 2012, *The Christian Science Monitor*, p. 34.

Water Pollution

Water covers about 75% of the Earth's surface and supports almost all aspects of life on our planet. We derive our drinking water from two sources: surface-level fresh water, and more than 1 million cubic miles of **groundwater** found beneath our feet.[23]

groundwater The supply of fresh water beneath the Earth's surface, which is a major source of drinking water.

Although water may seem like an endlessly available and renewable resource, only about 1% of the planet's entire water supply is accessible. As populations grow and global warming alters weather patterns, water shortages loom. Currently, about 1.2 billion people live in areas of water scarcity.[41] In addition to overpopulation and climate change, contamination reduces the amount of usable water.

Types of Pollutants Found in Water

Many of the pollutants released into our environment can enter our water supplies, reducing water quality and creating significant health risks. One form of this pollution is infectious microorganisms spread by a lack of basic sanitation. According to the World Health Organization, about 1.5 million children worldwide die from illnesses related to contaminated water. About 2.5 million people lack access to improved sanitation, and more than 880 million people lack access to safe drinking water.[42]

In the developed world, too, water supplies can be contaminated by harmful microbes. However, a more common source of contamination is a variety of chemical and industrial pollutants. These include:

- **Petroleum products,** such as gasoline and motor oil. Petroleum products contain a wide variety of toxins, such as benzene, which is linked to cancer.
- **Polychlorinated biphenyls (PCBs),** which were used as insulating materials in electrical equipment and in paints, motor oils, floor finishes, and many other products until they were banned in the United States in 1979. They are highly stable and persist for many years in the environment.[43] PCBs have been linked to birth defects and cancer.
- **Dioxins,** chemicals found in herbicides and pesticides and also created during industrial combustion, such as when a power plant burns coal to generate electricity. Dioxins linger in the environment—and in the human body—for years, are extremely toxic, and have been linked to a wide variety of health problems, including immune disorders, liver damage, and cancer. Because dioxins accumulate in the fatty tissues of animals, more than 95% of dioxin exposure in humans is thought to occur through dietary intake of meat, dairy products, and seafood.[44]
- **Chemicals used in agriculture,** such as pesticides and herbicides. According to the Environmental Protection Agency, more than 1,055 active ingredients are registered in the United States as pesticides, used everywhere from the fields that grow our food to our own backyards.[45] Pesticides have been linked to a wide variety of health concerns, including birth defects and nervous system disorders.

"As populations grow and global warming alters weather patterns, water shortages loom. Currently, about 1.2 billion people live in areas of water scarcity."

Some common sources of water pollution are identified in **Table 21.2** on the next page. Many of us try to protect ourselves from such pollutants by choosing to drink bottled water. Before you reach for your next bottle, however, it's worth looking at how healthful bottled water really is.

Is Bottled Water Worth It?

In the developed world, most of us have access to a ready supply of clean water. According to national estimates, about 85% of the U.S. population gets its drinking water from a community water system, and the rest from private wells.[46] Still, over the last decade, many of us have also opted for another source of water—from bottles. In 2009, bottled water represented the second largest category of all beverage sales, pulling in more than $10 billion. Americans now drink about 28 gallons of bottled water per person each year, about twice what we drank a decade ago.[47]

Many of us choose bottled water because we assume it is more healthful or more pure. But those assumptions aren't necessarily true. Contrary to what many people believe, bottled water is not required to exceed most health and safety standards set for drinking water from the tap. Federal environmental and health regulators do not certify bottled water, and do not require that bottled water come from a particular source. Some brands are actually made from tap water.

Don't assume that bottled water is always free from contaminants. In one study of bottled water sold in the Houston, Texas, area, 4 of the 35 brands analyzed were found to be contaminated with bacteria.[48] A federal study found that safety and consumer protections for bottled water are often less stringent than those applied to tap water.[49]

Federal rules, however, do require that bottlers use certain terms and definitions when labeling their water, including:

- **Artesian, ground, spring, or well water.** Water from an underground source, which may or may not be treated.
- **Distilled water.** Water that has been boiled and recondensed, a process that kills microbes and removes natural minerals.
- **Drinking water.** Water intended for human consumption and sealed in containers with no additional ingredients except for disinfectants.

Table 21.2: Common Types of Water Pollution

Pollutant	Source	Health Risks
Bacteria	Inadequate sanitation. According to the World Health Organization, about 2.6 million people lack access to adequate sanitation.[1]	A wide variety of waterborne diseases, such as cholera and trachoma.
Lead	Older plumbing that uses leaded pipes. About 15–20% of lead exposure in the United States comes from drinking water affected by leaded pipes.[2]	A variety of health problems. This heavy metal poses an especially serious risk of developmental delay and brain damage in young children.
Petroleum products	Leaking underground gasoline storage tanks. In 2009, more than 100,000 underground storage tanks awaited cleanup.[3] Used motor oil poured down storm drains.	Contain a number of toxins, such as benzene, which is linked to cancer.
Chemical contaminants	Industrial and home use of chemicals and improper disposal into waterways. Leaky underground storage containers. Worldwide, the extent of industrial water pollution is too vast to tally accurately. In the United States, the Great Lakes region alone has 43 polluted zones officially deemed "areas of concern."[4]	A wide variety of health problems, including cancers, thyroid disorders, and developmental disorders.
Pesticides and fertilizers	Crop production and horticulture that cause irrigation runoff or use aerial spraying. More than 1,000 pesticides are registered in the United States. Since 1960, the use of fertilizers in the United States has increased sharply, with combined use of three common fertilizers climbing from 46 pounds per acre in 1960 to 138 pounds per acre in 2005.[5]	A wide variety of health problems, including nervous system disorders and cancers. Fertilizers flow into runoff and contaminate waterways, stripping water of oxygen and leading to hazardous algae blooms and death of aquatic life.
Raw animal sewage; antibiotics and hormones given to livestock	Industrial meat production facilities and feed lots, where animals and their wastes are kept in confined areas. The United States has about 450,000 feedlot operations.[6] Leaky or inadequate storage facilities for waste or improper waste disposal spread this waste into the water supply.	Infectious disease; development of strains of microbes resistant to conventional antibiotics; exposure to hormones. One study found that standard livestock waste management practices do not adequately protect nearby water resources.[7]
Pharmaceuticals	Discarding medications and health and beauty products improperly, such as pouring them down the drain or flushing them down the toilet; wastewater treatment doesn't yet address these substances. Traces of more than 100 different pharmaceuticals have been detected in drinking water in the United States and Europe.[8]	Studies of health effects are still under way. Concerns have prompted increased regulation to keep these substances out of water supplies.

References: **1.** "Climate Change and Human Health: Water Services for Health," by the World Health Organization, 2010, retrieved from http://www.who.int/globalchange/ecosystems/water/en/index.html. **2.** "Reducing Lead Exposure from Drinking Water: Recent History and Current Events," by R. Mass, S. Patch, D. Morgan, & T. Pandolo, 2005, *Public Health Reports, 120*, pp. 316–321. **3.** *American Recovery and Reinvestment Act of 2009 – Environmental Protection Agency Recovery Act Program Plan: Underground Storage Tanks Program*, by the Environmental Protection Agency, May 15, 2009, retrieved from http://www.epa.gov/recovery/plans/oust.pdf. **4.** *Great Lakes*, by the Environmental Protection Agency, 2009, retrieved from http://www.epa.gov/greatlakes/index.html. **5.** *EPA's 2008 Report on the Environment: Highlights of National Trends*, by the Environmental Protection Agency, 2008, pp. 1–37, retrieved from http://oaspub.epa.gov/hd/downloads. **6.** *Animal Feeding Operations Unified Strategy*, by the Environmental Protection Agency, National Pollutant Discharge Elimination System, 2002, retrieved from http://cfpub.epa.gov/npdes/afo/ustrategy.cfm. **7.** "Impacts of Waste from Concentrated Animal Feeding Operations on Water Quality," by J. Burkholder, B. Libra, P. Weyer, S. Heathcote, D. Kolpin, P. Thorne, & M. Wichman, 2007, *Environmental Health Perspectives, 2*, pp. 308–312. **8.** "Damming the Flow of Drugs into Drinking Water," by Pat Hemminger, 2005, *Environmental Health Perspectives, 113*, retrieved from http://www.ehponline.org/members/2005/113-10/spheres.html.

- **Mineral water.** Groundwater containing certain levels of dissolved mineral solids.
- **Purified water.** Water from any source that has been treated to be essentially free of chemicals, and possibly microbes.
- **Sterile water.** Water from any source that has been sterilized to remove microbes.[50]

If you decide to purchase bottled water, check the label for these terms. For more help interpreting the label on bottled waters, check out the nearby **Consumer Corner.**

The convenience of bottled water also presents its own environmental challenges. Every year, more than 300 million tons of plastics are produced worldwide, and only about 10% of these are ever recycled. Plastic water bottles are a considerable part of this waste. Plastics that are not recycled wind up in landfills or incinerated, or they make their way into our oceans. Studies of a "debris convergence region" of the northern Pacific Ocean called the North Pacific Gyre have found an average of more than 334,000 items of plastic debris per square kilometer of ocean water.[51]

Watch a video about the efforts of Project Kaisei to clean up the North Pacific Gyre at www.projectkaisei.org.

What Can You Do to Reduce Water Pollution?

The choices you make each day have a direct effect on your ability to enjoy access to clean water. To reduce water pollution, take the following actions:

- Dispose of motor oil and similar products properly. Yes, it's a little more inconvenient to save used oil and take it to a disposal site, but it's worth the effort.
- Throw old soaps, lotions, and cosmetics away in the trash. Don't pour them down the drain or flush them down the toilet.
- Bring outdated medications to a medication or hazardous waste drop-off site, the location of which can be found by using the search tool at **http://earth911.com.** If such a program is not available in your community, ask your health-care provider for tips for proper disposal. And don't forget to recycle the plastic container!
- Limit the use of pesticides, herbicides, and fertilizers around your home.
- Choose environmentally friendly soaps and cleaning products. Check the label to ensure that they're made with ingredients that are biodegradable. These don't necessarily cost more, as many national brands have switched to "green" formulas in the past few years.
- Take your dirty car to the local car wash rather than cleaning it yourself. Most car washes are better equipped to treat such wastewater properly.

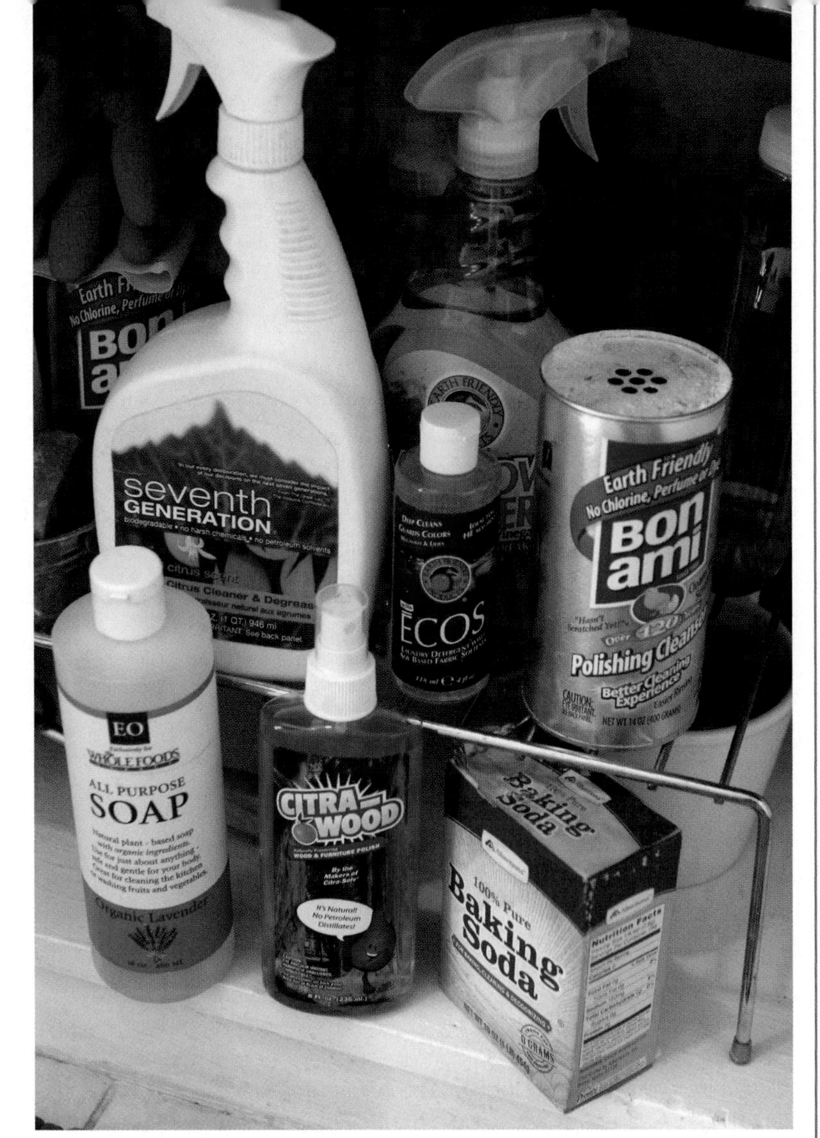

Environmentally friendly cleaners can help reduce water pollution.

- Whenever possible opt for foods produced without pesticides. As more consumers choose organic foods, the level of pesticides entering our waterways will decline.

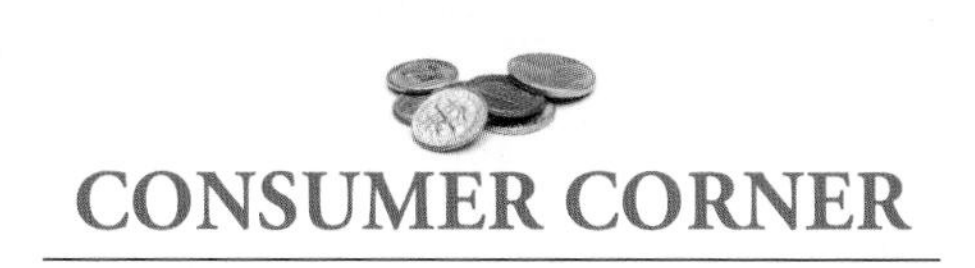

CONSUMER CORNER

What's in That Bottle?

Because one brand of bottled water can be very different from the one next to it on the store shelf, it pays to take a look at the label before you buy. Reading the label may help you understand where the water came from, how it was processed, what health benefits it claims to offer, and how those claims are backed up. You may also find that the label doesn't provide direct answers—if so, switch brands or contact the company for more information.

Before taking a bottle of water to the register, ask yourself the following questions:

- What is the source of this water? Does it say artesian, ground, spring, or well water? Or does the label contain the abbreviation "P.W.S.," indicating that the water comes from a public (tap) water source?
- Even once you know the source, purity isn't guaranteed. Is the water labeled as purified? What processing, if any, has the water undergone? Two effective methods for removing microbes are *micron filtration* and *reverse osmosis* (also called ultrafiltration).
- Are there added sugars, as in the case of "vitamin" waters or energy waters? It is best to avoid waters with added sugars, which provide empty calories.

Finally, before spending money for any brand of bottled water, ask yourself if your cash couldn't be better spent on a reusable bottle that you fill yourself, straight from the tap.

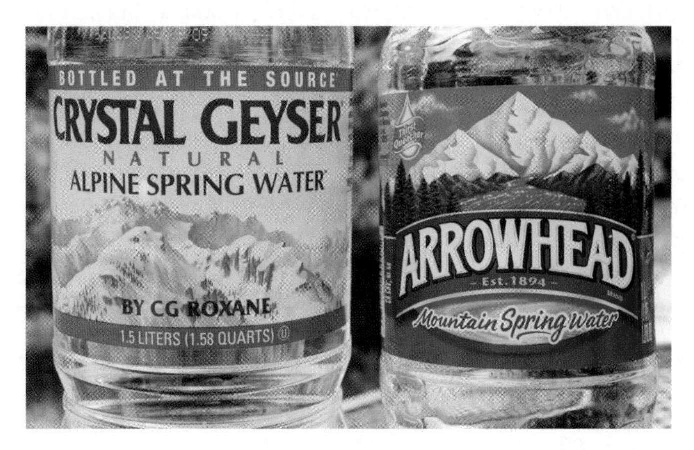

Land Pollution

Every day, the average person in the United States creates about 4.5 pounds of trash.[23] Two types of trash are of concern: municipal waste and hazardous waste.

Municipal Waste and Its Management

Formally referred to as **municipal solid waste (MSW),** this refuse typically consists of discarded food, packaging, yard clippings, paper, and plastics. People in the United States throw out more than 250 million tons of this garbage each year.[23]

Garbage requires a great deal of handling—and that handling is often far more complex than simply hauling it to a landfill or burning it in an incinerator. As landfill space becomes less available, more U.S. communities are encouraging residents to reduce, reuse, and recycle:

- *Reduction* is the altering of manufacturing and consumption processes to reduce the amount and toxicity of trash. For example, many food manufacturers are designing packaging that uses less plastic. For their part, consumers can choose to buy these products rather than versions with more plastic packaging. And there are other ways to reduce your trash as well. Switch to online bill payment wherever it's offered. And stop using a tray in the dining hall! By only choosing food and drink you can carry to your table without a tray, you can substantially cut food packaging, uneaten food waste, and other

municipal solid waste (MSW)
Nonhazardous garbage or trash generated by industries, businesses, institutions, and homes.

garbage. In addition, you will likely eat smaller meals and reduce the use of water for washing.[52]

- *Reuse* means switching from single-use items to versions that last. For instance, canvas shopping bags, cloth napkins, porcelain travel mugs, stainless steel water bottles, and rechargeable batteries are all multi-use items.
- *Recycling* is the processing of discarded paper, glass, metal, and plastics to turn these materials back into usable goods. Your role in recycling is twofold: First, stop and think each time you're tempted to throw an item into the trash. Can it be recycled? If you're not sure, contact your local recycling center and find out. Second, purchase goods made from recycled materials whenever possible: notebooks, tote bags, jewelry, wallets, door mats, lawn chairs . . . you name it, a recycled version is probably available.
- A related action is *composting,* the conversion of organic waste such as food scraps and yard trimmings into a natural fertilizer. Composting is now done in both residential backyards and on a large scale to provide soil boosters for organic farming. According to national estimates, about 33% of municipal solid waste is now composted or recycled.[23]

This video series shows you how to compost at home: www.ehow.com/video_4467169_composting.html.

See the **Choosing to Change Worksheet** on page 599 for more ideas about how to reduce, reuse, and recycle. If practiced consistently, these actions can make significant reductions in the amount of trash trucked to landfills. In 2003, for example, the city of San Francisco set aggressive goals of diverting 75% of the city's waste from landfills by 2010, and 100% by 2020.[53] Through the use of waste reduction measures, including a citywide composting program, the city reported in October 2012 that 80% of all waste was being diverted from landfills.[54]

To find recycling centers in your neighborhood, go to http://earth911.com.

> *"We all share in the generation of hazardous waste. Many household products, such as paint, cleaners, garden products, and batteries, are too hazardous to simply throw in the trash."*

Hazardous Waste and Its Management

Some waste is too toxic to be processed alongside regular trash. **Hazardous waste,** defined as refuse with characteristics or properties capable of harming human health or the environment, must be handled separately. This type of waste often consists of industrial chemicals or products containing heavy metals, which are difficult to treat or reuse safely.

hazardous waste Garbage or by-products that can pose a hazard to human health or the environment when improperly managed.

e-waste Hazardous waste generated by the production or disposal of electronic or digital devices.

Many of us equate hazardous waste with barrels of residue from factories. But we all share in the generation of hazardous waste. Many household products, such as paint, cleaners, garden products, and batteries, are too hazardous to simply throw in the trash. Many of the digital communication devices we use every day also generate toxic waste. Old computers, for example, can contain toxins and heavy metals. These machines, part of a category called **e-waste,** often end up dumped in developing countries, where people try to eke out a living by salvaging wires and other reusable parts amid the mountains of hazardous high-tech refuse.

Where does e-waste end up? These videos explain: www.youtube.com/watch?v=0JZey9GJQP0 and www.youtube.com/watch?v=ZHTWRYXy2gE&feature=related.

The nature of hazardous waste means that handlers are typically inclined to dispose of it as quickly as possible, even if that disposal isn't always safe. Then, when toxic components leak or spill at a site, handlers may simply let the problem sit, unsure of how to clean it up—or unwilling to bear the financial burden of doing so. As a result, the United States, along with many other countries, is dotted with hazardous waste "hotspots." U.S. environmental regulators started a concerted campaign to address hazardous waste sites in 1980 by passing the

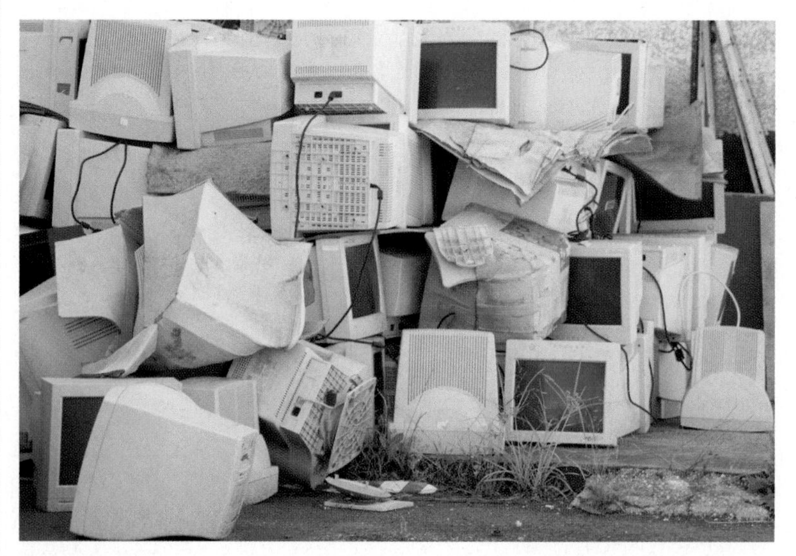

A new category of hazardous waste is "e-waste," items such as old cell phones and computers, which contain toxins and heavy metals.

Comprehensive Environmental Response and Liability Act, commonly referred to as the **Superfund.** This fund, financed largely by taxes on the chemical and petroleum industries, pays for ongoing hazardous waste cleanup of land, surface water, and groundwater. Although more than 32,000 potentially hazardous sites have been identified under the Superfund, and almost 1,500 have been listed as high priority, only a fraction of these have been fully cleaned up. The program has managed, however, to contain or control serious health risks emanating from most of these sites. According to federal statistics, human exposure to contaminants is under control at about 82% of high-priority Superfund sites; the rest either show no documented health exposure or remain unclassified.[23] Most states also keep track of hazardous waste sites, conduct or supervise cleanups, and monitor any possible environmental hazards.

Superfund A federal program that funds and carries out emergency and long-term identification, analysis, removal, and cleanup of toxic sites.

What Can You Do to Manage Household Hazardous Waste?

The average household in the United States generates 20 pounds of household hazardous waste (HHW) each year.[55] HHW includes products that contain corrosive, ignitable, toxic, or reactive ingredients. Any such product requires special care during disposal.

What can you do to reduce your contribution to HHW and clean up the HHW in your home and community? Try these ideas:

- First, don't purchase products with hazardous ingredients unless you have no alternative. For instance, skip the pesticides, switch to rechargeable batteries, and use common ingredients in your kitchen—such as baking soda and white vinegar—as cleaning solutions. See the **Get Connected** links at the end of this chapter for tips on how to make your own natural cleaning products.

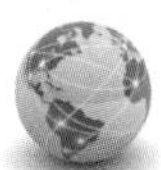

DIVERSITY & HEALTH

Working for Environmental Justice

Although we all feel the effects of environmental damage, its burden falls more heavily on some. In study after study, environmental regulators and researchers have noted that low-income and minority communities typically face increased health risks from the environment. Here are just a few recent examples documented by environmental scientists:

- Minority and low-income populations are more likely to live near high-priority Superfund sites, but are less likely to benefit from Superfund cleanup efforts, even after federal efforts to make the Superfund more equitable.[1]
- In North Carolina, schools with higher numbers of minority and low-income students were more likely to be located near large swine feedlots, which emit pollution that can affect air quality and water quality, and increase the prevalence of asthma symptoms.[2]
- Despite advances in the medical treatment of asthma, the condition continues to cause more sickness and death among African American and Hispanic children than Caucasian children, especially among those living in low-income urban areas.[3]

The reasons for these disparities are complex, but a few key factors stand out. Members of minority and low-income communities are more likely to live near businesses and industries that emit large amounts of pollutants, often because housing in these areas is more affordable, and zoning laws and tax incentives make such businesses more likely to locate in these areas.[4] Members of these communities are also more likely to live in poor-quality housing, which may increase exposure to environmental hazards such as inadequate ventilation or mold.

These disparities have given rise to the movement for *environmental justice*, a two-part process that works to ensure that everyone:

- Enjoys the same degree of protection from environmental and health hazards
- Has equal access to decision-making processes that influence the regional environment

Environmental justice can be very global in its focus, or extremely local. Some community groups, for example, work to help people half a world away attain access to clean drinking water. Others work in their own neighborhoods on issues such as trash pickup, tree planting, or the reduction of industrial emissions. If you are interested in helping to promote environmental justice, you can start by checking with your health instructor or environmental studies department on campus. These resources are likely to know of or be involved in efforts or research related to environmental equity.

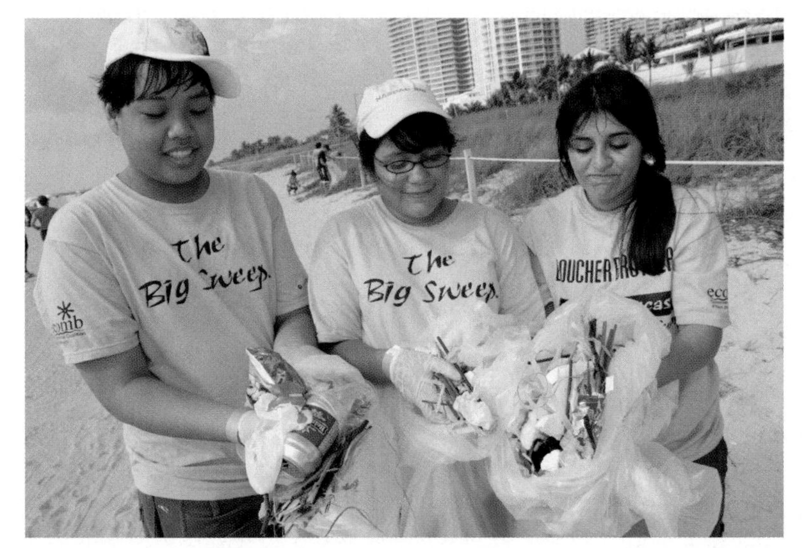

Participating in events like trash clean-ups can promote environmental justice.

References: **1.** "Superfund: Evaluating the Impact of Executive Order 12898," by S. O'Neal, 2007, *Environmental Health Perspectives, 115*, pp. 1087–1093. **2.** "Race, Poverty, and Potential Exposure of Middle-School Students to Air Emissions from Confined Swine Feeding Operations," by M. Mirabelli, S. Wing, S. Marshall, & T. Wilcosky, 2006, *Environmental Health Perspectives, 114*, pp. 591–596. **3.** "Asthma Disparities in Urban Environments," by T. Bryant-Stephens, 2009, *Journal of Allergy and Clinical Immunology, 123*, pp. 1199–1206. **4.** "Hazardous Waste Cleanup, Neighborhood Gentrification, and Environmental Justice: Evidence from Restricted Access Census Block Data," by S. Gamper-Rabindran & C. Timmons, 2011, *American Economic Review: Papers & Proceedings, 101*, pp. 620–624.

Recycling Cell Phones

STUDENT STORY

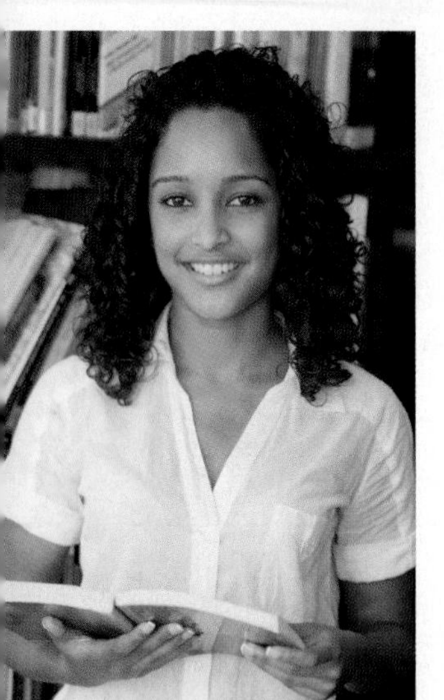

"Hi, I'm Camille. Like most of my fellow students, I feel like I'm pretty into the environment. But I recently got a new cell phone and when my boyfriend saw me throwing out my old one he told me that I should recycle it. Well, I didn't even know you could or should recycle cell phones and I didn't know how, or where I could take it. We looked up cell phone recycling and found a center, but it's all the way on the other side of town. I don't know if I want to travel that far just for a tiny little cell phone."

1: Have you ever recycled a cell phone or other electronic device? Where did you take it?

2: What's in a cell phone that would make you want to recycle it?

3: If you think about the fact that some cell phone plans let you get a new cell phone every 2 years, why might it seem more important to start recycling them?

Do you have a story similar to Camille's? Share your story at www.pearsonhighered.com/lynchelmore.

- Think before you toss. Recognize hazardous household waste and dispose of it properly. Don't throw batteries, paint, or other chemicals in the trash. Instead, take these products to the appropriate collection site on your campus or in your community.
- As suggested earlier, don't allow motor oil to flow into open drains. Collect it and take it to your local collection site. Alternatively, some local garages will accept used motor oil.
- Take your e-waste to an approved disposal center in your community. If your community waste-management facility doesn't accept e-waste, ask a staff member to identify the nearest collection site. Some local businesses have special drop-off days, and some campuses schedule e-waste collection days.
- Even empty containers of HHW can pose hazards because of residual chemicals that might remain. Keep the lid or cap on containers and take them to your campus or community collection site.
- Get involved! Identify the scope of the problem, the impact on the environment, the items that qualify as HHW, and the collection sites in your area. If you live in a dorm, for example, help organize a collection drive or collection center where students can turn in dead batteries, old fluorescent light bulbs, and other common HHW.

Pollution at Home

At home, you encounter pollutants in the foods and beverages you ingest and the indoor air you breathe. Let's take a closer look at how this occurs, as well as some changes you can make to reduce your exposure.

Pollutants in Foods and Beverages

When you eat an apple and drink a glass of milk, any pollutants present in your snack will enter your bloodstream and circulate through your body. Depending on their chemical makeup, some of these will then be quickly excreted. Others, however, are *fat soluble,* which means that they will be transported into your body's fat cells, where they can be stored for long periods of time, building up gradually in a process called **bioaccumulation.** The role of human beings at the top of the food chain exacerbates this process, because we also ingest contaminants that have built up in the fats found in the animal products we eat, including meats and dairy foods. In a process called **biomagnification,** these pollutants have become more and more concentrated as they've traveled up the food chain **(Figure 21.5).**

Mercury is a toxin that commonly bioaccumulates in fish (and in your own body if you eat contaminated seafood). Use this mercury calculator to see if you're consuming too much mercury: www.gotmercury.org.

If you're concerned about the buildup of pollutants in the foods you eat, a few simple steps can reduce your exposure. If you eat meat, choose lean cuts and trim off all visible fat. Drink skim milk, and buy lower-fat cheeses whenever possible. Purchase more organically grown foods. Because these can cost more than conventionally grown foods, shop sensibly if your budget is tight. Find out what types of conventionally grown foods tend to retain the highest pesticide residues, and spend your budget on organic versions of those. (Check out the **Consumer Corner** on page 131 of Chapter 5 for a list.)

We also ingest pollutants that were not originally present in the food itself, but have leached into it from the product packaging, or from plastic containers in which we've stored it. For example, a pollutant called bisphenol A, or BPA, is found in baby bottles, plastic dinnerware, plastic beverage and food storage containers, food can linings, and other products. Although the health effects of this chemical are still being researched, it's a form of synthetic estrogen, and scientists have linked it to breast cancer in both males and females, prostate cancer, miscarriage, reduced sperm count, genital abnormalities, heart disease, and diabetes.

The FDA began studying BPA in 2008, and in 2012 released its findings, which were supported by both animal studies and mathematical models. The FDA concluded that the level of BPA transmitted to humans from food containers was extremely low, and was quickly metabolized and excreted from the body. They noted that this is exactly opposite to certain other toxins, such as dioxins, that can build up and remain in the body's tissues for months or even years. Nevertheless, the FDA continues to support industry efforts to replace BPA, especially in containers, such as baby bottles and sippy cups, used by infants and young children.[56] The FDA also advises that you avoid carrying, storing, or microwave-heating foods or liquids in containers with the recycling code 3 or 7. Number 2, 4, 5, and

bioaccumulation The process by which substances increase in concentration in the fat tissues of living organisms as the organisms take in contaminated air, water, or food.

biomagnification The process by which certain contaminants become more concentrated in animal tissue as they move up the food chain.

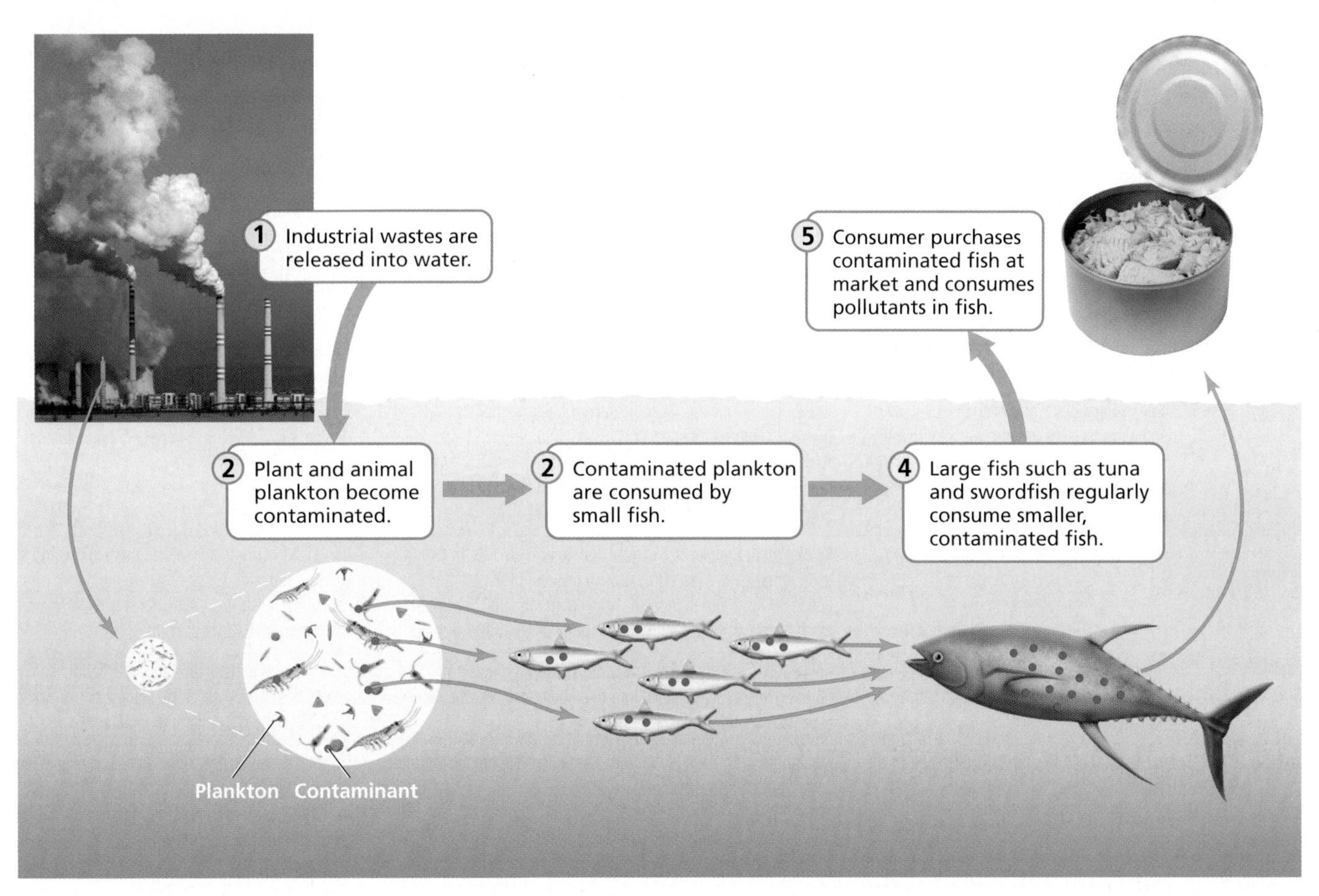

Figure 21.5 **Biomagnification.** In biomagnification, the concentration of contaminants increases as animals higher and higher in the food chain consume contaminated animal tissue. Biomagnification can increase the concentration of pollutants like mercury in fish that we commonly eat, like tuna.

6 plastics are BPA-free and are generally considered safe for carrying or storing food, water, and other beverages.

Pollutants in Indoor Air

Aspects of your home environment that you encounter every day—including paints, insulation materials, flooring, and furniture—may release toxic fumes or other contaminants into the indoor air. Other pollutants that may be found in homes, such as smoke from a woodstove or fireplace, tobacco smoke, mold spores, lead dust, rodent droppings, dust mites, or pet dander, can also build up in indoor air, especially in the winter when the windows are closed. When these pollutants are inhaled, they enter the bloodstream, travel throughout the body, and can be stored in fat tissues.

Asbestos is a microscopic mineral fiber that, until the 1970s, was used in insulation materials, floor and ceiling tiles, and other items in homes, schools, and other buildings. Breathing high levels of asbestos fibers can increase the risk of certain cancers and a condition called *asbestosis*, in which the fibers prompt scarring that reduces lung function. Asbestos in good condition should be left in place, as it is unlikely to release fibers.[57] In recent years, there have been several reports of asbestos concerns in cracked ceiling tiles and other features of aging campus buildings, including residence halls; if you're living in an older dorm and you notice cracks or other signs of deterioration, notify your campus office of residential services and request an inspection.

One indoor air pollutant of significant concern is radon. A radioactive gas released from uranium present naturally in rocks and soil, radon can leach into indoor air through a home's foundation. It can also enter groundwater and be released into the air as the water flows from faucets. The radioactive particles in radon are highly damaging to cells in the lungs. In fact, the National Cancer Institute lists radon exposure as second only to cigarette smoking as a cause of lung cancer.[58]

Another deadly indoor toxin is carbon monoxide (CO), which we mentioned earlier is a gas that impairs the ability of your bloodstream to carry oxygen. It is produced whenever any fuel such as gas, oil, wood, or charcoal is burned. If, for example, a wood-burning stove is not installed or maintained properly, dangerous levels of CO can be released. Unfortunately, CO is invisible and produces no odor, so its presence typically goes undetected. Low to moderate levels can produce headaches, nausea, confusion, and other symptoms, but can be fatal if allowed to persist. High levels can be fatal in minutes.[59]

Volatile organic compounds (VOCs) are a group of gases emitted from more than a thousand products, including paints, paint strippers, cleaning supplies, building materials, furnishings, glues, permanent markers, and office equipment. In addition to irritating the eyes, nose, throat, and skin, they can cause headaches, difficulty breathing, dizziness, nausea, and other symptoms, and some are known to cause cancer.[60]

For a closer look at sources of pollution at home, see **Table 21.3.**

Table 21.3: Common Types of Pollution at Home

Pollutant	Source	Pathway into Body	Health Effects
Pesticides and herbicides	Fruits, vegetables, meat, milk, and other foods. In annual surveys conducted since 1994, up to 71% of food samples have shown detectable amounts of pesticide residue.[1]	Consumed in the diet, either directly or as stored in the tissues of animal products. Public health officials are currently tracking the presence of more than 35 agricultural chemicals in the bodies of people in the United States.[2]	Varied. Some pesticides and herbicides are neurotoxins, while others are endocrine disruptors or have been linked to cancer.
Asbestos	Construction materials used until the early 1970s and designed to resist fire, including insulation, roofing, flooring, cement, and surface coatings; also natural sources[3]	Inhalation—asbestos fibers are light and small.	Asbestosis (scarring of lung tissue) and lung and other cancers
Lead	Old paint, gasoline, and pesticides containing lead. Lead paint was commonly used in the United States until 1978; lead-based pesticides were used even earlier but can remain in soil.	Inhalation or ingestion. Lead can be inhaled in dust or ingested through the mouth, especially by small children. Old lead paint flecks and chips can fall off surfaces and mix with soil outside homes or dust inside homes. Old lead-based pesticides can remain in soil for decades or longer.	Developmental delays and brain damage in children; reproductive problems and a variety of brain and nervous system disorders in adults[4]
Mercury	Fish; emissions from combustion	Inhalation or ingestion. Mercury, a heavy metal once commonly used in industry, bioaccumulates in tissues, including the tissues of fish, and is ingested when contaminated fish are eaten. It can also be inhaled from combustion emissions.	Varied. Mercury is a powerful neurotoxin, and at high levels, exposure is fatal. Large fish that are higher up in the food chain, such as tuna, Chilean sea bass, mackerel, and shark, carry more mercury than others.
Formaldehyde	Furniture made from plywood, particle board, or compressed wood; carpeting; some upholstery	Inhalation. Formaldehyde, a chemical found in glues and bonding agents, is released into the air and can be inhaled, especially in indoor spaces.	Coughing; eye, nose, and throat irritation; skin rashes; headaches; dizziness. Some people appear to be more sensitive to formaldehyde than others.[5]
Carbon monoxide (CO)	Indoor combustion units, including gas heaters, fireplaces, and gas stoves	Inhalation. Because it is colorless and odorless, people are often unaware of the presence of this gas.	Dizziness, headaches, confusion, and even death resulting from interference with the blood's ability to carry oxygen. About 500 people in the United States die each year from unintentional CO poisioning.[6]
Radon	Decay of uranium in rocks and soil beneath or surrounding a home	Inhalation of radioactive particles leached into indoor air or into well water. The particles become airborne when the water is used and are then inhaled.	Increased risk of lung cancer
Mold (fungus) and other biological pollutants	Damp spaces, including basements, bathrooms, ventilation systems, and spaces within walls; dander from cats and dogs; allergens from dust mites in bedding and furniture	Inhalation of airborne spores from mold, pet dander, or dust mite allergens	Allergies and other respiratory problems. Although it isn't possible to remove all traces of mold, dander, or dust mites from a home, regular cleaning and moisture control can usually keep these materials contained.[7] Regular bathing of pets and housecleaning can help reduce pet dander in the air.
Phthalates, bisphenol A (BPA), and other chemicals found in packaging	Plastic products, including drinking cups, baby bottles, food containers, and water bottles; cans lined with plastic	Ingested when food or drink that has touched plastic is consumed. In one study, people who used plastic bottles containing BPA showed a two-thirds increase in the level of the chemical in their urine after one week.[8]	Still being studied. However, a growing body of evidence indicates that these compounds may be endocrine disruptors, and BPA has also been linked to heart disease and diabetes.[9]
Volatile organic compounds (VOCs)	Cleaning products, paints, adhesives, solvents such as paint thinner and paint stripper, petroleum-based fuels	Inhalation. VOCs readily evaporate at room temperature and are inhaled, often as fumes that have a distinct chemical odor. Outdoors, they are a precursor to ground-level ozone.	Varied. Known immediate effects of some VOCs include eye and respiratory tract irritation, headaches, dizziness, visual disorders, and memory impairment. Many VOCs are known to cause cancer in animals. Some are suspected of causing, or are known to cause, cancer in humans.[10]

References: **1.** *EPA's 2008 Report on the Environment: Highlights of National Trends,* by the Environmental Protection Agency, 2008, pp. 1–37, retrieved from http://oaspub.epa.gov/hd/downloads. **2.** *Third National Report on Human Exposure to Environmental Chemicals,* by the Centers for Disease Control and Prevention, 2005, retrieved from http://www.cdc.gov/exposurereport/report.htm. **3.** *Understanding Asbestosis,* by the American Lung Association, 2010, retrieved from http://www.lungusa.org/lung-disease/asbestosis/understanding-asbestosis.html. **4.** *Lead in Paint, Dust, and Soil: Basic Information,* by the Environmental Protection Agency, 2009, retrieved from http://www.epa.gov/lead/pubs/leadinfo.htm. **5.** *An Introduction to Indoor Air Quality: Formaldehyde,* by the Environmental Protection Agency, 2009, retrieved from http://www.epa.gov/iaq/formalde.html. **6.** "Carbon Monoxide–Related Deaths: United States, 1999–2004," by M. King & C. Bailey, National Center for Environmental Health, 2007, *Morbidity and Mortality Weekly Report, 56,* pp. 1309–1312, retrieved from http://www.cdc.gov/mmwr/preview/mmwrhtml/mm5650a1.htm?s_cid=mm5650a1_e. **7.** *Mold and Moisture,* by the Environmental Protection Agency, 2008, retrieved from http://www.epa.gov/mold/index.html. **8.** "Polycarbonate Bottle Use and Urinary Bisphenol A Concentrations," by Jenny Carwile, Henry Luu, Laura Bassett, Daniel Driscoll, Caterina Yuan, Jennifer Chang, . . . & Karin Michels, 2009, *Environmental Health Perspectives, 117,* retrieved from http://www.ehponline.org/members/2009/0900604/0900604.pdf. **9.** "Association of Urinary Bisphenol A Concentration with Medical Disorders and Laboratory Abnormalities in Adults," by I. Lang, T. Galloway, A. Scarlett, W. Henley, M. Depledge, & R. Wallace, 2008, *Journal of the American Medical Association, 300,* pp. 1303–1310. **10.** *An Introduction to Indoor Air Quality: Volatile Organic Compounds (VOCs),* by the Environmental Protection Agency, 2009, retrieved from http://www.epa.gov/iaq/voc.html.

Health Effects of Pollutants at Home

Of course, we don't only eat or breathe indoor air when we're at home! The pollutants we encounter at school, work, shopping, or eating out can also influence our health. In fact, in parts of the world with a modern infrastructure, people spend more than 90% of their time indoors, giving indoor air quality significant potential to affect your well-being.[61]

Some of the effects of foodborne and indoor air pollutants have been researched for decades and are well understood.

- Some substances, such as certain pesticides found in fruits and vegetables, radon gas, some VOCs, and toxins found in wood and tobacco smoke, are known carcinogens, meaning that they are capable of causing cancer.

- Some substances, such as BPA and other compounds found in plastics or agricultural chemicals, are **endocrine disruptors,** meaning that they interfere with the body's hormones and endocrine system.
- Some substances, such as certain pesticides, mercury, and lead, are nervous system disruptors, or **neurotoxins,** meaning that they have the potential to harm the brain or nervous system or interfere with childhood development.
- Some substances, such as sulfites used as food preservatives, cigarette smoke, pet dander, dust mites, and rodent droppings, are *allergens*, substances capable of causing allergies and asthma. For example, many studies have implicated "mouse allergen" as a significant cause of asthma in inner-city children.[62, 63]

In other cases, the health effects of contaminants are not yet well understood. Just because a chemical is present in your body does not mean that it is harmful. Most contaminants must be present at a certain level before exerting any clear health effects. Scientists and medical experts are working to better define those thresholds. They are also trying to understand the cumulative effects of contaminants when they combine or are present together in a person's body.

Body burden is a person's cumulative exposure to and storage of chemicals and other pollutants. Scientists and health experts are assessing the effects of body burden through a process called **biomonitoring,** in which individuals' levels of certain contaminants are measured over time and then monitored to see what health effects develop. In the United States, biomonitoring is now a part of an ongoing national health survey, and some state and local governments have similar programs. Key findings from the most recent national biomonitoring survey include the following:

- Levels of lead in children's blood continue to decline, a positive sign that improved awareness and lead containment efforts are working.
- Levels of cotinine, a byproduct of the nicotine found in tobacco smoke, have dropped in the blood of nonsmokers over the past decade, a sign that efforts to ban smoking in indoor and outdoor spaces are working. But about 5% of U.S. adults have potentially risky levels of cadmium, with smoking the likely source, indicating that further research and smoking cessation efforts are needed.
- African American adults carry higher levels of potentially risky mercury than Caucasians or Mexican Americans. At elevated levels, mercury is a powerful neurotoxin that can affect adults, children, and developing babies.
- Many other chemicals were found in the blood of U.S. adults and children, including phthalates (plasticizers that make plastic materials flexible), PCBs, insecticides, herbicides, and heavy metals. However, it's important to note that the health effects of these exposures remain unclear in many cases.[64]

endocrine disruptor A substance that stops the production or blocks the use of hormones in the body and that can have harmful effects on health or development.

neurotoxin A substance that interferes with or harms the functioning of the brain and nervous system.

body burden The amount of a chemical stored in the body at a given time, especially a potential toxin in the body as the result of environmental exposure.

biomonitoring Analysis of blood, urine, tissues, and so forth to measure chemical exposure in humans.

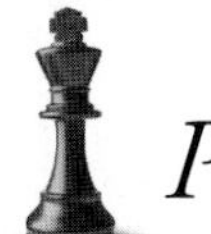

Practical Strategies for Change

Reducing Pollution at Home

When you eat:

- Choose organic when available and affordable.
- If you can't buy organic produce, scrub your fruits and vegetables thoroughly under cold running water. Remove the outer leaves of lettuce heads. For the inner leaves and other soft or small produce, rinse for several seconds under cold running water.
- Reduce the amount of meat and animal-based products in your diet.
- Opt for fresh, whole foods over processed foods. Read food labels—the more ingredients you don't recognize or can't pronounce, the more processed the item is.
- Limit your use of plastic containers and utensils. Be especially careful to avoid microwave-heating food in plastic containers with the recycling code 3 or 7.
- Choose the fish you eat carefully. The EPA recommends avoiding a few types of fish high in mercury, including swordfish, king mackerel, and shark, and limiting consumption of some types of tuna. To download a wallet card with specific recommendations, see the **Get Connected** links at the end of this chapter.

Where you live:

- Test your home for radon. To find out how, visit **www.epa.gov/radon/radontest.html**.
- Install a carbon monoxide detector.
- Learn whether or not your home has surfaces covered with lead paint, and repaint, remove, or contain them. If you do repaint, opt for zero- or low-VOC paint.
- Help prevent mold by making sure bathrooms, kitchens, and basements have good air circulation and are cleaned often.
- When purchasing new furniture, mattresses, rugs, or carpeting, look for low-VOC options and keep it outdoors (or in a room with the windows open) for a few days before using or installing it.
- Vacuum thoroughly and frequently to remove dust mites, pet hair and dander, and other potential allergens.
- If you smoke, take it outside. If a roommate smokes, insist that he or she do the same.
- A majority of U.S. states have banned smoking in all enclosed public spaces. If your state is in the minority, avoid bars and restaurants where you'll be exposed to secondhand smoke.
- In all indoor spaces, good ventilation is key to air quality. If you suspect a ventilation problem in a dorm or classroom building on campus, let the building supervisor know.
- Get involved in green efforts on your campus that encourage administrators to make changes such as using low-VOC paint, carpet, and other products.

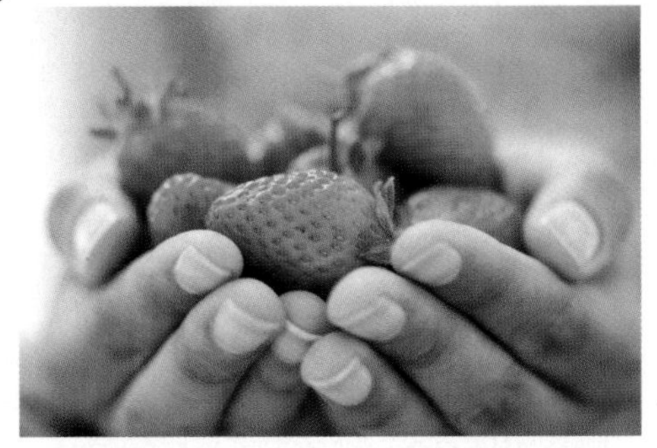

Choosing fresh, whole foods that have not been sprayed by pesticides can reduce your exposure to pollutants.

Now that you understand the potential health effects of pollutants that might be lurking in your home, you're probably wondering what you can do about them. Check out the **Practical Strategies for Change: Reducing Pollution at Home** on the previous page.

Noise Pollution

What did you say? Something about noise pollution? Hold on—I need to take out my earbuds first.

Noise is a fact of contemporary life, in the streets, on campus, and in our homes. But noise pollution takes a toll on our hearing: According to national estimates, the number of Americans with hearing loss has doubled over the last 30 years. About 30 million people in the United States are exposed to daily noise levels that are likely to lead to early hearing loss.[65] Of the 28 million individuals with impaired hearing, about half have hearing loss at least partly related to damage from noise. Noise pollution can also trigger other health effects, including elevated blood pressure, headaches, irritability, sleep disturbances, and increased heart rate.

The loudness—or amplitude—of sound is measured in **decibels,** and in many aspects of our lives, those decibels are high. Prolonged exposure to any sound over 85 decibels—the noise level of heavy city traffic—can damage the delicate hair cells of the inner ear and lead to gradual hearing loss. Sustained exposure to louder sounds can result in hearing loss more quickly. In fact, the surge in popularity of personal music devices such as MP3 players has resulted in a corresponding increase in hearing loss among people in their 20s.[66] If you turn the volume on your MP3 player all the way up, you'll be exposed to 120 decibels. Not only the volume, but the duration of exposure is important, too. More than 30 minutes of exposure to high-decibel noise—such as during a rock concert, or with an MP3 player set at more than three-quarters of maximum volume—can impair hearing. For a look at the decibel levels of some common sounds, see **Figure 21.6.**

decibel The unit of measurement used to express sound intensity.

MedlinePlus illustrates how we hear: www.nlm.nih.gov/medlineplus/ency/anatomyvideos/000063.htm.

Dangerous Decibels is an organization that provides information on hearing loss and protecting your ears: www.dangerousdecibels.org.

What can you do to limit your exposure to noise pollution and protect your hearing? Try the following:

- Give your ears a break from your earbuds. Switch to over-the-ear headphones, which block outside noise and provide fewer decibels at the same volume setting. And follow the 60/60 rule: Don't go past about 60% of the device's volume, and don't listen for more than 60 minutes a day. Consider downloading to your MP3 player an app that will enable you to limit the volume to safe levels.
- When you go to concerts, stay away from the speakers, and wear ear plugs. The music is usually so loud (about 105 decibels) that you'll still be able to hear through them just fine.
- If you go to bars and clubs with loud music, step outside every so often to give your ears a break.
- If you work around noise, use protective headphones. Most workplaces supply them.
- Loud music, movies, and TV can be fun. But pace yourself. By keeping the volume lower now, you'll be helping to make sure you can enjoy those same sounds later in life, too.

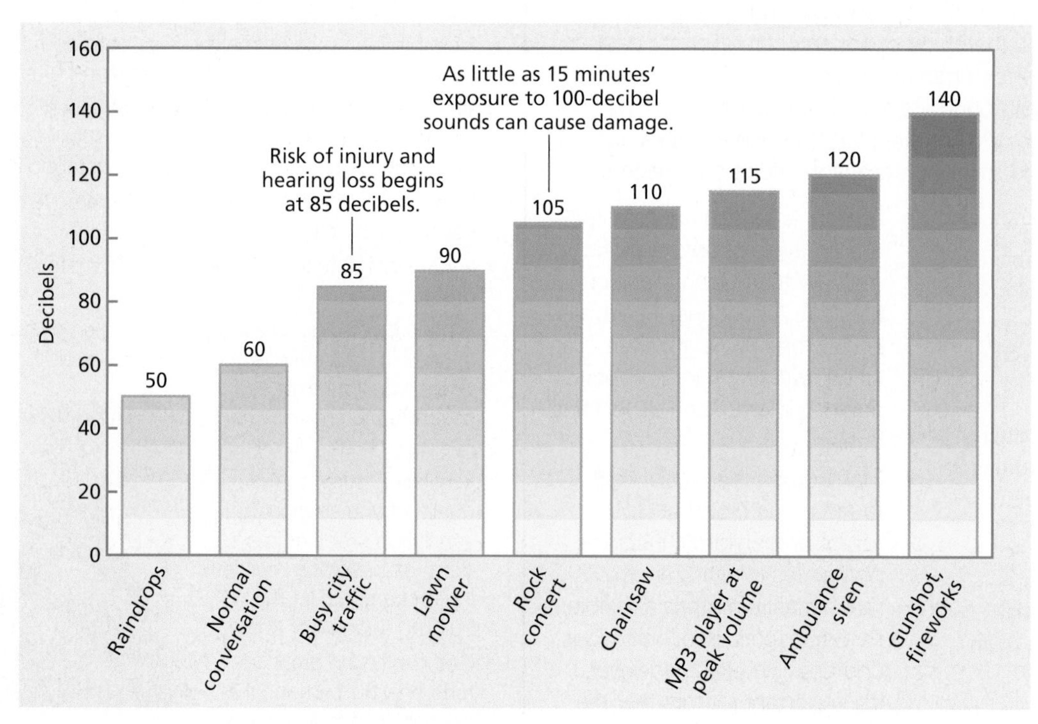

Figure 21.6 Decibel levels for common noises. Noise-related hearing damage can be caused not only by high decibel levels but also by prolonged exposure to noises above 85 decibels.

Source: Adapted from *Reduce Your Chance of Noise-Induced Hearing Loss,* by Emergency Medical Products, March 26, 2009, retrieved from http://www.buyempblog.com/2009/03/reduce-your-chance-of-noise-induced-hearing-loss/111, and *How Loud Is Too Loud? Bookmark,* by the National Institute on Deafness and Other Communication Disorders, 2009, retrieved from http://www.nidcd.nih.gov/health/hearing/ruler.asp.

SELF-ASSESSMENT

Is Loud Music Damaging Your Hearing?

Is your hearing at risk because of loud music? Answer these questions to find out.

1. Do you hear a ringing or buzzing in your ear (tinnitus) immediately after exposure to music? __ yes __ no
2. Do you experience slight muffling of sounds after exposure, making it difficult to understand people when you leave the area with loud music? __ yes __ no
3. While listening to music, do you experience difficulty understanding speech; that is, you can hear all the words, but you can't understand all of them? __ yes __ no
4. Do people who are only 3 feet away have to shout to be heard while you are listening to music? __ yes __ no

HOW TO INTERPRET YOUR SCORE

A "yes" on any item means the music may be too loud and pose a risk to your hearing. Wear ear plugs at clubs or concerts, and turn the music down on your MP3 player. If you think you may have hearing loss, make an appointment with an audiologist (a hearing professional who can measure hearing loss).

Source: Adapted from *Noise & Music Fact Sheet*, by the Center for Hearing and Communication, 2010,, retrieved from http://www.chchearing.org/noise-center-home/facts-noise/noise-music. Used with permission.

Take this Self-Assessment online at www.pearsonhighered.com/lynchelmore.

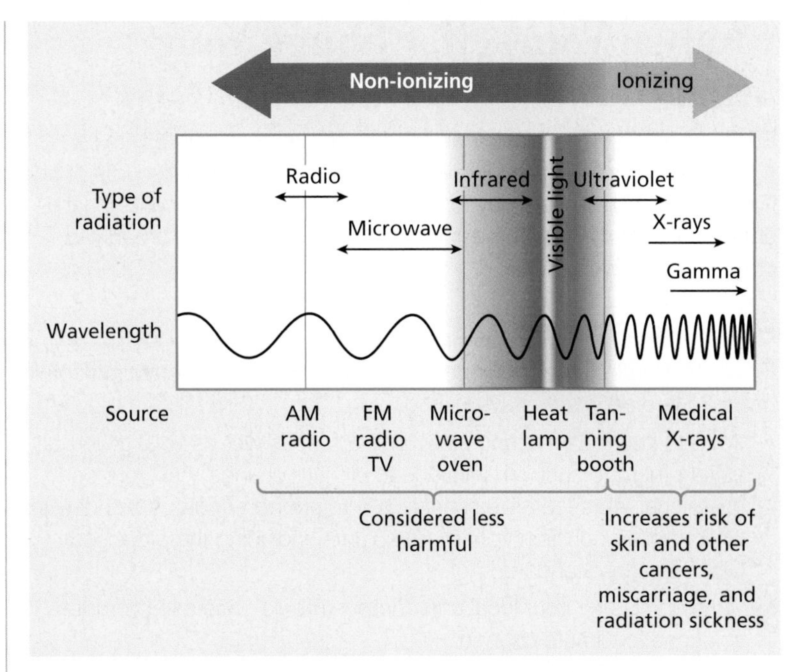

Figure 21.7 The electromagnetic spectrum and sources of radiation. Non-ionizing radiation is considered less harmful than ionizing radiation.

Source: Adapted from *Radiation Protection: Ionizing & Non-Ionizing Radiation*, by the Environmental Protection Agency, 2009, retrieved from http://www.epa.gov/radiation/understand/ionize_nonionize.html.

Radiation

Radiation, or energy that travels outward from a source in the form of invisible rays, waves, or particles, usually sounds like the stuff of warfare or science fiction. That's because radiation, in some cases, has the power to alter the molecular structure of living things, causing changes that can be harmful and even deadly. But the *electromagnetic spectrum*—the complete range of radiation from longest to shortest waves—is broad, and not all radiation is harmful **(Figure 21.7).** The trick is knowing the characteristics of different types, and avoiding or limiting exposure to those that are dangerous.

radiation Energy that travels in the form of rays, waves, or particles.

Types of Radiation and Their Health Effects

As you can see in Figure 21.7, radiation can be quite low in energy, like radio waves, which we typically don't even think of as a form of radiation. This is called non-ionizing radiation. In contrast, high-energy radiation, like medical and dental X-rays, is ionizing. The difference between the two has implications for your health:

- *Non-ionizing radiation* travels in the form of relatively long, shallow electromagnetic waves. It can cause molecules in matter to move, but can't alter them. Everyday examples include microwaves, radio waves, and visible light. In general, this form of radiation is considered less harmful, although questions have arisen about some electronic devices that rely on radio frequency (RF) waves, such as cell phones. See the **Myth or Fact?** box on the next page.
- *Ionizing radiation* carries enough energy to cause changes in molecules of matter, and exposure is considered more harmful, especially at higher or sustained levels. Ultraviolent (UV) rays from the sun or tanning beds, X-rays from medical diagnostic devices, radon, and the fuel found in nuclear weapons and nuclear power plants are common forms of ionizing radiation. Radiation exposure is measured in units called *radiation absorbed doses,* or *rads,* and can cause damage at relatively low levels. Health risks include cancer, such as skin cancer arising from prolonged exposure to UV sunlight, and miscarriages. At higher levels of exposure, radiation can lead to *radiation sickness,* a multisymptom condition that can cause nausea, fatigue, and hair loss. At very high levels, radiation destroys the body's ability to make white blood cells and is fatal.

What Can You Do to Reduce Your Exposure to Radiation?

You can reduce your exposure—and your health risks—with a few simple steps:

- Watch your sun exposure. Protect yourself with sunscreen, sunglasses, and a hat.
- Skip the tanning salon. That bronze glow is actually a sign of radiation-induced skin damage.
- Use a headset when talking on your cell phone, or put it on speaker and set it down.
- Work with your doctor and dentist to limit your exposure to X-rays and other imaging devices that use radiation.
- Test your home for radon. To find out how, visit **www.epa.gov/radon/radontest.html.**

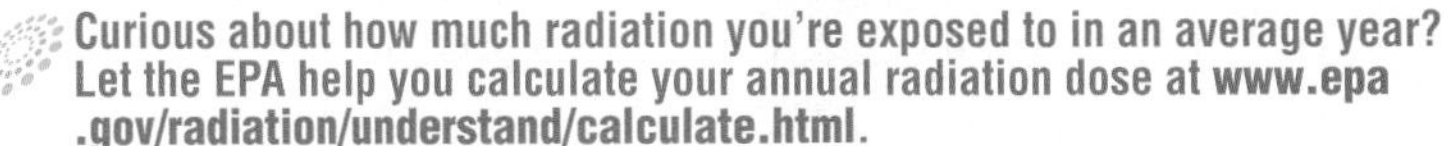

Curious about how much radiation you're exposed to in an average year? Let the EPA help you calculate your annual radiation dose at www.epa.gov/radiation/understand/calculate.html.

Change Yourself, Change Your World

Environmentalist David Orr reminds us that, "Hope is a verb with its sleeves rolled up."[67] Throughout this chapter, we've identified lots of actions you can take every day to help "save the planet"—and its inhabitants! Here, let's look at some ways you can commit more broadly to changing your world.

Personal Choices

Ready to plug into the "power of the people" to promote environmental health? Here are some ways to begin:

- Write to your national and state legislators, as well as your governor, asking them to support solutions to climate change. Ask your congressional representatives specifically to support rigorous standards to control air pollution from power plants, including the proposed Clean Energy Standards Act.
- Write articles for your local and campus media outlets to promote solutions to climate change.
- Host a movie night with friends and screen a film with an environmental theme such as *An Inconvenient Truth*, *Plastic Planet*, or *Food, Inc.* Afterward, share ideas for ways to get involved, and collect donations to an environmental action group such as the Natural Resources Defense Council or Greenpeace.
- Use your social networking sites to let friends know what you've been doing to clean up the Earth, and how they can get involved, too.

Campus Advocacy

Thousands of college campuses are "going green" with initiatives like offering low-emission shuttles to and from campus to cut down on driving, designing new buildings to be "green" or retrofitting older ones to be energy efficient, using energy-efficient appliances and light bulbs in residence halls, recycling paper in classrooms and offices, and composting food wastes in dining halls. Some schools have taken small steps, while others have set ambitious goals to become environmentally friendly fast. How green is your campus? The nonprofit Sustainable Endowments Institute publishes report cards on at least 300 public and private campuses. You can find out if your school is included, see its ranking, and compare schools at **www.greenreportcard.org.**

You should also know about the Association for the Advancement of Sustainability in Higher Education (AASHE). Its mission is to empower higher education to lead the sustainability transformation. Go to its website at www.aashe.org and click on Resources for Students. There, you'll find ways to get involved with AASHE and promote sustainability on your campus. A few of the AASHE's ideas include:[68]

- Organizing a dorm-versus-dorm sustainability competition hosted on the AASHE's YouTube channel
- Competing in the Campus Conservation Nationals
- Starting a campus farm and composting program
- Starting a peer outreach campaign

You'll also find an e-newsletter to which you can subscribe, and lots of other sources of information, including a blog and an archive of journal articles and other reports on sustainability.

Wondering whether or not your school is already a member of the AASHE? Find out at www.aashe.org/membership/member-directory.

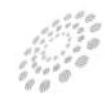
Watch videos of real students discussing environmental health at www.pearsonhighered.com/lynchelmore.

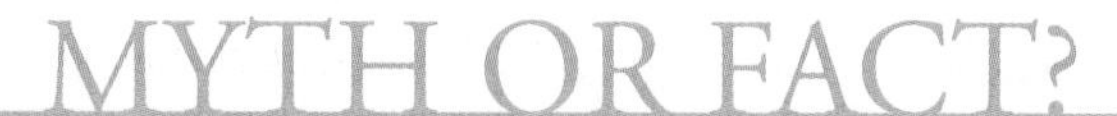

Does Using a Cell Phone Fry Your Brain?

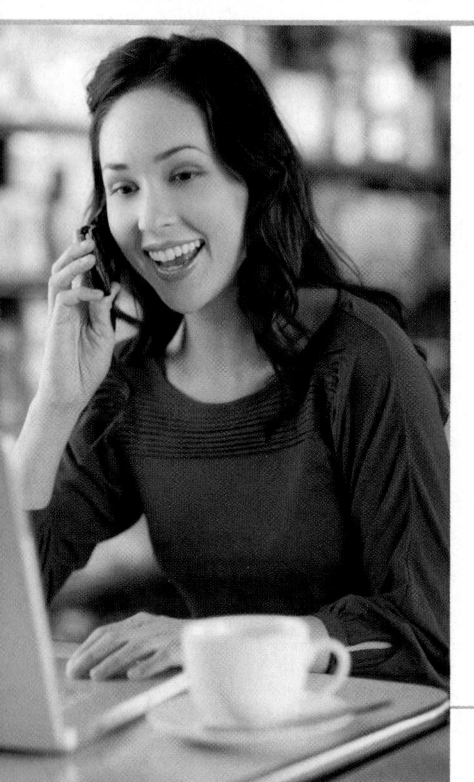

For most of us, cell phones are indispensable. But every time you use it, your cell phone emits radiation in the form of high-frequency electromagnetic waves. That fact has fueled a long-running controversy over whether this radiation exposure can damage your brain or lead to brain cancer, especially when you talk with your phone held close to your ear.

Numerous scientific studies have tackled this question, but so far, the jury is still out. While some evidence points to a correlation between cell phone use and an increased risk of brain cancer, scientists still aren't sure how significant this risk is. To find out, they'll need to track the health of cell phone users over long periods of time.[1] Only time will tell whether cell phones pose any real danger. In the meantime, you can play it safe by using a headset. Or put your cell on speaker and set it down. And remember that while the risk of brain cancer and cell phone use isn't yet clear, another risk *is* clear—driving while distracted. Going hands-free with your cell phone is not the solution. If your phone rings while you're driving, pull over before taking the call.

Reference: 1. "Review: The Controversy About a Possible Relationship Between Mobile Phone Use and Cancer," by M. Kundi, 2009, *Environmental Health Perspectives, 117*, pp. 316–324.

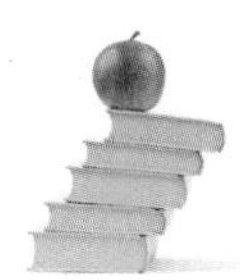

Choosing to Change Worksheet

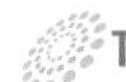

To complete this worksheet online, visit www.pearsonhighered.com/lynchelmore.

As you've learned from this chapter, many of your everyday actions can have an impact on the environment. While you may feel that you are just one person and nothing you do personally can make much difference in improving the environment, all the little things you do to "REDUCE, REUSE, RECYCLE" do add up.

Directions: Complete Part I. In Part II, determine your stage of behavior change and complete the rest of the worksheet with your stage of change in mind.

Part I. Assess Your Behaviors

Consider the following list of little things you can do to reduce, reuse, or recycle. Place a checkmark next to the items that you already do.

Reduce

- ❑ Raise (in the summer) or lower (in the winter) your thermostat 2 degrees.
- ❑ Cancel all junk mail. (Go to **www.dmachoice.org/dma/member/regist.action** to stop direct mail advertising and to **www.optoutprescreen.com** to stop credit card solicitations.)
- ❑ Switch to online bill payment.
- ❑ Turn off all TVs, computers, lights, printers, etc., when you aren't using them.
- ❑ Turn off the faucet when brushing your teeth.
- ❑ Commit to walking to one place you normally drive to.
- ❑ Replace incandescent light bulbs with compact fluorescent bulbs—or, even better, LEDs.
- ❑ Don't buy products with lots of packaging.
- ❑ Go "trayless" in the dining hall.
- ❑ Reduce your consumption of meats.

Reuse

- ❑ Bring your own reusable bags to stores.
- ❑ Use cloth napkins or dishtowels rather than disposable napkins or paper towels.
- ❑ Use a reusable bottle rather than buying bottled water or other drinks.
- ❑ Don't throw away items (clothing, furniture, appliances) that you don't want anymore. Take them to a center that collects donations or give them to your friends.
- ❑ Take your own cup to the coffee shop.
- ❑ Buy rechargeable batteries instead of using disposable ones.

Recycle

- ❑ Check with your local recycling company to find out what items can be easily recycled near you.
- ❑ Always put paper and other recyclable trash in an appropriate container.
- ❑ Buy products that contain recycled materials.
- ❑ Take any e-wastes (old computers, cell phones, MP3 players, or other electronics) to certified e-waste recyclers.

Part II. Take Action

Step 1: Your Stage of Behavior Change. Please check one of the following statements that best describes your readiness to improve your environmental health.

_____________ I do not intend to improve my environmental health in the next 6 months. (Precontemplation)

_____________ I am contemplating improving my environmental health in the next 6 months. (Contemplation)

_____________ I am planning on improving my environmental health in the next month. (Preparation)

_____________ I have been improving my environmental health for less than 6 months. (Action)

_____________ I have been improving my environmental health for 6 months or longer. (Maintenance)

Step 2: Set a Goal. Target one behavior from Part I that you currently don't do but would like to. Describe what next step you will take to make this change.

Example: *I will purchase an insulated water bottle to take to class with me instead of buying bottled water at the campus snack bar.*

Target behavior: ______________________________

Way to make this change: ______________________________

____

Timeline: ______________________________

Step 3: Overcome Obstacles. Describe what obstacles might get in your way and how you will address them.

Obstacle	How to Overcome
______________	______________
______________	______________
______________	______________
______________	______________

Chapter Summary

- Your environment has a direct effect on your health, and the choices you and others make help shape your environment and determine its quality. Environmental health is global—decisions made in one part of the world have the potential to affect all of us.
- Environmental health issues have changed over time, expanding from issues of hygiene and clean water to food production, industrial pollution, and global warming.
- The Earth's population is now more than 7 billion. Human population growth stresses our environment and can have effects that harm our health.
- Social reforms that have increased the availability and affordability of contraceptives and promoted equal access to education and career opportunities for women have had the greatest success in curbing population growth.
- Air pollution is primarily caused by the burning of fossil fuels. Some air pollutants cause smog or acid rain. Others lead to global warming or damage the Earth's protective ozone layer.
- Climate change includes not only warming of the Earth's atmosphere and oceans, but also changes in rainfall patterns, an increase in extreme weather events, and disruptions in ecosystems. The United States is the world's largest producer of greenhouse gas emissions.
- Water pollution can arise from biological contaminants, such as disease-causing microbes, or chemical contaminants, such as industrial compounds or pesticides and fertilizers.
- Although many of us reach for bottled water as a safer, more healthful choice, there is no guarantee that bottled water is any purer than tap water, and plastic bottles contribute to municipal waste.
- Land pollution is a result of our disposable society. The average person in the United States throws away about 4.5 pounds of solid waste each day. Some of this waste can be recycled or composted; some of it, however, contains toxins that make it too hazardous to dispose of without special containment or treatment.
- At home, we're exposed to pollution from the foods and beverages we ingest and the air we inhale. Some contaminants found in food can build up in our bodies' tissues over long periods of time, a process called bio-accumulation.
- Noise pollution damages hearing and causes other adverse health effects, including headaches, tension, and irritability. Exposure to about 85 decibels or lower is considered safe.
- We are all exposed to radiation on a regular basis, but only some forms are harmful, including UV radiation from the sun and ionizing radiation released by X-ray machines and other medical imaging devices.
- Through the personal decisions you make, you can improve both your own environmental health and that of those around you. Drive less. Carry reusable bags when you go shopping. Buy organic produce. Carry your own stainless steel water bottle and porcelain coffee mug, rather than getting a new disposable container every time you need a drink of water or buy a latte. These small choices add up to a healthier planet—and healthier people.
- You can get involved in improving environmental health by making small decisions every day to reduce your energy consumption and waste generation. You can also work to involve your friends and other students either individually or through an organization such as the Association for the Advancement of Sustainability in Higher Education.

Test Your Knowledge

1. Which of the following statements about population is true?
   a. No countries of the world have yet achieved negative population growth.
   b. By 2050, the United States will have achieved zero population growth.
   c. The world's population is expected to increase by about two billion before the year 2046.
   d. The world's population has doubled since the year 1804.

2. Which of these statements accurately characterizes global warming?
   a. Global warming harms wildlife, but hasn't hurt people yet.
   b. Global warming is a climate problem, not a health problem.
   c. Global warming is due to radon and stratospheric ozone.
   d. Global warming already has negatively affected human health.

3. Why is deforestation a problem?
   a. It reduces the Earth's ability to remove CO_2 from the atmosphere.
   b. It reduces the Earth's ability to remove ozone from the atmosphere.
   c. It releases too much oxygen into the atmosphere all at once.
   d. All of the above are problems of deforestation.

Get Critical

What happened:

In the fall of 2012, actress Darryl Hannah was arrested for protesting in Texas against approval of the Keystone XL pipeline, which would extract petroleum from tar sands in Alberta, Canada, and ship it to refineries on the coast of the Gulf of Mexico. A few months later, actor Mark Ruffalo was spotted protesting natural-gas drilling in New York state. Then it was Lucy Lawless who, with other members of Greenpeace, drew media attention to oil drilling in the Arctic by spending four days aboard an oil-drilling ship, preventing the ship from leaving port. Why do they do it? Lawless said she felt compelled to take a stand against oil drilling and global warming, not so much for herself, but for her children's future.

What do you think?

- **Do protests involving celebrities deserve more media coverage than protests involving people who aren't famous?**
- **Do celebrities have a greater moral or ethical responsibility than "ordinary people" to speak out against policies that they oppose—whether related to the environment, human rights, or any other issue?**
- **If celebrities are protesting to "save the planet," does that get you off the hook, or does it make you want to get involved, too?**

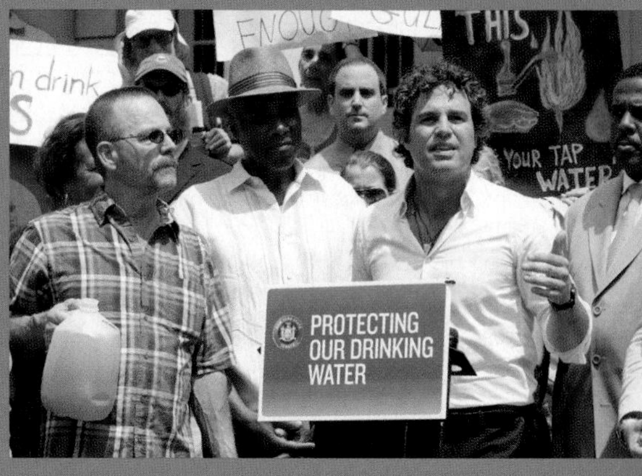

Marc Ruffalo protesting natural-gas drilling.

4. Which of these statements about bottled water is true?
   a. Bottled water is not necessarily more healthful than tap water.
   b. Bottled water has less environmental impact than tap water.
   c. Bottled water is cheaper than tap water.
   d. All of the above are true.

5. Why should you consider going trayless the next time you visit the dining hall?
   a. You'll probably generate less trash.
   b. You'll probably waste less food.
   c. You'll probably eat less.
   d. All of the above are possible outcomes.

6. Which common but potentially fatal indoor pollutant is released from the burning of fuels such as gas, oil, wood, or charcoal?
   a. carbon monoxide
   b. carbon dioxide
   c. radon
   d. mold spores

7. In modern societies, people spend about what percentage of their time indoors?
   a. 90%
   b. 75%
   c. 50%
   d. 40%

8. Which of these statements about endocrine disruptors is true?
   a. Endocrine disruptors are one way to clean up industrial air pollution.
   b. Endocrine disruptors have been linked to almost all glass, ceramic, and plastic containers.
   c. Endocrine disruptors only affect animals.
   d. Endocrine disruptors impair the functioning of the body's hormones.

9. What does biomonitoring refer to?
   a. ongoing studies that measure the levels of certain chemicals in people
   b. ongoing studies that measure the health of our biosphere
   c. ongoing studies that measure the amount of biofuels we burn
   d. none of the above

10. Which of these statements about radiation is true?
    a. Visible light is not part of the electromagnetic spectrum.
    b. Tanning beds emit ionizing radiation.
    c. Even low-dose exposure to the radiation emitted by radio waves can be fatal.
    d. All of the above are true.

Get Connected

Mobile Tips!

Scan this QR code with your mobile device to access additional tips about environmental health. Or, via your mobile device, go to **http://mobiletips.pearsoncmg.com** and navigate to Chapter 21.

Health Online Visit the following websites for further information about the topics in this chapter:

- National Center for Environmental Health (NCEH)
  www.cdc.gov/nceh
- Environmental Protection Agency
  www.epa.gov
- Natural Resources Defense Council, Mercury in Fish wallet card
  www.nrdc.org/health/effects/mercury/walletcard.PDF
- Centers for Disease Control and Prevention National Biomonitoring Program
  www.cdc.gov/biomonitoring
- Environmental Working Group Shopper's Guide to Pesticides in Produce
  www.ewg.org/foodnews
- Eartheasy Non-Toxic Home Cleaning
  http://eartheasy.com/live_nontoxic_solutions.htm

Website links are subject to change. To access updated web links, please visit *www.pearsonhighered.com/lynchelmore*.

References

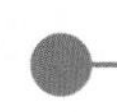

i. U.S. Census Bureau. (2012, March 28). U.S. and world population clocks. Retrieved from http://www.census.gov/main/www/popclock.html.

ii. Jacob, T., Wahr, J., Pfeffer, W. T., & Swenson, S. (2012). Recent contributions of glaciers and ice caps to sea level rise. *Nature*, DOI: 10.1038/nature10847.

iii. Environmental Protection Agency. (2008). *U.S. EPA's 2008 report on the environment: Highlights of national trends*,1–37. Retrieved from http://www.epa.gov/roe/docs/roe_hd/ROE_HD_Final_2008.pdf.

1. World Health Organization. (2010). *Environmental health.* Retrieved from http://www.who.int/topics/environmental_health/en.

2. World Health Organization. (2008). *10 facts on preventing disease through healthy environments.* Retrieved from http://www.who.int/features/factfiles/environmental_health/en/index.html.

3. Environmental Protection Agency. (2010). *About EPA: EPA's mission.* Retrieved from http://www.epa.gov/aboutepa/index.html.

4. World Health Organization. (2009). *Country profile of environmental burden of disease: China.* Retrieved from http://www.who.int/quantifying_ehimpacts/national/countryprofile/china.pdf.

5. Obrist, D., Hallar, A., McCubbin, I., Stephens, B., & Rahn, T. (2008). Measurements of atmospheric mercury at Storm Peak Laboratory in the Rocky Mountains: Evidence for long-range transport from Asia, boundary layer contributions, and plant mercury uptake. *Atmospheric Environment, 42* (33), 7579–7589.

6. Lewis, J. (1985, November). The birth of EPA. *EPA Journal*. Retrieved from http://www.epa.gov/history/topics/epa/15c.htm.

7. McMichael, A., Woodruff, R., & Hales, S. (2006). Climate change and human health: Present and future risks. *The Lancet, 367* (5), 859–869.

8. Ebi, K., Mills, D., Smith, J., & Grambach, A. (2006). Climate change and human health impacts in the United States: An update on the results of the U.S. national assessment. *Environmental Health Perspectives, 114* (9), 1318–1324.

9. World Health Organization. (2012). Climate change. *Health and Environment Linkages Initiative.* Retrieved from http://www.who.int/heli/risks/climate/climatechange/en.

10. U.S. Census Bureau. (2012, June 27). Expectation of life at birth, and projections. The 2012 statistical abstract. Retrieved from http://www.census.gov/compendia/statab/cats/births_deaths_marriages_divorces/life_expectancy.html.

11. Pimentel, D. (2011). World overpopulation. *Environmental Development and Sustainability*, DOI: 10.1007/s10668-011-9336-2. Online at http://www.springerlink.com/content/lr4065j08g702109.

12. Worldwatch Institute. (2011). *Worldwatch Institute's state of the world 2011*. Retrieved from http://www.worldwatch.org/sow11.

13. International Energy Agency. (2011). *World energy outlook 2011: Executive summary*. Retrieved from http://www.iea.org/Textbase/npsum/weo2011sum.pdf.

14. Worldwatch Institute. (2008). *State of the world 2008*. Retrieved from http://www.worldwatch.org/node/5568.

15. Energy Information Administration. (2006). *Energy kids.* Retrieved from http://www.eia.doe.gov/kids/classactivities/CrunchTheNumbers.pdf.

16. World Bank. (2012, March 9). *Data: Fertility rate.* Retrieved from http://data.worldbank.org/indicator/SP.DYN.TFRT.IN/countries.

17. United Nations Population Division. (2009). *World population prospects: The 2008 revision population database.* Retrieved from http://esa.un.org/unpp.

18. Population Reference Bureau. (2010). *Human population.* Retrieved from http://www.prb.org/Educators/TeachersGuides/HumanPopulation.aspx.

19. Eberstadt, N., & Shah, A. (2011, December 7). Fertility decline in the Muslim world: A veritable sea-change, still curiously unnoticed. *The American Enterprise Institute Working Paper Series on Development Policy*. Retrieved from http://www.aei.org/files/2011/12/19/-fertility-decline-in-the-muslim-world-a-veritable-seachange-still-curiously-unnoticed_103731477628.pdf.

20. Population Council. (2008, June). Knut Wicksell on the benefits of depopulation. *Population and Development Review, 34* (2), 347–355.

21. Kjellstrom, T., Hakansta, C., & Hogstedt, C. (2007). Globalisation and public health: Overview and a Swedish perspective. *Scandinavian Journal of Public Health, 70* (35), 2–68.

22. Energy Information Administration, Independent Statistics and Analysis. (2010). *Renewable energy consumption and electricity preliminary statistics 2009*. Retrieved from http://www.eia.doe.gov/cneaf/alternate/page/renew_energy_consump/rea_prereport.html.

23. Environmental Protection Agency. (2008). *U.S. EPA's 2008 report on the environment: Highlights of national trends,* 1–37. Retrieved from http://cfpub.epa.gov/ncea/cfm/recordisplay.cfm?deid=190806.

24. AIRNow. (2003). *AIRNOW air quality index: A guide to air quality and your health.* Retrieved from http://www.airnow.gov/index.cfm?action=aqibasics.aqi.

25. Environmental Protection Agency. (2009). *Bad nearby.* Retrieved from http://www.epa.gov/oar/oaqps/gooduphigh/bad.html.

26. American Lung Association. (2009). *State of the air 2009*. Retrieved from http://www.lungusa2.org/sota/2009/SOTA-2009-Full-Print.pdf.

27. Global Warming Policy Foundation. (2011, November 19). IPCC introduces new "climate change" definition. *GWPF Science News.* Retrieved from http://thegwpf.org/science-news/4374-ipcc-introduces-new-climate-change-definition.html.

28. Environmental Protection Agency. (2009). *Recent climate change: Temperature changes.* Retrieved from http://www.epa.gov/climatechange/science/recenttc.html.

29. Environmental Protection Agency. (2012, March 27). *Climate change indicators.* Retrieved from http://www.epa.gov/climatechange.

30. Energy Information Administration. (2008). *Emissions of greenhouse gases report.* Retrieved from http://www.eia.doe.gov/oiaf/1605/ggrpt.

31. Environmental Protection Agency. (2009). *Climate change—Greenhouse gas emissions: U.S. greenhouse gas inventory.* Retrieved from http://www.epa.gov/climatechange/emissions/usgginventory.html.

32. Nature Conservancy. (2009). *Rainforests at risk.* Retrieved from http://www.nature.org/rainforests/explore/threats.html.

33. Environmental Protection Agency. (2010). *Methane.* Retrieved from http://www.epa.gov/methane.

34. Food and Agriculture Organization. (2006). *Livestock impacts on the environment.* Retrieved from http://www.fao.org/ag/magazine/0612sp1.htm.

35. Eshel, G., & Martin, P. A. (2006). Diet, energy, and global warming. *Earth Interactions*, 10 (9). Retrieved from http://journals.ametsoc.org/doi/pdf/10.1175/EI167.1.

36. Environmental Protection Agency. (2010). *Health and environmental effects of ozone layer depletion.* Retrieved from http://www.epa.gov/ozone/science/effects.

37. Environmental Protection Agency. (2008). *Key elements of the Clean Air Act: Cars, trucks, buses, and "nonroad" equipment.* Retrieved from http://www.epa.gov/air/caa/peg/carstrucks.html.

38. Environmental Protection Agency. (2012, March). *Light-duty automotive technology, carbon dioxide emissions, and fuel economy trends, 1975 through 2011.* Retrieved from http://www.epa.gov/otaq/cert/mpg/fetrends/2012/420s12001.pdf.

39. United Nations Framework Convention on Climate Change. (2012). *The international response to climate change.* Retrieved from http://unfccc.int/essential_background/items/6031.php.

40. Global Carbon Project. (2011). *Carbon budget: Highlights: Emissions from fossil fuel and cement.* Retrieved from http://www.globalcarbonproject.org/carbonbudget/10/hl-full.htm#ffcement.

41. United Nations. (2012). *Water scarcity.* Retrieved from http://www.un.org/waterforlifedecade/scarcity.shtml.

42. World Health Organization/UNICEF Joint Monitoring Programme for Water Supply and Sanitation. (2009). *Millennium development goal assessment report.* Retrieved from http://mdgs.un.org/unsd/mdg/Resources/Static/Products/Progress2009/MDG_Report_2009_En.pdf.

43. Environmental Protection Agency. (2009). *Polychlorinated biphenyls (PCBs).* Retrieved from http://www.epa.gov/osw/hazard/tsd/pcbs/pubs/about.htm.

44. Food and Drug Administration. (2009). *Questions and answers about dioxins.* Retrieved from http://www.fda.gov/Food/FoodSafety/FoodContaminantsAdulteration/ChemicalContaminants/DioxinsPCBs/ucm077524.htm.

45. Environmental Protection Agency. (2007). *Assessing health risks from pesticides.* Retrieved from http://www.epa.gov/opp00001/factsheets/riskassess.htm.

46. Environmental Protection Agency. (2009). *Factoids: Drinking water and ground water statistics for 2009.* Retrieved from http://www.epa.gov/ogwdw000/databases/pdfs/data_factoids_2009.pdf.

47. Rodwan, J. G. (2009). *Bottled water 2009: Challenging circumstances persist: Future growth anticipated.* Retrieved from http://www.bottledwater.org/files/2009BWstats.pdf.

48. Saleha, M., Abdel-Rahmanb, F., Woodarda, B., Clarka, S., Wallacea, C., Aboabaa, A., . . . Nancea, J. (2008). Chemical, microbial, and physical evaluation of commercial bottled waters in the greater Houston area of Texas. *Journal of Environmental Science and Health, 43,* 335–347.

49. Government Accountability Office. (2009). *Bottled water: FDA safety and consumer protections are often less stringent than comparable EPA protections for tap water.* Retrieved from http://www.gao.gov/new.items/d09610.pdf.

50. Environmental Protection Agency. (2006). *Water health series: Bottled water basics.* Retrieved from http://www.epa.gov/safewater/faq/pdfs/fs_healthseries_bottlewater.pdf.

51. Allsopp, M., Walters, A., Santillo, D., & Johnston, P. (2007). Plastic debris in the world's oceans. *Greenpeace*. Retrieved from http://www.unep.org/regionalseas/marinelitter/publications/default.asp.

52. Foderaro, L. (2009, April 28). Without cafeteria trays, colleges find savings. *New York Times*. Retrieved from http://www.nytimes.com/2009/04/29/nyregion/29tray.html?_r=2.

53. San Francisco Department of the Environment. (2003). *Resolution setting zero waste date.* Retrieved from http://www.sfenvironment.org/downloads/library/resolutionzerowastedate.pdf.

54. City and County of San Francisco, Office of the Mayor. (October 5, 2012). *Mayor Lee announces San Francisco reaches 80 percent landfill waste diversion, leads all cities in North America*. News Release. Retrieved from http://sfmayor.org/index.aspx?recordid=113&page=846.

55. Environmental Protection Agency. (2012, February 23). *Household hazardous waste management: A manual for one-day community collection programs.* Retrieved from http://www.epa.gov/wastes/conserve/materials/pubs/manual.

56. Food and Drug Administration. (2012, March 30). *FDA continues to study BPA.* Retrieved from http://www.fda.gov/ForConsumers/ConsumerUpdates/ucm297954.htm.

57. Environmental Protection Agency. (2010, June 7). *Asbestos in your home.* Retrieved from http://www.epa.gov/asbestos/pubs/ashome.html#content.

58. National Cancer Institute. (2004). *Radon and cancer: Questions and answers.* Retrieved from http://www.cancer.gov/cancertopics/factsheet/Risk/radon.

59. Environmental Protection Agency. (2010). *Protect your family and yourself from carbon monoxide poisoning.* Retrieved from http://www.epa.gov/iaq/pubs/coftsht.html.

60. Environmental Protection Agency. (2010). *Volatile organic compounds (VOCs).* Retrieved from http://www.epa.gov/iaq/voc.html.

61. Wu, F., Jacobs, D., Mitchell, C., Miller, D., & Karol, M. (2007). Improving indoor environmental quality for public health: Impediments and policy recommendations. *Environmental Health Perspectives, (115)* 6, 953–957.

62. Matsui, E. C., Eggleston, P. A., Buckley, T. J., Krishnan, J. A., Breysse, P. N., Rand, C. S., & Diette, G. B. (2006, October). Household mouse allergen exposure and asthma morbidity in inner-city preschool children. *Annals of Allergy, Asthma & Immunology, 97* (4), 514–520.

63. Pongracic, J. A., Visness, C. M., Gruchella, R. S., Evans, R., & Mitchell, H. E. (2008, July). Effect of mouse allergen and rodent environmental intervention on asthma in inner-city children. *Annals of Allergy, Asthma & Immunology, 101* (1), 35–41.

64. Centers for Disease Control and Prevention. (2010). *Fourth national report on human exposure to environmental chemicals.* Retrieved from http://www.cdc.gov/exposurereport.

65. American Speech-Language-Hearing Association. (2012). *The prevalence and incidence of hearing loss in adults.* Retrieved from http://www.asha.org/public/hearing/Prevalence-and-Incidence-of-Hearing-Loss-in-Adults.

66. American Speech-Language-Hearing Association. (2010). *Unsafe usage of portable music players may damage your hearing.* Retrieved from http://www.asha.org/about/news/atitbtot/mp3players.htm.

67. Orr, D. W. (2007). Optimism and hope in a hotter time. *Conservation Biology, 21*(6), 1392–1395.

68. Association for the Advancement of Sustainability in Higher Education. (2012). *Resources for campus sustainability: Resources for students*. Retrieved from www.aashe.org/resources/general-resources-campus-sustainability/student-resources.

22

Embracing Change: The Gifts and Challenges of Aging

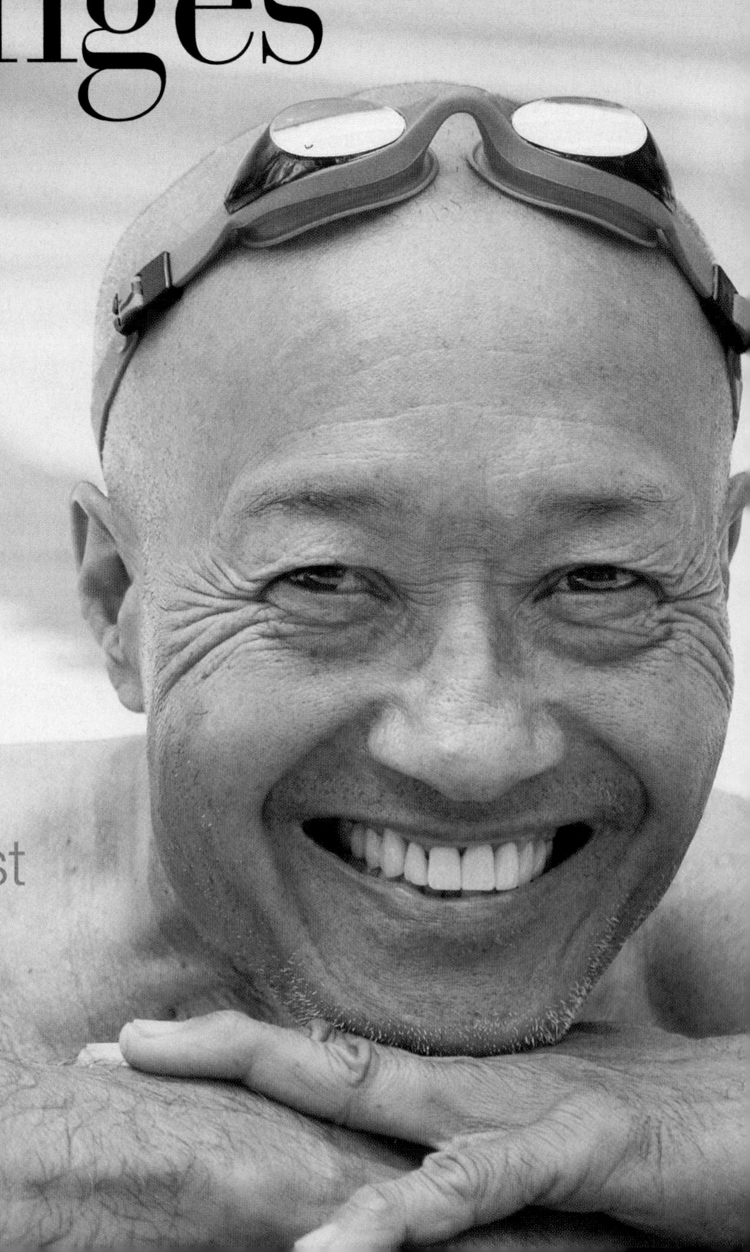

- More than 1 in 8 people in the United States is over age 65.[i]
- About 40% of noninstitutionalized older people in the United States rate their health as very good or excellent.[i]
- The 55-and-older crowd is the fastest growing age group on Facebook.[ii]

LEARNING OBJECTIVES

DISCUSS how life expectancy in the United States has increased in the past century.

DESCRIBE the physical and psychosocial changes that typically accompany aging.

IDENTIFY at least five key strategies for aging successfully.

COMPARE and contrast the available options when planning for the end of life.

EXPLAIN how people develop a concept of death.

DISCUSS care of the body after death.

IDENTIFY the stages of grief and the potential effects of grief on health.

EXPLAIN how to start aging well right now and how to support someone with a terminal diagnosis or someone who is grieving.

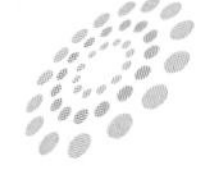

Health Online icons are found throughout the chapter, directing you to web links, videos, podcasts, and other useful online resources.

Aging brings many gifts:

a stronger sense of who you are and what you value; greater power to make your way in the world; and a broader range of experiences that, in turn, expands your appreciation for others and deepens your compassion. But aging also brings challenges. Your body starts to show the wear and tear of time. You experience the loss of loved ones. And you face the task of defining for yourself what is a good life, and a good death.

This chapter can help increase your awareness of the gifts of aging, and prepare you for its challenges. Whatever your age, the information here is relevant for you simply because aging and dying are part of the human experience.[1] What's more, the healthy choices you make today will help you to age with vitality. And finally, understanding end-of-life issues can help you cope with the death of loved ones, and clarify your thoughts and feelings about your own passing.

As with other aspects of health, aging is as social as it is personal. We'll start by looking at how America, as a whole, is growing older.

Aging in the United States

The United States is in the midst of a longevity revolution.[2] Between 2000 and 2010, the population of older Americans (aged 65 and above) increased more than 15%. Currently, more than one in eight Americans is over the age of 65. And people reaching the age of 65 have an average life expectancy of an additional 18.8 years. By the year 2050, according to federal government estimates, more than 88 million people in the United States will fall within this age category—about 20% of the population **(Figure 22.1).**[3] In another significant shift from the past, older Americans are becoming more racially and ethnically diverse. In 2000, about 83% of older adults in the United States were Caucasians. By 2050, that figure will fall to about 58%, with Hispanics, African Americans, and Asian Americans representing growing segments of the older population.[3]

Trends in Health and Health Care

As the number of older people in the United States grows, key aspects of aging—health and wellness—are changing:

- More older people are giving a positive report on their overall health. The number of people aged 65 to 74 rating their own health as only fair or poor has fallen from almost 28% in 1993 to just under 25% in 2010.[4] Older African Americans, Native Americans, and Hispanics are less likely to rate their own health as excellent or good than are Asian Americans or Caucasians.[2]
- At the same time, most older Americans have at least one chronic health condition. More than half—including both males and females—have hypertension, more than one-fourth have coronary heart disease, and nearly one-fifth have diabetes. Arthritis and lower respiratory diseases are also common, and many older adults have multiple chronic conditions.[5] But major contributors to poor health among older people are also preventable or reversible. Only 22% of older Americans report engaging in regular leisure-time physical activity and about 32% are obese.[5]
- Older Americans use more health care than any other age group; however, the costs vary dramatically by health status.[5] Older adults with no chronic conditions incur about one-fifth of the costs (an average of $5,186 annually) incurred by older adults with several chronic conditions (an average of $25,132 annually). It's clear, then, that improving the health of older people must be a priority if we're to curb our nation's increasing health-care spending.

The keys to avoiding chronic disease as you age—a balanced diet, regular exercise, and avoidance of tobacco and alcohol abuse—lie within the reach of most people. As we'll see next, these choices affect not only how well, but also how long you can expect to live.

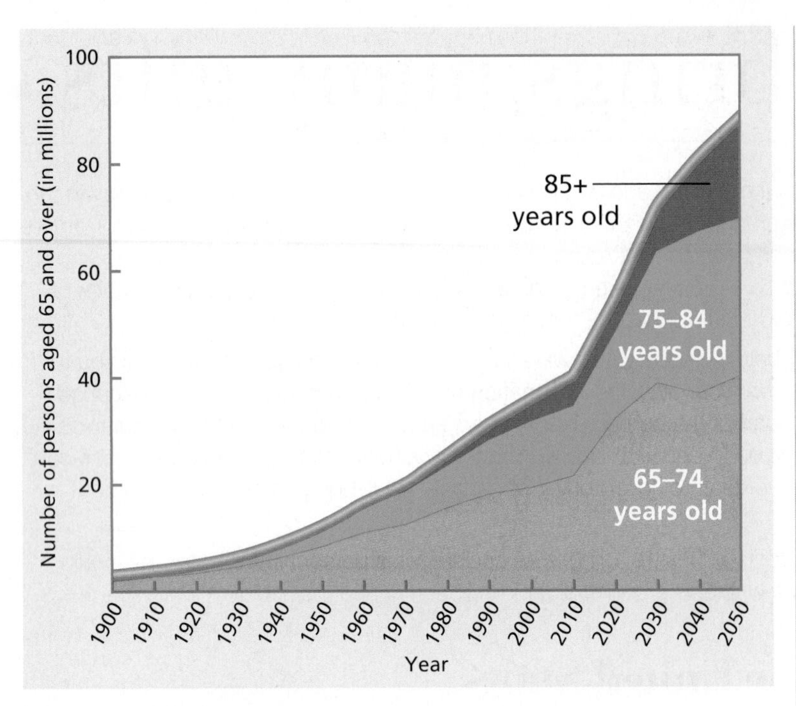

Figure 22.1 Number of older people in the U.S. population, 1900–2050.

Data from *Projected Future Growth of the Older Population – By Age: 1900–2050*. Administration on Aging, 2010, retrieved from http://www.aoa.gov/aoaroot/aging_statistics/future_growth/future_growth.aspx.

Life Expectancy

Life expectancy in the United States has climbed steadily over the last century along with improved nutrition, the growing availability of vaccines, advances in treatments such as surgery and medications, and public health campaigns, such as those that discourage smoking. Life expectancy for a person born in the United States in 2010 is now projected at 78.7 years.[6]

life expectancy The length of time a person can expect to live, usually measured in years.

Still, there is room for further improvement. Some of the leading causes of death, such as heart disease, stroke, and type 2 diabetes, can be prevented or moderated by maintaining a healthful weight, exercising, and not smoking. Some researchers are concerned that America's high rate of obesity, hypertension, and high blood glucose has already reduced U.S. life expectancy by at least 5 years, and could reduce it even further in coming decades.[7]

Troubling disparities in life expectancy also exist among racial groups and among populations with different levels of education. For example, a 2012 study found that Caucasian American men with at least a high school diploma had a life expectancy more than 14 years greater than that of African American men who did not complete high school. For women, the comparable gap was more than 10 years. The same study also reported that, although life expectancy among Americans overall rose modestly between 1990 and 2008, the least educated Caucasian men lost 3 years of life expectancy and the least educated women lost 5 years.[8]

Another research study has described the United States as a country of "eight Americas" in terms of longevity, distinguishing between these eight groups using a variety of racial, ethnic, economic, and geographic factors. According to this analysis, Asian Americans can expect to live the longest—almost 85 years. On the other end of the spectrum, African Americans living in the rural South or high-risk urban areas can expect to live about 71 years.[9] For an overview of the study's findings, see **Table 22.1.**

You might think that the United States is a world leader in life expectancy, but that's far from true. In the Central Intelligence Agency's ranking of the 221 countries of the world, the United States comes in at number 50, with the top 32 countries experiencing a life expectancy of 80 years or more. In

Table 22.1: **Longevity Gap in "8 Americas"**

America Number	General Description	Definition	Average Life Expectancy (years)
1	Asian American	Asians living in counties where Pacific Islanders make up less than 40% of the total Asian population	84.9
2	North Central, low-income, rural Caucasians	Caucasians living in Northern Plains and Dakotas with 1990 county-level per capita income below $11,775 and population density less than 100 persons per square kilometer	79.0
3	Caucasian Middle America	All other Caucasians not included in Americas 2 and 4, Asians not included in America 1, and Native Americans not included in America 5	77.9
4	Low-income Caucasians in Appalachia and the Mississippi Valley	Caucasians in Appalachia and the Mississippi Valley with 1990 county-level per capita income below $11,775	75.0
5	Western Native American	Native American populations in the mountain and plains areas, predominantly on reservations	72.7
6	African American Middle America	All other African American populations not included in counties in Americas 7 and 8	72.9
7	Southern, low-income, rural African Americans	African Americans living in counties in the Mississippi Valley and the Deep South with population density below 100 persons per square kilometer, 1990 county-level per capita income below $7,500, and total population size above 1,000 persons	71.2
8	High-risk urban African American	Urban populations of more than 150,000 African Americans living in counties with cumulative probability of homicide death between 15 and 74 years old greater than 1%	71.1

Source: Adapted from "Eight Americas: Investigating Mortality Disparities Across Races, Counties, and Race-Counties in the United States," by C. J. L. Murray, S. C. Kulkarni, C. Michaud, N. Tomijima, M. T. Bulzacchelli, T. J. Iandiorio, & M. Ezzati, 2006, *PloS Medicine, 3*, Table 1, retrieved from http://www.plosmedicine.org/article/slideshow.action?uri=info:doi/10.1371/journal.pmed.0030260&imageURI=info:doi/10.1371/journal.pmed.0030260.t001.

Monaco, the world leader, the average life expectancy is almost 90 years.[10]

> While nothing can predict how long you'll live, you can calculate your life expectancy based on your health, habits, and lifestyle at **www.longevitycentres.com/tools-agecalculator.html**.

Gender and Longevity

Men, in general, cannot expect to live as long as women. Life expectancy for U.S. males now stands at about 76.2 years, almost 5 years less than women, who have a life expectancy of about 81.1 years.[6] This gender-based longevity gap is not unique to the United States. Throughout the developed world, women tend to live several years longer than men.[11]

Although the factors at work in the gender longevity gap are complex and still under study, research has identified a few, including:

- **Delayed cardiovascular risks.** Women tend to develop cardiovascular conditions such as heart disease or stroke in their 70s and 80s, about 20 years later than men.
- **Sex chromosomes.** Human beings have one pair of sex chromosomes, which determine—along with many other traits—whether you are male or female. Women have two X chromosomes. Men have one X chromosome and one Y. The X chromosome is larger than the Y chromosome and holds many more genes, some of which perform important functions. Because they have two X chromosomes, women basically have a backup set of these genes, allowing their genomes to choose the best of the pair.
- **Fewer risk-taking behaviors.** Men are much more likely than women to die from unintentional injuries such as car crashes, or intentional injuries caused by violence (as described in Chapter 20).
- **Lower rate of smoking.** Although the difference in the rate of smoking among males and females is narrowing, especially among young smokers, men are still more likely than women to smoke at any given age.
- **More effective health management techniques.** Women are more likely to visit their health care provider regularly. They are also less likely to internalize stress, loneliness, or anger than men. These emotions can have powerful health effects, especially over time.[12]

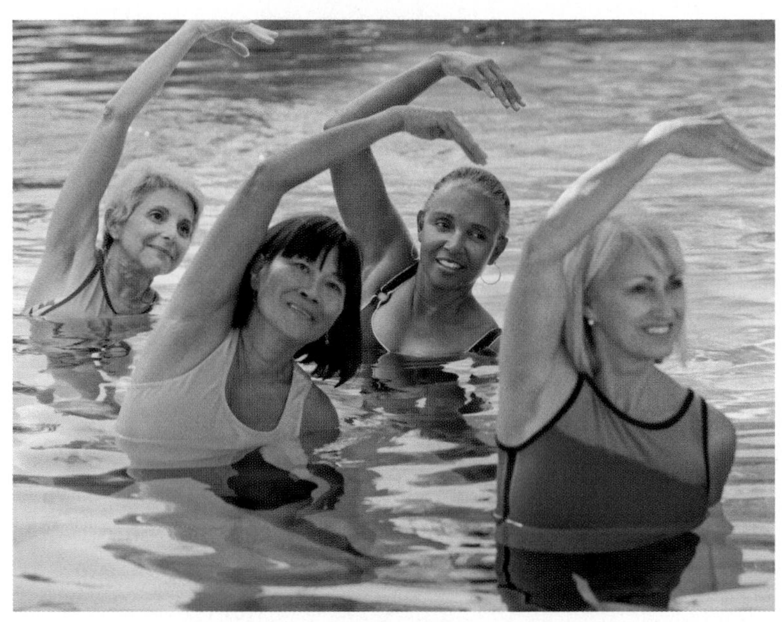

Women in the United States have a life expectancy almost 5 years longer than men's.

What Happens As You Age?

When they hear the term *aging*, most people think of biological aging—the physical changes that begin at birth and continue until death. But aging is also psychosocial, encompassing changes in cognition, memory, and mood as well as changes in relationships, career, and income. Not all of these changes happen to everyone, and if they do, the age at which they first occur varies widely. Moreover, they're interrelated: Physical limitations can affect mood and social life, and a reduction in work and income can influence physical and mental health.

Physical Changes

Have you ever heard the saying that, from the moment we're born, we begin to die? That's not physiologically true, since throughout childhood and adolescence, our cells are multiplying and our tissues and organs are growing. But at a certain point, cells reach their limit of replication. Telomeres, regions of DNA at the ends of our chromosomes, begin to shorten, until eventually the DNA can't be copied again and the cell dies. As more and more cells die, our tissues degrade. We age. Eventually, of course, the damage leads to an irreversible decline in our functioning, and we die. As you read the following discussion of the physical changes characteristic of aging **(Figure 22.2)**, bear in mind that you can delay and even reduce some of them. We'll explore how later in this chapter.

Changes in Body Composition

With aging, decreased production of certain hormones leads to a gradual decline in muscle tissue and a corresponding increase in body fat. At the same time, body fat shifts from subcutaneous stores, just below

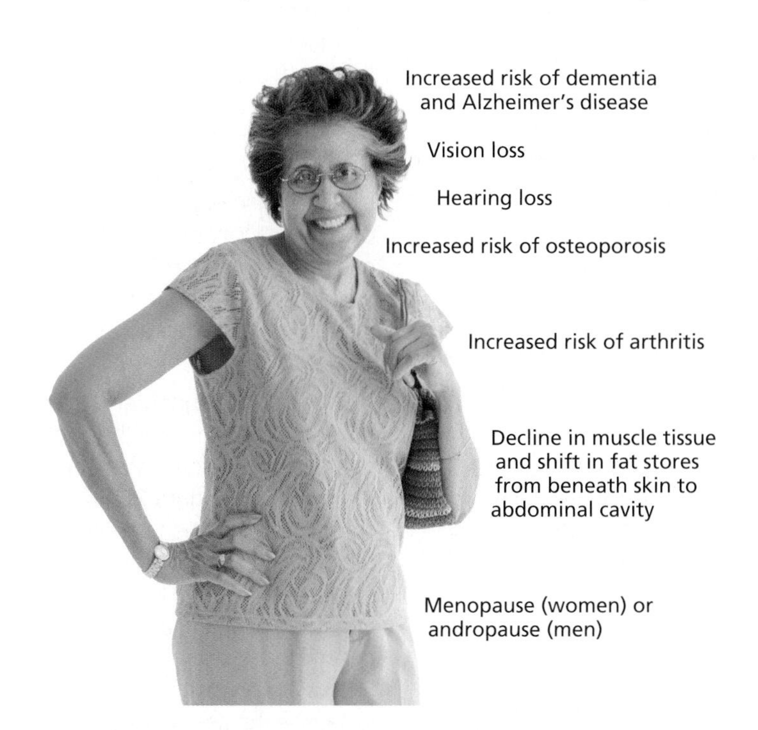

Figure 22.2 **Physical changes due to aging.**

the skin, to deeper stores, such as around the liver and other organs. The bones of the face, for example, appear more prominent, and the skin slackens. This shift coincides with an increased cardiometabolic risk. However, a diet low in nutrients and an inactive lifestyle greatly contribute to this loss of lean tissue and gain in fat; therefore, a nourishing diet and regular physical activity, including strength training, can help older adults maintain their muscle mass and strength.

Hearing Loss

Losing the ability to hear clearly is a common sign of aging, but that doesn't make the change any easier to accept. The reasons for age-related hearing loss, called **presbycusis,** vary from person to person, but the condition usually arises from damage to microscopic hair cells in the inner ear. Loss of the ability to hear conversation can cause the person to feel confused and frustrated and to withdraw from social contact. This in turn can lead to isolation.

Any hearing loss should be tested and treated. A variety of devices, such as hearing aids or phone amplifiers, may help. In severe cases, surgery may restore some hearing. When you are still young, do all you can to protect your hearing. For a refresher on basic hearing safety, see Chapter 20.

Vision Loss

Vision usually declines with age. By their mid-40s, many people have developed **presbyopia,** a gradual decline in the ability to focus on objects up close, especially in low light. This vision disorder can be addressed by wearing reading glasses when looking at objects at close range.

By age 80, more than half of all Americans develop **cataracts,** a clouding of the lens of the eye that dims vision **(Figure 22.3a).**[13] This condition can be treated successfully through surgery.

Glaucoma develops when fluid builds up in one or both eyes, increasing internal pressure and damaging the optic nerve **(Figure 22.3b).** Over 2 million Americans are thought to have glaucoma, but only about half of these cases have been diagnosed. Although the precise cause is not known, diabetes increases the risk. If untreated, glaucoma can result in a loss of peripheral vision or even total blindness. In fact, glaucoma is the second leading cause of blindness (after diabetic retinopathy). The condition can be detected through an eye exam, and is treated through medication, laser therapy, or surgery.[14]

Age-related macular degeneration (AMD) impairs the center of a person's vision rather than the periphery **(Figure 22.3c).** The disorder arises when the *macula,* a region of tissue at the center of the retina, deteriorates. It is somewhat common, affecting about 1.5% of Americans. Although no one knows the precise cause, smoking increases the risk. The condition can be detected through an eye

presbycusis Age-related hearing loss, which usually develops gradually, often due to damage to or changes in the inner ear.

presbyopia Age-related decline in the ability to focus on objects up close, especially in low light.

cataracts An age-related vision disorder marked by clouding of the lens of the eye.

glaucoma An age-related vision disorder arising from an increase in internal eye pressure that damages the optic nerve and reduces peripheral vision.

age-related macular degeneration (AMD) An age-related vision disorder caused by deterioration of the macula that reduces central vision.

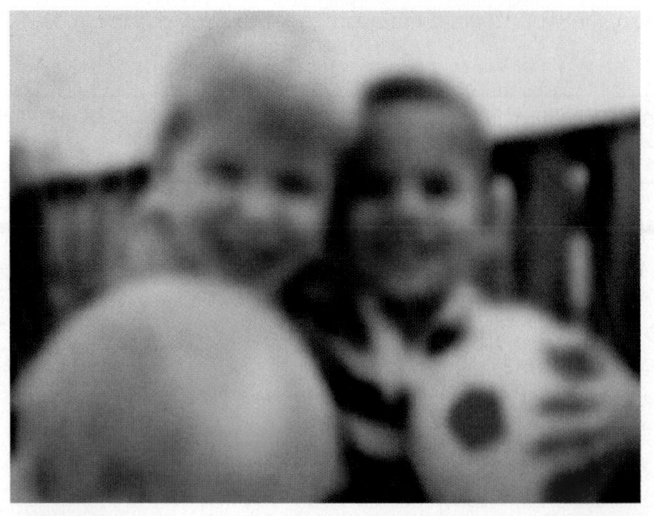

(a) Cataract

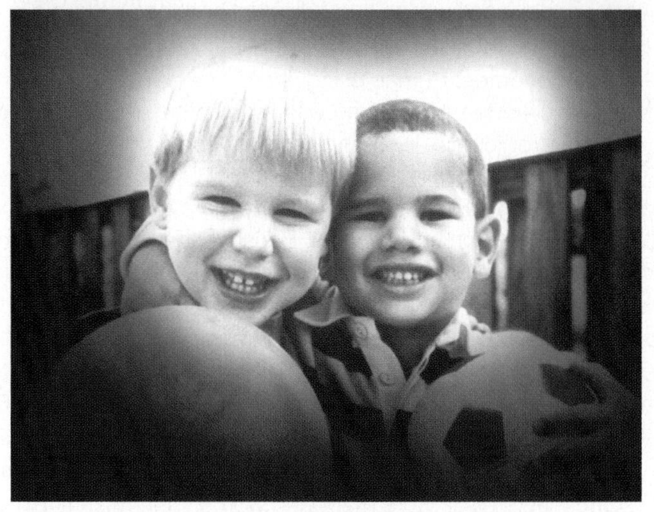

(b) Glaucoma

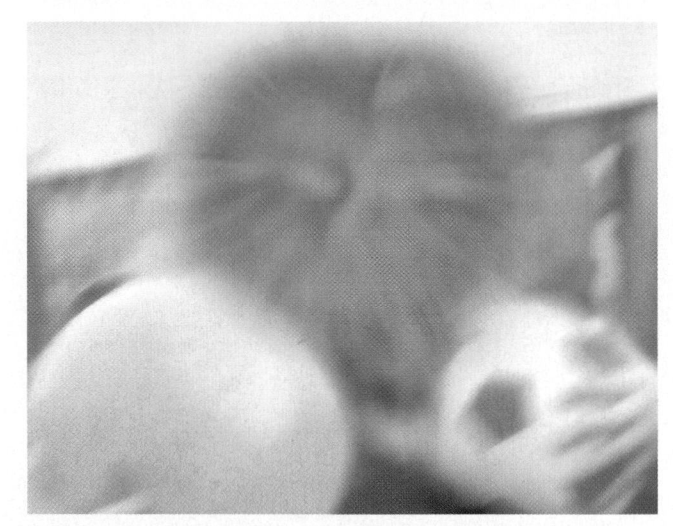

(c) Age-related macular degeneration

Figure 22.3 **Vision problems common to aging.**

exam, but is difficult to treat. Surgery or light therapy may help some patients. A study from the National Eye Institute indicates that taking a specific formulation of antioxidant vitamins and minerals may be able to slow the progression of the disease.[15]

Chronic Diseases

Aging increases your risk of many chronic diseases. Rates of cardiovascular disease, type 2 diabetes, and some cancers all rise significantly after age 65. For a review of these major chronic diseases and how to address them, see Chapters 11 and 12. Next we discuss two chronic bone disorders especially associated with aging: arthritis and osteoporosis.

arthritis Inflammation of one or more joints in the body, resulting in pain, swelling, and limited movement.

osteoporosis A disease characterized by low bone mass and deterioration of bone tissue, leading to fragile bones and an increased risk of fractures.

Arthritis. More than 50 million adults in the United States—about 22%—have some form of **arthritis.**[16] The disorder is characterized by repeated flare-ups of pain and stiffness affecting one or more joints, resulting in loss of motion. The condition usually arises from a breakdown of *cartilage,* protective tissue that lines the joints.

Although there are more than 100 forms of arthritis, affecting people of all ages, the most common form is *osteoarthritis,* a type that often arises with age. In people with osteoarthritis, cartilage wears away in the hands and weight-bearing joints of the body, such as the knees, hips, and ankles. Osteoarthritis often arises from a mix of genetic factors and damaging force, such as injury, repetitive motion, or excessive body weight.

There is no cure for osteoarthritis. But rest, physical therapy, and medication can all prevent further joint damage, reduce pain and swelling, and help restore daily activities. Low-impact exercises, such as swimming, walking, and gentler forms of yoga are all good options for staying physically active when diagnosed with osteoarthritis.

Osteoporosis. As you can see in **Figure 22.4, osteoporosis** is a disease characterized by excessively porous bones that are fragile and brittle, and therefore fracture easily. Osteoporosis arises when bone density decreases with age, and it is one of the leading disabling conditions among older people in the United States. According to the National Institutes of Health, about 40 million people already have osteoporosis or are at high risk because of low bone mass.[17]

Although 20% of people with osteoporosis are men, osteoporosis is more common in women for several reasons. Females reach their peak bone density earlier than males, and as adults have an absolute bone density lower than that of males. Women weigh less, on average, than men of the same height, and sociocultural expectations prompt many women to strive to maintain an unhealthfully thin body weight. This means that women's bones experience less of the weight-bearing stress that prompts bone building. Also, the female reproductive hormone estrogen helps maintain bone mass, and after menopause, the resulting drop in estrogen accelerates bone loss. Finally, women live an average of 5 years longer than

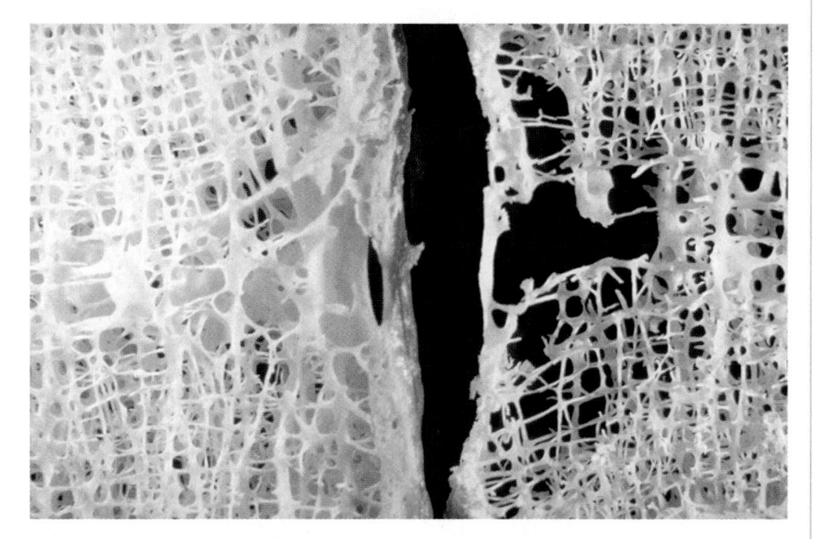

Figure 22.4 Effects of osteoporosis on the vertebrae of the spine. The vertebrae of a person with osteoporosis (right), and the vertebrae of a healthy person (left).

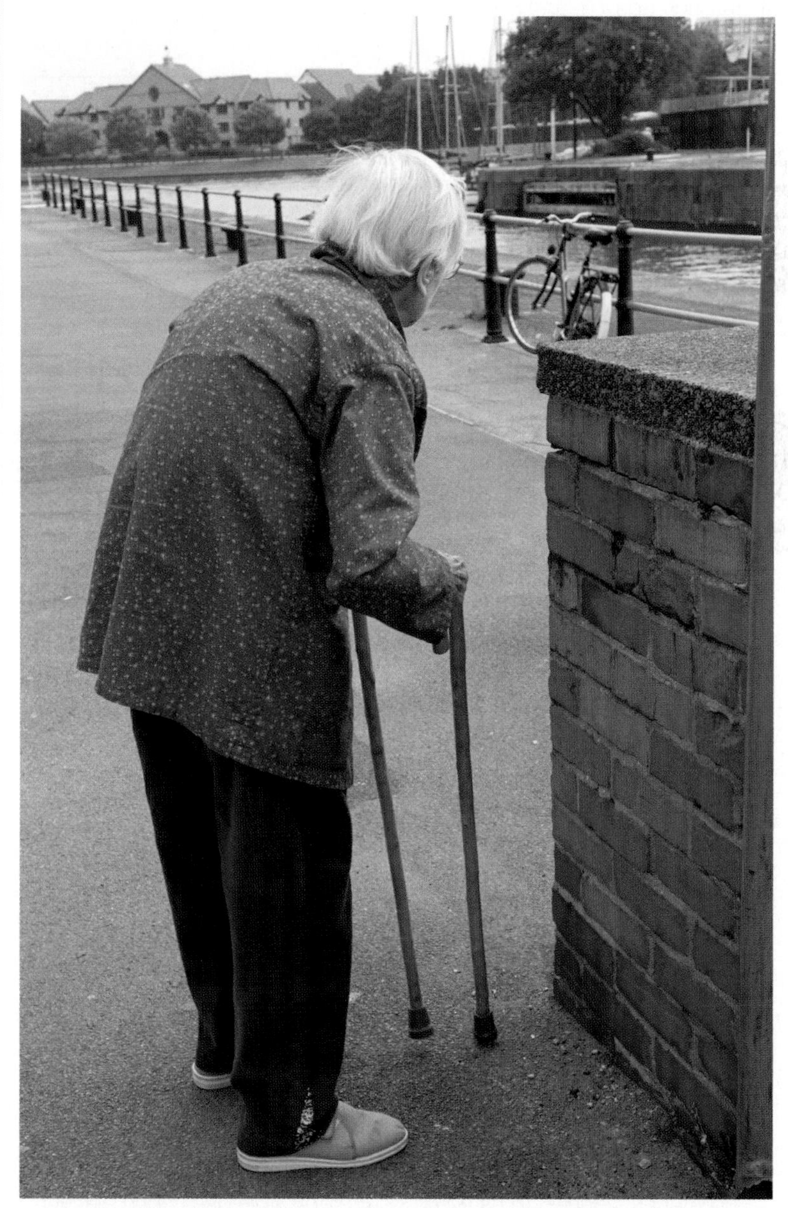

A hunched spine is a characteristic effect of osteoporosis.

men, and since bone loss increases with age, osteoporosis is more likely to show up in women.

Approximately 2 million fractures each year are due to osteoporosis. The bones of the wrist, spine, and hip are most at risk.[18] Hip fractures are especially debilitating—about 24% of people aged 50 and over who suffer a hip fracture die within a year of the injury.[19]

Some risk factors for osteoporosis, such as sex, age, and family history, can't be changed. Also, women with small bones and women of European and Asian descent are at higher risk. But other risk factors are within your control. Smoking, excessive alcohol consumption, a sedentary lifestyle, underweight, and a diet low in calcium and vitamin D all increase the risk of developing osteoporosis. Both males and females aged 14 to 18 years need 1,300 milligrams of calcium each day. Beginning at age 19, adults should consume 1,000 milligrams of calcium each day, and after age 50, that number goes up to 1,200 milligrams a day. The current vitamin D recommendation is 600 IU through age 70, and 800 IU thereafter.[20]

The Office of Dietary Supplements provides information on good food sources for calcium: http://ods.od.nih.gov/factsheets/Calcium-HealthProfessional.

Menopause

Menopause, or the permanent cessation of a woman's menstrual cycle and fertile years, is a normal, natural process, not an illness. But the hormonal changes that trigger menopause may cause temporary physical discomfort, as well as increase a woman's risk for cardiovascular disease and osteoporosis. For these reasons, some women turn to health remedies to address the effects of menopause.

menopause The permanent end of a woman's menstrual cycle and reproductive capacity.

andropause Period marked by a decline in the male reproductive hormone testosterone and its resultant physical and emotional effects; also referred to as *male menopause*.

Technically, menopause begins one year after a woman's last menstrual period. In the United States, that usually occurs in a woman's early 50s, but menopause-related changes often begin several years earlier. In *perimenopause,* women may notice changes in their periods, find they are more likely to build up stores of abdominal fat, have trouble sleeping, or start experiencing some of the classic symptoms of menopause, such as mood swings, vaginal dryness, bursts of perspiration known as hot flashes, and night sweats. These symptoms usually arise from the natural decline of reproductive hormones. Once a woman is 12 months past her last period, her ovaries produce much less estrogen and no progesterone, and no longer release eggs. The years that follow menopause are referred to as *postmenopause*.

After decades of the monthly hassles that having a period brings, some women welcome menopause. This is especially true if a woman experiences relatively few menopausal symptoms and side effects. For others, the process brings more mixed feelings. Some women may mourn the loss of their fertility, feel less feminine, or equate menopause with old age. Some may experience extremely uncomfortable or even debilitating physical or psychological symptoms. In these cases, treatments may include:

- **Psychotherapy to help combat fears surrounding menopause.** For instance, the end of menstruation doesn't mean that a woman is facing death: The average woman lives about 30 years after menopause.
- **Hormone therapy (HT).** Administration of synthetic reproductive hormones, referred to as *hormone therapy*, increases bone density and is an effective treatment for hot flashes and other menopausal symptoms. Combination HT, a mix of estrogen and progestin (synthetic progesterone), was once routinely prescribed, but a large study about 10 years ago linked long-term combination HT to an elevated risk of breast cancer in some women.[21] Estrogen-only HT, however, increases the risk for endometrial cancer, and both combination and estrogen-only HT confer an increased risk for blood clots, strokes, and dementia. Women considering HT should discuss the risks and benefits with their physician.[22]
- **Vaginal estrogen.** This topical medication relieves vaginal dryness and discomfort.
- **Bone-building medications.** These nonhormonal drugs, such as Fosamax or Boniva, are prescribed to prevent or decrease postmenopausal bone loss and reduce the risk of osteoporosis in older women. However, they are associated with some potentially serious side effects such as heartburn, chest pain, and difficulty swallowing, and in 2011, the U.S. Food and Drug Administration announced that it was reviewing the drugs for a potential increased risk for esophageal cancer.[23]
- **Antidepressants.** Some antidepressants may help with hot flashes or the mood swings surrounding menopause. In more severe cases, women may find that a combination of HT and antidepressants provides the greatest benefit.

Many women also have success with self-care measures, including:

- **Avoiding hot flash triggers.** Some women find that certain factors, such as spicy food, hot beverages, or sleeping quarters that are too warm, worsen the number and intensity of hot flashes.
- **Quitting cigarettes.** Smoking increases hot flashes and brings on earlier menopause.
- **Exercising regularly.** Exercise not only reduces the risk of postmenopausal health concerns such as osteoporosis and heart disease, but helps control weight and promotes healthful sleep.

Specific physical activity recommendations for older adults are discussed shortly.

Some women also turn to alternative remedies to try to address menopausal symptoms or promote their health after menopause. For a closer look at these alternatives, see the **Consumer Corner.**

Andropause

Levels of the male reproductive hormone testosterone begin to decline gradually around age 30. By about age 70, testosterone levels can have dropped by as much as half of what they were in young adulthood. This decline, and the physical and emotional changes that accompany it, are generally referred to as **andropause,** or *male menopause*. Men who experience andropause may report any of the following:[24]

- Changes in sexual functioning, including reduced desire, erectile dysfunction, and infertility
- Physical changes, including increased level of body fat and decreased muscle mass and strength, reduced bone density, and loss of body hair
- Disturbed sleep, including insomnia or hypersomnia
- Emotional disturbances, such as depression and difficulty concentrating

Some studies have also found a higher incidence of cardiovascular disease among men with low levels of testosterone; however, this link has not been definitively established.[25]

Of course, any of these signs and symptoms could be due to factors other than declining testosterone levels. Moreover, researchers are not unanimous in considering age-related testosterone decline a medical condition requiring treatment.[26] For these reasons, it's important that men experiencing signs and symptoms of andropause have a comprehensive clinical evaluation. Some physicians prescribe a course of testosterone supplementation, which has been shown to improve muscle mass and strength. However, whether supplementation can halt the progression of cardiovascular disease is unknown, and some studies suggest that, for men who already have hypertension, high blood cholesterol, or high blood sugar, testosterone supplementation can actually increase the risk for heart attack and stroke.[27] One thing we do know is that a program of medically supervised regular physical activity, including strength training, can preserve muscle mass and bone density, reduce levels of body fat and other risk factors for cardiovascular disease, promote healthful sleep, and relieve depression.

Sexuality

An active sex life is usually associated with the young, but older people are far from out of the game. As people age, sexual desire and activity may ebb and flow, but sexuality remains an important aspect of life. A substantial number of older people who are healthy and have a receptive partner remain sexually active. Moreover, an active sex life, as a reflection of social and emotional connections to others, may help increase longevity. Sexual desire, valuing sexuality, and high sexual self-esteem are important to a woman's sexual activity; for men, high sexual self-esteem, good health, and active sexual history make the most difference for sexual activity later in life.[28]

Changes Affecting Cognition and Memory

Issues once thought to be a routine part of aging, such as forgetfulness and confusion, are no longer considered inevitable. Instead, like the rest of the body, the brain appears to age quite well. Though brain mass

> *"Normal age-related changes include more difficulty in multitasking, remembering names . . . and learning new information quickly. Many of these skills can be boosted through 'brain fitness' activities."*

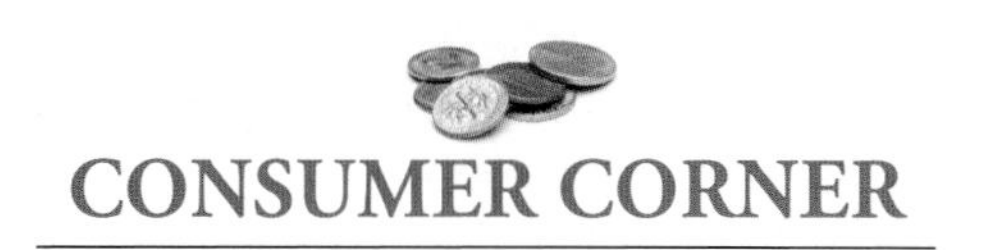

CONSUMER CORNER

Alternative Medications for Menopause?

Since a 2002 study linked pharmaceutical hormone therapy (HT) to an increased risk of breast cancer and other health problems, interest has surged in alternative therapies to treat menopause symptoms. Some women have switched to a form of treatment called bioidentical hormones, which are chemically identical to ovarian hormones, but are derived from plants. Others have tried herbs such as black cohosh or dong quai.

So far, evidence of any benefit is mixed at best. One large scientific analysis found that many alternatives to HT hadn't been studied at all, a few offered mixed results, and some showed no benefit.[1] In addition, many questions of safety remain unanswered. For example, bioidentical hormones are said to be superior to pharmaceutical HT because the prescription is precisely mixed to meet each woman's hormone needs, based on a test of her saliva. Unfortunately, the hormone levels in saliva don't correspond to those in the bloodstream, nor does a measurement of hormone levels correspond in any way to the menopause symptoms a woman experiences.[2] Moreover, the pharmacies used to produce these preparations are not subject to the same rigorous safety standards as conventional pharmaceutical manufacturers. In addition, neither black cohosh nor dong quai has been shown to be more effective than a placebo in reducing menopause symptoms, and in rare instances the use of black cohosh has been associated with liver failure.[3]

If you are considering an alternative treatment for menopause symptoms, research the therapy carefully, and talk to your doctor.

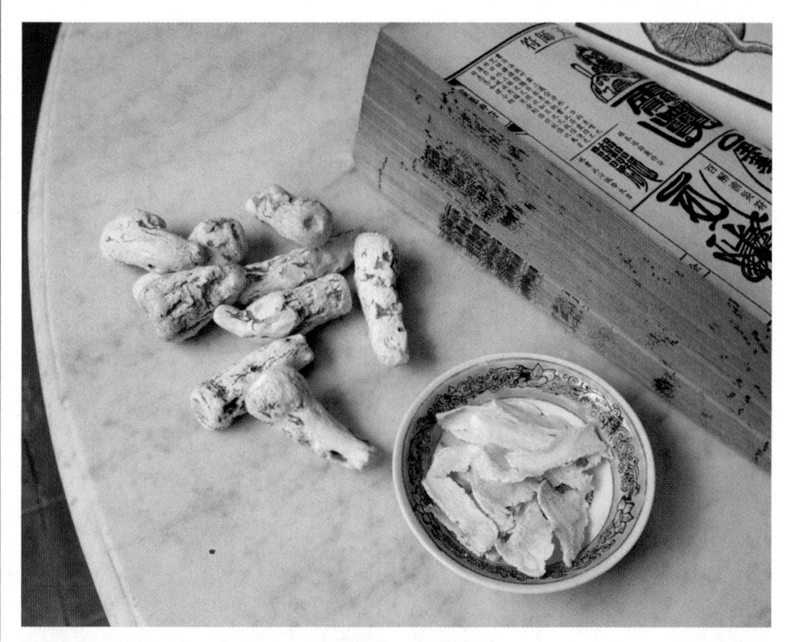

Dong quai, a common alternative to hormone therapy.

References: **1.** "Complementary and Alternative Therapies for the Management of Menopause-Related Symptoms: A Systematic Evidence Review," by A. Nedrow, J. Miller, M. Walker, P. Nygren, L. Huffman, & H. Nelson, 2007, *Archives of Internal Medicine, 166*, pp. 1453–1465. **2.** "Bioidentical Hormones: Are They Safer?" by Mary Gallenberg, 2009, retrieved from http://www.mayoclinic.com/health/bioidentical-hormones/AN01133. **3.** *Menopausal Symptoms and CAM* (NCCAM Publication No. D406), by the National Center for Complementary and Alternative Medicine, 2008, retrieved from http://nccam.nih.gov/health/menopause/menopausesymptoms.htm.

does decrease slightly, especially in areas related to complex memory and problem-solving, this change does not have to be debilitating.[29] In fact, many people become wiser with age, as their decades of accumulated experiences help them solve new problems.

dementia A decline in brain function.

Alzheimer's disease (AD) A progressive, fatal form of age-related dementia.

Normal age-related changes include more difficulty in multitasking, remembering names of people and places, and learning new information quickly. Many of these skills, however, can be boosted through "brain fitness" activities, which are discussed later in this chapter. It's also important to recognize that poor physical health overall appears to be a greater predictor of cognitive impairment in older adults than is age.[30]

Some older adults, however, do experience true degenerative neurological disorders. These include various forms of dementia, the most severe form of which is Alzheimer's disease.

Dementia. A broad term for a decline in brain functioning, **dementia** may arise at any point in life, but is much more common in people over the age of 80. It appears to arise from a variety of causes, only some of which are well understood. Genetics may play a role. People who suffer multiple brain-damaging strokes may also develop a form of dementia, and exposure to toxins, hormone imbalances, liver cirrhosis, malnutrition, and other factors may play a role.

Although there is no guaranteed path to preventing dementia, healthful behaviors may make a difference. Researchers are currently investigating the role of body weight, diet, exercise, and participation in socially and intellectually stimulating activities in preventing all forms of age-related dementia, including the most common form—Alzheimer's disease.[31]

Alzheimer's Disease. Few age-related illnesses are more feared than this progressive, fatal brain disorder. In **Alzheimer's disease (AD),** nerve cells in the brain stop functioning and disconnect from one another **(Figure 22.5).** Thus, their ability to transmit messages is lost. Affected nerve cells are found to be filled with abnormal collections of twisted protein threads called *tangles,* and deposits of apparently toxic protein fragments called *amyloid-beta plaques,* but it is still unclear whether these tangles and plaques cause the condition or are merely a sign.[32] Eventually, the affected nerve cells die. As the disorder progresses, entire regions of brain tissue atrophy (shrink), and brain mass is lost.

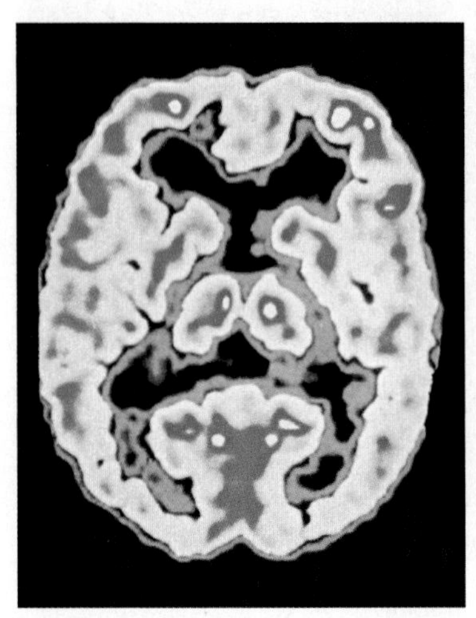

(a) Healthy brain

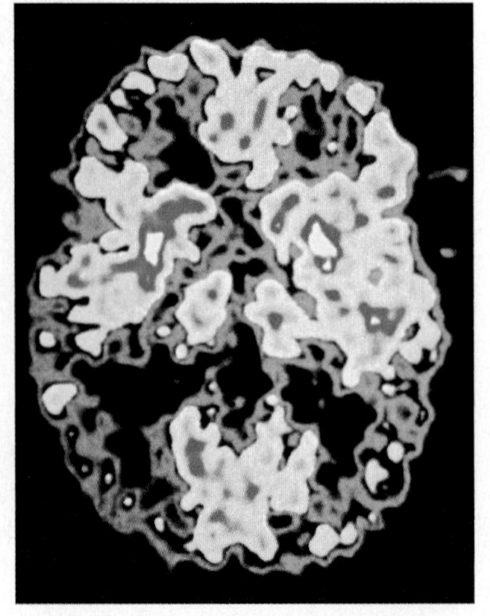

(b) Brain with Alzheimer's disease

Figure 22.5 **Brain activity and Alzheimer's disease.** Reds and yellows indicate high activity in tissues; blues and greens represent lower activity in tissues.

The damage is typically slow but progressive, and may begin as many as 10 to 20 years before any problems become evident. Eventually, however, the disease steals memory and concentration, and the ability to perform most daily tasks is lost. In normal age-related memory loss, the person typically forgets only certain details of an event. In contrast, in AD, all memory of an event vanishes. Recent memory is severely affected: For example, a person may watch a favorite television program, and a few minutes after it ends ask when the program is going to begin. Gradually, AD also affects mood and personality, leaving the person depressed, highly anxious, irritable, combative, and even paranoid and subject to delusions.

To view a video showing what happens to the brain in AD, go to www.nia.nih.gov/alzheimers/alzheimers-disease-video.

One in eight older Americans—more than 5 million adults—has Alzheimer's disease. This number is expected to escalate in the coming decades as more people live longer.[33] Alzheimer's is now the sixth leading cause of death in the United States. Leading risk factors include:[33]

- **Age.** Most cases of Alzheimer's disease occur in people older than 60, and risk jumps dramatically after the age of 80. This version of the condition, known as *late-onset Alzheimer's,* is the most common. A rarer form of the disease, known as *early-onset Alzheimer's,* has a strong genetic component and often begins in a person's 30s or 40s.
- **Genetics and family history.** If Alzheimer's runs in your family, you are at increased risk for developing the disease yourself. With the help of affected families, researchers are zeroing in on genetic factors linked to Alzheimer's risk. One such factor is related to a gene called *apolipoprotein E,* or *ApoE,* which codes for the assembly of a protein that helps the body regulate cholesterol. People with a particular variant of this gene have a substantially increased risk of Alzheimer's disease. Other genetic factors are now also the focus of intense scientific scrutiny.
- **Poor cardiovascular health.** A growing body of research indicates that factors that harm the cardiovascular system, such as a high-fat diet, high cholesterol, and a sedentary lifestyle, also increase Alzheimer's risk. Interestingly, the ApoE gene linked to Alzheimer's affects how the body processes cholesterol, another indication that vascular health and the body's ability to move blood through the brain plays a role in the disease. African Americans have an increased risk for Alzheimer's disease, and this is thought to be due to their increased rates of cardiovascular disease.
- **Head injury.** Any head injury severe enough to cause a loss of consciousness for 30 minutes or more increases the risk for developing Alzheimer's disease.

There are currently no treatments that alter the underlying course of Alzheimer's disease, although several prescription medications may ease some of the cognitive symptoms, such as memory loss, for a period of time. There are also no proven prevention strategies. However, maintaining a healthful body weight, keeping physically, socially, and intellectually active, and eating a healthful diet might reduce your risk. A diet rich in fruits, vegetables, whole grains, and healthy plant oils may be particularly beneficial, especially when combined with regular physical activity.[34]

The Alzheimer's Association provides information for people affected by Alzheimer's disease and their families and caregivers: www.alz.org.

Psychosocial Changes

As a college student, you are probably experiencing some powerful psychosocial changes. You may recently have moved from another town or state, leaving behind family members and friends. And you're probably already actively planning for your post-college career or graduate school—which may entail another move. If you think about the challenges that such shifts represent for you, you can begin to imagine how challenging similar changes can be in the lives of older adults.

Family Changes

After spending 18 years raising their children, day in and day out, older adults may welcome their newfound freedom as their kids head off to college or join a spouse in a distant state. Yet it's common for parents of adult children to struggle with feelings of loss and to question their worth. This so-called "empty nest syndrome" challenges older adults to rethink not only their day-to-day responsibilities, but also how they define their identities.

The empty nest syndrome also challenges couples. Older people who've raised children together will suddenly find themselves spending more time alone than they have in years, and will probably need to get to know each other again as individuals. Some couples, once their children have left home, find that the bonds that connected them as individuals have frayed, and they may separate. Others find that their connection is stronger than ever, and enjoy the extra time they have together.

At the same time that they are adjusting to their own aging, many older adults begin taking on significant caregiving tasks for very elderly parents. They may purchase a larger home that can accommodate a parent who can no longer live independently, or they may move into the parent's home. Even when living arrangements stay the same, older adults may find themselves spending many hours each week "parenting" their elderly parents, taking them to medical appointments, shopping for them, and making a variety of arrangements for their care. This change in family dynamics can be highly stressful, but it can also give older adults and their elderly parents precious opportunities to share memories and feelings, resolve conflicts, and affirm their love and caring.

Changes in Residence

Eighty percent of older Americans are homeowners, and 20% are renters; however, the size and type of dwelling that older adults own or rent often changes.[2] Empty nesters may discover that the four-bedroom house in which they raised their family now feels too large, or they may find the maintenance too burdensome. It's not uncommon, then, for older adults to move to a smaller house, a condominium, a mobile home, or an apartment. Some move in with a son or daughter, and may help with cooking and caring for their grandchildren. Others move to residential communities for older adults, where social activities and physical environments are arranged to promote fun and well-being, or to an assisted-living facility where meals and transportation are provided and health care is available round the clock.

At the same time, many older adults are embracing a concept called *aging in place*, which the U.S. Centers for Disease Control defines as the ability to live in one's own home and community safely, independently, and comfortably regardless of age, income, or ability level.[35] The National Aging in Place Council is a group of professional service providers, from elder specialists to financial planners to home and landscape contractors, whose aim is to support older adults who wish to live independently in their homes. They may help modify a home for a senior with limited mobility, for example, or arrange for in-home care. Adult children of seniors can also support their parents' desire to age in place by bringing meals, helping with house and yard work or bill paying, and driving their parents to health-care appointments. Even children who live a great distance from elder parents can help by maintaining daily phone or email contact and scheduling regular visits.

Changes in Employment

Most older adults have been working for decades, deriving a strong sense of identity and self-worth from their careers. And many—about 22% of men and 14% of women—continue to work past age 65.[2] For Americans born in 1960 or later, the "full" retirement age is 67. This means that people who delay retirement to age 67 will receive 100% of the Social Security benefits to which they are entitled. Retiring before age 67 reduces benefits by a percentage calculated according to the age at which benefits begin. This reduction takes into account the longer period of time during which benefits will be received. Older adults can also delay retirement until age 70, which means that the benefits received thereafter will be greater.[36]

Although retirement is meant to bring freedom from work, some seniors may find themselves unsure of who they are if they aren't attached to a profession. Having diverse interests outside of work earlier in life can help. Many seniors find that using their professional skills to volunteer or work part-time provides an easier transition from the professional world to retirement.

Economic Changes

Retirement may bring more free time—but reduced work translates into reduced income. Older adults who have no employer pension or retirement savings and find themselves living on their Social Security income may discover that they must reduce their spending, sometimes drastically, even as certain costs, such as medical expenses, may be rising. Unfortunately, 43% of single older adults and 22% of couples rely on Social Security benefits for 90–100% of their total income. In 2010, the average monthly Social Security benefit was just over $1,300 for men and $1,000 for women.[37] If you had to survive solely on Social Security benefits, could you do it?

Want a rough estimate of your Social Security retirement benefits? Check out www.socialsecurity.gov/estimator.

Clearly, personal retirement savings are critical—but people in the United States are notoriously poor at funding their retirement accounts. In a survey of the most common type of employer-based retirement account, the 401(k), most workers were contributing less than half of the federally allowed limit each year.[38] A recent analysis of federal data found that the average American household headed by a person with a 401(k) plan had less than one-quarter of the amount in the fund that would be needed—along with their Social Security and any pension funds—to maintain their standard of living in retirement.[39] Many 401(k) accounts

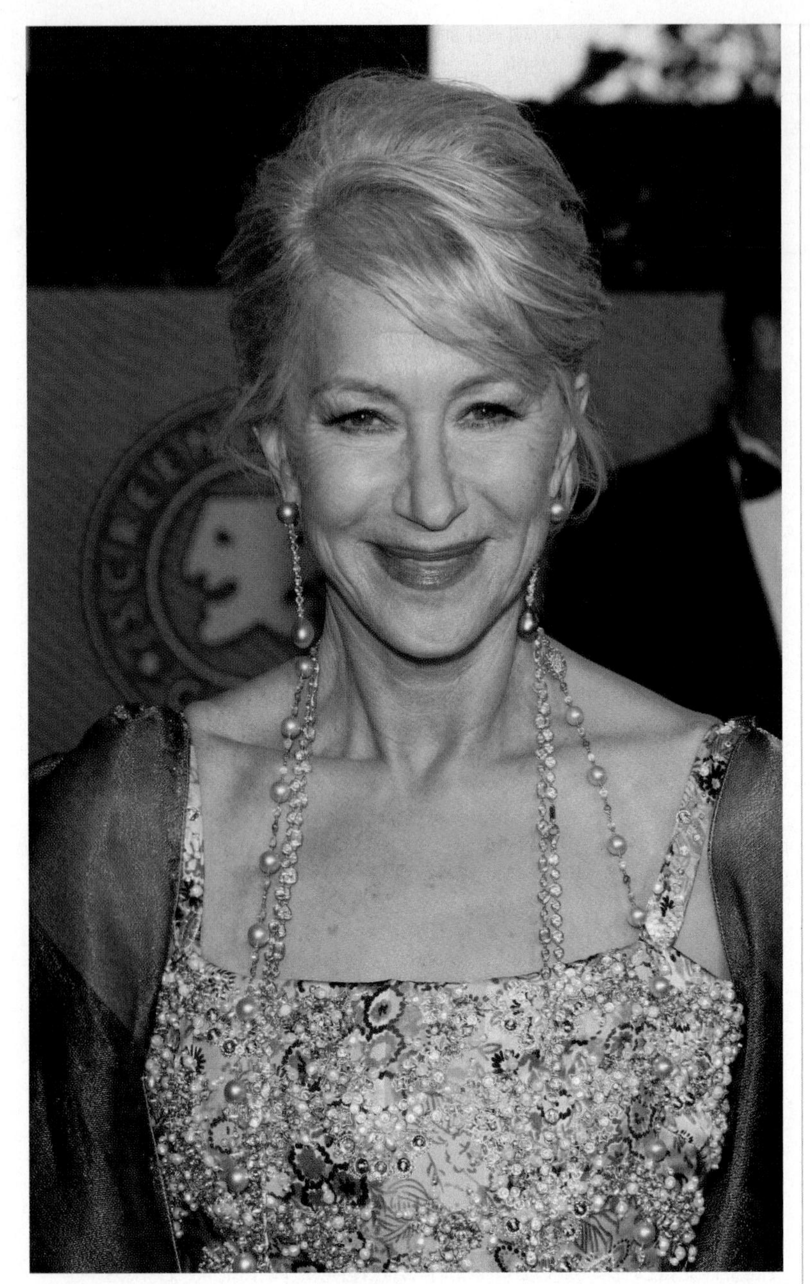

Helen Mirren, at age 68, is at a high point in her career.

are also invested in the stock market, which can fluctuate and, in some cases, substantially diminish the value of a person's retirement savings just as they are getting ready to leave the workforce.

As a result of these factors, the traditional view of retirement as a time of leisure has changed. Increased life expectancy means that people will need an income longer. As noted earlier, many U.S. workers are retiring later: In 2009, 14% of women and 24% of men age 70 to 74 were still working.[40] Many Americans try retirement for a while, then find themselves taking a part-time job or starting a small business to boost their income.

Mood Changes

Changing roles, such as leaving the workforce or having children move away, leave some men and women feeling unnecessary, even irrelevant. Vision and hearing losses, chronic pain, and functional limitations can further narrow an older adult's world. As friends and loved ones die, older adults may feel increasingly isolated in their grief.

As a result, rates of depression and suicide are relatively high among older adults. Whereas the suicide rate is about 11 per 100,000 in the general population, about 14 of every 100,000 people aged 65 and older die by suicide. Caucasian men aged 85 and older are most likely to take their own lives, with a rate of nearly 50 suicides per 100,000 persons in that age group.[41]

If an older relative or friend talks about feeling sad or hopeless, listen carefully and offer to help him or her find care. Many hospitals and senior centers offer support groups and mental health services designed for older adults. Above all, spend time with your loved one. Showing older adults that they are important to you can help them reject feelings of abandonment.

Substance Abuse and Polypharmacy

Despite the perception that substance abuse is an issue only for adolescents and young adults, it is a serious and growing health concern for older adults.[42] Research shows that illicit drug use among Americans aged 50 and older is increasing dramatically, leading researchers to estimate that the number of older adults with a substance use disorder will double by 2020. A 2011 federal study estimated that 5.8% of Americans aged 50 and older had used illicit drugs in the past year. The drugs most commonly abused are marijuana and prescription drugs, including prescription narcotics.[42]

Alcohol abuse is also a common problem among older adults. Approximately 40% of older Americans consume alcohol; however, precise statistics on alcohol abuse are difficult to gather.[43] We do know that older adults are more sensitive to alcohol's effects because they metabolize alcohol more slowly than younger people. As a result, alcohol stays in their bodies longer. Also, as we age, our body fluid level declines. Thus, older adults have a higher percentage of alcohol in their blood than younger people after drinking the same amount.[43] Alcohol consumption can also increase the symptoms of many diseases common to older adults, from hypertension and liver failure to memory problems and depression. Finally, alcohol and medications don't mix: Alcohol can reduce the actions of some medications, and increase the effects of others. Medication and alcohol interactions can even be fatal.

Another medication-related concern for older adults is **polypharmacy,** the use of a "cocktail" of several drugs that can interact in dangerous ways.[44] Older adults are especially vulnerable to polypharmacy because they often have several medical problems for which they see different doctors, each prescribing drugs, often without knowing what else the patient is taking. On average, individuals aged 65 to 69 take nearly 14 prescription medications a year. Polypharmacy is responsible for up to 28% of hospital admissions and is the fifth leading cause of death in the United States.[44]

polypharmacy Simultaneous use of several prescription medications that can interact in dangerous ways.

What Contributes to Successful Aging?

Although it might be difficult to imagine yourself as a senior citizen, you are aging! And the behaviors you establish right now can help you do it successfully. Wondering what that looks like? Experts agree that successful aging includes the following characteristics:

- An ability to maintain autonomy and independence
- The capability to function physically, cognitively, and socially
- A personal view of aging that is self-defined, individualistic, and reflects who you truly are
- An ability to continuously adapt to the changes that life brings
- A desire to live life fully and embrace all of its stages[45]

health preservation Performing activities that seek to maintain health, rather than simply responding to health crises as they occur.

Sounds good, right? So how do you get there? Genetic factors do appear to play some role in how long and how well a person lives. However, about 70% of life expectancy appears to be due to lifestyle, income, and other nongenetic influences.[46] Through consistent efforts at **health preservation,** you can help yourself grow older successfully. Let's start with a habit you've learned about throughout this book—exercise.

Physical Activity

As you age, you may not be able to run as fast as you could when you were 12, but that's no reason to stop moving. Regular physical activity is one of the most beneficial things you can do for your health, at any point in life. Consistent exercise greatly reduces your risk of dying from cardiovascular disease and of developing type 2 diabetes and several types of cancer. Physical activity also slows many of the physical aspects of aging, such as decreased bone density and muscle mass and increased body fat, helps relieve the pain of joint conditions such as arthritis, and eases mental health concerns such as anxiety and depression. Moreover, physical activity has been shown to boost *adult neurogenesis*—the generation of new neurons in certain regions of the brain.[47]

It's never too late to enjoy the benefits of exercise. For people who are 65 years of age or older, are generally fit, and have no limiting health conditions, public health experts recommend at least:

- Two hours and 30 minutes of moderate-intensity aerobic activity, such as brisk walking, each week AND muscle-strengthening activities that work all major muscle groups at least 2 days a week, OR
- One hour and 15 minutes of vigorous-intensity aerobic activity, such as jogging, every week AND muscle-strengthening activities that work all major muscle groups at least 2 days a week, OR
- An equivalent mix of moderate- and vigorous-intensity aerobic activity AND muscle-strengthening activities that work all major muscle groups at least 2 days a week[48]

For a refresher on physical activity, including aerobic exercise, muscle-strengthening fitness, and overall types and intensities of exercise, see Chapter 6.

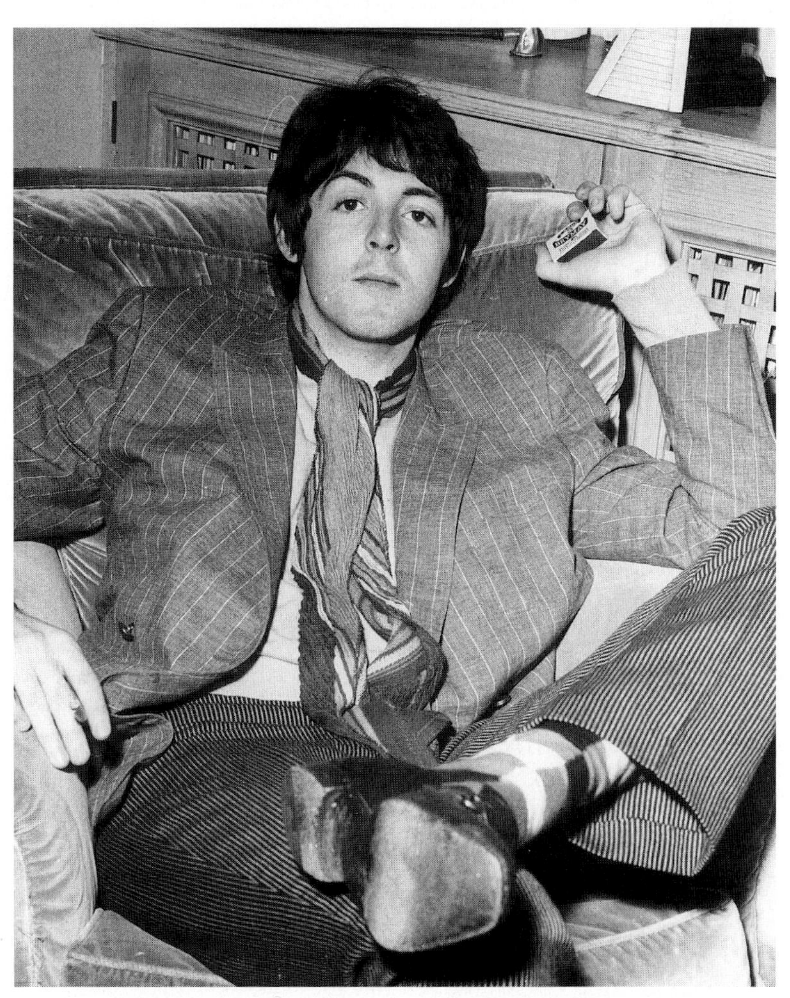

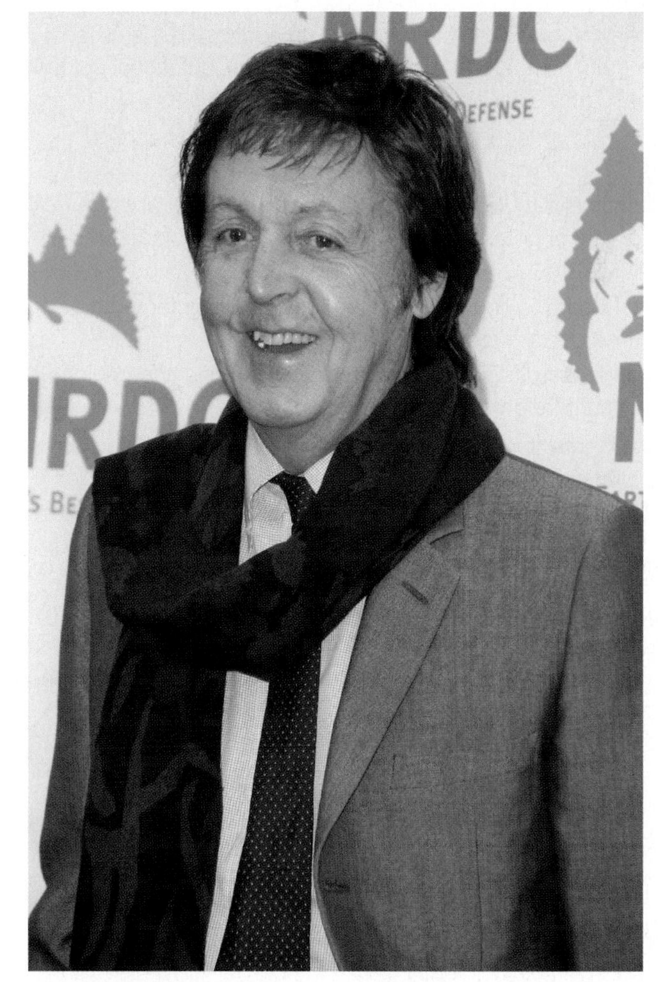

Aging happens to everyone. Beatle Paul McCartney in the 1960s and today.

SPOTLIGHT

Exercise: The Life Preserver

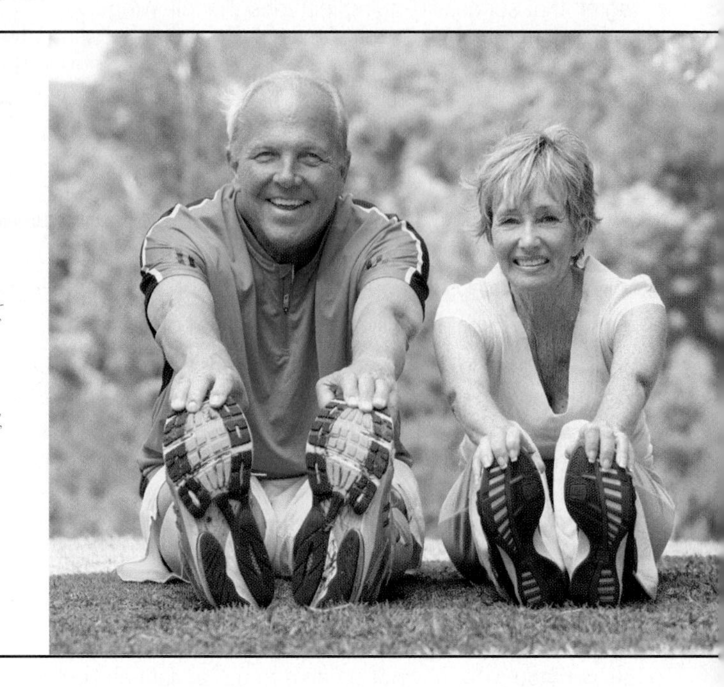

Want to live longer? Work out more.

Numerous studies show that fitness, especially higher levels of cardiorespiratory fitness, is among the best predictors of longevity. One set of research findings revealed that people with higher levels of cardiorespiratory fitness faced a lower risk of death even if they were overweight or carried a few extra pounds around their midsection.[1] Another study found that people between the ages of 70 and 88 were more likely to live longer if they either continued an existing exercise program or started a new one.[2]

Cardiorespiratory activities, such as brisk walking, biking, or running, matter most. But so do strength training and flexibility. At any age, we all need a regular mix of these types of activities. (For an overview of fitness and exercise options, see Chapter 6.)

References: **1.** "Cardiorespiratory Fitness and Adiposity as Mortality Predictors in Older Adults," by X. Sui, M. J. LaMonte, J. N. Laditka, J. W. Hardin, N. Chase, S. P. Hooker, & S. N. Blair, 2007, *Journal of the American Medical Association, 298*, pp. 2507–2516. **2.** "Physical Activity, Function, and Longevity Among the Very Old," by J. Stessman, R. Hammerman-Rozenberg, A. Cohen, E. Ein-Mor, & J. Jacobs, 2009, *Archives of Internal Medicine, 169*, pp. 1476–1483.

Good Nutrition

A healthful diet can extend your productive years and reduce your risk of chronic conditions such as cardiovascular disease, stroke, some types of cancer, diabetes, and osteoporosis. In addition to the essentials of good nutrition important for people of all ages, nutritional guidelines recommend that older adults:

- Get enough calcium and vitamins D and B_{12} from foods and/or supplements.
- Limit sodium intake to 1,500 milligrams per day and get at least 4,700 milligrams of potassium per day to help control blood pressure.
- Limit alcohol intake to no more than one drink per day for women and two drinks per day for men.
- Choose high-fiber fruits, vegetables, and whole grains and drink plenty of water to help prevent constipation.[49]

In 2011, the Center for Aging at Tufts University released a version of the United States Department of Agriculture's MyPlate modified for older adults (see **Figure 22.6**).

MyPlate for Older Adults

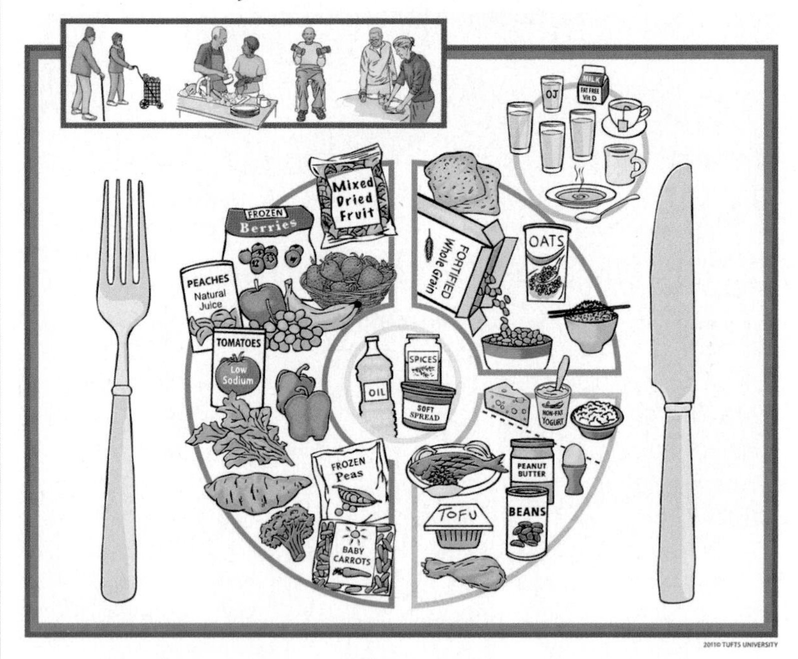

Figure 22.6 **MyPlate for Older Adults.** The icon illustrates the importance of fruits and vegetables, whole grains, and plant-based proteins such as tofu and beans. It also includes several examples of liquids, including soup, to encourage adequate hydration, and flavoring foods with spices instead of salt for reduced sodium intake. The plate is accompanied by icons depicting regular physical activity.

Source: MyPlate for Older Adults: Tufts University Nutrition Scientists Unveil MyPlate for Older Adults [News Release], November 1, 2011, Tufts University. © 2011, Tufts University. For details about the MyPlate for older adults, please see http://nutrition.tufts.edu/research/myplate-older-adults.

Weight Management

As we mentioned earlier in this chapter, almost a third of older adults are obese, and therefore at increased risk for cardiovascular disease, type 2 diabetes, many forms of cancer, sleep apnea, and arthritis. Obesity is also increasingly linked to a greater risk of Alzheimer's disease and other cognitive impairments as a person ages.

As you know, obesity develops as a consequence of an imbalance between energy intake (in food and beverages) and energy expenditure (in metabolism and physical activity). Stress is also a factor. The good news is, if you establish health habits that enable you to manage your weight now, you'll find it easier to maintain those habits—and your healthful weight—as you age. (For a review of how to maintain a healthful weight, see Chapter 7.)

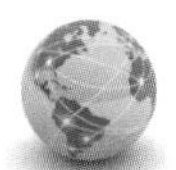

DIVERSITY & HEALTH

Old Age, Okinawa Style

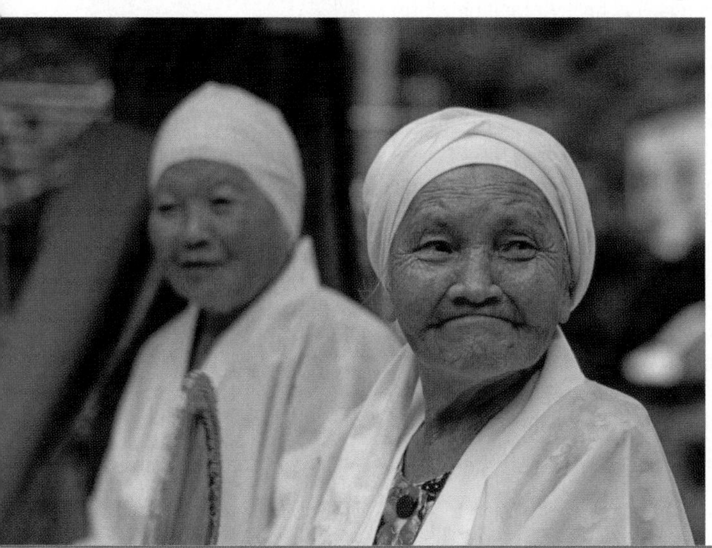

Okinawa, an island that is part of Japan, is at the center of current research on aging. More Okinawans live to see 100 than just about any other large population group in the world. And Okinawa's seniors age in remarkably good health, with clean arteries, low cholesterol levels, relatively few cases of cancer or serious osteoporosis, and low rates of dementia. Many remain active throughout their later years.

Part of the secret appears to lie in the traditional Okinawan diet, which centers around vegetables such as soybeans, leafy greens, and native gourds. This vegan diet provides protein and is high in protective nutrients such as folate and flavonoids. Older Okinawans also get a lot of physical activity each day. Genetics may also play some role.

As younger Okinawans are influenced by contemporary global lifestyles and adopt a less healthful, more Westernized diet and become more sedentary, researchers will see how life expectancy on the island changes.

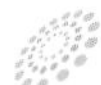

You can follow this ongoing research yourself, by visiting the Okinawa Centenarian Study at www.okicent.org/study.html.

Avoiding Dependence on Substances

When feeling sad, stressed, or unwell, resist the temptation to reach for a bottle, cigarette, or pill. Dependence on alcohol, tobacco, marijuana, and even nonessential medications and supplements can be harmful to you right now, and as you age. As we noted earlier, about 40% of older Americans drink alcohol. About 9% of older Americans smoke.[50] About 81% use at least one prescription medication, 42% take an over-the-counter medication, and 49% take at least one dietary supplement. Many older adults combine alcohol, tobacco, illicit drugs, medications, and supplements without informing their primary care provider, and without researching the potential effects of combining multiple substances.[51]

If you take multiple medications and supplements, with or without alcohol or tobacco, make an appointment to discuss this issue with your physician immediately. Bring to your appointment a complete list of all substances you use. Make sure to ask your doctor about their potential for harmful interactions. Also ask for advice and referrals to help you limit your dependence on these substances by making more healthful choices—a balanced diet, regular exercise, and techniques for managing stress.[52]

Of all substances, few shave more years off your life, and reduce the quality of the years you have, than tobacco. Someone who smokes one pack a day can expect to die about 10 years earlier than someone who has never smoked. Moreover, a person who smokes has a reduced quality of life: Smoking 20 or more cigarettes a day ages you by about 10 years, impairs the ability of your heart and lungs to function, and limits your ability to perform everyday tasks and enjoy your life.[53] Smoking has also been linked to premature balding, wrinkles, and osteoporosis. If you smoke, now is the time to quit.

brain fitness A person's ability to meet the cognitive requirements and demands of daily life, such as problem-solving and memory recall.

Mental Exercise

Just as exercise can maintain or restore your physical fitness, a daily "brain workout" can contribute to a state known as **brain fitness.** One study found that brain-engaging activities such as completing crossword puzzles, reading books, playing a musical instrument, or playing cards not only helped prevent cognitive decline overall, but slowed memory loss among those who had already developed dementia.[54] Religious or spiritual activities, such as scriptural studies, meditation, or participation in religious or spiritual services, may also have a positive effect on brain function.[55]

The key to beneficial activities lies in their interactivity. Any pastime that makes you think and requires that you connect with an object or another person—be it a musical instrument, an iPad, a grandchild, or a spiritual advisor—engages your brain and helps preserve thought and function. Staying connected through email, social networking sites, blogs, and Skype can also help. Conversely, activities that let you tune out and diminish your interactions with the world, such as watching television for extended periods of time on a regular basis, may have the opposite effect on brain fitness. So as you age, keep engaged!

Want to see how fast you can match squeaks, squawks, and croaking sounds to the animals that make them? Or decipher encrypted quotations? Have fun playing the American Association of Retired Persons' Brain Games at http://games.aarp.org.

Stress Management

You might think that, when you are older, you'll be retired, without any work obligations or a care in the world. You'll be able to spend your time however you'd like—what could be less stressful?

Playing a musical instrument is one way to keep your mind sharp as you age.

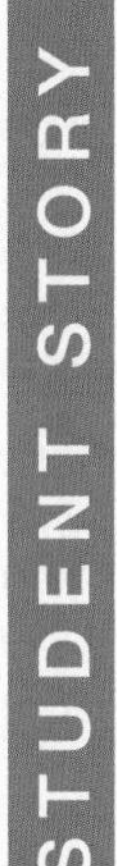

Handling Aging

"Hi, my name is Stephen. After having dropped out of college decades ago, I'm finally coming back to school and taking night classes to get my B.A. I'm 47, and a lot of my classmates are 20, 30 years younger than me. Compared to my first time in college, it's true that I'm not as athletic as I was, I have a few more aches and pains, and it's harder to keep weight off than when I was 20, but nowadays, I'm much more invested in my classes and I feel sharper than ever. Sometimes I feel like an old guy compared to my classmates, but then I think of my mom who's 73 and as active as ever. I guess we have good genes in our family that keep us young."

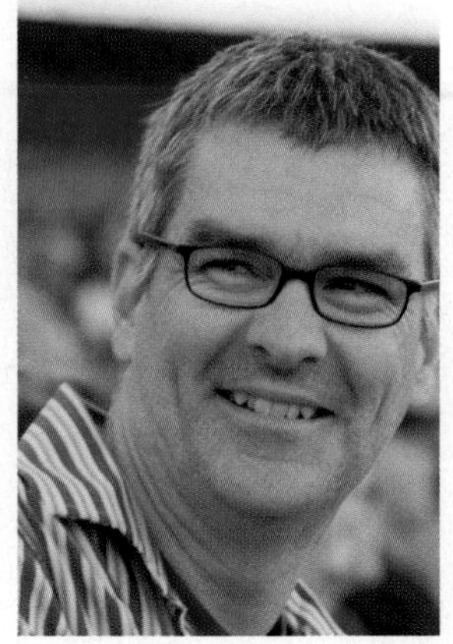

1: Stephen says he feels sharper than ever. Why do you think that is?

2: Why is it harder for Stephen to keep weight off now compared with when he was 20?

3: Do you think Stephen is right that "good genes" are keeping him young? What else will keep him healthy and aging well? Which do you think is most important, genes or lifestyle factors?

Do you have a story similar to Stephen's? Share your story at www.pearsonhighered.com/lynchelmore.

Tell that to an older adult, and watch them smile. While being older brings many benefits, it's hardly a stress-free time of life. Along with health concerns, there are also many practical changes to juggle. If you've worked all your life, the challenge of building a new identity after retirement can be stressful. Children may be grown and living on their own, but you're still concerned about them—and any grandchildren. And as noted earlier, the financial pressures of living on a reduced or fixed income can take a heavy toll.

So beginning today, challenge yourself to recognize signs of excessive stress in your life, and address them. Be sure to get enough sleep on a regular basis. Limit your consumption of alcohol, eat right, and exercise. Maintain a healthy network of personal relationships and friends who can serve as a sounding board and help you find your way through life's challenges. For a refresher on stress and stress management techniques, see Chapter 3.

Understanding Death and Dying

When was the last time you contemplated death? Or sat down with a friend or family member and talked about it? Not the death of a specific person, but the concept of death itself—your knowledge of the dying process, your beliefs about an afterlife, and even your fears? If you've rarely given death and dying much thought, you might find the following discussion helpful.

What Is Death?

Historically, a person was pronounced dead if he or she had stopped breathing and had no heartbeat. But because of advances in medical technologies that artificially sustain physiological functions, clinicians now recognize several different definitions of death.

- **Brain death** is the cessation of brain activity as indicated by various medical devices and diagnostic criteria.
- **Functional death** is the end of all vital physiological functions, including heartbeat, breathing, and blood flow.
- **Cellular death** is the end of all vital functions at the cellular level, such as cellular respiration and other metabolic processes.
- **Clinical death** is a medical determination that life has ceased,

brain death The cessation of brain activity as indicated by various medical devices and diagnostic criteria.

functional death The end of all vital physiological functions, including heartbeat, breathing, and blood flow.

cellular death The end of all vital functions at the cellular level, such as cellular respiration and other metabolic processes.

clinical death A medical determination that life has ceased according to medical criteria that often combine aspects of functional and neurological factors.

Grieving

STUDENT STORY

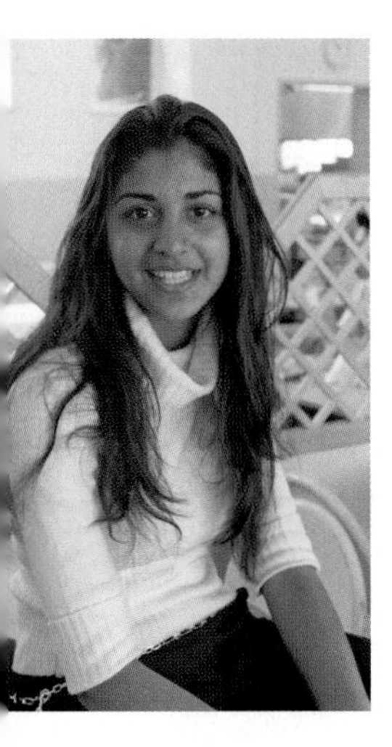

"Hi, I'm Michelle. When I was in high school, my uncle was killed in a car accident. It was a big shock to my family because he was still young and we weren't expecting it. I felt like a big part of what I had to do after it happened was support my mom and aunt, both of whom were really upset. Everyone felt so sad because we never had a chance to say good-bye. After the funeral, though, we all told stories and shared how he touched our lives. That made me feel a little better, and to this day I still try to talk about him and remember his spirit."

1: What types of things might Michelle have done to support her mom and aunt as they grieved for her uncle?

2: Why do you think telling stories about her uncle made Michelle feel better? What other types of things do people do to remember someone who's passed away?

3: What stage of grief do you think Michelle is in now?

Do you have a story similar to Michelle's? Share your story at www.pearsonhighered.com/lynchelmore.

- Anger, directed at everything from the death itself to the events surrounding the person's passing
- Depression, a persistent sadness that pervades daily life as the reality of the person's passing sets in
- Acceptance, blending together the joys of the person's life and the changes following his or her loss into a new perspective that reflects the totality of the experience[80]

Each person works through these stages in his or her own way, and some experiences of grief can be more complex than others. If a loved one has lived a long life and died after an illness, it may be easier to find peace with the death. If a person dies at a young age, commits suicide, or is a victim of a fatal injury or other unexpected, traumatic event, grief may be much more complex, intense, and long-lasting. Loved ones experiencing such *complicated grief* may benefit from the assistance of a grief counselor, therapist, or support group attended by others who have had a similar loss.

Grief in Children

Children who are grieving may cry, get angry, become depressed, have trouble sleeping, or regress in their behavior. These responses may be intermittent. Children may spend hours at play or in school and appear to be unconcerned about the loss. Experts on children's grief have identified three "burning issues" for grieving children:[81]

- Did I cause this loss?
- Is it going to happen to me?
- Who is going to take care of me?

Thus, children typically need reassurance that they are not to blame for the loved one's death, that they are not vulnerable to the same injury or illness, and that they will be cared for. Many children who lose a parent are especially concerned about the third of these issues, and may continue to talk to the absent parent to maintain the bond of caring and defend against the loss.

It is not uncommon for a child's grief to continue for longer than it might in an adult.[81] Children may need to work through their grief in each of their developmental stages; for example, graduating from high school may prompt a renewed sense of the loss—and a renewed anguish—in a teen whose mother died many years earlier.

Effects of Grief on Health

Death of a child, spouse, or other close family member is widely acknowledged as one of the top stressors that a human being can experience. People grieving a death, but especially those experiencing complicated grief, may suffer such severe stress that it becomes a risk to their own health. For example, one study found that loss of a spouse resulted in an immediate 12% reduction in life expectancy.[82] The

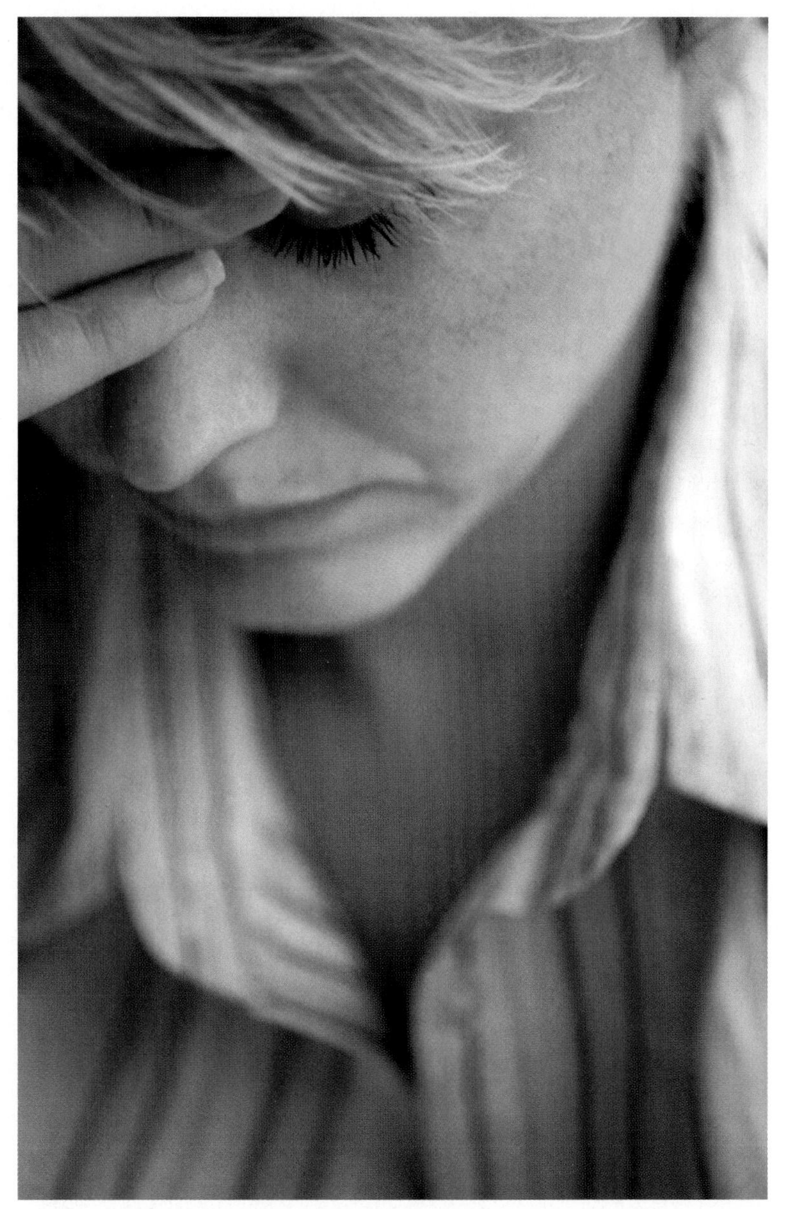

Grief can have a devastating effect on physical health.

effects of grief on health may include any of the following symptoms or conditions:

- External symptoms, such as digestive upset, changes in eating habits, headaches, fatigue, weakness, vague pain, and disturbed sleep
- Cardiac symptoms, such as higher blood pressure or irregular heartbeat
- Psychosocial symptoms, such as increased drinking, depression, suicidal thoughts, feelings of guilt, isolation from others, and significant spiritual conflict

Change Yourself, Change Your World

This chapter has of necessity included discussion of many unwelcome changes beyond your control. So let's look at things you *can* do to age with grace, to support loved ones as they face the end of life, and to cope with grief.

Personal Choices

If you find yourself feeling discouraged when thinking about the inevitable challenges of aging, bear in mind that aging is not a disease, but a normal, potentially vibrant and enriching stage of life. Two key approaches are to maintain six behaviors that slow aging, and to start living each moment fully now.

Make Six Smart Choices

A landmark study of aging from Harvard University followed more than 800 people for over five decades to determine the factors that best predict successful aging.[83] The results were surprising: Genetic and biological factors, such as the longevity of our parents or our cholesterol level, were not as important as six key lifestyle choices. Three of these are physical, and we mentioned them earlier in this chapter:

- Avoid tobacco, especially cigarettes.
- Maintain a healthful weight.
- Get regular exercise.

The other three are a little less obvious:

- Develop successful coping skills (the ability to make the best of a bad situation).
- Maintain strong social relationships.
- Pursue education throughout every life stage.

If these behaviors already characterize your life, congratulations! But if you're struggling with one or two, such as managing your weight, or coping with stress, don't despair. Review the chapters in this book that discuss your particular challenge. If the practical strategies provided don't seem to be working, seek help from health-care professionals promptly, without waiting for the problem or behavior to reach a crisis stage.

Start Living Fully Right Now

The American author and humorist Mark Twain wrote, "A man who lives fully is prepared to die at any time." Are you living fully? What does that mean? Earlier, we identified steps you can take to maintain your physical and intellectual health as you age. But there's more to life than mere preservation. Through the ages, spiritual teachers have advised that, to live fully, we focus our awareness, moment by moment, on the here and now. If you're eating an orange, you savor the orange: the color, the fragrance, the sweet taste. If you're talking with a friend, you attend to your friend's words, tone, face, and gestures. Such awareness can be demanding, as it requires that we cease our internal "chatter"—our stories, judgments, defenses, and desires. But even in challenging times, like the first few hours after a breakup, or while you're visiting a loved one who's seriously ill, *choiceless awareness*—a state of being in which you are present without self-reference—can awaken profound gratitude, even wonder, for the experience of life.

Let meditation expert Jon Kabat-Zinn guide you through an exercise in choiceless awareness. Visit www.oprah.com/spirit/Jon-Kabat-Zinns-Meditation-Mindfulness-as-Pure-Awareness.

Supporting a Loved One Who Is Dying

People's response to a terminal diagnosis is as unique as they are; still, certain reactions are more common than others. In her groundbreaking book *On Death and Dying*, psychiatrist Elisabeth Kübler-Ross, who worked with terminally ill patients in a Chicago hospital, proposed that individuals facing imminent death cycle back and forth through five overlapping and sometimes simultaneous states. You may notice that these are similar to the stages we identified for someone grieving the loss of a loved one, and indeed, Kübler-Ross's work has influenced grief research. The states are:[84]

- *Denial*, in which patients refuse to accept the validity of the diagnosis
- *Anger*, which may be directed at the diagnosis, the physician, family members, themselves, or God
- *Bargaining*, in which patients try to avoid or delay death in exchange for repentance or service to others
- *Depression*, which can be brief or prolonged, and may be marked by withdrawal from loved ones
- *Acceptance*, a stage in which patients stop rejecting or fighting the diagnosis, may be introspective but not withdrawn, and may seek out time with loved ones, especially those they have not seen recently and those with whom they have struggled, in order to make peace before death

When Kübler-Ross's work was published in 1969, it was the first comprehensive study of the psychology of the dying. In the decades since, many other researchers have refined and expanded our understanding of the experience. Some have emphasized the importance of understanding the unique way that the person has integrated the illness into his or her "life theme."[85] Others suggest identifying and trying to support the dying person's unique coping strategies, whether focused on appraisal or analysis of the situation, information-seeking and problem-solving, or emotional release.[86] In short, there is no "standard" way to experience dying, and no prescribed method of supporting the dying person.

If someone you love is diagnosed with a terminal illness, you may have several weeks or months to be with the person as he or she prepares for the end of life. You may welcome this opportunity to comfort and help, yet not know exactly how. In many cases, if you ask, the dying person will share with you quite candidly what he or she would find most helpful.

Many terminally ill people seek a "good death," or an exit handled on their own terms as much as possible. While everyone's definition of a good death may be a little different, researchers have identified six factors of high importance to the dying, their loved ones, and caregivers:

- **Pain and symptom management.** Most people are understandably anxious about spending the end of life in pain.

Chapter Summary

- The United States is heading toward a "longevity revolution," with life expectancy increasing and a growing percentage of the population falling into older age brackets.
- Not everyone, however, has the same life expectancy. Women tend to live at least 5 years longer than men, and life expectancy also correlates closely with a person's racial or ethnic background, income, and region of residence. Negative behaviors such as smoking, alcohol abuse, and failing to participate in regular physical activity also reduce life expectancy.
- Aging brings many physical changes, such as declines in vision and hearing. Hormonal changes cause women to experience menopause, and some men to experience andropause. Chronic diseases, including arthritis and osteoporosis, become more common.
- Some older adults experience impairments in cognition and memory. The more mild form of this condition is referred to as age-related dementia. The more severe, progressive, and fatal form is Alzheimer's disease.
- Aging also brings psychosocial changes. These might include shifts in family dynamics, a change of residence, retirement, reduced finances, and an increased risk of depression and substance abuse as the aging person is challenged to adapt to the changing circumstances.
- Through lifelong habits that promote health preservation, you can avoid or limit some of the challenges of aging, especially when it comes to reducing your risk of chronic conditions such as cardiovascular disease, type 2 diabetes, and osteoporosis.
- Key steps in healthy aging include engaging in regular physical activity, consuming a nutritious diet, maintaining a healthful weight, avoiding smoking, limiting use of alcohol and unnecessary medications and supplements, challenging your mind, and reducing stress. Put these healthy habits in place when you are young.
- Death is often defined by the cessation of heartbeat, breathing, and other vital functions, but may also be defined by other factors, such as the end of discernable brain-wave activity.
- Our concept of death evolves as we mature from childhood to adulthood, and is influenced by our life experiences as well as our beliefs and values. Increased publicity of near-death experiences has also influenced our society's understanding of death and dying.
- Numerous planning aids can help a person think through end-of-life issues ahead of time, state preferences, and make plans. These include advance directives for health, wills, and registration opportunities for organ/tissue donation.
- Options for end-of-life care include home care, hospital-based care, and hospice care in a hospice facility or in the person's home. In any setting, palliative care is a key aspect of care for the dying. The goal of palliative care is to decrease pain and suffering rather than to prolong the person's life.
- The ethics of rational suicide (including physician aid in dying), passive euthanasia, and end-of-life health-care spending are the subject of ongoing debate.
- After a death, a person's body may be subject to autopsy, a medical examination that may or may not lead to identification of the cause of death.
- By law, a body must be buried or cremated. In either case, family members may also choose to remember their loved one by holding a wake, funeral, and/or memorial service.
- Grieving is a natural part of and reaction to death, and those experiencing grief, especially complicated grief, need the support of friends and loved ones through the long process of coming to terms with their loss. Children experience grief differently from adults, but no matter their age, people experiencing grief often suffer physical and psychological effects.
- Key approaches for navigating the challenges of aging include maintaining six healthful behaviors, such as getting regular exercise and pursuing lifelong education, and living each moment fully now.
- Although people who are dying experience their situation in unique ways, some common responses have been identified, including stages of denial, anger, bargaining, depression, and acceptance. You can support the person by helping them think through questions such as where they want to die, and whether or not they'd like spiritual counseling, as well as affirming them as the complex, well-rounded people they have always been.
- You can support someone who is grieving in practical ways, as well as by simply being present.

Test Your Knowledge

1. Approximately what fraction of older U.S. adults are obese?
   a. about a tenth
   b. about a fourth
   c. about a third
   d. about half

2. What is the life expectancy for someone born in 2010 in the United States?
   a. about 68 years
   b. about 78 years
   c. about 88 years
   d. about 98 years

3. Which of the following accurately characterizes arthritis?
   a. Arthritis happens to everyone when they get older.
   b. Arthritis damages your ligaments.
   c. Arthritis is caused by loss of bone density.
   d. Arthritis typically affects the hands and weight-bearing joints.

4. What does Alzheimer's disease affect?
   a. how the brain functions
   b. how the body functions
   c. length of life
   d. all of the above

5. Physician aid in dying is a form of
   a. rational suicide.
   b. active euthanasia.
   c. passive euthanasia.
   d. autopsy.

6. What can people who smoke one pack of cigarettes a day expect?
   a. to experience reduced quality of life as they age
   b. to appear older than others who are the same age but have never smoked
   c. to die younger than those who have never smoked
   d. all of the above

7. What is the Five Wishes an example of?
   a. a health-care proxy
   b. a DNR order
   c. an advance directive
   d. a will

8. What percentage of American adults under age 35 have a will?
   a. less than 10%
   b. about 20%
   c. about 30%
   d. about 40%

9. What is the goal of palliative care?
   a. to prolong life
   b. to prevent further deterioration in the patient's condition
   c. to cure disease
   d. to relieve pain and suffering

10. If someone is grieving, what is the best way to help him or her?
   a. talk about something else
   b. be present and offer support, both in the moment and over the long term
   c. reassure him or her that you know how he or she feels
   d. talk about others who have died, to show that this particular death was a normal thing

Get Critical

What happened:

In 2012, the American Society of Clinical Oncology (ASCO), the nation's leading association of cancer physicians, advised doctors to stop offering three common diagnostic scans (PET, CT, and radionucleotide bone scans) and two drug therapies to patients with certain types of cancer. They noted that the tests and treatments had not been shown to improve quality of life or extend survival in the patient populations they identified, although physicians have been routinely prescribing them for such patients for many years. The scans cost as much as $5,000 each, and a round of chemotherapy treatments can cost $20,000 to $30,000 or more.

Some physicians and patients praised the announcement, noting that, because physicians profit from each intervention they prescribe, the ASCO was putting patient well-being above their own financial interests. Others disagreed, pointing out that, even if research suggests that 99% of patients do not benefit from a particular intervention (as was the case with the scans), that still means that 1% might.

What do you think?

- If you had been treated successfully for cancer 3 years ago, and subsequent annual scans had not revealed any further evidence of cancer, would you be pleased or outraged if your doctor said you didn't need any further scans?
- Let's say you currently have lung cancer. Two previous rounds of chemotherapy have not been beneficial, but you've just learned about an experimental form of chemotherapy being tried for your type of cancer. How would you feel if your oncologist told you that your previous poor responses disqualified you for any further chemo treatments? Should physicians be authorized to make such decisions independently? Or should they simply disclose all treatment information and allow patients to decide for themselves?
- In the above scenario, if your insurance carrier refused to pay for the chemotherapy treatments, and they were estimated to cost $40,000, would you pay for them yourself, even if they might only prolong your survival for a few months—or not at all?

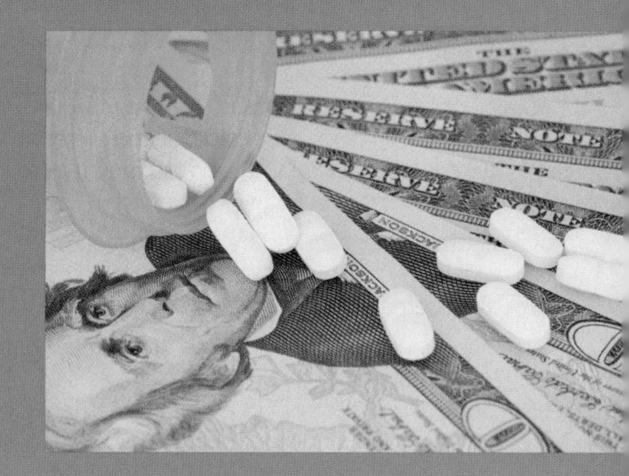

Get Connected

Mobile Tips!

Scan this QR code with your mobile device to access additional tips on aging well. Or, via your mobile device, go to **http://mobiletips.pearsoncmg.com** and navigate to Chapter 22.

Health Online Visit the following websites for further information about the topics in this chapter:

- Administration on Aging
  www.aoa.gov/AoARoot/index.aspx
- Alzheimer's Association
  www.alz.org
- American Association of Retired Persons (AARP)
  www.aarp.org
- Caring Connections Advance Directive Forms
  www.caringinfo.org
- National Institutes of Health Senior Health
  http://nihseniorhealth.gov
- RealAge Health Calculators and Assessments
  www.realage.com

Website links are subject to change. To access updated web links, please visit ***www.pearsonhighered.com/lynchelmore***.

References

i. Administration on Aging. (2012, February 10). *A profile of older Americans: 2011*. Retrieved from http://www.aoa.gov/AoARoot/Aging_Statistics/Profile/index.aspx.

ii. Rocheleau, M. (2010, July 26). Seniors get their tech on. *Christian Science Monitor, 102* (35), 29.

1. National Center for Education Statistics. (2011). Fast facts. U.S. Department of Education *Digest of Education Statistics, 2010* (NCES 2011-015). Retrieved from http://nces.ed.gov/fastfacts/display.asp?id=98.

2. Administration on Aging. (2012, February 10). *A profile of older Americans: 2011*. Retrieved from http://www.aoa.gov/AoARoot/Aging_Statistics/Profile/index.aspx.

3. Administration on Aging. (2010, June 23). *Projected future growth of the older population.* Retrieved from http://www.aoa.gov/AoARoot/Aging_Statistics/future_growth/future_growth.aspx.

4. Centers for Disease Control and Prevention. (2012, January 26). *Health-related quality of life: National trend – Percentage with fair or poor self-rated health: Age group.* Retrieved from http://apps.nccd.cdc.gov/HRQOL/TrendV.asp?State=1&Measure=1&Category=3&submit1=Go.

5. Federal Interagency Forum on Aging-Related Statistics. (2011). *Older Americans 2010: Key indicators of well-being.* Retrieved from http://www.agingstats.gov/agingstatsdotnet/Main_Site/Data/2010_Documents/Docs/OA_2010.pdf.

6. Murphy, S. L., Xu, J., & Kochanek, K. D. (2012, January 11). Abstract: Deaths: Preliminary data for 2010. *National Vital Statistics Reports, 60* (4). National Center for Health Statistics. Retrieved from http://www.cdc.gov/nchs/data/nvsr/nvsr60/nvsr60_04.pdf.

7. Kulkarni, S. C., Levin-Rector, A., Ezzati, M., & Murray, C. J. L. (2011). Falling behind: Life expectancy in US counties from 2000 to 2007 in an international context. *Population Health Metrics, 9*, 16. Retrieved from http://www.pophealthmetrics.com/content/pdf/1478-7954-9-16.pdf.

8. Olshansky, S. J., Antonucci, T., Berkman, L., Binstock, R. H., Boersch-Supan, A., Cacioppo, J. T. . . . Rowe, J. (2012, August). Differences in life expectancy due to race and educational differences are widening, and many may not catch up. *Health Affairs, 3*(8). 1803-1813.

9. Murray, C. J. L., Kulkarni, S. C., Michaud, C., Tomijima, N., Bulzacchelli, M. T., Iandiorio, T. J., & Ezzati, M. (2006, September). Eight Americas: Investigating mortality disparities across races, counties, and race-counties in the United States. *PLoS Medicine*. Retrieved from http://www.plosmedicine.org/article/info%3Adoi%2F10.1371%2Fjournal.pmed.0030260.

10. Central Intelligence Agency. (2012). Country comparison: Life expectancy at birth. In *The World Factbook*. Retrieved from https://www.cia.gov/library/publications/the-world-factbook/rankorder/2102rank.html.

11. Central Intelligence Agency. (2012). Field listing: Life expectancy at birth. In *The World Factbook*. Retrieved from https://www.cia.gov/library/publications/the-world-factbook/fields/2102.html.

12. Gorman, B. K., & Read, J. G. (2007). Why men die younger than women: The gender gap in mortality. *Geriatrics and Aging, 10* (3), 182–191.

13. American Academy of Ophthalmology. (2009, May). *Eye statistics at a glance*. Retrieved from http://www.aao.org/newsroom/press_kit/upload/Eye-Health-Statistics-June-2009.pdf.

14. Glaucoma Research Foundation. (2012, May 24). *Glaucoma facts and stats*. Retrieved from http://www.glaucoma.org/glaucoma/glaucoma-facts-and-stats.php.

15. National Eye Institute. (2010). *Facts about age-related macular degeneration.* Retrieved from http://www.nei.nih.gov/health/maculardegen/armd_facts.asp.

16. Centers for Disease Control and Prevention. (2011). *Arthritis: Data and statistics.* Retrieved from http://www.cdc.gov/arthritis/data_statistics.htm.

17. National Institutes of Health, Osteoporosis and Related Bone Diseases National Resource Center. (2011). *What is osteoporosis? Fast facts.* Retrieved from http://www.niams.nih.gov/Health_Info/Bone/Osteoporosis/default.asp.

18. National Osteoporosis Foundation. (2011). *About osteoporosis: Bone health basics.* Retrieved from http://www.nof.org/aboutosteoporosis/bonebasics/whybonehealth.

19. National Osteoporosis Foundation. (2011). *Fast facts on osteoporosis.* Retrieved from http://www.nof.org/node/40.

20. Institute of Medicine, Food and Nutrition Board. (2010). *Dietary reference intakes for calcium and vitamin D.* Washington, DC: National Academies Press.

21. Writing Group for the Women's Health Initiative Investigators. (2002). Risks and benefits of estrogen plus progestin in healthy postmenopausal women: Principal results from the Women's Health Initiative randomized controlled trial. *Journal of the American Medical Association, 288* (3), 321–333.

22. The North American Menopause Society. (2012). Position statement: The 2012 hormone therapy position statement of the North American Menopause Society. *Menopause: The Journal of the North American Menopause Society*, *19* (3), 257–271. DOI: 10.1097/gme.0b013e31824b970a.

23. U.S. Food and Drug Administration. (2011). *FDA drug safety communication: Ongoing safety review of oral osteoporosis drugs (bisphosphonates) and potential increased risk of esophageal cancer.* Retrieved from http://www.fda.gov/Drugs/DrugSafety/ucm263320.htm.

24. Mayo Foundation. (2011, July 23). *Male menopause: Myth or reality?* Retrieved from http://www.mayoclinic.com/health/male-menopause/MC00058.

25. Swartz, E. R., Phan, A., & Willix, R. D. (2011). Andropause and the development of cardiovascular disease presentation: More than an epi-phenomenon. *Journal of Geriatric Cardiology*, *8*, 35–43.

26. Coates, P. (2005, February). Androgen insufficiency in ageing men: How is it defined and should it be treated? *The Clinical Biochemist Reviews*, *26* (1), 37–41.

27. Basaria, S., Coviello, A. D., Travison, T. G., Storer, T. W., Farwell, W. R., Jette, A. M. . . . Bhasin, S. (2010). Adverse events associated with testosterone administration. *New England Journal of Medicine*, *363* (2), 109–122.

28. Kontula, O., & Haavio-Manilla, E. (2009). The impact of aging on human sexual activity and sexual desire. *Journal of Sex Research, 46* (1), 46–56.

29. Gunning-Dixon, F., Brickman, A., Cheng, J., & Alexopoulos, G. (2009). Aging of cerebral white matter: A review of MRI findings. *International Journal of Geriatric Psychiatry, 24*, 109–117.

30. Bergman, I., Blomberg, M., & Almkvist, O. (2007). The importance of impaired physical health and age in normal cognitive aging. *Scandinavian Journal of Psychology, 48*, 115–125.

31. National Institute on Aging. (2010). *The search for AD prevention strategies.* Retrieved from http://www.nia.nih.gov/Alzheimers/Publications/ADPrevented/strategies.htm.

32. National Institute on Aging. (2008). *The hallmarks of AD.* Retrieved from http://www.nia.nih.gov/Alzheimers/Publications/Unraveling/Part2/hallmarks.htm.

33. Alzheimer's Association. (2012). *2012 Alzheimer's disease facts and figures.* Retrieved from http://www.alz.org/downloads/Facts_Figures_2012.pdf.

34. Scarmeas, N., Luchsinger, J. A., Schupf, N., Brickman, A. M., Cosentino, S., Tang, M. X., & Stern, Y. (2009). Physical activity, diet, and risk of Alzheimer's disease. *Journal of the American Medical Association, 302* (6), 627–637.

35. Centers for Disease Control and Prevention. (2010, June 28). *Healthy places terminology*. Retrieved from http://www.cdc.gov/healthyplaces/terminology.htm.

36. Social Security Administration. (2012, April 23). *Retirement planner.* Retrieved from http://www.socialsecurity.gov/retire2/index.htm.

37. Social Security Administration. (2011). *Facts and figures about Social Security, 2011.* Retrieved from http://www.socialsecurity.gov/policy/docs/chartbooks/fast_facts/2011/fast_facts11.html#agedpop.

38. Middleton, T. (2007). Fixing the 5 biggest 401(k) blunders. *MSN Money: Personal Finance.* Retrieved from http://articles.moneycentral.msn.com/Investing/MutualFunds/The5biggest401kBlunders.aspx.

39. Browning, E. S. (2011, February 19). Retiring boomers find 401(k) plans fall short. *The Wall Street Journal*. Retrieved from http://online.wsj.com/article/SB10001424052748703959604576152792748707356.html.

40. Shattuck, A. (2010, Summer). Older Americans working more, retiring less. *Carsey Institute*. Issue Brief No. 16. Retrieved from http://www.carseyinstitute.unh.edu/publications/IB_Shattuck_Older_Workers.pdf.

41. National Institute of Mental Health. (2009). *Older adults: Depression and suicide facts (fact sheet).* Retrieved from http://www.nimh.nih.gov/health/publications/older-adults-depression-and-suicide-facts-fact-sheet/index.shtml.

42. Substance Abuse and Mental Health Services Administration. (2011, September 1). *Illicit drug use among older adults.* (NSDUH_013). National Survey on Drug Use and Health. Retrieved from http://oas.samhsa.gov/2k11/013/WEB_SR_013_HTML.pdf.

43. National Institutes of Health. (2010, August). Alcohol and aging. *NIH Senior Health*. Retrieved from http://nihseniorhealth.gov/alcoholuse/alcoholandaging/01.html.

44. American Society of Consultant Pharmacists. (2011). *Senior ASCP fact sheet.* Retrieved from https://www.ascp.com/articles/about-ascp/ascp-fact-sheet.

45. Hansen-Kyle, L. (2005). A concept analysis of healthy aging. *Nursing Forum, 40* (2), 45–57.

46. Barondess, J. (2008). Toward healthy aging: The preservation of health. *Journal of the American Geriatrics Society, 56* (1), 145–148.

47. Kempermann, G., Fabel, K., Ehninger, D., Babu, H., Leal-Galicia, P., Garthe, A., & Wolf, S. A. (2010). Why and how physical activity promotes experience-induced brain plasticity. *Frontiers in Neuroscience*, *4*, 189. DOI: 10.3389/fnins.2010.00189.

48. Centers for Disease Control and Prevention. (2011, December 1). *Physical activity for everyone: How much physical activity do older adults need?* Retrieved from http://www.cdc.gov/physicalactivity/everyone/guidelines/olderadults.html.

49. Lichtenstein, A., Rasmussen, H., Yu, W., Epstein, S., & Russell, R. (2008). Modified MyPyramid for older adults. *Journal of Nutrition, 138*, 78–82.

50. American Lung Association. (2010, February). *Smoking and older adults.* Retrieved from http://www.lung.org/stop-smoking/about-smoking/facts-figures/smoking-and-older-adults.html.

51. Qato, D. M., Alexander, G. C., Conti, R. M., Johnson, M., Schumm, P., & Lindau, S. T. (2008). Use of prescription and over-the-counter medications and dietary supplements among older adults in the United States. *Journal of the American Medical Association, 300* (24), 2867–2878.

52. Dominguez, L., Barbagallo, M., & Morley, J. (2009). Anti-aging medicine: Pitfalls and hopes. *The Aging Male, 12* (1), 13–20.

53. Strandberg, A., Strandberg, T. E., Pitkala, K., Salomaa, V. V., Tilvis, R. S., & Miettinen, T. A. (2008). The effect of smoking

in midlife on health-related quality of life in old age. *Archives of Internal Medicine, 168* (18), 1968–1974.

54. Hall, C. B., Lipton, R. B., Sliwinski, M., Katz, M. J., Derby, C. A., & Verghese, J. (2009). Cognitive activities delay onset of memory decline in persons who develop dementia. *Neurology, 73,* 356–361.

55. Hill, T. (2006). Religion, spirituality, and healthy cognitive aging. *Southern Medical Journal, 99* (10), 1176–1177.

56. Speece, M. W. (1995). Children's concepts of death. *Living and Dying: Family Decisions: Michigan Family Review, 15* (1), 1. Retrieved from http://quod.lib.umich.edu/m/mfr/4919087.0001.107?rgn=main;view=fulltext.

57. Howarth, G. (2011). Dying as a social relationship. In Oliviere, D., Monroe, B., & Payne, S., *Death, dying, and social differences.* London: Oxford University Press, 9–10.

58. Monroe, B., Oliviere, D., & Payne, S. (2011). Introduction: Social differences: The challenge for palliative care. In Oliviere, D., Monroe, B., & Payne, S., *Death, dying, and social differences.* London: Oxford University Press, 4.

59. International Association for Near-Death Studies. (2011, April 26). *Aftereffects of near-death states.* Retrieved from http://iands.org/about-ndes/common-aftereffects.html.

60. International Association for Near-Death Studies. (2011, April 26). *Impact of the near-death experience on grief and loss.* Retrieved from http://iands.org/impact-of-the-near-death-experience-on-grief-and-loss.html.

61. Greyson, B., Williams Kelly, E., & Kelly, E. F. (2009). Explanatory models of near-death experiences. In Greyson, B., & James, D., *Handbook of near-death experiences*. Santa Barbara: ABC-CLIO, LLC, 213–234.

62. Aging with Dignity. (2009). *Five wishes*. Retrieved from http://www.agingwithdignity.org/forms/5wishes.pdf.

63. Koenig, R., & Hyde, M. (2009). Be careful what you wish for: Analyzing the "Five Wishes" advance directive. *Illinois Bar Journal, 97* (5), 242–245.

64. U.S. Department of Health and Human Services. (2012). *Organ procurement and transplantation network: Transplant history.* Retrieved from http://optn.transplant.hrsa.gov/about/transplantation/history.asp.

65. Harris Interactive. (2007). *Most U.S. adults believe in the importance of organ donation but are ambivalent about how to increase the numbers of donors.* Retrieved from http://www.harrisinteractive.com/news/allnewsbydate.asp?NewsID=1226.

66. U.S. Department of Health and Human Services. (2012). *Organ procurement and transplantation network: Data.* Retrieved from http://optn.transplant.hrsa.gov.

67. Greenhough, J. (2011, March 31). 57% of adults don't have a will—Are you one of them? Estate planning survey results announced. *Rocket Lawyer Insider*. Retrieved from http://insider.rocketlawyer.com/2011-wills-estate-planning-survey-9524.

68. American Medical Association. (2006, September 20). Palliative care. *Journal of the American Medical Association, 296* (11). Retrieved from http://jama.ama-assn.org/cgi/reprint/296/11/1428.pdf.

69. Muramatsu, N., Hoyem, R. L., Yin, H., & Campbell, R. T. (2008). Place of death among older Americans: Does state spending on home- and community-based services promote home death? *Medical Care, 46* (8), 829–838.

70. National Hospice and Palliative Care Organization. (2012). *NHPCO facts and figures: Hospice care in America.* Retrieved from http://www.nhpco.org/files/public/statistics_research/2011_facts_figures.pdf.

71. Hospice Foundation of America. (2010). *Choosing hospice.* Retrieved from http://www.hospicefoundation.org/pages/page.asp?page_id=53053.

72. Messerli, J. (2012, January 7). Should an incurably ill patient be able to commit physician-assisted suicide? *BalancedPolitics.org.* Retrieved from http://www.balancedpolitics.org/assisted_suicide.htm.

73. Fox, E., Myers, S., & Pearlman, R. A. (2007). Ethics consultation in United States hospitals: A national survey. *American Journal of Bioethics, 7,* 13–25.

74. Perry, J. E. (2010). A missed opportunity: Health care reform, rhetoric, ethics, and economics at the end of life. *Mississippi College Law Review*, *29* (2), 409–426. Retrieved from http://papers.ssrn.com/sol3/papers.cfm?abstract_id=1594245.

75. U.S. Centers for Disease Control and Prevention/National Center for Health Statistics. (2011). *Health insurance coverage: Early release of estimates from the 2010 National Health Interview Survey*. Retrieved from http://www.cdc.gov/nchs/nhis/released201106.htm.

76. Yu, X. Q. (2009, October 14). Socioeconomic disparities in breast cancer survival: Relation to stage at diagnosis, treatment, and race. *BMC Cancer, 9*, 364. Retrieved from http://www.biomedcentral.com/1471-2407/9/364.

77. Stöppler, M. C. (2012). Autopsy (postmortem examination, obduction). *MedicineNet.com.* Retrieved from http://www.medicinenet.com/script/main/art.asp?articlekey=12217.

78. National Funeral Directors Association. (2012). *Statistics.* Retrieved from http://www.nfda.org/media-center/statisticsreports.html#cfacts.

79. Funeral Consumers Alliance. (2011, March 2). *Earth burial, tradition in simplicity.* Retrieved from http://www.funerals.org/faq/74-earth-burial-tradition-in-simplicity.

80. Maciejewski, P., Zhang, B., Block, S., & Prigerson, H. (2007). An empirical examination of the stage theory of grief. *Journal of the American Medical Association, 297* (7), 716–723.

81. Corr, C. A., Nabe, C. M., & Corr, D. M. (2009). *Death & dying, life & living*, 6th ed. Belmont, CA: Wadsworth, 340–343.

82. van den Berg, G. J., Lindeboom, M., & Portrait, F. (2006). *Conjugal bereavement effects on health and mortality at advanced ages.* Institute of Labor. IZA DP No. 2358. Retrieved from http://ftp.iza.org/dp2358.pdf.

83. Vaillant, G. E. (2002). *Aging well: Surprising guideposts to a happier life from the landmark Harvard study of adult development*. Boston: Little, Brown.

84. Kübler-Ross, E. (1997). *On death and dying*, reprint edition. New York: Collier Books.

85. Zlatin, D. M. (1995). Life themes: A method to understand terminal illness. *Omega: Journal of Death and Dying*, *31* (3), 189–206.

86. Corr, C. A., Nabe, C. M., & Corr, D. M. (2009). *Death & dying, life & living*, 6th ed. Belmont, CA: Wadsworth.

87. Steinhauser, K., Clipp, E., McNeilly, M., Christakis, N., McIntyre, L., & Tulsky, J. (2000). In search of a good death: Observations of patients, families, and providers. *Annals of Internal Medicine, 132* (10), 825–832.

88. Mayo Clinic. (2008). *Terminal illness: Supporting a terminally ill loved one.* Retrieved from http://www.mayoclinic.com/health/grief/CA00041.

89. U.S. Census Bureau. (2011, June 27). *Facts for features: Back to school.* Retrieved from http://www.census.gov/newsroom/releases/archives/facts_for_features_special_editions/cb11-ff15.html.

90. American Council on Education. (2007, October). *Framing new terrain: Older adults and higher education.* Retrieved from http://www.acenet.edu/Content/NavigationMenu/ProgramsServices/CLLL/Reinvesting/Reinvestingfinal.pdf.

91. Kvaavik, E., Batty, G. D., Ursin, G., Huxley, R., & Gale, C. R. (2010). Influence of individual and combined health behaviors on total and cause-specific mortality in men and women: The United Kingdom health and lifestyle survey. *Archives of Internal Medicine, 170* (8), 711–718.

Test Your Knowledge Answers

Chapter 1:
1. c 2. b 3. d 4. a 5. b 6. d 7. b 8. c
9. a 10. d

Chapter 2:
1. d 2. a 3. b 4. a 5. b 6. d 7. a 8. c
9. d 10. c

Chapter 3:
1. a 2. a 3. b 4. d 5. b 6. b 7. d 8. c
9. a 10. c

Chapter 4:
1. c 2. b 3. a 4. b 5. d 6. c 7. d 8. a
9. d 10. b

Chapter 5:
1. a 2. c 3. d 4. c 5. b 6. b 7. c 8. a
9. c 10. d

Chapter 6:
1. d 2. d 3. d 4. c 5. b 6. d 7. b 8. a
9. c 10. a

Chapter 7:
1. d 2. c 3. b 4. a 5. a 6. b 7. d 8. d
9. d 10. c

Chapter 8:
1. d 2. d 3. a 4. c 5. d 6. c 7. d 8. d
9. d 10. c

Chapter 9:
1. c 2. d 3. a 4. b 5. d 6. c 7. a 8. b
9. d 10. d

Chapter 10:
1. b 2. a 3. c 4. c 5. c 6. d 7. d 8. a
9. c 10. a

Chapter 11:
1. d 2. d 3. b 4. b 5. c 6. b 7. a 8. b
9. c 10. d

Chapter 12:
1. b 2. d 3. c 4. c 5. a 6. c 7. d 8. d
9. c 10. b

Chapter 13:
1. b 2. b 3. d 4. c 5. a 6. c 7. a 8. b
9. a 10. d

Chapter 14:
1. b 2. d 3. b 4. d 5. d 6. b 7. c 8. d
9. c 10. a

Chapter 15:
1. c 2. c 3. d 4. b 5. b 6. a 7. d 8. c
9. a 10. d

Chapter 16:
1. c 2. d 3. a 4. b 5. b 6. a 7. d 8. c
9. b 10. c

Chapter 17:
1. d 2. b 3. c 4. d 5. c 6. a 7. d 8. c
9. b 10. a

Chapter 18:
1. c 2. d 3. a 4. b 5. c 6. b 7. a 8. c
9. a 10. c

Chapter 19:
1. d 2. d 3. c 4. b 5. d 6. a 7.a 8. c
9. b 10. a

Chapter 20:
1. a 2. d 3. a 4. d 5. b 6. c 7. d 8. b
9. a 10. a

Chapter 21:
1. c 2. d 3. a 4. a 5. d 6. a 7. a 8. d
9. a 10. b

Chapter 22:
1. c 2. b 3. d 4. a 5. a 6. d 7. c 8. a
9. d 10. b

Credits

Photo Credits

Cover: George Doyle/Stockbyte/Getty Images; **Inside front cover:** EDHAR/Shutterstock; **Back cover:** Richard Drury/Photodisc/Getty Images; **Visual walkthrough, p. 2:** iofoto/Shutterstock; **Visual walkthrough, p. 5:** Yuri Arcurs/Shutterstock; **Visual walkthrough, p. 7:** Andresr/Shutterstock **p. i:** George Doyle/Stockbyte/Getty Images; **p. iv, top:** April Lynch; **p. iv, middle:** Barry Elmore; **p. iv, bottom:** Jerome Kotecki; **p. vii, top left:** Juice Images/Alamy; **p. vii, top right:** Bramalia/Dreamstime LLC; **p. vii, middle left:** Olivier Blondeau/iStockphoto; **p. vii, middle right:** Hill Street Studios/Blend Images/Getty Images; **p. vii, bottom left:** Neti Harnik/AP Wide World Photos; **p. vii, bottom right:** Jim West/ALAMY; **p. viii:** Shannon Fagan/The Image Bank/Getty Images; **p. ix, top:** Laura Doss/Corbis/Fancy; **p. ix, bottom:** Brand X Pictures/Jupiterimages/Getty Images; **p. x:** Bloom image/Getty Images; **p. xi, top:** Marnie Bukhart/Corbis Images; **p. xi, bottom:** Dennis Welsh/Getty Images; **p. xii:** Blend Images/Alamy; **p. xiii, top:** Chat Roberts/Corbis Images; **p. xiii, bottom:** George Doyle/Stockbyte/Getty Images; **p. xiv:** Robert Lawson/Photolibrary/Getty Images; **p. xv:** Purestock/Getty Images; **p. xvi, top:** Ian Hooton//SPL/Getty Images; **p. xvi, bottom:** Latin Stock Collection/Corbis Images; **p. xvii:** www.photo-chick.com/Getty Images; **p. xviii:** Image Source/Corbis; **p. xix, top:** uwe umstÃ¤tter/Getty Images; **p. xix, bottom:** Ian Hooton/SPL/Getty Images; **p. xx:** Suprijono Suharjoto/Fotolia; **p. xxi, top:** imagesource/Photolibrary Royalty Free; **p. xxi, bottom:** Don Mason/Blend Images/AGE Fotostock; **p. xxii:** Juice Images/Corbis; **p. xxiii:** Jupiterimages/Brand X Pictures/Getty Images

Chapter 1 opener: Shannon Fagan/The Image Bank/Getty Images; **p. 3:** Daniel Hurst Stock Connection Worldwide/Newscom; **p. 4:** John Dawson, Pearson Education; **p. 5:** Lane Erickson/Dreamstime; **p. 7:** Tetra Images/SuperStock; **p. 8:** Imagestate Media Partners Limited - Impact Photos/Alamy; **p. 9:** Friedrich Stark Alamy; **p. 10:** Fancy/Alamy; **p. 11:** Visions of America/SuperStock; **p. 12:** FOX Broadcasting Company/Album/Newscom; **p. 13:** alvarez/iStockphoto; **p. 14:** Cultura Creative/Alamy; **p. 15:** John Dawson, Pearson Education; **p. 16, top to bottom:** Lissandra/Shutterstock; Tom Mareschal/Alamy; Monkey Business Images/Shutterstock; Katrina Brown/Shutterstock; **p. 17:** Supri Suharjoto/Shutterstock; **p. 18:** Helen King/Lithium/AGE Fotostock; **p. 19:** Maridav/Shutterstock; **p. 24:** Press Association via AP Images

Chapter 2 opener: Laura Doss/Corbis/Fancy; **p. 29:** Glow Images/Newscom; **p. 30:** Dylan Ellis/Corbis; **p. 32, left to right:** RonTech2000/iStockphoto; Bennewitz/iStockphoto; Justin Horrocks/iStockphoto; Christopher Stewart/Alamy; **p. 33, left to right:** Christopher Stewart/Alamy; Benjamin Loo/iStockphoto; Neustockimages/iStockphoto; William Wang/Fotolia; **p. 34:** Pacificcoastnews/Newscom; **p. 36:** Design Pics Inc./Alamy; **p. 40:** Indeed/Getty Images; **p. 41:** Pearson Education; **p. 42:** catenarymedia/iStockphoto; **p. 43:** Stockbroker/MBI/Alamy; **p. 44, left:** John Bell/iStockphoto; **p. 44, right:** Marjorie Kamys Cotera/Bob Daemmrich Photography/Alamy; **p. 46:** Stockbroker/SuperStock; **p. 48:** John Dawson, Pearson Education; **p. 49:** Firefoxfoto/Alamy Images; **p. 50:** Sigrid Olsson/Altopress/Newscom; **p. 51:** Jeff Greenberg/Alamy Images; **p. 52:** Hill Street Studios/Blend Images/Alamy; **p. 56:** Heather Ainsworth/AP Wide World Photos

Chapter 3 opener: Brand X Pictures/Jupiterimages/Getty Images; **p. 61:** iStockphoto.com/Nikolay Suslov; **p. 62:** hektoR/Shutterstock; **p. 63:** Pearson Education; **p. 64:** Stockbyte/Getty Images; **p. 65:** AdamGregor/iStockphoto; **p. 67:** Radius Images/Alamy; **p. 68:** AFP PHOTO/ED KOSMICKI; **p. 69:** Adam Borkowski/iStockphoto; **p. 70:** mathieukor/iStockphoto; **p. 72, top:** Malyugin/Shutterstock; **p. 72, bottom:** Iakov Filimonov/iStockphoto; **p. 73:** Science Photo Library/Alamy; **p. 74:** AVAVA/iStockphoto; **p. 75:** Stígur Karlsson/iStockphoto; **p. 76:** Adrian Sherratt/Alamy; **p. 77:** Juice Images/Alamy; **p. 78:** Robert Kneschke/Shutterstock; **p. 82:** AFP PHOTO / OFICCIAL TV MINISTERY MINE/HANDOUT

Chapter 4 opener: BLOOM image/Getty Images; **p. 87:** Dmitriy Shironosov/Shutterstock; **p. 88, bottom:** WAVEBREAKMEDIA LTD/AGE Fotostock; **p. 88, top:** inspirestock/AGE Fotostock; **p. 91:** GoGo Images Corporation/Alamy; **p. 92, top:** Image Source/SuperStock; **p. 92, bottom:** CandyBox Photography/Alamy; **p. 93:** Bubbles Photolibrary/Alamy; **p. 95, top:** EDHAR/Shutterstock; **p. 95, bottom:** Anthony-Masterson/Foodpix/Getty Images; **p. 96:** Hank Morgan/Photo Researchers, Inc.; **p. 97:** JGI/Jamie Grill/Blend Images/Corbis; **p. 98:** Jeff Greenberg/AGE Fotostock; **p. 99:** Pearson Education; **p. 103:** Rick Friedman/Corbis

Chapter 5 opener: Marnie Bukhart/Corbis Images; **p. 107:** Tom Grill/Corbis; **p. 109:** wuttichok/Fotolia; **p. 110:** Feng Fu/Shutterstock; **p. 111, top:** Corbis Images; **p. 111, bottom:** Fotocrisis/Shutterstock; **p. 112:** Gustavo Caballero/Getty Images, Inc - Liaison; **p. 113:** Shutterstock; **p. 114, Figure 5.3, all photos:** Renn Sminkey CDV, Pearson Education; **p. 114, Table 5.1, all photos:** Corbis Images; **p. 115, Table 5.1, all photos except eggs:** Corbis Images; **p. 115, Table 5.1, eggs:** Barry Gregg/Corbis; **p. 116:** Regien Paassen/Shutterstock; **p. 117, Table 5.2, all photos except lobster:** Corbis Images; **p. 117, Table 5.2, lobster:** Morgan Lane Photography/Shutterstock; **p. 118:** Lana Langlois/Shutterstock; **p. 119:** Kati Molin/Shutterstock; **p. 120:** Jesse Kunerth/Alamy Images; **p. 125, Figure 5.6b:** Marie C Fields/Shutterstock; **p. 125, Figure 5.6a:** Pearson Learning Group Studo, Pearson Education; **p. 125, Figure 5.7, all photos:** Pearson Learning Group Studo, Pearson Education; **p. 126, top:** Pearson Education; **p. 126, bottom:** Don Smetzer / Alamy; **p. 127:** CDC/BSIP/AgeFotostock; **p. 128:** Bramalia/Dreamstime LLC; **p. 130:** age fotostock/SuperStock; **p. 131:** Taylor S Kennedy/Alamy Images; **p. 133:** Ariel Skelley/Blend Images/Alamy; **p. 134:** Michael Newman/PhotoEdit Inc.; **p. 137:** Mitchell/Mayer/Splash News/Newscom

Chapter 6 opener: Dennis Welsh/Getty Images; **p. 143:** Blue Jaen Images/Alamy Images Royalty Free; **p. 145:** Newscom; **p. 146:** djma/Fotolia LLC; **p. 147:** Renn Sminkey CDV, Pearson Education; **p. 148, left:** Maksim Šmeljov/Fotolia LLC; **p. 148, middle:** Doug Menuez/PhotoDisc/Getty Images Inc.; **p. 148, right:** Stockbyte/Getty Images; **p. 149:** Blue Jean Images/Getty Images; **p. 150, all photos:** Elena Dorfman, Pearson Education; **p. 151, all photos:** Elena Dorfman, Pearson Education; **p. 152:** Image Source/Getty Images; **p. 153, all photos:** Elena Dorfman, Pearson Education; **p. 154, all photos:** Elena Dorfman, Pearson Education; **p. 159:** Walter Lockwood/Corbis; **p. 160, left:** Olivier Blondeau/iStockphoto; **p. 160, right:** Jupiterimages/Getty Images; **p. 162, top:** RubberBall/Alamy Images Royalty Free; **p. 162, bottom:** PCN Black/Alamy; **p. 165:** Newscom; **p. 166, top:** motorolka/iStockphoto; **p. 166, bottom:** Pearson Education; **p. 170:** Tanned Maury/Newscom

Chapter 7 opener: Blend Images/Alamy; **p. 175:** Guilio Marcocchi/Newscom; **p. 177:** George Doyle/Getty Images; **p. 178, skinfold measurement:** Sean Aidan/Eye Ubiquitous/Alamy; **p. 178, hydrostatic weighing:** David Madison/Getty Images; **p. 178, Bod Pod:** ZUMA Wire Service/Alamy; **p. 178, bioelectrical impedance:** BSIP/SPL/Photo Researchers, Inc.; **p. 178, scanning technologies:** B. Boissonnet/BSIP SA/Alamy; **p. 179:** Frederiic J. Brown/Newscom; **p. 181:** ACE STOCK LIMITED/Alamy Images; **p. 183:** David R. Frazier Photolibrary, Inc./Alamy; **p. 184:** Newscom; **p. 185:** Pearson Education; **p. 186:** Jacek Chabraszewski/Fotolia; **p. 187, all photos:** Pearson Education; **p. 189, all photos:** Renn Sminkey CDV, Pearson Education; **p. 192:** OLJ Studio/Shutterstock; **p. 194:** Blake Little/Getty Images; **p. 195:** Asia Images Group/AGE Fotostock America Inc.; **p. 196:** Hisayoshi Osawa/Taxi Japan/Getty Images; **p. 199:** Pearson Education; **p. 202:** David Crane/La Daily News/Los Angeles Daily News/ZUMAPRESS/Alamy

Chapter 8 opener: Chat Roberts/Corbis Images; **p. 207:** Patrick Kosiniak Design Pics Inc./Alamy; **p. 208:** SGO/BSIP/AGE Fotostock; **p. 209:** Jamie Grill/Blend Images/Alamy; **p. 210:** Christopher Hudson/iStockphoto; **p. 212:** Robert Kneschke/Shutterstock; **p. 214:** Joy Scheller iPhoto Inc./Newscom; **p. 215:** Angela Maynard/Life File/Getty Images; **p. 217, top:** AJPhoto/Photo Researchers, Inc.; **p. 217, bottom:** J Marshall - Tribaleye Images/Alamy; **p. 218:** Jon Schulte/iStockphoto; **p. 219:** Multnomah County Sheriff/Splash/Newscom; **p. 221, left:** Nico Hermann/Westend61/Newscom; **p. 221, right:** DEA; **p. 223, Table 8.3, top:** nicholas belton/iStockphoto; **p. 223, Table 8.3, bottom:** DEA; **p. 223, top:** Ken Inness/iStockphoto; **p. 224, Table 8.3, top to bottom:** Joe Bird/Alamy; David Lee/Alamy Images; David Hoffman Photo Library/Alamy; DEA; DEA; **p. 227:** ZUMA Press/Newscom; **p. 228:** Pearson Education; **p. 230:** Liquorice Legs/Shutterstock; **p. 234:** Michael Germana/Everett Collection

Chapter 9 opener: George Doyle/Stockbyte/Getty Images; **p. 239:** Jamie Grill/Blend Images/Corbis; **p. 240:** Kristin Piljay, Pearson Education; **p. 243:** StockLite/Shutterstock; **p. 244:** Clark Brennan/Alamy; **p. 245:** MBI/Alamy; **p. 246:** Paul Piebinga/iStockphoto; **p. 247:** I52/ZUMA Press/Newscom; **p. 248:** Bochkarev Photography/Shutterstock; **p. 249:** ZUMA Press/Newscom; **p. 251:** Tatiana Popova/Shutterstock; **p. 252:** John Dawson, Pearson Education; **p. 257:** Jamie Grill Photography/Getty Images; **p. 258:** Pearson Education; **p. 262:** adharcimages.com/Alamy

Chapter 10 opener: Robert Lawson/Photolibrary/Getty Images; **p. 267:** iStockphoto; **p. 268:** Imagesource/Glow Images; **p. 270:** Hall Philip/SIPA/Newscom; **p. 271, top:** Mark Goddard/iStockphoto; **p. 271, bottom:** Alamogordo Daily News/AP Wide World Photos; **p. 272:** Image Source/Alamy Images; **p. 273, Figure 10.3a & b:** James Stevenson/Photo Researchers, Inc.; **p. 273, bottom:** Rayman/Getty; **p. 275:** SPL/Photo Researchers, Inc.; **p. 276, large photo:** Arman Zhenikeyev/Corbis Images; **p. 276, fingers:** Biophoto Associates/Photo Researchers, Inc.; **p. 276, lips:** Véronique Beranger/Corbis Cusp/Alamy; **p. 276, bad breath:** CREATISTA; **p. 276, cough:** Imaginechina/Corbis; **p. 276, impotence:** Andrey Popov/Shutterstock; **p. 277:** Martin Novak/Alamy; **p. 278:** INSADCO Photography/Alamy; **p. 279:** Oleg Zinkovetsky/Shutterstock; **p. 280:** US Food and Drug Administration FDA/http://www.fda.gov/TobaccoProducts/Labeling/Labeling/default.htm; **p. 283:** Pearson Education; **p. 284:** Milos Luzanin/Shutterstock; **p. 289:** AMC/courtesy Everett Collection

Chapter 11 opener: Purestock/Getty Images; **p. 296, top:** Jaimie Duplass/Shutterstock; **p. 296, bottom:** Digital Vision/Thinkstock; **p. 297:** twentyfree/Fotolia; **p. 298:** Adam Gault/Alamy; **p. 299, top:** Mark Hatfield/iStockphoto; **p. 299, bottom:** Pearson Education; **p. 301:** Toxawww/Dreamstime LLC -Royalty Free; **p. 302, left:** Science Photo Library/Photo Researchers, Inc.; **p. 302, right:** Ed Reschke/Alamy Images; **p. 304, left:** sumnersgraphicsinc/Fotolia; **p. 304, right:** Lisa F. Young/Alamy; **p. 307:** ZUMA Wire Service/Alamy; **p. 308:** Rudi Von Briel/Photolibrary/Getty Images; **p. 311:** Dreamstime; **p. 312:** picsfive/Fotolia; **p. 313, bottom:** Shutterstock; **p. 313, top:** Pearson Education; **p. 314:** Lana K/Shutterstock; **p. 315:** AndrewFurlongPhotography/iStockphoto; **p. 316:** Luis Santos/Shutterstock; **p. 319:** ST/Splash News/Newscom

Chapter 12 opener: Ian Hooton/SPL/Getty Images; **p. 327:** Jordan Siemens/Aurora Open/Alamy; **p. 328:** Pearson Education; **p. 329:** Kate Kunz/Fancy/Alamy; **p. 331:** National Cancer Institute/Photo Researchers; **p. 334:** Javier Larrea/AGE Fotostock; **p. 336:** P. Marazzi/Photo Researchers; **p. 337:** Mike Goldwater/Alamy; **p. 339:** Medical-on-Line/Alamy; **p. 340:** Image Source/Getty Images; **p. 342:** Westend61/Superstock; **p. 346:** Pearson Education; **p. 347:** Monkey Business Images/Shutterstock; **p. 354:** Latin Stock Collection/Corbis Images; **p. 351:** Chat Roberts/Corbis Premium RF/Alamy

Chapter 13 opener: Latin Stock Collection/Corbis Images; **p. 357, Table 13.1, left to right:** Dr. Linda Stannard, UCT/Photo Researchers; Ray Butler, Centers for Disease Control and Prevention (CDC); Libero Ajello, Centers for Disease Control and Prevention (CDC); Eye of Science/Photo Researchers; Andrew Syred/Photo Researchers; **p. 357, bottom:** Kletr/Fotolia; **p. 359:** detwo/Shutterstock; **p. 360:** John Dawson, Pearson Education; **p. 362:** JPC-PROD/Fotolia; **p. 364:** Mandel NGAN/Newscom; **p. 365:** Dr. Dan Kalman/Photo Researchers; **p. 366:** Polka Dot/Thinkstock; **p. 367:** Dani Vincek/Shutterstock; **p. 368:** Medical-on-Line/Alamy; **p. 369:** Ponir's Photography/Flickr/Getty Images; **p. 370:** Bruno Coignard &,Jeff Hageman, CDC; **p. 371:** James Gathany/Associated Press; **p. 373:** Michael A. Keller/AGE Fotostock; **p. 375:** Helen Sessions/Alamy; **p. 377:** Paul Bradbury/Alamy; **p. 380:** Don Emmert/AFP/Newscom

Chapter 14 opener: www.photo-chick.com/Getty Images; **p. 385:** Tom Chance/Alamy; **p. 386:** Datacraft - Sozaijiten/Alamy; **p. 387:** Putland Michael/Phototeque Oredia/AGE Fotostock; **p. 389:** Randy Faris/Corbis; **p. 390:** Laurence Mouton/PhotoAlto/Corbis; **p. 392:** John Dawson, Pearson Education; **p. 393:** Andres Rodriguez/Alamy; **p. 394:** Hill Street Studios/Blend Images/Getty Images; **p. 395:** Hill Street Studios/G/Blend Images/AGE Fotostock; **p. 397:** Yuri Arcurs/Shutterstock; **p. 398:** Ambient Images Inc./Alamy; **p. 399:** Image Source/Alamy; **p. 400:** Toru Hanai/REUTERS; **p. 402:** Ron Nickel/Design Pics/Newscom; **p. 403:** Corbis/AGE Fotostock; **p. 407:** HANDOUT/MCT/Newscom

Chapter 15 opener: Image Source/Corbis; **p. 412:** rubberball/AGE Fotostock; **p. 416:** Blend Images/Alamy; **p. 419:** Fancy/Alamy; **p. 421:** Tina Chang/Fancy/AGE Fotostock; **p. 423:** Ardelean Andreea/Shutterstock; **p. 424:** ZUMA Press/Newscom; **p. 425:** Rawdon Wyatt / Alamy; **p. 426:** momentimages/Tetra Images/AGE Fotostock; **p. 428:** Carin Baer / © Fox Television/Courtesy: Everett Collection; **p. 429:** John Dawson, Pearson Education; **p. 430:** Fancy/Alamy; **p. 433:** Emmanuel Dunand/AFP/Getty Images/Newscom

Chapter 16 opener: uwe umstÃ¤tter/Getty Images; **p. 438:** Stockbroker/Alamy Images Royalty Free; **p. 439:** Ian Miles-Flashpoint Pictures/Alamy; **p. 444:** Teh Eng Koon/AP Photo; **p. 445:** Rodger Bosch/AFP/Getty Images/Newscom; **p. 446, left:** Custom Medical Stock Photo; **p. 446, right:** Photo Researchers, Inc. / Biophoto Associates; **p. 447, both photos:** Centers for Disease Control and Prevention; **p. 448:** Gavin Hart, Centers for Disease Control and Prevention; **p. 449:** Jack Hollingsworth/Getty Images Royalty Free; **p. 450:** Meckes/Ottawa/Photo Researchers;

p. 451: Jose Luis Pelaez/Alamy Images Royalty Free; **p. 452:** sassyphotos/Fotolia; **p. 453:** Pearson Education; **p. 457:** nicolasjoseschirado/Fotolia

Chapter 17 opener: Ian Hooton/SPL/Getty Images; **p. 461:** mitgirl/Fotolia; **p. 465:** Sam Edwards/Alamy; **p. 466:** Reggie Casagrande/Getty Images; **p. 468, left:** Exactostock/SuperStock; **p. 468, right:** Peter Ardito/Photolibrary/Getty Images; **p. 470:** Gary Parker/Photo Researchers; **p. 471, bottom:** Christy Thompson/Shutterstock; **p. 471, top:** Pearson Education; **p. 472, left:** Agencja FREE/Alamy; **p. 472, right:** foto-begsteiger/vario images GmbH & Co.KG/Alamy; **p. 473:** Imagedoc/Alamy; **p. 475:** Jim West/Alamy; **p. 477:** David J. Green/Alamy; **p. 479, right:** Rido/Fotolia; **p. 479, left:** Fancy Collection/Superstock; **p. 482:** Marmaduke St. John/Alamy

Chapter 18 opener: Suprijono Suharjoto/Fotolia; **p. 486:** Exactostock/SuperStock; **p. 488:** Phanie/SuperStock; **p. 489, top:** Biophoto Associates / Science Source/Photo Researchers; **p. 489, bottom:** Stockbroker/MBI/Alamy; **p. 491, left:** GODONG/AGE Fotostock America; **p. 491, right:** IAN HOOTON/Alamy Images; **p. 493:** Monkey Business/Fotolia; **p. 494, top to bottom:** Lennart Nilsson/Scanpix; Lennart Nilsson/Scanpix; Neil Bromhall/Photo Researchers; Marc Kurschner/Getty Images; **p. 495:** Jose Luis Pelaez Inc/Blend Images/Alamy; **p. 496:** David Buffington/Blend Images/Alamy; **p. 497:** Science Photo Library/AGE Fotostock; **p. 499, bottom:** Ron Sutherland / Science Source/Photo Researchers; **p. 499, top:** stockyimages/Fotolia; **p. 500:** Odua Images/Fotolia; **p. 501, top:** Science Photo Library/AGE Fotostock; **p. 503:** Numjai/Kalium/Fotolia; **p. 504:** ROB & SAS/Corbis Flirt/Alamy; **p. 506:** Plus One Pix/Alamy; **p. 507:** JGI/Jamie Grill/Blend Images / Alamy; **p. 511:** Sony Pictures TV/Splash News/Newscom

Chapter 19 opener: imagesource/Photolibrary Royalty Free; **p. 516, top:** Jose Luis Pelaez/Alamy; **p. 516, bottom:** Raine Vara/Alamy; **p. 518:** Asher Welstead/iStockphoto; **p. 519:** moodboard/Cultura/Getty Images; **p. 522:** Bob Pardue/Alamy; **p. 523, bottom:** Simone van den Berg/Shutterstock; **p. 523, top:** Neti Harnik/AP Wide World Photos; **p. 524:** John Dawson, Pearson Education; **p. 525, right:** Dana Neely/The Image Bank/Getty Images; **p. 525, left:** Katrina Brown/Alamy; **p. 527:** Jupiter Images/Getty Images; **p. 528:** zilli/iStockphoto; **p. 529:** Mona Makela/Shutterstock; **p. 530:** Matthew Wakem/Digital Vision/Getty Images; **p. 532:** Jim West/Alamy; **p. 533:** CSPAN/AP Wide World Photos; **p. 535:** Siri Stafford/Photodisc/Getty Images; **p. 536, bottom:** Annuella Alexander, Pearson Education; **p. 536, top:** Digital Vision/Thinkstock; **p. 537:** Elnur/Shutterstock; **p. 538, top:** Westend61/Superstock; **p. 542:** ZUMA Wire Service/Alamy

Chapter 20 opener: Don Mason/Blend Images/AGE Fotostock; **p. 547:** Image Source/SuperStock; **p. 549, top:** John Dawson, Pearson Education; **p. 549, bottom:** Paul Conklin/PhotoEdit; **p. 551:** Mike Kemp RubberBal/Alamy; **p. 554:** David Stepheson/Newscom; **p. 555, top:** Radius Images Alamy; **p. 555, middle:** Sarah Fix Photography/Alamy; **p. 555, bottom:** University of California, Berkeley; **p. 556:** SuperStock/Purestock/Alamy; **p. 557:** Julia Nichols/iStockphoto; **p. 558:** Steve Olson/Alamy; **p. 559:** Roger L. Wollenberg/Newscom; **p. 561:** McPhoto/Alamy; **p. 563:** Martin Norris Studio Photography/Alamy; **p. 565:** moodboard/Alamy; **p. 566:** Mike Cherim/iStockphoto; **p. 571:** ZUMA Press/Newscom

Chapter 21 opener: Juice Images/Corbis; **p. 577:** Javier Larrea/age fotostock; **p. 579:** Ivan Vdovin/Alamy; **p. 580:** National Geographic Image Collection/Alamy; **p. 584:** RubberBall/Alamy; **p. 585:** Jim West/Alamy; **p. 586:** Car Culture/Getty Images; **p. 589, left:** Ciro Cesar/La Opinion/Newscom; **p. 589, right:** Kristen Piljay, Pearson Education; **p. 590:** Stephen Gibson/Shutterstock; **p. 591:** Jeff Greenberg/age fotostock; **p. 592:** MBI/Alamy; **p. 593, left:** tomas/fotolia; **p. 593, right:** Ronald Sumners/Shutterstock; **p. 595:** Pixland/Thinkstock; **p. 598:** JupiterImages/Thinkstock; **p. 601:** Mark Von Holden/WireImage/Getty Images

Chapter 22 opener: Jupiterimages/Brand X Pictures/Getty Images; **p. 607, right:** Jose Luis Pelaez/Alamy; **p. 607, left:** Ariel Skelley/Alamy; **p. 608, all photos:** National Eye Institute, NIH; **p. 609, left:** Michael Klein/Peter Arnold/Getty Images; **p. 609, right:** Charles Stirling/Alamy; **p. 611:** Luca Tettoni/Robert Harding Picture Library Ltd/Alamy; **p. 612:** Dr. Robert Friedland / Photo Researchers; **p. 614:** Newscom; **p. 615, left:** Mirrorpix/Newscom; **p. 615, right:** Newscom; **p. 616:** Monkey Business Images/Shutterstock; **p. 617:** Chris Willson/Alamy; **p. 618, right:** Ellen Isaacs/Alamy; **p. 618, left:** Stockbyte/Thinkstock; **p. 619:** Karen Gentry/Shutterstock; **p. 620:** David Hiser/Getty Images; **p. 622:** iceteaimages/Alamy; **p. 625, left:** Mike Booth/Alamy; **p. 625, right:** Graham Monro/gm photographics/Getty Images; **p. 627:** Purestock/Getty Images; **p. 628:** Dream Pictures/Photolibrary; **p. 632:** Bruce MacQueen/Shutterstock

Figure Credits

Figure 6.2: Text from Hopson, Janet, Donatelle, Rebecca, and Littrell, Tanya, *Get Fit, Stay Well!,* 2nd ed., © 2013. Fig. 5.8, pp. 127–139. Reprinted and electronically reproduced by permission of Pearson Education, Inc., Upper Saddle River, New Jersey. **Figure 6.3:** Text from Hopson, Janet, Donatelle, Rebecca, and Littrell, Tanya, *Get Fit, Stay Well!,* 2nd ed., © 2013. Fig. 5.8, pp. 127–139. Reprinted and electronically reproduced by permission of Pearson Education, Inc., Upper Saddle River, New Jersey.

Glossary

12-step programs Addiction recovery self-help programs based on the principles of Alcoholics Anonymous.

A

abortion A medical or surgical procedure used to terminate a pregnancy.
absorption The process by which alcohol passes from the stomach or small intestine into the bloodstream.
abstinence The avoidance of sexual intercourse.
accessory glands Glands (seminal vesicles, prostate gland, and Cowper's gland) that lubricate the reproductive system and nourish sperm.
accommodation A practice of giving in to the other person's needs or wishes and denying one's own.
acid rain A phenomenon in which airborne pollutants are transformed by chemical processes into acidic compounds, then mix with rain, snow, or fog and are deposited on Earth.
acquired immunity The body's ability to quickly identify and attack a pathogen that it recognizes from previous exposure. In some cases acquired immunity leads to lifelong protection against the same infection.
acquired immunodeficiency syndrome (AIDS) The final stage of infection with the human immunodeficiency virus (HIV), which attacks the immune system, leaving the patient vulnerable to various infections and cancers.
active stretching A type of static stretching where you gently apply force to your body to create a stretch.
addiction A chronic, progressive disease of brain reward, motivation, memory, and related circuitry characterized by uncontrollable craving for a substance or behavior despite both negative consequences and diminishment or loss of pleasure associated with the activity.
adoption The social, emotional, and legal process in which children who will not be raised by their birth parents become full and permanent legal members of another family.
advance directives Formal documents that state a person's preferences regarding medical treatment and medical crisis management.
advocacy Working independently or with others to directly improve services in or other aspects of the environment, or to change related policies or legislation.
aerobic exercise Prolonged physical activity that raises the heart rate and works the large muscle groups.
age-related macular degeneration (AMD) An age-related vision disorder caused by deterioration of the macula that reduces central vision.
aggravated assault An attack intended to cause serious physical harm, often involving a weapon.
Air Quality Index (AQI) An index for measuring daily air quality according to a list of federal air criteria, published by city or region.
alcohol abuse Drinking alcohol to excess, either regularly or on individual occasions, resulting in disruption of work, school, or home life and causing interpersonal, social, or legal problems.
alcohol dependence (alcoholism) A physical dependence on alcohol characterized by intense craving and by withdrawal symptoms when the drinker stops drinking.
alcohol intoxication The state of physical and/or mental impairment brought on by excessive alcohol consumption (in legal terms, a BAC of 0.08% or greater).
alcohol poisoning A dangerously high blood alcohol level, resulting in depression of the central nervous system, slowed breathing and heart rate, and compromised gag reflex.
alcoholic cirrhosis A condition in which many years of heavy drinking produce such chronic stress to liver cells that they cease to function and are replaced with scar tissue.
alcoholic hepatitis Inflammation of the liver, which results in progressive liver damage and is marked by nausea, vomiting, fever, and jaundice.
allergies Abnormal immune system reactions to substances that are otherwise harmless.
allostatic overload A harmful state that develops as a consequence of chronic, excessive stress.
altruism The practice of helping and giving to others out of genuine concern for their well-being.
Alzheimer's disease (AD) A progressive, fatal form of age-related dementia.
amenorrhea Cessation of menstrual periods.
amino acids The building blocks of protein; 20 common amino acids are found in food.
amniotic fluid Fluid that surrounds the developing fetus that aids in temperature regulation and allows the baby to move freely.
amphetamines Central nervous system stimulants that are chemically similar to the natural stimulants adrenaline and noradrenaline.
anaerobic exercise Short, intense exercise that causes an oxygen deficit in the muscles.
anal intercourse Intercourse characterized by the insertion of the penis into a partner's anus and rectum.
anaphylactic shock A result of anaphylaxis in which the release of histamine and other chemicals into the body leads to a drop in blood pressure, tightening of airways, and possible unconsciousness and even death.
andropause Period marked by a decline in the male reproductive hormone testosterone and its resultant physical and emotional effects; also referred to as *male menopause*.
angina pectoris Chest pain due to coronary heart disease.
anorexia nervosa Mental disorder characterized by extremely low body weight, body image distortion, severe calorie restriction, and an obsessive fear of gaining weight.
antibiotic A drug used to fight bacterial infection.
antibodies Proteins released by B cells that bind tightly to infectious agents and mark them for destruction.
antigen Substance, usually a protein, capable of inducing a specific immune response.
antioxidants Compounds in food that help protect the body from harmful molecules called free radicals.
anxiety disorders A category of mental disorders characterized by persistent feelings of fear, dread, and worry.
Apgar score A measurement of how well a newborn tolerated the stresses of birth, as well as how well he or she is adapting to the new environment.
appetite The psychological response to the sight, smell, thought, or taste of food that prompts or postpones eating.
arable Suitable for cultivation of crops.
arrhythmia Any irregularity in the heart's rhythm.

arteries Vessels that transport blood away from the heart, delivering oxygen-rich blood to the body periphery and oxygen-poor blood to the lungs.
arthritis Inflammation of one or more joints in the body, resulting in pain, swelling, and limited movement.
assertiveness The ability to clearly express your needs and wants to others in an appropriate way.
assortative mating The tendency to be attracted to people who are similar to us.
asthma Chronic inflammatory disease characterized by bronchospasm, inflammation of the bronchial lining, and overproduction of mucus within the narrowed bronchi.
atherosclerosis Condition characterized by narrowing of the arteries because of inflammation, scarring, and the buildup of fatty deposits.
atria The two upper chambers of the heart, which receive blood from the body periphery and lungs.
attachment An enduring bond of love for another.
attachment theory The theory that the patterns of attachment in our earliest relationships with others form the template for attachment in later relationships.
attention deficit hyperactivity disorder (ADHD) A type of attention disorder characterized by inattention, hyperactive behavior, fidgeting, and a tendency toward impulsive behavior.
attention disorders A category of mental disorders characterized by problems with mental focus.
autoimmune disease General term for any of a number of disorders characterized by inflammation and other immune responses against the body's own tissues.
autonomy The capacity to make informed, un-coerced decisions.
autopsy Medical examination of a corpse.

B

bacteria (singular: *bacterium*) Single-celled microorganisms that can be beneficial, harmless, or harmful, invading and damaging body cells and sometimes releasing toxins.
ballistic stretching Performing rhythmic bouncing movements in a stretch to increase the intensity of the stretch.
balloon angioplasty An arterial treatment that uses a small balloon to flatten plaque deposits against the arterial wall.
barbiturates A type of central nervous system depressant often prescribed to induce sleep.
bariatric surgery Weight-loss surgery using various procedures to modify the stomach or other sections of the gastrointestinal tract in order to reduce calorie intake or absorption.
basal metabolic rate (BMR) The rate at which the body expends energy for only the basic functioning of vital organs.
behavior change A sustained change in a habit or pattern of behavior that affects health.
behavior therapy A type of therapy that focuses on changing a patient's behavior and thereby achieving psychological health.
behavioral addiction A form of addiction involving a compulsion to engage in an activity such as gambling, sex, or shopping rather than a compulsion to use a substance.
benign tumor A tumor that grows slowly, does not spread, and is not cancerous.
benzodiazepines Medications commonly prescribed to treat anxiety and panic attacks.
binge drinking An episode of alcohol consumption that results in a blood alcohol concentration of 0.08% or above.
binge eating The rapid consumption of an excessive amount of food.
bioaccumulation The process by which substances increase in concentration in the fat tissues of living organisms as the organisms take in contaminated air, water, or food.
biomagnification The process by which certain contaminants become more concentrated in animal tissue as they move up the food chain.
biomonitoring Analysis of blood, urine, tissues, and so forth to measure chemical exposure in humans.
biopsy A test for cancer in which a small sample of the abnormal growth is removed and studied.
bipolar disorder (manic-depressive disorder) A mental disorder characterized by occurrences of abnormally elevated mood (or mania), often alternating with depressive episodes, with periods of normal mood in between.
birth control pills Pills containing combinations of hormones that prevent pregnancy when taken regularly as directed.
bisexuals People who are attracted to partners of both the same and the opposite sex.
blastocyst Early stage of embryonic development in which multiple cell divisions have produced an initial cell mass.
blood alcohol concentration (BAC) The amount of alcohol present in blood, measured in grams of alcohol per deciliter of blood.
blood pressure The force of the blood moving against the arterial walls.
body burden The amount of a chemical stored in the body at a given time, especially a potential toxin in the body as the result of environmental exposure.
body composition The relative proportions of the body's lean tissue and fat tissue.
body dysmorphic disorder Mental disorder characterized by obsessive thoughts about a perceived flaw in appearance.
body image A person's perceptions, feelings, and critiques of his or her own body.
body mass index (BMI) A numerical measurement, calculated from height and weight measurements, that provides an indicator of health risk categories.
bradycardia A slow arrhythmia.
brain death The cessation of brain activity as indicated by various medical devices and diagnostic criteria.
brain fitness A person's ability to meet the cognitive requirements and demands of daily life, such as problem-solving and memory recall.
brand-name drugs Patent-protected prescription drugs that can only be manufactured by one drug company and which usually carry a higher cost.
bulimia nervosa Mental disorder characterized by episodes of binge eating followed by a purge behavior such as vomiting, laxative abuse, or extreme exercise.
burnout Phenomenon in which increased feelings of stress and decreased feelings of accomplishment lead to frustration, exhaustion, lack of motivation, and disengagement.
bypass surgery A procedure to build new pathways for blood to flow around areas of arterial blockage.

C

caffeine A widely used stimulant found in coffee, tea, soft drinks, chocolate, and some medicines.
calorie Common term for *kilocalorie*. The amount of energy required to raise the temperature of 1 kilogram of water by 1 degree Celsius.

cancer A group of diseases marked by the uncontrolled multiplication of abnormal cells.
capillaries The smallest blood vessels, delivering blood and nutrients to individual cells and picking up wastes.
carbohydrates A macronutrient class composed of carbon, hydrogen, and oxygen, that is the body's universal energy source.
carbon monoxide A gas that inhibits the delivery of oxygen to the body's vital organs.
carcinogen A substance known to trigger DNA mutations that can lead to cancer.
carcinogenic Cancer causing.
carcinoma Cancer of tissues that line or cover the body.
cardiometabolic risk (CMR) A cluster of nine modifiable factors that identify individuals at risk for type 2 diabetes and cardiovascular disease.
cardiorespiratory fitness The ability of your heart and lungs to effectively deliver oxygen to your muscles during prolonged physical activity.
cardiovascular disease (CVD) Diseases of the heart or blood vessels.
carpal tunnel syndrome (CTS) A repetitive strain injury of the hand or wrist, often linked to computer keyboard use or other types of repetitive motion.
carrier A person infected with a pathogen who does not show symptoms, but who can transmit the pathogen to others. In genetics, a person with no genetic disease who has one normal copy and one defective copy of a gene associated with a recessive genetic disorder.
carrying capacity The number of organisms of one species that an environment can support indefinitely.
cataracts An age-related vision disorder marked by clouding of the lens of the eye.
cellular death The end of all vital functions at the cellular level, such as cellular respiration and other metabolic processes.
central nervous system cancer Cancer of the brain or spinal cord.
cervical cap A flexible silicone cap that is filled with spermicide and inserted in the vagina prior to sex to prevent pregnancy.
cervix The neck, or narrowed lower entrance, of the uterus that serves as a passageway to and from the vagina.
cesarean birth (c-section) Birth of an infant through a surgical incision in the mother's abdominal and uterine walls.
chain of infection Group of factors necessary for the spread of infection.
cholesterol An animal sterol found in the fatty part of animal-based foods such as meat and whole milk.
chronic obstructive pulmonary disease (COPD) A group of diseases characterized by a reduced flow of air into and out of the lungs. COPD includes emphysema, chronic bronchitis, and chronic asthmatic bronchitis.
circadian rhythm Pattern of physical, emotional, and behavioral changes that follows a roughly 24-hour cycle in accordance with the hours of darkness and light in the individual's environment.
circumcision The surgical removal of the foreskin.
climate change A change in the state of the climate that can be identified by changes in the average and/or variability of its properties that persist for an extended period.
clinical death A medical determination that life has ceased according to medical criteria that often combine aspects of functional and neurological factors.
clinical trials Tests of proposed new drugs using human subjects.
clitoris An organ composed of spongy tissue and nerve endings which is very sensitive to sexual stimulation.
club drugs Illicit substances, including MDMA (ecstasy), GHB, and ketamine that are most commonly encountered at nightclubs and raves.
co-pay A flat fee charged at the time of a medical service or when receiving a medication.
cocaine A potent and addictive stimulant derived from leaves of the coca shrub.
codependency When a friend or family member is part of a pattern that may perpetuate behaviors that sustain addiction.
cognitive-behavioral therapy (CBT) A form of psychotherapy that emphasizes the role of thinking (cognition) in how we feel and what we do.
cohabitation The state of living together in the same household; usually refers to unmarried couples.
collaboration An approach to conflict in which all parties work together to achieve a mutually acceptable resolution.
competition An approach to conflict in which the parties involved strive to fulfill their own needs or desires at the expense of the needs and desires of the others involved.
complementary and alternative medicine (CAM) Health practices and traditions not typically part of conventional Western medicine, either used alone (alternative medicine) or in conjunction with conventional medicine (complementary medicine).
complex carbohydrates Carbohydrates that contain chains of multiple sugar molecules; commonly called *starches* but also come in two non-starch forms: *glycogen* and *fiber.*
compromise An approach to conflict in which each party agrees to accept less than what they had fully wanted so that a resolution can be reached.
conception The combination of the genetic material (DNA) of a woman's ovum and a man's sperm.
condom (male condom) A thin sheath typically made of latex that is unrolled over the erect penis prior to vaginal penetration and serves as a barrier to conception.
conflict An experience prompted by a difference of opinion, principles, needs, or desires in which the partners involved perceive a threat to their self-interest.
conflict avoidance The active avoidance of discussing concerns, annoyances, needs, or other potential sources of conflict with another person.
conflict resolution Process in which a solution to a conflict is reached in a manner that both people can accept and that minimizes future occurrences of the conflict.
congestive heart failure A gradual loss of heart function.
conjunctivitis Inflammation of the conjunctiva of the eye.
consumer health An umbrella term encompassing topics related to the purchase and consumption of health-related products and services.
contagious Spread from one person to another via direct or indirect contact.
continuation rate The percentage of couples who continue to practice a given form of birth control.
contraception Any method used to prevent pregnancy.
contraceptive sponge A flexible foam disk containing spermicide that is inserted in the vagina prior to sex.
conventional medicine Commonly called Western medicine, this system of care is based on the principles of the scientific method; the belief that diseases are caused by identifiable physical factors and have a characteristic set of symptoms; and the treatment of physical causes through drugs, surgery, or other physical interventions.
coronary heart disease (coronary artery disease) Atherosclerosis of the arteries that feed the heart.

cortisol Adrenal gland hormone that is secreted at high levels during the stress response.
counter-conditioning A behavior-change technique in which the individual learns to substitute a healthful or neutral behavior for an unwanted behavior triggered by a cue beyond his or her control.
cramp An involuntary contracted muscle that does not relax, resulting in localized intense pain.
Crohn's disease Painful intestinal disorder characterized by inflammation and ulceration of one or more regions of the intestinal wall.
cue control A behavior-change technique in which the individual learns to change the stimuli that provoked the lapse.
cunnilingus Oral stimulation of the vulva or clitoris.
cyber crime Any criminal activity using a network or computer.

D

danger zone Range of temperatures between 40° and 140° Fahrenheit at which bacteria responsible for foodborne illness thrive.
date (acquaintance) rape Coerced, forceful, or threatening sexual activity in which the victim knows the attacker.
date rape drugs Drugs used to assist in a sexual assault, often given to the victim without his or her knowledge or consent.
dating Spending time with another person one on one to determine whether there is an attraction or a desire to see more of each other.
decibel The unit of measurement used to express sound intensity.
deductible The total amount of out-of-pocket health care expenses that a patient must pay before health insurance begins to cover health-care costs.
dementia A decline in brain function.
dentist A conventional medicine practitioner who specializes in care of the teeth, gums, and mouth.
depressants Substances that depress the activity of the central nervous system and include barbiturates, benzodiazepines, and alcohol.
depressive disorder A mental disorder usually characterized by profound, persistent sadness or loss of interest that interferes with daily life and normal functioning.
determinants of health The range of personal, social, economic, and environmental factors that influence health status.
diabetes mellitus A group of diseases in which the body does not make or use insulin properly, resulting in elevated blood glucose.
diaphragm A flexible shallow cup with a spring in the rim; it is filled with spermicide and inserted in the vagina prior to sex to prevent pregnancy.
diet The food you regularly consume.
Dietary Reference Intakes (DRIs) A set of energy and nutrient recommendations for supporting good health.
dietary supplements Products taken by mouth that include ingredients such as vitamins, minerals, amino acids, herbs, botanicals, or other compounds that could supplement the diet.
dilation and evacuation (D&E) A multistep method of surgical abortion that may be used in pregnancies that have progressed beyond 12 weeks.
disordered eating A range of unhealthful eating behaviors used to deal with emotional issues that does not warrant a diagnosis of a specific eating disorder.
dissociative drug A medication that distorts perceptions of sight and sound and produces feelings of detachment from the environment and self.
distress Stress resulting from negative stressors.
domestic partnership A legal arrangement in which a couple lives together in a long-term committed relationship and receives some, but not all, of the rights of married couples.
domestic violence An abusive situation in which a family member physically, psychologically, or sexually abuses one or more other family members.
dopamine A neurotransmitter that stimulates feelings of pleasure.
drug A chemical substance that alters the body physically or mentally for a non-nutritional purpose.
drug abuse The use (most often the excessive use) of any legal or illegal drug in a way that is detrimental to your health.
drug misuse The inappropriate use of a legal drug, either for a reason for which it was not medically intended, or by a person without a prescription.
dynamic flexibility The ability to move quickly and fluidly through a joint's entire range of motion with little resistance.
dynamic stretching A type of slow movement stretching in which activities from a workout or sport are mimicked in a controlled manner, often to help "warm up" for a game or event.
dyslipidemia Disorder characterized by abnormal levels of blood lipids, such as high LDL cholesterol or low HDL cholesterol.
dysmenorrhea Pain during menstruation that is severe enough to limit normal activities or require medication.
dysthymic disorder (dysthymia) A milder, chronic type of depressive disorder that lasts 2 years or more.

E

e-waste Hazardous waste generated by the production or disposal of electronic or digital devices.
eating disorders A group of mental disorders, including anorexia nervosa, bulimia nervosa, and binge eating disorder, that is characterized by physiological and psychological disturbances in appetite or food intake.
ecological footprint The collective impact of an entity on its resources, ecosystems, and other key environmental features.
ecological model Any of a variety of behavior-change models that acknowledge the creation of a supportive environment as equally important to achieving change as an individual's acquisition of health information and development of personal skills.
ecosystem A dynamic collection of organisms and their nonliving surroundings that function as a unit.
ectopic pregnancy A pregnancy that occurs when a fertilized egg implants outside the uterus, often within one of the fallopian tubes; considered a medical emergency.
elective surgery A nonessential surgery. The patient can decide when and if to undergo the procedure.
electrocardiogram (ECG) A test that measures the heart's electrical activity.
electroencephalograph (EEG) Device that monitors the electrical activity of different regions of the cerebral cortex of the brain using electrodes placed on or in the scalp; a tracing of brain activity is called an *electroencephalogram*.
embryo The growing collection of cells that ultimately becomes a baby.
emergency contraception (EC; morning after pill) A pill or pills containing a synthetic form of the hormone progesterone and used to prevent pregnancy after unprotected sex.
emotional health The "feeling" component of psychological health that influences your interpretation of and response to events.

emotional intelligence (EI) The ability to accurately monitor, assess, and manage your emotions and those of others.
empty calories Calories from solid fats, alcohol, and/or added sugars that provide few or no nutrients.
enablers People who protect addicts from the negative consequences of their behavior.
enabling factor A skill, asset, or capacity that influences an individual's ability to make and sustain behavior change.
endocrine disruptor A substance that stops the production or blocks the use of hormones in the body and that can have harmful effects on health or development.
endometriosis A condition in which endometrial tissue grows in areas outside of the uterus.
endorphins Hormones that act as neurotransmitters and bind to opiate receptors, stimulating pleasure and relieving pain.
energy balance The state achieved when energy consumed from food is equal to energy expended, maintaining body weight.
environmental health The discipline that addresses all the physical, chemical, and biological factors external to individual human beings, especially those that influence human health.
environmental mastery The ability to choose or create environments that suit you.
epidemiologist A scientist who studies the patterns of disease in populations.
epididymis A coiled tube on top of each testicle where sperm are held until they mature.
erectile dysfunction (ED) The inability of a male to obtain or maintain an erection.
erection The process of the penis filling up with blood as a result of sexual stimulation.
erogenous zones Areas of the body likely to cause sexual arousal when touched.
essential fatty acids (EFAs) Polyunsaturated fatty acids that cannot be synthesized by the body but are essential to body functioning.
essential nutrients Nutrients you must obtain from food or supplements because your body either cannot produce them or cannot make them in sufficient quantities to maintain health.
estate A person's personal holdings, including money, property, and other possessions.
ethyl alcohol (ethanol) The intoxicating ingredient in beer, wine, and distilled liquor.
euphoria A feeling of intense pleasure.
eustress Stress resulting from positive stressors.
evidence-based medicine Health-care policies and practices based on systematic, scientific study.
excitement The first phase of the sexual response cycle, marked by erection in men and by lubrication and clitoral swelling in women.
exercise A type of physical activity that is planned and structured.
expedited partner therapy (EPT) Provision of prescriptions or medications to the partner of a patient with gonorrhea or chlamydia without the physician first examining the partner.

F

failure rate The percentage of women who typically get pregnant after using a given contraceptive method for one year.
fallopian tubes A pair of tubes that connect the ovaries to the uterus.
family health history A detailed record of health issues in one's family that presents a picture of shared health risks.
fats (triglycerides) Lipids made up of three fatty acid chains attached to a molecule of glycerol; the most common types of food lipid.
fatty liver A buildup of fat cells in the liver that can occur after heavy drinking.
fee-for-service plan A type of health insurance in which you choose your providers, and you and your insurer share the costs of care.
fellatio Oral stimulation of the penis.
female condom A thin sheath with flexible rings that is inserted into the vagina prior to vaginal penetration and serves as a barrier to conception.
fertility awareness methods (FAM) Any of a variety of methods of avoiding pregnancy that require tracking of changes that occur in a woman's body throughout her monthly cycle, with periods of abstinence when the woman is fertile. Also known as natural family planning.
fertility rate Within a given population, the average number of births per woman.
fetal adaptation Theory proposing that nutrient deprivation during fetal development may trigger genetic, hormonal, and other mechanisms that favor storage of calories and excessive body fat in childhood and adulthood.
fetal alcohol spectrum disorders (FASDs) A range of complications seen in children whose mothers consumed alcohol during pregnancy.
fetal alcohol syndrome (FAS) A pattern of mental and physical birth defects found in some children of mothers who drank excessively during pregnancy.
fetus The term for the developing embryo eight weeks after fertilization.
fiber A nondigestible complex carbohydrate that aids in digestion.
fight-or-flight response A set of physiological reactions to a stressor designed to enable the body to stand and fight or to flee.
FITT Exercise variables that can be modified in order to accomplish progressive overload: frequency, intensity, time, and type.
flexibility The ability of joints to move through their full ranges of motion.
flexible spending account (FSA) A consumer-controlled account, usually offered through employers, that uses pre-tax dollars to cover approved health-related purchases.
food additive A substance added to foods during processing to improve color, texture, flavor, aroma, nutrition content, or shelf life.
food allergy An adverse reaction of the body's immune system to a food or food component.
food intolerance An adverse food reaction that doesn't involve the immune system.
foodborne illness (food poisoning) Illness caused by pathogenic microorganisms consumed through food or beverages.
functional death The end of all vital physiological functions, including heartbeat, breathing, and blood flow.
fungi Multicellular or single-celled organisms that obtain their food from organic matter, in some cases human tissue.

G

gang An economic or social group that forms to intimidate and control members and outsiders through threats and violence.
gastroesophageal reflux (GER) Condition in which stomach acid leaks back into the lower portion of the esophagus, causing irritation and burning.
gender roles Behaviors and tasks considered appropriate by society based on whether someone is a man or a woman

gene therapy Any of a variety of techniques used for correcting defective genes responsible for the development of diseases.
general adaptation syndrome (GAS) Theory explaining the stress response as a series of three phases (alarm, resistance, exhaustion) with characteristic physiologic events.
generalized anxiety disorder (GAD) An anxiety disorder characterized by chronic worry and pessimism about everyday events that lasts at least 6 months and may be accompanied by physical symptoms.
generic drugs Copies of brand-name drugs that can be created by other drug companies after a drug developer's patent expires. These drugs are required by law to contain the same active ingredients as the brand-name drugs they replicate.
genetic modification Altering a plant's or animal's genetic material in order to produce desirable traits such as resistance to pests, poor soil tolerance, or lower fat.
genome sequencing The full decoding and readout of an entire genome.
genome The genetic material of any living organism.
genomics The study of genomes and their effects on health and development.
gestational diabetes Form of diabetes that develops during pregnancy in women with no prior history of diabetes.
GHB (gamma-hydroxybutyric acid) A central nervous system depressant known as a "date rape drug" because of its use to impair potential victims of sexual assault.
glaucoma An age-related vision disorder arising from an increase in internal eye pressure that damages the optic nerve and reduces peripheral vision.
global warming A sustained increase in the Earth's temperature due to an increase in the greenhouse effect resulting from pollution.
globalization The interaction and integration of regional phenomena globally.
glycemic index Value indicating the potential of a food to raise blood glucose.
groundwater The supply of fresh water beneath the Earth's surface, which is a major source of drinking water.

H

hallucinogens Drugs that alter perception and are capable of causing auditory and visual hallucinations.
hangover Alcohol withdrawal symptoms, including headache and nausea, caused by an earlier bout of heavy drinking.
hate crime A crime fueled by bias against another person's or group's race or ethnicity, religion, national origin, sexual orientation, or disability.
hazardous waste Garbage or byproducts that can pose a hazard to human health or the environment when improperly managed.
hazing Initiation rituals to enter a fraternity or other group that can be humiliating, hazardous, or physically or emotionally abusive, regardless of the person's willingness to participate.
health More than merely the absence of illness or injury, a state of well-being that encompasses physical, social, psychological, and other dimensions and is a resource for everyday life.
health belief model A model of behavior change emphasizing the influence of personal beliefs on the process of creating effective change.
health discount program A system of health discounts given to members of groups, such as employees of a particular company or students attending a particular college.
health disparities Gaps in the rate and burden of disease and the access to and quality of health care among various population groups.
Health Insurance Portability and Accountability Act (HIPAA) Legislation that protects your medical privacy.
health insurance A contract between an insurance company and a group or individual who pays a fee to have some or all health costs covered by the insurer.
health literacy The ability to evaluate and understand health information and to make informed choices for your health care.
health maintenance organization (HMO) A type of managed care in which most health care is funneled through and must be approved by the primary care doctor.
health preservation Performing activities that seek to maintain health, rather than simply responding to health crises as they occur.
health savings account (HSA) A consumer-controlled savings account that can be used to pay the deductible costs of a high-deductible health insurance policy. Money in HSAs earns a tax benefit.
health-related fitness The ability to perform activities of daily living with vigor.
healthful weight The weight at which health risks are lowest for an individual; usually a weight that will result in a BMI between 18.5 and 24.9.
Healthy Campus An offshoot of the Healthy People initiative, specifically geared toward college students.
Healthy People initiative A federal initiative to facilitate broad, positive health changes in large segments of the U.S. population every 10 years.
heat exhaustion A mild form of heat-related illness that usually occurs as the result of exercising in hot weather without adequate hydration.
heatstroke A life-threatening heat-related illness that occurs when your core temperature rises above 105 degrees Fahrenheit.
heavy drinking The consumption of five or more drinks on the same occasion on each of five or more days in the past 30 days.
hemorrhagic stroke A stroke caused by a ruptured blood vessel.
hepatitis Inflammation of the liver that affects liver function.
herd immunity The condition in which greater than 90% of a community is vaccinated against a disease, giving the disease little ability to spread through the community, providing some protection against the disease to members of the community who are not vaccinated.
heroin The most widely abused of opioids; typically sold as a white or brown powder or as a sticky black substance known as "black tar heroin."
heterosexual A person sexually attracted to someone of the opposite sex.
high-density lipoprotein (HDL) A cholesterol-containing compound that removes excess cholesterol from the bloodstream; often referred to as "good cholesterol."
high-risk drinking An episode or pattern of alcohol consumption that is likely to result in harm to the drinker and/or to others.
homeostasis A physiologic ability to maintain the body's internal conditions within a normal, healthful range, usually achieved via hormonal and neurological mechanisms.
homophobia The irrational fear of, aversion to, or discrimination against homosexuals or homosexuality.
homosexual A person sexually attracted to someone of the same sex.
hooking up Casual, noncommittal, physical encounters that typically range from kissing to oral sex but may involve intercourse.
hormone Chemical secreted by a gland and transported through the bloodstream to a distant target organ, the activity of which it then regulates.

recovery The period necessary for the body to recover from exercise demands and adapt to higher levels of fitness.
recurrence The return of cancer after a period during which no cancer was detected.
registered nurse (RN) A certified health care professional who provides a wide range of health-care services and supports the work of medical doctors.
reinforcement A motivational behavior-change technique that rewards steps toward positive change.
reinforcing factor An encouragement or a reward that promotes positive behavior change, or a barrier that opposes change.
relapse A return to the previous state or pattern of behavior.
relative risk A measure of the strength of the relationship between known risk factors and a particular disorder.
relaxation response A set of physiological responses—including decreased heart rate, respiratory rate, and metabolism—regulated by the peripheral nervous system and inductive of rest; can be activated through relaxation techniques.
religion A system of beliefs and practices related to the existence of a transcendent power.
REM behavior disorder (RBD) Parasomnia characterized by failure of inhibition of muscle movement during REM sleep.
REM sleep Type of wakeful sleep during which rapid eye movement and dreaming occur.
repetitions The number of times you perform an exercise repeatedly.
repetitive strain injury (RSI) An injury that damages joints, nerves, or connective tissue caused by repeated motions that put strain on one part of the body.
replacement-level fertility The level of fertility at which a population exactly replaces itself from one generation to the next.
reservoir An environment in which a pathogen is able to multiply in large numbers.
resistance The ability of a bacterium to overcome the effects of an antibiotic through a random mutation, or change in the bacterium's genetic code.
resolution The stage of the response cycle in which the body returns to normal functioning.
restless legs syndrome (RLS) Nervous system disorder characterized by a strong urge to move the legs, accompanied by creeping, burning, or other unpleasant sensations.
retained placenta Condition in which expulsion of the placenta does not occur within 30 minutes of childbirth.
retrovirus A virus that contains a single strand of RNA and uses the enzyme reverse transcriptase to transcribe its RNA into a double strand of DNA.
reversibility The principle that fitness levels decline when the demand placed on the body is decreased.
Rohypnol A powerful sedative known as a "date rape drug" because of its use to impair potential victims of sexual assault.

S

sarcoma Cancer of muscle or connective tissues.
satiety Physical fullness; the state in which there is no longer the desire to eat.
saturated fats Fats that typically are solid at room temperature; generally found in animal products, dairy products, and tropical oils.
schizophrenia A severe mental disorder characterized by inaccurate perceptions of reality, an altered sense of self, and radical changes in emotions, movements, and behaviors.
scrotum The skin sac at the base of the penis that contains the testes.
seasonal affective disorder (SAD) A type of depressive disorder caused by fewer hours of daylight during the winter months.
secondhand smoke (environmental tobacco smoke) The smoke nonsmokers are exposed to when someone has been smoking nearby; a combination of sidestream smoke and mainstream smoke.
secretory phase Phase of the menstrual cycle characterized by the degeneration of the follicle sac, rising levels of progesterone in the bloodstream, and further increase of the endometrial lining.
self-acceptance A sense of positive and realistic self-regard, resulting in elevated levels of self-confidence and self-respect.
self-actualization The pinnacle of Maslow's hierarchy of needs, which indicates truly fulfilling your potential.
self-care Actions you take to keep yourself healthy.
self-disclosure The sharing of honest feelings and personal information about yourself with another person.
self-efficacy The conviction that you can make successful changes and the ability to take appropriate action to do so.
self-medicating Using alcohol or drugs to cope with problems and/or emotional distress.
self-monitoring A behavior-change technique in which the individual observes and records aspects of his or her behavior-change process.
self-talk A person's internal dialogue.
semen The male ejaculate consisting of sperm and other fluids from the accessory glands.
sets Separate groups of repetitions.
sexting The use of cell phones or similar electronic devices to send sexually explicit text, photos, or videos.
sexual dysfunctions Problems occurring during any stage of the sexual response cycle.
sexual harassment Unwelcome language or contact of a sexual nature that explicitly or implicitly affects academic or employment situations, unreasonably interferes with work or school performance, or creates an intimidating, hostile, or offensive work or school environment.
sexual orientation Romantic and physical attraction toward others.
sexual violence Any form of nonconsensual sexual activity.
sexuality The biological, physical, emotional, and psychosocial aspects of sexual attraction and expression.
sexually transmitted infections (STIs) Infections transmitted mainly through sexual activity, such as vaginal, anal, or oral sex.
shaping A behavior-change technique based on breaking broad goals into more manageable steps.
shyness The feeling of apprehension or intimidation in social situations, especially in reaction to unfamiliar people or new environments.
sidestream smoke Smoke emanating from the burning end of a cigarette or pipe.
simple carbohydrates The most basic unit of carbohydrates, consisting of one or two sugar molecules.
skills-related fitness The capacity to perform specific physical skills related to a sport or other physically demanding activity.
sleep A physiologically prompted, dynamic, and readily reversible state of reduced consciousness essential to human survival.
sleep apnea Disorder in which one or more pauses in breathing occur during sleep.
sleep bruxism Clenching or grinding the teeth during sleep.
sleep debt An accumulated amount of sleep loss that develops when the amount of sleep you routinely obtain is less than the amount you need.

sleep hygiene The behaviors and environmental factors that together influence the quantity and quality of sleep.
sleep terror Parasomnia characterized by the appearance of awakening in terror during a stage of NREM sleep.
sleepwalking Parasomnia in which a person walks or performs another complex activity while still asleep.
snoring A ragged, hoarse sound that occurs during sleep when breathing is obstructed.
social anxiety disorder (social phobia) An anxiety disorder characterized by an intense fear of being judged by others and of being humiliated by your own actions, which may be accompanied by physical symptoms.
social physique anxiety Mental disorder characterized by extreme fear of having one's body judged by others.
social support A sufficient quantity of relationships that provide emotional concern, help with appraisal, information, and even goods and services.
specificity The principle that a fitness component is improved only by exercises that address that component.
spermicide A substance containing a chemical that immobilizes sperm.
spirituality That which is in total harmony with the perceptual and nonperceptual environment.
stalking A pattern of harassment and threats directed at a specific person that is intended to cause intimidation and fear, often through repeated, unwanted contact.
standard drink A drink containing about 14 grams pure alcohol (one 12-oz. can of beer, one 5-oz. glass of wine, or 1.5 oz. of 80-proof liquor).
static flexibility The ability to reach and hold a stretch at one endpoint of a joint's range of motion.
static stretching Gradually lengthening a muscle to an elongated position and sustaining that position.
status syndrome The disparity in health status and rates of premature mortality between the impoverished and the affluent within any given society.
statutory rape Any sexual activity with a person younger than the legally defined "age of consent," regardless of whether any coercion or force was involved.
stimulants A class of drugs that stimulate the central nervous system, causing acceleration of mental and physical processes in the body.
stress The collective psychobiological state that develops in response to a disruptive, unexpected, or exciting stimulus.
stressor Any physical or psychological condition, event, or factor that causes positive or negative stress.
stroke A medical emergency in which blood flow to or in the brain is impaired. Also called a *cerebral vascular accident* (*CVA*).
suction curettage A method of surgical abortion characterized by vacuum aspiration; typically used in the first 6 to 12 weeks of pregnancy.
sudden cardiac arrest A life-threatening cardiac crisis marked by loss of heartbeat and unconsciousness.
sudden infant death syndrome (SIDS) The sudden death of a seemingly healthy infant while sleeping.
Superfund A federal program that funds and carries out emergency and long-term identification, analysis, removal, and cleanup of toxic sites.
surgery A procedure that treats injuries, disease, or disorders by physically cutting into and manipulating the body.
surrogate childbearing A complex legal arrangement in which a fertile woman agrees to carry a pregnancy for another, usually infertile, woman.
sustainability The ability to meet society's current needs without compromising future generations' abilities to meet their own needs; includes policies for ensuring that certain components of the environment are not depleted or destroyed.

T

tachycardia A fast arrhythmia.
tar A sticky, thick brown residue that forms when tobacco is burned and its chemical particles condense.
target heart rate range The heart rate range to aim for during exercise. A target heart rate range of 64–91% of your maximum heart rate is recommended.
terminal illness Term used to describe a disease for which treatment options have been exhausted and which is expected to cause the patient's death within a discrete period of time, often identified as 6 months.
terrorism Premeditated, politically motivated violence against noncombatant individuals, usually as a means of influence.
testes (testicles) The two reproductive glands that manufacture sperm.
tetanus A disorder caused by infection with *Clostridium tetani* and characterized by persistent muscle contraction.
thirdhand smoke Deposits of toxic chemicals generated from smoking that build up on environmental surfaces.
tolerance A condition in which the body becomes so accustomed to a drug (such as alcohol) that increasing amounts of the drug are required to achieve the same physical effects as when the drug was first taken.
toxic shock syndrome A rare, serious illness caused by staph bacteria that begins with severe flu symptoms but can quickly progress to a medical emergency.
toxicity The dosage level at which a drug becomes poisonous to the body.
***trans* fat** A type of fat that is produced when liquid fat (oil) is turned into solid fat during food processing.
transgenderism The state in which someone's gender identity or gender expression is different from his or her assigned sex at birth.
transient ischemic attack (TIA) A temporary episode of strokelike symptoms, indicative of high stroke risk.
transition The final phase of the first stage of labor, characterized by the dilation of the cervix and strong, prolonged contractions.
transsexual A transgendered individual who lives as the gender opposite to her or his assigned sex.
transtheoretical model of behavior change A model of behavior change that focuses on decision-making steps and abilities. Also called the *stages of change* model.
traumatic brain injury (TBI) An injury that disrupts normal functioning of the brain, caused by a jolt or blow to the brain or a penetrating head wound.
tubal ligation Form of permanent surgical sterilization that seals off the fallopian tubes, preventing sperm and ovum from making contact.
tuberculosis Disease caused by infection with *Mycobacterium tuberculosis* in which the immune response produces characteristic walled-off tubercles (nodules) in the lungs.
tumor An abnormal growth of tissue with no physiological function.

type 1 diabetes A form of diabetes that usually begins early in life and arises when the pancreas produces insufficient insulin.
type 2 diabetes A form of diabetes that usually begins later in life and arises when cells resist the effects of insulin.

U

umbilical cord A vessel linking the bloodstream of the placenta to that of the baby and enabling the exchange of gases, nutrients, and wastes.
underage drinking The drinking of an alcoholic beverage by a person who is under the age of 21.
underweight A weight resulting in a BMI below 18.5.
unintended pregnancy A pregnancy that is either mistimed or unwanted at the time of conception.
unintentional injury (accidents) Bodily damage that is not deliberately caused.
unsaturated fats (oils) Fats that typically are liquid at room temperature; generally come from plant sources.
urethra A duct that travels from the bladder through the shaft of the penis, carrying fluids to the outside of the body.
uterus (womb) The pear-shaped organ where a growing fetus is nurtured.

V

vagina The tube that connects a woman's external sex organs with her uterus.
vaginal intercourse Intercourse characterized by the insertion of the penis into the vagina.
values Internal guidelines used to make decisions and evaluate the world around you.
vas deferens A tube ascending from the epididymis that transports sperm.
vasectomy Form of permanent surgical sterilization that seals off the vas deferens, preventing sperm from reaching ejaculate.
vector An animal or insect that transports pathogens from one point to another.
vegetarian A person who avoids some or all foods from animal sources: red meat, poultry, seafood, eggs, and dairy products.
veins Vessels that transport blood toward the heart, delivering oxygen-poor blood from the body periphery or oxygen-rich blood from the lungs.
ventricles The two lower chambers of the heart, which pump blood to the body and lungs.
violence Use of physical force—threatened or actual—with the intent of causing harm.
violent crime One of four offenses involving force or the threat or force: murder and non-negligent manslaughter, forcible rape, robbery, and aggravated assault.
virus A microscopic organism that cannot multiply without invading body cells.
vitamins Compounds, with no energy value of their own, needed by the body in small amounts for normal growth and function.
vulva All of the female external organs, collectively. Also called *genitals*.

W

water A liquid composed of hydrogen and oxygen that is necessary for life.
wellness The process of actively making choices to achieve optimal health.
whole grains Unrefined grains that contain bran, germ, and endosperm.
whole-genome scanning A form of genetic testing that looks for variants within a person's genome.
will A legally binding document stating what should be done with a person's property after death.
withdrawal Physical symptoms that develop when a person stops using a drug. In sex, the withdrawal of the penis from the vagina before ejaculation.

Z

zygote A fertilized ovum.

Index

A

B

C

D

E

F

G

H

N

O

P

T

U

V

W

Y

Z